AF773653

Small bowel disorders

Edited by

Ranjit N Ratnaike MD, FRACP, FAFPHM
Senior Visiting Medical Specialist, and Head, Acute Geriatric Service, Department of Medicine, University of Adelaide, The Queen Elizabeth Hospital, Woodville, South Australia, Australia

ARNOLD

A member of the Hodder Headline Group
LONDON
Co-published in the USA by
Oxford University Press, Inc., New York

First published in Great Britain in 2000 by
Arnold, a member of the Hodder Headline Group,
338 Euston Road, London NWI 3BH

http://www.arnoldpublishers.com

Co-published in the USA by
Oxford University Press, Inc.,
198 Madison Avenue, New York, NY 10016
Oxford is a registered trademark of Oxford University Press

© 2000 Arnold

All rights reserved. No part of this publication may be reproduced or transmitted in any form or by any means, electronically or mechanically, including photocopying, recording or any information storage or retrieval system, without either prior permission in writing from the publisher or a licence permitting restricted copying. In the United Kingdom such licences are issued by the Copyright Licensing Agency: 90 Tottenham Court Road, London WIP 0LP.

Whilst the advice and information in this book is believed to be true and accurate at the date of going to press, neither the author[s] nor the publisher can accept any legal responsibility or liability for any errors or omissions that may be made. In particular (but without limiting the generality of the preceding disclaimer) every effort has been made to check drug dosages; however, it is still possible that errors have been missed. Furthermore, dosage schedules are constantly being revised and new side-effects recognized. For these reasons the reader is strongly urged to consult the drug companies' printed instructions before administering any of the drugs recommended in this book.

British Library Cataloguing in Publication Data
A catalogue record for this book is available from the British Library

Library of Congress Cataloging-in-Publication Data
A catalog record for this book is available from the Library of Congress

ISBN 0 340 76008 7

1 2 3 4 5 6 7 8 9 10

Commissioning Editor: Nick Dunton
Project Editor: Sarah de Souza
Production Editor: Wendy Rooke
Production Controller: Iain McWilliams

Typeset in 10/12 pt Minion by
Scribe Design, Gillingham, Kent, UK
Printed and bound in Great Britain by The Bath Press, Bath

What do you think about this book? Or any other Arnold title?
Please send your comments to feedback.arnold@hodder.co.uk

Dedication

To

Alan Kerr Grant

Inspired teacher, mentor and valued friend

Contents

Contributors

Heikki Arola MD, PhD
Physician, Tampere Occupational Health Center, Kauppakatu 9 D, Tampere, Finland

Angela H Barbour MBBS, PhD, FRCPA
Senior Lecturer in Pathology, University of Adelaide, Adelaide, South Australia, Australia

F Dylan L Bartholomeusz MBBS, FRACP, MD
Senior Consultant, Departments of Gastrointestinal Medicine and Nuclear Medicine, The Royal Adelaide Hospital, Adelaide, South Australia, Australia

Dave L Bigam MD, FRCSC
Assistant Professor of Surgery, University of Alberta Hospital, Edmonton, Alberta, Canada

Ross Butler PhD
Chief Medical Scientist, Gastroenterology Department, Women's and Children's Hospital, North Adelaide, South Australia, Australia

Grace Chandi MBBS, MS
Department of Anatomy, Christian Medical College, Vellore, Tamilnadu, India

Paul J Ciclitira MD, PhD, FRCP
Gastroenterology Unit, The Rayne Institute, Guy's and St Thomas' Hospital Trust, St Thomas' Hospital, Lambeth Palace Road, London, UK

Adrian G Cummins MD, PhD, FRACP
Senior Consultant, Gastroenterology Unit, The Queen Elizabeth Hospital, Woodville, South Australia, Australia

Geoffrey Davidson PSM, MD, FRACP
Director, Gastroenterology Unit, Women's and Children's Hospital, North Adelaide, South Australia, Australia

Ipatia Doussis-Anagnostopoulou MD
Division de Pathologie Clinique, Centre Medical Universitaire, 1211 Geneve 4, Switzerland

R Logan Faust, MD
Consultant Gastroenterologist, 1210 Sonoma Avenue, Suite B, Santa Rosa, California, USA

Andreas Frenzer MD
Facharzt FMH für Innere Medizin und Gastroenterologie, Leitender Arzt Medizinische Abteilung, Spital Oberengadin, Samedan, Switzerland

David R Grant MD, FRCSC
Professor of Surgery, University of Western Ontario, London Health Sciences Center, London, Ontario, Canada

David I Grove MD, FRACP, FRCPA, DTM&H
Clinical Professor, Department of Clinical Microbiology and Infectious Diseases, The Queen Elizabeth Hospital, Woodville, South Australia, Australia

Nadim Y Haboubi MD, FRCP
Consultant Physician, Department of Adult Medicine, Neville Hall Hospital, Gwent, UK

Najib Y Haboubi DPath, FRCPath
Consultant Histopathologist and Head, Department of Histopathology, Withington Hospital, Manchester, UK

BS Harsha MBBS
Christian Medical College, Vellore, Tamilnadu, India

Paul Hoadley MBBS
Resident Medical Officer, Division of Medicine, Flinders Medical Centre, Bedford Park, South Australia, Australia

Jens J Holst MD
Professor of Medical Physiology, Department of Medical Physiology, The Panum Institute, University of Copenhagen, Copenhagen, Denmark

Peter R Holt MD
Professor of Medicine, Department of Medicine, College of Physicians and Surgeons, Columbia University, Chief, Gastroenterology Division, St Luke's–Roosevelt Hospital Center, New York, USA

Peter Lawson FAIMS
Principal Hospital Scientist, Department of Clinical Microbiology and Infectious Diseases, The Queen Elizabeth Hospital, Woodville, South Australia, Australia

Emile Levy PhD
Director, Research Centre, Hôpital Sainte-Justine, Chemin Côte Sainte-Catherine, Montreal, Quebec, Canada

Minnie M Mathan MD, PhD, FRCPath, FNA
Consultant Pathologist, Division of Laboratory Science, International Centre for Diarrheal Disease Research, Mohakhali, Dhaka, Bangladesh

VI Mathan MD, PLP, FRCP, FNA
Division Director, Division of Laboratory Sciences, International Centre for Diarrheal Disease Research, Mohakhali, Dhaka, Bangladesh

Austin G Milton BSc (Hons), Dip Comp Sci
Medical Scientist, Department of Medicine, University of Adelaide, The Queen Elizabeth Hospital, Woodville, South Australia, Australia

Booshanam V Moses MS, FACS, FICS
Professor and Chairperson, Surgery Unit-III, Christian Medical College and Hospital, Vellore, Tamilnadu, India

Kelly Papanaoum MBBS, FRACP, FRCPA
Consultant Physician, Infectious Diseases Unit, The Royal Adelaide Hospital, Adelaide, South Australia, Australia

Gitanjali Pawar MBBS, MD, DM
Department of Gastroenterology, The Queen Elizabeth Hospital, Woodville, South Australia, Australia

Mrinalini C Rao PhD
Department of Physiology and Biophysics, College of Medicine, University of Illinois at Chicago, South Wolcott Avenue, Chicago, Illinois, USA

Ranjit N Ratnaike MD, FRACP, FAFPHM
Senior Visiting Medical Specialist, and Head, Acute Geriatric Service, Department of Medicine, University of Adelaide, The Queen Elizabeth Hospital, Woodville, South Australia, Australia

Ian C Roberts-Thomson MD, FRACP
Director and Clinical Professor, Department of Gastroenterology, The Queen Elizabeth Hospital, Woodville, South Australia, Australia

David R Shaw MBBS, FRACP
Director, Infectious Diseases Unit, The Royal Adelaide Hospital, Adelaide, South Australia, Australia

Wei Ming Sun MD, PhD
Director, GI Motility Laboratory, Division of Gastroenterology, Department of Internal Medicine, Taubman Center, Ann Arbor, Michigan, USA

Fiona Thompson BSc (Hons), PhD
Visiting Research Fellow, Department of Medicine, University of Adelaide, The Queen Elizabeth Hospital, Woodville, South Australia, Australia

Anil B Utturkar MD, MBBS, DMRE, FRACR
Consultant Radiologist, Radiology Department, The Queen Elizabeth Hospital, Woodville, South Australia, Australia

Nicholas Wickham MA, MBBChir, MRCP, FRCPath, FRCPA
Head, Haematology–Oncology Research, Clinical Senior Lecturer in Medicine, University of Adelaide, The Queen Elizabeth Hospital, Woodville, South Australia, Australia

Sven Widgren MD
Reader in Pathology, Consultant Pathologist, Institut Neuchâtelois d'Anatomie Pathologique, Neuchâtel, Switzerland

Peter D. Zalewski PhD
Research Fellow, Department of Medicine, University of Adelaide, The Queen Elizabeth Hospital, Woodville, South Australia, Australia

Foreword

The small bowel is formed from a tube that is the source of all digestive organs and appears during the fourth week of gestation. Our concept of the small intestine has evolved in a similar fashion during the twentieth century from the view of the bowel as a relatively simple tube, which processes what we eat, into a body of knowledge that defines a marvellously complex organ. We now understand that the small intestine produces messenger molecules, which signal and coordinate a multiplicity of functions. We recognize it as the largest immune organ of the body, which sorts the vast array of antigens we eat and drink, in order to protect us from infections and maintain a helpful flora. Although digestion of food remains the cardinal role of the small bowel, there is a growing appreciation as we move into the twenty-first century of the collateral but crucial functions of regulating metabolism, defending against diseases, and processing a large quantity of water and solutes along with nutrients.

Each of the normal functions of the small bowel can be perturbed by either external influences or internal disturbances. Thus, disease and disorders of function are manifested by altered intrinsic processes of the intestine. One of the most dramatic examples of disordered function may be seen in cholera. We now know that a potent, soluble exotoxin produced by a bacteria, *Vibrio cholerae*, attaches to any cell which possesses a specific GM gangloside receptor. The B subunit of the toxin provides a means of inserting the toxic A moiety into the cell. It then acts as a 'nonsense' hormone, which increases cyclic AMP maximally. This 'second messenger' signals a function characteristic of the affected cell type. In the case of the absorptive and secretory epithelium of the small bowel, the absorption of sodium and chloride is blocked at the villous tips, and secretion from crypt cells is turned up to maximum. In addition, neuroendocrine cells of the gut are affected, altering neural signals, which also increase fluid losses. Other affected cells signal other measurable changes. Fortunately, in the case of cholera, the toxin is bound entirely by the cells lining the gut and does not enter the body proper, hence the only treatment needed to cure a cholera patient is replacement of salts and water of the correct composition and volume at an appropriate rate. A redundant absorptive mechanism of the small bowel – the co-transport pathway by which sodium is linked to glucose, amino acids or peptides – is not affected by the cholera toxin, cytokines or other regulating substances, and can be used for oral rehydration therapy, not only in cholera, but also in essentially all instances of intestinal fluid loss where there is no obstruction.

We have defined many new processes of the small bowel during the twentieth century and have identified many others that still require further elucidation. One of the areas in which we can expect advances is improved identification of infections affecting the intestine. Whipple's disease now has a proven microbial cause in *T. whippelii*. Dr David Relman used a specific gene sequence and amplification techniques, rather than traditional microbiologic methods, to define the cause of Whipple's disease. We hope pursuit of other inflammatory diseases may also yield to such new methodologies. Knowledge of the signalling substances, which govern development of the small bowel and its accessory organs embryologically, may help us understand and utilize those factors that govern growth and development, to allow us to hasten repair of intestinal epithelium, restoring normal function and replacing lost functions. Improved non-invasive imaging, together with specific tests on secretions or stool for altered genes or gene products, can revolutionize early diagnosis and reduce reliance on more invasive methods. Such methods can help in the early detection of neoplasms as well as infections.

This book displays the state of our current knowledge and the methods we currently use to attain this knowledge. It also gives insight into what we may expect in the future to improve our ability to diagnose and treat disturbances of structure and function of the small bowel – an organ critical to our survival and good health.

William B. Greenough III, MD
Johns Hopkins Geriatrics Center,
Johns Hopkins University,
Baltimore, Maryland, USA

Preface

Small Bowel Disorders is a text for clinicians involved in the practice of gastroenterology, for postgraduate students and for undergraduate medical students as a reference text. It provides detailed and up-to-date evidence-based information on the small intestine.

The text complements existing larger reference works, and provides updates in key areas where advances have occurred. The material is presented in an easy-to-read format, allowing for easy and rapid access to information.

The small bowel is the powerhouse of the gastrointestinal tract. The first part of this text discusses the morphology and the functional diversity of the small bowel. The chapters on small bowel function discuss extensive recent information relating to defence mechanisms in host protection, the processes of fluid and electrolyte absorption and secretion, and the digestion and absorption of nutrients. These chapters provide a platform to more fully appreciate the pathogenesis and manifestations of the diseases subsequently discussed.

The text then deals with disorders of the small bowel that are most commonly seen in everyday practice. Rarer conditions are also discussed, for example Whipple's disease, which, due to its associated high mortality, needs to be diagnosed rapidly and treated effectively using recent diagnostic techniques and current treatment regimes. The chapters on infectious diseases acknowledge the wide prevalence of problems such as infectious diarrhoea in less industrialized regions of the world. These problems are also relevant to the industrialized world because of the increasing risk of transmission due to the ease of fast international travel. HIV and AIDS is extensively discussed in relation to the small bowel.

As far as possible, the contributors have provided information based on current 'best evidence' to assist the reader in clinical decision-making rather than relying upon strategies (such as personal experience) that have not been subjected to rigorous examination.

The text has been reviewed extensively to obtain input from gastroenterologists and others with an interest in specific topics. It is hoped that the incorporation of their comments and criticisms have enhanced the relevance and readability of the text.

Reviewers of texts sometimes raise the issue of repetition of information. If this has occurred, it is hoped that it would be regarded as 'reinforcement' rather than poor editing. Since most readers may not read a text book from cover to cover at one sitting, but return to it as need arises, some repetition of information is considered helpful. It is of course equally important for irritating repetitiousness not to occur. Therefore, clear cross-references are provided for the rapid access of information.

It is hoped that *Small Bowel Disorders* will present a comprehensive, up-to-date and practical resource for clinicians and students of gastroenterology with an interest in the small bowel to confidently diagnose and treat a variety of conditions based on a sound understanding of the functions of the small intestine.

Ranjit N. Ratnaike
16 November 1999

Acknowledgements

I am indebted to a large number of colleagues at The Queen Elizabeth Hospital, Woodville, South Australia who assisted me in a variety of ways. Members of the Department of Histopathology were particularly helpful to clarify to my satisfaction a variety of issues. I thank Dr Robert Dymock, Dr John Cooper and Dr John Pierides.

I was provided with invaluable assistance with typing, collating material and manuscript checking, in addition to a variety of other tasks, by Mr Austin G. Milton, Mrs Mary Denys, Ms Vanessa Kuipers and Mrs Ellie Giardini.

I am grateful to my contributors who, by and large, honoured their promise to deliver the chapters on time. A highlight of my experience editing this text was to receive a wedding invitation from a contributor instead of the chapter (which did arrive in due course!).

My wife, Stephanie, and our children, Alinta and Christen, are accustomed now to my cantankerousness as deadlines for manuscripts approached. They have been unfailing in their forbearance and kindness to me.

I consider it a privilege and a pleasure to have worked with Mr Nicholas Dunton and his staff at Arnold (Publishers) Limited, London. I had most contact (by almost daily email) with Ms Sarah de Souza, the Project Editor. Her continuous graciousness and helpfulness did much to make this project a pleasurable task. I am also grateful to Ms Wendy Rooke, the Production Editor, who, despite the great inconvenience, was agreeable to update the text to include several new advances in the field. It was a great pleasure working with Ms Clare Freeman, the Copy-editor and Sue Nicholls, the Proofreader.

Ranjit N. Ratnaike

1

The morphology and development of the small intestine

GRACE CHANDI, BS HARSHA, BOOSHANAM V MOSES

MORPHOLOGY: INTRODUCTION

The small intestine is a coiled part of the tubular alimentary tract which extends from the pylorus to the ileo-caecal junction. Its average length is 5 m, but is variable and correlates with the height of the individual. It appears longer after death because of the loss of muscle tone. The small intestine occupies the central part of the abdominal cavity and is surrounded by the large intestine (Williams, 1995).

Divisions of the small intestine

It is divided into three parts. The short, upper fixed part is the duodenum, which continues as the long mobile proximal two-fifths, known as the jejunum, and the distal three-fifths, the ileum.

DUODENUM (Fig. 1.1)

This is the fixed part of the small intestine, extending from the pylorus to the duodenojejunal flexure. It is C-shaped and, within its C-curve, it encloses the head of the pancreas. It consists of four parts. The superior part or first part is 5 cm long and is directed upwards and to the right, ending at the neck of the gallbladder. It then takes a sharp turn and descends as the descending part or second part, 8–10 cm long, into which opens the ampulla of Vater. It then takes a turn to the left, passing in front of the third lumbar vertebra. This is called the horizontal part, or third part, and is about 10 cm long with the superior mesenteric vessels lying in front of it. The ascending part, or fourth part, 2.5 cm long, ascends to the left of the aorta and at the level of the second lumbar vertebra continues as the jejunum.

JEJUNUM

The jejunum, which is about 4 cm in diameter, occupies the upper and left part of the abdomen, and is thicker because of the frequent permanent thick circular folds or plicae circulares, or valves of Kerckring.

ILEUM

The ileum feels much thinner than the jejunum and its circular folds are fewer in number. It occupies the right lower part of the abdominal cavity. Its terminal part

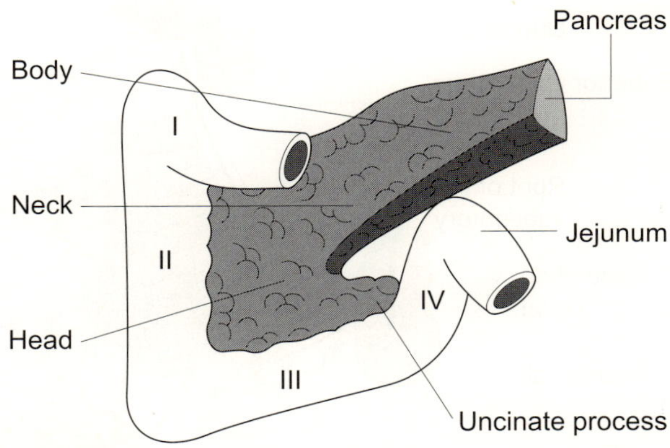

Figure 1.1 *Parts of the duodenum.*

usually lies in the pelvis but ascends upwards and to the right to join the caecum.

Mesentery (Fig. 1.2)

The mesentery consists of two folds of parietal peritoneum, which suspends the jejunum and ileum. The root of the mesentery, which is about 15 cm long, is attached to the posterior abdominal wall extending from the duodenojejunal junction on the left side of the second lumbar vertebral body to the upper part of the right sacro-iliac joint. It crosses, from the left to the right, the third part of the duodenum, aorta, inferior vena cava, right testicular or ovarian vessels, right ureter and right psoas major. The superior mesenteric vessels, nerves, lymph nodes, lymph vessels and a variable amount of fat lie between the two layers of the mesentery.

The jejunal and ileal branches of the superior mesenteric artery divide and form a series of arterial arcades, which increase in number towards the ileum (Fig. 1.3).

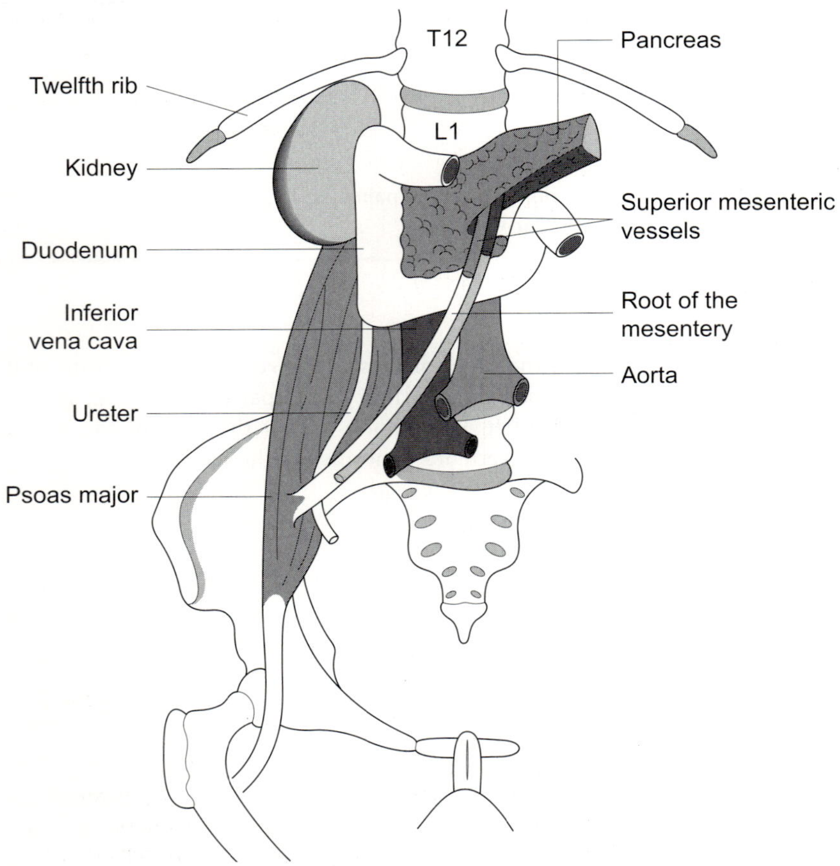

Figure 1.2 *Structures crossed by the root of the mesentery.*

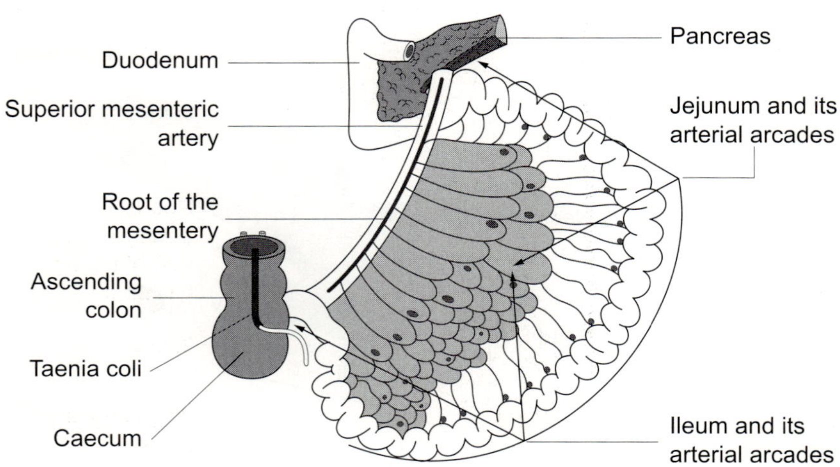

Figure 1.3 *The jejunum and ileum and their arterial arcades. Note the increase in the arterial arcades from jejunum to ileum.*

Blood supply of the small intestine

ARTERIAL SUPPLY (Fig. 1.4)

The first and second parts of the duodenum up to the opening of the ampulla of Vater, which are derived from the foregut, are supplied by the superior pancreatico-duodenal artery, a branch of gastroduodenal artery which arises from the artery of the foregut (coeliac artery), namely the coeliac trunk. The rest of the duodenum, derived from midgut, is supplied by the inferior pancreatico-duodenal artery, a branch of the artery of the midgut or the superior mesenteric artery. Arterial anastomoses between the artery of the foregut (the coeliac) and the artery of the midgut (the superior mesenteric) are established via superior and inferior pancreatic duodenal arteries. A variable number of jejunal and ileal branches arise from the convexity of the superior mesenteric artery. These divide to form a series of arterial arcades in the mesentery.

The arterial arcades are fewer in number proximally but increase distally (and may be up to five in number) in the lower part of the ileum (Fig. 1.5). Straight arteries from the most peripheral arcades run distally to the gut without any anastomoses with each other. At the inner border of the gut they divide and run on either side of the gut. This pattern of arterial supply prevents interference with the circulation during the movement

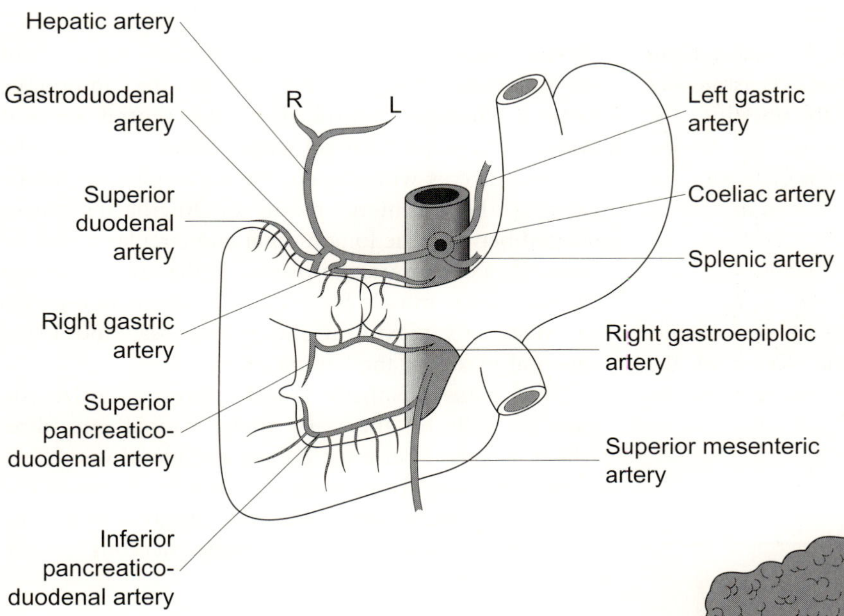

Figure 1.4 *The arterial supply to the duodenum.*

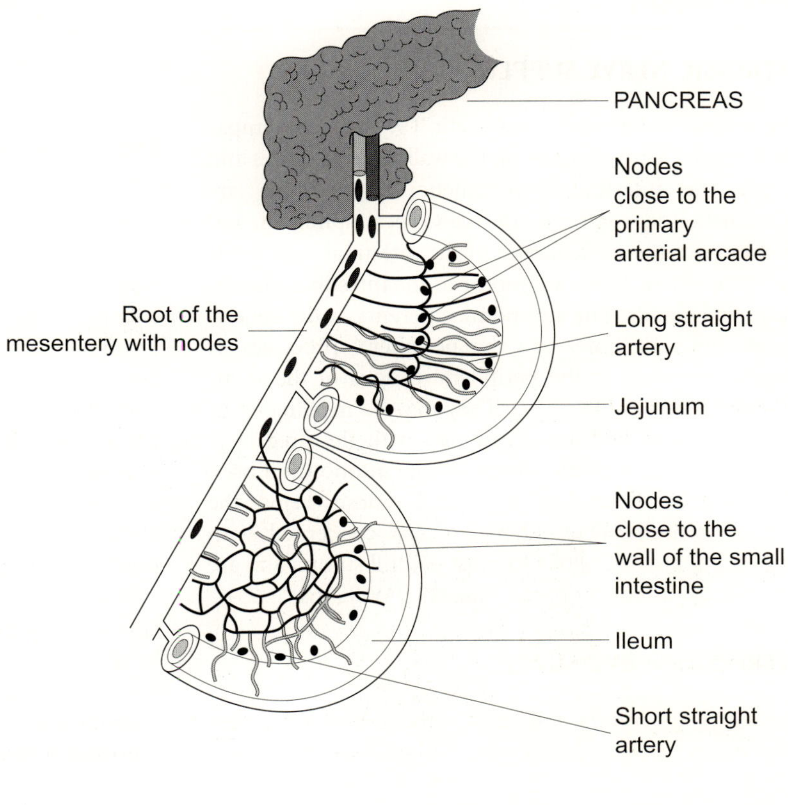

Figure 1.5 *Schematic illustration showing the decrease in the length of the straight arteries from jejunum to ileum.*

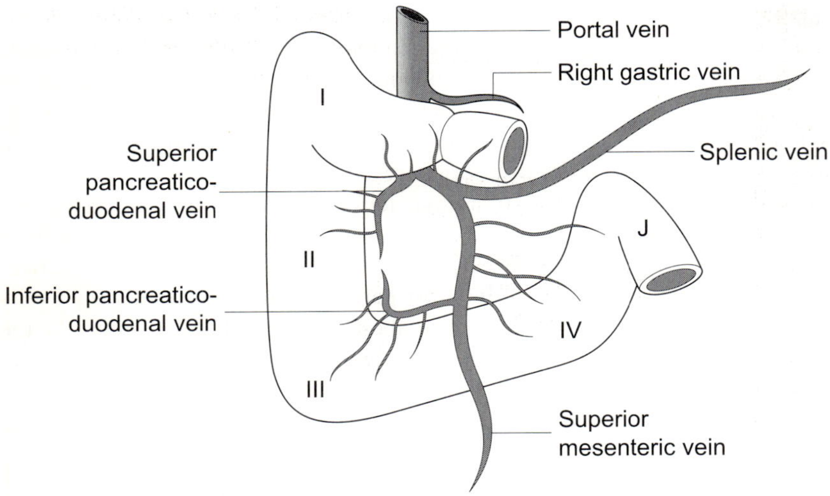

Figure 1.6 *Venous drainage of the duodenum.*

of the gut. Within the wall of the gut, the vessels form an anastomosing network of small vessels. Anastomoses are few in the antimesenteric border of the intestine. The intramural anastomoses are able to sustain several centimetres of intestine, but when there is distension, its circulation can become impaired (Gardner *et al.*, 1975).

VENOUS DRAINAGE (Fig. 1.6)

The veins draining the duodenum join the splenic, superior mesenteric and portal veins. Veins of the jejunum and ileum drain into the portal vein via the superior mesenteric vein.

Nerve supply

EXTRINSIC NERVE SUPPLY

The autonomic nerves (sympathetic T9, T10, parasympathetic vagus) form plexuses on the walls of the arteries and supply the intestine. Sympathetic nerve fibres are vasoconstrictor, motor to the ileo-caecal sphincter and inhibitory to the musculature of the intestinal wall, while parasympathetic fibres are motor to the intestinal musculature and glands. The autonomic afferents or the general visceral afferent fibres are the peripheral processes of unipolar neurons in the peripheral ganglia of the vagus and spinal nerves (T9, T10). They may be myelinated or non-myelinated and are distributed with the preganglionic and postganglionic fibres of the autonomic fibres. These afferent fibres initiate visceral reflexes below the level of consciousness. They are also concerned with nausea, but are insensitive to most painful stimuli and are sensitive to distension of the intestine (Williams, 1995).

INTRINSIC NERVE SUPPLY

The enteric nervous system (or the intrinsic nerves) consists of ganglia interconnecting nerve fibres and plexuses within the gut wall, and can carry out many of its functions independently, unlike the autonomic system, which is controlled by the central nervous system. The superficial subserous plexus connects the extrinsic nerves with the enteric nerve plexuses which are: (1) the myenteric plexus or Auerbach's plexus located between the longitudinal and circular muscular layer; (2) a deep muscular plexus on the mucosal aspect of the circular muscle layer; (3) the submucosal plexus or Meissner's plexus in the submucosa; and (4) a mucosal plexus in the lamina propria.

The parasympathetic vagal fibres arborize on ganglion cells on the wall, unlike sympathetic fibres which terminate on muscle layer and blood vessels.

Studies using histochemical, neurophysiological and pharmacological experiments are in progress to increase our understanding of the enteric nervous system (Fawcett, 1994).

Lymphatic drainage (Fig. 1.7)

Lymphatics from the duodenum drain into the hepatic and coeliac group of lymph nodes. Some lymphatics also go to the superior mesenteric nodes. Lymph from the jejunum and ileum drains into lymph nodes in the mesentery. Each mucosal villus contains in its centre a lymphatic capillary, termed the central lacteal, which drains into an intramural plexus, which in turn drains into lymph vessels that accompany mesenteric blood vessels. Lymph nodes are abundant in the mesentery and lie along the blood vessels. The lymph finally drains into the thoracic duct via intestinal trunks.

The liver is frequently the first organ involved in the spread of cancer from the intestine. Lymphatic vessels in the wall of the small intestine run at right angles to its long axis, and therefore cancer or tuberculosis spreads along them and tends to encircle the gut and constrict it (Gardner *et al.*, 1975).

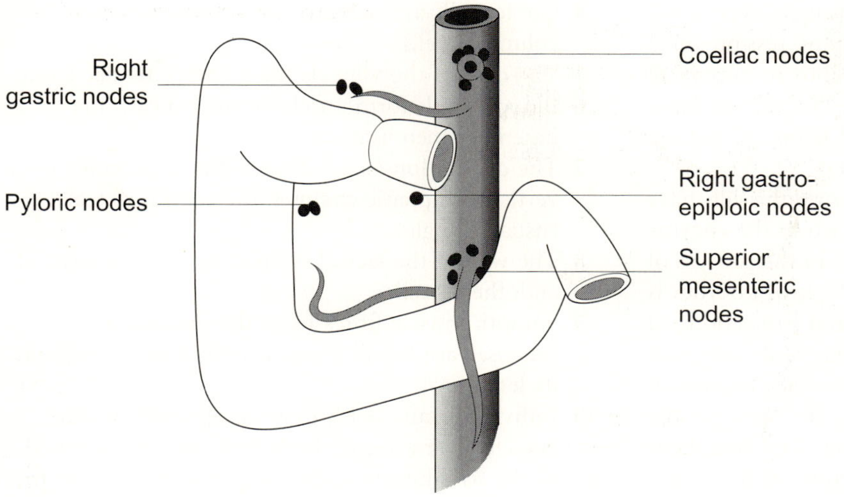

Figure 1.7 *Schematic illustration showing the arrangement of the lymph nodes.*

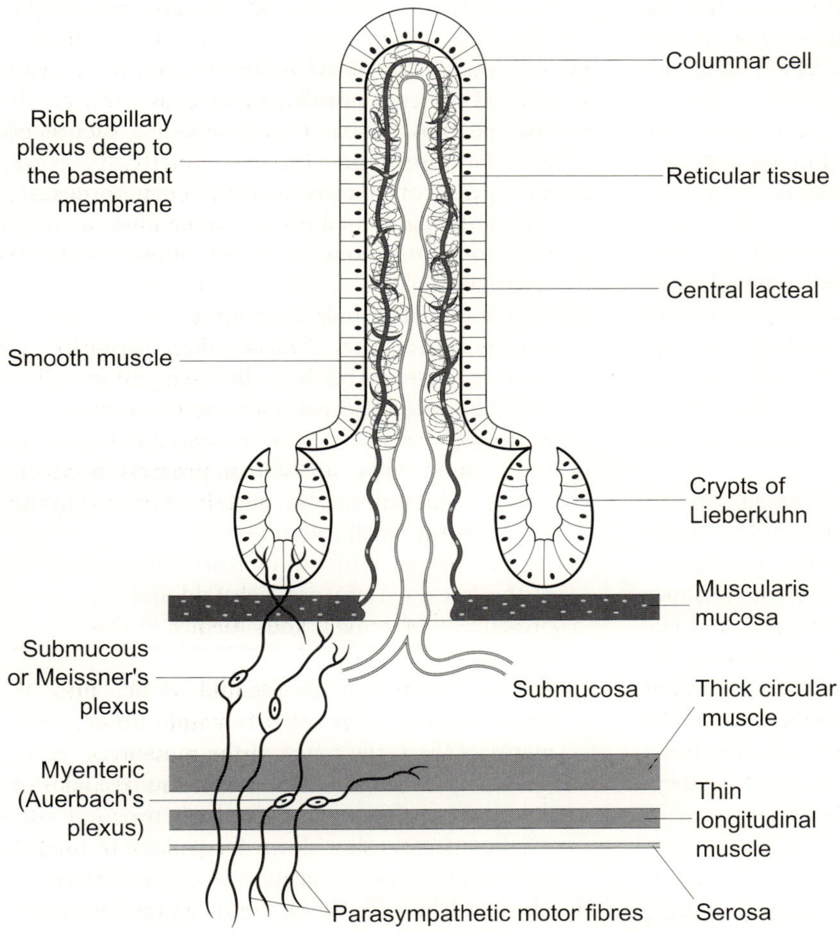

Figure 1.8 *Layers of the small intestine and the structure of a villus.*

Layers of the small intestine (Fig. 1.8)

1 Outermost = serosa = peritoneal covering
2 Muscular layer
  - Outer – thin and longitudinal
  - Inner – thick and circular
3 Submucous layer
4 Mucosa highly vascular and consists of:
  - Epithelial lining = tall columnar cells resting on a basement membrane
  - Lamina propria = connective tissue: blood vessels, nerves, lymphoid follicles
  - Muscularis mucosae – outer longitudinal and inner circular.

The mucous membrane is lined by a single layer of tall columnar epithelial cells or enterocytes resting on a basement membrane and is thrown into innumerable finger-like projections known as villi. The villi are large and numerous in the duodenum and jejunum, but are smaller and fewer in the ileum.

The columnar epithelial cells covering the villi have a striated or brush border. It is very rich in the enzyme alkaline phosphatase and is concerned in the process of active absorption. Ultrastructurally, the brush border is composed of minute parallel cylindrical projections of cytoplasm known as microvilli. Goblet cells occur at regular intervals between the columnar cells. Individual lymphocytes and lymphoid follicles are seen in the lamina propria of the small intestine. The lymphoid follicles are larger and more numerous in the ileum than in the jejunum, and are called Peyer's patches. They are usually located in the antimesenteric mucosa of the intestine. Villi or crypts of Lieberkuhn are not present over the Peyer's patches. The epithelium over the Peyer's patches, or dome area, or follicle-associated epithelium (FAE) has specialized cells that lack microvilli. The cell membrane on the luminal aspect of these cells has undulations or microfolds. Numerous vesicles and mitochondria are seen in the apical cytoplasm. These cells are closely related to the lymphocytes. These cells are called microfold cells (M cells) (Owen and Jones, 1974). Single, tubular intestinal glands, or the crypts of Lieberkuhn, open by circular apertures between the villi. These do not penetrate the muscularis mucosa. Additionally, in the duodenum, there are Brunner's glands in the submucosa and these open into the lumen.

The mucosa has innumerable permanent circular folds, which are either complete or incomplete circles that begin in the duodenum below the duodenal papillae, are closely set in the proximal half of the jejunum and diminish progressively in its distal half and the proximal half of the ileum, and are almost absent in the distal half of the ileum. These circular folds are called the valves of Kerckring, and serve to slow down the passage of food to facilitate its digestion and absorption as well as to increase the surface area available for these functions.

Structure of the villus

Some important points concerning the structure of the villus are listed below.

1. The villi are highly vascular, finger-like projections of mucous membrane in the small intestine.
2. They are numerous in the duodenum and jejunum, but are fewer and smaller in the ileum.
3. The villi are covered by a basement membrane, which supports a single layer of columnar epithelial cells (enterocytes).
4. Goblet cells are scattered among the rows of columnar cells.
5. The core of the villus is filled with reticular tissue.
6. Blood vessels form a rich plexus beneath the basement membrane.
7. The central long axis of the villus is occupied by a vertical lymphatic channel, the central lacteal (usually single).
8. The wall of the lacteal is lined by a single layer of endothelial cells.
9. Smooth muscle fibres from the muscularis mucosae are found around the lacteal throughout its length.
10. Individual muscle fibres are given off from the muscle layer around the lacteal, and are attached to the basement membrane at one end and to the wall of the central lacteal at the other end. Contraction of these has the effect of milking the lacteal.
11. The free surface of the columnar cells has a highly striated or brush border, which is very rich in alkaline phosphatase and concerned in the process of active absorption.
12. Using electron microscopy, the brush border is seen to be composed of minute parallel cylindrical projections of cytoplasm called the microvilli.
13. Simple tubular glands or intestinal glands, also known as the crypts of Lieberkuhn, open by circular apertures between the bases of the villi. They do not penetrate the muscularis mucosae.
14. In the duodenum, in addition, there are Brunner's glands in the submucosa, and these open into the lumen of the small intestine.
15. (a) The presence of villi increases the surface area of the intestinal mucosa eightfold and the presence of microvilli adds further to this increase.
    (b) The presence of circular folds of mucous membrane, i.e. valves of Kerckring, further increases the surface area of the mucosa.
    (c) The great length of the small intestine adds to the increase of its mucosal surface area.
    All these factors slow down the passage of food and facilitate easy absorption of digested food.
16. The epithelial cells lining the small intestine are frequently replaced by mitotic activity of the epithelium in the intestinal glands. This process is known as cell turnover. It takes 3–6 days for the upward migration of the cell from the crypt to the tip of the villus.
17. The M cells or microfold cells are seen in the epithelium over aggregates of lymphoid tissue. These are the antigen-presenting or antigen-sensitive cells concerned with the initiation of the sequential immune responses.

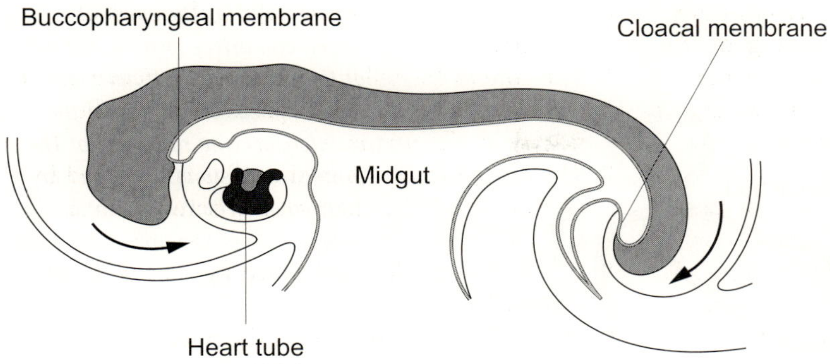

Figure 1.9 *Drawing of a midline sagittal section of an embryo showing the effect of cephalocaudal folding. (Adapted from* Langman's medical embryology, *Fig. 5.14C, p. 74.)*

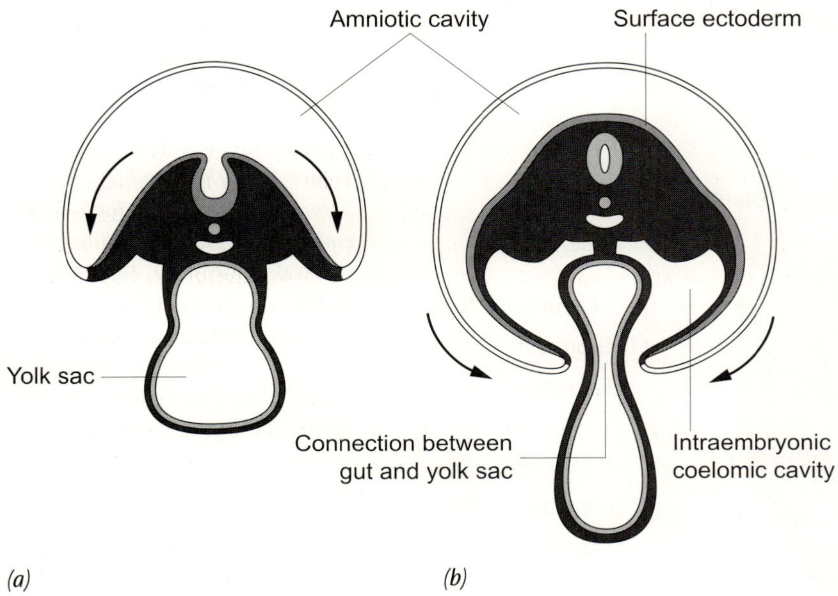

Figure 1.10 *(a) and (b) Drawing of a transverse section through the embryo to show the effect of lateral folding on the endoderm-lined cavity. (Adapted from* Langman's medical embryology, *Fig. 5.15A,B, p. 75.)*

DEVELOPMENT OF THE SMALL INTESTINE

Introduction

The small intestine is developed from the endoderm germ layer (Figs 1.9 and 1.10a,b). With cephalocaudal and lateral folding of the embryo, the endodermal gut tube is created from the yolk sac and becomes demarcated into a cranial part or foregut, a middle part or midgut which communicates with the rest of the yolk sac, and a caudal part or hindgut.

Foregut

The foregut gives rise to the oesophagus, stomach and proximal part of the duodenum until the opening of the bile duct.

Midgut

The midgut begins distal to the opening of the bile duct into the duodenum and ends at the junction of the proximal two-thirds with the distal one-third of the transverse colon. The midgut communicates with the yolk sac by a broad channel called the vitellointestinal duct, which becomes narrower and is eventually obliterated, following which the midgut comes to lie free within the abdominal cavity.

The midgut is suspended by its dorsal mesentery and is supplied by the superior mesenteric artery. It lengthens rapidly and forms the primary intestinal loop (Fig. 1.11). The cephalic part of the loop becomes the distal duodenum, jejunum and proximal ileum, while the distal part of the loop becomes the distal ileum, caecum, appendix, ascending colon and proximal two-thirds of the transverse colon (Figs 1.12 and 1.13). The junction between the proximal and distal limbs of the loop is

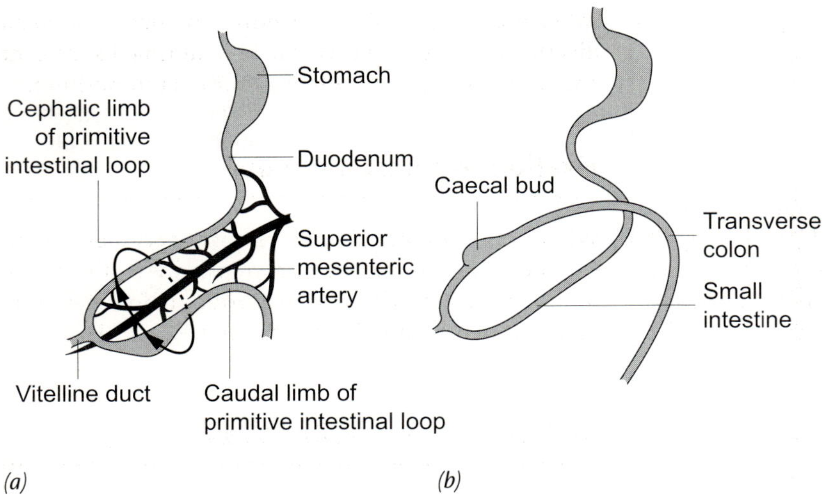

Figure 1.11 *(a) The superior mesenteric artery forming the axis of the primitive intestinal loop. The arrow indicates direction of the counterclockwise rotation. (b) The primitive intestinal loop after a 180° counterclockwise rotation. (Adapted from* Langman's Medical Embryology, *Fig. 14.13A, p. 248.)*

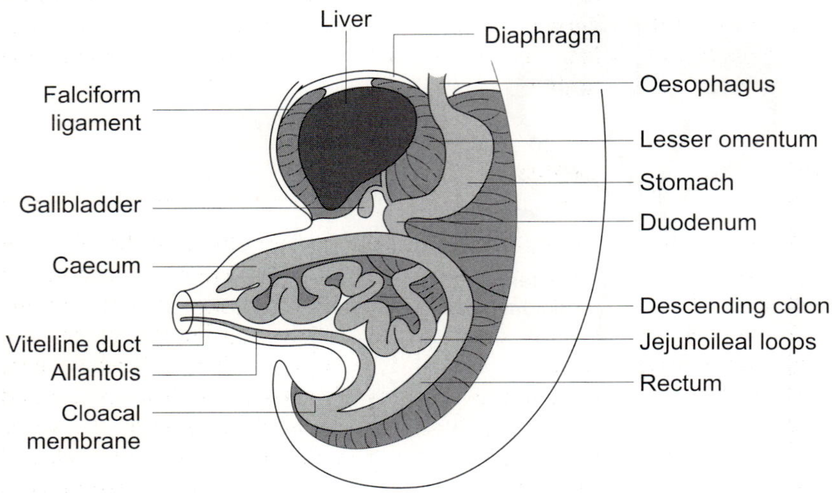

Figure 1.12 *The umbilical herniation of intestinal loops in an embryo. (Adapted from* Langman's medical embryology, *Fig. 14.14, p. 249.)*

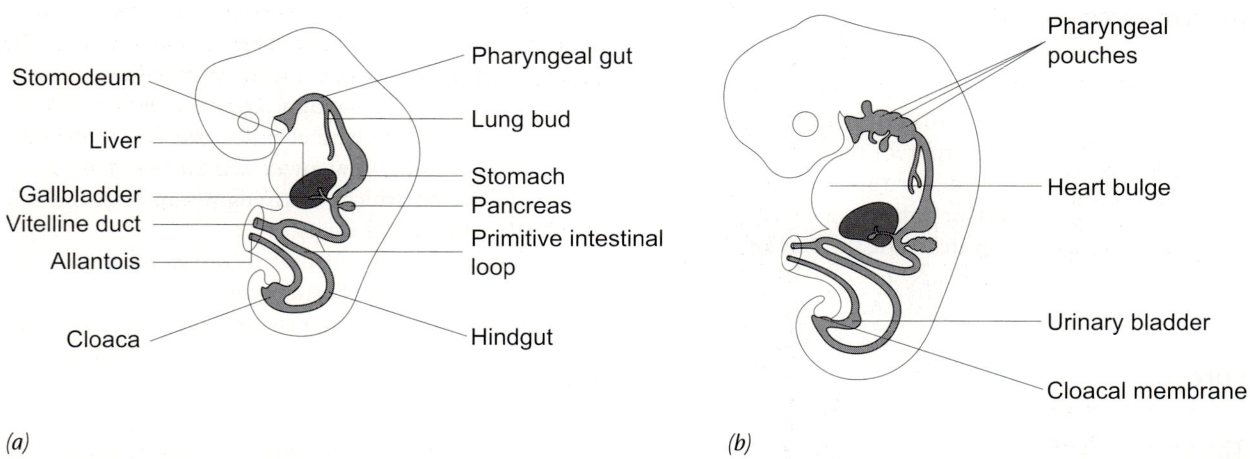

Figure 1.13 *(a) and (b) Schematic drawings of sagittal sections through embryos at various stages of development to show the derivatives of endodermal germ layer. (Adapted from* Langman's medical embryology, *Fig. 5.16, p. 76.)*

marked by the vitelline duct, which, if persistent, is called Meckel's diverticulum (Fig. 1.12).

Physiological herniation

The abdominal cavity becomes inadequate owing to expansion of the liver bud and the rapid lengthening of the intestine. This results in the formation of a primary intestinal loop that later herniates into the umbilical cord during the sixth week of intrauterine life (Fig. 1.12).

Rotation of midgut

The intestinal loop rotates in a counterclockwise direction around the axis formed by the superior mesenteric artery. The rotation is approximately 270°, of which 90° occurs during herniation and 180° during reduction of the hernia into the abdominal cavity. Even during the rotational process, the small and large bowel elongates resulting in coiling of the small bowel.

Retraction of the herniated loops

The abdominal cavity expands and, probably as a result of this expansion, the herniated intestine re-enters the abdominal cavity at the end of 3 months gestation. As the intestine re-enters, the jejunum comes to lie on the left side of the abdomen and the succeeding loops to the right side of the abdomen. The caecal bud, which is the last to re-enter the abdominal cavity, comes to lie in the right hypochondrium, but soon descends down to the right iliac fossa as the hepatic flexure and ascending colon are formed. The appendix develops as a small diverticulum from the caecal bud during its descent and, as such, it is most often retrocaecal in position.

Fixation of intestinal loops

While the intestine after its re-entry occupies certain specific places within the abdominal cavity, the dorsal mesentery fuses with the posterior abdominal wall, fixing it permanently in that position (Fig. 1.14).

DEVELOPMENTAL ANOMALIES

Congenital umbilical hernia

Congenital umbilical hernia occurs when the intestine that has re-entered the abdominal cavity once again herniates through the umbilicus and out of the abdominal cavity covered by amnion and skin around the umbilicus.

Exomphalos

Exomphalos (omphalocoele) results from the failure of all or part of the midgut to re-enter the abdominal cavity (Plate 1.1). It is covered by amniotic membrane on the outside, and peritoneum on the inner side, separated by a middle layer of Wharton's jelly. There are two types of exomphalos – exomphalos major and exomphalos minor. In exomphalos minor, the sac is very small and may contain loops of small bowel, and the umbilicus is attached to the centre. In exomphalos

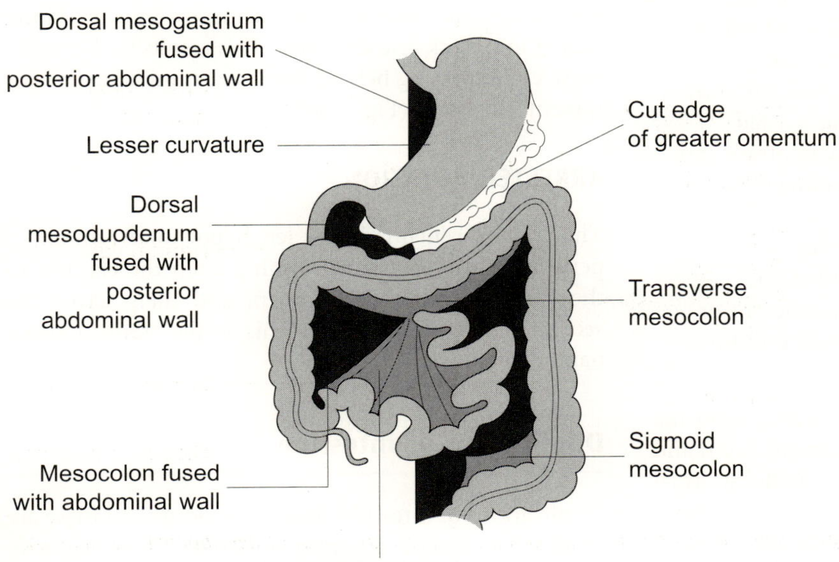

Figure 1.14 *Frontal view of the intestinal loops after the removal of the greater omentum. Note the line of attachment of the mesentery. The dark shaded areas indicate the parts of the dorsal mesentery that fuse with the posterior abdominal wall. (Adapted from* Langman's Medical Embryology, *Fig. 11.14B, p. 176.)*

major, the sac is large and usually contains large bowel and a segment of liver, in addition to loops of small bowel, and the umbilical cord is attached to the inferior aspect of the sac.

In its severe form, the entire anterior abdominal wall may be absent and all the abdominal viscera may be found outside the abdominal cavity. This condition is called eventration of the abdominal viscera (gastroschisis) and it is usually associated with extrophy of the urinary bladder.

Persistent vitellointestinal duct (Fig. 1.15a–d)

This can occur in five different ways, which are listed below.

1 The vitellointestinal duct remains patent and the tract is lined by intestinal epithelium. It extends from the terminal ileum to the umbilicus. The resultant umbilical fistula discharges mucus and, rarely, faeces when there is distal intestinal obstruction.
2 Often only a small part of the duct near the umbilicus remains unobliterated and this gives rise to umbilical sinus that discharges mucus (Plate 1.2). The epithelial lining of the sinus often becomes everted to form an adenoma (umbilical adenoma), or umbilical polyp or enteroteratoma. The child is brought with a cherry red polypoidal mass projecting from the umbilicus with blood-stained mucous discharge.
3 Sometimes both the umbilical and the intestinal ends of the duct close with a patent intervening portion which develops into an intra-abdominal cyst, an enterocystoma.
4 The vitellointestinal duct, whether obliterated or not, can become an intraperitoneal band which often leads to intestinal obstruction. The obstruction results from a coil of small intestine passing under or over, or becoming twisted around the band. Such a band may contract and pull the Meckel's diverticulum, resulting in a congenital umbilical hernia.
5 Sometimes a vitellointestinal cord that is connected to the Meckel's diverticulum but not attached to the umbilicus becomes adherent or knotted around another loop of small intestine and causes intestinal obstruction.

Occasionally, there may be a band extending from the umbilicus to the mesentery near the terminal ileum and this band probably is the obliterated vitellointestinal artery (superior mesenteric artery). If this band connects the Meckel's diverticulum to the ileal mesentery, it is called a mesodiverticular band.

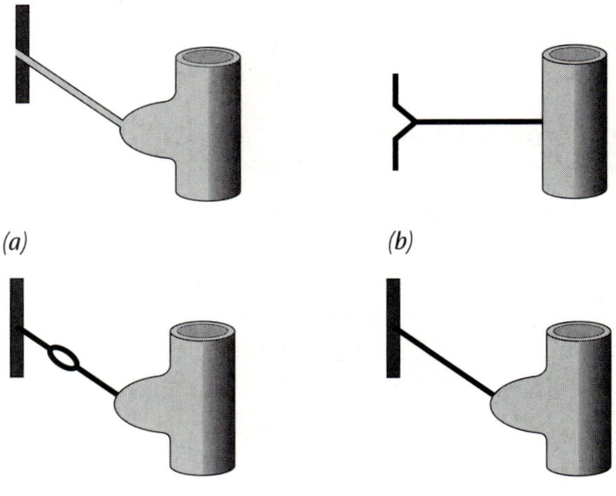

(a) (b) (c) (d)

Figure 1.15 *Schematic diagrams of the various forms of persistent vitellointestinal duct.*

Abnormalities of rotation and fixation

The gut herniates into the umbilical cord and later it re-enters the abdominal cavity. During this process it undergoes a series of rotations totalling 270° counter-clockwise – 90° during herniation and 180° during re-entry. Sometimes the rotation is only 90° and, in such instances, the colon and caecum, which are the first to return to the abdominal cavity, occupy the left side of the colon while the small bowel loops are on the right side. This is called left-sided colon (Fig. 1.16a).

There are congenital bands associated with malrotation and these bands may cause intestinal obstruction by direct compression.

REVERSED ROTATION

Sometimes the rotation of the primitive intestinal loop occurs in a clockwise direction. This results in the transverse colon passing behind the duodenum and superior mesenteric artery (Fig. 1.16b).

ARRESTED ROTATION

The caecum remains in the left hypochondrium and a peritoneal band is found running from the caecum to the right side of the abdomen, and then across the second part of duodenum. This is the transduodenal band of Ladd (Fig. 1.17).

Duplication of intestine

Duplications of intestinal loops may occur and these are usually found near the terminal ileum. They may vary from a small diverticulum to a large cyst. The dupli-

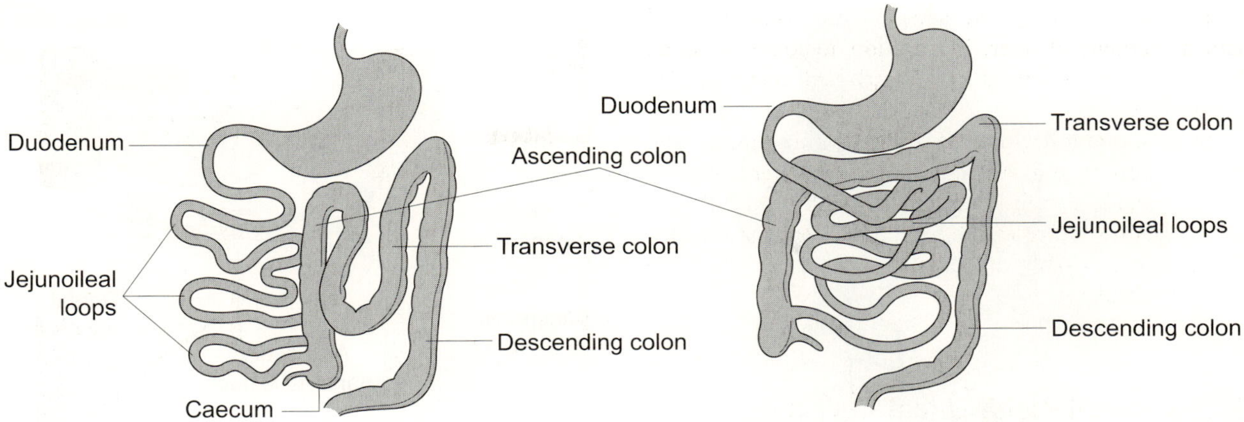

Figure 1.16 *(a) The colon is located on the left side owing to abnormal rotation of the primitive intestinal loop. (b) Reversed rotation of the primitive intestinal loop. (Adapted from* Langman's medical embryology, *Fig. 14.20, p. 253.)*

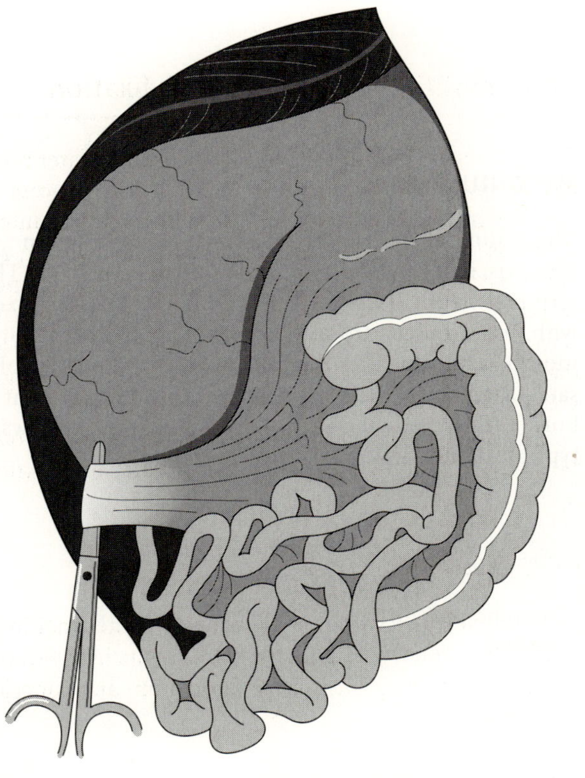

Figure 1.17 *Incomplete rotation of the caecum and Ladd's transduodenal band. (Courtesy of* Bailey & Love's short practice of surgery, *1968, Fig. 1202, p. 938.)*

cated cyst always remains attached to the segment of its origin but the mucosa may not be the same.

The intestine is a solid tube initially and the intestinal lumen develops by canalization. During the process some recanalized area may not join with the main lumen and duplication results. If the duplicated part remains in continuity with the main lumen, a diverticulum results, otherwise it becomes a cyst. These cysts are usually found on the mesenteric borders.

Congenital diverticula

MECKEL'S DIVERTICULUM

Meckel's diverticulum is present in 2 per cent of cases, is 60 cm (2 ft) from the ileocaecal valve and is 5 cm (2 in) long. In nearly 90 per cent of cases, it arises from the antimesenteric border of the intestine and possesses all three coats of the intestinal wall. It has its own blood supply, and is liable to obstuction and infection. In 20 per cent of cases the proximal part of the mucosa contains heterotrophic epithelium, namely, gastric, colonic or pancreatic tissue.

Atresia and stenosis of the jejunum

Atresia and stenosis are thought to be caused by interruption of blood supply to the bowel during development. Ischaemia in a short segment only produces stenosis, while a larger and more extensive ischaemic necrosis produces a fibrous cord between adjacent loops of bowel, and the bowel may be completely separated.

Vascular malformation

Haemangiomas are believed to be embryologically sequestrated mesoangial tissue. These can occur in the bowel wall, in the lumen or in the mesentery. They can be either cavernous, capillary or of mixed type.

Miscellaneous

VOLVULUS NEONATORUM

The gut herniates into the umbilical cord during the sixth week of intrauterine life. When the gut re-enters

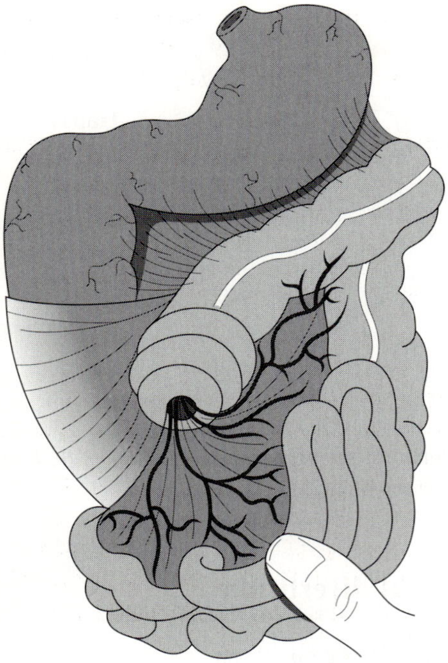

Figure 1.18 *Volvulus of the midgut. (Courtesy of* Bailey & Love's short practice of surgery, *1968, Fig. 1203, p. 938.)*

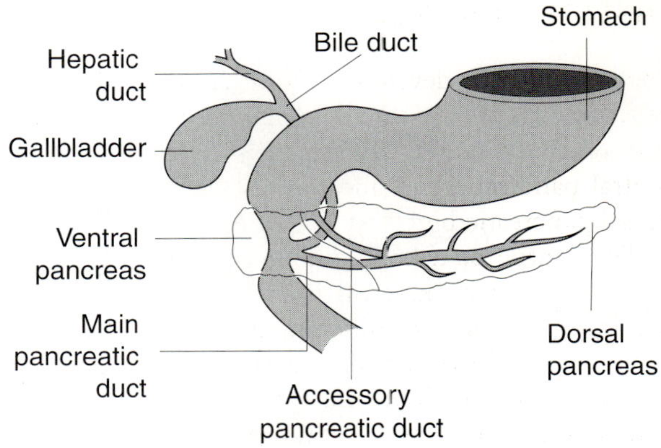

Figure 1.19 *Annular pancreas. The ventral pancreas forms a ring around the duodenum, occasionally resulting in duodenal stenosis. (Adapted from* Langman's medical embryology, *Fig. 14.12, p. 247.)*

the abdominal cavity, it undergoes a series of rotations. Failure of this process leads to various rotational abnormalities. The small bowel may be entirely on the right side with the caecum in the left iliac fossa. In these cases, the small bowel has a long narrow mesentery that has a tendency to rotate, producing a volvulus of the midgut (volvulus neonatorum) (Fig. 1.18).

MECONIUM ILEUS

Meconium ileus is the neonatal manifestation of mucoviscidosis-fibrocystic disease of the pancreas. The terminal ileum becomes filled with meconium mixed with viscid mucus from the pancreas. During the later months of foetal life, this meconium becomes inspissated, leading to intestinal obstruction, and the infant is born with intestinal obstruction. Radiography shows a typical matted distended small bowel.

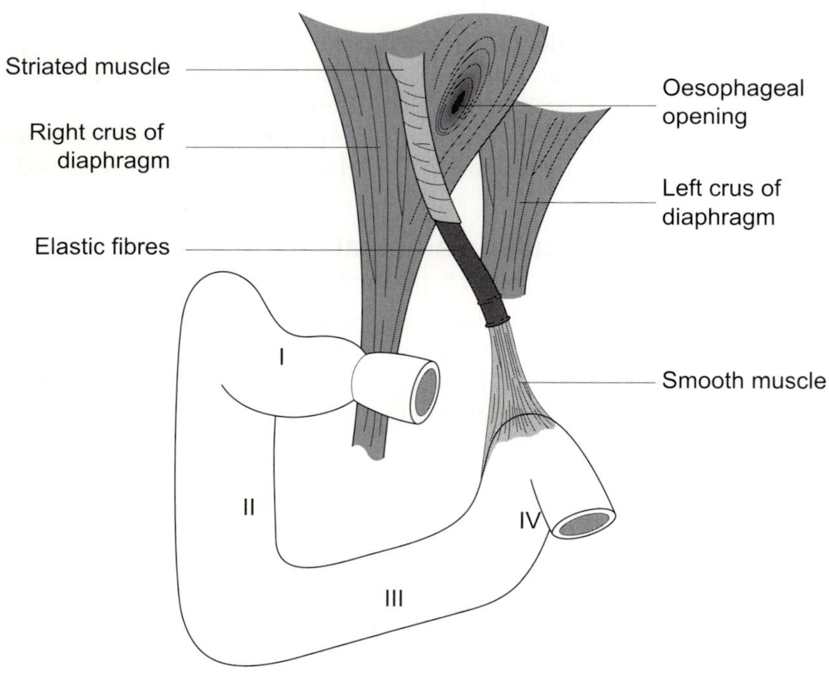

Figure 1.20 *The suspensory ligament of the duodenum.*

ANNULAR PANCREAS

The pancreas is developed from dorsal and ventral pancreatic buds. The uncinate process and the inferior part of the head of the pancreas develop from the ventral pancreatic bud and the rest develops from the dorsal pancreatic bud.

The ventral pancreatic bud consists of two components. An annular pancreas is the result of non-fusion and migration in two different directions of the two components of the ventral pancreatic bud around the second part of the duodenum (Fig. 1.19). This malformation may constrict the duodenum and can cause obstruction.

LIGAMENT OF TREITZ

A suspensory ligament of the duodenum, or ligament of Treitz, extends from the duodenojejunal flexure to the right crus of the diaphragm (Fig. 1.20). The ligament of Treitz limits the descent of the duodenum. It may contain smooth muscle fibres and variation in its attachment to the duodenum is not uncommon. It may be attached only to the duodenojejunal flexure, or to the flexure and the third and fourth parts of the duodenum or to the third and fourth parts alone. If its attachment to the duodenojejunal flexure is narrow, the contraction of the smooth muscle fibres in the ligament can decrease the angulation at the flexure, which may cause obstruction (Hollinshead, 1956).

Acknowledgements The authors express their gratitude to the artist Mr Samuel R. Sargunar DFA for the colour reproduction of Dr B.S. Harsha's diagrams, to Professor K.E. Mammen and Dr A. Pavai for the photographs, and to publishers Williams & Wilkins as well as H.K. Lewis & Co. Ltd for permission to use their illustrations.

REFERENCES

Fawcett, D.W. 1994: *A text book of histology*, 12th edn. New York: Chapman & Hall, 644–9.

Gardner, E., Gray, D.J., O'Rahilly, R. 1975: *Anatomy*, 4th edn. Philadelphia: W.B. Saunders Company, 386–7.

Hollinshead, H., 1956: *Anatomy for surgeons*, Vol. 2. New York: Hoeber-Harper, 415–16.

Owen, R.L., Jones, A.L. 1974: Epithelial cell specialization within human Peyer's patches. An ultrastructural study of intestinal lymphoid follicles. *Gastroenterology* 66, 184–203.

Williams, P.L. 1995: *Gray's anatomy*. 38th edn. London: Churchill Livingstone, 1763, 1297, 1306–8.

2

The small intestinal mucosa

MINNIE M MATHAN

THE NORMAL SMALL INTESTINE

The small intestine connects the gastric pylorus to the caecum of the large intestine and is about 3–6 m in length in postmortem specimens (Underhill, 1955). In life, the length may be considerably shorter owing to the tone of the longitudinal musculature. The general organization of the small intestinal wall, mucosa, submucosa, muscularis and serosa is similar throughout its length. It is divided into three anatomical regions. The first approximately 20 cm from the gastric pylorus, mainly retroperitoneal around the head and body of the pancreas, is the duodenum. The next region is the jejunum, the proximal two-fifths of the remainder, while the ileum is the distal three-fifths ending at the ileocaecal valve.

A well-recognized function of the small intestine is to digest and absorb nutrients and water. The end products of luminal digestion may undergo further membrane digestion at the surface of enterocytes, especially carbohydrates and proteins (disaccharidases, dipeptidases). A variety of transport processes, active transport involving receptors and requiring expenditure of energy, passive diffusion, diffusion down an electrochemical gradient and solvent drag are involved in transport by enterocytes. Some nutrients are resynthesized by the enterocyte before further transport (e.g. triglycerides) and others are transported to the rest of the body without resynthesis, e.g. glucose and amino acids. An equally important but less well-recognized function of the small intestine is as a primary barrier between the external environment in the lumen of the gut and the internal environment of the body. The lumen of the small intestine contains ingested food and gastrointestinal secretions and has an abundant microflora. The intestinal mucosa is not a passive physical barrier but has one of the largest collections of immunocytes, designated the gut-associated lymphoid tissue, which is specialized to provide appropriate immunological defence against invasion by microbes from the lumen (Brandtzaeg *et al.*, 1989; Kato and Owen, 1994; Marsh and Ensari, 1995).

The mucosa

The small intestinal mucosa has an epithelial lining, consisting mainly of enterocytes, supported by the lamina propria, which is separated from the submucosa by the muscularis mucosa. The effective mucosal surface area is increased by the provision of primary circular folds of the mucosa, the folds of Kerckring (plica circularis or valvulae conniventes), which are most prominent in the distal duodenum and proximal jejunum, being absent after about the mid-ileum. The surface area of the mucosa is further increased 7–15-fold by finger- or leaf-like projections of the mucosa called villi, about 10–40 per mm^2. The final increase in effective surface area is provided by the microvilli on the luminal surface of enterocytes giving approximately 200 000 mm^2 of enterocyte surface. It is therefore estimated that the functional surface area of the small intestine available for absorption is approximately 300 m^2 or roughly the size of a tennis court! (Moog, 1981).

The epithelium is organized into a mature functional compartment covering the villi and an immature regenerative compartment lining the crypts of Lieberkuhn. The openings of several crypts surround the base of

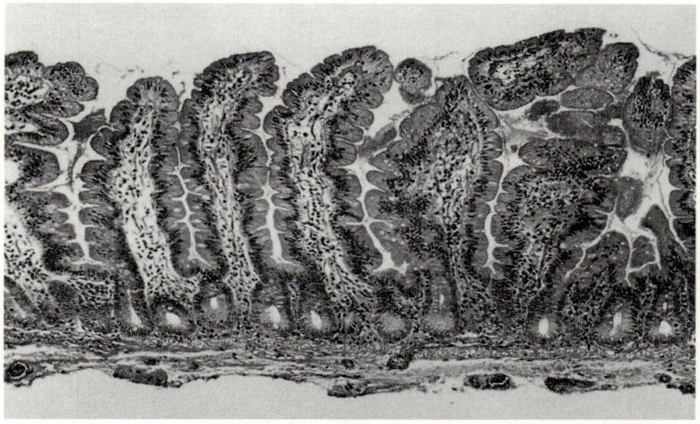

Figure 2.1 *Jejunal mucosal biopsy. Tropical control (haematoxylin and eosin (H&E), ×100).*

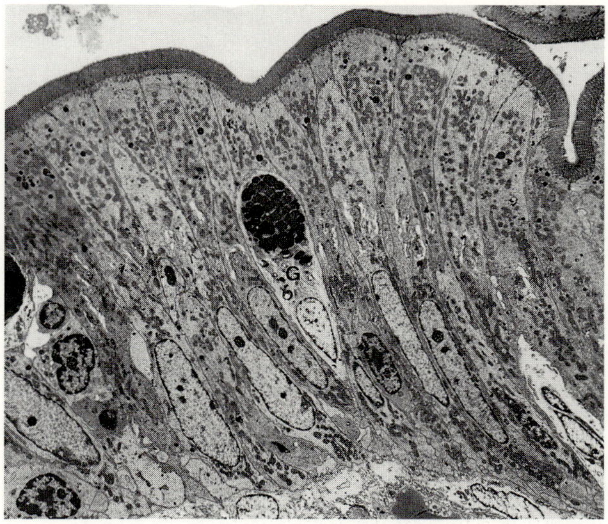

Figure 2.2 *Electron micrograph of normal villus enterocytes. A portion of a goblet cell (G) is also seen (×2000).*

each villus. The epithelial lining is a single layer consisting of several types of columnar cells, enterocytes and goblet cells on the villus epithelium, undifferentiated stem cells, immature crypt enterocytes, Paneth cells and endocrine cells in the crypts, all of which are derived from the endoderm (Fig. 2.1). This single layer usually contains epithelial lymphocytes, mast cells and few macrophages.

The enterocytes or specialized absorptive cells are polarized tall columnar cells with a single basal oval nucleus, resting on a basement membrane (Fig. 2.2). The luminal border of the enterocyte bears closely packed microvilli, slender cylinders approximately 1–1.5 μm in length and 0.1 μm in diameter covered by glycocalyx (Fig. 2.3) (Trier, 1969). The glycocalyx, synthesized continuously by the enterocytes, contains a variety of enzymes and transport proteins necessary for membrane digestion and absorption (Trier and Madara, 1981). Each microvillus has a core of actin filaments connected with the apical network of microfilaments to give stability and to facilitate movement of the microvilli. The apical borders of adjacent enterocytes are interconnected by a junctional complex composed of tight junction, intermediate junction and desmosomes. The junctional complexes regulate epithelial permeability through paracellular pathways and maintain the polarity of the enterocyte by restricting movement of integral membrane proteins (Claude and Goodenough, 1973; Pisam and Ripoche, 1976). Intercellular communication occurs through cell adhesion molecules, gap junctions and interdigitations of the lateral cell walls (Boyer and Thiery, 1989). The cytoplasm of the enterocyte contains mitochondria, Golgi apparatus, smooth and rough endoplasmic reticulum, ribosomes and lysosomes (Trier and Madara, 1981).

Goblet cells are mucus-secreting cells. Their proportion in the epithelial compartment increases from the duodenum to the distal ileum. The upper two-thirds of this cell with a basal nucleus is distended with mucin

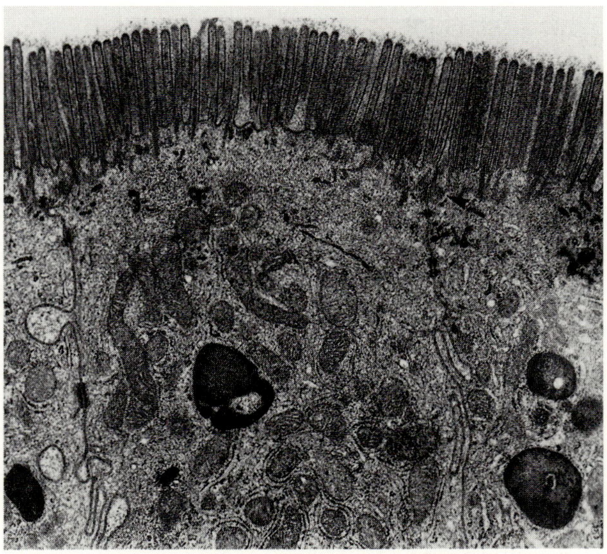

Figure 2.3 *Electron micrograph of apical part of enterocytes. Note the regularly arranged microvilli with glycocalyx, the junctional complex (arrowhead), and the mitochondria, endoplasmic reticulum and lysosomes (L) (×11 000).*

granules forming the theca, which is shaped like a wine glass. Mucin release may be stimulated by noxious agents or immune mechanisms and has a protective role (Lake *et al.*, 1980; Lamont, 1992).

In the upper two-thirds of the crypt, enterocytes are immature with less developed microvilli and apical secretory granules. Undifferentiated pluripotential stem cells, present in the base of crypts, are also columnar with basal nuclei, short sparse microvilli, less developed glycocalyx and scanty cellular organelles, but abundant ribosomes and polysomes. Dividing undifferentiated

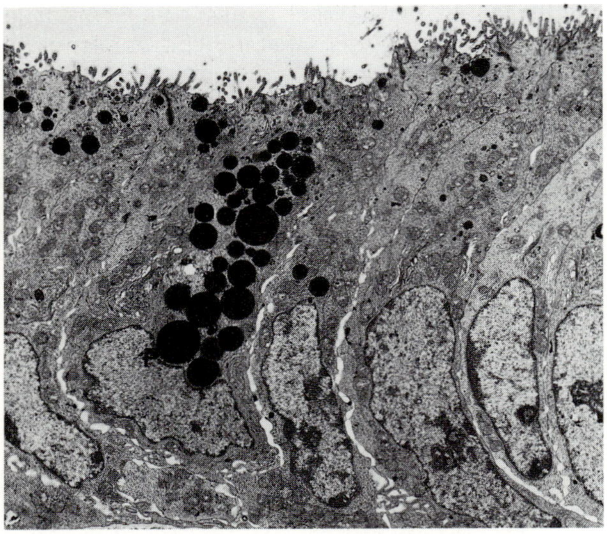

Figure 2.4 *Electron micrograph of crypt enterocytes with shorter, sparser microvilli. A Paneth cell (P) with supranuclear dense spherical granules is also present (×4000).*

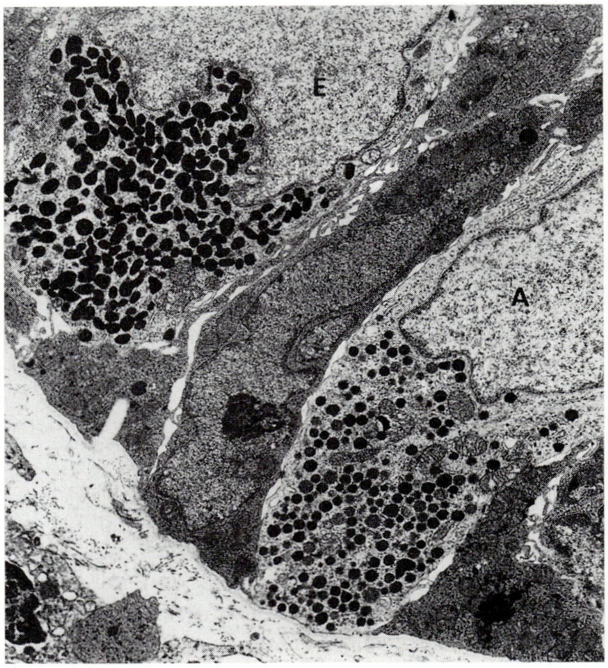

Figure 2.5 *Electron micrograph of a jejunal crypt. Note the enterochromaffin cell with pleomorphic granules (E) and an endocrine cell (A) with spherical infranuclear secretory granules (×6600).*

cells have rounded nuclei with indistinct nuclear membrane.

Paneth cells found up to the seventh cell position from the base of the crypt are wider at their base, narrower luminally and contain eosinophilic secretory granules supranuclearly. These granules contain antimicrobial peptides (defensins), growth factors and enzymes (Ouellette and Selsted, 1996). Ultrastructurally, these cells have a rich array of endoplasmic reticulum and large round electron-dense granules (Fig. 2.4).

The small intestinal epithelium has an abundant supply of specialized endocrine cells. These cells are also designated amine precursor uptake and decarboxylation (APUD) cells because of their ability for amine precursor uptake and decarboxylation (Pearse, 1980). They are not easily identifiable on routine haematoxylin–eosin-stained paraffin sections but can readily be detected by silver stains (Grimelius and Wilander, 1980), panendocrine markers like neuron-specific enolase, chromogranin, synaptophysin or specific antibodies, and by electron microscopy (Pearse, 1969; Facer *et al.*, 1976). Generally, they fall into one of two morphological types – open and closed (Solcia *et al.*, 1981). Triangular cells with a broad base on the basement membrane and infranuclear granules are of the closed type (Fig. 2.5), whereas the open type of cells are flask shaped with apices reaching the lumen with few microvilli (Fig. 2.6). The type of hormones secreted can be identified only by specific antisera to the hormones. Endocrine cells have also been described in the lamina propria and submucosa (Lundqvist and Wilander, 1986).

Two other specialized types of epithelial cells are found scattered throughout the small intestine. The

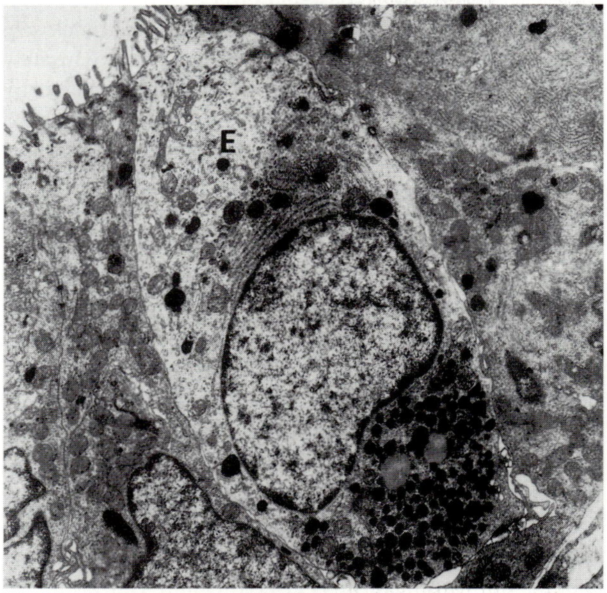

Figure 2.6 *Electron micrograph of a jejunal crypt. This shows an open type of endocrine cell (E), the apex of the cell extending to the lumen, with sparse microvilli and infranuclear secretory granules (×3600).*

epithelial lining over lymphoid follicles in the lamina propria consists of specialized cells with flattened nuclei and short ridges or microfolds on their luminal surface instead of microvilli (Fig. 2.7). Many lymphocytes

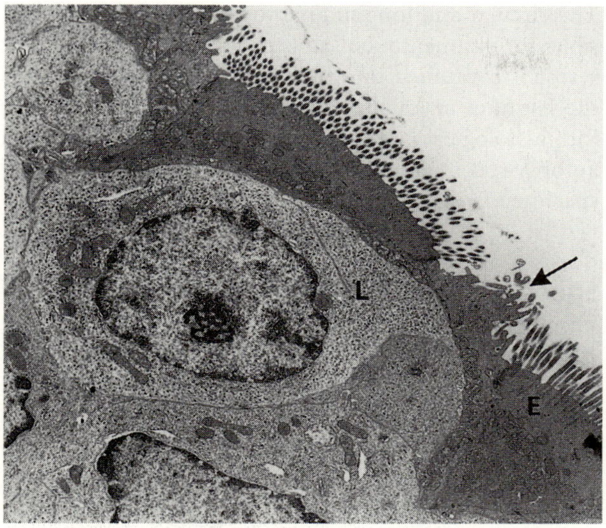

Figure 2.7 *Electron micrograph of epithelium covering a lymphoid follicle. Note the enterocytes (E) with long microvilli. The thinned out apical cytoplasm of an M cell enfolds lymphocytes (L) and has microfolds (arrow) (×5500).*

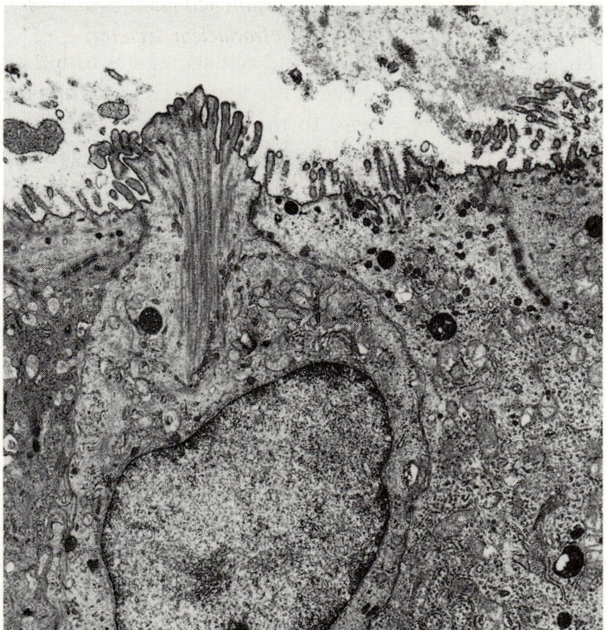

Figure 2.8 *Electron micrograph of a jejunal crypt. Note a tuft cell with longer and wider microvilli, and bundles of microfilaments extending deep into the cytoplasm (×7000).*

invaginate their lateral walls. These cells, designated M cells, are specialized antigen sampling and presenting cells that play a key role in mucosal immunity (Owen and Jones, 1974; Trier, 1991b; Neutra and Kraehenbuhl, 1993; Borghesi *et al.*, 1996). Caveolated cells or tuft cells, are pear-shaped cells present in the crypts and villi of the small intestine with narrow apices bearing wider and longer microvilli (Fig. 2.8). The core filaments of the microvilli extend deep into the apical cytoplasm and end near vesicles or deep irregular tubules called caveoli. The function of these infrequently present cells is not known (Nabeyama and Leblond, 1974).

Intraepithelial lymphocytes (IEL), scattered throughout the surface epithelium, are CD3-positive T cells. A total of 80 per cent of them are CD8 (cytotoxic/suppressor) positive and 5–15 per cent are of the CD4 (helper/inducer) type. Normally, less than 20 IEL are present per 100 epithelial cells above the basement membrane in the intercellular spaces. Their function is not fully understood (Ferguson and Murray, 1971; Austin and Dobbins, 1982; Brandtzaeg *et al.*, 1989).

The functions of the lamina propria are primarily structural and immunological. It extends from the muscularis mucosa, surrounding the crypts and forming the core of the villi, up to the basement membrane. The basement membrane is the interphase between the epithelium and the lamina propria. It allows passage of lymphocytes and nutrients. Beneath the basement membrane there is a subepithelial fibroblast sheath surrounded by collagen fibres. These mesenchymal cells are important for epithelial differentiation and function (Mathan *et al.*, 1972; Kedinger *et al.*, 1988; Berschneider, 1992). The matrix of the lamina propria contains blood vessels, lymphatics and nerve fibrils and consists of collagen bundles, other connective tissue fibres, fibroblasts, fibrocytes, smooth muscle cells and a large number of immunocytes (Brandborg, 1969).

The immunocytes are characterized by constant activation, migration and homing of cells in response to luminal environmental challenges and interaction with resident endothelial cells, fibroblasts, smooth muscles, nerves and epithelial cells (Targan, 1992). T and B lymphocytes and mature plasma cells, containing predominantly immunoglobulin A (IgA), are the dominant immunocytes of the lamina propria (Kett *et al.*, 1986; Mowat, 1987). CD4-positive (helper/inducer) T lymphocytes are the predominant T-lymphocyte type found throughout the lamina, but they often form dense collections just above the muscularis mucosa and also aggregate as nodules with germinal centres organized as Peyer's patches (see 'special structures'). A smaller number of macrophages and dendritic cells are present, usually located near the tips of villi, and have phagocytic, T-cell regulation and antigen-presenting function (Selby *et al.*, 1983; Mahida *et al.*, 1989; Steinman, 1991).

Eosinophils and mast cells are the only granulocytes normally found in the lamina propria. Eosinophils can be readily identified by their bilobed nuclei and the large eosinophilic granules in the cytoplasm. Although their exact role in the mucosa is not known, their ability to produce a variety of mediators and their dynamic interaction with other cells suggest a key role in host defence against infectious agents in addition to a role in allergic inflammation (Weller, 1991). Mucosal mast cells are distinct from connective tissue mast cells and basophils. The ability of the mast cells to secrete a variety of preformed and inducible mediators suggests a role in chronic inflammatory conditions and anaphylaxis, and in coordinating host inflammatory and immune response (Heatley, 1983; Wershil, 1995; Abraham and Malaviya, 1997). The intimate morphological relationship of mast cells to nerve fibrils indicates a mutual interaction (Stead *et al.*, 1989). Mast cells are best demonstrated with special techniques such as staining with toluidine blue, sulphated alcian blue or Geimsa stain (Strobel *et al.*, 1981).

The rich vascular and lymphatic network (Bark *et al.*, 1967) in the lamina propria is responsible for the provision of metabolites and oxygen to the enterocytes, and the transport of absorbed nutrients. Small arterioles course up to the tips of the villi and break up into a subepithelial capillary network that lines the villi and surrounds the crypts. The small venules empty into the submucosal venous plexus (Lundgren, 1974; Gannon and Cavati, 1990). The endothelial cells lining these blood vessels play an active role in determining vascular tone by secreting vasodilators (prostacyclins, nitric oxide) and vasoconstrictors (endothelin-1) (Griffith *et al.*, 1984; Katusic *et al.*, 1988). Endothelial factors also play a role in leucocyte recruitment and vascular permeability (Osborne, 1990; Kirkpatrick *et al.*, 1996) and are now increasingly recognized as important in the reaction of the gut to infection (Choudari *et al.*, 1985; Mathan and Mathan, 1985b).

The enteric nervous system is a distinct division of the autonomic nervous system. The other two divisions of the autonomic nerves, the sympathetic and parasympathetic, also supply the gut. The enteric nervous system functions independently of the central nervous system and is based on ganglia and neuronal plexuses at several levels in the intestinal wall. At least ten pharmacologically and functionally different types of neurones have been identified, including inhibitory, excitatory and secretory neurones (Furness and Costa, 1980; Jodal *et al.*, 1988).

The muscularis mucosa is the structural foundation of the mucosa. A few smooth muscle fibres, arranged longitudinally (outer) and circularly (inner), and elastic fibres form this layer. Some of the smooth muscle fibres may extend into the villi and may be attached to the epithelial basement membrane. It is also of particular importance in helping to orient mucosal biopsies properly for sectioning.

Submucosa, muscularis and serosa

These three layers sheath the mucosa, and contain the vascular and lymphatic plexuses and two neural ganglion layers (Auerbach's and Meissner's plexuses). The circular and longitudinal muscle layers are responsible for segmentation and propulsive motility. The serosa is continued into the mesentery, which suspends the jejunum and ileum. These layers become available for histological examination only in surgical and autopsy specimens, as in diagnostic peroral biopsies the specimen is confined to the mucosa.

Special structures

BRUNNER'S GLANDS

These are tubuloalveolar submucosal glands, located just distal to the gastroduodenal junction, and they become sparse in the second part of the duodenum, distal to the ampulla of Vater, the entrance of the bile and pancreatic ducts. The cuboidal to columnar Brunner's gland cells contain neutral mucins that are periodic acid–Schiff (PAS) positive and diastase resistant. The presence of Brunner's gland tissue positively identifies a biopsy from the proximal duodenum.

PEYER'S PATCHES

These are specialized lymphoid cell aggregates found on the antemesenteric aspect of the ileum. They occupy the mucosa and may extend to the submucosa. The patch has four distinct components: follicle, dome, follicle-associated epithelium and parafollicular regions. The follicles contain germinal centres with many surface IgA-positive B lymphocytes and occasional CD4-positive T cells and macrophages, and a mantle zone with small IgD- and IgM-positive B cells. The dome separates the follicle from the overlying specialized epithelium. The follicle-associated epithelium contains specialized M cells, which have already been described, and a greater proportion of CD4-positive T-helper/inducer cells. The parafollicular region is similar to that in lymph nodes with a predominance of CD4-positive T lymphocytes. Plasma cells are relatively few in Peyer's patches except in the dome area. The Peyer's patches play a key role in mucosal immunity (Wolf and Bye, 1984; Spencer *et al.*, 1986; Segal and Petras, 1992).

Geographic variations in mucosal morphology

An increase in the depth of crypts with a corresponding reduction in villus height, associated with an absence of finger-shaped villi, and with the mucosa folded into leaf-shaped or longer ridge-like structures has been reported in jejunal biopsies from apparently healthy asymptomatic volunteers from several tropical developing countries in Africa, Asia and Latin America (Chacko *et al.*, 1969; Baker and Mathan, 1972; Cook *et al.*, 1969). These changes are associated with exposure to the local, usually heavily microbially contaminated, environment and result also in an increase in the immunocyte population of the epithelium and lamina propria (Baker, 1973). Similar changes develop in expatriates from the temperate zones resident in such countries (Lindenbaum *et al.*, 1971). The changes revert back on transfer of residence to more temperate climates with lower levels of environmental contamination (Gerson *et al.*, 1971). It is essential to keep this normal pattern in mind when interpreting biopsies in individuals who may have developed these changes. Based on their prevalence, they have been designated tropical enteropathy (Mathan *et al.*, 1981) and similar features of a tropical colonopathy have also been reported (Mathan and Mathan, 1985a).

HISTOPATHOLOGY OF THE SMALL INTESTINAL MUCOSA

The small intestinal mucosa and its epithelial lining can respond to injury or infection only in relatively limited ways. Infiltration by neutrophil polymorphs is infrequent, but increase in mononuclear cells, especially epithelial lymphocytes, can be quite striking. In addition there is a reduction in villus height and an increase in the depth of the crypt layer. These changes have been designated as villus atrophy (partial, subtotal and total). More recent studies involving *in vitro* organ culture techniques using labelled tracers to follow stem cell turnover, maturation and migration of enterocytes to the villi suggest that the reduction in villus height is secondary to alterations in the regenerative compartment, the crypts (Mathan *et al.*, 1986). It therefore appears more appropriate to grade the overall mucosal architectural changes as mild, moderate and severe (Fig. 2.9). This morphologic grading is also based on enterocyte abnormalities and cellularity of the lamina propria (Perera *et al.*, 1975), but is only a morphologic description and not a specific diagnosis of a disease. Such a grading system also does not prejudge whether it is a villus atrophy or a crypt hypertrophy that is the main change. Marsh (1989, 1992a) has suggested an alternative nomenclature for mucosal pathology, especially in coeliac sprue. This defined infiltrative, hyperplastic, destructive and hypoplastic phases based on damage caused by cell-mediated immune mechanisms. While the model appears relevant to coeliac sprue and other situations of food antigen hypersensitivity, it is probably not applicable to many other conditions.

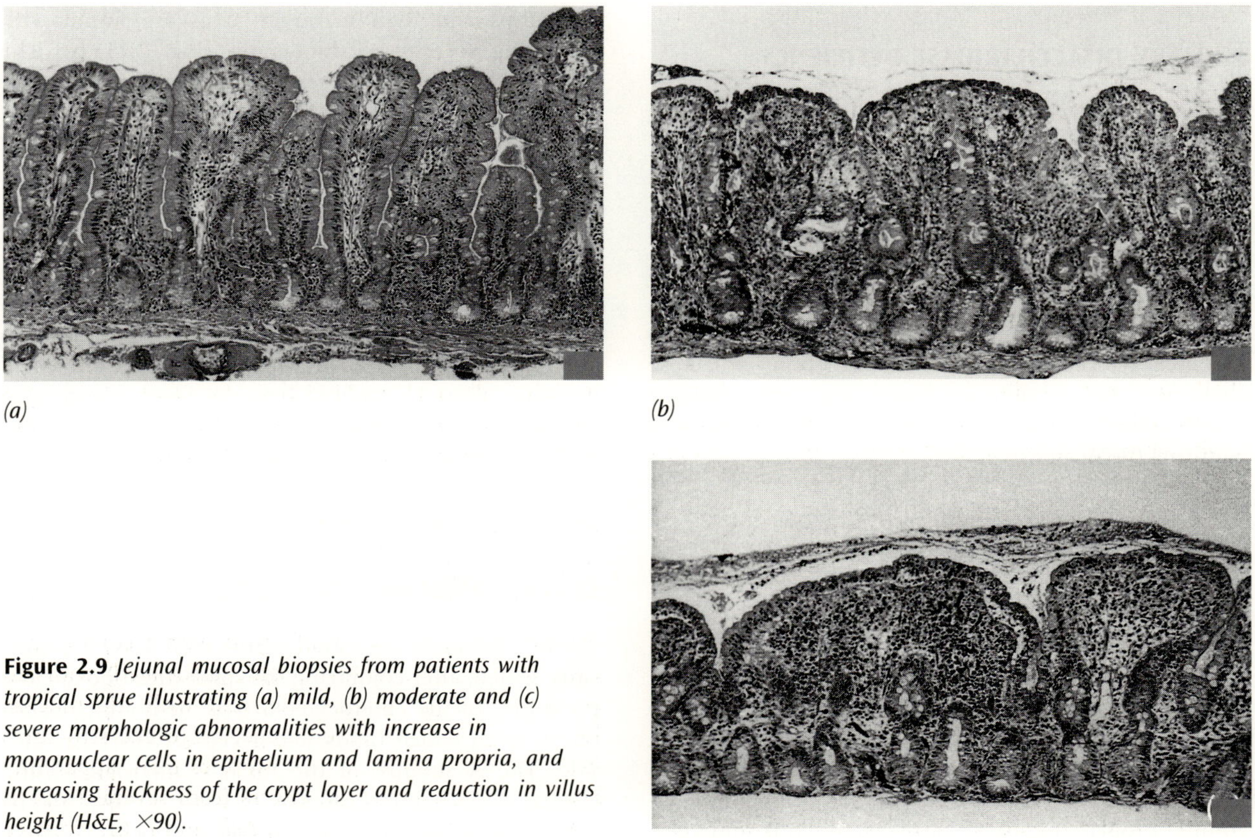

(a) *(b)* *(c)*

Figure 2.9 *Jejunal mucosal biopsies from patients with tropical sprue illustrating (a) mild, (b) moderate and (c) severe morphologic abnormalities with increase in mononuclear cells in epithelium and lamina propria, and increasing thickness of the crypt layer and reduction in villus height (H&E, ×90).*

Congenital mucosal abnormalities

MICROVILLUS INCLUSION DISEASE

Children with this disorder present with intractable diarrhoea, which is usually fatal, within 3 weeks of birth. Villus height is reduced without an increase in crypt depth or cellularity of the lamina propria. A PAS stain does not show a brush border or glycocalyx, but prominent PAS-positive inclusions are found at the luminal border of enterocytes and colonocytes. These inclusions, at electron microscopy, are cytoplasmic vesicles lined by intact microvilli. An abnormality of enterocyte microfilaments and the consequent inability to transport microvillus membrane to the luminal border has been suggested as a possible mechanism (Cutz *et al.*, 1989; Bell *et al.*, 1991; Phillips and Schmitz, 1992).

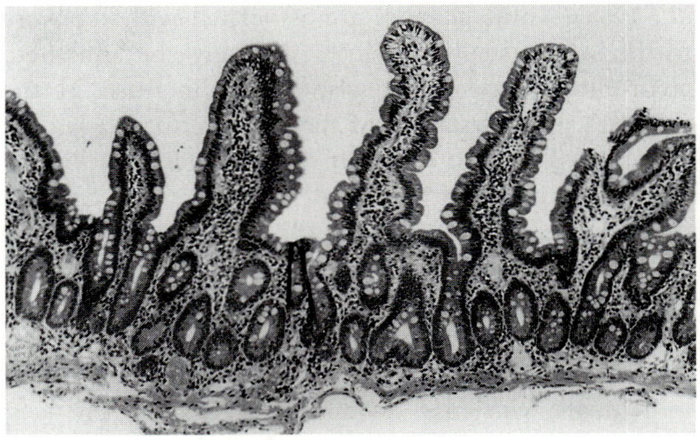

Figure 2.10 *Normal mucosal biopsy from the first part of the duodenum. The villi are shorter and the cellular infiltrate more compared to normal jejunal mucosa (H&E, ×90).*

TUFTING ENTEROPATHY

Duodenal biopsies from infants presenting with intractable neonatal diarrhoea reveal a severe reduction in villus height with normal or hypoplastic crypts. There is focal crowding and disorganization of enterocytes, which may involve 80–90 per cent of the epithelium. These disorganized areas are called tufts. Enterocytes are normal at the ultrastructural level. This disorder is thought to be due to abnormal epithelial mesenchymal interaction (Reifen *et al.*, 1994).

PRIMARY DISACCHARIDASE DEFICIENCY

Inherited brush border enzyme deficiency involving disaccharidases is fairly prevalent, especially lactose deficiency in certain tropical populations. The deficiency can also manifest in infancy, usually after an episode of infective diarrhoea. There may be episodes of diarrhoea and non-specific mucosal abnormalities related to milk ingestion (Harrison and Walker-Smith, 1977). The more common lactose deficiency in adults becomes symptomatic only when there is a lactose challenge and is not associated with morphologic abnormalities. An assay of enzyme levels in biopsies confirms the diagnosis.

Non-specific inflammation

In the proximal duodenum, which is most often sampled in endoscopic biopsies, in contrast to the distal duodenum and the jejunum, there is often a mild degree of injury (Fig. 2.10) characterized by an increase in mononuclear cells, some reactive crypt hyperplasia and shorter villi (Goldman and Antonioli, 1982). An increase in mononuclear cells in the epithelium and lamina propria indicates non-specific inflammation. Acute inflammatory changes are present in the mucosa surrounding duodenal ulcers (McCarty, 1924). Similar changes may also be found in patients with dyspepsia without duodenal ulcers (Judd and Nagel, 1927).

Duodenitis is characterized by changes in villous architecture, with oedema and congestion, and increased infiltration of the lamina propria by mononuclear cells, with activity of the inflammatory process being shown by infiltration by neutrophil polymorphs (Whitehead *et al.*, 1975; Jenkins *et al.*, 1985). Epithelial damage, Brunner's gland hyperplasia and gastric metaplastic changes with gastric-type cells initially at villus tips and then in larger areas are found with increasing severity of duodenites (Fig. 2.11a,b). The precise relationship between chronic duodenitis, active duodenitis and duodenal ulcer is not yet clear.

Acute infections

Acute bacterial or viral infections of the small intestine result in diarrhoea, which is usually watery in nature. The invasive pathogens associated with dysentery, especially *Shigellae*, do not appear to invade the small intestine, although typhoid (enteric) fever is associated with an infection of the Peyer's patches by *S. typhi*. The bacterial agents that infect the small bowel and cause diarrhoea either elaborate an enterotoxin, or adhere to and alter the luminal border of enterocytes.

ENTEROTOXIGENIC ORGANISMS

Vibrio cholerae is the paradigm of this class of organisms, which, after colonizing the small intestine in close proximity to the enterocyte surface membrane, elaborate a toxin which binds to a receptor, GM1 ganglioside. The A subunit of the toxin is internalized and triggers a biochemical cascade, resulting in secretion by the small intestinal mucosa and a profuse watery diarrhoea. It was originally thought that the small

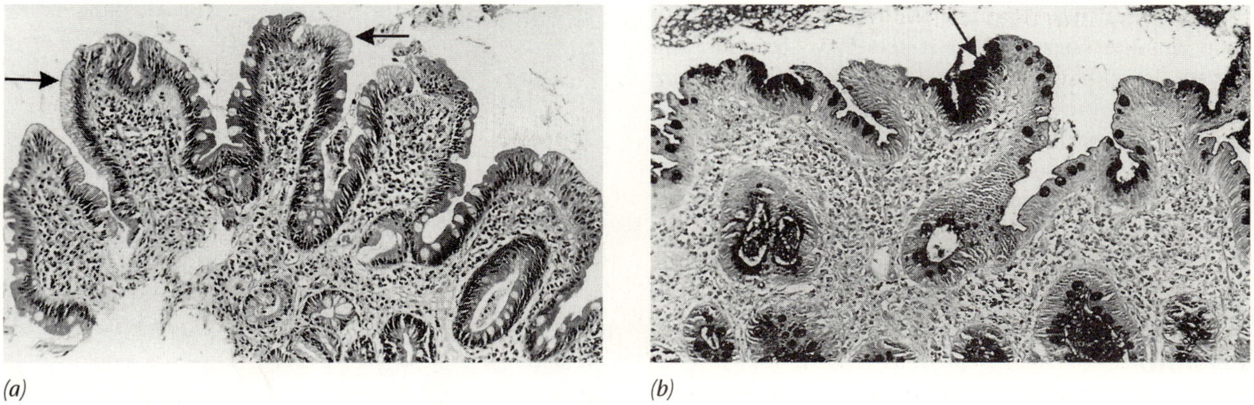

Figure 2.11 *(a) Duodenal mucosal biopsy. The increased cellularity of the lamina propria and focal gastric metaplasia (arrow) indicates chronic duodenitis (H&E, ×100). (b) The metaplastic gastric epithelium associated with chronic duodenitis stains positive for neutral mucin (arrow) (Alican blue periodic acid–Schiff, ×100).*

intestinal epithelium was denuded, based on postmortem observations, but Gangarosa and colleagues (1960) clearly showed that, at light microscopic examination, the epithelium and mucosa were apparently normal. The earlier suggestions (Asakura *et al.*, 1974) that there are apparently ultrastructural abnormalities in jejunal biopsies in patients with cholera has now been confirmed and extended (Mathan *et al.*, 1995). Electron microscopic examination of duodenal mucosal biopsies from 19 patients with cholera showed that widening of intercellular spaces and alteration of apical junctional complexes were prominent in the villous epithelium, whereas blebbing of the microvillous border and mitochondrial changes were more prominent in the crypt epithelium. In addition, degranulation of argentaffin cells, mucosal mast cells and eosinophils; increases in neutrophil polymorphs; and changes in enteric nerve fibres and microvasculature were also present. These ultrastructural changes suggest that the pathogenesis of cholera is not just a simple biochemical reaction, but that it also involves immunocytes, endocrine cells, blood vessels and nerves. A clear understanding of the pathogenesis of this mucosal lesion is essential, especially because it is now known that cholera affects not only the small intestine but also the colon (Ramakrishna and Mathan, 1993). There are as yet no published studies on the pathology of the gut in diarrhoea associated with enterotoxigenic organisms other than *V. cholerae*, but similar mechanisms are likely to be operative.

ADHERENT ORGANISMS

A variety of *Escherichia coli* are associated with diarrhoea and all of them, including the enteropathogenic *E. coli*, adhere to the luminal surface of enterocytes and bring about changes (Nataro and Kaper, 1998). Enteroaggregative *E. coli* appear to form a biofilm on the enterocyte surface using goblet cell mucus, and cause cytotoxicity in cell culture, organ culture and in experimental models (Tzipori *et al.*, 1992; Nataro *et al.*, 1996). Diffusely adherent *E. coli* stimulate elongation of microvilli and appear to be niched among them. Enteropathogenic *E. coli* have the ability to produce a lesion designated the attachment/effacement lesion with destruction of microvilli and a pedestal formation at the luminal border of enterocytes (Rothbaum *et al.*, 1982) (Fig. 2.12).

VIRAL DIARRHOEAS

Rotavirus is a major cause of acute diarrhoea in children under 3 years of age in both temperate and

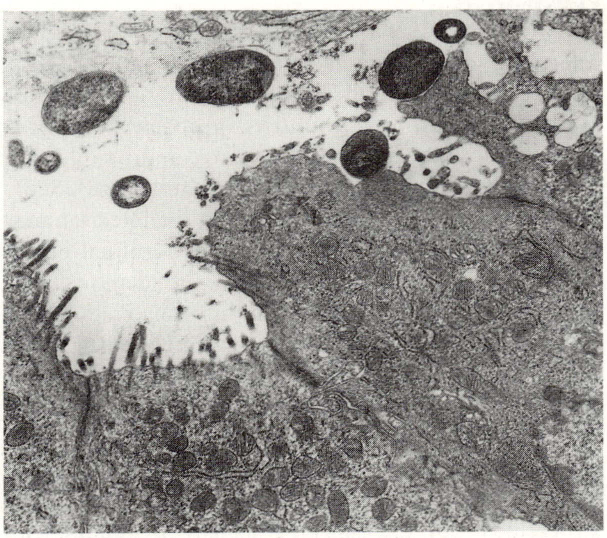

Figure 2.12 *Low-power electron micrograph of small intestinal mucosa. Note bacterial bodies and their attachment to the enterocyte by a 'pedestal' (×6000).*

tropical countries. Limited studies in children with rotavirus diarrhoea (Bishop *et al.*, 1973; Davidson and Barnes, 1979) have shown that the virus infects mature enterocytes, which are shed, shortening the villi, and are replaced by relatively immature cells. The loss of absorptive surface area and the immaturity of new enterocytes may contribute to secretion (Osborne *et al.*, 1988). Norwalk and related viral agents also damage absorptive enterocytes and shorten villi (Agus *et al.*, 1973).

TYPHOID

The Peyer's patches in the ileum are the entry point for this faecally–orally spread infection by *Salmonella typhi* or *paratyphi* A and B. After entry the organisms produce a febrile illness and infect the reticuloendothelial cells. They are then excreted in the bile and re-enter the Peyer's patches again from the lumen of the gut. The Peyer's patches then become markedly inflamed and ulcerate in the second and third week of the illness. Erosion of blood vessels may produce haemorrhage and the ulcers may perforate. Microscopically typical typhoid macrophages, which often contain ingested bacilli, red blood cells and nuclear debris, are the characteristic feature in infected Peyer's patches (Smith, 1976). Proximal jejunum is not affected and biopsies are normal (Chuttani *et al.*, 1971).

Chronic infections of the small intestine

Ulceration and stricture formation as well as involvement of the mesenteric lymph nodes are common in a variety of bacterial, viral and mycotic infections.

YERSINIOSIS

Infection with *Yersinia enterocolitica* and *Yersinia pseudotuberculosis* occurs more frequently in temperate zones than in tropical countries, probably because of the preference for lower temperatures and predilection of the organism to infect iron-replete individuals. Starting usually as an acute terminal ileitis, the infection may persist with longitudinal ulcers in the terminal ileum. Large colonies of coccobacilli can be demonstrated below the surface exudate and in microabscesses, which may be surrounded by neutrophil polymorphs and macrophages (Bradford *et al.*, 1974; Cover and Aber, 1989).

TUBERCULOSIS

Tuberculosis of the intestine usually manifests with strictures and intestinal obstruction, and can cause malabsorption owing to intraluminal enteric bacterial overgrowth. Massive enlargement of the mesenteric lymph nodes and tuberculous peritonitis may be associated. Intestinal tuberculosis commonly affects the ileum. It is associated with pulmonary tuberculosis in over 50 per cent of patients. Tuberculous intestinal ulcers are placed transversely and may be annular as infection spreads through the lymphatic channels in the intestinal wall. Caseating granuloma may be frequently found at the edges and below the floor of the ulcer. These ulcers seldom result in perforation, owing to extensive fibrosis. The tuberculous granuloma is characteristically an agglomeration of many tubercles with oval or spindle-shaped epithelioid cells, Langhans-type giant cells and a cuff of lymphocytes with central caseation, a homogeneous pink-staining material containing nuclear debris (Fig. 2.13). It may be possible to demonstrate tubercle bacilli using a Ziehl–Nielsen stain or DNA amplification techniques. It is important to distinguish tuberculous enteritis and Crohn's disease

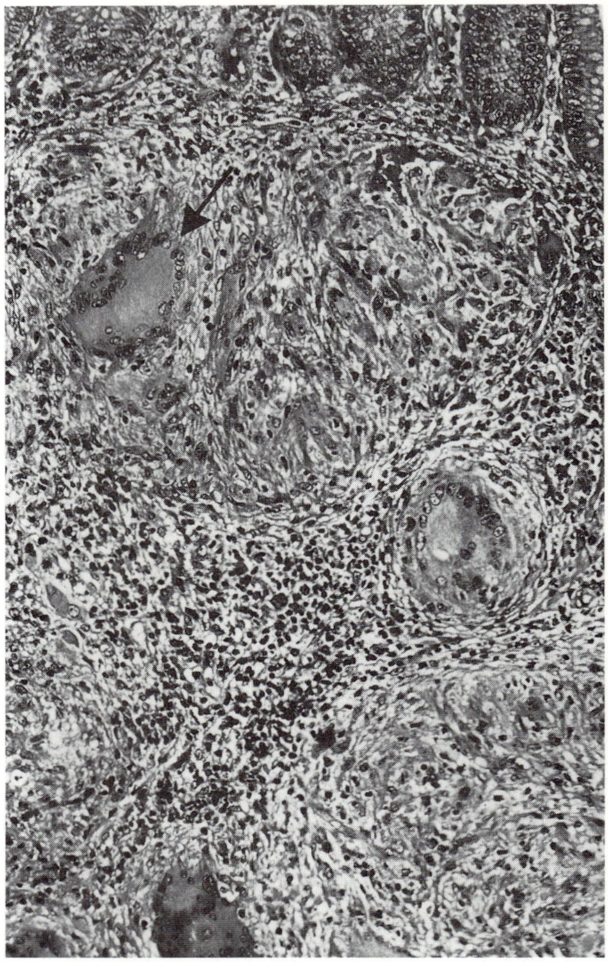

Figure 2.13 *Submucosa of the ileocaecal region in a patient with tuberculosis. Note several coalescing granulomas consisting of epithelioid cells, the Langhans-type of giant cells (arrow) surrounded by a cuff of lymphocytes and fibroblasts (H&E, ×160).*

because the management and prognosis of the two conditions are distinctly different (Tandon and Prakash, 1972; Tonghua *et al.*, 1981).

MYCOBACTERIUM AVIUM-INTERCELLULARE

The importance of non-tuberculous mycobacterial infections of the small intestine has been recognized with the increasing prevalence of immunocompromised individuals. These mycobacteria are ingested from the environment and may also cause systemic infections. The characteristic histopathological feature is a poorly defined granuloma with pale blue striated histocytes containing large numbers of mycobacteria, easily identifiable with the Ziehl–Nielsen stain (Pitchenik and Fertel, 1992).

CHRONIC VIRAL INFECTIONS

Asymptomatic infection by cytomegalovirus is widespread in the normal population (Weller, 1971; Mukundan *et al.*, 1977). Symptomatic infection with mucosal ulceration occurs rarely in immunocompetent individuals, but can be a problem in the immunocompromised, particularly in the oesophagus and the large intestine. Small intestinal infection can be confined to single epithelial cells without inflammatory response or causing ulceration. Characteristic cytomegaly and acidophilic intranuclear inclusions with a clear halo (Cowdry body), giving an owl's eye morphology (Henson, 1972) or atypical inclusions (Schwartz and Wilcox, 1992) in macrophages, endothelial cells and stromal cells, enables a clear diagnosis (Fig. 2.14).

WHIPPLE'S DISEASE

Small bowel biopsy can be diagnostic in this rare multisystem infection. The patients usually present with malabsorption syndrome and may also have extraintestinal manifestations. Endoscopic examination of the duodenum shows thickened granular or plaque-bearing mucosa due to the infiltration of the villus lamina propria by infected macrophages (Mayberry *et al.*, 1986). Histologically the lamina propria is expanded by numerous macrophages with granular greyish cytoplasm. The macrophages contain PAS-positive, diastase-resistant, round or sickle-shaped bacilli in the cytoplasm. These macrophages have to be distinguished from *Mycobacterium avium-intercellulare* infection. Examination of epon-embedded 1-μm sections on electron microscopy will enable better recognition of the bacilli, especially following therapy (Dobbins and Kawanishi, 1981; Fleming *et al.*, 1988). These uncultivable organisms have been characterized by DNA amplification techniques, and are apparently related to the actinomycetes and have been named *Tropheryma whippelii* (Relman *et al.*, 1992; Herbay *et al.*, 1996).

FUNGAL INFECTIONS

Fungal pathogens (*Candida albicans*, mucormycosis, *Histoplasma capsulatum*, *Aspergillus*) are often present in the bowel lumen and can cause infections in immunocompromised individuals and diabetics, and when prolonged antibiotic therapy is given. *Candida* infection is usually superficial and produces a white coating. It may also infect duodenal ulcers (Peters *et al.*, 1980) or produce penetrating ulcerated lesions (Walsh and Merz, 1986). Mucormycosis and aspergillosis can cause ulcerative lesions. Their predilection to invade blood vessels can cause ischaemia and infarction. Intestinal involvement with *Histoplasma* may result from haematogenous spread from pulmonary infection. The characteristic histological appearance of vacuolated macrophages in the lamina propria containing numerous spherical organisms is diagnostic (Fig. 2.15). PAS and Gomori's methenamine–silver stains are useful in

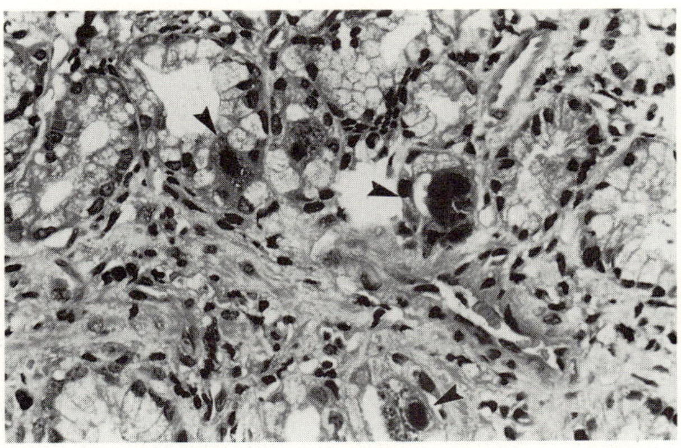

Figure 2.14 *Duodenal mucosal biopsy. Note the characteristic nuclear inclusion of cytomegalovirus infection in Brunner's gland epithelium (arrowhead). An inflammatory response is characteristically absent (H&E, ×380).*

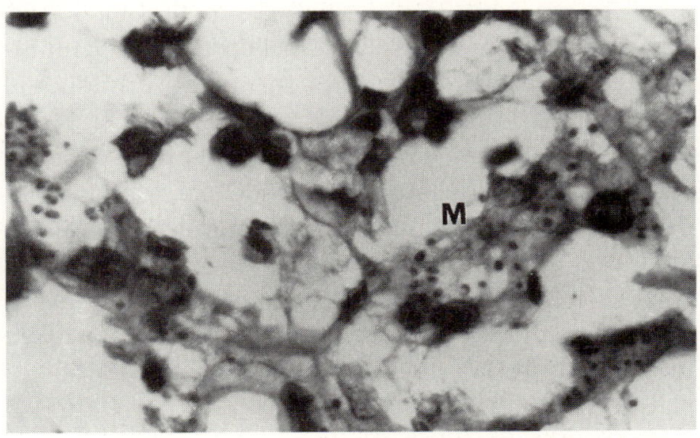

Figure 2.15 *Mesenteric lymph node with vacuolated macrophages (M) containing numerous spherical 1–5 μm* Histoplasma *organisms (H&E, ×800).*

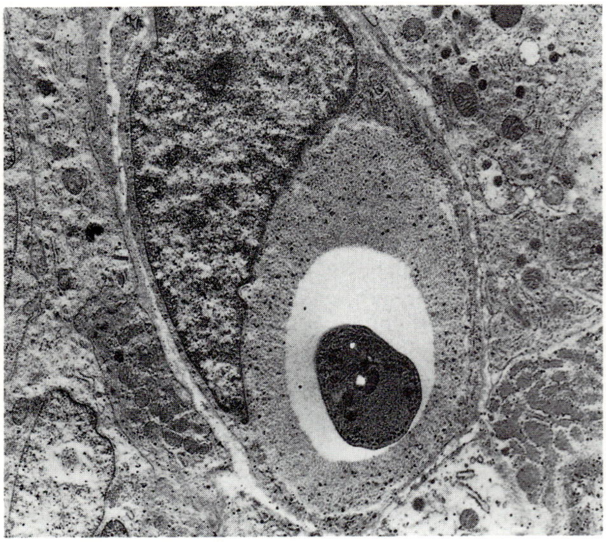

Figure 2.16 *Electron micrograph of a duodenal mucosal lamina propria macrophage from a patient with AIDS with intact* Histoplasma capsulatum *in cytoplasmic space (×12 500).*

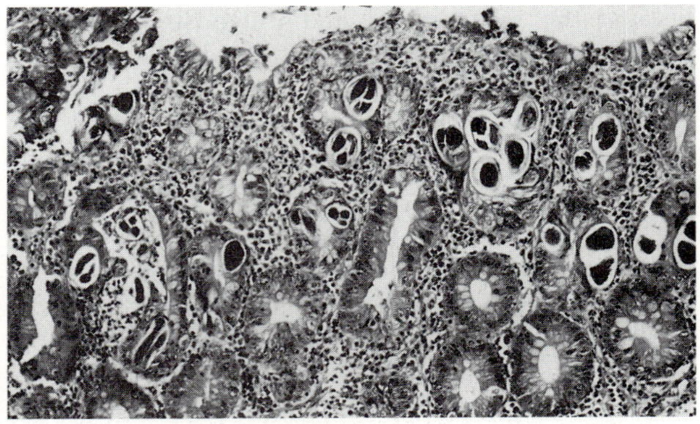

Figure 2.17 Strongyloides stercoralis *infection of jejunal mucosa. Adult worms, larvae and segmented eggs are present within enterocytic tunnels. The mucosa shows increased cellularity of the lamina propria (H&E, ×120).*

confirming the diagnosis (Bank *et al.*, 1965). Effective host response is dependent on the interaction between CD4-positive T cells and macrophages. In immunocompromised patients, disseminated infection may occur (Mandell *et al.*, 1986) (Fig. 2.16).

Parasitic infections

The wide prevalence of intestinal parasites has long been recognized, but the presence of large numbers of immunocompromised patients, especially patients infected with human immunodeficiency virus (HIV), has focused attention on intracytoplasmic parasites belonging to the *Coccidia*.

STRONGYLOIDES STERCORALIS

Asymptomatic infections are widely prevalent. Symptomatic infection with diarrhoea and malabsorption and disseminated hyperinfection can occur (Milder *et al.*, 1981; Igra-Siegman *et al.*, 1981). Larvae of the parasites can be detected in stools or duodenal aspirates. In duodenal biopsies, adult female worms, eggs and larvae are found within epithelial tunnels (Fig. 2.17) (Grove *et al.*, 1987). They damage enterocytes with shortening of villi, crypt hypertrophy, ulceration and marked increase in lamina propria cellularity (Marcial-Rojas, 1975).

CAPILLARIA PHILIPPINENSIS

Infection with this nematode causes diarrhoea and malabsorption and was first recognized in an epidemic in the Philippines. It has been reported from south Asia and the Middle East (Cross, 1992; Kang *et al.*, 1994). Proximal small intestinal mucosa contains the adult worm in epithelial tunnels, causing shortening of villi and infiltration of the lamina propria by plasma cells, lymphocytes, eosinophils and neutrophil polymorphs (Figs 2.18 and 2.19). There may be degenerative changes in enterocytes (Fig. 2.20). The abnormalities revert on successful therapy.

GIARDIA LAMBLIA

This protozoan parasite is found world-wide. In many tropical countries it is primarily a pathogen of children with acute watery or persistent diarrhoea, while adults are usually asymptomatic sporadic cyst passers. In temperate climates it has been associated with water-borne or institution-associated epidemics. In immunocompetent individuals the diarrhoea is often self-limiting but occasionally may be persistent. *Giardia* are an important cause of chronic diarrhoea in the

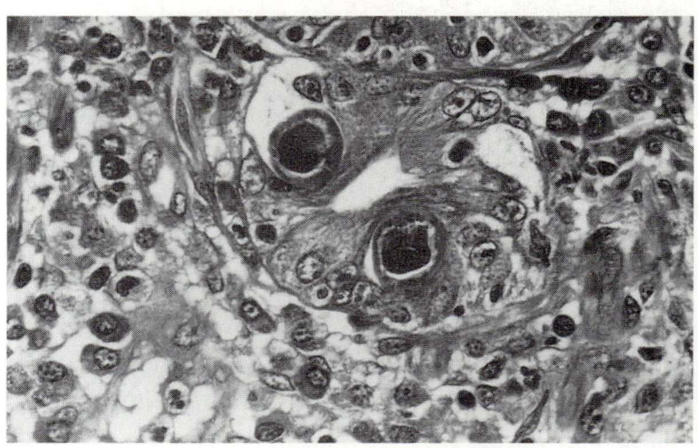

Figure 2.18 *Duodenal biopsy of a patient with capillariasis. The section of the adult worm is present in an enterocytic tunnel in the crypt epithelium (H&E, ×700).*

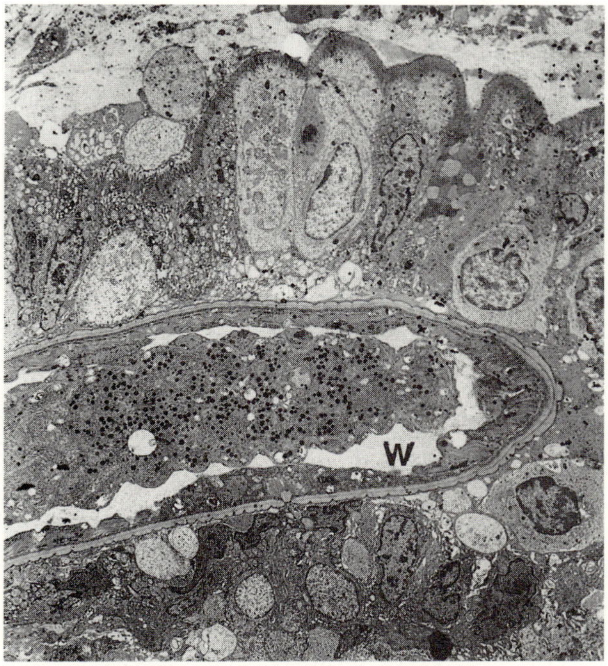

Figure 2.19 *Electron micrograph of a duodenal biopsy with longitudinal section of adult capillaria worm (W). The adjacent epithelial cells show degenerative changes (×1200).*

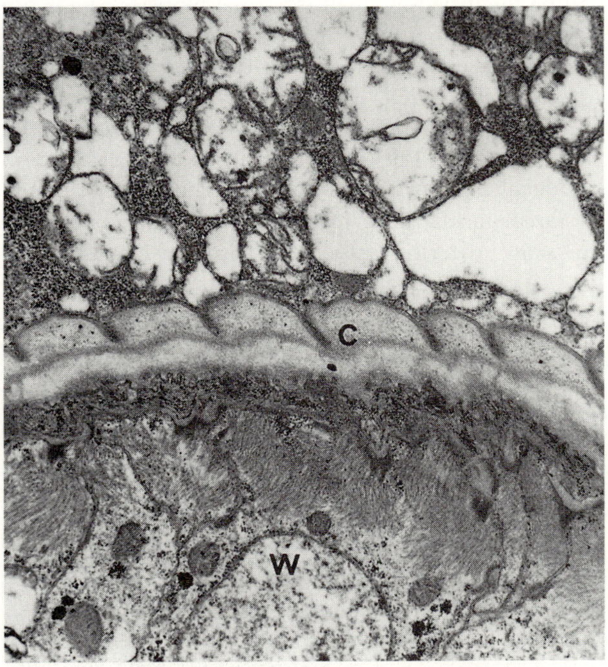

Figure 2.20 *Higher power electron micrograph of the section show in Fig. 2.19. The cuticle (C) of the worm (W) is in direct contact with the enterocyte cytoplasm with swollen damaged mitochondria (×22 000).*

immunocompromised (Farthing, 1997). The proximal small intestine is the preferred site of infection, and diagnosis can be made by detecting the parasites in

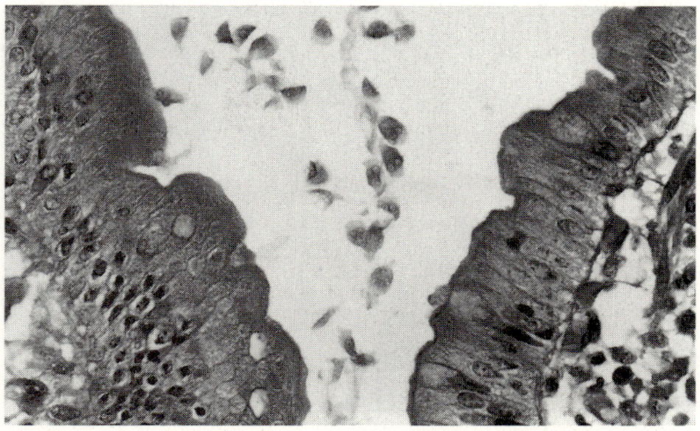

Figure 2.21 *Jejunal biopsy with many pear- and sickle-shaped* Giardia lamblia *trophozoites with their characteristic two nuclei at the broader end in the space between villi (×600).*

aspirates or biopsies, by immunoassay or microscopy or detection of cysts in stool (Mank *et al.*, 1997). Pear- or sickle-shaped parasites can be detected in paraffin sections (Fig. 2.21). In smears they are flat and pear-shaped with two nuclei at the broad end and up to four flagellae attached to the narrow end. Electron microscopic examination reveals a suction disc on the ventral surface (Fig. 2.22). The jejunal mucosa may be apparently normal, have increased intraepithelial lymphocytes and plasma cells or, especially in immunocompromised subjects, show more severe changes with villus atrophy and crypt hypertrophy (Oberhuber *et al.*, 1997).

COCCIDIA

Intracellular parasites belonging to the *Coccidia* group are now recognized as a significant problem in immunocompromised individuals who present with

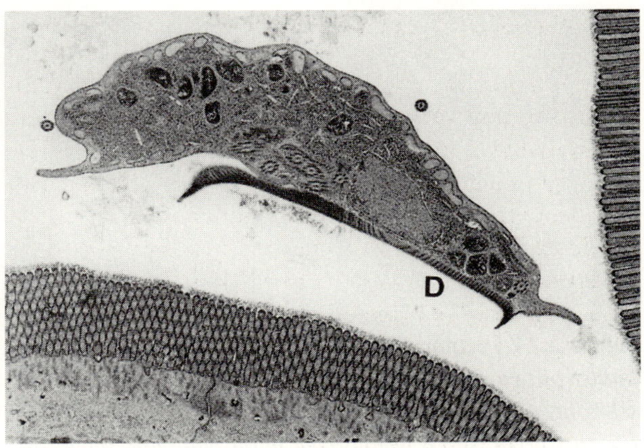

Figure 2.21 *Electron micrograph of section of* Giardia lamblia *trophozoite in the intervillus space. The ventral suction disc (D) is clearly identifiable (×8400).*

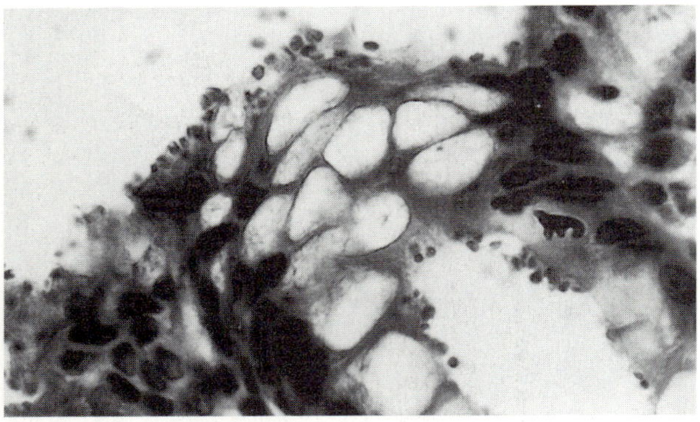

Figure 2.23 *Cryptosporidia attached to the luminal border of enterocytes (H&E, ×1000).*

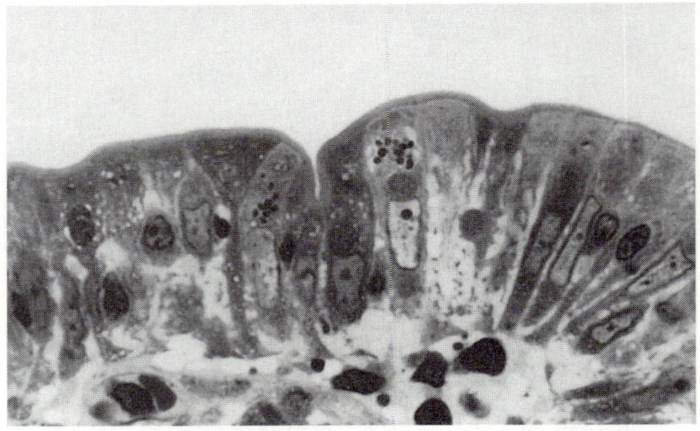

Figure 2.25 *A 1-μm section of jejunal mucosal biopsy stained with toluidene blue. The spores of microsporidia are seen supranuclearly in two enterocytes (×1000).*

chronic diarrhoea and malabsorption (Curry *et al.*, 1991; Gellin and Soave, 1992). They can also infect immunocompetent individuals.

Cryptosporidia can infect immunocompetent individuals and cause a self-limiting watery diarrhoea or no symptoms (Mathan *et al.*, 1985). More disseminated infection occurs in immunocompromised patients (Godwin, 1991; Navin and Juranck, 1984). In biopsies the organisms can be identified as faintly basophilic, 2–4 μm spherical structures on the luminal border of enterocytes in haematoxylin–eosin-stained paraffin sections (Fig. 2.23). Villus shortening and increased cellularity of the lamina propria may be seen (Lefkowitch *et al.*, 1984). Ultrastructurally, the parasite is located at the luminal surface of the enterocyte within the apical cell membrane (Fig. 2.24) (Bird and Smith, 1980).

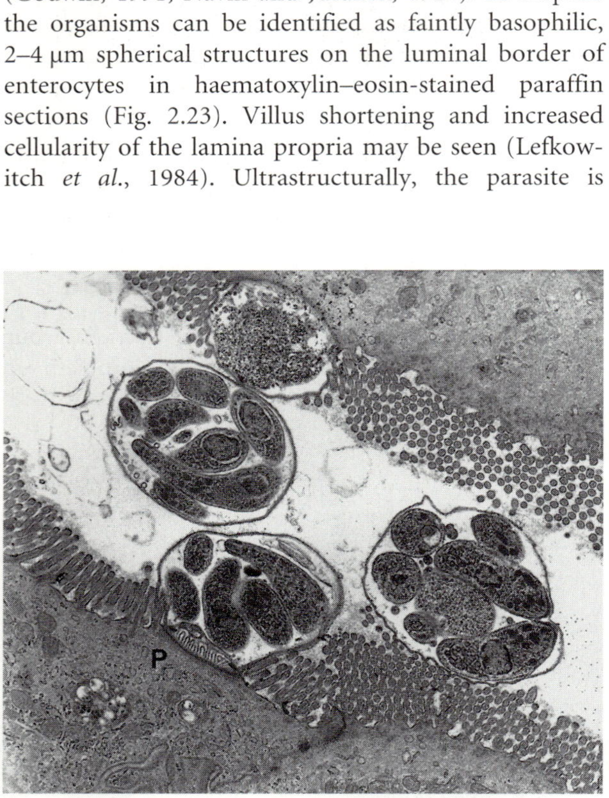

Figure 2.24 *Electron micrograph showing the microvillus border of two enterocytes. Two mature* Cryptosporidium *schizonts are seen in the lumen. One schizont is attached to the enterocyte with a well-formed basal plate and shows the loss of microvilli at the site of attachment (P). The parasitophorous vacuole is formed by the enterocyte apical cell membrane (×9000).*

Microsporidia are obligate intracellular parasites causing a wide variety of illness, including chronic diarrhoea and malabsorption in immunocompetent and immunodeficient patients (Canning and Hollister, 1987; Weber and Bryan, 1994). Intracellular organisms can be identified in small intestinal biopsies as 4–5 μm intracellular meronts and sporonts with multiple 1.5 μm spores in the supranuclear cytoplasm in villus tip cells (Fig. 2.25). Electron microscopy is useful in identifying the species (Fig. 2.26) (Bryan *et al.*, 1991; Michiels *et al.*, 1993). Spores can also be detected in duodenal aspirate and stools (Orenstein *et al.*, 1990).

Sarcosporidia have recently been reported to cause an acute enteritis associated with the ingestion of

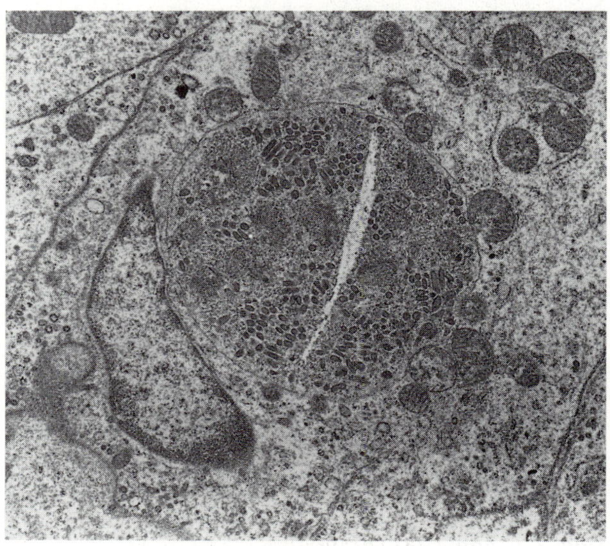

Figure 2.26 *Electron micrograph of an enterocyte. Note the microsporidium sporont(s) adjacent to the nucleus (×12 500).*

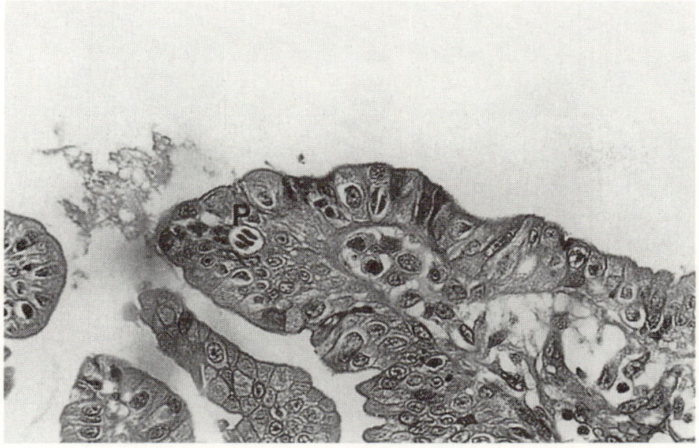

Figure 2.27 *Duodenal biopsy. Note the merozoites of* Isospora *in parasitophorous vacuole in enterocytes (P) (H&E, ×400).*

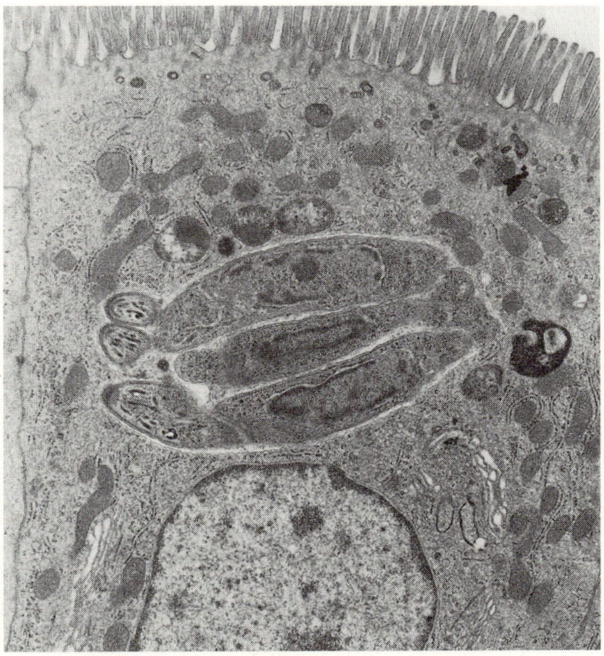

Figure 2.28 *Electron micrograph of a duodenal enterocyte containing three merozoites in the supranuclear cytoplasm (×8000).*

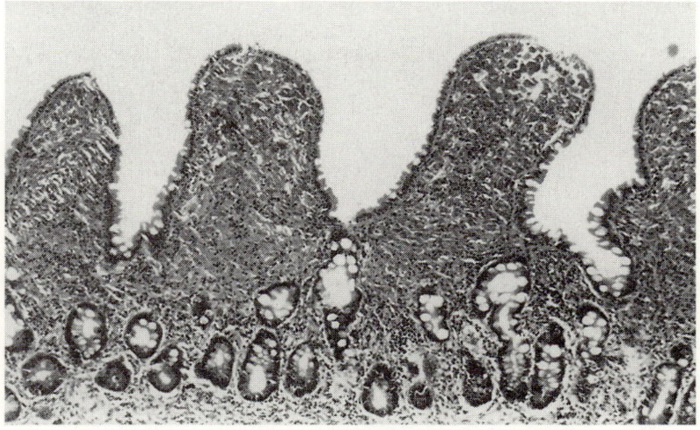

(a)

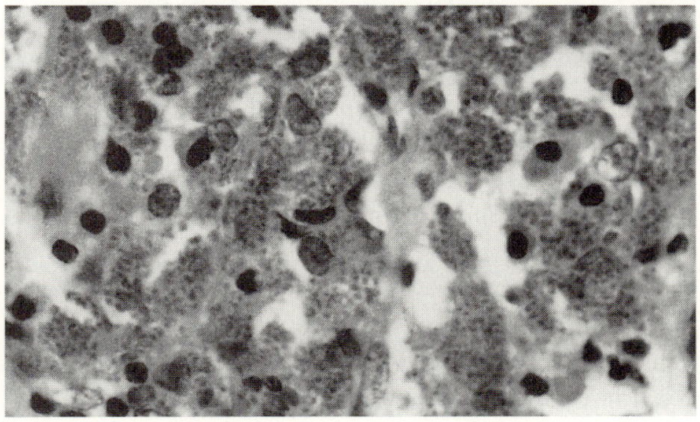

(b)

Figure 2.29 *(a) Duodenal mucosal biopsy in a patient with kala-azar. Note blunted villi and marked infiltration of the lamina propria (H&E, ×120). (b) High-power view of the lamina propria in (a) showing numerous macrophages with Leishman–Donovan bodies (H&E, ×1000).*

uncooked beef (Bunyaratvej *et al.*, 1982). Intracellular sexual forms of sarcosporidia were seen in epithelial cells in segments of intestine with eosinophilic or necrotizing enteritis.

Isospora belli, another coccidian parasite, is found world-wide (Pape and Johnson, 1991). Ingested sporulated oocysts excyst in the intestinal lumen and sporozoites invade enterocytes where various stages of schizogony (asexual) or gametogony can be identified (Fig. 2.27 and 2.28) (Brandborg *et al.*, 1970; Trier *et al.*, 1974). Villus atrophy, crypt hyperplasia and increased lamina propria cellularity may be seen. Prolonged and invasive infection has been reported in patients with the aquired immunodeficiency syndrome (AIDS) (Michiels *et al.*, 1994).

Cyclospora is another coccidian parasite which can cause self-limiting or prolonged diarrhoea and malabsorption (Bendall *et al.*, 1993; Pape *et al.*, 1994). In mucosal biopsies, the intracellular parasite is present in vacuoles in enterocytes (Connor *et al.*, 1993; Ortega *et al.*, 1993). Diagnosis is facilitated by the detection in the stools of 8–10 μm-sized oocysts that are larger and have a variable staining pattern compared to *Cryptosporidium* (Soave, 1996).

LEISHMANIASIS

Intestinal manifestations of visceral leishmaniasis have been reported from areas where kala-azar is endemic (Datry *et al.*, 1990; Altes *et al.*, 1991). Villous atrophy is present in the duodenal mucosa with the lamina propria of the villous tip densely packed with macrophages containing Leishman–Donovan bodies.

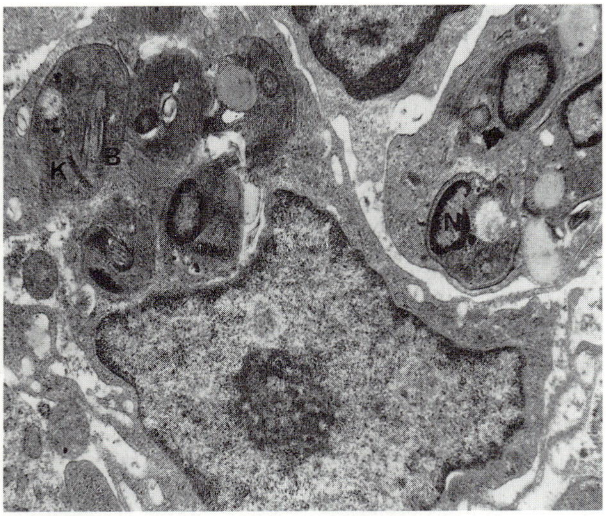

Figure 2.30 *Electron micrograph of a macrophage in the duodenal lamina propria of a patient with kala-azar. The Leishman–Donovan body with nucleus (N), kinetoplast (K) and basal body (B) are clearly identifiable (×18 000).*

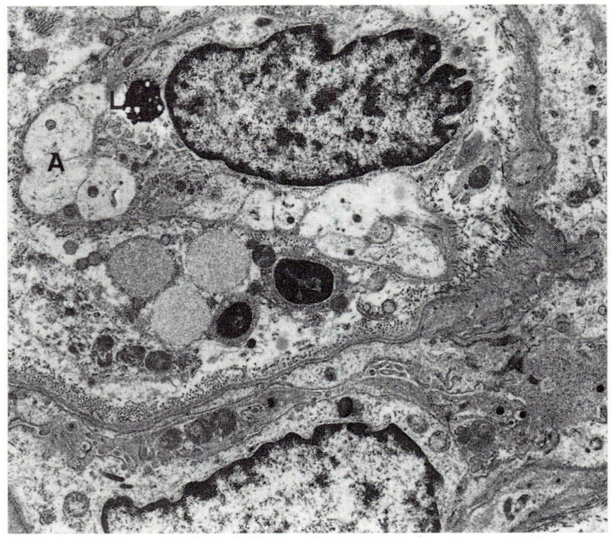

Figure 2.31 *Electron micrograph of a Schwann cell in the duodenal mucosal lamina propria in a patient with AIDS. Note increase in lysosomes (L) and degenerated axons (A) (×3600).*

They are 2–3 μm long and can be seen in haematoxylin–eosin-stained paraffin sections (Fig. 2.29a,b). Giemsa stain brings out the details of a large red nucleus, deep violet rod-like kinetoplast and a dot-like basal body. Electron microscopy helps in identifying the different *Leishmania* species (Manson-Bhar and Bell, 1987) (Fig. 2.30).

HIV infection

Persistent diarrhoea and malabsorption has been a frequent finding in many patients with AIDS due to HIV infection. A large number of opportunistic infections of the intestine have a high prevalence in these patients (Dworkin *et al.*, 1985; Sewankambo *et al.*, 1987; Greenson *et al.*, 1991). The HIV virus can infect epithelial cells (Nelson *et al.*, 1988) and cells in the lamina propria (Ehrenpreis *et al.*, 1992), and an enteropathy associated with HIV infection with histological changes and malabsorption has been reported (Kotler *et al.*, 1984; Ullrich *et al.*, 1989; Clayton *et al.*, 1992). In jejunal biopsies from HIV-affected individuals without any opportunistic infection, at the ultrastructural level, degenerative changes in enterocytes and enteric nerves (Fig. 2.31) and proliferative changes in the microvasculature were present. There was marked proliferation of the smooth endoplasmic reticulum with dilated tubules and supranuclear vacuolation of enterocytes, suggesting a primary HIV enteropathy (Griffin *et al.*, 1988; Mathan *et al.*, 1990). Kaposi's sarcoma, lymphomas and other malignancies also occur with higher frequency in HIV infections (Danzig *et al.*, 1991; Beral *et al.*, 1992).

Malabsorption syndromes

Failure of the primary function of the small intestine results in malabsorption of nutrients, usually associated with histological changes in the small intestinal mucosa.

COELIAC SPRUE

Surface enterocyte damage and loss owing to a reaction to the gliadin fraction of the gluten of wheat, rye or barley is the key to the pathogenesis of this syndrome, also known as gluten-sensitive enteropathy. The underlying metabolic defect in the patient is not known but genetic, immunological, infectious and environmental factors have been suggested (Marsh, 1992b). Biopsies from the duodenum or upper jejunum have a markedly distorted architecture with almost total loss of villi and crypt hypertrophy (Rubin, 1960). There is a marked increase in epithelial lymphocytes in the surface epithelium and increased lymphocytes, plasma cells, mast cells and eosinophils in the lamina propria. Total exclusion of gluten from the diet leads to an improvement in symptoms and recovery of the mucosal architecture, which relapses if gluten is reintroduced in the diet (Trier, 1991a). This sequence of response is diagnostic, while the basic morphological appearance is shared by other conditions. Untreated long-standing coeliac sprue may lead to the development of neoplasms (carcinoma or T-cell lymphoma) of the small intestine (Swinson *et al.*, 1983; Isaacson *et al.*, 1985). Patients with dermatitis herpetiformis may also have a gluten-sensitive enteropathy and respond to gluten withdrawal. In some patients with apparent coeliac disease, there might be no response to gluten withdrawal (refractory sprue) and some of them may have a thick band of collagen at the base of the epithelium (collagenous sprue) (Weinstein *et al.*, 1970; Trier *et al.*, 1978).

BLIND LOOP (STAGNANT BOWEL) SYNDROME

Strictures, fistulae or diverticulae of the small intestine enable the proliferation of a faecal-type bacterial flora in the lumen of the small intestine with resultant malabsorption. Biopsies of upper small bowel mucosa may be relatively normal, although the loop with bacterial proliferation may show non-specific changes in architecture, and increase in the mononuclear infiltrate in the lamina propria and the epithelium. The malabsorption is the result of bacterial competition for nutrients and breakdown of enzymes or bile salts (Ament *et al.*, 1972).

ABETALIPOPROTEINAEMIA

This is a rare disorder of failure of triglyceride transfer protein synthesis leading to defective assembly of chylomicrons and very low density lipoprotein (Wetterau *et al.*, 1992; Rader and Brewer, 1993). The architecture of the mucosa is normal but large vacuoles are present in the supranuclear cytoplasm of enterocytes, which, using special stains (Oil red O) or electron microscopy, can be shown to be triglyceride droplets (Fig. 2.32). The resynthesis of absorbed fat into triglyceride molecules is not affected but there is defective production of betalipoprotein, which is necessary for triglyceride transport. The patient may develop essential fatty acid deficiencies and neurological abnormalities. Ultrastructural studies show lipid in supranuclear cytoplasm and Golgi but not in intercellular spaces or lacteals (Kayden, 1972) (Fig. 2.33).

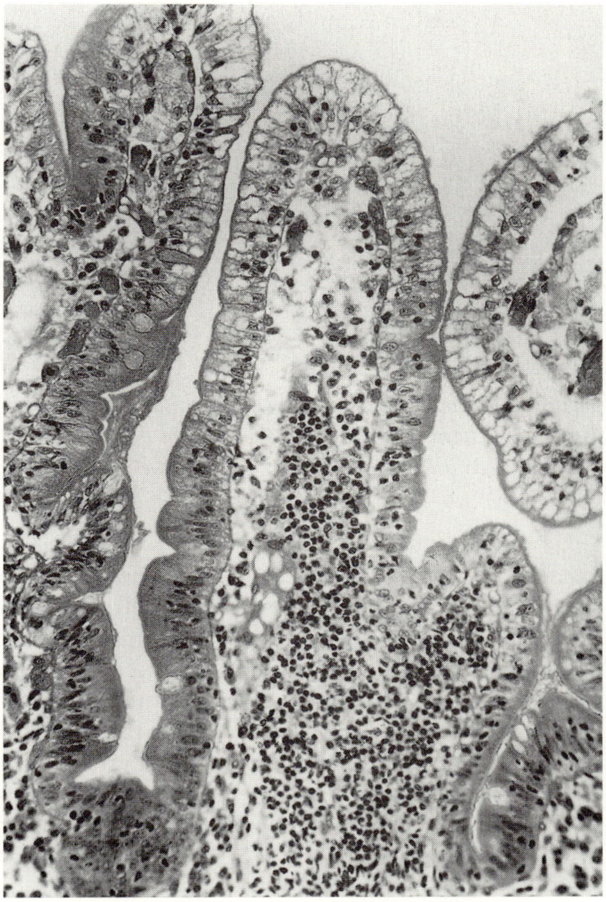

Figure 2.32 *Duodenal biopsy in a patient with abetalipoproteinaemia. Note the supranuclear vacuolization of enterocytes on the upper third of villi (H&E, ×180).*

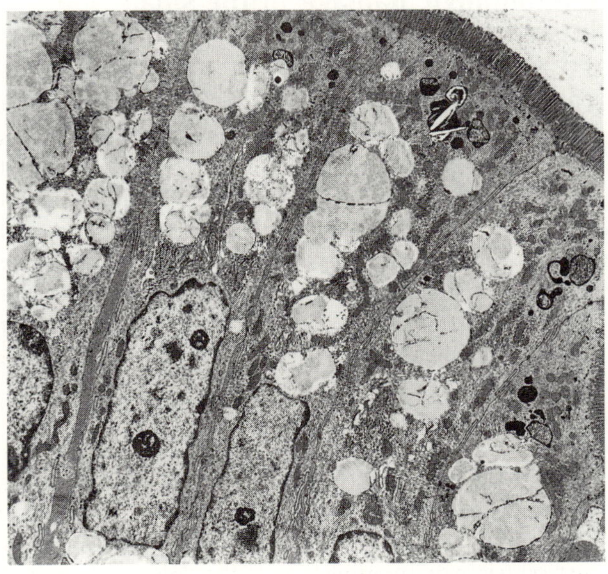

Figure 2.33 *Electron micrograph of villus enterocytes in the duodenal biopsy of a patient with abetalipoproteinaemia. Many fat droplets are present in the supranuclear cytoplasm of enterocytes (×3700).*

INTESTINAL LYMPHANGIECTASIA

Patients may present with hypoalbuminaemia and a protein-losing enteropathy and may have dilated lymphatics in one or more segments of the small intestine (Pomerantz and Waldmann, 1963). This may be a primary heritable disorder or secondary to a variety of conditions that can give rise to obstruction of lymph flow. Dilated lymphatics are present in the mucosa with distortion of architecture but an intact epithelium (Fig. 2.34) (Dobbins, 1966).

TROPICAL SPRUE

This is primary malabsorption syndrome affecting residents of, or visitors to, several tropical regions and is due to damage to enterocytes. The morphological alterations are non-specific, with a reduction in villous height, increase in the thickness of crypts and an

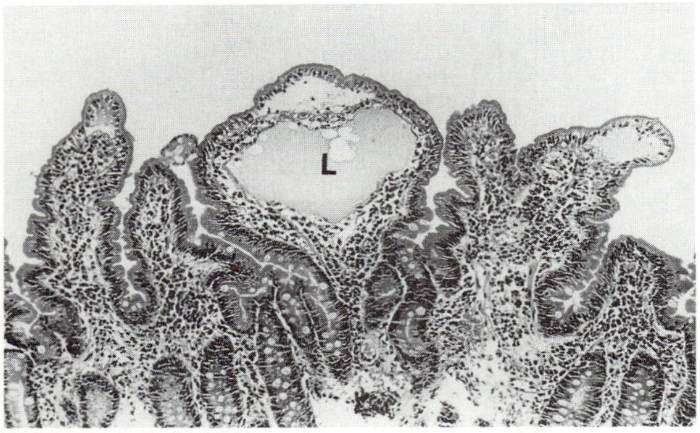

Figure 2.34 *Duodenal mucosal biopsy from a patient with lymphangiectasia. The villi are distorted with dilated lymphatics (L) (H&E, ×80).*

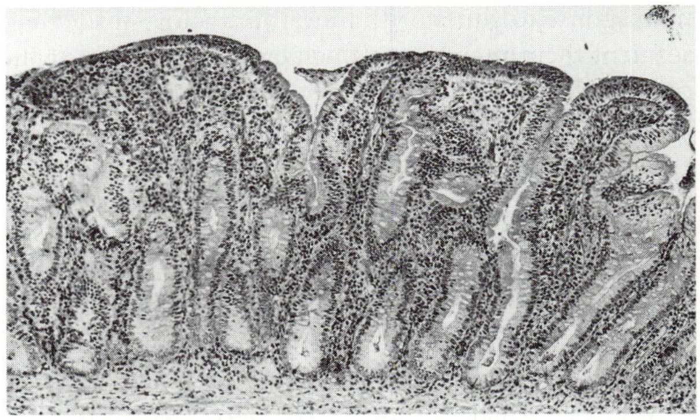

Figure 2.35 *Jejunal biopsy from a patient with tropical sprue with moderately severe changes. The crypt villus ratio is 1:1. The villus enterocytes are short with an increase in intraepithelial lymphocytes. The crypt layer is thickened with increased mitosis. The cellularity of the lamina propria is increased (H&E, ×90).*

increase in mononuclear cell infiltrate in the lamina propria (Fig. 2.35) (Mathan *et al.*, 1975). Ultrastructural studies and pulse labelling of *in vitro* organ cultures following the migration of labelled cells to the villi has suggested that the enterocyte stem cells produce defective progeny, which are extruded from the epithelial layer well before they reach the zone of extrusion at villous tips. This leads to accelerated cell turnover in an attempt to compensate for the cell loss. The balance between cell loss, increased cell production and the nutritional status of the patient, influenced by the malabsorption, determine the ultimate architectural changes in the upper small intestinal mucosa (Mathan *et al.*, 1986).

Immunologic damage to the small intestine

The gut-associated lymphoid tissue is one of the largest immunological organs in the body, situated in a primary barrier between the internal environment of the body and the external environment in the lumen of the intestine. Immunological damage to the intestinal mucosa may occur as part of graft versus host disease (GVHD) in bone marrow transplant recipients, as a manifestation of various immune deficiency states or due to food allergy.

GRAFT VERSUS HOST DISEASE

In the acute phase of GVHD, starting about 3 weeks post-transplant, immunocompetent donor T cells are involved. The patient may present with diarrhoea or gastrointestinal bleeding, and the histopathological changes may range from single cell apoptosis in the crypts to confluent ulcers (Fig. 2.36). The GVHD changes have to be identified against the background of the effects of prior radiation, chemotherapy and opportunistic infections such as cytomegalovirus (Beschorner, 1984; Snover *et al.*, 1985). In the chronic phase, starting 40–400 days post-transplant, small intestinal involvement is relatively rare, although ulcers, strictures and submucosal fibrosis may occur (Snover, 1990).

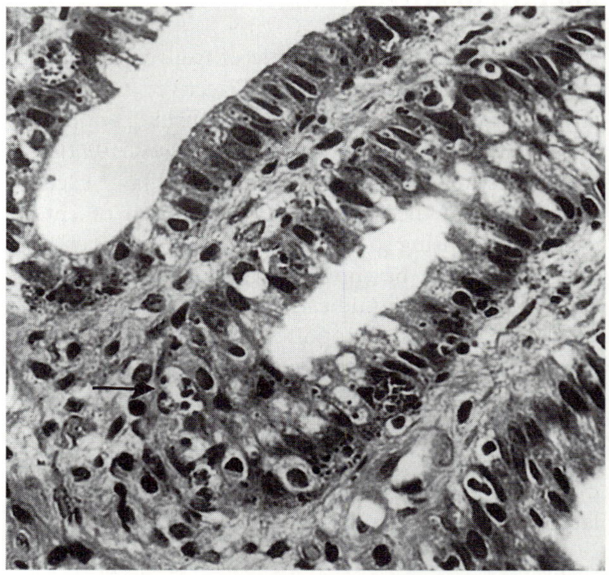

Figure 2.36 *Duodenal crypts in an endoscopic biopsy from a patient with acute graft versus host disease. There are many vacuolated apoptotic enterocytes with nuclear fragments (arrow). Intraepithelial lymphocytes are increased (H&E, ×600).*

IMMUNODEFICIENCY SYNDROMES

Immunodeficiency states that have an effect on the small intestine may be predominantly antibody deficient (X-linked agammaglobulinaemia, common variable hypogammaglobulinaemia, selective IgA deficiency), predominantly defects in cell-mediated immunity (severe combined immunodeficiency) or immunodeficiency associated with other defects, such as the DiGeorge syndrome. The gastrointestinal manifestations are usually related to opportunistic infections and malabsorption. Immunocytochemical techniques can demonstrate paucity or absence of specific immunocyte subtypes in small intestinal mucosal biopsies. Multiple lymphoid nodules may be present in the mucosa in association with any of the immunodeficiency states (Hermans *et al.*, 1966; Amman and Hunj, 1971; Rosen *et al.*, 1984; Ament, 1985).

NODULAR LYMPHOID HYPERPLASIA (NLH)

Multiple lymphoid nodules involving the entire small bowel and sometimes the colon are found in 20–60 per cent of patients with common variable hypogammaglobulinaemia, but are less common in those suffering from selective IgA deficiency (Ament *et al.*, 1973). This condition may also be present in the ileum and/or colon of some children and adults, and is often an incidental finding. The mucosa affected with NLH may be nodular and large collections may distort neighbouring villi. Histologically, they resemble a benign or reactive lymphoid collection, with no specialization of the overlying epithelium, proliferating B cells in the germinal centre with a mantle zone containing B and T cells. The surrounding lamina propria may not contain any plasma cells in immunodeficient subjects (Fig. 2.37a,b).

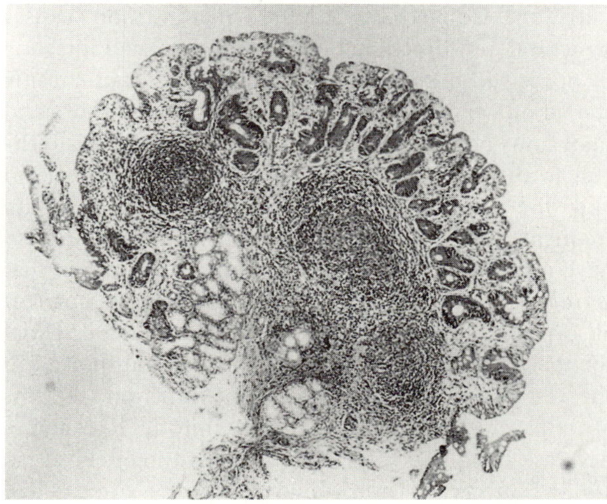

(a)

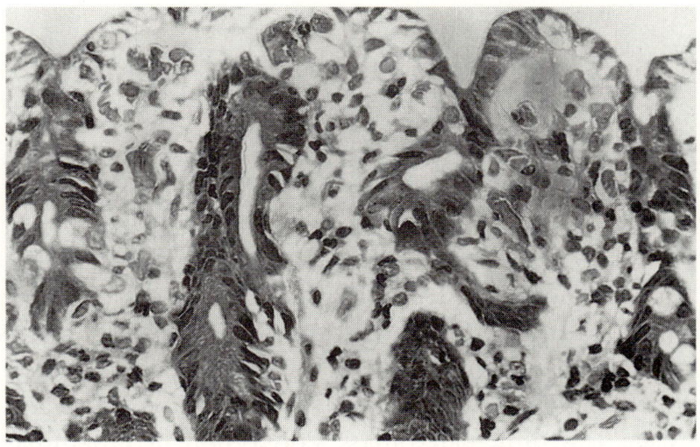

(b)

Figure 2.37 *(a) Duodenal mucosa with prominent lymphoid follicles with germinal centres in the deeper mucosa and submucosa. Biopsy from a patient with nodular lymphoid hyperplasia and hypogammaglobulinaemia (H&E, ×50). (b) Higher power view of biopsy in (a). Note paucity of plasma cells in the lamina propria (H&E, ×400).*

FOOD ALLERGY

In spite of the variety of foreign proteins ingested into the gastrointestinal tract, the relatively low occurrence of food allergy is a tribute to the efficiency of the intestinal mucosa as a primary barrier. Nevertheless, there are certain conditions where there is an immune response to normal constituents of food with significant damage to the mucosal lining. Cow's milk protein allergy, a temporary disorder of small children usually triggered by an episode of acute infective diarrhoea, presents with continuing diarrhoea and failure to thrive. Mucosal biopsies resemble that of coeliac sprue (Iyngkaran *et al.*, 1978; Kosnai *et al.*, 1984). Exclusion of cow's milk from the diet leads to rapid recovery. It is notable that such children lose their intolerance by about 18 months of age. A similar intolerance to soy protein may also occur (Ament and Rubin, 1978). There are also isolated reports of intolerance to other animal or vegetable proteins.

EOSINOPHILIC ENTERITIS

Acute eosinophilic enteritis may result from an allergic response to a food item, with mast cell degranulation and acute gastrointestinal symptoms including diarrhoea (Min and Metcalfe, 1991). Chronic eosinophilic enteritis may be part of an atopic reaction or may occur as a result of hidden food allergies. It is associated with massive infiltration of the mucosa, especially of the gastric antrum and duodenum by eosinophils with peripheral eosinophilia. The infiltration may extend to the submucosa and muscularis (Talley *et al.*, 1990).

Malnutrition and the small bowel

Since virtually all nutrients enter the body via the gastrointestinal tract, the functional integrity of the small intestine is essential for the maintenance of nutrition. Conversely, whether malnutrition causes structural and functional damage in the small intestine or not is still not clearly established. Studies of chronic starvation and in children with kwarshiorkor and marasmus have produced conflicting results: it is difficult to distinguish between the effects of malnutrition and the many gastrointestinal infections that are frequent in such individuals. Animal experiments also have not fully clarified the situation. The question that is raised is whether, during the process of nutrient absorption, enterocytes ensure that nutrients essential for their survival are kept back and not transported to the rest of the body. In severe malnutrition, there is atrophy of the mucosa, a lower mitotic rate and a decrease in IgA-secreting plasma cells (Stanfield *et al.*, 1965). Effects of nutritional deficiency are rapidly corrected by refeeding (Cook and Lee, 1966; Nassar *et al.*, 1980).

Neoplastic lesions of the small intestine

Primary or secondary tumours of the small intestine are relatively rare and account for less than 6 per cent of the tumours of the gastrointestinal tract (Darling and Welch, 1959; Herbsman *et al.*, 1980). Benign and malignant tumours could be of epithelial, mesenchymal or lymphoid origin. Often the tumours present as polyps, a descriptive term for any circumscribed elevation above the apparently normal surrounding mucosa as a sessile or pedunculated mass. Polyps may be inflammatory, hamartomatous or neoplastic. Even heterotopic gastric mucosa in the duodenum can present as polyps (Fig. 2.38) (Franzin *et al.*, 1982).

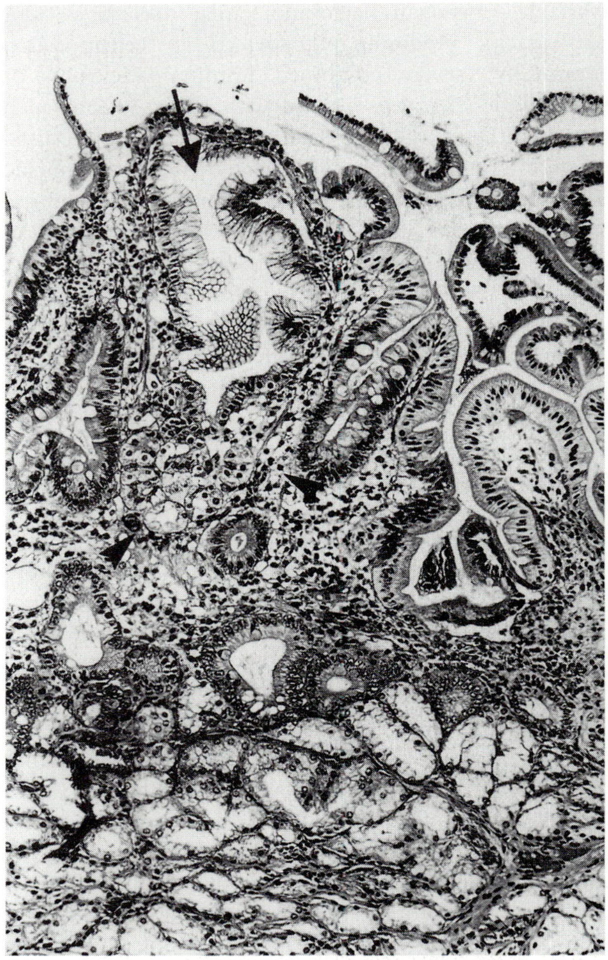

Figure 2.38 *Duodenal biopsy. Mucosa shows foci of gastric heterotopia. Gastric surface cells (arrow) and oxyntic glands (arrowhead) are seen in deeper areas (H&E, ×100).*

BENIGN EPITHELIAL TUMOURS

Adenomas are the most common epithelial tumour and occur mainly in the duodenum. Histologically they may be villous or tubular adenomas, similar to the more frequent colonic lesions, and have the potential to turn malignant (Perzin and Bridge, 1981). Other epithelial lesions include hamartomas of the Brunner's glands (Goldman, 1963) and hereditary and non-hereditary polyposis, such as Peutz–Jeghers syndrome (Bartholomew *et al.*, 1957), Cronkhite–Canada syndrome (Johnson *et al.*, 1972) and Cowden's disease (Weinstock and Kawanishi, 1978).

MALIGNANT EPITHELIAL TUMOURS

Adenocarcinomas of the small intestine are rare and occur mainly in the duodenum, and are therefore easily accessible to the endoscopist for biopsy (Treadwell and White, 1975). Small intestinal adenocarcinomas can occur through adenoma–carcinoma sequence, as in the colon (Perzin and Bridge, 1981, 1982), and they are similar grossly and histologically to colonic lesions with moderate differentiation (Fig. 2.39) (Blackman and Nash, 1985). Although small intestinal adenocarcinomas are well differentiated, the 5-year survival is only 20 per cent because they are usually detected late owing to the late onset of obstructive symptoms as the intestinal contents are fluid.

Neoplastic transformation to form adenocarcinoma has been reported in Crohn's disease (Lashner, 1992) coeliac disease (Javier and Lukie, 1980) and in long-standing ileostomies (Suarez *et al.*, 1988).

ENDOCRINE CELL TUMORS

Endocrine cell tumors arise from endocrine cells of the small intestine. Nearly 40 different types of endocrine cells are now recognized, derived either from the endoderm or the neural crest with endocrine, neuroendocrine and paracrine function. These tumours are generally called carcinoids (carcinoma-like). Histo-

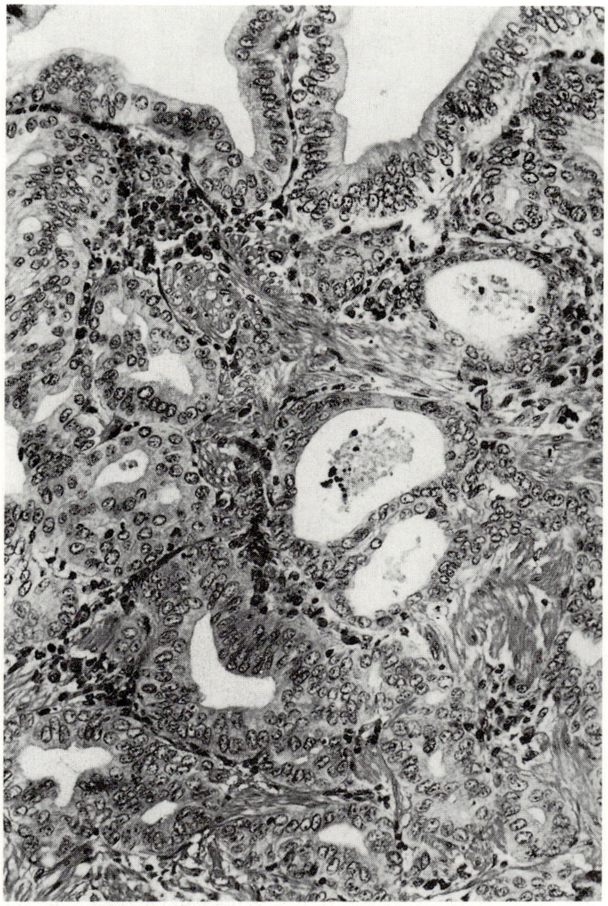

Figure 2.39 *Biopsy of duodenal mucosa with moderately differentiated tumor cells arranged in glandular pattern. A rare case of adenocarcinoma of the duodenum (H&E, ×200).*

chemical staining techniques (Wilander *et al.*, 1977; Lundqvist and Wilander, 1986; Rindi *et al.*, 1986; Wiedenmann *et al.*, 1986), electron microscopy (Solcia *et al.*, 1979) and hormone-specific immunohistochemistry can be used to specify the cell types. A total of 50 per cent of the carcinoid tumours of the gut occur in the small intestine. Histologically the carcinoid pattern consists of solid clumps, nests, cords or trabeculae of uniform cells with peripheral palisading, surrounded by prominent fibrovascular stroma (Fig. 2.40). Although they appear benign histologically and are slow growing, infiltration and metastasis can occur. Owing to their submucosal location and extension to the mucosa, they may be accessible to biopsy.

MESENCHYMAL TUMOURS

Tumours arising from the smooth muscle, fibroblasts, adipocytes, vessels or nerves are rare in the small intestine. Leiomyomas are the most common and arise from the muscularis mucosae, muscle coat or wall of blood vessels. Intraluminal lesions are accessible to biopsy

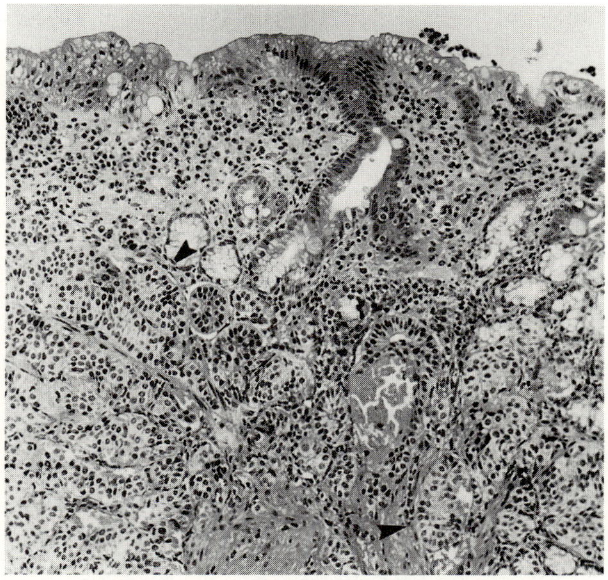

Figure 2.40 *Clumps of uniform cells with peripheral palisading deep in the mucosa are diagnostic of carcinoid tumour in this duodenal biopsy (H&E, ×100).*

(Fig. 2.41). The characteristic appearance of interlacing of smooth muscle cells in a whorled pattern is diagnostic (Herbsman *et al.*, 1980). Leiomyosarcomas are the most common malignant mesenchymal tumour of small intestine (Treadwell and White, 1975).

LYMPHOID TUMOURS

Although small bowel neoplasms are relatively rare, one in five is likely to be a lymphomatous tumour. Lymphomas of the B-cell lineage include mucosa-associated lymphoid tissue (MALT) lymphomas, which may be low-grade or high-grade B-cell tumours, immunoproliferative small intestinal disorder (IPSID),

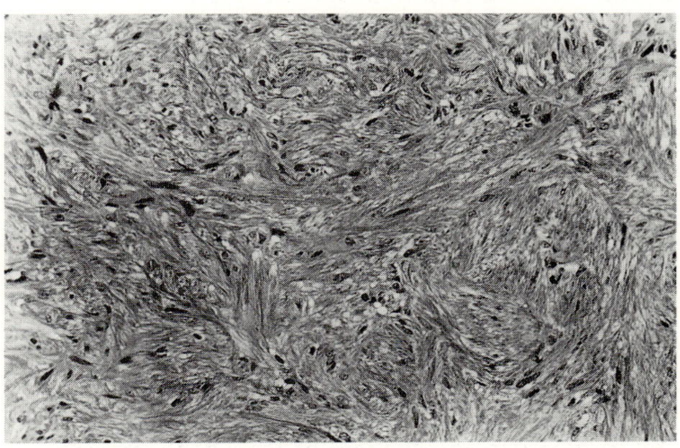

Figure 2.41 *The interlacing bundles of smooth muscle cells in a whorled pattern is diagnostic of leiomyoma. This tumour in the duodenum was diagnosed in an endoscopic biopsy (H&E, ×200).*

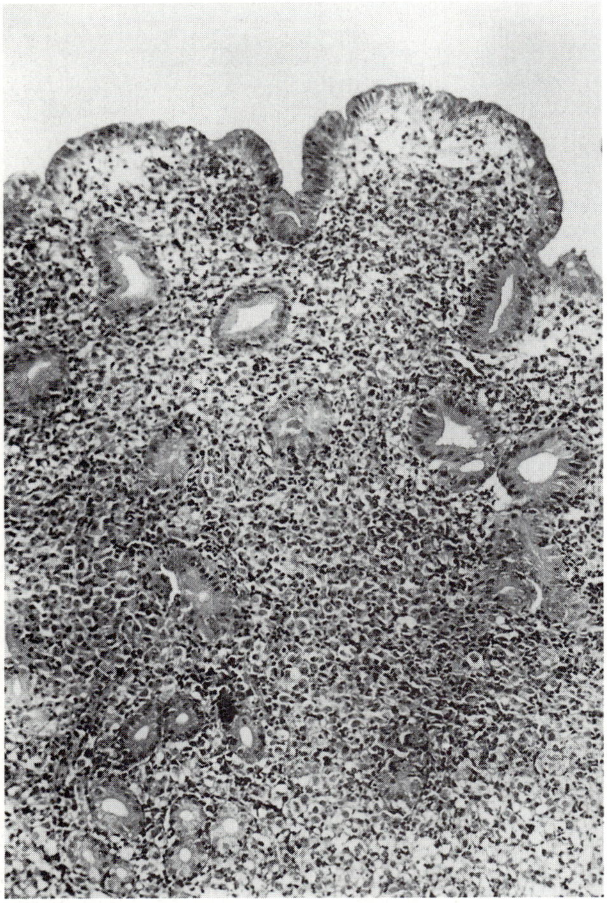

(a)

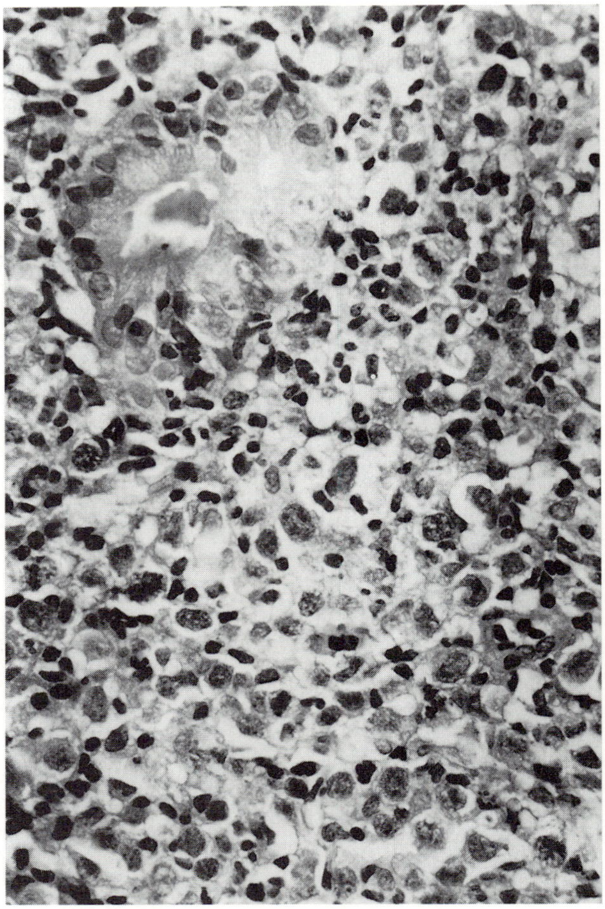

(b)

Figure 2.42 *(a) Duodenal mucosal biopsy from a case of primary lymphoma with a dense cellular infiltrate in the lamina propria, short wide villi and effacement of crypts (H&E, ×90). (b) This high power view of the infiltrate in (a) shows that it is made up of many blast cells and lymphocytes (×400).*

mantle cell type malignant lymphoma or Burkitt's lymphoma. T-cell lymphomas are rare and usually associated with enteropathies such as coeliac or Crohn's disease (Wotherspoon *et al.*, 1998). A characteristic feature of B-cell lymphomas is the lymphoepithelial lesion, the invasion of individual crypts by centrocyte-like (CCL) cells. CCL cells are transformed blast cells with plasma cell differentiation resembling the centrocyte cells of lymphoid follicles. IPSID (alpha-chain disease, Mediterranean lymphoma) was initially described in the Middle East and has now been reported from several tropical countries. Patients present with a history of long-standing diarrhoea and malabsorption. These precede the development of frank lymphoma by several years. There is a clonal expansion of plasma cells, which produces an abnormal α-heavy chain. In the early stages, the changes of IPSID are reversible by prolonged antibiotic therapy, although, once neoplastic changes are established, antibiotics alone are unlikely to be effective. Histological examination of the affected tissues shows the lamina propria expanded by a heavy infiltrate of plasma cells with relatively normal surface epithelial cells (Figs 2.42a,b and Fig. 43a,b).

Miscellaneous conditions

THE SMALL INTESTINE IN SYSTEMIC ILLNESSES

Histologic abnormalities can occur in the small intestine in a wide variety of conditions that are not primarily considered to be gastrointestinal illnesses. These include cystic fibrosis, mastocytosis, amyloidosis, scleroderma and a variety of storage diseases. In the storage diseases, it may be possible to demonstrate the abnormal stored material in lamina propria macrophages in many of the conditions. In systemic amyloidosis, there is small intestinal involvement in 90 per cent of cases, which manifests as abnormal intestinal motility, malabsorption or chronic ulceration. Amyloid deposits can be visualized in mucosal biopsies subendothelially, initially in small and medium vessels,

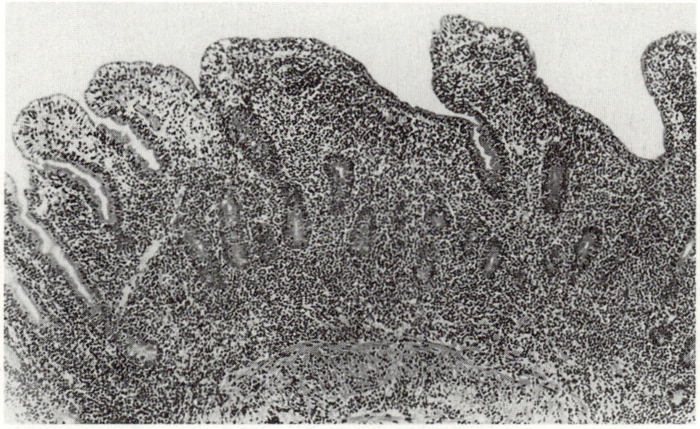

(a)

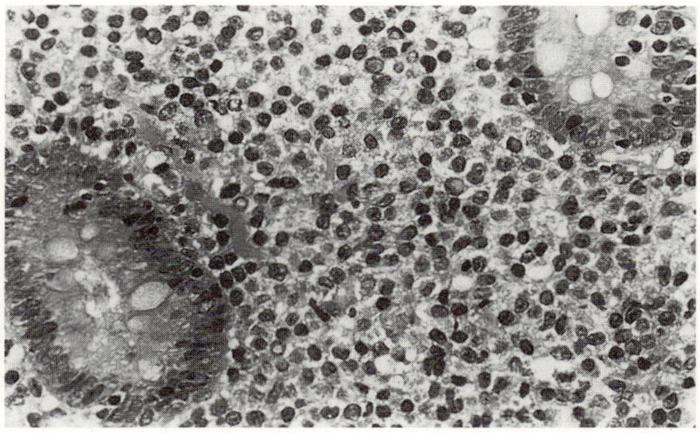

(b)

Figure 2.43 *(a) Jejunal biopsy with short widened villi and effacement of crypts, and a dense cellular infiltrate (H&E, ×90). (b) higher power view of infiltrate in (a) shows mature plasma cells. IPSID stage A is confined to the mucosa (H&E, ×390).*

and interstitially in the muscularis mucosa. Characteristic birefringent staining of the homogeneous pink material can be demonstrated with Congo red or crystal violet stains (Fig. 2.44). In hereditary amyloidosis, muscle layers and nerve plexuses are involved (Green *et al.*, 1961; Cohen, 1967; Tada *et al.*, 1990).

ISCHAEMIA AND RADIATION DAMAGE

Enteric vasculature may be affected in many types of systemic vasculitis. Acute infarction of the small intestine may be caused by dissecting aneurysm, emboli or atherosclerosis, and can present as an abdominal surgical emergency (Swerdlow *et al.*, 1981). Chronic ischaemia leads to mucosal atrophy and is one of the factors in radiation damage. The small intestinal epithelium with its rapid turnover is very sensitive to the effects of ionizing radiation. Reduction of villus height, focal hypereosinophilia of collagen and atypical dendritic fibroblasts in the lamina propria may all be indicators of radiation enteritis (Berthong, 1986).

CROHN'S DISEASE

Crohn's disease is a chronic, relapsing inflammatory condition characterized by the presence of non-caseating granulomas, which may affect the small or large intestine with skip areas (Crohn *et al.*, 1932; Williams, 1964; Rotterdam *et al.*, 1977; Bozdechs and Farmer, 1990). Its prevalence is increasing in most temperate zone industrialized countries and Crohn's disease is now diagnosed more frequently in several tropical countries. The aetiology of this disease is unknown, although environmental, infective, immunologic, genetic and other factors have been suggested (Mayberry and Rhodes, 1984). The small intestine is involved in about 60 per cent of the patients, in half of whom the disease is confined to the small intestine (Mekhijian *et al.*, 1979). The most commonly affected area is the terminal ileum and ileocolitis is associated with the highest recurrence rate after surgery. Duodenal mucosal biopsies (Schmitz-Moormann *et al.*, 1985; Gad, 1989; Alcantara *et al.*, 1993) and rectal biopsies (Rotterdam *et al.*, 1977) can help in diagnosis even if the mucosa appears macroscopically normal.

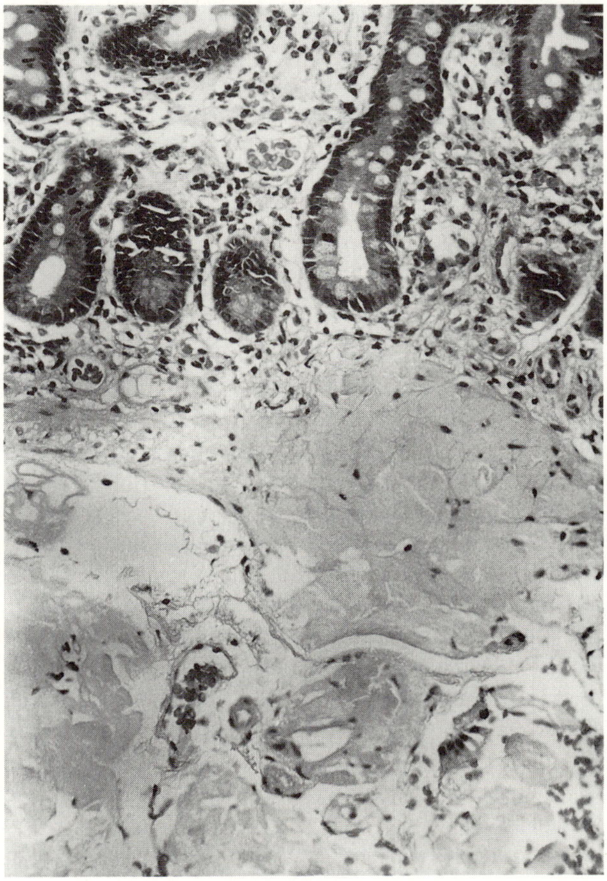

Figure 2.44 *Homogeneous cellular amyloid deposit in the submucosa of the duodenum (H&E, ×200).*

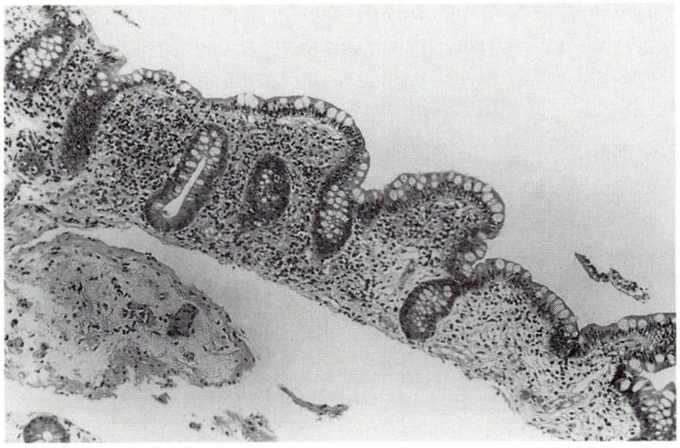

Figure 2.45 *Ileal mucosal biopsy in a patient with Crohn's disease. Villi are shortened with patchy increase in lamina propria cellularity (H&E, ×80).*

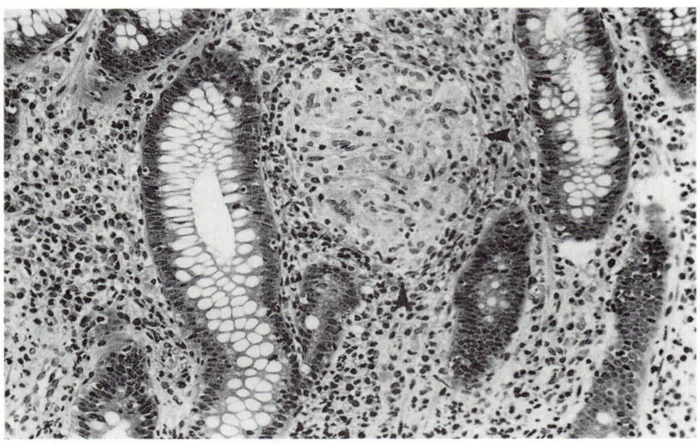

Figure 2.46 *Lamina propria of the ileal mucosa in a patient with Crohn's disease. Note the non-caseating granuloma composed of compactly arranged epithelioid cells and a few lymphocytes (arrowhead) (H&E, ×200).*

Two cardinal pathologic features of Crohn's disease are transmural inflammation and skip areas. There is mucosal 'cobblestoning', linear or serpiginous ulcers, and deep fissures of the mucosa. Fistulae, between bowel loops and to the skin, are common. Patchy mucosal inflammation with microscopic skip areas (Fig. 2.45), sarcoid-like non-caseating granulomas (Fig. 2.46), microgranulomas (Fig. 2.47) or areas of focal non-specific inflammation as well as aphthous ulcers are characteristic diagnostic features in mucosal biopsies. Damage to muscularis mucosa with splaying of muscle fibres and infiltration by collagen can be quite characteristic (Morson and Dawson, 1990). Focally enhanced inflammation has been emphasized (Yardley, 1997) as a diagnostic criterion in Crohn's disease of the gastric mucosa.

In areas where tuberculosis is endemic, it is essential to distinguish between Crohn's disease and intestinal tuberculosis. The natural history, management and prognosis of these two granulomatous inflammations are strikingly different. A retrospective analysis of endoscopic mucosal biopsies from patients with these two conditions showed that tuberculous enterocolitis was associated with large, usually caseating and well-defined granulomas, ulcers lined by conglomerate epithelioid histocytes and disproportionate submucosal inflammation. The granulomas were scantier, poorly organized and smaller in Crohn's disease, and there were microgranulomas as well as areas of focally enhanced inflammation.

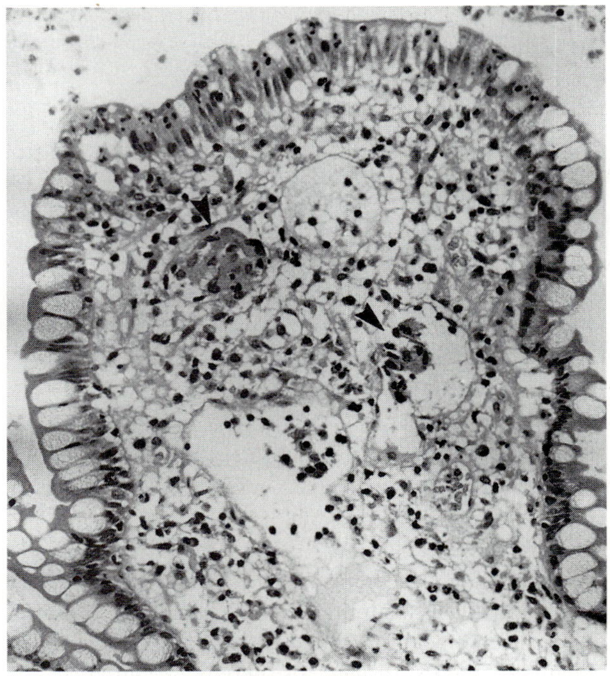

Figure 2.47 *Ileal mucosa from a patient with Crohn's disease. Note the loose collections of epithelioid cells (arrowhead) (microgranuloma) near the lumen of lymphatics (H&E, ×300).*

REFERENCES

Abraham, S.N., Malaviya, R. 1997: Mast cells in infection and immunity. *Infection and Immunity* 65, 3501–8.

Agus, S.G., Dolin, R., Wyatt, R.G., Tousimis, A.J., Northrup, R.S. 1973: Acute infectious nonbacterial gastroenteritis: intestinal histopathology. Histological enzymatic alterations during illness produced by the Norwalk agent in man. *Annals of Internal Medicine* 79, 18–25.

Alcantara, M., Rodriguez, R., Potenciano, J.L.M., Carrobles, J.L., Munoz, C., Gomez, R. 1993: Endoscopic and bioptic findings in the upper gastrointestinal tract in patients with Crohn's disease. *Endoscopy* 25, 282–6.

Altes, J., Slas, A., Rivera, M. 1991: Visceral leishmaniasis. Another HIV-associated opportunistic infection. Report of eight cases and review of literature. *AIDS* 5, 201–7.

Ament, M.E. 1985: Immuno deficiency syndromes of the gut. *Scandinavian Journal of Gastroenterology* 114, 127–35.

Ament, M.E., Rubin, C.E. 1978: Soy protein, another cause of the flat intestinal lesion. *Gastroenterology* 62, 227–33.

Ament, M.E., Shimoda, S., Saunders, D. 1972: Pathogenesis of steatorrhea in 3 cases of small intestinal stasis syndrome. *Gastroenterology* 63, 28–37.

Ament, M.E., Ochs, H.D., Dairs, S.D. 1973: Structure and functions of the gastrointestinal tract in primary immunodeficiency syndromes. A study of 39 patients. *Medicine* 52, 227–48.

Amman, A.J., Hunj, F. 1971: Selective IgA deficiency: presentation of 30 cases and a review of the literature. *Medicine* 50, 223–45.

Asakura, H., Tsuchiya, M., Watanabe, Y., Enomoto, Y., Morita, A., Morishita, T., Fukumi, H., Ohashi, M., Castro, A., Uylaanogc, C. 1974: Electron microscopic study on the jejunal mucosa in human cholera. *Gut* 15, 531–44.

Austin, L.L., Dobbins, W.O. III 1982: Intraepithelial leukocytes of the intestinal mucosa in normal man and Whipple's disease. *Digestive Diseases and Sciences* 27, 301–2.

Baker, S.J. 1973: Geographical variations in the morphology of the small intestinal mucosa in apparently healthy individuals. *Pathologic Microbiology* 39, 222–31.

Baker, S.J., Mathan, V.I. 1972: Tropical enteropathy and tropical sprue. *American Journal of Clinical Nutrition* 25, 1047–55.

Bank, S., Trey, C., Gans, G., Marks, G.N., Groll, A. 1965: Histoplasmosis of the small bowel with 'giant' intestinal villi and secondary protein-losing enteropathy. *American Journal of Medicine* 39, 492–501.

Bark, S., Fisher, G., Marks, I.N., Groll, A. 1967: The lymphatics of the intestinal mucosa. A clinical and experimental study. *American Journal of Digestive Diseases* 12, 619–27.

Bartholomew, L.G., Dahlin, D., Waugh, J.M. 1957: Intestinal polyposis associated with mucocutaneous melanin pigmentation (Peutz–Jeghers syndrome). *Gastroenterology* 32, 434–51.

Bell, S.W., Kernev, J.A., Sibley, R.K. 1991: Microvillus inclusion disease: the importance of electron microscopy for diagnosis. *American Journal of Surgical Pathology* 15, 1157–64.

Bendall, R.P., Lucas, S., Moody, A., Tovey, G., Chiodini, P.L. 1993: Diarrhoea associated with Cyanobacterium-like bodies. *Lancet* 341, 590–2.

Beral, V., Bull, D., Darby, S., Welles, I., Carne, C., Beecham, M., Jaffe, H. 1992: Risk of v-aposis sarcoma and sexual practices associated with faecal contact in homosexual or bisexual men with AIDS. *Lancet* 339, 632–5.

Berschneider, H.M. 1992: Fibroblast modulation of intestinal secretory response. *Annals of the New York Academy of Sciences* 664, 140–7.

Berthong, M. 1986: Pathologic changes secondary to radiation. *World Journal of Surgery* 10, 155–70.

Beschorner, W.E. 1984: Destruction of the intestinal mucosa after bone marrow transplantation and graft-versus-host disease. *Survey and Synthesis of Pathology Research* 3, 264–74.

Bird, R.G., Smith, M.D. 1980: Cryptosporidiosis in man. Parasite life cycle and fine structural pathology. *Journal of Pathology* 132, 217–33.

Bishop, R.F., Davidson, G.P., Holmes, I.H., Ruch, B.J. 1973: Virus particles in epithelial cells of duodenal mucosa from children with acute non-bacterial gastroenteritis. *Lancet* 2, 1281–3.

Blackman, E., Nash, S.V. 1985: Diagnosis of duodenal and ampullary epithelial neoplasms by endoscopic biopsy: a clinicopathologic and immunohistochemical study. *Human Pathology* 10, 901–10.

Borghesi, C., Regoli, M., Bertelli, E., Nicoletti, C. 1996: M cell: the main entrance of the mucosal immune system. *Fundamental and Clinical Immunology* 4, 87–94.

Boyer, B., Thiery, J.P. 1989: Epithelial cell adhesion mechanisms [review]. *Journal of Membrane Biology* 112, 97–108.

Bozdechs, J.M., Farmer, R.G. 1990: Diagnosis of Crohn's disease. *Hepato Gastroenterology* 37, 8–17.

Bradford, W.D., Noce, P.S., Gutman, L.T., Durham, N.C. 1974: Pathologic features of enteric infection with Yersinia enterocolitica. *Archives of Pathology* 89, 17–21.

Brandborg, L.L. 1969: The lamina propria: orphan of the gut. *Gastroenterology* 576, 191–205.

Brandborg, L.L., Goldberg, S.B., Breidenbach, W.C. 1970: Human coccidiosis – a possible cause of malabsorption. The life cycle in small bowel mucosal biopsies as a diagnostic feature. *New England Journal of Medicine* 283, 1306–13.

Brandtzaeg, P., Halstensen, T.S., Kett, K., Krajci, P., Kvale, D., Rognum, T.O., Scott, H., Sollid, L.M. 1989: Immunobiology and immunopathology of human gut mucosa: humoral immunity and intraepithelial lymphocytes. *Gastroenterology* 97, 1562–84.

Bryan, R.T., Cali, A. Owen, R.L., Spencer, H.C. 1991: Microsporida: opportunistic pathogens in patients with AIDS. *Progress in Clinical Parasitology* 2, 1–26.

Bunyaratvej, S., Bunyawongwiroj, P., Nitiyanant, P. 1982: Human intestinal sarcosporidiosis: report of six cases. *American Journal of Tropical Medicine and Hygiene* 31, 36–41.

Canning, E., Hollister, W.S. 1987: Microsporida of mammals – widespread pathogens or opportunistic curiosities. *Parasitology Today* 3, 267–73.

Chacko, C.G.J., Paulson, K.A., Mathan, V.I., Baker, S.J. 1969: The villus architecture of the small intestine in the tropics. A necropsy study. *Journal of Pathology* 98, 146–51.

Choudari, C.P., Mathan, M., Rajan, D.P., Raghavan, R., Mathan, V.I. 1985: A correlative study of etiology, clinical features and rectal mucosal pathology in adults with acute infectious diarrhoea in southern India. *Pathology* 17, 443–50.

Chuttani, H.K., Jain, K., Misra, C. 1971: Small bowel in typhoid fever. *Gut* 12, 709–14.

Claude, P., Goodenough, D.A. 1973: Fracture faces of zonulae occludentes from 'tight' and 'leaky' epithelia. *Journal of Cell Biology* 58, 390–400.

Clayton, F., Reka, S., Cronin, W.J., Tolakovic, E., Sigal, S.H., Kotler, D.P. 1992: Rectal mucosal pathology varies with human immunodeficiency virus antigen content and disease stage. *Gastoenterology* 103, 919–33.

Cohen, A.S. 1967: Amyloidosis. *New England Journal of Medicine* 277, 628–37.

Connor, B.A., Shlim, D.R., Scholes, J.V., Raybarn, J.L., Reidy, J., Rajah, R. 1993: Pathological changes in the small bowel in nine patients with diarrhoea associated with a coccidia-like body. *Annals of Internal Medicine* 119, 377–82.

Cook, G.C., Lee, F.D. 1966: The jejunum after kwashiorkor. *Lancet* 11, 1263–4.

Cook, G.C., Kajubi, S.K., Lee, F.D. 1969: Jejunal morphology of the African in Uganda. *Journal of Pathology* 98, 157–69.

Cover, T.L., Aber, R.C. 1989: Yersinia enterocolitica. *New England Journal of Medicine* 321, 16–24.

Crohn, B.B., Ginzburg, L., Oppenheimer, G.D. 1932: Regional ileitis: a pathological and clinical entity. *Journal of the American Medical Association* 99, 1323–31.

Cross, J.H. 1992: Intestinal capillariasis. *Clinical Microbiology Reviews* 5, 120–9.

Curry, A., Turner, A.J., Lucas, S. 1991: Opportunistic protozoan infections in human immunodeficiency virus disease: review highlighting diagnosis and therapeutic aspects. *Journal of Clinical Pathology* 1, 182–93.

Cutz, E., Rhoads, J.M., Drumm, B., Sherman, P.M., Durie, P.R., Forstner, G.G. 1989: Microvillus inclusion disease: an inherited defect of brush-border assembly and differentiation. *New England Journal of Medicine* 320, 646–51.

Danzig, J.B., Brandt, L.J., Reinus, J.F., Klein, R.S. 1991: Gastrointestinal malignancy in patients with AIDS. *American Journal of Gastroenterology* 86, 715–18.

Darling, R.C., Welch, C.E. 1959: Tumours of the small intestine. *New England Journal of Medicine* 260, 397–408.

Datry, A., Similourski, J.P., Rosenheim, M., Katlama, C., Maheu, E., Kazaz, S., Fassin, D., Danis, M., Gentilini, M. 1990: AIDS-associated leishmaniasis: an unusual gastroduodenal presentation. *Transactions of the Royal Society of Medicine and Hygiene* 84, 239–40.

Davidson, G.P., Barnes, G.L. 1979: Structural and functional abnormalities of the small intestine in infants and young children with rotavirus enteritis. *Acta Paediatrica Scandinavica* 68, 181–6.

Dobbins, W.O. 1966: Electron microscope study of the intestinal mucosa in intestinal lymphangiectasia. *Gastroenterology* 51, 1004–17.

Dobbins, W.O. III, Kawanishi, H. 1981: Bacillary charecteristics in Whipple's disease: an electron microscopic study. *Gastroenterology* 80, 1468–75.

Dworkin, B., Wormser, G.P., Rosenthal, W.S., Heier, S.K., Braunstein, M., Weiss, L., Jankowski, R., Levy, D., Weisberg, S. 1985: Gastrointestinal manifestations of the acquired immunodeficiency syndrome: a review of 22 cases. *American Journal of Gastroenterology* 80, 774–8.

Ehrenpreis, E.D., Patterson, B.K., Brainer, J.A., Yokoo, H., Rademaker, A.W., Geogowski, W., Noskin, G.A.S., Craig, R.M. 1992: Histopathologic findings of duodenal biopsy specimens in HIV infected patients with and without diarrhoea and malabsorption. *American Journal of Clinical Pathology* 97, 21–8.

Facer, P., Polak, J.M., Marangas, P.J., Pearse, A.G.E. 1976: Immunohistochemical localisation of neurone specific enolase (NSE) in the gastrointestinal tract. *Proceedings of the Microscopic Society (London)* 15, 113–14.

Farthing, M.J.G. 1997: The molecular pathogenesis of giardiasis. *Journal of Pediatric Gastroenterology and Nutrition* 24, 79–88.

Ferguson, A., Murray. D. 1971: Quantitation of intraepithelial lymphocytes in human jejunum. *Gut* 12, 988–99.

Fleming, J.L., Wiesner, R.H., Shorter, R.G. 1988: Whipple's disease: clinical, biochemical and histopathological features and assessment of treatment in 29 patients. *Mayo Clinic Proceedings* 63, 539–51.

Franzin, G., Musola, R., Negri, A., Mencarelli, R., Fratton, A. 1982: Hetrotopic gastric (fundic) mucosa in the duodenum. *Endoscopy* 14, 166–7.

Furness, J.B., Costa, M. 1980: Types of nerves in the enteric nervous system. *Neurological Science* 5, 1–20.

Gad, A. 1989: The diagnosis of gastroduodenal Crohn's disease by endoscopic biopsy. *Scandinavian Journal of Gastroenterology* 24, 23–8.

Gangarosa, E.J., Beisel, W.R., Benyati, C., Sprinz, H., Piyaratan, P. 1960: The nature of the gastrointestinal lesion in Asiatic cholera and its relation to pathogenesis: a biopsy study. *American Journal of Tropical Medicine and Hygiene* 9, 125–35.

Gannon, B.J., Cavati, C.J. 1990: Intestinal microvascular organisation. In Messmen K., Hammersen F. (eds) *Gastrointestinal microcirculation*, Vol. 17. Basel: Karger, 55–89.

Gellin, G.B., Soave, R. 1992: Coccidian infections in AIDS. Toxoplasmosis, cryptosporidiosis and isosporiasis. *Medical Clinics of North America* 76, 205–34.

Gerson, C.D., Kent, T.H., Saha, J., Siddiqi, N., Lindenbaum, J. 1971: Recovery of small intestinal structure and function after residence in the tropics. Studies in Indians and Pakistanis living in New York City. *Annals of Internal Medicine* 75, 41–8.

Godwin, T.A. 1991: Cryptosporidiosis in the acquired immunodeficiency syndrome: a study of 15 autopsy cases. *Human Pathology* 22, 1215–24.

Goldman, H., Antonioli, D.A. 1982: Mucosal biopsy of the esophagus, stomach and proximal duodenum. *Human Pathology* 13, 423–48.

Goldman, R.L. 1963: Hamartomatous polyp of Brunner's glands. *Gastroenterology* 44, 57–62.

Green, P.A., Higgins, J.A., Brown, A.L. Jr. Hoffman, H.N., Sommerville, R.L. 1961: Amyloidosis. *Gastroenterology* 41, 452–6.

Greenson, J.K., Betitsos, P.C., Yardley, J.H., Bartlett, J.G. 1991: AIDS enteropathy: occult enteric infections and duodenal mucosal alterations in chronic diarrhoea. *Annals of Internal Medicine* 114, 366–372.

Griffin, G.E., Miller, A., Batman, P., Forster, S.M., Pinching, A.J., Harris, J.R.W., Mathan, M.M. 1988: Damage to jejunal intrinsic autonomic nerves in HIV infection. *AIDS* 2, 379–82.

Griffith, T.M., Edward, D.H., Lewis, M.J., Newby, A.C., Henderson, A.H. 1984: The nature of endothelium-derived vascular relaxant factor. *Nature* 308, 645–7.

Grimelius, L., Wilander, E. 1980: Silver stains in the study of endocrine cells of the gut and pancreas. *Investigative Cell Pathology* 3, 3–12.

Grove, D.I., Warton, A., Yu, L.L., Northern, C., Papadimitriou, 1987: Light and electron microscopical studies of the location of Strongyloides stercoralis in the jejunum of the immuno suppressed dog. *International Journal of Parasitology* 17, 1257–65.

Harrison, M., Walker-Smith, J.A. 1977: Reinvestigation of lactose intolerant children. *Gut* 18, 48–52.

Heatley, R.V. 1983: The gastrointestinal mast cell. *Scandinavian Journal of Gastroenterology* 18, 449–53.

Henson, D. 1972: Cytomegalovirus inclusion bodies in gastrointestinal tract. *Archives of Pathology* 93, 477–82.

Herbay, A.V., Ditton, H., Maiwald, M. 1996: Diagnostic application of a polymerase chain reaction assay for the Whipple's disease bacterium to intestinal biopsies. *Gastroenterology* 110, 1735–43.

Herbsman, H., Wetstein, L., Rosen, Y., Srces, H., Aifon, S.O., Iyer, S.K., Gardner, B. 1980: Tumours of the small intestine. *Current Problems in Surgery* 17, 126–83.

Hermans, P.E., Huizenga, K.A., Hoffman, H.N., Brown, H.L., Markowitz, H. 1966: Dysgammaglobulinemia associated with nodular lymphoid hyperplasia of the small intestine. *American Journal of Medicine* 40, 78–89.

Igra-Siegman, Y., Kapila, R., Sen, P., Kaminski, Z.C., Louria, D.B. 1981: Syndrome of hyperinfection with Strongyloides stercoralis. *Review of Infectious Diseases* 3, 397–407.

Isaacson, P.G., O'Connor, N.T., Spencer, J., Bevan, D.H., Connally, C.E., Kirkham, N., Pollock, D.J., Wainscot, S.S., Stein, H., Mason, D.Y. 1985: Malignant histiocytosis of the intestine: a T cell lymphoma. *Lancet* 2, 688–91.

Iyngkaran, N., Robinson, M.J., Prathap, K., Sumithran, E., Yadav, M. 1978: Cow's milk protein sensitive enteropathy: combined clinical and histological criteria for diagnosis. *Archives of Diseases of Children* 53, 20–6.

Javier, J., Lukie, B. 1980: Duodenal adenocarcinoma complicating celiac sprue. *Digestive Diseases and Sciences* 25, 150–3.

Jenkins, D., Goodall, A., Gillet, F.R., Scott, B.B. 1985: Defining duodenites: quantitative histological study of mucosal responses and their correlations. *Journal of Clinical Pathology* 38, 1119–26.

Jodal, M., Eklund, S., Sjövall, H. 1988: Enteric nerves and function of intestinal mucosa. *Digestive Diseases and Sciences* 6, 203–15.

Johnson, G.K., Soergel, K.H., Hensley, G.T., Dodds, W.J., Hogan, W.J. 1972: Cronkhite-Canada syndrome. *Gastroenterology* 63, 140–51.

Judd, E.D., Nagel, G.W. 1927: Excision of ulcer of the duodenum. *Surgery, Gynaecology and Obstetrics* 45, 17–23.

Kang, G., Mathan, M., Ramakrishna, B.S., Mathai, E., Sarada, V. 1994: Human intestinal capillariasis: first report from India. *Transactions of the Royal Society of Tropical Medicine and Hygiene* 88, 204.

Kato, T., Owen, R.L. 1994: Structure and function of intestinal mucosal epithelium. In Ogra, P.L., Strober, W., Mestecky, J., McGhee, J.R., Lamm, M.E., Binenstock, J. (eds) *Handbook of mucosal immunology*. New York: Academic Press, 11–26.

Katusic, Z.S., Shepherd, J.T., Vanhoutte, P.M. 1988: Endothelium dependent contractions to calcium ionophore A23187, arachidonic acid and acetylcholine in canine basilar arteries. *Stroke* 19, 476–9.

Kayden, H.J. 1972: Abetalipoproteinemia. *Annual Review of Medicine* 23, 285–96.

Kedinger, M.P., Simon-Assmann, F., Haffen, K. 1988: Epithelial mesenchymal interactions in intestinal epithelial differentiation. *Scandinavian Journal of Gastroenterology* 23, 62–9.

Kett, K., Brandtzaeg, P., Radl, J., Haaijman, J.F. 1986: Different subclass distribution of IgA-producing cells in human lymphoid organs and various secretory tissues. *Journal of Immunology* 136, 3631–5.

Kirkpatrick, C.J., Bittinger, F., Klein, C.L., Hauptman, S., Klosterhaifen, B. 1996: The role of the microcirculation in multiple organ dysfunction syndrome (MODS): a review and perspective. *Virchows Archiv* 427, 461–76.

Kosnai, I., Kuitonen, P., Savilabte, E., Sipponen, P. 1984: Mast cells, and eosinophils in the jejunal mucosa of patients with intestinal cow's milk allergy and coeliac disease of childhood. *Journal of Pediatric Gastroenterology and Nutrition* 3, 368–80.

Kotler, D.P., Gaetz, H.O., Lange, M., Klein, E.D., Holt, P.R. 1984: Enteropathy associated with the acquired immunodeficiency syndrome. *Annals of Internal Medicine* 101, 421–8.

Lake, A.M., Bloch, K.J., Sinclair, K.J., Walker, W.A. 1980: Anaphylactic release of intestinal goblet cell mucus. *Immunology* 39, 173–8.

Lamont, J.T. 1992: Mucus: the front line of intestinal mucosal defense. *Annals of the New York Academy of Sciences* 664, 190–201.

Lashner, B.A. 1992: Risk factors for small bowel cancer in Crohn's disease. *Digestive Diseases and Sciences* 37, 1179–84.

Lefkowitch, J.H., Krumholz, S., Feng-Chen, K.C., Griffin, P., Despommier, D., Brasitus, T.A. 1984: Cryptosporidiosis of the human small intestine: a light and electron microscopic study. *Human Pathology* 15, 746–52.

Lindenbaum, J., Gerson, C.D., Kent, T.H. 1971: Recovery of small intestinal structure and function after residence in the tropics. Studies in Peace Corps Volunteers. *Annals of Internal Medicine* 74, 218–22.

Lundgren, O. 1974: The circulation of the small bowel mucosa. *Gut* 15, 1005–12.

Lundqvist, M., Wilander, E. 1986: Subepithelial neuroendocrine cells and carcinoid tumours of the small intestine and appendix. A comparative immunohistochemical study with regard to serotonin, neuron specific enolase and S-100 protein reactivity. *Journal of Pathology* 48,141–7.

Mahida, Y.R., Patel, S., Jewel, D.P. 1989: Mononuclear phagocyte system of human Peyer's patches: an immunohistochemical study using monoclonal antibodies. *Clinical and Experimental Immunology* 75, 82–6.

Mandell, W., Goldberg, D.M., Neu, H.C. 1986: Histoplasmosis in patients with the acquired immune deficiency syndrome. *American Journal of Medicine* 81, 974–8.

Mank, T.G., Zaat, J.O., Dcelder, A.M., VanEijk, J.T., Polderman, A.M. 1997: Sensitivity of microscopy versus enzyme immuno assay in the laboratory diagnosis of giardiasis. *European Journal of Clinical Microbiology and Infectious Diseases* 16, 615–19.

Manson-Bhar, P.E.C., Bell, D.R. 1987: *Manson's tropical diseases*, 19th edn. London: Bailliere Tindall, 1298–301.

Marcial-Rojas, R.A. 1975: Strongyloidiasis. In Marcial-Rojas, R.A. (ed.) *Pathology of protozoal and helminthic diseases.* New York: Krieger, 711–23.

Marsh, M.N. 1989: Studies of intestinal lymphoid tissue XV. Histopathologic features suggestive of cell-mediated reactivity in jejunal mucosa of patients with dermatitis herpetiformis. *Virchows Archiv A: Pathologic Anatomy* 416, 125–32.

Marsh, M.N. 1992a: Celiac and allied sprue syndromes. *Seminars in Gastrointestinal Diseases* 4, 214–23.

Marsh, M.N. 1992b: Gluten, major histocompatibility complex and the small intestine. A molecular and immunobiologic approach to the spectrum of gluten sensitivity ('celiac sprue'). *Gastroenterology* 102, 330–54.

Marsh, M.N., Ensari, A. 1995: The gut-associated lymphoid tissue and immune system. In Whitehead, R. (ed.) *Gastrointestinal and oesophageal pathology*. London: Churchill Livingstone, 201–25.

Mathan, M.M., Mathan, V.I. 1985a: Rectal mucosal morphologic abnormalities in normal subjects in southern India: a tropical colonopathy. *Gut* 26, 710–17.

Mathan, M.M., Mathan, V.I. 1985b: Local Schwartzman reaction in the rectal mucosa in acute diarrhoea. *Journal of Pathology* 146, 179–87.

Mathan, M.M., Hermos, J.A., Trier, J.S. 1972: Structural features of the epithelio-mesenchymal interface of rat duodenal mucosa during development. *Journal of Cell Biology* 52, 577–88.

Mathan, M.M., Mathan V.I., Baker, S.J. 1975: An electron microscopic study of jejunal mucosal morphology in control subjects and in patients with tropical sprue in Southern India. *Gastroenterology* 68, 17–32.

Mathan, M., Venkatesan, S., George, R., Mathew, M., Mathan, V.I. 1985: *Cryptosporidium* and diarrhoea in Southern Indian children. *Lancet* 2, 172–5.

Mathan, M.M., Ponniah, J., Mathan, V.I. 1986: Epithelial cell renewal and turnover and its relationship to the morphological abnormalities in the jejunal mucosa in tropical sprue. *Digestive Diseases and Sciences* 31, 586–93.

Mathan, M.M., Griffin, G.E., Miller, A., Batgman, P., Forster, S.M., Pinching, A.J. and Harvis, J.R.W. 1990: Ultrastructure of the jejunal mucosa in human immunodeficiency virus infection. *Journal of Pathology* 161, 119–27.

Mathan, M.M., Chandy, G., Mathan, V.I. 1995: Ultra-structural changes in the upper small intestinal mucosa in patients with cholera. *Gastroenterology* 109, 422–30.

Mathan, V.I., Mathan, M., Ponniah, J. 1981: Tropical enteropathy: an adaptation of the small intestine to accelerated cell loss in contaminated environments. In Robinson, J.W.I., Dowling, R.H., Riecken, E.O. (eds) *Mechanisms of intestinal adaptation*. Lancaster: MTP Press, 609–10.

Mayberry, J.F., Rhodes, J. 1984: Epidemiological aspects of Crohn's disease: a review of the literature. *Gut* 25, 886–99.

Mayberry, J.F., Furness, P., Austin, B., Toghell, P. 1986: Endoscopic appearances in Whipple's disease. *Transactions of the Royal Society of Medicine* 79, 483–5.

McCarty, W.C. 1924: Excised duodenal ulcers, a report of 420 specimens. *Journal of the American Medical Association* 83, 1894–8.

Mekhijian, H.S., Butler, J.J., Oshorne, B.M., Manning, J.T. 1979: Clinical features and natural history of Crohn's disease. *Gastroenterology* 77, 898–906.

Michiels, J.F., Hofman, P., Saint Paul, M.C., Loubiere, R., Bernard, E., Lefichoux, Y. 1993: Pathological features of intestinal microsporidiosis in HIV positive patients. *Pathology Research and Practice* 189, 377–83.

Michiels, J.F., Hofman, P., Bernard, E., Saint Paul, M.C., Boissy, C., Mondain, V., Lefichoux, Y., Loubiere, R. 1994: Intestinal and extraintestinal Isospora belli infection in an Aids patient. *Pathology Research and Practice* 190, 1089–93.

Milder, J.E., Walzer, P.D., Kilgore, G., Rutherford, J., Klein, M. 1981: Clinical features of Strongyloides stercoralis infection in an endemic area of the United States. *Gastroenterology* 80; 1481–8.

Min, K.U., Metcalfe, D.D. 1991: Eosinophilic gastroenteritis. *Immunology and Allergy Clinics of North America* 11, 799–814.

Moog, F. 1981: The lining of the small intestine. *Scientific American* 245, 154–78.

Morson, B.C., Dawson, I.M.P. (eds) 1990: *Morson and Dawson's gastrointestinal pathology*, 3rd edn. Oxford: Blackwell Scientific, 258–76.

Mowat, A. McI. 1987: The cellular basis of gastrointestinal immunity. In Marsh M.N. (ed.) *Immunopathology of the small intestine.* London: Wiley, 41–72.

Mukundan, P., Jadhav, M., John, T.J. 1977: Prevalence of cytomegalovirus antibody in young children in Vellore. *Indian Journal of Medical Research* 65, 584–92.

Nabeyama, A., Leblond, C.P. 1974: Caveolated cells characterised by deep surface invaginations and abundant filaments in mouse gastrointestinal epithelia. *American Journal of Anatomy* 140, 147–66.

Nassar, A.M., Tantawy, S.A., Khalifa, S., Abdel-Fattah, S., Abdel-Hamid, J. 1980: Ultrastructural changes in the mucosa of the small intestine due to protein calorie malnutrition. *Journal of Tropical Paediatrics* 26, 62–9.

Nataro, J.P., Kaper, J.B. 1998: Diarrheagenic *Escherichia coli*. *Clinical Microbiology Reviews* 11, 142–201.

Nataro, J.P., Hicks, S., Philips, A.D., Vial, P.A., Sears, C.L. 1996: T 84 cells in culture as a model for enteroaggregative *Escherichia coli* pathogenesis. *Infection and Immunity* 64, 4761–8.

Navin, T.R., Juranck, D.D. 1984: Cryptosporidiosis: clinical, epidemiologic and parasitologic review. *Review of Infectious Diseases* 66, 313–27.

Nelson, J.A., Wiley, C.A., Reynolds-Kohler, C., Reese, C.E., Margaretten, W., Levy, J.A. 1988: Human immunodeficiency virus detected in bowel epithelium from patients with gastrointestinal symptoms. *Lancet* 1, 259–62.

Neutra, M.R., Kraehenbuhl, J.P. 1993: The role of transepithelial transport by M cells in microbial invasion and host defense. *Journal of Cell Science* 17, 209–15.

Oberhuber, G., Kastner, N., Stolte, M. 1997: Giardiasis: a histologic analysis of 567 cases. *Scandinavian Journal of Gastroenterology* 32, 48–51.

Orenstein, J.M., Zierdt, W., Zierdt, C., Kotley, D.P. 1990: Identification of spores of Enterocytozoon binieusi in stool and duodenal fluid from AIDs patients. *Lancet* 2, 1289–900.

Ortega, Y.R., Sterling C.R., Gilman, R.H., Cama, B.A., Diaz, F. 1993: Cyclospora species – a new protozoan pathogen of humans. *New England Journal of Medicine* 328, 1308–12.

Osborne, L. 1990: Leukocyte adhesion to endothelium in inflammation. *Cell* 62, 3–6.

Osborne, M.P., Haddon, S.J., Spencer, A.J., Collins, J., Starkey, W.G., Wallis, T.S., Clark, G.J., Worton, K.J., Candy, D.C., Stephen, J. 1988: An electron microscopic investigation of time-related changes in the intestine of neonatal mice infected with murine rotavirus. *Journal of Pediatric Gastroenterology and Nutrition* 7, 236–48.

Ouellette, A., Selsted, M.E. 1996: Paneth cell defensins: endogenous components of intestinal host defence. *FASEB Journal* 10, 180–9.

Owen, R.L., Jones, A.L., 1974: Epithelial cell specialisation within human Peyer's patches: an ultrastructural study of intestinal lymphoid follicles. *Gastroenterology* 82, 232–42.

Pape, J.W., Johnson, W.D. 1991: Isospora belli infections. *Progress in Clinical Parasitology* 2, 119–27.

Pape, J.W., Verdiev, R.I., Boncy, M., Boncy, J., Johnson, W.D. Jr. 1994: Cyclospora infection in adults infected with HIV. Clinical manifestations, treatment and prophylaxis. *Annals of Internal Medicine* 121, 654–7.

Pearse, A.G.E. 1969: The cytochemistry and ultrastructure of polypeptide hormone producing cells of the APUD series and the embryonic physiologic and pathologic implications of the concept. *Journal of Histochemistry and Cytochemistry* 17, 303–13.

Pearse, A.G.E. 1980: The APUD concept and hormone production. *Clinics in Endocrinology and Metabolism* 9, 211–22.

Perera, D.R., Weinstein, W.M., Rubin, C.E. 1975: Small intestinal biopsy. *Human Pathology* 6, 157–217.

Perzin, K.H., Bridge, M.F. 1981: Adenomas of the small intestine: a clinicopathologic review of 51 cases and a study of their relationship to carcinoma. *Cancer* 48, 799–819.

Perzin, K.H., Bridge, M.F. 1982: Adenomatous and carcinomatous changes in hamartomatous polyps of the small intestine (Peutz–Jeghers syndrome). *Cancer* 49, 971–83.

Peters, M., Weiner, J., Whelan, G. 1980: Fungal infection associated with gastroduodenal ulceration: endoscopic and pathologic appearances. *Gastroenterology* 78, 350–8.

Phillips, A.D., Schmitz, J. 1992: Familial microvillus atrophy: a clinico pathological survey of 23 cases. *Journal of Paediatric Gastroenterology and Nutrition* 14, 380–96.

Pisam, M., Ripoche, P. 1976: Redistribution of surface macromolecules in dissociated epithelial cells. *Journal of Cell Biology* 71, 907–20.

Pitchenik, A.E., Fertel, D. 1992: Tuberculous and nontuberculous mycobacterial disease. *Medical Clinics of North America* 76, 121–71.

Pomerantz, M., Waldmann, J.A. 1963: Systemic lymphatic abnormalities associated with gastrointestinal protein loss secondary to intestinal lymphangiectasia. *Gastroenterology* 45, 703–11.

Rader, D.J., Brewer, H.B. 1993: Abetalipoproteinemia. New insights into lipoprotein assembly and Vit E metabolism from a rare genetic disease. *Journal of the American Medical Association* 271, 865–9.

Ramakrishna, B.S., Mathan, V.I. 1993: Colonic dysfunction in acute diarrhoea: the role of short chain fatty acids. *Gut* 34, 1215–18.

Reifen, R.M., Cutz, E., Griffiths, A., Ngan, B.Y., Sherman, P.M. 1994: Tufting enteropathy: a newly recognized clinicopathological entity associated with refractory diarrhoea in infants. *Journal of Paediatric Gastroenterology and Nutrition* 18, 379–85.

Relman, D.A., Schmidt, T.M., McDermott, R.P., Falkow, S.

1992: Identification of uncultured bacillus of Whipple's disease. *New England Journal of Medicine* 32, 297–301.

Rindi, G., Buffa R., Sessa, F., Tortora, O., Solcia, E. 1986: Chromogranin A, B and C immunoreactivities of mammalian endocrine cells. *Histochemistry* 85, 19–28.

Rosen, F.S., Cooper, M.D., Wedgewood R.T.P. 1984: The primary immunodeficiencies. *New England Journal of Medicine* 311, 300–10.

Rothbaum, R., McAdams, J., Giannella, R., Partin, J.C., 1982: A clinicopathological study of enterocyte adherent *Escherichia coli*: a cause of protracted diarrhea in infants. *Gastroenterology* 83, 441–54.

Rotterdam, H., Korelitz, B.I., Sommers, S.C. 1977: Microgranulomas in grossly normal rectal mucosa in Crohn's disease. *American Journal of Clinical Pathology* 67, 550–4.

Rubin, C.E. 1960: Celiac disease and idiopathic sprue. *Gastroenterology* 39, 260–1.

Schmitz-Moormann, P., Malchow, H., Pittner, P.M. 1985: Endoscopic and bioptic study of the upper gastrointestinal tract in Crohn's disease patients. *Pathology Research and Practice* 179, 377–8.

Schwartz, D.A., Wilcox, C.M. 1992: Atypical CMV inclusions in gastrointestinal biopsy specimens from patients with AIDS. *Human Pathology* 23, 1019–26.

Segal, G.H., Petras, R.E. 1992: Small intestine. In Stennberg, S.S. (ed.) *Histology for pathologists.* New York: Raven Press, 547–71.

Selby, W.S., Poulter, L.W., Hobbs, S., Jewell, D.P., Janossy, G. 1983: Heterogeneity of HLA. DR-positive histiocytes in human intestinal lamina propria: a combined histochemical and immunohistological analysis. *Journal of Clinical Pathology* 36, 379–84.

Sewankambo, N., Mugerwa, R.D., Goodgame, R., Carswell, J.W., Moody, A., Lloyd, G., Lucas, S.B. 1987: Enteropathic AIDS in Uganda. An endoscopic, histological and microbiological study. *AIDS* 1, 9–13.

Smith, J.H. 1976: Typhoid fever. In Binford, C.H., Connar, D.H. (eds) *Pathology of tropical and extraordinary diseases.* Washington DC: Armed Forces Institute of Pathology, 123–34.

Snover, D.C. 1990: Graft versus host disease of gastrointestinal tract. *American Journal of Surgical Pathology* 14, 101–8.

Snover, D.C., Weinsdorf, J.A., Vercellottz, G.M., Rank, B., Hutton, S., McGlave, P. 1985: A histopathologic study of gastric and small intestinal graft-versus-host disease following allogenic bone marrow transplantation. *Human Pathology* 16, 387–92.

Soave, R. 1996: Cyclospora: an overview. *Clinical Infectious Diseases* 23, 429–37.

Solcia, E., Capella, C., Buffa, R., Usellini, L., Frigerio, B., Fontana, P. 1979: Endocrine cells of the gastrointestinal tract and related tumours. In Joachim, H.L. (ed.) *Pathology annual.* New York: Raven Press, 163–204.

Solcia, E., Polak, J.M., Larsson, L.I., Buchan, A.M.J., Capella, C. 1981: Update on Lausanne classification on endocrine cells. In Bloom, S.R., Polak, J.M. (eds) *Gut hormones.* Edinburgh: Churchill Livingstone, 96–100.

Spencer, J., Finn, T., Isaacson, P.G. 1986: Human Peyer's patches: an immunohistochemical study. *Gut* 27, 405–10.

Stanfield, J.P., Hutt, M.S.R., Tunnicliffe, R. 1965: Intestinal biopsy in kwashiorkor. *Lancet* 2, 519–23.

Stead, R.H., Dison, M.F., Bramwell, N.H., Riddell, R.H., Bienenstock, J. 1989: Mast cells are closely opposed to nerves in the human gastrointestinal mucosa. *Gastroenterology* 97, 575–85.

Steinman, R.M. 1991: The dendritic cell system and its role in immunogenicity. *Annual Review of Immunology* 9, 271–96.

Strobel, S., Milles, H.R.P, Ferguson, A. 1981: Human intestinal mucosal mast cells: evaluation of fixation and staining techniques. *Journal of Clinical Pathology* 34, 851–8.

Suarez, V., Alexander-Williams, J., O'Connor, H.J., Campus, A., Fuggle, W.J., Thompson, H., Enker, W.E., Grenstein, A.J. 1988: Carcinoma developing in ileostomies after 25 or more years. *Gastroenterology* 95, 205–8.

Swerdlow, S.H., Antonioli, D.A., Goldman, H. 1981: Intestinal infarctions: a new classification. *Archives of Pathology and Laboratory Medicine* 105, 218–31.

Swinson, C.M., Coles, E.C., Slavin, G., Booth, C.C. 1983: Celiac disease and malignancy. *Lancet* 1, 111–15.

Tada, S., Iida, M., Iwashita, A., Matsui, T., Fuchigami, T., Yamamoto, Y.T., Fujushima, M. 1990: Endoscopic and biopsy findings of the upper digestive tract in patients with amyloidosis. *Gastrointestinal Endoscopy* 36, 10–14.

Talley, N.H., Shorter, R.G., Philips, S.F. 1990: Eosinophilic gastroenteritis, a clinicopathological study of patients with diseases of the mucosa, muscle layer and submucosal tissue. *Gut* 31, 54–8.

Tandon, H.D., Prakash, A. 1972: Pathology of intestinal tuberculosis and its distinction from Crohn's disease. *Gut* 13, 260–9.

Targan, S.R. 1992: The lamina propria: a dynamic, complex mucosal compartment. An overview. *Annals of the New York Academy of Sciences* 664, 61–8.

Tonghua, L., Guozong, P., Minzhang, C. 1981: Crohn's disease: clinicopathologic manifestations and differential diagnosis from enterocolonic tuberculosis. *Chinese Medical Journal* 94, 431–40.

Treadwell, T.A., White, R.R. 1975: Primary tumours of the small bowel. *American Journal of Surgery* 130, 749–55.

Trier, J.S. 1969: The surface coat of gastrointestinal epithelial cells. *Gastroenterology* 56, 618–22.

Trier, J.S. 1991a: Celiac sprue. *New England Journal of Medicine* 325, 1709–19.

Trier, J.S., 1991b: Structure and function of intestinal M cells. *Gastroenterology Clinics of North America* 20, 531–47.

Trier, J.S., Madara, J.L. 1981: Functional morphology of the mucosa of the small intestine. In Johnson, L.R. (ed.) *Physiology of the gastrointestinal tract.* New York: Raven Press, 925–61.

Trier, J.S., Moxey, P.C., Schimmel, E.M., Robles, E. 1974: Chronic intestinal coccidiosis in man: intestinal morphology and response to treatment. *Gastroenterology* 66, 923–35.

Trier, J.S., Falchuk, Z.M., Carey, M.C., Schreiber, D.S. 1978: Celiac sprue and refractory sprue. *Gastroenterology* 75, 307–16.

Tzipori, S., Montanaro, J., Robins-Browne, R.M., Vial, P., Gibson, R., Levine, M.M. 1992: Studies with enteroaggregative *Escherichia coli* in the gnotobiotic piglet gastroenteritis model. *Infection and Immunity* 60, 5302–6.

Ullrich, R., Zertz, M., Heise, W., L'Age, M., Hoffken, G., Riecken, E.O. 1989: Small intestinal structure and function in patients with human immunodeficiency virus (HIV): evidence for HIV induced enteropathy. *Annals of Internal Medicine* 111, 15–21.

Underhill, B.M.L. 1955: Intestinal length in man. *British Medical Journal* 2, 1243–6.

Walsh, T.J., Merz, W.G. 1986: Pathologic features in the human alimentary tract associated with invasiveness of Candida tropicalis. *American Journal of Clinical Pathology* 85, 498–502.

Weber, R., Bryan, R.T. 1994: Microsporidial infections in immunodeficient and immunocompetent patients. *Clinical Infectious Diseases* 19, 517–21.

Weinstein, W.M., Saunders, D.R., Tytgat, G.N., Rubin, C.E. 1970: Collagenous sprue, an unrecognized type of malabsorption. *New England Journal of Medicine* 283, 1297–301.

Weinstock, J.V., Kawanishi, H. 1978: Gastrointestinal polyposis with orocutaneous hamartomas (Cowden's disease). *Gastroenterology* 74, 890–5.

Weller, P.F. 1991: The immunobiology of eosinophils. *New England Journal of Medicine* 324, 1110–18.

Weller, T.H. 1971: The cytomegalovirus, ubiquitous agents with protean clinical manifestations. *New England Journal of Medicine* 285, 267–74.

Wershil, B.K. 1995: Role of mast cells and basophils in gastrointestinal inflammations. In Marone, G. (ed.) *Human basophils and mast cells: clinical aspects. Chemical immunology*. Basel: Karger, 187–203.

Wetterau, J.R., Aggerbeck, L.P., Bouma, M.E., Eisenberg, C., Munck, A., Michel, H., Jaeques, S., Gerard, G. 1992: Absence of microsomal triglyceride transfer protein in individuals with abetalipoproteinaemias. *Science* 258, 999–1001.

Whitehead, R., Roca, M., Meikle, D.D., Skinner, J., Truelove, S.C. 1975: The histological classification of duodenitis in fibreoptic biopsy specimens. *Digestion* 13, 129–36.

Wiedenmann, B., Franke, W.W., Khun, C., Moll, R., Gould, V.E. 1986: A marker protein for neuroendocrine cells and neoplasms. *Proceedings of the National Academy of Sciences USA* 83, 3500–4.

Wilander, E., Partela-Gomes, G., Westermark, P. 1977: Argentafin and argyrophil reaction of human gastrointestinal carcinoids. *Gastroenterology* 73, 733–6.

Williams, J.W. 1964: Histology of Crohn's syndrome. *Gut* 5, 510–16.

Wolf, J.L., Bye, W.A. 1984: The membraneous epithelial (M) cell and the mucosal immune system. *Annual Review of Medicine* 35, 95–112.

Wotherspoon, A.C., MacDonald, T.T., Spener, J. 1998: Gastrointestinal lymphoma. In Ogray, P.L., Mestecky, J., Lamma, M.E., Strober, W., Binenstrock, J., Macghee, J.R. (eds) *Mucosal immunology*. New York: Academic Press, 1025–34.

Yardley, J.H. 1997: Gastroduodenal Crohn's disease. The focus is on focality. *Gastroenterology* 112, 1031–43.

3

Growth and maintenance of the intestinal mucosa

FIONA THOMPSON, ADRIAN G CUMMINS

FOETAL GROWTH OF THE SMALL INTESTINE

The growth of the small intestine during foetal life differs between species, with the human small intestine being further developed at birth than that of rodents (Colony, 1983; Klein, 1987). It is important to distinguish two types of intestinal growth: cylindrical whole organ growth in length and diameter, and luminal mucosal growth (Fig. 3.1). During foetal life in humans, the intestine grows in length and width. At 4 weeks gestation, the intestine is a simple tube. By the fifth week, it begins rotating, with the cranial limb moving from the midline to the right and the caudal limb moving to the left. Separate circular and longitudinal muscle layers in both small and large intestine are recognizable in 10-week-old foetuses, although at this age the the longitudinal muscle appears as essentially undifferentiated mesenchyme. By 13 weeks, the longitudinal muscle can be more definitely identified. In humans, cylindrical organ growth occurs with lengthening of the intestinal tube, which is linear during the first half of pregnancy. Intestinal length doubles prenatally during the third trimester as growth accelerates during the last 15 weeks of gestation (Weaver *et al.*, 1991). The average length of the small intestine is 275 cm at birth. Growth in intestinal length continues during early postnatal life but from about 1 year onwards it slows and remains linear with increasing age up to adulthood. An increase in width would be associated with this change in length but this has not been measured. The primary surface area of the small intestine is that of a long cylinder. This pattern of growth occurs with maintenance of an immature mucosa, as the epithelium grows by longitudinal fission of intestinal crypts that individually maintain a low rate of proliferation until postnatal life (Sullivan *et al.*, 1991).

The secondary surface area of the small intestine is made up of submucosal folds and villi, which amplify the primary surface area by a factor of four in the proximal small intestine, decreasing to two in the distal small intestine (Wilson, 1967). This mucosal amplification of the cylindrical surface area means that 50 per cent of the total intestinal surface area is present in the first 25 per cent of the small intestine. Villi form at approximately 10 weeks of gestation and crypts slightly later at 12 weeks of gestation. The formation of villi has been studied using foetal mouse duodenal tissue in explant culture (Ménard and Calvert, 1991). This has shown that small islands of mesenchymal cells first aggregate under the stratified epithelium, which gradually becomes cuboidal or columnar. This only occurs if the culture medium contains glutamine. Thus, the formation of villi seems to be dependent on underlying mesenchymal cells and on the presence of glutamine. While the epithelium is stratified, the proliferative pool

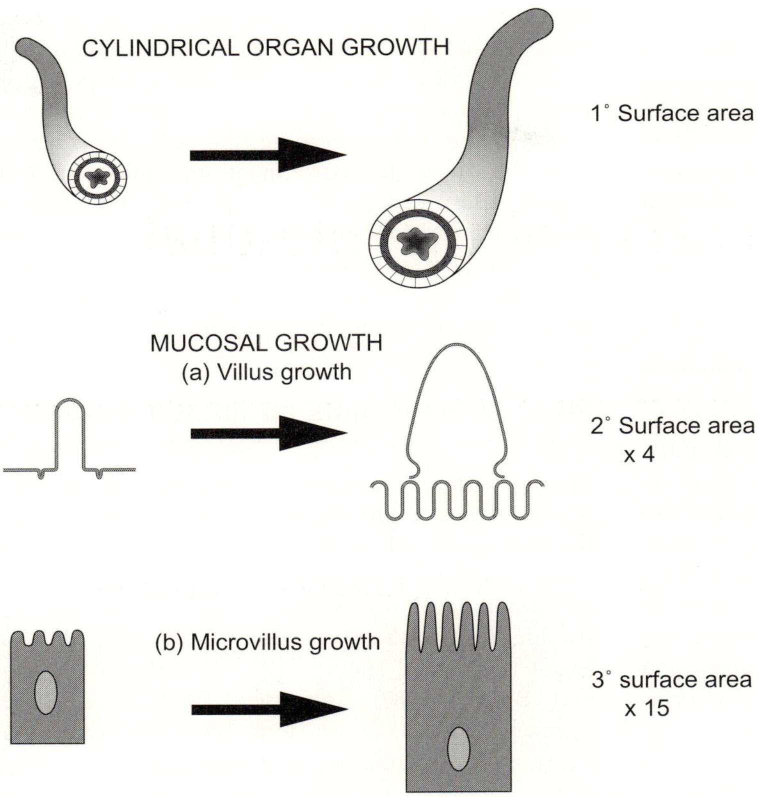

Figure 3.1 *Intestinal growth occurs in two ways. There is cylindrical organ growth in length and width. Mucosal growth occurs inwards towards the lumen and the surface area is amplified by the presence of submucosal folds, villi and microvilli.*

exists throughout the epithelial layer. Crypts form as downwards growth of the epithelium into which the proliferating cells increasingly localize. Crypt formation is again dependent on the mesenchyme (Kedinger *et al.*, 1986). Normal foetal small intestinal development has been shown to be dependent on swallowing of amniotic fluid *in utero* (Trahair *et al.*, 1986, 1987; Trahair, 1993). Interestingly, there seems to be a specific factor in amniotic fluid that promotes formation of crypts (Calvert *et al.*, 1983). Crypts increase by binary longitudinal fission (Fig. 3.2).

FUNCTIONAL DEVELOPMENT OF THE SMALL INTESTINE

Functional maturation of the small intestine in humans occurs much earlier in foetal life as compared to laboratory rodents so some care must be taken when extrapolating from one species to another. In the human small intestine, intestinal digestive enzyme activities (e.g. sucrase, maltase) at 14 weeks gestation are 70–100 per cent of levels found in adult intestines (Antonowicz *et al.*, 1974; Antonowicz and Lebenthal, 1977; Ménard and Calvert, 1991). Lactase activity, a key enzyme in the hydrolysis of milk, is present as early as 10 weeks gestation but, unlike other disaccharidases, lactase activity remains around 30 per cent of the levels of newborns (Ménard and Calvert, 1991). Lactase activity increases towards the end of gestation and peaks early in postnatal life at 2–4 times the activity of older infants and

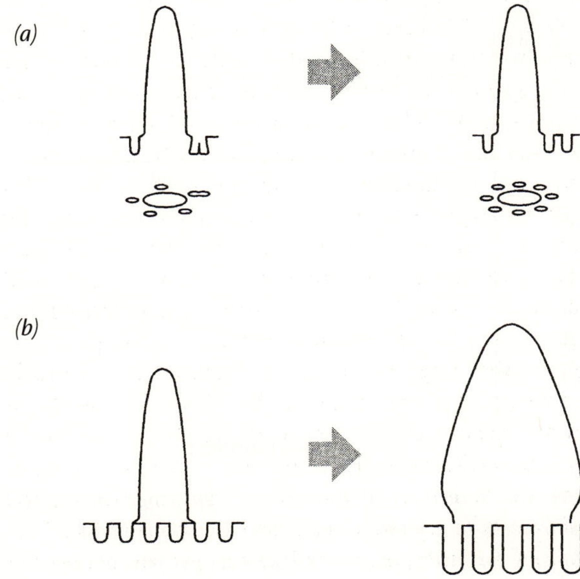

Figure 3.2 *The two patterns of intestinal mucosal growth. (a) How intestinal crypts divide by longitudinal binary fission and (b) how individual crypts proliferate.*

adults (Auricchio and Sebastio, 1989). Intestinal motility has been observed in the intestines of 11-week-old foetuses. This observation has been questioned, however, as it was made in asphyxiated foetuses and may not represent normal intestinal activity. Studies in cats and guinea pigs would suggest that mid-gestation would be a more reasonable period at which to expect peristalsis to occur normally.

POSTNATAL GROWTH

Once the foetus is born, the gastrointestinal tract of the newborn must change to accommodate enteral nutrition and bacterial colonization. The villi of neonates are initially finger-like, but these widen to broader leaf-like forms during childhood (5 months to 5 years), and then become finger-like again in older children and adults (Walker-Smith, 1972). The crypts during infancy are also hyperplastic (Thompson *et al.*, 1998). During this time, individual crypts show increased proliferation (Fig. 3.2). Crypts are longer (means of 270 μm versus 206 μm) and have higher proliferation (means of 4.2 versus 2.5 mitotic figures per crypt) in infants from 6 weeks to 2 years compared with adults. Crypt hyperplasia peaks at around 4–6 months, which is approximately at the time of weaning (Fig. 3.3). This suggests that the luminal environment promotes mucosal growth. Our work would suggest that this stage of development is promoted by an immunomesenchymal interaction that increases crypt proliferation. Functionally, infants have lower absorption of fat and carbohydrate as determined by xylose absorption.

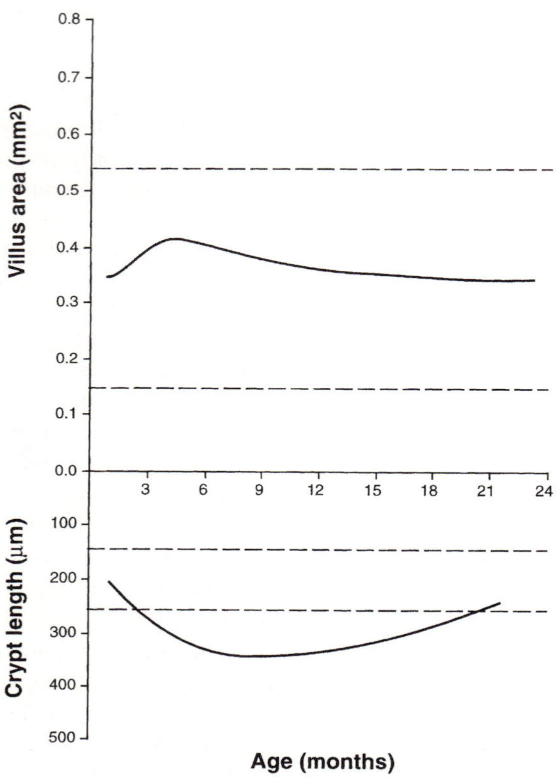

Figure 3.3 *Changes in villus area and crypt length in infants from 6 weeks to 2 years of age. These 74 infants had endoscopy for investigation of irritability and possible reflux oesophagitis and were otherwise normal. The horizontal lines are the 95 per cent limits of the confidence interval for 77 adult subjects. The graph is redrawn from data given by Thompson* et al. *(1998).*

Effect of breast milk on intestinal growth

The newborn's natural source of nutrition is breast milk. It is important to emphasize that breast milk feeding is the normal physiology of humans, even though human infants can survive and grow on infant formula feeds. A popular notion has been that breast milk has a specific trophic effect on the gastrointestinal tract of the human infant (Heird and Hansen, 1977; Berseth, 1987; Corps and Brown, 1987; Koldovsky, 1989; Read, 1989; Zumkeller, 1992). It has long been established that breast milk contains many growth factors in varying concentrations, along with the necessary antibodies and viable immune cells the neonate needs to minimize the infectious threat of its new environment (Cummins and Thompson, 1997). Other studies in rodents have shown intestinal growth occurs during weaning, i.e. when milk feeding is being withdrawn (Hruby, 1966; Herbst and Sunshine, 1969; Cummins *et al.*, 1988; Thompson *et al.*, 1996). It has also been shown that the artificial rearing of rat pups on a substitute formula or early weaning actually leads to precocious growth of the small intestine (Lee and Lebenthal, 1983). Also formula-fed infants have larger villi and longer crypts compared to breast-fed infants (Thompson *et al.*, 1998). These seemingly contradictory effects of breast milk on intestinal growth can be explained. What many studies have failed to do is to distinguish between whole-organ intestinal growth (with an immature mucosa) and specific inward growth of the mucosa (Figs 3.1 and 3.2). It would to reasonable to expect that these two distinct patterns of growth are mediated by different factors. We suspect that breast milk promotes intestinal organ growth in length and width, but that the mucosa remains immature, and that weaning promotes specific mucosal inward growth that prepares the intestine to digest and absorb diverse nutrients.

CLOSURE TO MACROMOLECULES

Cessation of absorption of macromolecules is called 'closure'. The time of closure has been well defined for various animal species but less so for humans (Klein, 1989b). It has been shown that there is increased penetration of the gut by intraluminal, immunologically recognizable proteins during the early postnatal period (Beach *et al.*, 1982; Roberton *et al.*, 1982). In the case of food antigens, premature and newborn infants can absorb proteins such as bovine serum albumin and produce antibodies to food proteins, whereas older children are less capable of antigen absorption. The actual mechanism of closure appears to differ between species and the mechanism involved in man is not known (Klein, 1989b). However, it would appear that the human intestinal mucosa undergoes closure after the 1–2 weeks of postnatal life and that this is promoted by breast feeding (Catassi *et al.*, 1995).

EPITHELIAL MESENCHYMAL INTERACTION

The intestinal epithelium is derived from embryonic endodermal tissue, while intestinal connective tissue in the mucosal lamina propria and submucosa, and muscularis mucosae and surrounding submucosal circular and longitudinal muscular layers are derived from embryonic mesenchymal tissue. A variety of studies have indicated that the ontogeny and differentiation of the endodermal-derived intestinal epithelium is influenced by the adjacent mesenchymal tissue (Haffen *et al.*, 1987, 1989). Techniques such as *in vitro* culture, explant culture, *in ovo* culture or growth of transplanted intestinal tissue under the kidney capsule have been used to study the interaction of the intestinal epithelium (endoderm) and mesenchymal tissue. Various tissues used include endoderm and mesenchyme dissected from chick or rat embryos, or human foetal tissue (derived from therapeutic abortion). These results showed that intestinal rather than other tissue-derived mesenchyme was important for intestinal epithelial development. Thus, the mesenchyme of a specific regional tissue (small intestine) preferentially supports development of the epithelium of the same regional tissue. Although the mesenchyme directs epithelial growth and development, it does not affect the timing of ontogeny of digestive enzyme expression (e.g. disaccharidases), which remains characteristic of the species from which the epithelium (endoderm) was derived (Kedinger *et al.*, 1981; Lacroix *et al.*, 1984). Thus, chick intestine does not express lactase, and rat intestine showed characteristic late sucrase expression. A third finding was that the epithelial mesenchymal interaction is reciprocal with the endoderm affecting differentiation of the mesenchyme. Thus, chick intestinal endoderm influences rat and human skin fibroblasts to differentiate into connective tissue of villi and into intestinal muscular layers (Lacroix *et al.*, 1985; Arnold *et al.*, 1987).

Although these previously described studies pertain to foetal intestinal development, it is also likely that an epithelial mesenchymal interaction continues during postnatal life. The mesenchyme is represented by pericryptal fibroblasts and perhaps other elements of the connective tissue, and the endoderm is represented by the intestinal crypt and villus. Studies have shown that intestinal mucosal fibroblasts cultured from infant rats support the growth and intestinal differentiation of both the chick gizzard (stomach) or the crypt cell intestinal epithelial cell IEC-17, when transplanted under the kidney capsule of rats (Haffen *et al.*, 1983, 1987). These demonstrate that there is an epithelial–mesenchymal interaction in the postnatal intestine just as there is in the foetal intestine.

In summary, studies have shown that, in foetal and postnatal intestine, there is an epithelial–mesenchymal interaction that is mutually reciprocal, and that this interaction influences and directs the growth and development of the epithelium and of the underlying connective tissue and muscle.

IMMUNOMODULATION OF THE EPITHELIUM

Ferguson and Jarrett (1975) were the first to show that intestinal structure is altered by activation of thymus-derived T cells. They showed that partial villous atrophy of the small intestine only occurred in rats with an intact immune system and did not occur in hypothymic 'nude' animals with *Nippostrongylus* worm infection. Various studies have since shown that the epithelium of the small intestine is modulated by the immune system. While this might seem mutually exclusive to the concept of the epithelial–mesenchymal interaction, and indeed both lines of enquiry have largely proceeded in ignorance or defiance of each other, it is possible to reconcile these concepts into a three-way interaction of the epithelium, the mucosal immune system and the mesenchyme that will be discussed below.

The evidence for immunomodulation of the epithelium is that pathologically activated T cells are associated with epithelial crypt hyperplasia as best demonstrated in coeliac disease (Halstensen and Brandtzaeg, 1993). This is also present in models of experimental immunologically mediated intestinal damage (e.g. graft versus host reaction, intestinal allograft rejection) (Ferguson, 1987; Marsh and Cummins, 1993) and in human foetal intestinal explant cultures stimulated by T-cell mitogens (MacDonald and Spencer, 1988). Conversely, immunosuppression leads to reduced crypt hyperplasia in these experimental models (Cummins *et al.*, 1989a), in foetal intestinal explant cultures (MacDonald and Spencer, 1988) and in the immunodeficiency syndrome of human immunodeficiency virus (HIV) (Ullrich *et al.*, 1989; Cummins *et al.*, 1990b). While these mainly pathological or experimental diseases result in tissue damage, there is also evidence that immunomodulation is important in normal epithelial growth postnatally. Crypt hyperplasia is present in human small intestine during the first 2 years of life as compared to adult intestine, and this is associated with a physiological peak of immunological activity (Cummins *et al.*, 1994; Thompson *et al.*, 1998). In rats, this physiological T-cell activity is localized to the gut-associated lymphoid tissue with expression of the T-cell activation marker, interleukin-2 receptors (Thompson *et al.*, 1996). Thus, immunological activity and crypt hyperplasia coincide in time and place. Perhaps the main evidence for immunomodulation of the epithelium is that immunosuppression delays growth of the small intestine in healthy infant rats.

Cyclosporin A treatment causes relative crypt and villus hypoplasia (Cummins *et al.*, 1989b) and selective treatment with anti-interleukin-2 receptor antibody similarly causes both crypt and villus hypoplasia (Thompson *et al.*, 1996). While γδ T cells in the epithelium have been suggested to mediate this effect in mice (Komano *et al.*, 1995), this is very unlikely in rats and humans, as there are low (< 10 per cent of T cells) numbers of mucosal γδ T cells present in these species and it is difficult to envisage how intraepithelial lymphocytes could affect intestinal crypts as these are anatomically separated compartments. Our studies have shown that there are immune cells expressing interleukin-2 receptors in mesenteric lymph nodes and jejunal Peyer's patches, but particularly in the lamina propria, where they would be available to influence pericryptal fibroblasts and thereby affect proliferation of intestinal crypts.

EFFECT OF THE IMMUNE SYSTEM ON THE MESENCHYME

The immune system is a specialized mesenchymal tissue and therefore it is likely to interact with other mesenchymal cells but particularly with pericryptal fibroblasts to influence epithelial crypt proliferation. At the present time, this link is still circumstantial but the evidence is suggestive. Interleukin-1 (IL-1) (an immune cytokine) has been shown to stimulate cyclooxygenase *in vitro* in myofibroblasts (Hinterleitner *et al.*, 1996) that could then potentially stimulate epithelial proliferation through prostaglandins (Uribe *et al.*, 1992). IL-1 and lipopolysaccharide stimulate isolated intestinal fibroblasts to secrete various immune cytokines such as granulocyte–macrophage colony-stimulating factor (GM-CSF, IL-6 and IL-8. Both transforming growth factor-β (TGFβ) and IL-2 influence isolated intestinal fibroblasts to promote *in vitro* cell growth and differentiation of intestinal epithelial endoderm (Fritsch *et al.*, 1997). Cross-talk also exists between the mesenchyme and the immune system: for example, insulin-like growth factor-1 (IGF-1) has a synergistic effect with IL-2 on lymphocyte proliferation (Schillaci *et al.*, 1995), and conversely IGF-1 receptors are expressed on lymphocytes (Xu *et al.*, 1995). When overexpressed in transgenic mice, IGF-1 caused muscular hyperplasia with intestinal lengthening, but apparently not specific epithelial growth (Wang *et al.*, 1997; Lund, 1998).

TROPHIC FACTORS

Establishing a causal role for any trophic factor of the small intestine

There have been many purported growth factors for the gastrointestinal tract (Podolsky, 1993). The majority of studies have used exogenous growth factors at pharmacological levels and shown an effect on intestinal length and weight. Some have shown changes in DNA and others changes in function. Some studies have demonstrated the presence of growth factor receptors and used this as support for a physiological role of the growth factor in question. Despite a plethora of work, no definitive growth factor has been demonstrated at a physiological level to promote intestinal growth.

Henning *et al.* (1994) suggested that a number of factors need to be met before a convincing role for any factor could be be considered to promote intestinal growth. While these criteria were written in consideration of endocrine factors, we have generalized these criteria for any growth factor or activity. Four minimum criteria were described:

1. The proposed factor should have increased activity at the time of intestinal growth.
2. Earlier administration of the factor (preferably in physiological and not pharmacological doses) should cause precocious intestinal growth.
3. The effect of the factor *in vivo* should be reproduced *in vitro*.
4. Ablation or blockade of the endogenous source of the factor should retard intestinal growth.

Vanderhoof (1993) has proposed essentially the same criteria: (1) to administer an exogenous agent; (2) to increase endogenous production; and (3) to block endogenous production. We particularly support the notions that any putative growth factor should have demonstrated increased levels at the time it is meant to be causing intestinal growth, and that blockade of the growth factor, especially *in vivo*, should inhibit intestinal growth. We would additionally emphasize that it is important to define what is meant by intestinal growth, i.e. whole-organ intestinal growth or mucosal epithelial growth. Many studies have investigated administration

Table 3.1 *Comparison of various growth factors for the small intestine according to the Henning criteria*

Factor	Activity	Pharmacology	*In vitro*	Blockade/ knockout	References
Corticosteroids[a]	Yes	A	Yes	Yes	Wright *et al.* (1978), Henning (1981), Berseth (1987), Koldovsky (1989), Ichiba *et al.* (1992), Henning *et al.* (1994)
EGF	ND	Yes[c]	Yes	Yes	Corps and Brown (1987), Miettinen *et al.* (1995)
FGF	ND	ND	Yes	Yes	Liu *et al.* (1990), Dignass *et al.* (1994b)
GLP-2	ND	Yes	ND	ND	Drucker *et al.* (1996)
HGF	ND	Yes	Yes	No	Dignass *et al.* (1994a), Fukamachi *et al.* (1994), Kato *et al.* (1997)
Insulin	Yes	Yes	Yes	ND	Blazquez *et al.* (1970, 1975), Gallo-Payet *et al.* (1987)
KGF	ND	Yes	Yes	ND	Housely *et al.* (1994)
IGF-1	ND	Yes	Yes	No	Steer (1980), Corps and Brown (1987), Steeb *et al.* (1995), Yang *et al.* (1997)
PGE_2	ND	Yes	ND	Yes	Uribe *et al.* (1987, 1992)
T cells	Yes	Yes	Yes	Yes	Lund *et al.* (1986), Ferreira *et al.* (1990), Thompson *et al.* (1996)
TGFα	ND	Yes	ND	ND	Hormi and Lehy (1996)
Thyroxine[b]	Yes	Yes	Var	Var	Henning (1987)

[a]While corticosteroids promote intestinal maturation, they are antitrophic to the intestine.
[b]Many of the actions of thyroxine are mediated via corticosteroids.
EGF, epidermal growth factor; FGF, fibroblast growth factor; GLP-2, glucagon-like peptide-2; HGF, hepatocyte growth factor; KGF, keratinocyte growth factor; IGF-1, insulin-like growth factor-1; PGE_2, prostaglandin E_2; TGFα, transforming growth factor-α; Yes, has been determined; ND, not determined; No, no effect observed; A, antitrophic effect; Var, variable.
[c]Only demonstrated systemically and not luminally.

of exogenous hormones or growth factors in pharmacologically large doses to young animals and, although this is a good first step in investigating any potential growth factor, the interpretation of such data must be taken with caution until the remaining criteria are investigated. Table 3.1 lists a number of possible growth factors for the small intestine.

Peptide growth factors

There are a number of peptide growth factors that include epidermal growth factor (EGF), acidic and basic fibroblast growth factor (FGF), hepatocyte growth factor (HGF), insulin-like growth factor (IGF) and keratinocyte growth factor (KGF). These growth factors are generally produced by mesenchymal tissues. As well as producing growth of mesenchymal tissues, they also affect epithelial tissues to varying extents. Some such as KGF only cause epithelial growth, others such as IGF-1 cause mesenchymal growth (e.g. intestinal submucosal and muscle growth), and both IGF-1 and HGF may be expressed predominantly in foetal life.

EPIDERMAL GROWTH FACTOR

EGF was initially thought to be a major growth factor for the intestine (Berseth, 1987), and has been used therapeutically to promote postnatal intestinal growth in a human neonate (Sullivan *et al.*, 1991). Various studies, however, have shown that, while it is active pharmacologically when administered systemically (Goodlad *et al.*, 1987), it is not active luminally even though EGF is present in breast milk physiologically. Also, EGF receptors are present on the basal lateral membrane of enterocytes and not on the expected apical luminal membrane, if EGF was active physiologically (Playford *et al.*, 1996). The EGF receptor knockout mouse has reduced intestinal development but this depends on the genetic background of the mouse (Miettinen *et al.*, 1995). It is also known that TGFα interacts with the EGF receptor, but once again the physiological significance is difficult to discern as to why the distribution of the receptor is basal rather than apical whatever the ligand. Taken together, there seems to be inconclusive evidence that EGF or TGFα are physiological trophic factors for the intestine but they may have some other role, such as in tissue repair.

FIBROBLAST GROWTH FACTOR

FGFs are peptides that affect mesenchymal growth. Both acidic and basic FGFs cause growth of the IEC-6 non-transformed rat intestinal cell line *in vitro*. This effect is further enhanced by the addition of heparin, which perhaps mimics the *in vivo* situation of growth factors binding to the extracellular matrix (Dignass *et al.*, 1994b). The IEC-6 cell line has similarities to normal rat crypt epithelial cells. Importantly, infusion of blocking anti-FGF antibody slows the growth of transplanted rodent intestine under the kidney capsule (Liu *et al.*, 1990). The blocking antibody was administered into the renal artery of recipient animals.

HEPATOCYTE GROWTH FACTOR

HGF is a further mesenchymal growth factor that increases epithelial growth at least when administered in pharmacological doses (Fukamachi *et al.*, 1994; Kato *et al.*, 1997). HGF stimulates *in vitro* intestinal IEC-6 epithelial cells and rat foetal intestinal cells in primary culture (Dignass *et al.*, 1994a; Fukamachi *et al.*, 1994) and is more potent in stimulating proliferation than either EGF or IGF-1 (Kato *et al.*, 1997).What is intriguing is that HGF is strongly expressed by intestinal crypts in foetal life, which suggest that it may be a more prominent growth factor for intestinal epithelial foetal growth (Wang *et al.*, 1994). It would be interesting to study whether HGF causes longitudinal fission of intestinal crypts, as this is a pattern of growth that is more important at this stage. The HGF knockout mouse apparently does not show any decreased intestinal growth (Drucker, 1997), which would be against a major role for HGF physiologically.

INSULIN-LIKE GROWTH FACTOR-1

IGF-1 is another candidate hormone for which there is experimental evidence that it acts as a growth factor for the intestine. It is produced by cultured intestinal mesenchymal cells, at least in rats, and can be demonstrated to increase proliferation of the IEC-6 intestinal cell line (MacDonald *et al.*, 1998). When given pharmacologically and systemically to neonatal or adult rats, it increases intestinal growth (Steeb *et al.*, 1994, 1995) or, where overexpressed (20–30-fold overexpression of mRNA for IGF-1) transgenically, it increases intestinal growth particularly of the muscle layers (Wang *et al.*, 1997). We are not aware of any study that has shown that IGF-1 activity is increased at the relevant time of accelerated mucosal growth postnatally. There is, however, a major technical problem in that *in situ* hybridization in rodent models of gut injury with increased crypt proliferation may show increased mRNA for IGF-1 but immunostaining using a variety of antibodies has been remarkably ineffective in demonstrating protein levels (Winesett *et al.*, 1995). In addition, a number of IGF binding proteins may regulate the effectiveness of IGF-1 activity. Apparently, the IGF-1 knockout mouse does not show any defect of intestinal growth which would indicate that IGF-1 is not a principal physiological factor for intestinal growth (Drucker, 1997).

KERATINOCYTE GROWTH FACTOR

KGF is another factor that has been recently reported to be involved in the maintenance and repair of the gastrointestinal tract. KGF is a known epithelial mitogen that is found throughout the gastrointestinal tract (Mason *et al.*, 1994; Finch *et al.*, 1995). It is unique in that it does not affect mesenchymal growth and is exclusively an epithelial mitogen. Thus, KGF is expressed by underlying mesenchymal cells, whereas the responding epithelial cells express the KGF receptor. The mRNA for KGF is present in mesenchymal cells underlying the mature villous cells but mRNA for KGF receptor is most abundant in the crypt stem cell region (Housely *et al.*, 1994). This suggests that intestinal stem cells are responsive to KGF in a paracrine manner. When administered pharmacologically it produces increased cell proliferation of the gastrointestinal tract, including the small intestine, but especially goblet cell hyperplasia (Housely *et al.*, 1994). It also causes growth of the rat IEC-6 intestinal cell line *in vitro* (Dignass *et al.*, 1994b). It is produced from mesenchymal cells, especially pericryptal fibroblasts, at least in Crohn's disease (Bajaj-Elliott *et al.*, 1997). Thus, potentially, KGF could be produced physiologically by pericryptal fibroblasts, although this has not been studied. Pharmacological doses of KGF help maintain mainly distal ileal and colonic villous and crypt structure and proliferation during enteral hypocaloric feeding (Estívariz *et al.*, 1998).

Local and systemic hormones

GLUCOCORTICOIDS

Glucocorticoids have been extensively studied in laboratory rodents as a mediator of maturation of the gastrointestinal tract (Table 3.1). Their systemic levels rise in laboratory rats early in weaning (days 18–19). What has been overlooked is that corticosteroids are antitrophic to the intestine as they decrease proliferation of crypts at least in adult animals (Wright *et al.*, 1978), and so are likely to do the same to intestinal crypts in infant rats. Corticosteroids lead to precocious expression of certain enzymes, such as sucrase activity, which characterize the mature intestine. The question that still remains unresolved is whether the glucocorticoids act directly or indirectly through other mediators. The most likely physiological role of glucocorticoids in the human is to stimulate the maturational events that occur in the last 2 weeks of gestation.

GLUCAGON-LIKE PEPTIDE-2

The work on glucagon-like peptide-2 (GLP-2) comes originally from the clinical observation that an enteroglucagon-secreting tumour caused intestinal hyperplasia (Gleeson *et al.*, 1971). GLP-2 is a 33-amino-acid fragment of a larger proglucagon molecule and has a specific trophic effect on the small intestine. GLP-2 (and other proglucagon-derived peptides) are produced by the L-enteroendocrine cells of the small and large intestine. Studies in nude mice implanted with proglucagon-secreting tumours showed that intestinal weight was increased and particularly that intestinal growth occurred with larger villi (Drucker *et al.*, 1996). Mice treated with synthetic GLP-2 also had comparable intestinal growth. The effect of GLP-2 on the small intestine is relatively tissue specific (Drucker, 1997). These studies have not addressed whether GLP-2 is a trophic factor for physiological growth.

INSULIN

Insulin is another factor that has received extensive study. The binding of ^{125}I-labelled insulin to isolated intestinal epithelial cells of mice increases during infancy, suggesting that there is increased expression of insulin receptors (Gallo-Payet *et al.*, 1987). Data from rats, humans and pigs demonstrate that insulin levels increase just prior to ontogenic changes in disaccharidase activities. Other evidence also shows that insulin affects the maturation of the gut as measured by disaccharidase levels. Administration of insulin to 8-day-old mouse pups led to the early expression of sucrase activity and an increase of all other brush-border enzyme activities, resulting in a precocious pattern of hydrolytic enzyme expression. Epithelial cell proliferation was also increased (Ménard *et al.*, 1981). Similar results were found in explant tissue culture when insulin was added to the serum-free medium (Arsenault and Ménard, 1984). Some data have shown that other changes may occur independently of the disaccharidase shift.

THYROID HORMONE

Thyroid hormone has been extensively studied in the laboratory rodent with regard to intestinal maturation. Overall, there is less convincing evidence for a role for thyroid hormone in intestinal maturation than there is for glucocorticoids. This is complicated further by the fact that changes in thyroid status are always associated with concomitant changes in circulating glucocorticoids. In humans the situation is no clearer, although the evidence suggests that thyroid hormone may synergize with glucocorticoids late in the last trimester, resulting in maturation of the intestine.

Immunological promotion of epithelial growth

The mucosal immune system may also interact with other mesenchymal tissue, such as pericryptal fibroblasts, to promote the growth of the small intestine. This is based on evidence that mucosal T cells promote intestinal epithelial proliferation in such experimental models as the graft versus host reaction or intestinal allograft rejection (Mowat and Ferguson, 1981; Ferguson, 1987), *in vitro* in human foetal explant cultures (Ferreira *et al.*, 1990), and pathologically in certain diseases such as coeliac disease (Halstensen and Brandtzaeg, 1993). Conversely, epithelial proliferation is decreased in HIV infection in which there is T-cell deficiency (Cummins *et al.*, 1990b; Ullrich *et al.*, 1990). These might suggest that crypt proliferation could also be T-cell dependent. Our studies have shown that T-cell activity peaks both in rats and in humans during infancy, which is the time of physiologically postnatal crypt hyperplasia and intestinal epithelial growth (Henning criterion 1) (Thompson *et al.*, 1996, 1998). Heightened immunological activity, such as in neonatal graft versus host reaction, induces precocious intestinal growth before evolving into an enteropathy because of unrestrained immunological activity (Henning criterion 2) (Lund *et al.*, 1986). Mitogen-activated mucosal T cells in foetal human intestinal explant cultures cause crypt hyperplasia (Henning criterion 3) (Ferreira *et al.*, 1990). Immunosuppression with either cyclosporin A or anti-IL-2 receptor antibody delays intestinal growth (Henning criterion 4) (Cummins *et al.*, 1989b; Mengheri *et al.*, 1996; Thompson *et al.*, 1996).

ADAPTATION OF THE GASTROINTESTINAL TRACT

General

Intestinal adaptation has been extensively reviewed previously (Williams, 1978a,b; Dowling, 1982). Once the initial development of the small intestine has been established, a steady state must be maintained. The first period of adaptation is during weaning, when breast milk is gradually replaced by food. This is associated with mucosal epithelial growth inwards into the lumen. Crypt proliferation is relatively increased during weaning in both rats (Koldovsky *et al.*, 1966; Herbst and Sunshine, 1969) and in human infants (Thompson *et al.*, 1998). After weaning, a new steady state is achieved that is more or less lifelong. There are only two pertubations to this steady state: physiological or pathological. Physiological villous and crypt hyperplasia may occur in association with lactation or cold adaptation, although both have only been characterized in rodents (Dowling, 1982). There are two forms of pathological adaptation. Traditionally, these have been divided into hypoplastic villous atrophy and hyperplastic villous atrophy. This is probably too simplistic a notion as villous atrophy can be seen with normal crypt proliferation or with relatively mild crypt hyperplasia. The mechanism of villous atrophy seems to be collapse of the extracellular matrix in the lamina propria from activated immune cells (especially macrophages), perhaps after a certain threshold level of immunological activity (Murch *et al.*, 1993; Murch, 1995; Pender *et al.*, 1996), whereas crypt hyperplasia has been known for a long time to occur at a lower threshold of immunological activation of T cells (Ferguson, 1987).

Dissociation of villous atrophy from crypt hyperplasia

The spectrum of responses of intestinal crypts from hypoplasia to hyperplasia in association with villous atrophy suggests that the response of villi and that of crypts may be either totally or partially independent events with possibly different mediating factors. Hypoplastic villous atrophy is associated with malnutrition (particularly kwashiorkor) and total parenteral nutrition (Brunser *et al.*, 1968; Shiner *et al.*, 1973; Lo and Walker, 1989). In animal models such as the weanling rat, deprivation of intraluminal nutrients leads to decreased intestinal length and mucosal mass, but this rapidly reverses on refeeding (Castillo *et al.*, 1991), and similarly total parenteral nutrition in pigs causes intestinal atrophy with villous and crypt hypoplasia (Goldstein *et al.*, 1985). Malnutrition in humans with marasmus causes thinning of the mucosa with relative hypoplastic villous atrophy, but kwashiorkor causes blunting and further fusion of villi. Normoplastic villous atrophy is seen in chronic enteral feeding and in cirrhosis (Cummins and Wilson, 1996). HIV enteropathy was originally described by Kotler as villous atrophy with crypt hyperplasia associated with malabsorption (Kotler *et al.*, 1984) but subsequent studies have shown that crypt hyperplasia is relatively deficient (Ullrich *et al.*, 1989, 1990; Cummins *et al.*, 1990b).

Figure 3.4 shows intestinal morphometry in which biopsies from patients with the acquired immunodeficiency syndrome (AIDS) have been individually matched for villous atrophy using biopsies from coeliac patients. This comparison shows that crypt hyperplasia in HIV enteropathy is relatively deficient in comparison with coeliac disease. This is taken as some evidence that crypt hyperplasia is T-cell dependent (Marsh and Cummins, 1993). Hyperplastic villous atrophy is seen in various disease states including coeliac disease, cow's milk allergy, giardiasis and tropical sprue (Ferguson, 1987), and occurs as an adaptation to intestinal resection (Brunser *et al.*, 1968). Coeliac disease (Chapter 23) is certainly the classical example of hyperplastic villous atrophy (Cummins *et al.*, 1990a) and this is associated with markers of mucosal T-cell activation (Halstensen and Brandtzaeg, 1993). Similar T-cell activation and vigorous crypt hyperplasia is seen in cow's milk sensitive enteropathy (Walker-Smith *et al.*, 1998) and to a lesser extent in tropical sprue (Veitch *et al.*, 1998).

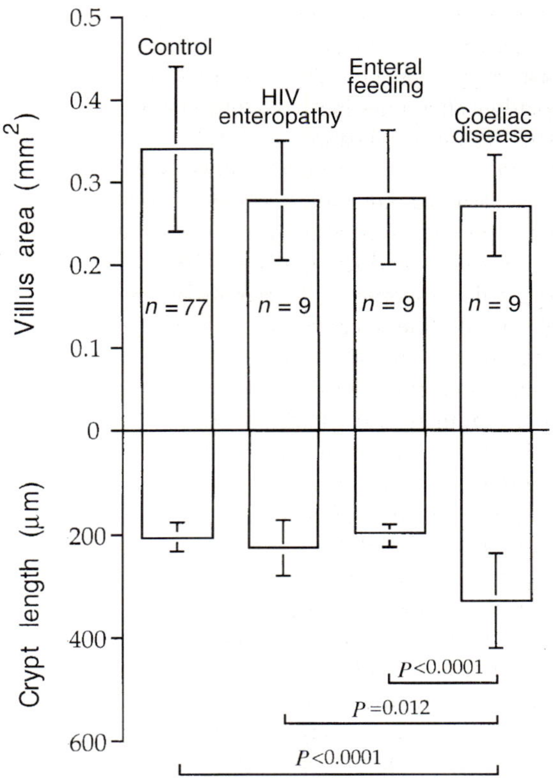

Figure 3.4 *Comparison of patients on enteral feeding, patients with HIV enteropathy and those with coeliac disease. Biopsies were individually matched for villus area to allow comparison of crypt hyperplasia between groups. Note that patients with untreated coeliac disease usually have more severe villous atrophy and crypt hyperplasia than depicted if biopsies are not matched. Data are given as mean ± SD.*

Short bowel sydrome

Short bowel syndrome (Chapter 29) is an important clinical problem and is used experimentally as a paradigm of intestinal adapatation. It occurs during infancy from a variety of conditions (e.g. necrotizing enterocolitis, intestinal volvulus, intestinal atresia) and in adults in whom there is usually advanced atherosclerosis with mesenteric ischaemia, or less often from Crohn's disease. It has been known for some time that, if the patients are supported on parenteral nutrition, then intestinal adaptation occurs, especially if enteral feeds are introduced gradually (Bohane *et al.*, 1979). Intestinal adaptation after surgical resection has been studied extensively in experimental animals. Epithelial proliferation is stimulated by partial intestinal resection (Brunser *et al.*, 1968). Part of the response is mediated systemically (Biller *et al.*, 1986) but adaptation is also dependent on luminal food (Menge *et al.*, 1975).

Survival of both animals and humans is possible after loss of most of the small bowel, and the associated diarrhoea and malabsorption tend to improve with time. Thus, the small intestine has both a functional reserve and a capacity to regenerate. The general features of intestinal adaptation after intestinal resection are mucosal hyperplasia, intestinal dilatation and submucosal muscular hypertrophy. Mucosal hyperplasia consists of villous and crypt hyperplasia. Adaptation is always greater after proximal as opposed to distal resection, and is maximal near the anastomosis and tapers distally. The intensity of the hyperplastic response is directly proportional to the length of intestine resected. Bacterial overgrowth may be present in the intestinal remnant and may adversely prolong parenteral nutrition, if it is not identified and treated (Kaufman *et al.*, 1997). A variety of interventions have been tried in humans or experimentally in animals to improve intestinal adaptation, including glutamine, EGF, growth hormone, IGF-1, GLP-2 and octreotide with varying success (Sullivan *et al.*, 1991; Drucker, 1997; Scolapio *et al.*, 1997). Octreotide treats the secretory diarrhoea and also may improve splanchnic blood flow, which is more important generally for adults with short bowel syndrome in whom there may be vascular disease. It is also known that luminal food, especially polymeric protein, as well as carbohydrate and long-chain triglycerides, promote intestinal adaptation.

CELL PROLIFERATION IN DISEASE STATES

Diseases with crypt hyperplasia

Coeliac disease (Chapter 23) results in malabsorption of nutrients and diarrhoea, with morphological and functional abnormalities when the diet contains wheat, barley and oats. The characteristic histological appearance involves epithelial effacement, villous atrophy, crypt hyperplasia and lymphocytic infiltration of both the epithelium and the lamina propria. Paneth cells are decreased in number (Klein, 1989a). Immune cells have been shown to have a higher level of activation than those in normal controls (Halstensen and Brandtzaeg, 1993). Cell kinetics are dramatically altered during active disease with an increased crypt depth and mitotic count (Cummins *et al.*, 1990a). In addition the proliferative compartment is enlarged.

Cow's milk intolerance is another condition where proliferation and structure have been examined. In general, mucosal changes in cow's milk allergy are milder than in coeliac disease, although the changes in cell kinetics are strikingly similar (Kosnai *et al.*, 1980; Klein, 1989a). In both cases there is a loss of enterocytes and a subsequent crypt hyperplasia. The similarities between these two conditions is not surprising given the pathogenesis is immunological in both diseases.

In giardiasis a shortening of the villi and a varying degree of inflammation has been reported (Yardley *et al.*, 1964; Duncombe *et al.*, 1978). There is associated villous atrophy and crypt hyperplasia, but to a lesser extent than that seen in coeliac disease (Farthing, 1997). Only about 10 per cent of patients with giardiasis have total villous atrophy on intestinal biopsy. The mitotic index is directly proportional to the degree of inflammation. An inter-relationship between the events in the lamina propria and the crypts occurs under normal conditions and pathological states such as graft versus host disease. In this condition the gut is considered an innocent bystander to the action of lymphokines produced by local T cells. Tropical sprue also has partial villous atrophy and crypt hyperplasia with increased mitotic count in crypts. This is associated with increased activation of mucosal T cells (Veitch *et al.*, 1998).

Intestinal mucositis after chemotherapy

It has been known for some considerable time that cytotoxic drugs given for cancer cause crypt hypoproliferation (Trier, 1962). Interestingly, pyknotic bodies were also observed in intestinal crypts that could well have been apoptotic bodies (Trier, 1962). Our studies have indicated that apoptosis of crypt cells peaks within 1 day after cancer chemotherapy in both humans and rats, whereas villous atrophy and crypt hypoplasia peaks at 3 days after treatment (unpublished data). Moreover, the intestine of rats, at least, seems to be more sensitive than a tumour to apoptosis because apoptosis increased 29-fold in intestinal crypts after methotrexate, but only threefold in a subcutaneously implanted breast cancer.

In humans, our studies have shown apoptosis increases 11-fold in intestinal crypts at day 1 after chemotherapy. Mucositis after chemotherapy is just being investigated again, after many decades of neglect, with trials of various factors to ameliorate intestinal damage. A clinical trial of misoprostil failed to show any benefit (Duenas-Gonsalez *et al.*, 1996). Interleukin-11 is one promising agent that reduces apoptosis of intestinal crypts at least experimentally in rodents (Orazi *et al.*, 1996). Another agent that has demonstrated benefit at least experimentally is KGF (Farrell *et al.*, 1998). The worry with KGF is that it may accelerate growth of a cancer but alternatively this could also sensitize the tumour to chemotherapy. Ideally, an agent is needed that acts locally only on the small intestine and does not have any systemic action. Unfortunately, this will still not be beneficial for gastrointestinal tumours that require chemotherapy.

CONCLUDING REMARKS

The small intestine is remarkable in having such a large internal surface area for absorption of dietary nutrients.

It grows longitudinally and in width as a cylinder during foetal and postnatal life, and has a relatively immature mucosa in which intestinal crypts divide by binary fission. In humans, the inner epithelial surface starts to grow even in foetal life by developing villi, and these in turn have microvilli, both of which magnify the surface area. This mucosal growth continues postnatally, with relative crypt hyperplasia in humans during infancy that prepares the small intestine for weaning. These different processes of cylindrical growth and mucosal growth are presumably mediated by different factors, but include a clear mesenchymal dependence during foetal life and an immunological dependence during postnatal life. We suggest that there is a continuing immune reaction that integrates with other mesenchymal growth factors. This mesenchymal–immune interaction is likely to be mediated by immunological modulation of pericryptal fibroblasts that directly influence intestinal crypt cell proliferation. A dynamic equilibrium may exist that maintains the structure and function of the small intestine with a continuing imperative to regulate and control physiological inflammation of the small intestine to prevent progression on to pathological inflammation.

REFERENCES

Antonowicz, I., Lebenthal, E. 1977: Developmental pattern of small intestinal enterokinase and disaccharidase activities in the human fetus. *Gastroenterology* 72, 1299–303.

Antonowicz, I., Chang, S., Grand, R. 1974: Development and distribution of lysosomal enzymes and disaccharidases in human fetal intestine. *Gastroenterology* 67, 51–8.

Arnold, C., Haffen, K., Kedinger, M., Rochette-Egly, C., Simon-Assmann, P. 1987: Immunohistological localization of smooth-muscle actin during morphogenesis of normal rat and chimaeric (rat/chick and human/chick) intestines. *Journal of Physiology (London)* 396, 29P.

Arsenault, P., Ménard, D. 1984: Insulin influences the maturation and proliferation of suckling mouse intestinal mucosa in serum-free organ culture. *Biology of the Neonate* 46, 229–36.

Auricchio, S., Sebastio, G. 1989: Development of disaccharidases. In Lebenthal, E. (ed.) *Human gastrointestinal development*. New York: Raven Press, 451–70.

Bajaj-Elliott, M., Bresse, E., Poulsom, R., MacDonald, T. 1997: Increased expression of keratinocyte growth factor (KGF) in inflammatory bowel disease (IBD). Possible role in epithelial restitution after tissue injury. *Immunology and Cell Biology* 75, A113.

Beach, R., Menzies, I., Clayden, G., Scopes, J. 1982: Gastrointestinal permeability changes in the preterm neonate. *Archives of Disease in Childhood* 57, 141–5.

Berseth, C.L. 1987: Enhancement of intestinal growth in neonatal rats by epidermal growth factor in milk. *American Journal of Physiology* 253, G662–5.

Biller, J.A., Montgomery, R.K., Grand, R.J., Klagsbrun, M., Rosenthal, A. 1986: Use of a 3T3 cell growth factor assay for the delineation and characterization of humoral trophic factors involved in intestinal adaptation in the rat. *Gastroenterology* 91, 448–55.

Blazquez, E., Montoya, E., Quijada, C.L. 1970: Relationship between insulin concentration in plasma and pancreas of foetal and weanling rats. *Journal of Endocrinology* 48, 553–61.

Blazquez, E., Lipshaw, L.A., Blazquez, M., Foa, P.P. 1975: The synthesis and release of insulin in fetal, nursing, and young adult rats: studies *in vivo* and *in vitro*. *Pediatric Research* 9, 17–25.

Bohane, T.D., Haka-Ikse, K., Biggar, W.D., Hamilton, J.R., Gall, D.G. 1979: A clinical study of young infants after small intestinal resection. *Journal of Pediatrics* 94, 552–8.

Brunser, O., Reid, A., Mönckeberg, F., Maccioni, A., Contreras, I. 1968: Jejunal mucosa in infant malnutrition. *American Journal of Clinical Research* 21, 976–83.

Calvert, R., Lehoux, J.-C., Arsenault, P., Ménard, D. 1983: Extracts of rat amniotic fluid contains a potent inducer of intestinal crypt formation. *Anatomical Record* 205, 27–37.

Castillo, R.O., Feng, J.J., Stevenson, D.K., Kwong, L.K. 1991: Altered maturation of small intestinal function in the absence of intraluminal nutrients: rapid normalization with refeeding. *American Journal of Clinical Research* 53, 558–61.

Catassi, C., Bonucci, A., Coppa, G.V., Carlucci, A., Giorgi, P.L. 1995: Intestinal permeability changes during the first month: effect of natural versus artifical feeding. *Journal of Parenteral and Enteral Nutrition* 21, 383–6.

Colony, P. 1983: Successive phases of human fetal intestinal development. In Kretchner, N., Minkowski, A. (eds) *Nutritional adaption of the gastrointestinal tract of the newborn*. Vevey: Nestle/New York: Raven Press, 3–28.

Corps, A., Brown, K. 1987: Stimulation of intestinal epithelial cell proliferation in culture by growth factors in human and ruminant mammary secretions. *Journal of Endocrinology* 113, 285–90.

Cummins, A.G., Thompson, F.M. 1997: Postnatal changes in mucosal immune response: a physiological perspective of breast feeding and weaning. *Immunology and Cell Biology* 75, 419–29.

Cummins, A.G., Wilson, P.C. 1996: Enteral feeding maintains but does not improve villous atrophy in malnourished patients. In Vellas, B., Russel, R., Dyard, F., Garry, P., Albarede, J. (eds) *Facts and research in gerontology*. Paris: Serdi Publisher, 167–72.

Cummins, A.G., Steele, T.W., LaBrooy, J.T., Shearman, D.J.C. 1988: Maturation of the rat small intestine at weaning: changes in epithelial cell kinetics, bacterial flora and mucosal immune activity. *Gut* 29, 1672–9.

Cummins, A.G., Munro, G.H., Miller, H.R.P., Ferguson, A. 1989a: Effect of cyclosporin A on the enteropathy of graft-versus-host reaction in the rat: a quantitative study of intestinal morphology, epithelial cell kinetics and mucosal immune activity. *Immunology and Cell Biology* 67, 153–60.

Cummins, A.G., LaBrooy, J.T., Shearman, D.J.C. 1989b: Effect of cyclosporin A in delaying maturation of the small intestine during weaning in the rat. *Clinical and Experimental Immunology* 75, 451–6.

Cummins, A.G., Penttila, I.A., LaBrooy, J.T., Shearman, D.J.C., Robb, T.A., Davidson, G.P. 1990a: Recovery of the small intestine in coeliac disease on a gluten-free diet: changes in intestinal permeability, small bowel morphology and T-cell activity. *Journal of Gastroenterology and Hepatology* 6, 53–7.

Cummins, A.G., LaBrooy, J.T., Stanley, D.P., Rowland, D.P., Shearman, D.J.C. 1990b: Quantitative histological study of enteropathy associated with HIV infection. *Gut* 31, 317–21.

Cummins, A.G., Eglinton, B.A., Gonsalez, A., Roberton, D.M. 1994: Immune activation during infancy in healthy humans. *Journal of Clinical Immunology* 14, 107–15.

Dignass, A., Lynch-Devaney, K., Podolsky, D. 1994a: Hepatocyte growth factor/scatter factor modulates intestinal epithelial proliferation and migration. *Biochemical and Biophysical Research Communications* 202, 701–9.

Dignass, A., Tsunekawa, S., Podolsky, D.K. 1994b: Fibroblast growth factors modulate intestinal epithelial cell growth and migration. *Gastroenterology* 106, 1254–62.

Dowling, H. 1982: Small bowel adaptation and its regulation. *Scandinavian Journal of Gastroenterology* 74, 53–65.

Drucker, D.J. 1997: Epithelial cell growth and differentiation. I. Intestinal growth factors. *American Journal of Physiology* 273, G3–6.

Drucker, D.J., Ehrlich, P., Asa, S.L., Brubaker, P.L. 1996: Induction of intestinal epithelial proliferation by glucagon-like peptide 2. *Proceedings of the National Academy of Sciences USA* 93, 7911–16.

Duenas-Gonsalez, A., Sobrevilla-Calvo, P., Frias-Mendivil, M. *et al.* 1996: Misoprostil prophylaxis for high-dose chemotherapy-induced mucositis: a randomized double-blind study. *Bone Marrow Transplantation* 17, 809–12.

Duncombe, V.M., Bolin, T.D., Davis, A.E., Cummins, A.G., Crouch, R.L. 1978: Histopathology in giardiasis: a correlation with diarrhoea. *Australian and New Zealand Journal of Medicine* 8, 392–6.

Estívariz, C., Jonas, C.R., Gu, L.H. *et al.* 1998: Gut-trophic effects of keratinocyte growth factor in rat small intestine and colon during enteral refeeding. *Journal of Parenteral and Enteral Nutrition* 22, 259–67.

Farrell, C.L., Bready, J.V., Rex, K.L. *et al.* 1998: KGF protects from chemotherapy and radiation-induced gastrointestinal injury and mortality. *Cancer Research* 58, 933–9.

Farthing, M.J.G. 1997: Invited review. The molecular pathogenesis of giardiasis. *Journal of Pediatric Gastroenterology and Nutrition* 24: 79–88.

Ferguson, A. 1987: Models of immunologically driven small intestinal damage. In Marsh, M. (ed.), *Immunopathology of the small intestine*. Chichester: John Wiley, 225–52.

Ferguson, A., Jarrett, E.E.E. 1975: Hypersensitivity reactions in the small intestine. 3. Thymus dependency of experimental 'partial' villous atrophy'. *Gut* 16, 114–17.

Ferreira, R.D.C., Forsyth, L., Richman, P., Wells, C., Spencer, J., MacDonald, T. 1990: Changes in the rate of crypt epithelial cell proliferation and mucosal morphology induced by a T-cell-mediated response in human small intestine. *Gastroenterology* 98, 1255–63.

Finch, P.W., Cunha, G.R., Rubin, J.S., Wong, J., Ron, D. 1995: Pattern of keratinocyte growth factor and keratinocyte growth factor receptor expression during mouse fetal development suggests a role in mediating morphogenetic mesenchymal–epithelial interactions. *Developmental Dynamics* 203, 223–40.

Fritsch, C., Simon-Assmann, P., Kedinger, M., Evans, G.S. 1997: Cytokines modulate fibroblast phenotype and epithelial–stroma interactions in rat intestine. *Gastroenterology* 112, 826–38.

Fukamachi, H., Ichinose, M., Tsukada, S., Kakei, N., Suzuki, T., Miki, K., Kurokawa, K., Masui, T. 1994: Hepatocyte growth factor region specifically stimulates gastro-intestinal epithelial growth in primary culture. *Biochemical and Biophysical Research Communciations* 205, 1445–51.

Gallo-Payet, N., Pothier, P., Hugon, J.S. 1987: Ontogeny of EGF receptors during postnatal development of mouse small intestine. *Journal of Pediatric Gastroenterology and Nutrition* 6, 114–20.

Gleeson, H.M., Bloom, S.R., Polak, J.M., Henry, K., Dowling, R.H. 1971: Endocrine tumour in kidney affecting small bowel structure, motility, and absorptive function. *Gut* 12, 773–82.

Goldstein, R.M., Hebiguichi, T., Luk, G.D., Taqi, F., Guilarte, T.R., Niemiec, P.W., Dudgeon, D.L. 1985: The effects of total parenteral nutrition on gastrointestinal growth and development. *Journal of Pediatric Surgery* 20, 785–91.

Goodlad, R.A., Wislon, T.J., Lenton, W., Gregory, H., McCullagh, K.G., Wright, N.A. 1987: Intravenous but not intragastric urogastrone-EGF is trophic to the intestine of parenterally fed rats. *Gut* 28, 573–82.

Haffen, K., Kedinger, M., Simon-Assmann, P. 1987: Mesenchyme-dependent differentation of epithelial progenitor cells in the gut. *Journal of Pediatric Gastroenterology and Nutrition* 6, 14–23.

Haffen, K., Kedinger, M., Simon-Assmann, P. 1989: Cell contact dependent regulation of enterocyte differentiation. In Lebenthal, E. (ed.), *Human gastrointestinal development*. New York: Raven Press, 19–39.

Haffen, K., Lacroix, B., Kedinger, M., Simon-Assmann, P.M. 1983: Inductive properties of fibroblastic cell cultures derived from rat intestinal mucosa on epithelial differentiation. *Differentiation* 23, 226–33.

Halstensen, T.S., Brandtzaeg, P. 1993: Activated T lymphocytes in the celiac lesion: non proliferative activation (CD25) of CD4+ $\alpha\beta$ cells in the lamina propria but proliferation (Ki-67) of $\alpha\beta$ and $\gamma\delta$ cells in the epithelium. *European Journal of Immunology* 23, 505–10.

Heird, W.C., Hansen, I.H. 1977: Effect of colostrum on growth of intestinal mucosa. *Pediatric Research* 11, 406A.

Henning, S.J. 1981: Postnatal development: coordination of feeding, digestion and metabolism. *American Journal of Physiology* 241, 199–214.

Henning, S.J. 1987: Functional development of the gastro-intestinal tract. In Johnson, L. (ed.), *Physiology of the gastrointestinal tract*. New York: Raven Press, 285–300.

Henning, S.J., Rubin, D.C., Shulman, R.J. 1994: Ontogeny of the intestinal mucosa. In Johnson, L. (ed.), *Physiology of the gastrointestinal tract*. New York: Raven Press, 571–610.

Herbst, J.J., Sunshine, P. 1969: Postnatal development of the small intestine of the rat. Changes in mucosal morphology at weaning. *Pediatric Research* 3, 27–33.

Hinterleitner, T.A., Saada, J.I., Berschneider, H.M., Powell, D.W., Valentich, J.D. 1996: IL-1 stimulates intestinal myofibroblast COX gene expression and augments activation of Cl-secretion in T84 cells. *American Journal of Physiology* 271, C1262–8.

Hormi, K., Lehy, T. 1996: Transforming growth factor-α *in vivo* stimulates epithelial cell proliferation in digestive tissues of suckling rats. *Gut* 39, 532–8.

Housely, R.M., Morris, C.F., Boyle, W. *et al.* 1994: Keratinocyte growth factor induces proliferation of hepatocytes and epithelial cells throughout the rat gastrointestinal tract. *Journal of Clinical Investigation* 94, 1764–77.

Hruby, L. 1966: A quantitative study of the relative growth of the small intestine of the rat during the period of suckling. *Folia Morphologica* 15, 308–14.

Ichiba, H., Kusuda, S., Itagane, Y., Fujita, K., Issiki, G. 1992: Measurement of growth promoting activity in human milk using a fetal small intestinal cell line. *Biology of the Neonate* 61, 47–53.

Kato, Y., Yu, D., Lukish, J.R., Schwartz, M.Z. 1997: Influence of luminal hepatocyte growth factor on small intestine mucosa *in vivo*. *Journal of Surgical Research* 71, 49–53.

Kaufman, S.S., Loseke, C.A., Lupo, J.V., Young, R.J., Murray, N.D., Pinch, L.W., Vanderhoof, J.A. 1997: Influence of bacterial overgrowth and intestinal inflammation on duration of parenteral nutrition in children with short bowel syndrome. *Journal of Pediatrics* 131, 356–61.

Kedinger, M., Simon, P.M., Grenier, J.F., Haffen, K. 1981: Role of epithelial–mesenchymal interactions in the ontogenesis of intestinal brush-border enzymes. *Developmental Biology* 86, 339–47.

Kedinger, M., Simon-Assmann, P.M., Lacroix, B., Marxer, A., Hauri, H.P., Haffen, K. 1986: Fetal gut mesenchyme induces differentiation of cultured intestinal endodermal and crypt cells. *Developmental Biology* 113, 474–83.

Klein, R.M. 1987: Models for the study of cell proliferation in the developing gastrointestinal tract. *Journal of Pediatric Gastroenterology and Nutrition* 5, 513–17.

Klein, R.M. 1989a: Cell proliferative regulation in developing small intestine. In Lebenthal, E. (ed.), *Human gastrointestinal development*. New York: Raven Press, 393–436.

Klein, R.M. 1989b: Small intestinal cell proliferation during development. In Lebenthal, E. (ed.), *Human gastrointestinal development*. New York: Raven Press, 367–92.

Koldovsky, O. 1989: Search for role of milk-borne biologically active peptides for the suckling. *Journal of Nutrition* 119, 1543–51.

Koldovsky, O., Sunshine, P., Kretchmer, N. 1966: Cellular migration of intestinal epithelia in suckling and weaned rats. *Nature* 212, 1389–90.

Komano, H., Fujiura, Y., Kawaguchi, M. *et al.* 1995: Homeostatic regulation of intestinal epithelia by intraepithelial $\gamma\delta$ T cells. *Proceedings of the National Academy of Sciences USA* 92, 6147–51.

Kosnai, I., Kuitunen, P., Savilahti, E., Rapola, J., Kohegyi, J. 1980: Cell kinetics in the jejunal crypt epithelium in malabsorption syndrome with cow's milk protein intolerance and in coeliac disease of childhood. *Gut* 21, 1041–6.

Kotler, D.P., Gaetz, H.P., Lange, M.E.A. 1984: Enteropathy associated with the acquired immunodeficiency syndrome. *Annals of Internal Medicine* 101, 421–8.

Lacroix, B., Kedinger, M., Simon-Assmann, P., Haffen, K. 1984: Effects of human fetal gastroenteric mesenchymal cells on some developmental aspects of animal gut endoderm. *Differentiation* 28, 129–35.

Lacroix, B., Kedinger, M., Simon-Assmann, P., Haffen, K. 1985: Enzymatic response to glucocorticoids of the chick intestinal endoderm associated with various mesenchymal cell types. *Biology of the Cell* 54, 235–40.

Lee, P.C., Lebenthal, E. 1983: Early weaning and precocious development of small intestine in rats: genetic, dietary or hormonal control. *Pediatric Research* 17, 645–50.

Liu, L., Russell, S.M., Nicoll, C.S. 1990: Analysis of the role of basic fibroblast growth factor in growth and differentiation of transplanted fetal rat paws and intestines. *Endocrinology* 126, 1764–70.

Lo, C.W., Walker, W.A. 1989: Changes in the gastrointestinal tract during enteral or parenteral feeding. *Nutrition Reviews* 47, 193–8.

Lund, E.K., Bruce, M.G., Smith, M.W., Ferguson, A. 1986: Selective effects of graft-versus-host reaction on disaccharidase expression by mouse enterocytes. *Clinical Science* 71, 189–98.

Lund, P.K. 1998: The alpha-smooth muscle actin promoter: a useful tool to analyse autocrine and paracrine roles of mesenchymal cells in normal and diseased bowel. *Gut* 42, 320–2.

MacDonald, R.G., McCusker, R.H., Blackwood, D.J., Vanderhoof, J.A., Park, J.H.Y. 1998: Production of insulin-like growth factor (IGF-1) and IGF-binding proteins by rat intestinal stromal cells *in vitro*. *Cellular and Molecular Life Sciences* 54, 158–66.

MacDonald, T.T., Spencer, J. 1988: Evidence that activated mucosal T-cells play a role in the pathogenesis of enteropathy in human small intestine. *Journal of Experimental Medicine* 167, 1341–9.

Marsh, M.N., Cummins, A.G. 1993: The interactive role of mucosal T lymphocytes in intestinal growth, development and enteropathy. *Journal of Gastroenterology and Hepatology* 8, 270–8.

Mason, I., Fuller-Pace, F., Smith, R., Dickson, C. 1994: FGF-7 (keratinocyte growth factor) expression during mouse development suggests roles in myogenesis, forebrain development and epithelial–mesenchymal interactions. *Mechanisms of Development* 45, 15–30.

Ménard, D., Calvert, R. 1991: Fetal and postnatal development of the small and large intestine: patterns and regulation. In Morisset, J., Solomon, T.E. (eds), *Growth of the gastrointestinal tract*. Boca Raton: CRC Press Inc., 159–74.

Ménard, D., Malo, C., Calvert, R. 1981: Insulin accelerates the development of intestinal brush border hydrolytic activities of suckling mice. *Developmental Biology* 85, 150–5.

Menge, H., Werner, H., Lorenz-Meyer, H., Riecken, E.O. 1975: The nutritive effect of glucose on the structure and function of self-emptying blind loops in the rat. *Gut* 16, 462–7.

Mengheri, E., Ciapponi, L., Vignolini, F., Nobili, F. 1996: Cytokine gene expression in intestine of rat during the postnatal development period: increased IL-1 expression at weaning. *Life Sciences* 59, 1227–36.

Miettinen, P.J., Berger, J.E., Meneses, J., Phung, Y., Pedersen, R.A., Werb, Z., Derynck, R. 1995: Epithelial immaturity and multiorgan failure in mice lacking epidermal growth factor receptor. *Nature* 376, 337–41.

Mowat, A.M., Ferguson, A. 1981: Hypersensitivity in the small intestine. V. Induction of cell-mediated immunity to a dietary antigen. *Clinical and Experimental Immunology* 43, 574–82.

Murch, S.H. 1995: Sulphation of proteoglycans and intestinal function. *Journal of Gastroenterology and Hepatology* 10, 210–12.

Murch, S.H., MacDonald, T.T., Walker-Smith, J.A., Levin, M., Lionetti, P., Klein, N.J. 1993: Disruption of sulphated glycosaminoglycans in intestinal inflammation. *Lancet* 341, 711–14.

Orazi, A., Du, X., Yang, Z., Kashai, M., Williams, D.A. 1996: Interleukin-11 prevents apoptosis and accelerates recovery of small intestinal mucosa in mice treated with combined chemotherapy. *Laboratory Investigation* 75, 33–42.

Pender, S.L.F., Lionetti, P., Murch, S.H., Wathan, N., MacDonald, T.T. 1996: Proteolytic degradation of intestinal mucosal extracellular matrix after lamina propria T cell activation. *Gut* 39, 284–90.

Playford, R.J., Hanby, A.M., Gschmeissner, S., Peiffer, L.P., Wright, N.A., McGarrity, T. 1996: The epidermal growth factor receptor (EGF-R) is present on the basolateral, but not on the apical surface of enterocytes in the human gastrointestinal tract. *Gut* 39, 262–6.

Podolsky, D. 1993: Regulation of intestinal epithelial proliferation: a few answers, many questions. *American Journal of Physiology* 264, G179–86.

Read, L.C. 1989: Milk-derived epidermal growth factor (EGF): is it important to the suckling infant? *Breastfeeding Reviews* 13, 33–4.

Roberton, D.M., Paganelli, R., Dinwiddie, R., Levinsky, R.J. 1982: Milk antigen absorption in the preterm and term neonate. *Archives of Disease in Childhood* 57, 369–72.

Schillaci, R., Brocardo, M., Roldan, A. 1995: Co-operative effect between insulin-like growth factor-1 and interleukin-2 on DNA synthesis and interleukin-2 receptor-α chain expression in human lymphocytes. *Immunology and Cell Biology* 73, 340–5.

Scolapio, J.S., Camilleri, M., Fleming, C.R. *et al.* 1997: Effect of growth hormone, glutamine and diet on adaptation in short-bowel syndrome: a randomised, controlled study. *Gastroenterology* 113, 1074–81.

Shiner, M., Redmond, O.B., Hansen, J.D.L. 1973: The jejunal mucosa in protein energy malnutrition. A clinical, histological and ultrastructural study. *Experimental and Molecular Pathology* 19, 61–78.

Steeb, C.-B., Trahair, J.F., Tomas, F.M., Read, L.C. 1994: Prolonged administration of IGF peptides enhances growth of gastrointestinal tissues in normal rats. *American Journal of Physiology* 266, G1090–8.

Steeb, C.-B., Trahair, J.F., Read, L.C. 1995: Administration of insulin-like growth factor-1 (IGF-1) peptides for three days stimulates proliferation of the small intestinal epithelium in rats. *Gut* 37, 630–8.

Steer, H.W. 1980: An analysis of the lymphocyte content of rat lacteals. *Journal of Immunology* 125, 1845–8.

Sullivan, P.B., Brueton, M.J., Tabara, Z.B., Goodlad, R.A., Lee, C.Y., Wright, N.A. 1991: Epidermal growth factor in necrotising enteritis. *Lancet* 338, 53–4.

Thompson, F.M., Mayrhofer, G., Cummins, A.G. 1996: Dependence of epithelial growth of the small intestine on T cell activation during weaning in the rat. *Gastroenterology* 111, 37–44.

Thompson, F.M., Catto-Smith, A.G., Moore, D., Davidson, G., Cummins, A. 1998: Epithelial growth of the small intestine in human infants. *Journal of Pediatric Gastroenterology and Nutrition* 26, 506–12.

Trahair, J.F. 1993: Is fetal enteral nutrition important for normal gastrointestinal growth? A discussion. *Journal of Enteral and Parenteral Nutrition* 17, 82–5.

Trahair, J.F., Harding, R., Bocking, A.D., Silver, M., Robinson, P.M. 1986: The role of ingestion in the development of the small intestine in fetal sheep. *Advances in Pediatrics* 71, 99–104.

Trahair, J.F., Perry, R.A., Silver, M., Robinson, P.M. 1987: Studies on the maturation of the small intestine of the fetal sheep. I. The effects of bilateral adrenalectomy. *Quarterly Journal of Experimental Biology* 72, 61–9.

Trier, J.S. 1962: Morphological alteration induced by methrexate in the mucosa of the proximal small intestine. *Gastroenterology* 42, 295–305.

Ullrich, R., Zeitz, M., Heise, W., L'Age, M., Höffen, G., Riecken, E.O. 1989: Small intestinal structure and function in patients infected with human immunodeficiency virus (HIV): evidence for HIV-induced enteropathy. *Annals of Internal Medicine* 111, 15–21.

Ullrich, R., Zeitz, M., Heise, W. *et al.* 1990: Mucosal atrophy is associated with loss of activated T cells in the duodenal mucosa of human immunodeficiency syndrome. *Digestion* 46(Suppl), 302–7.

Uribe, A., Johansson, C., Rubio, C. 1987: Cell proliferation of the rat gastrointestinal tract mucosa after treatment with E_2 prostaglandins and indomethacin. *Digestion* 36, 238–45.

Uribe, A., Alam, M., Midtvedt, T. 1992: E_2 prostaglandins modulate cell proliferation in the small intestinal epithelium of the rat. *Digestion* 52, 157–64.

Vanderhoof, J.A. 1993: Editorial. Regulatory peptides and intestinal growth. *Gastroenterology* 104, 1205–8.

Veitch, A.M., Kelly, P., Luo, N., Segal, I., Spies, S.K., Farthing, M.J.G. 1998: Small intestinal crypt hyperplasia and T cell activation in African tropical sprue. *Gastroenterology* 114, A1108 (G4536).

Walker-Smith, J.A. 1972: Variation of small intestinal morphology with age. *Archives of Disease in Childhood* 47, 80–3.

Walker-Smith, J.A., Jones, A., Murch, S.H., Philip, A.D. 1998: T-cell activation markers in small intestinal mucosa in chronic diarrhoea of childhood. *Journal of Pediatric Gastroenterology and Nutrition* 27, 254A.

Wang, J., Niu, W., Nikiforov, Y. *et al.* 1997: Targeted overexpression of IGF-1 evokes distinct patterns of organ remodelling in smooth muscle cell tissue beds of transgenic mice. *Journal of Clinical Investigation* 1000, 1425–39.

Wang, Y., Selden, C., Farnaud, S., Calnan, D., Hodgson, H.J.F. 1994: Hepatocyte growth factor (HGF/SF) is expressed in human epithelial cells during embryonic development; studies by *in situ* hybridization and Northern blot analysis. *Journal of Anatomy* 185, 543–51.

Weaver, L.T., Austin, S., Cole, T.J. 1991: Small intestinal length: a factor essential for gut adaption. *Gut* 32, 1321–3.

Williams, R.C.N. 1978a: Intestinal adaptation. Mechanism of control. *New England Journal of Medicine* 278, 1444–50.

Williams, R.C.N. 1978b: Intestinal adaptation. Structural, functional and cytokinetic changes. *New England Journal of Medicine* 298, 1393–402.

Wilson, J.P. 1967: Surface area of the small intestine in man. *Gut* 8, 618–21.

Winesett, D.E., Ulshen, M.H., Hoyt, E.C., Mohapata, N.K., Fuller, R., Lund, P.K. 1995: Regulation and localization of the insulin-like growth factor system in small bowel during altered nutrient status. *American Journal of Physiology* 268, G631–40.

Wright, N.A., Al-Dewachi, H.S., Appleton, D.R., Watson, A. 1978: The effect of single and multiple doses of prednisolone tertiary butyl acetate on cell population kinetics in the small bowel mucosa of the rat. *Virchows Archiv Cell Pathology* 28, 339–50.

Xu, X., Mardell, C., Xian, C.J., Zola, H., Read, L.C. 1995: Expression of functional insulin-like growth factor-1 receptor on lymphoid cell subsets of rats. *Immunology* 85, 395–9.

Yang, H., Ney, D.M., Peterson, C.A., Lo, H.-C., Carey, H.V., Adamo, M.L. 1997: Stimulation of intestinal growth is associated with increased insulin-like growth factor-binding protein 5 mRNA in the jejunal mucosa of insulin-like growth factor-1-treated parenterally fed rats. *Proceedings of the Society for Experimental Biology and Medicine* 216, 438–45.

Yardley, J.H., Takano, J., Hendrix, T. 1964: Epithelial and other mucosal lesions of the jejunum in giardiasis. Jejunal biopsy studies. *Bulletin of the Johns Hopkins Hospital* 115, 389–406.

Zumkeller, W. 1992: Relationship between insulin-like growth factor-I and -II and IGF-binding proteins in milk and the gastrointestinal tract: growth and development of the gut. *Journal of Pediatric Gastroenterology and Nutrition* 15, 357–69.

4

The structure and function of the gastrointestinal immune system

R LOGAN FAUST

The gastrointestinal tract is in contact with hundreds of grams per day of bacterial, dietary and enzymatic antigens over an area estimated to be between 200 and 400 m^2 (Brandtzaeg *et al.*, 1987; Kato and Owen, 1994; McGowan *et al.*, 1997). A selective immune defense over this area is required to prevent harmful responses to these antigens and yet allow the absorption of the macromolecules necessary for nutrition (Walker, 1986). An immune defense localized to this tissue and functioning partly independent of the systemic immune system was first demonstrated in the early 1900s. The enormity of the gastrointestinal immune system becomes apparent when one realises that 80 per cent of all immunoglobulin-producing cells in the body are located there and that, in animal models, there are twice as many lymphocytes present in the gastrointestinal mucosa as there are in the spleen, with at least equal amounts in these tissues in humans (Brandtzaeg *et al.*, 1989; Pabst and Trepel, 1975).

OVERVIEW

The gastrointestinal immune system is a portion of the mucosa-associated lymphoid tissue (MALT). MALT provides immunity to areas that possess mucosal surfaces directly exposed to the environment. While spread over the length of the gastrointestinal tract, gut-associated lymphoid tissue (GALT) is confined to the lamina propria and epithelium, and its immune response is largely humoral (Blumberg and Stenson, 1995). The predominant immunoglobulin (Ig) that affects this response is IgA and, appropriately, IgA is the most prevalent immunoglobulin in human intestinal secretions. The same is not true in serum, where IgA makes up only 10–15 per cent of the total immunoglobulin pool. It is secreted as a complex of two monomers joined by a polypeptide known as the S chain. In its secreted form, this dimeric IgA accounts for nearly 95 per cent of the IgA in normal intestinal fluid (Brandtzaeg *et al.*, 1987).

The immune system of the gut is composed of various cells, each of which performs a specialized function. The lymphoid tissue itself is divided into three major groups: Peyer's patches, lamina propria lymphoid cells and intraepithelial lymphocytes (Kagnoff, 1993). Antigen reception by cells in the Peyer's patches provides the initial stimulus to B cells, which, so primed, migrate via blood and lymphatics to the lamina propria. Here terminal differentiation to IgA-secreting plasma cells occurs. These plasma cells produce S-chain-containing dimeric IgA, which is then transported across the intestinal cell to be secreted into the lumen of the gut as secretory IgA (sIgA). The function of intraepithelial lymphocytes is less clearly understood but it is thought to be cytolytic (Klein and Kagnoff, 1984). Their location between the epithelial cells in the mucosa suggests an early role in immune defense.

This chapter reviews the various components and features of the intestinal immune system and their interaction.

DEVELOPMENT OF THE GASTROINTESTINAL IMMUNE SYSTEM

The intestine anatomically begins to differentiate at 10–11 weeks' gestation with the development of villi and crypts. Paneth cells also appear at this time, followed by goblet and endocrine cells at 12–13 weeks (Insoft *et al.*, 1996).

In the fetus, Peyer's patches develop initially at 11 weeks' gestation as clusters of subepithelial cells expressing CD4 antigen, which are located largely in the ileum (Spencer and MacDonald, 1990). By 16–18 weeks, larger collections of cells can be distinguished immunohistochemically as containing both T and B cells, and by 18–20 weeks these cells separate into discrete areas within the Peyer's patches. Fetal B cells are able to secrete cytoplasmic IgM and surface IgD by 16 weeks (Spencer *et al.*, 1986). The numbers of Peyer's patches increase from 45 at 24 weeks to 80–120 at gestation and peak in the mid-teens at about 200 per intestine (Spencer and MacDonald, 1990).

Lymphocytes can be found within the lamina propria by about 14 weeks' gestation. These are largely B and T cells as opposed to a predominance of IgA-secreting plasma cells in this location in the adult (Insoft *et al.*, 1996). This difference is due to the relative lack of antigenic stimulation in the fetus, although there is evidence in fetal life of a low-grade immune reaction to food antigens derived from the mother and present in the amniotic fluid (Matsumura *et al.*, 1967; Dahl *et al.*, 1984). Appendectomy in neonatal rabbits markedly reduces the number of IgA-secreting plasma cells later developing in the lamina propria, suggesting that the appendix may play a role in seeding plasma cell precursors to this area (Dasso and Howell, 1997).

Intraepithelial lymphocytes are found by 11–12 weeks' gestation. These largely express CD3 antigen, which then gradually with time gives way to CD4 and CD8 expression, before becoming almost completely a population of CD8-expressing cells postnatally (Insoft *et al.*, 1996).

Breast feeding links the maternal and infant mucosal immune systems with the fully breast-fed infant receiving up to 0.5–1 g of secretory IgA per day. Additionally, IgA is found earlier and in larger quantities in the feces of breast-fed infants than in those who receive formula (Hanson *et al.*, 1994). This passive immunization is felt to result in the lower incidence of gastrointestinal and respiratory infections as well as the lower morbidity seen in breast-fed infants. Cytokines present in breast milk may be responsible for the enhanced immunization responses in breast-fed infants. Exposure to bacterial antigens postnatally also occurs, leading to increased levels of serum and fecal immunoglobulins, increased numbers of B cells throughout the gastrointestinal tract and expansion of the Peyer's patches (Cummins and Thompson, 1997).

Weaning produces a high point in immune activation in the infant. During this time, there is expansion and degranulation of intestinal mast cells, which are associated with a transient increase in mucosal permeability. Intestinal T-cell activity is increased and there is also the expression of the DR loci of the human leukocyte antigen (HLA) system on intestinal epithelial cells. Finally, there is an increase in the population of intraepithelial lymphocytes at this time as well (Cummins and Thompson, 1997).

COMPONENTS OF THE ADULT GASTROINTESTINAL IMMUNE SYSTEM

Peyer's patches, M cells and antigen recognition

Recognition of intestinal antigen and the initiation of the intestinal immune response take place in the Peyer's patches. These are aggregates of lymphoid cells that extend through the mucosa into the submucosa of the small intestine. Most of these are located in the terminal ileum. As mentioned previously, the number of patches increases through puberty to a peak of about 200 per intestine. From age 20, there is a gradual decline to a plateau of approximately 100 in persons aged 70–95 years (Cornes, 1965). This is not related to a change in the surface area of the small intestine as jejunal biopsies have shown no reduction in area and no change in morphology as a consequence of aging (Corazza *et al.*, 1986). Every Peyer's patch has five or more follicles each of which has a characteristic structure with a central B-cell-rich zone and a surrounding area of mixed cellularity. T cells, predominantly CD4+, accumulate in the interfollicular zones (McGowan *et al.*, 1997). The number of follicles in each Peyer's patch decreases with advancing age and a similar age-related loss of follicles can be seen in the human large intestine.

The uptake of antigen by the epithelium of the Peyer's patches in the small intestine and the solitary follicles of the large intestine provides the initial stimulus to lymphoid cells which begin the immune response (Fig. 4.1). Antigen uptake occurs in the small intestine through a specialized follicle-associated epithelium that overlies the surface or dome of the Peyer's patches. This epithelium is relatively deficient in mucus-producing goblet cells and has no-IgA-transporting capacity, which leaves it more accessible to contact with antigen (Bjerke *et al.*, 1988).

Follicle-associated epithelium also contains specialized cells, known as microfold (M) cells, which facilitate the entry of luminal antigens into the lymphoid follicle (Owen and Jones, 1974). Structurally they have fewer, shorter and wider microvilli, less overlying mucus and fewer intracellular organelles, thus allowing them to be

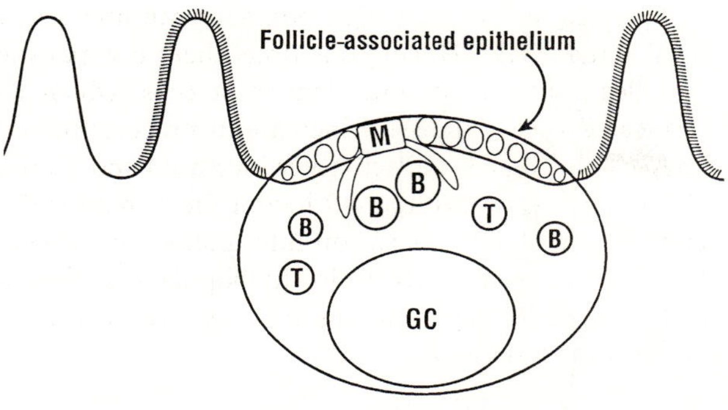

Figure 4.1 *Diagrammatic representation of a Peyer's patch with overlying follicle-associated epithelium. M cells (M) are in close proximity to immature lymphocytes (B and T) and present antigen, thereby priming the immune response. The germinal center (GC) is also shown.*

more easily traversed by antigen macromolecules in the gut (Wolf *et al.*, 1981; Sanderson and Walker, 1993). A deep invagination in the basal membrane of the M cell allows close proximity to the underlying lymphoid cells (Bockman and Cooper, 1973). Via pinocytosis, M cells transport luminal antigens inward to within 0.3 μm of lymphocytes in the Peyer's patches. B cells and T cells are thus 'primed' – the former by direct recognition of antigenic determinants on the antigen itself and the latter by recognition of antigenic determinants in association with major histocompatibility complex molecules. The transport of luminal antigens by M cells is selective. Infectious agents known to be taken up include the human immunodeficiency virus, *Vibrio cholera*, reoviruses and mycobacteria (Wolf *et al.*, 1981). In contrast, normal enteric flora and heat-killed organisms are not taken up (Owen *et al.*, 1986).

Intraepithelial lymphocytes

A fraction of Peyer's patch cells in mice migrate to the spaces between the columnar epithelial cells that line the villi of the bowel and are termed intraepithelial lymphocytes (IEL). The majority of these cells in humans are T lymphocytes, 75–80 per cent of which express the CD8 surface marker and 5–15 per cent being CD4+ (Janossy *et al.*, 1980; Cerf-Bensussan *et al.*, 1983). Exactly what percentage of these cells actually arise from Peyer's patches is unknown for man or rodents. There is a ratio of 20 IEL per 100 epithelial cells in the jejunum and 13 per 100 in the ileum (Dobbins, 1986). Their function has not been well elucidated. In rodents they mediate direct cytotoxic activities and have natural killer (NK) cell activity (Flexman *et al.*, 1983; Mowat *et al.*, 1983). In humans, they are presumed to have cytolytic activity as well, but not NK cell activity (Cerf-Bensussan *et al.*, 1985).

The population of intraepithelial lymphocytes is subdivided into two main groups based on T-cell receptor (TCR) status. Seventy-five per cent have a TCR with α and β subunits while less than 10 per cent have a TCR with a γ and a δ chain (Jarry and Cerf-Bensussan, 1990). Little is known about the latter TCR-expressing cells, but the α/β T cells recognize foreign antigen in conjunction with 'self' HLA molecules and become activated, secreting a number of cytokines such as perforin, interferons, tumor necrosis factor and proteoglycans (Kagnoff, 1993). This cocktail of cytokines may generate a humoral response, a cell-mediated response or may be directly cytolytic (McGowan *et al.*, 1997). Additionally, the majority of α/β-positive cells also have a marker, CD45RO, which suggests the presence of a memory of previously encountered intestinal antigens (Jarry and Cerf-Bensussan, 1990). Correspondingly, there is a marked increase in the IEL population in the first few years of life, when new antigenic exposure is greatest (Spencer *et al.*, 1989) and in the setting of celiac disease (*see* Chapter 23). Removal of gluten from the diet results in a decline in the number of these cells (McGowan *et al.*, 1997).

The lamina propria

If the Peyer's patches are considered the afferent limb of the gastrointestinal immune system, then the efferent limb would be the lamina propria cells, which are postulated to respond to epithelial cell injury. Here B and T cells, plasma cells, macrophages, mast cells and eosinophils are present and are all felt to have a role in the immune response.

Nearly 60 per cent of the cells of the lamina propria are T cells with a CD4+ to CD8+ ratio of 2:1, similar to peripheral blood (Cerf-Bensussan *et al.*, 1983). Ninety-five per cent have the α/β TCR and the CD4+ cells lack the Leu 8 antigen thought to be consistent with a role in activation and differentiation of lamina propria B cells (Berg *et al.*, 1991; James, 1991). There is also an abundance of T cells expressing CD25 and CD71, both antigens characteristically associated with T-cell activation. These activated T cells may also play a role in responding to epithelial injury by secreting cytokines such as interleukin-4 (IL-4) and IL-5, as well as interferon (IFN) α, β and γ (Fiocchi *et al.*, 1984; James and Kwan, 1990; Youngman *et al.*, 1993). Overproduction of these inflammatory mediators may also be important in the production of tissue injury in the bowel (MacDonald and Spencer, 1988; Deem *et al.*, 1991).

Forty per cent of the lymphoid cells of the lamina propria are B cells. These B cells are unique among B cells of the immune system in that 80 per cent secrete IgA, with only 15–20 per cent secreting IgG and two per cent producing IgE. In the spleen and peripheral lymph nodes >50 per cent of B cells secrete IgG (Kagnoff, 1987). Interleukins produced by T cells in the lamina propria are critical for the terminal differentiation of B cells into IgA-secreting cells. IL-4 and IL-5 activate B cells and then induce their growth and maturation (Mestecky and McGhee, 1987; Lebman and Coffman, 1988). IL-6 is responsible for the terminal differentiation of these cells (Kunimoto *et al.*, 1989).

Macrophages, along with dendritic cells, are the primary antigen presenting cells of the GALT. Macrophages also perform characteristic functions of phagocytosis as well as synthesis and secretion of a variety of inflammatory mediators, which are important in T-cell activation (McGowan *et al.*, 1997). Mast cells demonstrate both a direct and indirect effect on immunity (Befus *et al.*, 1987; Bienenstock *et al.*, 1988). The direct effect is best seen in parasitic infection, where products of degranulation are able to kill parasites directly and also promote vasodilatation, which in turn allows a more rapid response from the antibody-mediated host defense. Indirect effects are seen by products of these cells that act as chemoattractants, recruiting granulocytes, eosinophils, macrophages and lymphocytes. Steroid therapy results in a loss of these cells and an increased propensity for parasitic infection. Eosinophils in the lamina propria are thought to have similar functions (Kagnoff, 1993).

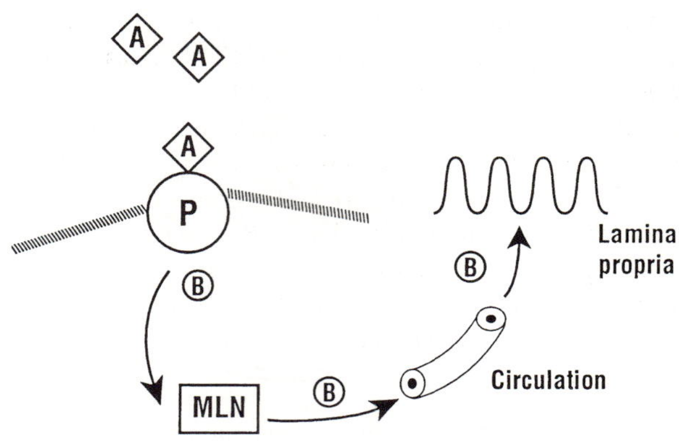

Figure 4.2 *Migration and homing of B lymphocytes. Antigen (A) is presented at the Peyer's patch and primed B lymphocytes (B) then migrate via the mesenteric lymph nodes (MLN) to the circulation and eventually to specific tissues.*

FEATURES OF THE ADULT GASTROINTESTINAL IMMUNE SYSTEM

Lymphocyte migration

Commitment of the B cells to the IgA class occurs predominantly in the germinal center of the lymphoid follicle. This is regulated in an incompletely understood fashion by T lymphocytes present in Peyer's patches and also perhaps by continual antigen-driven division in the absence of signals for further differentiation. With aging, a reduction in the ratio of helper to suppressor T cells in the Peyer's patches has been shown. This is postulated to explain the decline in *in vitro* immunoglobulin production and proliferative responses seen in aged cells taken from the Peyer's patches and mesenteric lymph nodes during stimulation by T-cell-dependent B-cell mitogens (Kawanishi, 1993).

B lymphocytes primed in Peyer's patches do not mature into antibody-secreting plasma cells there but rather leave the lymphoid follicle and travel via mesenteric lymph nodes to the thoracic duct and peripheral circulation (Fig. 4.2). A proportion then return to the gastrointestinal mucosa where they mature into IgA-secreting plasma cells and provide protective immunity in the lamina propria. The return of the cells to the location of their priming is important in providing antigen-specific antibodies for that region. Additionally, some of the cells travel to mucosal secretory sites away from their site of priming, such as the bronchus-associated lymphoid tissue, mammary gland and female genital tract. For cells primed in the gastrointestinal tract, this allows antibodies directed against antigens in the gastrointestinal tract to be secreted in the lung, breast, genital and even eye fluid (Bienenstock *et al.*, 1978; Mestecky, 1987). It is the interaction of proteins on the lymphocyte surface with ligands on endothelial cells that control this 'homing' of lymphocyte populations (Butcher and Picker, 1996).

Homing antigens on the surface of immature lymphocytes interact with specific receptors called 'addressins' found on the surface of specialized blood vessels known as high endothelial venules (Stoolman, 1989). This interaction leads to the extravasation of lymphocytes from the blood into tissues in a multistep process of tethering, adhesion and transmigration. At the tissue site, T-lymphocyte-dependent maturation and terminal differentiation then occurs yielding immunoglobulin-secreting plasma cells. In response to inflammation, there is an upregulation of high endothelial venules. Cytokines released during an inflammatory response, such as IL-1, IFN-γ and tumor necrosis factor, enhance the expression of addressins and also increase the adherence of lymphocytes to these areas (Jalkanen *et al.*, 1988). This results in an influx of antigen-specific lymphocytes to areas in need of increased host defense mechanisms (Lewis *et al.*, 1989).

The homing antigens on the surface of lymphocytes are known as integrins. Integrins are glycoproteins integral to the lymphocyte membrane. There are two important integrins on lymphocytes in the GALT system, $\alpha_4\beta_7$ and $\alpha^E\beta_7$. The $\alpha_4\beta_7$ integrins have an affinity for the mucosal vascular addressin MAdCAM-1. This addressin is expressed only on Peyer's patch high endothelial venules and on lamina propria venules, thus drawing lymphocytes specifically to these areas (Berlin *et al.*, 1993). $\alpha^E\beta_7$ integrins are found on 95 per cent of IEL in a variety of locations including the gut. They are also found on approximately 40 per cent of lamina propria lymphocytes but this molecule is not expressed by circulating lymphocytes. The $\alpha^E\beta_7$ integrin's expression appears to be induced locally by transforming growth factor-β1 and leads to the recruitment of the lymphocytes to the epithelial tissue (Cerf-Bensussan *et al.*, 1987).

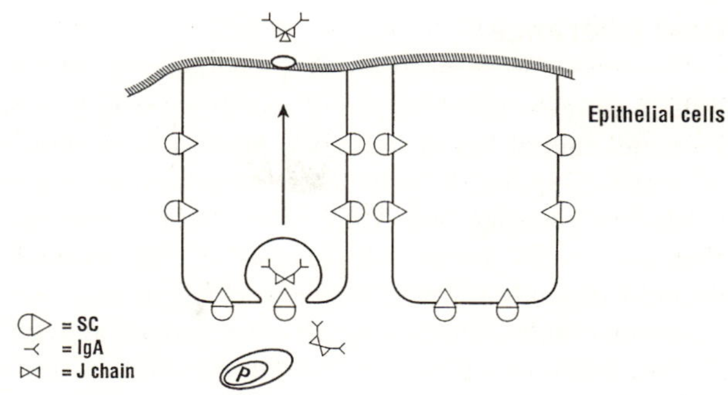

Figure 4.3 *Production and transport of sIgA. Plasma cells (P) secrete dimeric IgA, which is bound to SC molecules on the basal and lateral surface of gastrointestinal epithelial cells. This complex is then transported across the cell and out into the intestinal lumen. A portion of the SC molecule remains attached to the epithelium.*

Immunoglobulin secretion

While IgA, IgM and IgG are all secreted by the lamina propria B lymphocytes, the primary immunoglobulin in immune defense is IgA (Mestecky and McGhee, 1987). Its production marks the terminal step in the differentiation of the B lymphocyte. IgA serves as the first line of defense in preventing the translocation of dietary antigens across the mucosa, and also inhibits the attachment and invasion of bacteria and toxins (Sanderson and Walker, 1994; Insoft *et al.*, 1996).

The compound is composed of two IgA monomers and two important additional polypeptides – SC, or secretory component, and the J chain. The importance of SC lies in the non-covalent interaction between it and the IgA dimer, which has been shown to decrease the susceptibility of the antibody to dissolution on passage through the gut (Colombel *et al.*, 1988). J chain is a polypeptide produced by plasma cells and B lymphocytes. It links two IgA monomers into a dimer and is essential for the external transport of dimeric IgA through the epithelial cells of the intestinal border as its incorporation creates the binding sites for the molecule to these cells (Brandtzaeg, 1985).

SC is a glycoprotein encoded on chromosome 1 and produced predominantly by columnar cells of the crypts of Lieberkuhn (Colombel *et al.*, 1988). It is expressed on the basal and lateral surface of secretory epithelial cells, which are also largely found in the crypts. It acts as the epithelial cell surface receptor with the dimeric IgA–J chain complex. Bound SC–immunoglobulin complexes are endocytosed and transported across the cell to the apical membrane where the SC molecule is proteolytically split. A portion remains bound to the apical membrane and the remainder is covalently bound to the IgA–J chain complex forming the complete sIgA molecule (Fig. 4.3) (Kagnoff, 1993).

The human intestinal IgA system is fully developed by 2 years of age. In mice, there is a small but significant decline in the gut IgA content with aging, while in the serum of both mice and humans, a slight increase is noted with age. However, in human whole-gut lavage fluid, there was no demonstrable difference in the concentration of IgA, IgM or IgG in subjects greater than 70 years of age as compared with those less than 50 (Watson *et al.*, 1985; Arranz *et al.*, 1992). As in humans, in a rhesus monkey model, total IgA concentration in whole-gut lavage fluid is independent of age. However, antigen-specific IgA antibody levels were markedly reduced in old as compared to young animals. Additionally, flow cytometry has shown that the relative number of peripheral blood lymphocytes expressing surface IgA or cholera toxin antigens after intraduodenal immunization with cholera toxin is reduced in older animals. It has been suggested that a decrease in the pool of antigen-specific B lymphocytes decreases the number of cells migrating back to the lamina propria of the intestine and thereby decreases specific IgA antibody production (Taylor *et al.*, 1992).

Secretory IgA has its main function in 'immune exclusion': that is, protection of the surface of epithelial cells against dietary antigens and infectious agents. Deficiency of sIgA leads to increased titers of serum antibodies and immune complexes against food antigens, which may lead to allergic responses such as those seen with cow's milk protein (Cunningham-Rundles *et al.*, 1979). The secretory form of the immunoglobulin has been shown to have a more broad antibody specificity than the corresponding systemic form and this may be useful in coping with the variability in the antigenic makeup of microorganisms. sIgA binds directly to bacteria, such as *Vibrio cholera*, and prevents their adherence to and subsequent colonization of intestinal epithelial cells (Williams and Gibbons, 1972). sIgA has also been reported to neutralize toxins secreted by these microorganisms (Sanderson and Walker, 1994). There is even a role for sIgA in the inhibition of viral replication and passive protective immunity (Hanson *et al.*, 1980; Mestecky and McGhee, 1987).

Oral tolerance

Enteric antigens not only play a role in eliciting a local immune response but they also may produce some degree of systemic response. Whether enteric exposure to antigen results in priming and stimulation of the systemic immune system or to suppression of the systemic response depends on many factors such as prior antigen exposure, health of the host, genetic background and age.

The ability of antigens in the intestine to activate a mucosal immune response while suppressing the systemic response is the basis of oral tolerance (Kagnoff, 1988). Suppression of the systemic immune system is antigen specific and may be useful to the host in two ways. Firstly, by preventing innocuous, widespread, non-pathogenic antigens from stimulating systemic allergic reactions and, secondly, by avoiding cross-reactions with self-proteins leading to autoimmune phenomena.

Two mechanisms of oral tolerance have been proposed depending on the amount of antigen delivered to the intestine (Miller *et al.*, 1992; Weiner *et al.*, 1994). Antigen delivery in low dose provokes the development of T cells capable of producing transforming growth factor-β, IL-4 and IL-10. These cytokines inhibit the production of antigen-specific lymphocytes. At high doses antigen delivery induces clonal anergy or death of antigen-specific cells that would otherwise cause a systemic immune response. Clinically, the concept of tolerance has been preliminarily studied as a treatment for two chronic disease states, rheumatoid arthritis (Trentham *et al.*, 1993) and multiple sclerosis (Weiner *et al.*, 1993). The thought is that the chronic, exuberant systemic immune response in these disease states could be ameliorated by induction of oral tolerance to the appropriate antigens. Some benefit has been derived by the oral administration of type II collagen to rheumatoid arthritis patients and myelin antigens to subjects with multiple sclerosis.

Tolerance induction has been studied in young and aged mice by oral administration of sheep red blood cells. Young (2 months old) mice given sheep red blood cells orally for 2 weeks become tolerant to a subsequent systemic sheep red blood cell challenge. However, older (1 year) mice resisted tolerance induction and produced a prominent systemic IgA response. This implies that the tolerance-inducing function of the GALT declines with age. This may partially explain the increase in autoimmune markers noted in the elderly as reactions to denatured self-proteins (Hosokawa *et al.*, 1988).

NUTRITION AND THE MUCOSAL IMMUNE SYSTEM

Protein-calorie malnutrition is associated with diminished levels of sIgA and reversal of the condition reverses the immunoglobulin deficiency. In addition to the quantity and type of nutrients ingested, the route of administration of nutrients is proving to be an important determinant of mucosal integrity. Multiple studies have demonstrated impaired mucosal immunity in patients receiving total parenteral nutrition (TPN) (*see* Chapter 29). Among the defects noted are: a decrease in GALT mass; a depletion of Peyer's patches, IEL and lamina propria lymphocyte populations; reduced intestinal IgA levels; and a reversal of the CD4+/CD8+ ratio in the lamina propria (Li *et al.*, 1995).

Enteral feeding is not associated with similar changes and in, fact, can produce a reversal in many of the defects induced by TPN. Mice with immune defects induced by TPN achieve a near-complete reversal of cell counts within the Peyer's patches in 1 day, and shortly thereafter cells in the lamina propria also return to their pre-TPN levels. Intraepithelial lymphocyte levels remained depressed despite a change to enteral nutrition (Janu *et al.*, 1997b). Clinically, this improvement in immune function is evidenced by a reduced incidence of pneumonia and intra-abdominal abscesses in patients who are critically ill and fed enterally rather than parenterally (Moore *et al.*, 1992).

Recently, there has been considerable interest in glutamine, which is a fuel for enterocytes and colonocytes (LeLeiko and Walsh, 1996). It has been demonstrated that the addition of glutamine to TPN prevents many of the immune defects seen with TPN (Li *et al.*, 1997). Another compound trophic for cells of the gastrointestinal tract is bombesin and this also has been shown to prevent the immune degradation associated with TPN (Janu *et al.*, 1997a). Use of these agents may lead to immune recovery in TPN-fed states and help to reduce infectious complications in these patients.

The gastrointestinal immune system is a complex aggregation of numerous cells and soluble factors. Humoral defense appears to predominate but it should be kept in mind that little is known concerning the effect of the T lymphocyte and cell-mediated immunity in the gut. This chapter has reviewed the important components of the gastrointestinal immune system in health, and examined their interrelationships and some of the features of gastrointestinal mucosal immunity. Application of molecular techniques will continue to fuel the advances in our understanding of this complex field.

REFERENCES

Arranz, E., O'Mahony, S., Barton, J.R., Ferguson, A. 1992: Immunosenescence and mucosal immunity: significant effects of old age on secretory IgA concentrations and intraepithelial lymphocyte counts. *Gut* 33, 882–6.

Befus, A., Dyck, N., Goodacre, R., Bienenstock, J. 1987: Mast cell from the human intestinal lamina propria. Isolation, histochemical subtypes, and functional characterization. *Immunology* 138, 2604–10.

Berg, M., Murakawa, Y., Camerini, D, James, S.P. 1991: Lamina propria lymphocytes are derived from circulating cells that lack the Leu-8 lymph node homing receptor. *Gastroenterology* 101, 90–9.

Berlin, C., Berg, E., Briskin, M., Andrew, D.P., Kilshaw, P.J., Holzmann, B. 1993: Alpha 4 beta 7 integrin mediates lymphocyte binding to the mucosal vascular addressin MAdCAM-1. *Cell* 74, 185.

Bienenstock, J., McDermott, M., Befus, D., O'Neill, M. 1978: A common mucosal immunologic system involving the bronchus, breast and bowel. *Advances in Experimental Medicine and Biology* 107, 53–9.

Bienenstock, K., Denburg, J., Scicchitano, R., Stead, R., Perdue, M., Stanisz, A. 1988: Role of neuropeptides, nerves and mast cells in intestinal immunity and physiology. *Monographs in Allergy* 24, 134–43.

Bjerke, K., Brandtzaeg, P., Fausa, O. 1988: T cell distribution is different in follicle-associated epithelium of human Peyer's patches and villous epithelium. *Clinical and Experimental Immunology* 74, 270–5.

Blumberg, R., Stenson, W. 1995: The immune system. In Yamada, T. (ed.), *Textbook of gastroenterology.* Philadelphia: J.P. Lippincott, 111–40.

Bockman, D., Cooper, M., 1973: Pinocytosis by epithelium associated with lymphoid follicles in the bursa of fabricius, appendix, and Peyer's patches. An electron microscopic study. *American Journal of Anatomy* 136, 455–77.

Brandtzaeg, P. 1985: Role of J chain and secretory component in receptor-mediated glandular and hepatic transport of immunoglobulins in man. *Scandinavian Journal of Immunology* 22, 111–46.

Brandtzaeg, P., Baklien, K., Bjerke, K. *et al.* 1987: Nature and properties of the human gastrointestinal immune system. In Miller, K., Nicklin, S. (eds), *Immunology of the gastrointestinal tract*, Vol. 1. Boca Raton: CRC Press, 1–85.

Brandtzaeg, P., Halstensen, T., Kett, K. *et al.* 1989: Immunobiology and immunopathology of human gut mucosa: humoral immunity and intraepithelial lymphocytes. *Gastroenterology* 97, 1562–84.

Butcher, E., Picker, L. 1996: Lymphocyte homing and hemostasis. *Science* 272, 60–6.

Cerf-Bensussan, N., Schneeberger, E., Bhan, A. 1983: Immunohistologic and immunoelectron microscopic characterization of the mucosal lymphocytes of human small intestine by the use of monoclonal antibodies. *Journal of Immunology* 130, 2615–22.

Cerf-Bensussan, N., Guy-Grand, D., Griscelli, C. 1985: Intraepithelial lymphocytes of human gut: isolation, characterization and study of natural killer activity. *Gut* 26, 81–8.

Cerf-Bensussan, N., Jarry, A., Brousse, N., Lisowska-Grospierre, B., Guy-Grand, D., Griscelli, C. 1987: A monoclonal antibody (HML-1) defining a novel membrane molecule present on human intestinal lymphocytes. *European Journal of Immunology* 17, 1279–85.

Colombel, J., Rambaud, J., Vaerman, J. *et al.* 1988: Massive plasma cell infiltration of the digestive tract. Secretory component as the rate-limiting factor of immunoglobulin secretion in external fluids. *Gastroenterology* 95, 1106–13.

Corazza, G., Frazzoni, M., Gatto, M., Gasbarrini, G. 1986: Aging and small bowel mucosa: a morphometric study. *Gerontology* 32, 60–5.

Cornes, J. 1965: Number, size, and distribution of Peyer's patches in the human small intestine. *Gut* 6, 225–59.

Cummins, A., Thompson, F. 1997: Postnatal changes in mucosal immune response: a physiological perspective of breast feeding and weaning. *Immunology and Cell Biology* 75, 419–29.

Cunningham-Rundles, C., Brandeis, W., Good, R., Day, N.K. 1979: Bovine antigens and the formation of circulating immune complexes in selective immunoglobulin A deficiency. *Journal of Clinical Investigation* 64, 272–9.

Dahl, G., Telemo, E., Westrom, B., Jakobsson, I., Lindberg, T., Karlsson, B.W. 1984: The passage of orally fed proteins from mother to fetus in the rat. *Comparative Biochemistry and Physiology. A: Comparative Physiology* 77, 199–201.

Dasso, J., Howell, M. 1997: Neonatal appendectomy impairs mucosal immunity in rabbits. *Cellular Immunology* 182, 29–37.

Deem, R., Shanahan, F., Targan, S. 1991: Triggered human mucosal T cells release tumor necrosis factor-alpha and interferon-gamma which kill human colonic epithelial cells. *Clinical and Experimental Immunology* 83, 79–84.

Dobbins, W. 1986: Human intestinal intraepithelial lymphocytes. *Gut* 27, 972–85.

Fiocchi, C., Hilfiker, M., Youngman, K., Doerder, N.C., Finke, J.H. 1984: Interleukin 2 activity of human intestinal mucosa mononuclear cells: decreased levels in inflammatory bowel disease. *Gastroenterology* 86, 734–42.

Flexman, J., Shellam, G., Mayrhofer, G. 1983: Natural cytotoxicity, responsiveness to interferon and morphology of intraepithelial lymphocytes from the small intestine of the rat. *Immunology* 48, 733–41.

Hanson, L., Ahlstedt, S., Anderson, B. *et al.* 1980: The biologic properties of secretory IgA. *Journal of the Reticuloendothelial Society.* 28(Suppl), 1S–S.

Hanson, L.A., Hahn-Zoric, M., Berndes, M. *et al.* 1994: Breast feeding: overview and breast milk immunology. *Acta Paediatrica Japonica* 36, 557–61.

Hosokawa, T., Motoi, S., Aoike, A., Koyama, K., Rokutan, K., Nishi, Y., Kawai, K. 1988: Effect of aging on immunological memory in gastrointestinal tract induced by sheep red blood cells in mice. *Gastroenterologia Japonica* 23, 13–17.

Insoft, R., Sanderson, I., Walker, W. 1996: Development of

immune function in the intestine and its role in neonatal diseases. *Pediatric Clinics of North America* 43, 551–71.

Jalkanen, S., Streeter, P., Lakey, E., Bargatze, R., Butcher, E.C. 1988: Lymphocyte and endothelial cell recognition elements that control lymphocyte traffic to mucosa-associated lymphatic tissues. *Monographs in Allergy* 24, 144–9.

James, S. 1991: Mucosal T-cell function. *Gastroenterology Clinics of North America* 20, 597–612.

James, S., Kwan, W. 1990: T cells in inductive and effector compartments of the intestinal mucosal immune system of nonhuman primates differ in lymphokine mRNA expression, lymphokine utilization, and regulatory function. *Journal of Immunology* 144, 1251–6.

Janossy, G., Tidman, N., Selby, W., Thomas, J.A., Granger, S., Kung, P.C., Goldstein, G. 1980: Human T lymphocytes of inducer and suppressor type occupy different microenvironments. *Nature* 288, 81–4.

Janu, P., Kudsk, K., Li, J., Renegar, K.B. 1997a: Effect of bombesin on TPN-induced impairment of upper respiratory tract immunity. *Archives of Surgery* 132, 89–93.

Janu, P., Li, J., Renegar, K., Kudsk, K.A. 1997b: Recovery of gut-associated lymphoid tissue and upper respiratory tract immunity after parenteral nutrition. *Annals of Surgery* 225, 707–17.

Jarry, A., Cerf-Bensussan, N. 1990: Subsets of CD3+ and CD3– lymphocytes isolated from normal human gut epithelium display phenotypical features different from their counterparts in peripheral blood. *European Journal of Immunology* 20, 1097–103.

Kagnoff, M. 1987: Immunology of the digestive system. In Johnson, L. (ed.), *Physiology of the gastrointestinal tract.* New York: Raven Press, 1699–28.

Kagnoff, M. 1988: Oral tolerance. *Monographs in Allergy* 24, 222–6.

Kagnoff, M. 1993: Immunology and inflammation of the gastrointestinal tract. In Sleisenger, M., Fordtran, J. (eds), *Gastrointestinal disease.* Philadelphia: W.B. Saunders, 45–86.

Kato, T., Owen, R. 1994: Structure and function of intestinal mucosal epithelium. In Ogra, P., Mestecky, J., Lamm, M. *et al.* (eds), *Handbook of mucosal immunology.* San Diego: Academic Press, 11–26.

Kawanishi, H. 1993: Recent progress in senescence-associated gut mucosal immunity. *Digestive Diseases* 11, 157–72.

Klein, J., Kagnoff, M. 1984: Nonspecific recruitment of cytotoxic effector cells in the intestinal mucosa of antigen-primed mice. *Journal of Experimental Medicine* 160, 1931–6.

Kunimoto, D., Nordan, R., Strober, W. 1989: IL-6 is a potent cofactor of IL-1 in IgM synthesis and of IL-5 in IgA synthesis. *Journal of Immunology* 143, 2230–5.

Lebman, D., Coffman, R. 1988: The effects of IL-4 and IL-5 on the IgA response by murine Peyer's patch B cell subpopulations. *Journal of Immunology* 141, 2050–6.

LeLeiko, N., Walsh M. 1996: The role of glutamine, short chain fatty acids, and nucleotides in intestinal adaptation to gastrointestinal disease. *Pediatric Clinics of North America* 43, 451–69.

Lewis, R., Buchsbaum, M., Whitaker, D., Murphy, G.F. 1989: Intercellular adhesion molecule expression in the evolving human cutaneous delayed hypersensitivity reaction. *Journal of Investigative Dermatology* 93, 672–7.

Li, J., Kudsk, K.A., Gocinski, B., Dent, D., Glezer, J., Langkamp-Henken, B. 1995: Effects of parenteral nutrition on gut-associated lymphoid tissue. *Journal of Trauma* 39, 44–51.

Li, J., Kudsk, K., Janu, P., Renegar, K.B. 1997: Effect of glutamine-enriched total parenteral nutrition on small intestinal gut-associated lymphoid tissue and upper respiratory tract immunity. *Surgery* 121, 542–9.

MacDonald, T., Spencer, J. 1988: Evidence that activated mucosal T cells play a role in the pathogenesis of enteropathy in human small intestine. *Journal of Experimental Medicine* 167, 1341–9.

Matsumura, T., Kuroume, T., Iwasaki, I., Oguri, M., Matsumoto, T. 1967: Studies on congenital sensitization. 1. Detection of food antigens and antibodies in the maternal serum, umbilical cord serum, the serum and the first voided urine of newborn infants, amniotic fluid and meconium. *Arerugi. Japanese Journal of Allergology* 16, 858–65.

McGowan, I., Chalmers, A., Smith, G., Jewell, D. 1997: Advances in mucosal immunology. *Gastroenterology Clinics of North America* 26, 145–73.

Mestecky, J. 1987: The common mucosal immune system and current strategies for induction of immune responses in external secretions. *Journal of Clinical Immunology* 7, 265–76.

Mestecky, J., McGhee, J. 1987: Immunoglobulin A (IgA): molecular and cellular interactions involved in IgA biosynthesis and immune response. *Advances in Immunology* 40, 153–245.

Miller, A., Lider, O., Roberts, A., Sporn, M.B., Weiner, H.L. 1992: Suppressor T cells generated by oral tolerization to myelin basic protein suppress both in vitro and in vivo immune responses by the release of transforming growth factor β after antigen-specific triggering. *Proceedings of the National Academy of Sciences USA.* 89, 421–5.

Moore, F., Feliciano, D., Andrassay, R. 1992: Early enteral feeding compared with parenteral reduces postoperative septic complications: results of a meta-analysis. *Annals of Surgery* 216, 172–83.

Mowat, A., Tait, R., MacKenzie, S., Davies, M.D., Parrott, D.M. 1983: Analysis of natural killer effector and suppressor activity by intraepithelial lymphocytes from mouse small intestine. *Clinical and Experimental Immunology* 52, 191–8.

Owen, R., Jones, A. 1974: Epithelial cell specialization within human Peyer's patches: an ultrastructural study of intestinal lymphoid follicles. *Gastroenterology* 66, 189–203.

Owen, R., Pierce, N., Apple, R., Cray, W.C., Jr 1986: M cell transport of *Vibrio cholerae* from the intestinal lumen into Peyer's patches: a mechanism for antigen sampling and for microbial transepithelial migration. *Journal of Infectious Disease* 153, 1108–18.

Pabst, R., Trepel, F. 1975: Quantitative evaluation of the total number and distribution of lymphocytes in young pigs. *Blut* 31, 77–86.

Sanderson, I., Walker, W. 1993: Uptake and transport of macromolecules by the intestine: possible role in clinical disorders (an update). *Gastroenterology* 104, 622–39.

Sanderson, I., Walker, W. 1994: The mucosal barrier. In Ogra, P., Mestecky, J., Lamm, M. (eds), *Handbook of mucosal immunology*. San Diego: Academic Press, 41.

Spencer, J., MacDonald, T. 1990: Ontogeny of human mucosal immunity. In MacDonald, T. (ed.), *Ontogeny of the immune system of the gut*. Boca Raton: CRC Press, 23–50.

Spencer, J., MacDonald, T., Finn, T., Isaacson, P.G. 1986: Development of Peyer's patches in human fetal terminal ileum. *Clinical and Experimental Immunology* 64, 536–43.

Spencer, J., Isaacson, P., Walker-Smith, J., MacDonald, T.T. 1989: Heterogeneity in intraepithelial lymphocyte subpopulations in fetal and postnatal human small intestine. *Journal of Pediatric Gastroenterology and Nutrition* 9, 173–7.

Stoolman, L. 1989: Adhesion molecules controlling lymphocyte migration. *Cell* 56, 907–10.

Taylor, L., Daniels, C., Schmucker, D. 1992: Aging compromises gastrointestinal mucosal immune response in the rhesus monkey. *Immunology* 75, 614–18.

Trentham, D., Dynesius-Trentham, R., Orav, E. *et al.* 1993: Effects of oral administration of type II collagen on rheumatoid arthritis. *Science* 261, 1727–30.

Walker, W. 1986: Antigen handling by the small intestine. *Clinical Gastroenterology* 15, 1–20.

Watson, R., McMurray, D., Martin, P., Reyes, M.A. 1985: Effect of age, malnutrition and renutrition on free secretory component and IgA in secretion. *American Journal of Clinical Nutrition* 42, 281–8.

Weiner, H., Friedman, A., Miller, A. *et al.* 1993: Double-blind pilot trial of oral tolerization with myelin antigens in multiple sclerosis. *Science* 259, 1321–4.

Weiner, J., Friedman, A., Miller, A. *et al.* 1994: Oral tolerance: immunologic mechanisms and treatment of murine and human organ specific autoimmune diseases by oral administration of autoantigens. *Annual Review of Immunology* 12, 809–37.

Williams, R., Gibbons, R. 1972: Inhibition of bacterial adherence by secretory immunoglobulin A: a mechanism of antigen disposal. *Science* 177, 697–9.

Wolf, J., Rubin, D., Finberg, R., Kauffman, R.S., Sharpe, A.H., Trier, S., Fields, B.N. 1981: Intestinal M cells: a pathway for entry of reovirus into the host. *Science* 212, 471–2.

Youngman, K., Simon, P., West, G., Cominelli, F., Rachmilewitz, D., Klein, J.S., Fiocchi, C. 1993: Localization of intestinal interleukin 1 activity and protein and gene expression to lamina propria cells. *Gastroenterology* 104, 749–58.

5

Non-immunological defence mechanisms

RANJIT N RATNAIKE

The human gastrointestinal tract is potentially vulnerable to a range of extensive and complex external agents that can harm the host. In most instances, the damage is mild and limited to the mucosa of the gastrointestinal tract. Less often, the structural integrity of the mucosa and intrinsic intestinal function can be significantly altered, resulting in serious derangement to ultimately harm the host. The deleterious influences on the gastrointestinal tract are wide-ranging. They include viruses, bacteria, protozoa, worms and flukes, toxic substances in the diet, chemicals and antigens, and other agents that may be ingested knowingly or unknowingly. Most therapeutic agents for illnesses are taken orally and therefore come into close contact with the mucosa of the upper gastrointestinal tract. Iatrogenic alteration of normal gastrointestinal function is not uncommon (Ratnaike and Jones, 1998) and the numerous consequences are discussed in Chapters 15, 16 and 29.

The non-immunological defences of the gastrointestinal tract provide protective mechanisms that involve the stomach, small intestine and colon. These defences are effective predominantly against enteric viral, bacterial and protozoan pathogens. They are, however, not omnipotent. The human gastrointestinal tract may not successfully overcome all the challenges offered to it. For example, in the less industrialized countries where diarrhoea is a major health problem, especially in children under 5 years old, the massive inoculum of bacteria ingested in food and water overwhelms the immunological defences (*see* Chapter 4) and the powerful chemical sterilizing action of gastric acid, and the other non-immunological defence mechanisms. A number of influences, some iatrogenic, others physiological, including the ageing process, can also alter the effectiveness of these defence mechanisms. However, most threats to disrupt the structure and functions of the gastrointestinal tract are foiled or at least minimized by a range of mechanisms, some simple, others complex, but which all act in concert to protect the host.

GASTRIC DEFENCES

Vomiting

Vomiting is the most primitive defence mechanism of the gastrointestinal tract. Gastric contents are expelled by vigorous retrograde propulsion (*see* Chapter 14). In toxin-associated food poisoning, for example, with the emetic toxin of *Bacillus cereus* (*see* Chapter 18) and in viral gastroenteritis (*see* Chapter 17), vomiting is an important protective mechanism. Chemoreceptors in the first part of the duodenum are sensitive to emetic substances and transmit messages to the vomiting centre in the medulla. Another specialized area of the brain, the area postrema or chemoreceptor trigger zone (CTZ), is sensitive to substances circulating in the blood that cause vomiting.

Gastric acid

The gastric acid barrier is a critical defence mechanism against a variety of viral, bacterial and parasitic infections that cause diarrhoea (*see* Chapters 17–19). Gastric juice consists of water, hydrochloric acid (HCl), bicarbonate, inorganic ions (mainly sodium and potassium), and mucus, diluted with swallowed salivary juice. In normal subjects, the gastric pH is usually below 4.0 and prevents the survival of pathogens that may cause diarrhoea (Giannella *et al.*, 1972; Axon, 1986). This bacteriocidal activity is due to the actual pH change rather than other factors contained in gastric juice (Giannella *et al.*, 1972). In healthy persons, fewer than 10^4 organisms per millilitre are present in the stomach and the majority are oral flora swallowed with food or saliva. Gastric acid kills most of these organisms. There is a strong correlation between the pH of gastric acid and bacterial counts in the stomach (Morris *et al.*, 1984). As the pH of the stomach falls and becomes more acidic, the bacterial count declines and, at a pH of 3.0, the stomach is virtually sterile (Hunt, 1988). On an empty stomach, the pH is maintained between 1 and 2 for long periods of time (Pounder *et al.*, 1976).

At pH 4–5, bacteria normally found in saliva are present in the stomach. A pH greater than 5 allows bacterial, viral and protozoan pathogens to survive. The bactericidal activity of HCl on different species of bacteria has been evaluated. At various pH values, depending on the duration of contact between acid and pathogen, the bactericidal activity of HCl is highest at pH 2 and pH 3 on strains of *Campylobacter jejuni, Aeromonas hydrophila, Plesiomonas shigelloides, Yersinia enterocolitica, Salmonella* species and *Shigella* species, with complete killing after 60 minutes of incubation (Rotimi *et al.*, 1990). Gram-negative bacteria are most susceptible and the spore-forming anaerobes are least vulnerable. Compared to other bacteria, Lactobacilli are more resistant to the action of gastric juice and therefore survive longer in the stomach. Strains of *Shigella* and *Salmonella* were most sensitive to HCl. At pH 4 and above, these organisms survive *and* multiply rapidly. In 28 patients in an intensive care unit on ventilation, in whom the gastric pH was above 4.0, quantitative and qualitative bacteriological examination of daily gastric aspirates showed rapid colonization with high counts of bacteria, especially coliforms (Hillman *et al.*, 1982).

Patients with normal gastric acidity should not suffer from gastroenteritis caused by these intestinal pathogens unless overwhelmed by the inoculum of the pathogen. However, infections due to *Shigella* may occur despite a 'normal' gastric acid barrier. This is because the number of organisms that need to survive the acid barrier to cause an infection of the small intestine is as few as 10 bacteria (Levine *et al.*, 1973). Decreased acid production significantly increases the risk of diarrhoea in immunocompromised patients (Belitsos *et al.*, 1992).

The risk of diarrhoea due to enteric pathogens increases as the pH of gastric acid rises. In rats, surgical procedures that reduce gastric acidity increase bacterial counts in the proximal small intestine (Lambert *et al.*, 1967). Experiments on human volunteers also demonstrate this important relationship between gastric acidity and bacterial survival. The simultaneous ingestion of the attenuated vaccine of *Shigella flexneri* and sodium bicarbonate causes a threefold increase in the rate of enteric multiplication (Dupont *et al.*, 1972). Susceptibility to *V. cholerae* increases 10 000-fold when 2 g of sodium bicarbonate are administered with the bacterial dose (Cash *et al.*, 1974). Individuals may be susceptible to chronic tropical sprue due to achlorhydria, as about a third of Indian subjects with this condition were achlorhydric (Baker and Mathan, 1971). Achlorhydria due to cannabis use in overland travellers in India predisposes to cholera infection (Nalin *et al.*, 1978). In conditions of achlorhydria and hypochlorhydria, the increased risk of infection occurs not only from bacteria but also from intestinal parasites, e.g. *Giardia lamblia* (Giannella et *al.*, 1973).

Iatrogenic causes are common and important in decreasing gastric acidity. In several conditions, for example, peptic ulcer, gastro-oesophageal reflux and the Zollinger–Ellison syndrome, the therapeutic goal is to decrease gastric acid production or neutralize acid by increasing pH. Cimetidine, a H-2 receptor blocker, causes diarrhoea in 3–12 per cent of patients (Papadopoulos *et al.*, 1985; Hamilton *et al.*, 1986) and is also a significant risk factor for carriage of *Clostridium difficile* with the potential to develop pseudomembraneous colitis (Walker *et al.*, 1993). A prospective study of critical care patients on cimetidine and antacids showed that 59 per cent of 236 patients with a gastric pH of 4.0 or greater were positive for Gram-negative rods (GNR), although only 12 of 88 (14 per cent) cultures with pH < 4 were positive for GNR (Donowitz *et al.*, 1986). In a patient on cimetidine, diarrhoea due to bacterial overgrowth with large numbers of enterococci, *Streptococcus viridans,* coliforms and *Bacteroides* resolved with withdrawal of the drug alone (Ruddell and Losowsky, 1980). In a group of neonates on ranitidine, the mean pH was 5.6 compared to 4.4 in the control group, and gastric colonization was also higher in the treated group (Cothran *et al.*, 1997).

The use of omeprazole, the powerful proton pump inhibitor, resulted in bacterial overgrowth in 53 per cent of patients in a study by Thorens *et al.* (1996). Short-term treatment with omeprazole transiently increases gastric colony counts in healthy human volunteers but resolves 3 days after treatment is stopped (Sharma *et al.*, 1984). *Salmonella* infections occur in conditions of reduced gastric acidity (Giannella *et al.*, 1973). In patients with hypochlorhydria, salmonella gastroenteritis is much more serious and is associated with severe diarrhoea (Gray and Trueman, 1971).

Another iatrogenic cause that breaches the non-immune defences is surgery for peptic ulcer to decrease gastric acidity. Before the era of effective oral therapy, the surgical procedures for peptic ulceration often resulted in both significant gastric and jejunal colonization as early as a week after surgery and which persisted for 6 months (Muscroft *et al.*, 1981). The association between partial gastrectomy, bacterial overgrowth of pathogens in the stomach and upper small intestine, and diarrhoea is well documented. Hypochlorhydria as a result of gastric surgery predisposes the elderly to salmonellosis (Waddell and Kuntz, 1956). After partial gastrectomy (and in patients with pernicious anaemia), there is an increased incidence of gastric cancer, which could be due to the large numbers of nitrate-reducing bacteria in the achlorhydric stomach (Muscroft *et al.*, 1981). These organisms produce nitrites and *N*-nitroso compounds, which are known carcinogens (Axon, 1986; Sarker and Gyr, 1992). After total gastrectomy for malignancy, small bowel bacterial overgrowth is a frequent occurrence attributed to decreased gastric secretion and intestinal motility (Lock *et al.*, 1995; Brägelmann *et al.*, 1997).

In the elderly, decreased acid production may be part of the ageing process. Up to 80 per cent of healthy elderly subjects (mean age of 84 years, range 80–91 years) are hypochlorhydric and have gastric bacterial colonization dominated by Gram-positive flora (Husebye *et al.*, 1992). The traditional view is that gastric acid production decreases with age (Blackman *et al.*, 1970) and that it is associated with a decreased parietal cell mass (Andrews *et al.*, 1967; Kekki *et al.*, 1982). A recent report on a large study on elderly non-hospitalized persons by Hurwitz *et al.* (1997) found that 90 per cent were able to acidify gastric contents even in the basal unstimulated state. In this study those who were 'consistent hyposecretors had serum markers of atrophic gastritis'.

Conditions which are more common in the elderly, associated with hypochlorhydria or achlorhydria, are gastric carcinoma, chronic atrophic gastritis, pernicious anaemia, and the WDHA syndrome (watery diarrhoea, hypokalaemia and achlorhydria) and gastroparesis in patients with diabetes mellitus treated with insulin over a long term (Katz and Spiro, 1966; Stockbrügger, 1985; Armbrecht *et al.*, 1987). In atrophic gastritis the proximal small intestinal pH is significantly higher, as are bacterial counts in this part of the intestine (Russell *et al.*, 1986). In seven patients with pernicious anaemia, the mean pH of gastric juice was 7.3 and as high as 8.2 in six subjects with hypogammaglobulinaemia (Borriello *et al.*, 1985).

Helicobacter pylori infection may be associated with atrophic gastritis, which would decrease the parietal cell mass and reduce acid output (Eidt *et al.*, 1996; Sipponen *et al.*, 1996; Annibale *et al.*, 1997). Decreased gastric acidity has also been documented in marijuana smokers (Nalin *et al.*, 1978).

In protein-energy malnutrition, a persistent major problem in the developing world, the high prevalence of bacterial and parasitic infections is attributed to decreased gastric acidity (Yardley and Bayless, 1967; Webster, 1980). In Bangladesh, a group of 35 malnourished children were compared with 20 'better nourished' children before and after betazole stimulation in regard to basal gastric acid output (Gilman *et al.*, 1988). The malnourished children were then tested after 3 weeks of nutritional supplementation. Before nutritional supplementation, both the basal and betazole-stimulated acid output was significantly lower than that of the control children. Serum gastrin concentrations were not significantly different. Eighty-one per cent of the malnourished children had bacterial colonization of the stomach compared to none of the control group. After nutritional supplementation over 3 weeks, there was marked improvement in weight-for-height (comparable to the 20 'better nourished' children), although gastric acid concentration continued to be depressed. An interesting finding was that, among the 'better nourished' children, only 45 per cent (nine out of 20) had a gastric pH below 4.0. However, none showed evidence of bacterial contamination of the stomach. The authors suggested that the gastric acid barrier may be an intermittent defence factor in Bangladeshi children. The association of malnutrition and decreased gastric acid production increases the risk of many millions of malnourished children in less industrialized countries to acquire infections such as diarrhoea.

In a study of preterm infants, pH tended to decrease with increasing age, reflecting the development of acidity as the stomach matured (Usowicz *et al.*, 1988). These workers also showed that the gastric pH was also significantly lower in infants fed exclusively with breast milk, which suggests that human milk may influence gastric acid production. This observation strengthens the vigorous advocacy of the protective effect of breast feeding against diarrhoea in infants by the World Health Organization Diarrhoeal Diseases Control Programme. This protective action of breast milk through gastric acidity may be due to the cytokines present either in the breast milk or in maternal cells present in milk (Srivastava *et al.*, 1996).

Recent studies have focused beyond bacterial contamination of the stomach to investigate the bacterial composition of the small intestine in states of reduced gastric acidity.

In a study of 18 patients with gastric ulcers treated with H-2 receptor antagonists, expired breath samples showed a significant increase in $^{14}CO_2$ activity compared with samples before administration of H-2 receptor antagonists and those of normal controls (Shindo and Fukumura, 1995). Significant correlations were present between the $^{14}CO_2$ activity and gastric pH before and after administration of the H-2 receptor antagonist. Bacterial overgrowth occurred in the jejunal fluid of all these patients and oral tetracycline reduced the $^{14}CO_2$ activity significantly. The species identified in the jejunal fluid samples included *Escherichia coli*, *Pseudomonas aeruginosa*, enterococci, *Lactobacillus bifidus*, *Bacteroides vulgatus*, *Bacteroides uniformis*, *Eubacterium lentum*, *Eubacterium parvum* and *Candida albicans*. All the species identified except *Escherichia coli*, *Pseudomonas aeruginosa* and *Candida albicans* deconjugated bile acids. In 53 healthy volunteers, a shift to neutral pH in gastric juice due to cimetidine therapy resulted in bacterial overgrowth and deconjugation of bile salts (Shindo *et al.*, 1996). Small intestinal bacterial overgrowth and subsequent bile salt deconjugation can lead to diarrhoea and steatorrhoea (Tabaqchali *et al.*, 1968).

Gastric motility and mucus

Gastric motility enhances the protective role of gastric acid against pathogens. The adequate mixing of gastric contents with gastric juice contributes to the efficient killing of pathogens. This activity may be compromised by conditions that increase the rate of gastric emptying, such as gastric surgery, pancreatic exocrine deficiency and 'early' non-insulin-dependent diabetes mellitus (Horowitz and Camilleri, 1997). Certain drugs also increase gastric emptying. Metoclopramide, domperidone, cisapride, erythromycin and diazepam are gastrointestinal tract prokinetic agents (Weber *et al.*, 1993; Patterson, 1994).

Mucus secreted by the cells of the gastric epithelium forms a continuous protective layer over the gastric mucosa of varying thickness. The mucus protects the mucosa against ingested toxins, organisms and other substances such as carcinogens harmful to the host. The mucus layer is possibly another protective factor to prevent stomach cancer, in addition to the absence of, or low number of, bacteria in the stomach. The protective effects of mucus warrants further study.

SMALL INTESTINAL DEFENCES

The small intestine is an organ with numerous complex functions. It receives gastric juice, bile and pancreatic juice, secretes enzymes, and is responsible for food digestion and absorption and for the movement of luminal contents to the colon. An important role is in host defence. The small intestine uses a variety of mechanisms against agents that may adversely affect the mucosa and, ultimately, the host.

In health, the environment of the normal small intestine is not conducive to providing a permanent habitat for gut flora. This is in contrast to the colon where bacteria are normally resident and are of great benefit to the host, as discussed below. However, bacterial overgrowth may occur in the small intestine when the mechanisms of host defence are absent or compromised (*see also* Chapters 4 and 12). Increased gastric acidity parallels decreased bacterial counts in the jejunum and also influences the composition of bacteria (Pollak *et al.*, 1986). The preventive action of gastric acid on bacterial colonization is demonstrable not only in the stomach but also in the small intestine (Shindo *et al.*, 1996). However, despite the powerful action of the gastric defence mechanism discussed above, the small intestine is not invariably a sterile organ (Simon and Gorbach, 1984). In the upper small intestine, flora, if present, reflect their ability to survive multiple host defences. The composition and distribution of small intestinal flora vary from individual to individual and reflect geographical commonalities (Baker and Mathan, 1971).

In the fasting state, the upper small intestine of normal subjects in industrialized countries is usually sterile or the bacterial count seldom is greater than 10^4 per millilitre of the intestinal aspirate. Bacteria, if present, are few in number, from ingested food or are oral bacteria swallowed with saliva, having survived destruction by gastric acid (Savage, 1977). The greatest bacterial contamination is in the distal ileum and may reflect the close proximity to the large intestine. Decreased motility in this region may be a contributory factor (Vantrappen *et al.*, 1977).

At present, it is possible that the precise ecology of the small intestine may be incomplete owing to technical limitations in cultivating and identifying organisms.

Motility

Motility of the small intestine is a primary defence mechanism to protect the host against enteric pathogens and harmful substances. This protection is achieved by minimizing the contact between toxic substances or organisms that may cause damage and the small bowel mucosa. The environment of the small intestine is continuously changing and presents a hostile milieu to pathogens. Motility ensures adequate mixing of the digestive secretions with food, and the digestive enzymes and secretions that are continuously produced are harmful to pathogens. Motility also exposes the products of digestion to the surface of the small intestine for absorption and propels the digested food products to the colon. Enterocytes on to which bacteria may adhere are constantly shed and replaced.

Intestinal motility is associated with migrating myoelectric complexes (MMC). The MMC consists of three phases of activity (the motility of the small intestine is discussed in detail in Chapter 11), which are detailed below.

- Phase 1: the quiescent phase. There is no spiking activity.
- Phase 2: irregular contractive activity is initiated and increases in intensity.

- Phase 3: the dominant phase. Bursts of constant, intense intestinal contractions occur at the maximal frequency. Peristalsis of consecutive intestinal segments takes place. During this phase, propulsion of the intestinal contents is at a peak and they are swept away in an aboral direction. This phase of the MMC has been aptly described as the 'gastrointestinal housekeeper' (Code and Schlegel, 1974). These activity fronts migrate over a 90–120-min period from the antrum of the stomach to the terminal ileum in continuous succession.

Besides transporting digested food products, the MMC removes the mucus layer that is continuously replenished, preventing prolonged contact between enteric pathogens, toxins and the mucosa of the intestine (Dixon, 1960; Kent *et al.*, 1966). Laboratory studies on rats show that, if the MMC is abolished with morphine and phenylephrine for more than 6–15 hours, bacterial overgrowth develops (Scott and Cahall, 1982). On cessation of the drugs and the return of the MMC, bacterial overgrowth is abolished. Similar effects were seen in human studies, where five patients with disordered or absent MMC also showed bacterial overgrowth (Vantrappen *et al.*, 1977). When motility decreases, stasis occurs, resulting in bacterial overgrowth, as the products of digestion are an ideal milieu for bacteria to multiply and cause diarrhoea.

When diarrhoea occurs, the propulsive functions of the intestine are exaggerated. Increased fluid within the lumen increases motility and the rapid evacuation of intestinal contents prevents or minimizes contact between the mucosal surface of the intestine and the pathogens themselves or their toxins. This raises the question of the role of antimotility agents in the treatment of infective diarrhoea. For example, with shigellosis, the infection is prolonged if the patients are treated with Lomotil (Dupont and Hornick, 1973).

A variety of systemic diseases and local conditions listed in Table 5.1, which involve the small intestine, decrease motility, leading to bacterial overgrowth and diarrhoea. There is no evidence of significantly altered small intestinal motility associated with the ageing process (Anuras and Sutherland, 1984; Husebye and Engedal, 1992).

Autonomic neuropathy in patients with diabetes mellitus causes a decrease in both gastric and small intestinal motility. Despite the wide range in intestinal transit time, most patients with diabetes mellitus have decreased motility resulting in increased transit time (Scarpello *et al.*, 1976). This leads to bacterial colonization and diarrhoea. Indeed, in the largest epidemic of *Salmonella enteritidis* in a hospital in the USA, diabetics on treatment were at an increased risk of infection (Telzak *et al.*, 1991).

Drug therapy may cause decreased intestinal motility. Although anticholinergic drugs have as their most frequent side-effect the problem of constipation, these drugs have the potential to reduce intestinal motility and may as a result of stasis cause bacterial proliferation leading to diarrhoea. Anticholinergic drugs are now no longer widely used, with the exception of propantheline (urinary incontinence), benztropine (Parkinson's disease) and tricyclic antidepressants (Ratnaike and Jones, 1998). Most of the major pharmacological ingredients of marijuana decrease both the rate of gastric emptying and small intestinal transit times in rodents, thus inhibiting gastrointestinal motility (Shook and Burks, 1989).

Table 5.1 *Causes of decreased small intestinal motility*

Diabetic autonomic neuropathy
Hypothyroidism
Amyloidosis
Scleroderma
Myotonia dystrophica[a]
Lymphoma
Intestinal pseudo-obstruction
Radiation enteritis
Drug therapy

[a]A hereditary condition characterized by myotonia, muscular wasting, cataracts, testicular atrophy and frontal baldness.

Mucus

A thick layer of mucus covers the epithelial surface of the intestine to protect the mucosa and lubricate the movement of digested food. Mucus is synthesized and secreted by goblet cells in the gastrointestinal tract. Mucus consists of 95 per cent water, linked glycoprotein molecules with a high carbohydrate content, small amounts of proteins and lipids, cells, cell debris, products of digestion, protein from gastrointestinal secretions and enmeshed microorganisms. Its most important ingredient is the high molecular weight polymer of glycoprotein molecules linked by disulphide bonds (Pearson *et al.*, 1980). The layer of mucus is percolated from beneath by bicarbonate ions secreted by the underlying epithelial cells to protect the epithelium from the acidic contents of the stomach (Allen *et al.*, 1993).

As with intestinal motility, mucus also serves to minimize contact between the intestinal mucosa and harmful animate and inanimate agents. The mucus layer protects the mucosa from enteric pathogens and bacterial toxins, antigens, dietary chemicals and injurious components of bile, pancreatic juice and intestinal secretions. Owing to its structural composition, the mucus layer excludes molecules larger than 20 000 molecular weight, such as external antigens and toxins, and also pepsin and trypsin, all of which have the capacity to damage the mucosa (Clamp, 1986).

Mucus provides a barrier, especially to pathogens that adhere to the mucosa, and is also a lubricant that coats pathogens to assist in their removal by intestinal motility. A more sophisticated form of protection by the mucus is directed against bacteria. The carbohydrate composition of the glycoprotein mimics the surface of the epithelial cell and entraps bacteria that damage the cell by adherence, such as *Pseudomonas aeruginosa* (Ramphal and Pyle, 1983), *Escherichia coli* (Cohen *et al.*, 1983) and *Vibrio cholerae* (Schrank and Verwey, 1976).

Increased mucus production occurs to deal with toxins produced by bacteria, such as *Vibrio cholerae* and *Escherichia coli* (Moon *et al.*, 1971; Strombeck and Harrold, 1974; Adler *et al.*, 1981). Mucus binds the toxin and decreases diffusion to the intestinal mucosal cells. The mucus layer is continuously replaced and the motility of the small bowel helps remove this mucus along with any pathogens it may have trapped.

Other factors

Bile salts and pancreatic secretions within the lumen of the small intestine provide a protective function owing to their antibacterial properties. Proteolytic enzymes cause bacterial lysis and some viruses *in vitro* are susceptible to the action of trypsin. Another protective mechanism is lysozyme, a protein within the mucus layer that kills bacteria (Waker, 1976). Breast milk also contains lysozyme, which may contribute to its protective action against enteric bacteria in breast-fed infants (Hanson *et al.*, 1994).

The constant shedding and renewal of the enterocytes of the small intestine provide further protection against injury to the mucosa by bacterial adherence. This rapid cell turnover is also a protective factor against small bowel cancer, as are the absent or small number of bacteria in the small bowel, the alkaline environment and low levels of enzymes with the capacity to activate precarcinogens (Neugut *et al.*, 1998). Nitrate-reducing bacteria in the gut can produce nitrites and *N*-nitroso compounds that are carcinogens (Axon, 1986).

The ileo-caecal valve

The ileo-caecal valve (ICV) may have a defensive role in protecting the gastrointestinal tract. The ICV between the small intestine and the colon regulates the passage of digested food, preventing the reflux of contaminated large bowel contents to the relatively sterile small intestine. Bacterial colony counts in the ileal region adjacent to the ICV are significantly lower compared to counts in the caecum. The functions of the ICV are still in question as ileo-caecal resection does not lead to altered motility of the bowel or derangement of luminal contents, nor bacterial colonization of the small intestine. Thus the precise role of the ICV needs more study.

COLONIC DEFENCES

The colonic defences, which rely primarily upon the normal flora inhabiting the colon, are briefly set out here. Although large intestinal infection is minimized by the mechanisms discussed above, many pathogens may survive and reach the colon where the 'normal' bacterial flora provides a further 'line' of defence. The resident colonic bacteria are diverse. A study of over 200 faecal specimens identified 300 species of bacteria (Moore and Holdeman, 1975). The diversity of the colonic flora was also reported by Finegold *et al.* (1975) who identified *Bacteroides* (18 species), *Eubacterium* (42 species), *Clostridium* (55 species) and 11 species of *Bifidobacter*.

The bacterial composition of the colon is unique for each individual and is determined early in life by interactions between the host and the bacteria, and between bacteria themselves. The number and types of colonic bacteria are relatively constant throughout life (Simon and Gorbach, 1986). Even a major change from a non-vegetarian to a vegetarian diet does not significantly alter the species mix or number of colonic flora.

The commensal bacteria in the colon form a complex well-balanced ecological system to protect the host against infection by a variety of mechanisms. Many normal commensal bacteria attach to the colonic mucosal surface and their presence therefore hinders the attachment of pathogenic strains to mucosal adhesion sites. Other mechanisms include: modification of bile acids; stimulation of peristalsis; induction of immunological responses; depletion of essential substrates from the environment; competition for adhesion sites; creation of restrictive metabolic environments; and elaboration of antibiotic-like substances (Rolfe, 1984). The antibiotic-like substances bacteria produce include colicins and short-chain fatty acids, which have bacteriocidal or bacteriostatic properties (Byrne and Danker, 1979). The protective activity of the colon is often disrupted by antibiotics, allowing other bacteria harmful to the host, such as *Clostridium difficile*, to proliferate.

The non-immunological mechanisms involving the stomach, small intestine and colon, together with the immunological defences (*see* Chapter 4), provide a formidable barrier to protect the host from a variety of external deleterious challenges.

REFERENCES

Adler, K.B., Hardwick, D.H., Craighead, J.E. 1981: Effect of cholera toxin on secretion of mucin by explants of guinea pig trachea. *Laboratory Investigations* 45, 372–7.

Allen, A., Flemstrom, G., Garner, A., Kivilaakso, E. 1993: Gastroduodenal mucosal protection. *Physiological Reviews* 73, 823–57.

Andrews, G.R., Haneman, B., Arnold, B.J., Booth, J.C., Taylor, K. 1967: Atrophic gastritis in the aged. *Australasian Annals of Medicine* 16, 230–5.

Annibale, B., Marignani, M., Azzoni, C. *et al.* 1997: Atrophic body gastritis: distinct features associated with Helicobacter pylori infection. *Helicobacter* 2, 57–64.

Anuras, S., Sutherland, J. 1984: Small intestinal manometry in healthy elderly subjects. *Journal of the American Geriatrics Society* 32, 581–3.

Armbrecht, U., Eden, S., Seeberg, S., Stockbrügger, R.W. 1987: The value of the hydrogen (H2) breath test for the diagnosis of bacterial overgrowth in gastric achlorhydria. *Hepato-Gastroenterology* 34, 219–22.

Axon, A.T. 1986: Potential hazards of hypochlorhydria in the treatment of peptic ulcer. *Scandinavian Journal of Gastroenterology* (Suppl.) 122, 17–21.

Baker, S.J.M., Mathan, V.I. 1971: Tropical sprue in Southern India. In The Wellcome Trust (ed.), *Tropical sprue and megaloblastic anaemia*. London: Churchill Livingstone, 189–260.

Belitsos, P.C., Greenson, J.K., Yardley, J.H. 1992: Association of gastric hypoacidity with opportunistic enteric infections in patients with AIDS. *Journal of Infectious Diseases* 166, 277–84.

Blackman, A.H., Lambert, D.L., Thayer, W.R., Martin, H.F. 1970: Computed normal values for peak acid output based on age, sex and body weight. *American Journal of Digestive Diseases* 15, 783–9.

Borriello, S.P., Reed, P.J., Dolby, J.M., Barclay, F.P., Webster, A.D. 1985: Microbiological and metabolic profile of achlorhydric stomach: comparison of pernicious anaemia and hypogammaglobulinaemia. *Journal of Clinical Pathology* 38, 946–53.

Brägelmann, R., Armbrecht, U., Rosemeyer, D., Schneider, B., Zilly, W., Stockbrügger, R.W. 1997: Small bowel bacterial overgrowth in patients after total gastrectomy. *European Journal of Clinical Investigations* 27, 409–16.

Byrne, B.M., Danker, T.J. 1979: Volatile fatty acids and aerobic flora in gastrointestinal tract of mice under various conditions. *Infection and Immunity* 23, 559–63.

Cash, R.A., Music, S.T., Libonati, J.P., Snyder, M.J.J., Wenzel, R.P., Hornick, R.B. 1974: Response of man to infection with vibrio cholera. I. Clinical, serologic and bacteriologic responses to known inoculum. *Journal of Infectious Diseases* 129, 45–52.

Clamp, J. 1986: The role of mucus in human intestinal defence. In Losowsky, M.S., Heatley, R.V. (eds), *Gut defences in clinical practice*. Edinburgh: Churchill Livingstone, 83–94.

Code, C.F., Schlegel, J.F. 1974: The gastrointestinal housekeeper. In Daniel, E.E. (ed.), *Gastrointestinal motility*. Vancouver: Mitchell Press, 631–3.

Cohen, P.S., Rossoll, R., Cabelli, V.J., Yang, S.L., Laux, D.C. 1983: Relationship between the mouse-colonizing ability of a human faecal Escherichia coli strain and its ability to bind a specific mouse colonic gel protein. *Infection and Immunity* 40, 62–9.

Cothran, D.S., Borowitz, S.M., Sutphen, J.L., Dudley, S.M., Donowitz, L.G. 1997: Alteration of normal gastric flora in neonates receiving ranitidine. *Journal of Perinatology* 17, 383–8.

Dixon, J.M.S. 1960: The fate of bacteria in the small intestine. *Journal of Pathology and Bacteriology* 79, 131–40.

Donowitz, L.G., Page, M.C., Mileur, B.L., Guenthner, S.H. 1986: Alteration of normal gastric flora in critical care patients receiving antacid and cimetidine therapy. *Infection Control* 7, 23–6.

Dupont, H.L., Hornick, R.B. 1973: Adverse effect of lomotil therapy in shigellosis. *Journal of the American Medical Association* 226, 1525–8.

Dupont, H.L., Hornick, R.B., Snyder, M.J., Libonati, J.P., Formal, S.B., Gangarosa, E.J. 1972: Immunity in shigellosis: I. Response of man to attenuated strains of shigella. *Journal of Infectious Diseases* 125, 5–11.

Eidt, S., Oberhuber, G., Schneider, A., Stolte, M. 1996: The histopathological spectrum of type A gastritis. *Pathology Research and Practice* 192, 101–6.

Finegold, S.M., Sutter, V.L., Boyle, J.D., Shimada, K. 1975: The normal flora of ileostomy and transverse colostomy effluents. *Journal of Infectious Diseases* 122, 376–81.

Giannella, R.A., Broitman, S.A., Zamchek, N. 1972: Gastric acid barrier to ingested microorganisms in man: studies in vivo and in vitro. *Gut* 13, 251–6.

Giannella, R.A., Broitman, S.A., Zamchek, N. 1973: Influence of gastric acidity on bacterial and parasitic enteric infections. A perspective. *Annals of Internal Medicine* 78, 271–6.

Gilman, R.H., Partanen, R., Brown, K.H. *et al.* 1988: Decreased gastric acid secretion and bacterial colonization of the stomach in severely malnourished Bangladeshi children. *Gastroenterology* 94, 1308–14.

Gray, J.A., Trueman, A.M. 1971: Severe salmonella gastroenteritis associated with hypochlorhydria. *Scottish Medical Journal* 16, 255–8.

Hamilton, I., O'Connor, H.J., Wood, N.C., Bradbury, I., Axon, A.T. 1986: Healing and recurrence of duodenal ulcer after treatment with tripotassium dicitrate bismuthate (TDB) tablets or cimetidine. *Gut* 27, 106–10.

Hanson, L.A., Hahn-Zoric, M., Berndes, M. *et al.* 1994: Breast feeding: overview and breast milk immunology. *Acta Paediatrica Japonica* 36, 557–61.

Hillman, K.M., Riordan, T., O'Farrell, S.M., Tabaqchali, S. 1982: Colonization of the gastric contents in critically ill patients. *Critical Care Medicine* 10, 444–7.

Horowitz, M., Camilleri, M. 1997: Gastric and intestinal motility disorders. In Shearman, D.J.C., Finlayson, N., Camilleri, M., Carter, D. (eds), *Diseases of the gastrointestinal tract and liver*. New York: Churchill Livingstone, 423–50.

Hunt R.H. 1988: The protective role of gastric acid. *Scandinavian Journal of Gastroenterology* 23, 34–9.

Hurwitz, A., Brady, D.A., Schaal, S.E., Samloff, I.M., Dedon, J., Ruhl, C.E. 1997: Gastric acidity in older adults. *Journal of the American Medical Association* 278, 659–62.

Husebye, E., Engedal, K. 1992: The patterns of motility are maintained in the human small intestine throughout the process of aging. *Scandinavian Journal of Gastroenterology* 27, 397–404.

Husebye, E., Skar, V., Hoverstad, T., Melby, K. 1992: Fasting hypochlorhydria with gram positive gastric flora is highly prevalent in healthy old people. *Gut* 33, 1331–7.

Katz, L.A., Spiro, H.M. 1966: Gastrointestinal manifestations in diabetes. *New England Journal of Medicine* 275, 1350–61.

Kekki, M., Samloff, I.M., Ihamaki, T., Varis, K., Siurala, M. 1982: Age and sex-related behaviour of gastric acid secretion at the population level. *Scandinavian Journal of Gastroenterology* 17, 737–43.

Kent, T.H., Formal, S.B., LaBrec, E.H. 1966: Acute enteritis due to Salmonella typhimurium in opium-treated guinea pigs. *Archives of Pathology* 81, 501–8.

Lambert, R., Chassignol, S., Sedallian, A., Descos, L., Martin, F. 1967: Influence of gastrectomy and by-passing of the stomach on the intestinal flora of the rat. *Journal of Pathology and Bacteriology* 94, 183–9.

Levine, M.M., DuPont, H.L., Formal, S.B., Hornick, R.B., Takeuchi, A., Gangarosa, E.J., Snyder, M.J., Libonati, J.P. 1973: Pathogenesis of Shigella dysenteriae 1 (Shiga) dysentery. *Journal of Infectious Diseases* 127, 261–70.

Lock, G., Hollerbach, S., Linde, H.J., Vogt, W., Andus, T., Schölmerich, J., Holstege A. 1995: Bacterial overgrowth after gastric surgery: comparison of endoscopic aspiration and glucose H2-breath test. *Gastroenterology* 110A (Suppl.), 343.

Moon, H.W., Whipp, S.C., Baetz, A.L. 1971: Comparative effects of enterotoxins from Escherichia coli and Vibrio cholerae on rabbit and swine small intestine. *Laboratory Investigations* 25, 133–40.

Moore, W.E., Holdeman, L.V. 1975: Some newer concepts of the human intestinal flora. *American Journal of Medical Technology* 41, 427–30.

Morris, D.L., Youngs, D., Muscroft, T.J., Cooper, J., Rojinski, C., Burdon, D.W., Keighley, M.R.B. 1984: Mutagenicity in gastric juice. *Gut* 25, 723–7.

Muscroft, T.J., Deane, S.A., Youngs, D., Burdon, D.W., Keighley, M.R.B. 1981: The microflora of the postoperative stomach. *British Journal of Surgery* 68: 560–4.

Nalin, D.R., Levine, M.M., Rhead, J. *et al.* 1978: Cannabis, hypochlorhydria and cholera. *Lancet* 2, 859–62.

Neugut, A.I., Jacobson, J.S., Suh, S., Mukherjee, R., Arber, N. 1998: The epidemiology of cancer of the small bowel. *Cancer Epidemiology, Biomarkers and Prevention* 7, 243–51.

Papadopoulos, C., Kalantzis, N., Rekoumis, G., Kanaghinis, T. 1985: A comparative trial of 400 mg cimetidine twice daily and 100 mg daily in the short-term treatment of duodenal ulceration. *Current Medical Research and Opinion* 9, 511–15.

Patterson, D.J. 1994: Prokinetic agents in post gastrectomy patients. *Gastroenterology Clinics of North America* 23, 313–25.

Pearson, J., Allen, A., Venables, C. 1980: Gastric mucus: isolation and polymeric structure of the undegraded glycoprotein: its breakdown by pepsin. *Gastroenterology* 78, 709–15.

Pollak, R., Varkonyi, T., Nagy, E., Varro, V. 1986: Gastric acidity: an important factor regulating the composition of the bacterial flora in the small intestine. *Acta Medica Hungarica* 43, 365–8.

Pounder, R.E., Williams, J.G., Milton-Thompson, G.J., Misiewicz, J.J. 1976: Effect of cimetidine on 24-hour intragastric acidity in normal subjects. *Gut* 17, 133–8.

Ramphal, R., Pyle, M. 1983: Evidence for mucins and sialic acid as receptors for Pseudomonas aeruginosa in the lower respiratory tract. *Infection and Immunity* 41, 339–44.

Ratnaike, R.N., Jones, T.E. 1998: Mechanisms of drug-induced diarrhoea in the elderly. *Drugs and Aging* 13, 245–53.

Rolfe, D.R. 1984: Interactions among micro-organisms of the indigenous intestinal flora and their influence on the host. *Reviews of Infectious Diseases* 6 (Suppl.), 73–9S.

Rotimi, V.O., Egwari, L., Akande, B. 1990: Acidity and intestinal bacteria: an in-vitro assessment of the bactericidal activity of hydrochloric acid on intestinal pathogens. *African Journal of Medicine and Medical Sciences* 19, 275–80.

Ruddell, W.S., Losowsky, M.S. 1980: Severe diarrhoea due to small intestinal bacterial colonization during cimetidine treatment. *British Medical Journal* 281, 273.

Russell, R.M., Krasinski, S.D., Samloff, I.M., Jacob, R.A., Hartz, S.C., Brovender, S.R. 1986: Folic acid malabsorption in atrophic gastritis. Possible compensation by bacterial folate synthesis. *Gastroenterology* 91, 1476–82.

Sarker, S.A., Gyr, K. 1992: Non-immunological defence mechanisms of the gut. *Gut* 33, 987–93.

Savage, D.C. 1977: Microbial ecology of the gastrointestinal tract. *Annual Review of Microbiology* 31, 107–33.

Scarpello, H.B., Greaves, M., Sladen, G.E. 1976: Small intestinal transit in diabetes. *British Medical Journal* 2, 1225–6.

Schrank, G.D., Verwey, W.F. 1976: Distribution of cholera organisms in experimental Vibrio cholerae infections: proposed mechanisms of pathogenesis and antibacterial immunity. *Infection and Immunity* 13, 195–203.

Scott, L.D., Cahall, D.L. 1982: Influence of the interdigestive myoelectric complex on enteric flora in the rat. *Gastroenterology* 82, 737–45.

Sharma, B.K., Santana, I.A., Wood, E.C. *et al.* 1984: Intragastric bacterial activity and nitrosation before, during and after treatment with omeprazole. *British Medical Journal Clinical Research Education* 289, 717–19.

Shindo, K., Fukumura, M. 1995: Effect of H2-receptor antagonists on bile acid metabolism. *Journal of Investigative Medicine* 43, 170–7.

Shindo, K., Yamazaki, R., Koide, K., Fukumura, M., Hirai, Y. 1996: Alteration of bile acid metabolism by cimetidine in healthy humans. *Journal of Investigative Medicine* 44, 462–9.

Shook, J.E., Burks, T.F. 1989: Psychoactive cannabinoids reduce gastrointestinal propulsion and motility in rodents. *Journal of Pharmacology and Experimental Therapeutics* 249, 444–9.

Simon, G.L., Gorbach, S.L. 1984: Intestinal flora in health and disease. *Gastroenterology* 86, 174–93.

Simon, G.L., Gorbach, S.L. 1986: The human intestinal microflora. *Digestive Diseases and Sciences* 31, 147–62S.

Sipponen, P., Kekki, M., Seppala, K., Siurala, M. 1996: The relationships between chronic gastritis and gastric acid secretion. *Alimentary Pharmacology and Therapeutics* 10 (Suppl. 1), 103–18.

Srivastava, M.D., Srivastava, A., Brouhard, B., Saneto, R., Groh-Wargo, S., Kubit, J. 1996: Cytokines in human milk. *Research Communication in Molecular Pathology and Pharmacology* 93, 263–87.

Stockbrügger, R.W. 1985: Bacterial overgrowth as a cause of reduced gastric acidity. *Scandinavian Journal of Gastroenterology* (Suppl.) 111, 7–16.

Strombeck, D.R., Harrold, D. 1974: Binding of cholera toxin to mucins and inhibition by gastric mucin. *Infection and Immunity* 10, 1266–72.

Tabaqchali, S., Hatgioannou, J., Booth, C.C. 1968: Bile salt deconjugation and steatorrhoea in patients with stagnant loop syndrome. *Lancet* 2, 12–16.

Telzak, E.E., Greenberg, M.S., Budnick, L.D., Singh, T., Blum, S. 1991: Diabetes mellitus – a newly described risk factor for infection from Salmonella enteritidis. *Journal of Infectious Diseases* 164, 538–41.

Thorens, J., Froehlich, F., Schwizer, W. *et al.* 1996: Bacterial overgrowth during treatment with omeprazole compared with cimetidine: a prospective randomised double blind study. *Gut* 39, 54–9.

Usowicz, A.G., Dab, S.B., Emery, J.R., McCann, E.M., Brady, J.P. 1988: Does gastric acid protect the preterm infant from bacteria in unheated human milk? *Early Human Development* 16, 27–33.

Vantrappen, G., Janssens, J., Hellemans, J., Ghoos, Y. 1977: The interdigestive motor complex of normal subjects and patients with bacterial overgrowth of the small intestine. *Journal of Clinical Investigation* 59, 1158–66.

Waddell, W.R., Kuntz, L.J. 1956: Association of Salmonella enteritis with operation in the stomach. *New England Journal of Medicine* 255, 555–9.

Waker, W.A. 1976: Host defense mechanisms in gastrointestinal tract. *Paediatrics* 57, 901–6.

Walker, K.J., Gilliland, S.S., Vance-Bryan, K., Moody, J.A., Larsson A.J., Rotschafer, J.C., Guay, D.R. 1993: Clostridium difficile colonization in residents of long-term care facilities: prevalence and risk factors. *Journal of the American Geriatrics Society* 41, 940–6.

Weber, F.H., Richards, R.D., McCallum, R.W. 1993: Erthyromycin: a motilin agonist and gastrointestinal prokinetic agent. *American Journal of Gastroenterology* 88, 485–90.

Webster, A.B.D. 1980: Giardiasis and immunodeficiency diseases. *Transcripts of the Royal Society of Tropical Medicine and Hygiene* 74, 440–3.

Yardley, J.H., Bayless, T.M. 1967: Giardiasis. *Gastroenterology* 52, 301–4.

6

The process of aging and small bowel diseases in the elderly

PETER R. HOLT

INTRODUCTION

The specialty of gastroenterology, when compared to cardiology and neurology, is thought of as one that deals more with diseases of the young than of the old. As a result, gastrointestinal diseases of the elderly, including disorders of the small bowel, have received little attention. Well-researched information is difficult to find. A number of factors make it important to consider gastrointestinal disorders in older individuals. First, the population of the world is aging rapidly. By the year 2025, it has been estimated that more than three-quarters of a billion persons over the age of 65 will be alive in the world. The health needs of the elderly have only recently received attention and may be the most important health care question that faces society in the twenty-first century.

The frequency and dramatic, overt manifestations of cardiovascular and central nervous system diseases in the old have overshadowed the importance of diseases in the gastrointestinal tract in this age group. Furthermore, some of the most important general issues in diseases that affect older individuals are prejudices and misconceptions. Generalized misconceptions include the fact that aging is inevitably associated with a progressive deterioration of function. This prejudice often has led to physicians ignoring early signs of disease in the old by rejecting them as 'normal deterioration with age'. It is crucial to define, therefore, what we know about normal changes that occur in the small intestine and ancillary organs that may lead to disorders of small bowel function in the absence of overt disease. Put another way, knowing the borders of normal physiology will alert the astute physician to the presence of a potentially treatable disease in an older individual.

This review will provide information that is available to the author regarding changes with age in anatomy, histology, blood and nerve supply, as well as the consequent physiologic changes that might accrue and alter digestion, absorption, intestinal proliferation, motor function and motility, as well as the defense mechanisms that protect the milieu interior of Claude Bernard from being disturbed. For a fuller and more detailed description of the anatomic and physiologic changes that occur with age, the reader is directed to a chapter in a book that focuses upon the elderly (Holt, 1995).

ANATOMIC CHANGES

Anatomy and blood supply

Early studies of the structure of small bowel villi and microvilli all reported progressive pathologic changes with age (Mathis, 1928; Suntzeff and Angeletti, 1951; Van Lennep, 1962; Baker *et al.*, 1963) due to 'exposure to toxic intestinal contents'. Subsequent authors described only modest reduction in villus height in advanced age (Clarke, 1972, 1977) restricted to the jejunum (Hohn *et al.*, 1978). In contrast, two investigators reported increased jejunal cell numbers (Moog, 1977; Ecknauer *et al.*, 1982).

Our studies, using carefully standardized experimental conditions, showed that upper intestinal villus dimension remained constant (Holt *et al.*, 1984), crypt depth was greater and ileal height increased starting at 21 months in mice fed *ad libitum* (Heller *et al.*, 1990). Food restriction at 60 per cent of usual caloric intake reverted these changes (Heller *et al.*, 1990).

Villus height also appeared to increase with age in the ileum (Heller *et al.*, 1990). In human biopsies, Corrazza and coworkers (1988) found no change in villus cellularity in subjects up to 75 years, an observation that contradicted earlier studies (Webster and Leeming, 1975b; Warren *et al.*, 1978).

PANCREAS

The size and weight of the pancreas decreases after the seventh decade of life (Andrew, 1944; Schmitz-Moorman *et al.*, 1985), and ductal epithelial hyperplasia, intralobular fibrosis, acinar cell degranulation and fat accumulation also have been described (Houcke *et al.*, 1964; Kreel and Sandin, 1973). Changes in parenchymal mass are responsible for the relative dilatation of the pancreatic duct system in the elderly (Aoyama *et al.*, 1979). The size of the human liver decreases progressively with age (Howell, 1978; Wynne *et al.*, 1989) accompanied by some reduction in hepatic blood flow (Zoli *et al.*, 1989) and several histologic changes (Sato and Tauchi, 1975; David and Reinke, 1988).

Splanchnic blood and nerve supply

Splanchnic blood flow declines with cardiac output (Texter and Jordan, 1983) and also may fall as a fraction of cardiac output in the elderly (Varga and Csaky, 1976). The fact that infarcts in the mesenteric vessels occur much more commonly in the elderly than in the young indicates that the mesenteric collateral circulation is impaired with age. Much research has been directed to understanding age-related changes in the central nervous system, but little study has been directed to evaluating changes in the nerve supply to the intestine. Much of the available data was summarized after an National Institutes of Health meeting (Szurszewski *et al.*, 1989).

PHYSIOLOGIC CHANGES

At one time it was believed that the process of aging was accompanied by a progressive reduction in the digestion and absorption of both macronutrients and micronutrients. In fact, many of the elderly who lost weight and showed evidence of malnutrition were believed to be suffering from progressive impaired absorption. Since such 'physiologic' decrements in function were believed not to be susceptible to change or treatment, these patients were often allowed to 'dwindle' slowly. It now is recognized that there are relatively few age-dependent decrements of gastrointestinal function that are due to the aging process itself, and that most disorders resulting in impaired digestion and absorption are due to diseases, and thus are potentially treatable.

Nutrient digestion (*see also* Chapter 10)

Digestion, involving hydrolysis of complex nutrients into smaller molecular weight compounds that can be absorbed by the small intestine, occurs both within the intestinal lumen and at the mucosal luminal membrane of epithelial cells. Since macronutrient digestion remains unaffected when pancreatic enzyme production is no more than 10–20 per cent of normal (DiMagno and Summerskill, 1977), little evidence for digestive abnormalities during aging has been found. The responsiveness of the pancreas of aging animals to stimulant peptides such as cholecystokinin or cerulein is reduced (Greenberg and Holt, 1986; Miyasaka and Kitani, 1987). Furthermore, adaptation of pancreatic enzyme secretion to abrupt changes in diet composition is muted (Greenberg *et al.*, 1988). Since protein synthesis is very large and is reduced with age, it is not surprising that amino acid incorporation into pancreatic protein is impaired (Kim *et al.*, 1981).

Carbohydrate digestion is initiated within the intestinal lumen and completed by enzymes present on the intestinal mucosal membrane. Minor changes in brush-border membrane staining by antibodies to intestinal alkaline phosphatase have been described (Moog, 1977). Although the percentage of individuals with lactase deficiency increases with age (Welsh *et al.*, 1978), this probably represents a gradual increase in the number who lose the lactase enzyme during adulthood as a result of a genetic defect in lactase formation or assembly.

Intestinal absorption

It once was believed that many biological functions slowed with age, including the intestinal absorption of lipids, carbohydrates and vitamins (Texter, 1983). Such malabsorption was thought to result in progressive weight loss but most elderly patients lose weight because of reduced caloric intake. However, a review of over 500 healthy ambulatory elderly people, evaluated in a geriatric care facility, showed that 12 per cent were malnourished and, of these cases, 40 per cent involved intestinal malabsorption (McEvoy *et al.*, 1983).

Early studies of carbohydrate absorption in the elderly used xylose as a probe molecule and emphasized

Table 6.1 *Studies of glucose absorption*

Human	
Glucose absorptive capacity reduced	
Xylose absorption shifted distally	
Brush-border uptake reduced	
Animal	
In vivo	
	Glucose absorption reduced
	Galactose absorption reduced
	Shift to distal absorption
In vitro	
	Glucose absorption reduced between 2 and 12 months
	Glucose absorption reduced at 30 months
	Brush-border uptake reduced

how frequently urinary xylose excretion was decreased. However, xylose excretion is exquisitely dependent upon renal function. Careful dual studies of intravenous and orally administered xylose have shown only a slight reduction in absorptive capacity as a function of age (Kendall, 1970; Webster and Leeming, 1975a), which often involves a shift of absorption to more distal intestinal sites (Weiner *et al.*, 1984). Studying carbohydrate absorption by breath hydrogen testing (Feibush and Holt, 1982), showed that young control volunteers were able to consume up to 200 g of carbohydrate without the detection of any excess breath hydrogen, whereas one-third of the over-65 year group excreted excess breath hydrogen after a mixed meal containing 100 g of carbohydrate.

In animals, a moderate fall in intestinal glucose transport with age has been described by several investigators. Carrier-mediated glucose uptake was impaired in jejunal inverted sacs (Doubek and Armbracht, 1987) and during intestinal perfusion (Thompson, 1979; Beaumont *et al.*, 1987; Chen *et al.*, 1990) (Table 6.1).

Limited studies of brush-border uptake in human intestine also suggested a disturbance of sodium-dependent active glucose transport (Vincenzini *et al.*, 1989; Wallis *et al.*, 1993).

The important studies of Ferraris and co-workers (Ferraris *et al.*, 1993) demonstrated a reduction in glucose transporter site density in old animals; however, since these rats showed mucosal hyperplasia, the total number of glucose transporters was no less than in the young. Caloric restriction delayed age-related decreases in nutrient transport. Importantly, observations that ileal villus mass in older animals fed *ad libitum* is greater than in younger animals (Raul *et al.*, 1988; Reville *et al.*, 1991) strongly support a reduction in the duodenal uptake of carbohydrates and increased luminal substrates reaching the distal small intestine.

There is little information about protein absorption in the elderly. Most suggest some decrement in active transport may occur (Penzes *et al.*, 1968; Penzes, 1970, 1974; Navah and Winter, 1988). Ferraris' group suggests that decreased amino-acid uptake may reflect a change in intestinal active transport, related to reduced carrier density (Casirola *et al.*, 1996).

Lipids

The available information concerning changes in the intestinal digestion and absorption of lipids as a function of aging has been summarized by Holt and Balint (1993). The capacity for the intestinal absorption of long-chain triglycerides in humans is very large and greatly exceeds the usual dietary intake. Early studies used techniques that no longer are accepted as accurate (Becker *et al.*, 1950; Webster *et al.*, 1977) and recent studies using disease-free volunteers demonstrated no differences in fecal fat excretion throughout the life span when up to 100 g of fat were eaten (Arora *et al.*, 1989). When emulsified formulas containing high fat concentrations were perfused into the intestine of undernourished older individuals, no diarrhea occurred with as much as 400 g of fat (Simko and Michael, 1989).

In aging rats, Hollander's group described greater intestinal absorption of oleic acid (Hollander and Dadufalza, 1983), cholesterol (Hollander and Morgan, 1979a), cholesterol and vitamin A (Hollander and Morgan, 1979b), vitamin D (Hollander and Tarnawski, 1984) and vitamin E (Hollander and Dadufalza, 1989) in older rats per 100 cm of small intestine when perfusing micellar lipids. Emulsified triglyceride perfusion, however, did demonstrate lower lipid absorption in older rats (Holt and Dominguez, 1981).

There appear to be no significant overall changes in intestinal lipid transport with age. However, physiologic changes in intestinal mucosal lipid transfer and lipoprotein formation have not been extensively explored.

Micronutrient absorption (*see also* Chapter 9)

There is little evidence for any age-related effects on intestinal electrolyte absorption, and only minor changes in the absorption of metals. However, calcium absorption clearly falls with advancing age (Bullamore *et al.*, 1970; Gallagher *et al.*, 1979). The current hypothesis is that reduced calcium absorption in the elderly results from alteration of vitamin D metabolites or their effects (Bullamore *et al.*, 1970; Morris *et al.*, 1985). Plasma 1,25-dihydroxy vitamin D levels are low in elderly subjects and calcium absorption in older individuals fails to respond appropriately to changes in calcium intake (Ireland and Fordtran, 1973). In animal studies, the number of calcium transporters in the basolateral membrane of intestinal cells may fall (Armbrecht *et al.*, 1988) and mucosal vitamin D-dependent calbindin concentrations are reduced. The stimulation of calbindin mRNA by 1,25-dihydroxy vitamin D is unaltered, suggesting a translational defect. Changes in intestinal 1,25-dihydroxy vitamin D receptor sites also have been described (Horst *et al.*, 1990; Takamoto *et al.*, 1990). The colon also may play a role in calcium absorption independent of 1,25-dihydroxy vitamin D. Since achlorhydria is more common in older than younger persons, calcium absorption in the fasting state may be impaired in such individuals (Recker, 1985). However, calcium absorption is maintained normally, even with achlorhydria, when calcium is provided with a meal (Heaney *et al.*, 1989; Axelson *et al.*, 1991). Milk lactose may specifically increase intestinal calcium absorption (Buchowski and Miller, 1991; Schuette *et al.*, 1991), providing a reason for encouraging elderly individuals to consume greater amounts of dairy products. There also is a reduced capacity of the human skin to produce vitamin D_3 from sunlight in advanced age (MacLaughlin and Hollock, 1985).

Vitamins

Water-soluble vitamin absorption is unaltered as a function of age but folate absorption may fall with achlorhydria. Folate is converted to a neutral unionized species in the acidic microenvironment of the glycocalyx, where uptake then occurs by passive diffusion. Reduced folate absorption has been demonstrated in achlorhydric elderly subjects given a test meal of ^{3}H-labeled folic acid ± HCl (Russell *et al.*, 1986) and a reduction in intestinal folate conjugase activity may occur (Baker *et al.*, 1978).

VITAMIN B_{12} ABSORPTION

Serum vitamin B_{12} levels generally are lower in advanced age than in the young (Kilpatrick and Withey, 1965). The intestinal uptake of a test dose of cobalt-labeled vitamin B_{12} is similar to that for younger controls (Hyams, 1964). However, important mechanisms affecting vitamin B_{12} absorption in the elderly include reduced acid and intrinsic factor secretion that may accompany atrophic gastritis and intestinal bacterial overgrowth. Subtle cobalamin deficiency occurs commonly in older free-living and institutionalized individuals when tested by the accumulation of methylmalonic acid and homocysteine (Lindenbaum *et al.*, 1990). The application of these tests showed that the levels of vitamin B_{12} previously accepted as demonstrating depletion were set too low (Pennypacker *et al.*, 1992). Serum vitamin B_{12} concentrations of as high as 220–250 μg/mL may be accompanied by accumulation of these metabolites (Carmel, 1996, 1997). Abnormal deoxyuridine suppression tests responding to vitamin B_{12} administration also occur (Carmel and Karanaze, 1985) and electrophysiologic–neurologic abnormalities have been demonstrated (Carmel, 1994).

Gastric dysfunction is the commonest reason for vitamin B_{12} malabsorption in the elderly. Atrophic gastritis and drugs that suppress gastric acid secretion may cause food cobalamin malabsorption (Walton *et al.*, 1954; Doscherholmen and Swaim, 1973; van Asselt *et al.*, 1998) by impairing release of the vitamin from food proteins. Some authors have even suggested that vitamin B_{12} deficiency may be more frequent in elderly patients with Alzheimer's disease (Joosten *et al.*, 1997; Pennypacker *et al.*, 1992). Physicians have become increasingly aware of vitamin B_{12} depletion in older subjects and some are treating patients at risk with oral crystalline vitamin B_{12}.

The data for aging and malabsorption of fat-soluble vitamins also have been summarized by Holt and Balint (1993). The evidence for age-related vitamin D malabsorption has led increasing numbers of geriatricians to recommend supplemental vitamin D of up to 800 IU/day. No changes in vitamin A and vitamin K absorption occurs except in the presence of gastrointestinal diseases.

Proliferation

In 1993, our group summarized available data on proliferation in the small intestine as a function of age (Atillasoy and Holt, 1993). The information on small intestinal proliferation appears to fly in the face of established concepts of the effect of aging on cellular reproduction. These concepts followed upon the classical work of Hayflick and Moorehead (1961) showing loss of proliferation after a fixed number of fibroblast doubling in culture *in vitro*. Changes in proliferation can have profound effect on the morphology and functions of the small intestine because cell production and migration are so rapid.

Although early studies suggested reduced proliferation of the small bowel in aged animals (Lesher *et al.*, 1961; Fry *et al.*, 1962), more recent studies demonstrated that there are no changes in proliferation (Cullan *et al.*, 1982; Ecknauer *et al.*, 1982). Greater proliferative activities have been detected (Holt and Yeh, 1988). Starvation and refeeding induced major impairment of adaptive response in older rats (Holt *et al.*, 1988; Holt and Luk, 1990). Increased small intestinal polyamine concentrations have also been found (Poston *et al.*, 1990; Yoshinaga *et al.*, 1993). Importantly, restoration of normal gut mucosal mass following intestinal resection takes longer to return to normal in older animals than in younger animals (Dimri and Campisi, 1994).

The precise molecular and biochemical reasons for changes in proliferation as a function of age still are not understood. Data from studies of senescent fibroblasts demonstrate a block in the G1 phase of the cell cycle. Data on genes involved in G1 have shown reduced transcription factor binding activities, e.g. to AP1 and CREBP (Robetorye *et al.*, 1996), and overexpression of CDK inhibitor genes encoding P21 and P16 accompanied by impaired phosphorylation of the retinoblastoma (RB) tumor suppressor protein (Greider, 1990; Stein *et al.*, 1990).

A new approach to understanding the effect of senescence involves studies of telomeres and the enzyme, telomerase. In cultured human fibroblasts, the mean length of the terminal restriction fragment of chromosomes was decreased in a replication-dependent manner accompanied by a reduction in the expression of the enzyme telomerase (Broccoli *et al.*, 1995). Changes in telomeres and telomerase during aging now have been extended to studies of tumors that fail to suppress proliferation. The relationship of aging to the development of epithelial tumors has raised the question of whether proliferative changes may be related to tumorigenesis (Atillasoy and Holt, 1993). Certainly, failure of cell-cycle checkpoint proteins and tumor suppressor genes suggests that aging may be an indirect effect of the cell's attempt to suppress tumorigenesis (Moss *et al.*, 1996).

APOPTOSIS

Another defect that could account for an age-related change in intestinal proliferation is altered cell death. We have recently measured apoptosis in the small intestine of young and aging animals who were fed *ad libitum* and calorie restricted (Holt *et al.*, 1998), and found that restriction in aging rats was associated with a significantly higher intestinal apoptotic rate. These studies imply that enhanced apoptosis with caloric restriction might protect the gastrointestinal tract from accumulation of DNA altered cells during the aging process.

Motor function and motility

There are a number of reasons why motor function might be altered in the elderly. However, older, healthy volunteers may not differ in their rate of intestinal transit from that measured in the young (Varga, 1976; Melkersson *et al.*, 1983; Haboubi *et al.*, 1988). Little difference in small intestinal transit also was detected in aging animals (McDougal *et al.*, 1980). Overall, small intestinal motor patterns are maintained in old age. Early studies concluded that fasting motor patterns were unchanged, but that the frequency and strength of contractions were less in older subjects (Anuras and Sutherland, 1984; Fich *et al.*, 1989). Normal findings also were confirmed in a small number of healthy older volunteers (Husebye and Engedal, 1992). Preliminary studies found changes in interdigestive motor motility patterns, accompanied by elevated serum motilin concentrations without the normal cyclical fluctuations seen in younger subjects (Bortolotti *et al.*, 1987). Altered fasting motor patterns have been described in patients with intestinal bacterial overgrowth (Vantrappen *et al.*, 1977), but whether this is a major factor for this syndrome presently is unclear.

Defense mechanisms

CHANGES IN IMMUNE FUNCTIONS

Aging generally is characterized by an overall decline in the effectiveness of the immune system (Makinodan and Kay, 1990). However, studies of immune function in older individuals generally have only tested effects on systemic immune defenses. The gut-associated lymphoid tissue (GALT) consists of cells in Peyer's patches, mesenteric lymph nodes as well as effector lymphocytes, and plasma cells within the lamina propria and intraepithelial cells. There is some evidence that the functional size of Peyer's patches decreases in the elderly, probably starting in middle age (Goodman and Makinodan, 1975). In humans over the age of 70, more immunoglobulin secretion and higher intraepithelial IgA plasma cell counts were described (Arranz *et al.*, 1992). The responses of the GALT to stimulant has been shown to be lower in older than in young animals (Kawanishi *et al.*, 1990; Kawanishi and Joseph, 1992). In addition, changes in the secretion of dimeric IgA that passes from the liver through the biliary system into the gastrointestinal tract were described in rodents (Taylor *et al.*, 1990) but the application of this observation to humans is less clear (Dooley *et al.*, 1982).

RESPONSES TO STRESS

A general physiologic phenomenon that frequently is described during the aging process is that, although basal organ functions may be maintained as well as in the young, the responses to stress, i.e. adaptation to a new stimulus, generally are impaired. This appears to apply to the intestine as well.

Classically, small intestinal responses to stress are evaluated by determining the effect of intestinal resection in rodents or by evaluating the responses to abrupt changes in food intake. As described above, aging did delay the small intestine recovery from partial intestinal resection and alter the responses to changes in nutrient intake.

Hormonal response

The gastrointestinal tract is the largest endocrine organ of the body and is specialized for the production of a wide variety of peptides, which can alter the function of the gastrointestinal tract itself or other tissues in the body. Changes in gastrointestinal peptide activity could result from altered tissue production (synthesis, molecular peptide processing or peptide release), circulating levels or a change in end-organ cellular effects (such as altered receptor number, or binding, intracellular signaling or gene activation). Furthermore, circadian rhythms of peptide actions also may be changed as a function of age. Despite the potential importance of such changes in peptide secretion and action in the elderly, relatively few studies have been performed. The response of pancreatic growth to gastrin is blunted (Majumdar and Dubick, 1991), changes in pancreatic receptors occur (Poston *et al.*, 1989), and trophic responses to cerulein (Greenberg *et al.*, 1988) and bombesin (Poston *et al.*, 1988) have been described.

A dramatic increase in fasting and postprandial concentrations of serum pancreatic polypeptide have been shown to be present in 60–84-year-old non-diabetic volunteers (Khalil *et al.*, 1985). The precise reasons and effects of these changes are unknown. Circulating motilin and neurotensin concentrations also may be high in the elderly (Khalil and Thompson, 1987). Hyperglucagonemia occurs in some elderly subjects (Marco *et al.*, 1977). These changes have been ascribed to altered end-organ receptor number or affinity, which does occur in the gallbladder (Murakami *et al.*, 1991). Whether this is an adequate explanation for the elevated serum levels of peptides described above is not known.

DISEASE STATES

General issues

Many gastrointestinal symptoms are reported by older patients to their physicians yet, in contrast to those in young patients, usually relatively little is known about the etiology. Two studies have focused on the frequency of gastrointestinal symptoms in older individuals. A study from the UK suggested that one-third of elderly symptomatic patients had a history consistent with some sort of functional bowel disorder (Thompson and Heaton, 1980). In a study of non-institutionalized Olmstead County, Minnesota residents aged between 65 and 93 years, about 25 per cent of respondents reported the presence of frequent abdominal pain, 25 per cent complained of constipation and 14 per cent of chronic diarrhea (Talley *et al.*, 1992). Over 10 per cent had symptoms compatible with the irritable bowel syndrome using the Manning criteria. However, most of the surveyed individuals had not seen a physician for these symptoms. These data suggest that abdominal complaints are common in the older population, and generally are underdiagnosed and probably undertreated. The reasons for complaints of chronic diarrhea were not analysed.

The diagnosis of an acute abdominal emergency often is erroneous in the older patient. An accurate history may be difficult to obtain because of a patient's failing memory or fear of medical care. Physical signs of acute abdominal diseases may be altered by central or peripheral nervous system disorders. Thus, tenderness, pain, muscle rigidity and guarding may be minimal or absent. The common use of non-steroidal anti-inflammatory drugs for chronic diseases also impairs the patient's responses. Furthermore, multiple abdominal disease processes may be present simultaneously. For example, gallstones and diverticulosis are common, so that acute mesenteric ischemia or intestinal obstruction may be misdiagnosed. Furthermore, acute appendicitis often does not present classically with anorexia, fever and right lower quadrant pain, so that many older individuals have a long delay prior to surgery. As a result, frank perforation is much more common in older than younger patients (Horattas *et al.*, 1990).

Abdominal surgery for intestinal disorders in the elderly

Small bowel disorders can lead to major abdominal surgery, which can present more problems in elderly patients harboring other serious illnesses. Equality of access to surgery is an issue because surgeons believe that age alone increases mortality and morbidity; however, this occurs as a result of associated cardiovascular and respiratory disease, and not age. With careful attention to these disorders there is no greater risk of surgery in the elderly than in the young. Recent development in gastrointestinal surgery, such as the widespread introduction of laparoscopic surgery, has improved the prognosis of the older patient. Fear of complications can delay necessary abdominal exploration. Emergency surgery then results in a far greater risk of serious complications than elective surgery. The perioperative diagnostic accuracy of the acute abdomen is poorest in the older patient (Koruda and Sheldon, 1991).

Diarrhea

Although acute diarrheal disorders usually affect young children, over 50 per cent of deaths occur amongst individuals aged 74 and more than one-quarter occur in the 55–74-year age range (Lew *et al.*, 1991). The old may be at increased risk of dying from diarrhea because they may develop dehydration and electrolyte problems; they have impaired immunity and often are institutionalized in hospitals and nursing homes. Over 85 per cent of patients over age 55 with diarrhea have a reported diagnosis of non-infectious gastroenteritis (Lew *et al.*, 1991). Most deaths occur in the winter and in patients in long-term care facilities. It seems likely that defects in both immune and non-immune defenses may play an important role in gastrointestinal infections in the elderly (Ratnaike, 1990).

Chronic diarrhea occurs quite commonly in older patients (Holt, 1990). Physicians must specifically ask about diarrhea. The elderly often complain freely of constipation but are less likely to volunteer complaints of diarrhea because they are fastidious, and because diarrhea frequently produces incontinence. Infectious causes of diarrhea should always be considered even if prolonged symptoms are present. One report emphasized the presence of unexpected infection with *Giardia lamblia* in older persons with diarrhea and failure to thrive (Beaumont and James, 1986).

C. difficile-associated colitis occurs commonly in elderly patients. The diagnosis may be difficult to make with certainty because *C. difficile* toxin is found in the feces in elderly patients in over 30 per cent of nursing-home residents. Elimination of the organism with antibiotics can be difficult and the mortality rate of elderly patients in whom *C. difficile* toxin is found was described as over 40 per cent (Bender *et al.*, 1986). Thus, the finding of *C. difficile* toxin in elderly patients with diarrhea may not necessarily indicate the presence of *C. difficile* colitis.

Drugs are a common cause of chronic diarrhea in the elderly, principally because they consume so many medications (Table 6.2). Drugs may cause diarrhea either because of a direct effect upon receptors on the intestinal mucosa, because of damage to mucosal cells and altered intestinal motility (see below), or because of increased sodium and water secretion by the gut. Many drugs have been incriminated as causing diarrhea in older individuals and one approach to diagnosis is to eliminate many of the medications the patient is taking.

Diarrhea occurs very commonly in patients with diabetes mellitus. Classically, such diarrhea occurs nocturnally, often with incontinence, but it can occur at other times and frequently is intermittent (Feldman and Schiller, 1983) and may not be correlated with neuropathy. Diabetic diarrhea may be very severe or mild (Schiller *et al.*, 1982). Owing to the clinical association with neuropathic findings elsewhere in some patients, damage to the autonomic nervous system is believed to be responsible for severe diarrhea (Fedorak *et al.*, 1985). Alpha-2 agonists such as clonidine can reduce stool output (Schiller *et al.*, 1985) but only in large doses, which may induce unacceptable hypotension and somnolence. Symptomatic relief can result from administration of broad-spectrum antibiotics to reduce bacterial overgrowth. Treatment with bile salt-sequestering resins also may be successful.

Table 6.2 *Drugs that may cause small bowel diarrhea*

Antimetabolites (e.g. 5-fluorouracil)
Cardiovascular drugs including diuretics and antiarrhythmics
Gastrointestinal agents, e.g. bile salts, misoprostol, lactulose, magnesium-containing antacids
Cholesterol-lowering drugs, such as cholestyramine
Colchicine
Antibiotics, e.g. neomycin

Malabsorption syndromes

The diseases resulting in malabsorption in the elderly are very similar to those seen in younger patients (Montgomery *et al.*, 1986). Malabsorption often results from pancreatic disease and from celiac disease, or is associated with past surgery for peptic ulcer disease (Price *et al.*, 1977). Malabsorption syndromes whose prevalence is common in older patients include bacterial overgrowth syndrome (Roberts *et al.*, 1977) and, occasionally, chronic intestinal vascular disease (Shaw and Maynard, 1958).

Pancreatic insufficiency without a history of acute pancreatitis or alcoholism is a peculiar feature in the elderly. One study of chronic pancreatitis of unknown etiology found that three-quarters of the patients were elderly (Ammann and Sulser, 1976). Pancreatic calcification and exocrine pancreatic failure of unknown cause has been described in France (Laugier and Sarles, 1985) and Japan (Nagai and Ohtsubo, 1984). However, macronutrient malabsorption resulting from pancreatic insufficiency is quite rare.

CELIAC DISEASE

The incidence of new cases of celiac (non-tropical) sprue is bimodal with a first peak in the fourth decade and a second in the seventh decade. Up to one-third of patients newly diagnosed with celiac disease are older then 60 years of age (Campbell *et al.*, 1977; Kirby and Fielding, 1984; Logan *et al.*, 1986).

The clinical presentation of sprue in elderly patients may be quite different from that seen in the young: only 25 per cent have diarrhea and weight loss as major clinical symptoms (Swinson and Levi, 1980). Most older patients present with vague symptoms of dyspepsia and ill health (Table 6.3). Micronutrient depletion presenting with low serum folate concentration or low serum iron without gastrointestinal bleeding should suggest the diagnosis of sprue (McIntyre and Long, 1993). Patients with unusually severe osteopenia or osteomalacia may have this disease; patients also may present with associated autoimmune diseases. The frequency of

Table 6.3 *Common manifestations of celiac disease that may be misdiagnosed in the elderly*

Weight loss
Anemia (iron-deficient, folate-deficient)
Osteopenia (or fractures with minimal trauma)
Weakness
Muscular atrophy
Central nervous system disturbances
Impotence
Peripheral edema

Table 6.4 *Possible mediators of drug-induced malabsorption*

1. Direct toxic effect causing morphologic changes in the intestinal mucosa, e.g. by neomycin or colchicine.
2. The inhibition of mucosal enzymes with or without morphologic evidence of mucosal damage, e.g. azulfidine or colchicine.
3. Binding and precipitation of micellar compounds, such as bile acids, e.g. neomycin cholestyramine.
4. Alterations of the physiochemical state of another drug, e.g. dietary iron by antacids.
5. Interfering with intestinal transit, e.g. tricyclic antidepressants.

making the diagnosis of celiac disease in the elderly is directly related to how often small intestinal biopsies are performed (Swinson and Levi, 1980; Gillberg *et al.*, 1984). An abnormal small bowel biopsy has the same diagnostic accuracy in older as in the younger patients, i.e. aging does not alter small bowel histology. Serologic tests have similar sensitivity and specificity in old and young individuals (Attia and Holt, 1995).

The clinical presentation of elderly patients with malabsorption can be subtle because symptoms often result from the effects of unabsorbed nutrients entering the colon. The colon appears to be less reactive in older individuals. In addition, lymphoma of the small intestine may be particularly common when celiac disease appears late in life (Swinson *et al.*, 1983). The clinical features of intestinal lymphoma complicating celiac disease are covert and lymphoma may specifically need to be excluded. Conversely, T-cell lymphomas may present as sprue (Isaacson, 1995). The incidence of several other malignancies in patients with sprue increases with duration of clinical follow-up. Extra-intestinal malignancies, particularly of the reticuloendothelial system and squamous cell cancers of the skin, occur more commonly as sprue patients grow older. Some patients may develop diffuse intestinal ulceration, which may be very difficult to distinguish from classical celiac disease (Robertson *et al.*, 1983). Splenic atrophy associated with cavitation of mesenteric lymph nodes and accompanied by atrophy of the upper intestinal mucosa occurs in older patients and may occasionally respond to a gluten-free diet. Some elderly sprue patients may develop subacute intestinal pseudo-obstruction syndrome (Dawson *et al.*, 1984). Older patients do not adapt easily to a dramatic change in diet, so that treatment with a gluten-free diet must be accompanied by intensive nutritional advice. Close supervision of the levels of micronutrients during follow-up is mandatory.

BACTERIAL OVERGROWTH

Bacterial overgrowth occurs far more commonly in the elderly than in the young (Hellemans *et al.*, 1984). One study of healthy, ambulatory elderly people found that, of 20 per cent with malnutrition, 35 per cent were found to have malabsorption, the majority of whom had bacterial overgrowth (McEvoy *et al.*, 1983). The factors that contribute to bacterial overgrowth become more prominent with age. The phase III migrating interdigestive motor complex may be disturbed, gastric acid secretion may be less and anatomic changes that lead to bacterial overgrowth, such as jejunal diverticulosis, are much more common.

The degree to which such bacterial accumulation results in clinical or metabolic changes is quite variable. In the classical small bowel overgrowth syndrome, diarrhea and steatorrhea are prominent, but in older patients only nutritional depletion may occur. Opposing conclusions were reached in two studies of the elderly from England (Haboubi and Montgomery, 1992; Lipski *et al.*, 1992). A recent study also emphasized the frequency of evidence of upper intestinal overgrowth with colonic-type bacteria in elderly patients with chronic diarrhea, anorexia or nausea even without overt signs (Riordan *et al.*, 1997). Most elderly patients with small bowel bacterial overgrowth have normal bowel anatomy.

There is also evidence that fecal bacteria, as well as their enzymes, may change in type as a function of age (Goldin *et al.*, 1978). In humans, the influence of the environment, including the diet, probably is more important than the effect of age (Mitsuoka, 1992).

Drugs may cause malabsorption by several different mechanisms (Table 6.4). Fortunately, few drugs taken by older patients cause malabsorption.

Motility disorders

INTESTINAL PSEUDO-OBSTRUCTION SYNDROMES

Intestinal pseudo-obstruction is a clinical syndrome in which the signs or symptoms of intestinal obstruction are found, but without any demonstrable obstructing lesion (Faulk *et al.*, 1978; Quigley, 1996). Pseudo-obstruction can involve any part of the gastrointestinal tract, may be isolated, or may be part of a more generalized process. Clinically, there is an acute form that often presents as a transit disorder occurring in older patients who are chronically ill. In addition, there is a chronic variety that is recurrent and can occur in patients of all ages.

Primary intestinal pseudo-obstruction occurs in the absence of an association with other diseases. Patients typically have recurrent attacks of nausea, vomiting, abdominal discomfort and abdominal distension (Verne and Snisky, 1995). With time, there is an increase in the frequency of the obstructive symptoms measured, followed by a chronic state with bacterial overgrowth. Radiologic abnormalities occur in the esophagus, stomach and/or the colon, showing dilatation and abnormal transit. Abnormalities of esophageal manometry are often found. Disorders can affect the smooth muscle, the nerve supply or the collagen of the small intestine (Krishnamurthy and Schuffler, 1987).

Transient acute pseudo-obstruction (or ileus) usually occurs in elderly patients with other diseases, including congestive heart failure, uremia, acute infections and sepsis (Table 6.5). Acute pseudo-obstruction may be associated with low serum levels of potassium, calcium and/or magnesium, and correction of metabolic abnormalities can return normal function. Impaired small bowel propulsive function from drugs can lead to the clinical picture of intestinal obstruction.

Megaduodenum is a localized form of intestinal dilatation. Rarely, mechanical megaduodenum occurs with the superior mesenteric artery syndrome resulting from prolonged immobility. Vomiting and abdominal discomfort are common complaints reflecting upper intestinal obstruction. Megaduodenum also may be seen as part of a generalized pseudo-obstruction syndrome.

Chronic intestinal pseudo-obstruction, due to myopathy or neuropathy, occurs when recurrent attacks of clinical acute obstruction cease to have any remissions. This syndrome occurs mostly in the elderly, since the conditions that are causative occur commonly in that age group (Table 6.5). Whether changes in autonomic nerve supply and/or intestinal smooth muscle and collagen, which may occur with aging, contribute to this frequency is unknown.

Amyloidosis affects either muscle or nerve supply or both, and dermatomyositis or polymyositis occasionally involves the small bowel. Important in the elderly is paraneoplastic visceral neuropathy (DiBaise and Quigley, 1998), resulting not only from carcinoma of the lung (Schuffler *et al.*, 1992) but also a wide variety of other tumors (Chin and Schuffler, 1988). Recently, antienteric neuronal antibodies associated with myenteric plexus degeneration have been described (Lennon *et al.*, 1991; Condom *et al.*, 1993). Other antibodies occur (Gerl *et al.*, 1992). This syndrome may precede the discovery of the cancer and thus may be initially diagnosed as pseudo-obstruction of unknown etiology.

Agents used to treat patients with cancer, such as vinca alkaloids and opiates, may all be associated with chronic pseudo-obstruction syndrome.

Table 6.5 *Causes of intestinal pseudo-obstruction in the elderly*

Acute intestinal pseudo-obstruction
Infections, e.g. sepsis, pneumonia
Inflammatory, e.g. pancreatitis
Miscellaneous
Electrolyte disturbances
Congestive heart failure
Drugs, e.g. anticholinergics, colchicine, vincristine, antidepressants
Clinical intestinal pseudo-obstruction
Renal failure
Diabetes, myxedema, hypoparathyroidism
Neuromuscular – parkinsonism
Radiation
Collagen vascular disorders, e.g. scleroderma, dermatomyositis, polymyositis
Amyloidosis
Infections, e.g. herpes zoster, Epstein–Barr virus, cytomegalovirus
Paraneoplastic visceral neuropathy

Small bowel diverticulosis

In the absence of congenital abnormalities and systemic disorders involving intestinal collagen or smooth muscle, diverticulosis of the small intestine is diagnosed mainly in older patients. Evidence of small bowel diverticulosis is seen in 1–2 per cent of barium x-ray studies (Eggert *et al.*, 1982), usually as an incidental finding, but several metabolic disturbances can occur. Diverticula of the small bowel frequently are multiple in the upper jejunum but may be found diffusely throughout the entire small intestine. They are 'pseudodiverticula' lacking a muscular coat and are atonic, filling easily with small intestinal contents during peristalsis, but emptying slowly.

Small bowel diverticulosis can produce local complications including perforation, hemorrhage or inflammation, just as in other diverticulae of the gastrointestinal tract. Occasionally, hemorrhage may be arterial and can be fatal. Small bowel diverticula may be demonstrated during the radiologic evaluation of patients with symptoms of obscure abdominal pain, but such symptoms rarely should be ascribed to the presence of diverticulosis. Multiple small bowel diverticulosis may also result in extensive bacterial overgrowth. The number and size of diverticulae do not necessarily correlate with the degree of metabolic changes consequent upon bacterial overgrowth, although, in general, more proximal diverticulae produce the greatest disorder.

Solitary duodenal diverticulae without diverticulosis of the remainder of the small intestine can be identified in up to 5 per cent of routine radiologic studies and up to 20 per cent of autopsies, but rarely cause symptoms. They do not occur in the first part of the duodenum where pseudodiverticulosis from peptic ulcer disease is found. Diverticulae in the region of the ampulla of Vater are associated with an increased incidence of biliary calculi and biliary symptoms, especially in the elderly (Kennedy and Thompson, 1988). Benign duodenal diverticulae can be associated with obstruction of the common bile duct or the pancreatic duct. Occasionally, intestinal contents may stagnate in a diverticulum forming a concretion (enterolith), which can obstruct the intestine (Shocket and Simon, 1982). This intraluminal diverticulum presents with obstruction extending distally into the duodenum and does not fill with barium, but has a radiologic picture resembling a pedunculated polyp (Fleming *et al.*, 1975).

Inflammatory bowel disease (*see also* Chapter 25)

Non-specific inflammatory bowel disease is thought of as a disorder of the young, yet both ulcerative colitis and Crohn's disease increasingly is first diagnosed in the elderly, or continues its course and requires treatment in patients in whom the diagnosis was made at an earlier age. The prevalence of Crohn's disease has changed over time. In 1958, Crohn and Yarnis (1958) reported that only 4.3 per cent of their 530 patients had the onset of illness after age 50. In striking contrast, a recent study described that over 30 per cent of their patients diagnosed in the 1960s were over age 50 (Smith *et al.*, 1975). The reported incidence of Crohn's disease in Cardiff, Wales, increased 50-fold between 1931 and 1985, with a similar incidence in those over 70 and in their 20s (Rose *et al.*, 1988). A summary of the incidence of late-onset Crohn's disease has been published (Grimm and Friedman, 1990). It is unclear whether the peak incidence in older patients represents a different disease or the same disease altered by age-related factors. Overall, the data in the elderly suggests that ulcerative colitis is commoner in males, whereas Crohn's disease is commoner in females (Shapiro *et al.*, 1981; Farmer *et al.*, 1985). In a survey of 2657 inflammatory bowel disease patients that comprised the Organization Mondiale de Gastroenterologie (OMGE) study material, Softley *et al.* (1988) found that less than 10 per cent were over the age of 60 at the time of registration into the survey.

The clinical features of older Crohn's disease patients differ somewhat from those of their younger counterparts. Most patients report diarrhea, weight loss and abdominal pain. Acute Crohn's disease of the terminal ileum (acute regional enteritis) occurs more commonly in children than adults but has been described in the elderly. Older patients may have a more gradual onset of the disease but this may be due to a failure to make an early diagnosis. Elderly patients with ileal involvement clinically may present acutely with peritonitis, massive intestinal bleeding or small bowel obstruction (Fabricus *et al.*, 1985; Lee and Gaiffer, 1987), or the symptoms may be confused with distal intestinal ulceration associated with non-steroidal anti-inflammatory drug use. Occasionally, the illness may be quite atypical (Eisen *et al.*, 1993). Crohn's disease in the elderly commonly affects the distal colon (Truelove and Pena, 1976; Carr and Schofield, 1982); however, proximal small bowel, gastroduodenal and even esophageal involvement has been described. Concomitant illness may confuse the clinical picture. For example, if anemia develops, it may present with angina in a patient with cardiovascular disease.

The elderly are prone to nutritional deficiencies and may present with spontaneous fractures, fractures from minor trauma or with vertebral collapse because of calcium malabsorption. Extraintestinal manifestations of the disease probably occur with similar frequently at all ages but may not be recognized quickly. Elderly patients presenting with arthritis, ankylosing spondylitis or pyoderma gangrenosa are usually misdiagnosed.

Carcinoma of the small bowel does not occur more commonly as a function of age but rather develops with prolonged duration of the disease. Furthermore, extraintestinal malignancies occur more commonly in the elderly, including esophageal tumors, squamous cell skin cancers (Ekbom *et al.*, 1991) and reticuloendothelial neoplasms (Greenstein *et al.*, 1985).

Laboratory abnormalities and radiologic findings are similar at all ages, and the endoscopic appearance also is similar. A prolonged course and a delay in diagnosis is very common in the elderly. One report stated that a diagnosis of Crohn's disease was made about 6.4 years after the onset of symptoms in older patients compared to 2.4 years in younger patients (Harper *et al.*, 1986).

DIFFERENTIAL DIAGNOSIS

The differential diagnosis of elderly patients with Crohn's disease is more difficult than in younger individuals. Non-specific symptoms of ill health may be misinterpreted because of the high incidence of other diseases. Gastrointestinal infections occur commonly, and may be confusing (Table 6.6). *Shigella*, infection with the *C. difficile* organism, and *E. coli* O157:H7 are seen. *Yersinia* and tuberculosis affect the terminal ileum, and present difficulty in diagnosis. Small bowel obstructive symptoms in the elderly are usually attributed to postsurgical adhesions and not to Crohn's disease.

Table 6.6 *Differential diagnosis of small bowel Crohn's disease*

1 Infections (usually affect the colon)
Yersinia
Shigella, Salmonella
C. difficile
E. coli 0157:A7
Tuberculosis
2 Tumors
Ileo-cecal carcinoma
Lymphoma, carcinoid
3 Drugs
Non-steroidal anti-inflammatory drugs
Potassium
4 Enteropathic arthropathies
5 Radiation, ischemia
6 Vasculitides

Other diagnoses that can cause confusion include ileo-cecal carcinoma and carcinoid tumors (Table 6.6) presenting as a mass lesion or intestinal obstruction. Tuberculosis may perfectly mimic Crohn's disease.

Drugs, particularly non-steroidal anti-inflammatory drugs, which cause inflammation of the terminal ileum (Bjarnason *et al.*, 1993) and consequent potassium chloride ulceration, are in the differential diagnosis. Radiation damage to the small bowel should not be missed if an adequate history is obtained. Ischemia may produce chronic symptoms and fibrotic strictures of the colon, but will usually present with an acute event in the small bowel. Enteropathic arthropathies with inflammation in biopsies of the terminal ileum can mimic Crohn's disease.

PROGNOSIS AND OUTCOME

Early studies suggested a poor prognosis for attacks of Crohn's disease in the elderly. More recently, the overall prognosis of Crohn's disease in the elderly has been established as perhaps being even better than in the young (Softley *et al.*, 1988). However, older patients with ileo-colonic or ileal Crohn's disease may benefit more from earlier surgery than younger patients. The reasons for this are that recurrences are less common or occur at longer intervals in elderly patients, so that recurrences are less likely in their lifetime (Cooke *et al.*, 1980; Aimerman *et al.*, 1985), and there may be concerns about diagnoses such as ileo-cecal cancer. One study has demonstrated no recurrences of Crohn's disease for 10 years in older patients (Harper *et al.*, 1986).

MEDICAL MANAGEMENT

Treatment with large doses of antidiarrheal agents must be carefully monitored because of the risk of central nervous depression. There is no evidence that azulfidine or 5-aminosalicylic acid compounds are poorly tolerated in the elderly, permitting administration of full doses. Antibiotics also have no special risks in the elderly.

Corticosteroid therapy, however, is accompanied by serious side-effects in older patients. Bone loss, added to underlying age-associated osteopenia, and the additional bone loss accompanying active inflammatory bowel disease can lead rapidly to fractures or vertebral collapse. Corticosteroid treatment results in changes in mood, and dementia and rapid progression of cataract formation are hazards. Corticosteroids can be used to bring an acute attack of Crohn's disease under control, but the drug should be discontinued as rapidly as possible.

Because of the side-effects of corticosteroid therapy, the immunomodulators, azathioprine and 6-mercaptopurine, should be introduced rapidly into the therapy of older patients with active Crohn's disease. There is no evidence that these agents produce any more side-effects in the elderly than in the young. Indeed, the potential concern of physicians for the development of lymphoma with long-term use of 6-mercaptopurine or azathioprine is modulated in patients whose life expectancy is shorter. Whether older patients can tolerate the newer immunomodulators, such as tumor necrosis factor antibodies, presently is unknown.

SURGICAL MANAGEMENT

Older studies of surgery in elderly patients with Crohn's disease suggested that the mortality rate was very high. This probably resulted from the fact that surgery was delayed until patients were too ill to tolerate major bowel resection well. Recent data indicate the risks of surgery for inflammatory bowel disease relate to the severity of the primary illness and to comorbid conditions, and not to patient age. When surgery is necessary for strictures, stricturoplasty rather than intestinal resection is particularly useful. The development of laparoscopic intestinal surgery also has improved the postoperative care of older patients.

Cancer

More than half of all gastrointestinal cancers occur in people older than 65 years of age, and most mortality occurs in this group (Kennedy, 1992). Physiologic factors invoked to explain the rapid increase in gastrointestinal epithelial tumors with age include the accumulation of DNA damage (Ebbesen, 1984), dysregulation of growth control (Martin, 1993), decreased apoptosis (Laderoute, 1994), errors in the synthesis of DNA, postmitotic damage induced by free radicals and/or glycosylation amongst others

(Cohen, 1974; Hart and Turturro, 1992), decreased DNA repair (Neidermuller, 1983), and the induction of telomerase.

Whether the clinical course of cancer in older individuals is more or less benign than in the young is unclear. Important potential factors in the increasing mortality from cancer seen in elderly patients are changes in the pattern of care and treatment decisions (Samet *et al.*, 1986; Newcomb and Carbone, 1993). Physicians undertreat elderly patients with chemotherapy because of fear of toxicity (Fentiman *et al.*, 1990). Most data indicate that the elderly tolerate the usual regimens as well as younger patients (Begg and Carbone, 1983; Giovanazi-Bannon *et al.*, 1994). Fear of the side-effects of radiation probably results in increased mortality in patients with intestinal tumors (Yuhas *et al.*, 1969; Steinfeld *et al.*, 1989; Farniok and Levitt, 1994). Although some studies suggest that the intestine of older mice is more sensitive to radiation injury than that of younger animals, other studies of repeated radiation showed essentially no difference in intestinal proliferative responses (Hamilton and Franks, 1979).

SMALL BOWEL TUMORS

Small intestinal malignancies account for just over 1 per cent of gastrointestinal cancers and 0.8 per cent of digestive tract cancer deaths in the USA (Boring *et al.*, 1992), and most occur in the elderly (Neugut *et al.*, 1998). Most benign adenomas and malignant carcinomas occur in the proximal intestine close to the entry of the bile duct, suggesting that bile components such as bile acids are pathogenic. Adenomas pass through the same series of sequential histological changes as adenomas in the large intestine, including progressive dysplasia, leading to villous changes. Villous adenomas have a high prevalence of developing cancer and often contain invasive cancer (Bjork *et al.*, 1990).

Lymphomas and carcinoid tumors also occur mainly in the elderly, usually in the distal small intestine, presenting with intestinal obstruction and/or acute gastrointestinal bleeding. Chronic blood loss with iron-deficiency anemia is occasionally seen. The diagnosis is often made only at the time of surgery (Weingrad *et al.*, 1982). Malignant carcinoid tumors may present with metastases and the symptoms and signs of classical carcinoid syndrome. About 10 per cent of non-Hodgkin's lymphomas have gastrointestinal involvement. Many patients with small bowel lymphomas have tumors that involve several segments of the digestive tract simultaneously at the time of diagnosis (Ruskone-Fourmestraux, 1993).

Metastatic tumors also may present as tumors of the small intestine. An unusual but classical small bowel metastatic tumor is malignant melanoma.

Vascular disease involving the small bowel

Vascular diseases affecting the small bowel induce varying degrees of ischemia depending upon the degree of vascular occlusion and the adequacy of blood supply through anastomoses. The clinical manifestation depends upon the severity and duration of the ischemic insult, and the degree of clinical suspicion determines the rapidity of diagnosis and prognosis. Occlusive ischemic disease may affect either the mesenteric arteries or mesenteric veins, or the ischemia may be non-occlusive.

Acute ischemic syndromes result from temporary or permanent reduction in the vascular flow, inducing gut wall ischemia. Spasm of the vessels and reduced perfusion pressure aggravates the ischemic insult, resulting in tissue infarction and gangrene, often with perforation or peritonitis. Because older patients have cardiovascular, renal or other systemic disorders, mortality rates of up to 70 per cent are reported (Boley *et al.*, 1977). About half of all acute mesenteric infarction is caused by embolic or thrombotic occlusion of the superior mesenteric artery, and the remainder from non-occlusive infarction (Ottinger, 1982). The gut ischemia results in loss of fluid into the gut, hyperkalemia and late metabolic acidosis. Radiologic bowel wall thickening, thumbprinting and loop separation are relatively late features. Rapid evaluation of the mesenteric vascular system is mandatory in order to make an early diagnosis.

The existence of chronic ischemic syndromes of the bowel is controversial (Rogers and Cohen, 1985), since extensive collateral flow usually develops. The classical syndrome of postprandial abdominal pain, similar to exercise-induced angina, is rarely found. Some patients may complain of weight loss and diarrhea or non-specific gastrointestinal complaints. The diagnosis of chronic mesenteric ischemia is a major challenge: abdominal symptoms are common in elderly individuals, laboratory findings are unrevealing, and angiographic examination may not help because obstruction to two or even all three major mesenteric arteries occurs without any abdominal symptoms. Thus, arteriosclerotic occlusions are commonly seen amongst the elderly population but intestinal angina is very rare. Enthusiastic surgical reports have been published (Stanton *et al.*, 1986) but the mortality rate has been high (Cunningham *et al.*, 1991). Intravascular balloon angioplasty of arterioscleroticlemias in major mesenteric vessels might allow for better testing of the potential results of more extensive surgical treatment.

Focal ischemic disease of the small bowel also may occur. The majority of these represent the result of collagen vascular disease, including systemic lupus erythematosus, polyarteritis nodosa in which 50 per cent of patients have involvement of the gastrointestinal tract, rheumatoid arthritis and Sjogren's syndrome.

Angiitis syndromes also may affect the mesenteric vessels, although, in most situations, the systemic manifestations of these conditions may be readily diagnosed.

SUMMARY

During the aging process, the function of the small bowel appears to be well maintained. Whether the reserve capacity for the absorption of nutrients is somewhat diminished has not been established. Most of the diseases that affect the small bowel in the elderly are the same as those seen in the young. However, the manifestation of ischemic disease, acute abdominal emergencies and diseases that result in malabsorption may be modified, usually with a less overt clinical picture. The disorders that must be considered as primarily affecting the gut of the elderly include bacterial overgrowth syndrome, vascular disease of the small intestine and cancer.

Acknowledgment I should like to acknowledge the careful and persistent efforts of Karol Winslow in the preparation of this manuscript.

REFERENCES

Andrew, W. 1944: Senile changes in the pancreas of Wistar Institute rats and of man with special regard to the similarity of locule and cavity formation. *American Journal of Anatomy* 74, 97–127.

Aimerman, J., Gavish, D., Rachmilewitz, D. 1985: Early and late onset ulcerative colitis: distinct clinical features. *Journal of Clinical Gastroenterology* 7, 492–8.

Ammann, R., Sulser, H. 1976: Die 'senile' chronische Pankreatitis-eine neue nosologische Eiheit? *Schweiz Med Wochenschr.* 106, 429–37.

Anuras, S., Sutherland, J. 1984: Small intestinal manometry in healthy elderly subjects. *Journal of the American Geriatric Society* 32, 581–3.

Aoyama, S., Kawamura, S., Nishio, K., Harima, K., Aibe, T., Takemoto. T. 1979: Histopathological study on aging of the pancreas from 423 autopsy cases. *Nippon Ronen Igakkai Zasshi* 6, 574–9.

Armbrecht, H.J., Doubek, W.G., Porter, S.B. 1988: Calcium transport by basal lateral membrane vesicles from rat small intestine decreases with age. *Biochimica et Biophysica Acta* 944, 367–73.

Arora, S., Hassarjian, S., Krasinski, S.D., Croffey, B., Kaplan, M.M., Russell, R.M. 1989: Effect of age on tests of intestinal and hepatic function in healthy humans. *Gastroenterology* 96, 1560–5.

Arranz, E., O'Mahony, S., Barton, J.R., Ferguson, A. 1992: Immunosenescence and mucosal immunity: significant effects of old age on secretory IgA concentrations and intraepithelial lymphocyte counts. *Gut* 33: 882–6.

Atillasoy, E., Holt, P.R. 1993: Gastrointestinal proliferation and aging. *Journal of Gerontology* 8, B43–9.

Attia, L., Holt, P.R. 1995: Serologic testing for celiac disease in the elderly. *Gastroenterology* 109, 2053.

Axelson, J., Person, P., Gagnermo-Persson, R., Kakanson, R. 1991: Importance of the stomach in maintaining calcium homeostasis in the rat. *Gut* 32, 1298–302.

Baker, H., Jaslow, S.P., Frank, O. 1978: Severe impairment of dietary folate utilization in the elderly. *Journal of the American Geriatric Society* 26, 218–21.

Baker, S.J., Mathan, V.I., Cherian, V. 1963: The nature of the villi in the small intestine of the rat. *Lancet* i, 860.

Beaumont, D.M., James, O.F.W. 1986: Unsuspected giardiasis, a cause of malnutrition and diarrhea in the elderly. *British Medical Journal* 293, 554–5.

Beaumont, D.M., Cobden, L., Sheldon, W.L., Laker, M.F., James, O.W.F. 1987: Passive and active carbohydrate absorption by the ageing gut. *Age and Ageing* 16, 294–300.

Becker, G.H., Meyer, J., Necheles, H. 1950: Fat absorption in young and old age. *Gastroenterology* 14, 80–92.

Begg, C.B., Carbone, P.P. 1983: Clinical trials and drug toxicity in the elderly. The experience of the Eastern Cooperative Oncology Group. *Cancer* 52, 1986–92.

Bender, B.S., Bennett, R., Laughon, B.E. *et al.* 1986: Is Clostridium difficile endemic in chronic care facilities? *Lancet* 88, 11–13.

Bjarnason, I., Hayllar, J., Macpherson, J., Russell, A.S. 1993: Side effects of nonsteroidal anti-inflammatory drugs on the small and large intestine in humans. *Gastroenterology* 104, 1832–47.

Bjork, K.J., Davis, C.J., Nagorney, D.M. *et al.* 1990: Duodenal villous tumors. *Archives of Surgery* 125, 961–5.

Boley, S.J., Sprayregan, S., Seigelman, S.S., Veith, F.J. 1977: Initial results from an aggressive roentgenological and surgical approach to acute mesenteric ischemia. *Surgery* 82, 848–55.

Boring, C.C., Squires, T.S., Tong, T. 1992: Cancer statistics 1991. *Cancer* 42, 19–38.

Bortolotti, M., Frada, G., Vezzadini, P., Bonora, G., Barbagallo-Sangiorgi G., Labb, G. 1987: Influence of gastric acid secretion on interdigestive gastric motor activity and serum motilin in the elderly. *Digestion* 38, 226–33.

Broccoli, D., Young, J.W., DeLange, T. 1995: Telomerase activity in normal and malignant hematopoietic cells. *Proceedings of the National Academy of Sciences USA* 92, 9082–6.

Buchowski, M.S., Miller, D.D. 1991: Lactose, calcium source and age affect calcium bioavailability in rats. *Journal of Nutrition* 121, 1746–54.

Bullamore, J.R., Wilkinson, K., Gallagher, J.C., Nordin, B.E.C., Marshall, D.H. 1970: Effect of age on calcium absorption. *Lancet* ii, 535–7.

Campbell, C.B., Roberts, R.M., Cowen, A.E. 1977: The changing clinical presentation of coeliac disease in adults. *Medical Journal of Australia* 1, 89–93.

Carmel, R. 1994: Food-cobalamin malabsorption. In Bhatt, H.R., James, V.H.T., Besser, G.M., Bottazzo, G.F., Keen, H. (eds), *Advances in Thomas Addison's diseases. Vol. 2. Clinical developments in adrenal cortical disease and vitamin B_{12} deficiency*. Bristol: Thomas Addison Society and Journal of Endocrinology Ltd, 149–61.

Carmel, R. 1996: Subtle cobalamin deficiency. *Annals of Internal Medicine* 124, 338–40.

Carmel, R. 1997: Cobalamin, the stomach, and aging. *American Journal of Clinical Nutrition* 66, 750–9.

Carmel, R., Karanaze, D.S. 1985: The deoxyuridine suppression test identifies subtle cobalamin deficiency in patients without typical megaloblastic anemia. *JAMA* 253, 1284–7.

Carr, N., Schofield, P.F. 1982: Inflammatory bowel disease in the older patient. *British Journal of Surgery* 69, 223–9.

Casirola, D.M., Rifkin, B., Tsai, W., Ferraris, R.P. 1996: Adaptations of intestinal nutrient transport to chronic caloric restriction in mice. *American Journal of Physiology* 34, G192–200.

Chen, T.S., Currier, G.J., Wabner, C.L. 1990: Intestinal transport during the life span of the mouse. *Journal of Gerontology* 45, B129–33.

Chin, J.S., Schuffler, M.D. 1988: Paraneoplastic visceral neuropathy as a cause of severe gastrointestinal motor dysfunction. *Gastroenterology* 95, 1279–85.

Clarke, R.M. 1972: The effect of growth and of fasting on the number of villi and crypts in the small intestine of the albino rat. *Journal of Anatomy* 112, 27–33.

Clarke, R.M. 1977: The effects of age on mucosal morphology and epithelial cell production in rat small intestine. *Journal of Anatomy* 123, 805–11.

Cohen, H.J. 1974: Biology of aging as related to cancer. *Cancer* 74, 2092–100.

Condom, E., Vidal, A., Rota, R., Graus, F., Dalman. J., Ferrer, I. 1993: Paraneoplastic intestinal pseudo-obstruction associated with high titer of Hu autoantibodies. *Virchows Archiv Pathological Anatomy* 423: 507–11.

Cooke, W.T., Mallas, E., Priori, P. 1980: Crohn's disease: course, treatment and longterm prognosis. *Quarterly Journal of Medicine* 49, 363–84.

Corraza, G.R., Strocchi, A., Rossi, R., Sirola, D., Gasbarrini, G. 1988: Sorbitol malabsorption in normal volunteers and in patients with coeliac disease. *Gut* 29, 44–8.

Crohn, B.B., Yarnis, H. 1958: *Regional ileitis*. Philadelphia: Grune and Stratton.

Cullan, C.E., Crouse, D.A., Sharp, T.G. 1982: Adaptive changes in intestinal cell proliferation studies *in situ* and in ectopic fetal intestinal grafts in ageing mice. In Robinson, J.W.L., Dowling, R.H., Riechen, E.O. (eds) *Mechanism of intestinal adaptation.* Falk Symposium 30. Lancaster: MTS Press, 29–46.

Cunningham, C.G., Reilly, L.M., Rapp, J.H., Schneider, P.A., Stoney, R.J. 1991: Chronic visceral ischemia: three decades of progress. *Annals of Surgery* 214, 276–88.

David, H., Reinke, P. 1988: Liver morphology with aging. In Bianchi, L., Holt, P.R., James, O.F.W., Butler, R.N. (eds), *Aging in liver and gastrointestinal tract* (Falk symp. No. 47, Titisee, 1987), Lancaster: MTP Press, 143–59.

Dawson, D.J., Sciberras, C.M., Whitewell, H. 1984: Coeliac disease presenting with intestinal pseudo-obstruction. *Gut* 25, 1003–8.

DiBaise, J.K., Quigley, E.M.M. 1998: Tumor-related dysmotility. Gastrointestinal dysmotility syndromes associated with tumors. *Digestive Diseases and Sciences* 43, 1369–401.

DiMagno E.P., Summerskill, W.H.J. 1977: Relations between pancreatic enzyme output and malabsorption in severe pancreatic insufficiency. *New England Journal of Medicine* 288, 813–15.

Dimri, G.P., Campisi, J. 1994: Altered profile of transcription factor-binding activities in senescent human fibroblasts. *Experimental Cell Research* 212, 132–40.

Dooley, J.S., Potter, B.J., Thomas, H.C. *et al.* 1982: A comparative study of the biliary secretion of human dimeric and monomeric IgA in rat and man. *Hepatology* 2, 232–7.

Doscherholmen, A., Swaim, W.R. 1973: Impaired assimilation of egg Co 57 vitamin B_{12} in patients with hypochlorhydria and achlorhydria and after gastric resection. *Gastroenterology* 64, 913–19.

Doubek, W.G., Armbrecht, H.J. 1987: Changes in intestinal glucose transport over the lifespan of the rat. *Mechanisms of Ageing and Development* 39, 91–102.

Ebbesen, P. 1984: Cancer and normal aging. *Mechanisms of Ageing and Development* 25, 269–83.

Ecknauer, R., Vadakel, T., Wepler, R. 1982: Intestinal morphology and cell production rate in aging rats. *Journal of Gerontology* 37, 151–5.

Eggert, A., Teichmann, W., Wittmann, D.H. 1982: The pathologic implication of duodenal diverticula. *Surgical Gynecology and Obstetrics* 154, 62–4.

Eisen, G.M., Schutz, S.M., Washington, M.K. *et al.* 1993: Atypical presentation of inflammatory bowel disease in the elderly. *American Journal of Gastroenterology* 88, 2098–101.

Ekbom, A., Helmick, C., Zack, M. *et al.* 1991: Extracolonic malignancies in inflammatory bowel disease. *Cancer* 67, 2015–19.

Fabricus, P.J., Gyde, S.N., Shouler, P. *et al.* 1985: Crohn's disease in the elderly. *Gut* 26, 461–5.

Farmer, R.G., Whelan, G., Fazio, V.W. 1985: Long-term follow-up of patients with Crohn's disease. Relationship between the clinical pattern and prognosis. *Gastroenterology* 88, 1818.

Farniok, K.E., Levitt, S.H. 1994: The role of radiation therapy in the treatment of colorectal cancer. Implications for the older patient. *Cancer* 74, 2154–9.

Faulk, D., Anuras, S., Christensen, J. 1978: Chronic intestinal pseudoobstruction. *Gastroenterology* 74, 422–31.

Fedorak, R.N., Field, M., Chang, E.B. 1985: Treatment of

diabetic diarrhea with clonidine. *Annals of Internal Medicine* 103: 197–9.

Feibush, J.M., Holt, P.R. 1982: Impaired absorptive capacity for carbohydrate in the aged. *Digestive Diseases and Sciences* 27, 1095–100.

Feldman, M., Schiller, L.R. 1983: Disorders of gastrointestinal motility associated with diabetes mellitus. *Annals of Internal Medicine* 98, 378–84.

Fentiman, I.S., Tirelli, U., Monfardini, S. *et al.* 1990: Cancer in the elderly: why so badly treated? *Lancet* 355, 1020–2.

Ferraris, R.P., Hsiao, J., Hernandez, R., Hirayama, B. 1993: Site density of mouse intestinal glucose transporters declines with age. *American Journal of Physiology* 264, Q285–93.

Fich, A., Camilleri, M., Phillips, S.F. 1989: Effect of age on human gastric and small bowel motility. *Journal of Clinical Gastroenterology* 11, 416–20.

Fleming, C.R., Newcomer, A.D., Stephens, D.H., Carlson, H.C. 1975: Intraluminal duodenal diverticulum: report of two cases and review of the literature. *Mayo Clinic Proceedings* 50, 244–7.

Fry, R.J.M., Lesher, S., Kohn, H.I. 1962: Influence of age on the transit time of cells of the mouse intestinal epithelium. *Laboratory Investigations* 11, 289–93.

Gallagher, J.C., Riggs, B.L., Eisman, J., Hamstra, A., Arnaud, S.B., DeLuca, H.F. 1979: Intestinal calcium absorption and serum vitamin D metabolites in normal subjects and osteoporotic patients. *Journal of Clinical Investigation* 54, 729–36.

Gerl, A., Storck, M., Schalhorn, A. 1992: Paraneoplastic chronic intestinal pseudoobstruction as a rare complication of bronchial carcinoid. *Gut* 33, 1000–3.

Gillberg, R., Dotevall, G., Kastrup, W. *et al.* 1984: Conventional malabsorption tests: do they detect the adult patient with villous atrophy? *Scandinavian Journal of Clinical Laboratory Investigation* 44, 91–8.

Giovanazi-Bannon, S., Rademaker, A., Lai, G. *et al.* 1994: Treatment tolerance of elderly cancer patients entered into phase II clinical trials: an Illinois Cancer Center study. *Journal of Clinical Oncology* 12, 2447–52.

Goldin, B., Dwyer, J. Sc.C., Gorbach, S.L., Gordon, W., Swenson, L. 1978: Influence of diet and age on fecal bacterial enzymes. *American Journal of Clinical Nutrition* 31, S136–40.

Goodman, S.A., Makinodan, T. 1975: Effect of age on cell-mediated immunity in long-lived mice. *Clinical Experimental Immunology* 19, 533–42.

Greenberg, R.E., Holt, P.R. 1986: Influence of aging upon pancreatic digestive enzymes. *Digestive Diseases and Sciences* 31, 970–7.

Greenberg, R.E., McCann, P.P., Holt, P.R. 1988: Trophic responses of the pancreas differ in aging rats. *Pancreas* 3, 311–16.

Greenstein, A., Gennuso, R., Sachar, D. *et al.* 1985: Extraintestinal cancers in inflammatory bowel disease. *Cancer* 56, 2914–21.

Greider, C.W. 1990: Telomeres, telomerase and senescence. *BioEssays* 12, 363–9.

Grimm, I.S., Friedman, L.S. 1990: Inflammatory bowel disease in the elderly patient. *Gastroenterology Clinics of North America* 19, 361.

Haboubi, N.Y., Montgomery, R.D. 1992: Small bowel bacterial overgrowth in elderly people: clinical significance and response to treatment. *Age and Ageing* 21: 13–19.

Haboubi, N.Y, Hudson, P., Rahman, Q., Lee, G.S., Ross, A. 1988: Small-intestinal transit time in the elderly. *Lancet* i, 933.

Hamilton, E., Franks, L.M. 1979: Cell proliferation and ageing in mouse colon. II. Late effects of repeated X-irradiation in young and old mice. *European Journal of Chemotherapy* 16, 663–9.

Harper, P., McAuliffe, T., Beeken, W. 1986: Crohn's disease in the elderly. A statistical comparison with younger patients matched for sex and duration of disease. *Archives of Internal Medicine* 146, 753–5.

Hart, R.W., Turturro, A. 1992: Overview of cancer and aging: a mechanistic perspective. *Experimental Gerontology* 27, 567–74.

Hayflick, L., Moorhead, P.S. 1961: The serial cultivation of human diploid cell strains. *Experimental Cell Research* 25, 585–21.

Heaney, R.P., Smith, K.T., Recker, R.R., Hinders, S.M. 1989: Meal effects on calcium absorption. *American Journal of Clinical Nutrition* 49, 372–4.

Hellemans, J., Joosten, E., Ghoos, Y. *et al.* 1984: Positive $^{14}CO_2$ bile acid breath test in elderly people. *Age and Ageing* 13, 138–43.

Heller, T.D., Holt, P.R., Richardson, A. 1990: Food restriction retards age-related histologic changes in rat small intestine. *Gastroenterology* 98, 387–91.

Hohn, P., Gabbert, H., Wagner, R. 1978: Differentiation and aging of the rat intestinal mucosa. II. Morphological, enzyme histochemical and disc electrophoretic aspects of the aging of the small intestinal mucosa. *Mechanisms of Ageing and Development* 7, 217–26.

Hollander, D., Dadufalza, V.D. 1983: Intestinal exsorption of oleic acid: influence of aging, bile, pH and ethanol. *Journal of Nutrition* 113, 511–18.

Hollander, D., Dadufalza, V.D. 1989: Lymphatic and portal absorption of vitamin E in aging rats. *Digestive Diseases and Sciences* 34, 768–72.

Hollander, E., Morgan, D. 1979a: Increase in cholesterol intestinal absorption with aging in the rat. *Experimental Gerontology* 14, 201–4.

Hollander, E., Morgan, D. 1979b: Aging: its influence on vitamin A intestinal absorption *in vivo* by rat. *Experimental Gerontology* 14, 301–5.

Hollander, D., Tarnawski, H. 1984: Influence of aging on vitamin D absorption and unstirred water layer dimensions in the rat. *Journal of Laboratory and Clinical Medicine* 103, 462–9.

Holt, P.R. 1990: Diarrhea and malabsorption in the elderly. *Gastrointestinal Disorders in the Elderly* 19, 345–59.

Holt, P.R. 1995: The gastrointestinal tract. In Masoro, E.J.

(ed.), *Handbook of physiology. Aging.* New York: Oxford University Press, 505–54.

Holt, P.R., Balint, J. 1993: The effects of aging upon intestinal lipid absorption. *American Journal of Physiology* 264, G1–6.

Holt, P.R., Dominguez, A.A. 1981: Intestinal absorption of triglyceride and vitamin D3 in aged and young rats. *Digestive Diseases and Sciences* 26, 1109–15.

Holt, P.R., Luk, G.D. 1990: Ageing intestinal polyamine metabolism in the rat. *Experimental Gerontology* 25, 173–81.

Holt, P.R., Yeh, K.Y. 1988: Small intestinal crypt cell proliferation rates are increased in senescent rats. *Journal of Gerontology* 44, B9–14.

Holt, P.R., Pascal, R.R., Kotler, D.P. 1984: Effect of aging upon small intestinal structure in the Fisher rat. *Journal of Gerontology* 39, 642–7.

Holt, P.R., Yeh, K.Y., Kotler, D.P. 1988: Altered controls of proliferation in proximal small intestine of the senescent rat. *Proceedings of the National Academy of Sciences USA* 85, 2771–5.

Holt, P.R., Moss, S.F., Heydari, A.R., Richardson, A. 1998: Diet restriction increases apoptosis in the gut of aging rats. *Journal of Gerontology: Biological Sciences* 53A, B168–72.

Horattas, M.C., Guyton, D.P., Wu, D. 1990: A reappraisal of appendicitis in the elderly. *American Journal of Surgery* 160, 291–3.

Horst, R.L., Goff, J.P., Reinhardt, T.A. 1990: Advancing age results in reduction of intestinal and bone 1,25-dihydroxyvitamin D receptor. *Endocrinology* 126: 1053–7.

Houcke, E., Houcke, M., Leblois, J. 1964: The pancreas of older adults: a histological study. *La Presse Medicale* 72, 1887–92.

Howell, T.H. 1978: Organ weights in nonagenarians. *Journal of the American Geriatric Society* 26, 385–90.

Husebye, E., Engedal, K. 1992: The patterns of motility are maintained in the human small intestine throughout the process of aging. *Scandinavian Journal of Gastroenterology* 27, 397–404.

Hyams, D.E. 1964: The absorption of vitamin B_{12} in the elderly. *Gerontology Clinics* 6, 193–206.

Ireland, P., Fordtran, J.S. 1973: Effect of dietary calcium and age on jejunal calcium absorption in humans studied by intestinal perfusion. *Journal of Clinical Investigation* 52, 2673–81.

Isaacson, P.G. 1995: Intestinal lymphoma and enteropathy. *Journal of Pathology* 177, 111–13.

Joosten, E., Lesaffre, E., Riezler, R., Ghekiere, V., Dereymaeker, L., Pelemans, W., Dejaeger, E. 1997: Is metabolic evidence for vitamin B-12 and folate deficiency more frequent in elderly patients with Alzheimer's disease? *Journal of Gerontology: Medical Sciences* 52A, M76–9.

Kawanishi, H., Joseph, K. 1992: Effects of phorbol myristate and ionomycin on in vitro growth of aged Peyer's patch T and B cells. *Mechanisms of Ageing and Development* 65, 289–300.

Kawanishi, H.H., Ajitsu, S., Mirabella, S. 1990: Impaired humoral immune responses to mycobacterial antigen in aged murine gut-associated lymphoid tissues. *Mechanisms of Ageing and Development* 54, 143–61.

Kendall, M.J. 1970: The influence of age on the xylose absorption test. *Gut* 11, 498–501.

Kennedy, B.J. 1992: Aging and cancer. In Balducci, L., Lyman, G.H., Ershler, W.B. (eds), *Geriatric oncology.* Philadelphia: J.B. Lippincott, 1–7.

Kennedy, R.H., Thompson, M.H. 1988: Are duodenal diverticula associated with choledocholithiasis? *Gut* 29, 1003.

Khalil, T., Thompson, J.C. 1987: Aging and gut peptides. In Thompson, J.C., Greeley, C.H., Jr, Rayford, P.L., Townsend, C.M., Jr, (eds), *Gastrointestinal endocrinology.* New York: McGraw-Hill, 147–57.

Khalil, T., Walkier, J.P., Greeley, G.H., Jr, Townsend, C.M., Jr, Thompson, J.C. 1985: Effect of aging on fasting and fat-stimulated plasma levels of pancreatic polypeptide in man. *Gastroenterology* 88, A1445.

Kilpatrick, G.S., Withey, J.L. 1965: The serum vitamin B_{12} concentration in the general population. *Scandinavian Journal of Haematology* 2, 220–9.

Kim, S.K., Weinhold, P.A., Calkins, D.W., Hartog, V.W. 1981: Comparative studies of the age-related changes in protein synthesis in the rat pancreas and parotid gland. *Experimental Gerontology* 16, 91–9.

Kirby, J., Fielding, J.F. 1984: Very adult coeliac disease! The need for jejunal biopsy in the middle aged and elderly. *Irish Medical Journal* 77, 35.

Koruda, M.J., Sheldon, G.F. 1991: Surgery in the aged. *Advances in Surgery* 24, 293–331.

Kreel, L., Sandin, B. 1973: Changes in pancreatic morphology associated with aging. *Gut* 14, 962–70.

Krishnamurthy, S., Schuffler, M. 1987: Pathology of neuromuscular disorders of the small intestine and colon. *Gastroenterology* 93, 610–39.

Laderoute, M.P. 1994: A new perspective on the nature of the cancer problem: anticellular senescence. *Molecular Carcinogenesis* 10, 125–33.

Laugier, R., Sarles, H. 1985: The pancreas: In James O.F.W. (ed.) *Clinics in gastroenterology.* Philadelphia: W.B. Saunders, 749–56.

Lee, F.I., Gaiffer, M. 1987: Crohn's disease of late onset in Blackpool. *Postgraduate Medical Journal* 63, 471–3.

Lennon, V.A., Sas, D.F., Busk, M.F. *et al.* 1991: Enteric neuronal antibodies in pseudoobstruction with small-cell lung cancer. *Gastroenterology* 100, 137–42.

Lesher, S., Fry, R.J.M., Kokn, H.I. 1961: Age and the generation time of the mouse duodenal epithelial cell. *Experimental Cell Research* 24, 335–43.

Lew, J.F., Glass, R.I., Gangarosa, R.E., Cohen, I.P., Bern, C., Moe, C.L. 1991: Diarrheal deaths in the United States 1979 through 1987. *JAMA* 265, 3280–4.

Lindenbaum, J., Savage, D.G., Stabler, S.P., Allen, R.H. 1990: Diagnosis of cobalamin deficiency: II. Relative sensitivities of serum cobalamin, methylmalonic acid and total homocysteine concentrations. *American Journal of Hematology* 34, 99–107.

Lipski, P.S., Kelly, P.J., James, O.F.W. 1992: Bacterial contamination of the small bowel in elderly people. Is it necessarily pathological? *Age and Ageing* 21, 5–12.

Logan, R.F.A., Rifkind, E.A., Busuttil, A. *et al.* 1986: Prevalence and 'incidence' of celiac disease in Edinburgh and the Lothian region of Scotland. *Gastroenterology* 90, 334–42.

MacLaughlin, J., Hollock, M.F. 1985: Aging decreases the capacity of human skin to produce vitamin D_3. *Journal of Clinical Investigation* 76, 1536–8.

Majumdar, A.P.N., Dubick, M.A. 1991: Gastrin affects enzyme activity and gene expression in the aging rat pancreas. *Experimental Gerontology* 26, 57–64.

Makinodan, T., Kay, M.M.B. 1990: Age influence on the immune system. *Advances in Immunology* 29, 287–330.

Marco, J., Hedo, J.A., Villanueva, M.L. 1977: Hyperglucagonism in the elderly. *Diabetes* 26, 381a.

Martin, G.H. 1993: Summation and synthesis: from the aging point of view. In Yang, S.S., Warner, H.R. (eds), *The underlying molecular, cellular and immunological factors in cancer and aging*. New York: Plenum Press, 321–7.

Mathis, J. 1928: Beitrage zur konntris das fledermaus darmes. *Zeitschrift für mikroskopische-anatomische. Forschung*. 12, 595–647.

McDougal, J.W., Miller, M.S., Burks, T.F. 1980: Intestinal transit and gastric emptying in young and senescent rats. *Digestive Diseases and Sciences* 25, A-15.

McEvoy, A., Dutton, J., James, O.F.W. 1983: Bacterial contamination of the small intestine is an important cause of occult malabsorption in the elderly. *British Medical Journal* 287, 789–93.

McIntyre, A.S., Long, R.G. 1993: Prospective survey of investigations in outpatients referred with iron deficiency anaemia. *Gut* 34, 1102–7.

Melkersson, M., Anderson, H., Bosaeus, J., Falkhenden, I. 1983: Intestinal transit time in constipated and non-constipated geriatric patients. *Scandinavian Journal of Gastroenterology* 18, 593–7.

Mitsuoka, T. 1992: Intestinal flora and aging. *Nutrition Reviews* 50, 438–46.

Miyasaka, K., Kitani, K. 1987: Aging and pancreatic exocrine function: studies in conscious male rats. *Pancreas* 2, 523–30.

Montgomery, R.D., Haboubi, N.Y., Mike, N.H. *et al.* 1986: Causes of malabsorption in the elderly. *Age and Ageing* 15, 235–40.

Moog, R. 1977: The small intestine in old mice: growth, alkaline phosphatase and disaccharidase activities, and deposition of amyloid. *Experimental Gerontology* 12, 223–34.

Morris, H.A., Nordin, B.E.C., Fraser, V., Hartley, T.F., Need, A.G., Horowitz, M. 1985: Calcium absorption and serum 1,25 dihydroxyvitamin D levels in normal and osteoporotic women. *Gastroenterology* 88: A1508.

Moss, S.F., Attia, L., Scholes, J.V., Walters, J.R.F., Holt, P.R. 1996: Increased small intestinal apoptosis in celiac disease. *Gut* 39, 811–17.

Murakami, M., Ishizuka, J., Yoshinaga, K. *et al.* 1991: Age-related changes in gallbladder contractility and cytoplasmic Ca^{++} concentration in the guinea pig. *Gastroenterology* 100, A539.

Nagai, H., Ohtsubo, K. 1984: Pancreatic lithiasis in the aged. *Gastroenterology* 86, 331–8.

Navah, F., Winter, C.G. 1988: Effect of aging on intestinal absorption of aromatic amino acids in vitro in the rat. *American Journal of Physiology* 254, G630–6.

Neidermuller, H. 1983: Age dependency of DNA repair in rats after DNA damage by carcinogens. *Mechanisms of Ageing and Development* 19, 259–71.

Neugut, A.I., Jacobson, J.S., Suh, S., Mukherjee, R., Arber, N. 1998: The epidemiology of cancer of the small bowel. *Cancer Epidemiology, Biomarkers and Prevention* 7, 243–51.

Newcomb, P.A., Carbone, P.P. 1993: Cancer treatment and age: patient perspectives. *Journal of the National Cancer Institute* 85, 1580–4.

Ottinger, L.W. 1982: Mesenteric ischemia. *New England Journal of Medicine* 307, 535–7.

Pennypacker, L.C., Allen, R.H., Kelly, J.P. *et al.* 1992: High prevalence of cobalamin deficiency in elderly outpatients. *Journal of the American Geriatric Society* 40, 1197–204.

Penzes L. 1970: Intestinal transfer of 1-Arg in relation to age. *Experimental Gerontology* 5, 193–201.

Penzes L. 1974: Intestinal absorption of glycine, L-alanine and L-leucine in the old rat. *Experimental Gerontology* 9, 245–52.

Penzes, L., Simon, G., Winter, M. 1968: Intestinal absorption and utilization of radiomethionine in old age. *Experimental Gerontology* 3, 257–63.

Poston, G.J., Singh, P., Draviam, E.J., Upp, J.R., Thompson, J.C. 1988: Development and age-related changes in pancreatic cholecystokinin receptors and duodenal cholecystokinin in guinea pigs. *Mechanisms of Ageing and Development* 46, 59–66.

Poston, G.J., Saydjari, R., Lawrence, J.P., Townsend, C.M., Jr., Thompson, J.C. 1989: Trophic effect of CCK bombesin and pentagastrin on the aged rat pancreas. *Pancreas* 4, A637.

Poston, G.J., Saydjari, R., Lawrence, J.P., Alexander, R.W., Townsend, C.M., Jr., Thompson, J.C. 1990: The effect of age on small bowel adaptation and growth after proximal enterectomy. *Journal of Gerontology* 45, B220–5.

Price, H.L., Gazzard, B.G., Dawson, A.M. 1977: Steatorrhoea in the elderly. *British Medical Journal* 1, 1582.

Quigley, E.M.M. 1996: Gastric and small intestinal motility in health and disease. *Gastroenterology Clinics of North America* 25, 113–45.

Ratnaike, R.N. 1990: Diarrhoea in the elderly: epidemiological and aetiological factors. *Journal of Gastroenterology and Hepatology* 5, 449–58.

Raul, F., Gosse, F., Doffoel, M., Darmenton, P., Wessely, J.Y. 1988: Age related increase of brush border enzyme activities along the small intestine. *Gut* 29, 1557–63.

Recker, R.R. 1985: Calcium absorption and achlorhydria. *New England Journal of Medicine* 313, 70–3.

Reville, M.F., Goose, F., Kachelhoffer, J., Doffoel, M., Raul, F. 1991: Ileal compensation for age-dependent loss of jejunal function in rats. *Journal of Nutrition* 121, 498–503.

Riordan, S.M., McIver, C.J., Wakefield, D., Bolin, T.D., Duncombe, V.M., Thomas, M.C. 1997: Small intestinal bacterial overgrowth in the symptomatic elderly. *American Journal of Gastroenterology* 92, 47–51.

Roberts, S.H., Janes, O., Jarvis, E.H. 1977: Bacterial contamination of the small intestine is an important cause of occult malabsorption in the elderly. *Lancet* 2, 1194–5.

Robertson, D.A.F., Dison, M.F., Scott, B.B. *et al.* 1983: Small intestinal ulceration: diagnostic difficulties in relation to coeliac disease. *Gut* 24, 565–74.

Robetorye, R.S., Nakanishi, M., Venable, S.F., Pereira-Smith, O.M., Smith, J.R. 1996: Regulation of p21 Sdi1/Cip1/Waf1/mda-6 and expression of other cyclin-dependent kinase inhibitors on senescent human cells. *Mole. Cell Differ.* 4, 113.

Rogers, A.I., Cohen, J.L. 1985: Ischemic bowel disease. In Bockus, H.L. (ed.), *Gastroenterology*, Vol. 3. Philadelphia: Saunders, 1915–36.

Rose, J.D., Roberts, G.M., Williams, G. *et al.* 1988: Cardiff Crohn's disease jubilee: the incidence of 50 years. *Gut* 29, 346.

Ruskone-Fourmestraux, A.R., Aegerter, P., Delmer, A., *et al.* 1993: Primary digestive tract lymphoma: a prospective multicentric study of 91 patients. *Gastroenterology* 105, 1662–71.

Russell, R.M., Krasinski, S.D., Samloff, I.H. *et al.* 1986: Folic acid malabsorption in atrophic gastritis. *Gastroenterology* 91, 1476–82.

Samet, J., Hunt, W.C., Key, C. *et al.* 1986: Choice of cancer therapy varies with age of patient. *JAMA* 255, 3385–90.

Sato, T., Tauchi, H. 1975: The formation of enlarged and giant mitochondria in the aging process of human hepatic cells. *Acta Pathologica Japonica* 25, 403–12.

Schiller, L.R., Schmulen, A.C., Santa Ana, C.A. *et al.* 1982: Pathogenesis of fecal incontinence in diabetes mellitus. *New England Journal of Medicine* 307, 1666–71.

Schiller, L.R., Morawak, S.F., Santa Ana, C.A. *et al.* 1985: Studies of antidiarrheal action of clonidine. Effects on motility and intestinal absorption. *Gastroenterology* 89, 982–8.

Schmitz-Moorman, P., Himmelmann, G.W., Brondes, J.W. *et al.* 1985: Comparative radiological and morphological study of human pancreas: pancreatitis-like changes in post-mortem ductograms and their morphological pattern. *Gut* 26, 406–14.

Schuette, S.A., Yasillo, N.J., Thompson, C.M. 1991: The effect of carbohydrates in milk on the absorption of calcium by postmenopausal women. *Journal of the American College of Nutrition* 10, 132–9.

Schuffler, M.D., Baird, W., Fleming, R. *et al.* 1992: Intestinal pseudo-obstruction as a rare complication of bronchial carcinoid. *Gut* 33, 1000–3.

Shapiro, P., Peppercorn, M., Antonioli, D. *et al.* 1981: Crohn's disease in the elderly. *American Journal of Gastroenterology* 76, 132–7.

Shaw, R.S., Maynard, E.P. III. 1958: Acute and chronic thrombosis of the mesenteric arteries associated with malabsorption: a report of two cases successfully treated by thromboendarterectomy. *New England Journal of Medicine* 258, 874.

Shocket, E., Simon, S.A. 1982: Small bowel obstruction due to enterolith (bezoar) formed in a duodenal diverticulum: a case report and review of the literature. *American Journal of Gastroenterology* 77: 621–4.

Simko, V., Michael, S. 1989: Absorptive capacity for dietary fat in elderly patients with debilitating disorders. *Archives of Internal Medicine* 149, 557–60.

Smith, I.S., Young, S., Gillespie, G. *et al.* 1975: Epidemiological aspects of Crohn's disease in Clydesdale, 1961–1970. *Gut* 16, 62.

Softley, A., Myren, J., Clamp, E. et al. 1988: Inflammatory bowel disease in the elderly patient. *Scandinavian Journal of Gastroenterology* 23(S144), 27–30.

Stanton, P.E., Jr, Hollier, P.A., Seidel, T.W., Rosenthal, D., Clark, M., Lamis, P.A. 1986: Chronic intestinal ischemia: diagnosis and therapy. *Journal of Vascular Surgery* 338–44.

Stein, G.H., Beeson, M., Gordon, L. 1990: Failure to phosphorylate the retinoblastoma gene product in senescent human fibroblasts. *Science* 249, 666–9.

Steinfeld, A.D., Diamond, J.J., Hanks, G.E. *et al.* 1989: Patient age as a factor in radiotherapy. Data from the Patterns of Care study. *Journal of the American Geriatric Society* 37, 355–8.

Suntzeff, V., Angeletti, P. 1951: Histological and histochemical changes in intestines of mice with aging. *Journal of Gerontology* 16, 225–9.

Swinson, C.M., Levi, A.J. 1980: Is coeliac disease underdiagnosed? *British Medical Journal* 281, 1258–60.

Swinson, C.M., Clavin, G., Coles, E.C., Booth, C.C. 1983: Coeliac disease and malignancy. *Lancet* 1, 111–15.

Szurszewski, J.H., Holt, P.R., Schuster, M. 1989: Neuromuscular function and dysfunction of the GI tract in aging. Mayo Clinic Workshop Proceedings, Nov. 2–3, 1987. *Digestive Diseases and Sciences* 34, 1135–46.

Takamoto, S., Seino, Y., Sackor, B., Liang, C.T. 1990: Effect of age on duodenal 1,25-dihydroxyvitamin D-3 receptors in Wistar rats. *Biochimica et Biophysica Acta* 1034, 22–8.

Talley, N.J., O'Keefe, E.A., Zinsmeister, A.R., Melton, L.J. III. 1992: Prevalence of gastrointestinal symptoms in the elderly: a population-based study. *Gastroenterology* 102, 895–901.

Taylor, L.D., Daniels, C.K., Schmucker, D.L. 1990: Does aging impair gastrointestinal mucosal immunity. *Aging* 2, 205–9.

Texter, E.C., Jr (ed.) 1983: *The aging gut: pathophysiology, diagnosis, and management*. New York: Masson, 105–15.

Texter E.C., Jordan H.J. 1983: The effect of vascular factors on nutrient absorption. In Rechcigl, M. (ed.), *Handbook of nutrition and food*. Boca Raton: CRC Press, 13–20.

Thompson, A.B.R. 1979: Unstirred water layer and age dependent changes in rabbit jejunal D glucose transport. *American Journal of Physiology* 236, E685–91.

Thompson, W.G., Heaton, K.W. 1980: Functional bowel disorders in apparently healthy people. *Gastroenterology* 79, 283–8.

Truelove, S.C., Pena, A.S. 1976: Course and prognosis of Crohn's disease. *Gut* 17, 192–201.

van Asselt, D.Z.B., de Groot, L.C.P.G.M., van Staveren, W.A., Blom, H.J., Wevers, R.A., Biemond, I., Hoefnagels, W.H.L. 1998: Role of cobalamin intake and atrophic gastritis in mild cobalamin deficiency in older Dutch subjects. *American Journal of Clinical Nutrition* 68, 328–34.

Van Lennep, E.W. 1962: The histology of the mucosa of the small intestine of the long-nosed bandicoot with special reference to the intestinal secretion. *Acta Anatomica* 50, 73–89.

Vantrappen, G., Janssens, J., Hellemans, J., Ghoos, Y. 1977: The interdigestive motor complex of normal subjects and patients with bacterial overgrowth of the small intestine. *Journal of Clinical Investigation* 59, 1158–66.

Varga, F. 1976: Transit time changes with age in the gastrointestinal tract of the rat. *Digestion* 14, 319–24.

Varga, F., Csaky, T.Z. 1976: Changes in the blood supply of the gastrointestinal tract in rats with age. *Pflugers Archiv* 364, 129–33.

Verne, G.N., Snisky, C.A. 1995: Chronic intestinal pseudoobstruction. *Digestive Diseases* 13, 163–81.

Vincenzini, M.T., Iantomasi, T., Stio, M., Favilli, F., Vanni, P., Tonelli, F., Treves, C. 1989: Glucose transport during ageing by human intestinal brush-border membrane vesicles. *Mechanisms of Ageing and Development* 48, 33–41.

Wallis, J.L., Lipski, P.S., Mathers, J.C., James, O.F.W., Hirst, B.H. 1993: Duodenal brush-border mucosal glucose transport and enzyme activities in ageing man and the effect of bacterial contamination of the small intestine. *Digestive Diseases and Sciences* 38, 403–9.

Walton, J.N., Kiloh, L.G., Osselton, J.W., Farral, J. 1954: The electroencephalogram in pernicious anaemia and subacute combined degeneration of the cord. *Electroencephalography in Clinical Neurophysiology* 6, 45–64.

Warren, P.M., Pepperman, M.A., Montgomery, R.D. 1978: Age changes in small intestinal mucosa. *Lancet* ii, 849.

Webster, S.G.P., Leeming, T.J. 1975a: Assessment of small bowel function in the elderly using a modified xylose tolerance test. *Gut* 16: 109–13.

Webster, S.G.P., Leeming, J.T. 1975b: The appearance of the small bowel mucosa in old age. *Age and Ageing* 4, 168–74.

Webster, S.G.P., Wilkinson, E.M., Gowland, E. 1977: A comparison of fat absorption in young and old subjects. *Age and Ageing* 6, 113–17.

Weiner, P.G., Dietze, F., Laue, R. 1984: Age-dependent alterations of intestinal absorption. II. A clinical study using a modified D-xylose absorption test. *Archives of Gerontology and Geriatrics* 3, 97–108.

Weingrad, D.N., Decosse, J.J., Sherlock, P., Straus, D., Lieberman, P.H., Filippa, D.A. 1982: Primary gastrointestinal lymphoma: a 30-year review. *Cancer* 49, 1258–65.

Welsh, J.D., Poley, J.R., Bhatia, M., Stevenson, D.E. 1978: Intestinal disaccharidase activities in relation to age, race and mucosal damage. *Gastroenterology* 75, 847–55.

Wynne, H.A., Cope, L.H., Mutch, E., Rawlins, M.D., Woodhouse, K.W., James, O.F.W. 1989: The effect of age upon liver volume and apparent liver blood flow in healthy men. *Hepatology* 9, 297–301.

Yoshinaga, K., Ishizuka, J., Saydjari, R., Townsend, C.M., Jr., Thompson, J.C. 1993: Effect of aging on polyamine pathway of small intestine in the rat. *Digestive Diseases and Sciences* 38, 410–16.

Yuhas, J.M., Huang, D., Strorer, J.B. 1969: Residual radiation injury: hematopoietic and gastrointestinal involvement in relation to age. *Radiation Research* 38, 501–12.

Zoli, M., Iervese, T., Abbati, S., Bianchi, G.P., Marchesini, G., Pisi, E. 1989: Portal blood velocity and flow in aging man. *Gerontology* 35, 61–5.

7

Regulatory peptides of the gastrointestinal tract

JENS J HOLST

BACKGROUND: HISTORY AND CHEMISTRY

The history of the regulatory peptides of the gut begins in January 1902, when Bayliss and Starling discovered secretin, the first hormone to be identified. They also made the first preparation of a gastrointestinal hormone, after having demonstrated for the first time that pancreatic secretion could be elicited by application of acid to the mucosa of a denervated segment of the small intestine. They scraped off the mucosa from the segment, ground it with hydrochloric acid and filtered the solution. This solution – the first preparation of secretin – when injected into a cervical vein, greatly augmented pancreatic secretion. Actually, the chemical information that could be derived from the experiment was limited. Clearly, what was discovered was the existence of a 'chemical reflex', necessarily transmitted via the blood stream (because of the denervation), and the fact that the responsible agent (the 'hormone': Greek 'arouse to activity') could be extracted from the mucosa. Bayliss and Starling called the agent secretin, but it took more than 60 years of additional intensive research to find out what secretin is: a polypeptide of 27 amino acids (Mutt *et al.*, 1970). After the discovery of secretin, a few additional hormones were identified mainly from physiological experimentation involving denervation or cross-circulation: gastrin in 1905 (Edkins, 1905), cholecystokinin in 1928 (Ivy and Oldberg, 1928), the incretins in the 1930s (Labarre, 1932) and pancreozymin in 1943 (Harper and Raper, 1943). Although cholecystokinin and pancreozymin were discovered as two separate entities, chemical isolation proved them to be one and the same peptide (Mutt and Jorpes, 1968).

In the 1970s, advances in biochemical techniques for the isolation and characterization of peptides led to a dramatic increase in the number of regulatory peptides that could be extracted from the gut and other tissues. The first of these (motilin, gastric inhibitory polypeptide (GIP), vasoactive intestinal polypeptide (VIP)) were isolated on the basis of their presumed biological activites as indicated by their names. Subsequent peptides were identified on the basis of their chemical properties: pancreatic polypeptide, as an impurity in insulin preparations; and peptide histidine isoleucine amide (PHI), peptide tyrosine tyrosine (PYY) and neuropeptide Y (NPY) because of the presence of a carboxy-terminal amidation, which could be identified biochemically (Tatemoto and Mutt, 1982). The amidation is a characteristic feature of many regulatory peptides, and this prompted a search for amidated peptides. For these chemically identified peptides, there were no *a priori* assumptions as to their function, and it has been a considerable research effort subsequently to find the physiological functions of these newer peptides.

In the era of molecular biology, the genes that encode most of the regulatory peptides have been cloned. In some instances, the precursors identified in this way could be demonstrated to contain other peptide sequences that turned out to be hormones or transmitters in their own right. Thus, by differential processing, the glucagon precursor was shown to release the two hormones glucagon-like peptide 1 and 2 (GLP-1 and 2), but not glucagon, when processed in gut endocrine cells, whereas in the pancreas, glucagon but not GLP-1 and 2 is formed (Ørskov *et al.*, 1986). By differential processing of the mRNA precursor (differential splicing), the gene encoding the calcium-regulating hormone calcitonin was demonstrated to lead to the expression of calcitonin in the thyroid C-cells, and to the formation of 'calcitonin gene-related peptide' (CGRP) in sensory afferent neurons throughout the body (Rosenfeld *et al.*, 1983). Molecular cloning of the receptors for the regulatory peptides revealed that most belong to the family of G-protein-coupled receptors. By homology screening for such receptors (Libert *et al.*, 1989), a number of orphan receptors were discovered. The most recent development in the field is to identify the natural ligands for such orphan receptors. This approach has identified new regulatory peptides such as nociceptin (Meunier *et al.*, 1995). The morphine receptors were, in fact, orphan receptors until the opioid peptides were discovered to be their natural ligands.

Chemically, some of the gut peptides form so-called *families*. Gastrin and cholecystokinin form a family because they have identical C-terminal sequences. Glucagon, secretin, GIP, VIP, PHI, PACAP (pituitary adenylate cyclase-activating polypeptide) and the glucagon-like peptides constitute a family because of marked sequence homology, particularly with respect to their N-terminal sequences (Bell, 1986). The pancreatic polypeptide was found to have two amidated counterparts with about 50 per cent sequence homology and remarkably similar crystal structures: neuropeptide Y and peptide YY (Mannon and Taylor, 1994).

Most of the gut regulatory peptides exhibit *molecular heterogeneity*. Thus, the gastrin precursor gives rise to several peptides ranging in size from 4 to 58 amino acids, all of which are capable of stimulating acid secretion, because their C-terminal sequences, the domains responsible for interaction with the gastrin receptor, are identical. The different forms represent varying degrees of proteolytic cleavage of the precursor (Wiborg *et al.*, 1981) but, because they are metabolized at different rates (the shortest forms usually most rapidly), the heterogeneity may have physiological relevance.

LOCALIZATION: ENDOCRINE, PARACRINE AND NEUROCRINE SYSTEMS

As discussed above, many of the gut regulatory peptides were originally extracted from the intestinal mucosa, and it was soon suspected that Feyrter's 'hellen Zellen' (Feyrter, 1938), cells that appeared clear upon histological examination because their granular content was washed out during preparation, could be the origin of the peptides. However, it was the new immunohistochemical techniques that finally provided information about their specific localization (Bishop *et al.*, 1988). As the peptides themselves eventually became isolated in pure form, and modern techniques for synthesis of replicas of the peptides became available, specific antibodies were raised against them. Not only were these antibodies suitable for radioimmunological determination of the peptides, a technique developed by, among others, Berson and Yalow (1967), but they could also be used for the specific demonstration of the peptides in tissue sections. Hence, it became possible to classify the gut endocrine cells, often already classified ultrastructurally, according to their hormone production (Solcia *et al.*, 1981). Thus, the cells responsible for gastrin production turned out to be the endocrine G-cells of the antral glands, and the secretin- and cholecystokinin-producing cells turned out to correspond to the previously classified S and I cells of the duodenal mucosa. Somatostatin was present in the D-cells of the gastric glands and the pancreatic islets. Most of these cells are pyramidal in shape with an apical process, equipped with microvilli, reaching the lumen of the gastrointestinal tract. Such cells are often called *open-type endocrine cells*, reflecting the notion that they may register chemical or other signals from the lumen by way of the microvilli. Other cells are more rounded in shape and do not seem to contact the lumen. Such cells are called *closed cells*.

In 1976, the immunohistochemical search for the cellular origin of the newly discovered intestinal polypeptide VIP revealed that this peptide of the glucagon/secretin family was not localized to endocrine cells at all, but to a dense network of nerve fibres in both the central and the peripheral nervous system (Larsson *et al.*, 1976). By immunoelectron microscopy the peptide could be localized to the dense granules of the nerve terminals, and subsequent physiological experiments revealed that the peptide could be released from the nerve terminals upon appropriate stimulation (Fahrenkrug *et al.*, 1978). Thus, the gut peptides belonged to a much larger system, the diffuse neuroendocrine system, which is responsible for intercellular communication in all complex organisms, dating back 1000 million years in evolution to the primitive animals like the hydra. Several of the newer peptides turned out to be neuropeptides rather than endocrine transmitters: NPY, PHI, CGRP, the tachykinins, the opioids, galanin, the mammalian bombesin (GRP). In keeping with their transmitter function in the diffuse neuroendocrine system, the regulatory peptides of the gut are found in many extraintestinal tissues. Cholecystokinin, for example, is a major neurotransmitter in the brain. VIP, NPY, galanin and CGRP also have a widespread distribution throughout the central and peripheral nervous system. Conversely, peptides like the tachykinins (substance P) and neurotensin, originally identified in the central nervous system, were now found to function also as intestinal transmitters or hormones.

In 1979, Larsson *et al.* noted that many of the gastric somatostatin-containing D-cells had a peculiar shape. These cells typically possess one or more dendrite-like cytoplasmic processes stretching out by 1–3 cell diameters, seemingly establishing close contacts with other cell types, e.g. the antral gastrin cells. In view of the finding that somatostatin powerfully influences (usually inhibits) the function of many other cells, this morphology was highly suggestive of a local, so-called paracrine interaction between the D-cell and supposed target cells. Subsequent research established that the cytoplasmic processes exhibit 'axonal transport' of the paracrine transmitter (somatostatin) and that it can be released from the cells. Immunoneutralization experiments confirmed the paracrine regulation, e.g. the gastrin cells by the D-cells (Holst *et al.*, 1992a,b).

Thus, the regulatory peptides of the gut, originally thought of as gastrointestinal hormones in the classical understanding of the term, are now recognized to be transmitters in endocrine, paracrine and neurocrine divisions of the diffuse neuroendocrine system (Polak and Bloom, 1979).

MOLECULAR BIOLOGY OF THE GUT REGULATORY PEPTIDES AND THEIR RECEPTORS

Molecular cloning techniques have greatly advanced our knowledge of the biology of the gut peptides and their receptors. One of the first areas to benefit from this new development was the study of the biosynthetic processing of the peptides. Following the pioneering work of Steiner and co-workers regarding the biosynthesis of insulin (Tager and Steiner, 1974), it was recognized that the gut peptides could be generated by cleavage of larger precursor molecules, but the ultrashort lifetime of these precursor molecules or 'prohormones' made it difficult to isolate them and precluded detailed studies. Progress was made when it became possible to translate enriched preparations of mRNA encoding the peptides in cell-free systems, in which the primary translation product could escape co-translational or post-translational proteolytic cleavage, but molecular cloning of the cDNAs encoding the peptides finally solved the problem of defining the precursor structures.

Typically, a pool of radiolabelled oligonucleotides, prepared to include all the different triplet variations that may arise as a consequence of the degenerate genetic code and corresponding to the sequence of small fragments of the peptide, were brought to hybridize with a library of cDNAs prepared by reverse transcription of mRNA from the endocrine tissue in question. Hybridizing clones were then sequenced and the structure of the encoded protein deduced by translation of the triplets of the cDNA sequence. The cDNAs thus identified were subsequently used to isolate the genes from genomic libraries by hybridization reactions. From such studies, a wealth of information was derived. The structure of the precursors of nearly all of the gut peptides was revealed (Brand *et al.*, 1994), and it was confirmed that they were all derived from proteolytic processing of larger precursor molecules. The precursor structure provided explanation for the molecular heterogeneity characterizing, e.g. gastrin and cholecystokinin, by proving that each of the molecular forms corresponds to a certain fragment of the precursor (Wiborg *et al.*, 1981; Takahashi *et al.*, 1985).

The unexpectedly large size of the peptide precursors brought up the question of the 'function' of the precursor apart from giving rise to the peptide itself. In some instances, as in the case of pro-enkephalin A, encoding the leu- and met-enkephalins, the precursor was shown to contain several copies (in this instance, seven) of the regulatory peptide, thereby boosting the number of transmitter molecules formed for each transcriptional cycle (Gubler *et al.*, 1982). In other cases, the precursor seemed to contain duplicated or triplicated but modified copies of the 'original' peptide. Thus, the highly homologous peptide PHI was found to constitute part of the VIP precursor (Itoh *et al.*, 1983), and PHI and VIP were found to be released in parallel from VIP-containing nerves upon appropriate stimulation (Holst *et al.*, 1987). Because their functions seem to be overlapping, this probably represents another way of enhancing the signal. The precursor for glucagon was shown to contain three copies of related peptides, namely glucagon itself and two highly homologous, so-called glucagon-like peptides, but these three peptides have completely distinct functions (Holst, 1997). For many precursors the functions of the surplus parts of the precursors are still not known, but it is often assumed that they may help direct the post-translational processing.

Correct processing of the precursors clearly plays an essential role in the biosynthetic process, and today the study of the enzymes involved, the so-called prohormone convertases, has been established as an important research field in its own right. Thus, mutations of the convertases have recently been demonstrated to result in often dramatic endocrine and metabolic disturbances (Furuta *et al.*, 1997; Jackson *et al.*, 1997; Leiter, 1997).

Investigations of the untranslated promotor regions of the genes encoding the gut peptides have established their functions as targets for DNA binding proteins (transcription factors) that up- or down-regulate transcription rates and are responsible for tissue specificity of expression. The study of the regulation of expression genes encoding the gut peptides is still in its infancy but information on the specific regulation of each of the numerous gut peptides is accumulating at great pace (Brand *et al.*, 1994). The precise mechanisms that regulate the tissue-specific expression of a given peptide at a given time may be accounted for in the not too distant future. This field of research has particular clinical relevance for the study of the tumours producing these peptides, such as the gastrin and VIP producing tumours (giving rise to the Zollinger–Ellison and Werner–Morrison syndromes).

The earliest studies of the receptors for the gut peptides mainly consisted of attempts to bind labelled preparations of the peptides to cell membranes or cells from target tissues. Positive binding was followed by attempts to isolate and characterize the receptors chemically. Because of their membrane localization and large size, these studies were complicated and progress was slow. The introduction of molecular cloning techniques quickly changed the picture. The cholecystokinin (CCK) receptors were among the first to be studied. During the tedious attempts to prepare sufficient material for biochemical characterization, several groups succeeded in isolating small proteolytic fragments of the receptor. Using a similar technique to that used for cloning the peptide precursors, oligonucleotides corresponding to these short amino-acid sequences could now be synthesized and appropriate libraries screened for hybridizing cDNAs. Using this technique, the primary structure of the CCK-A receptor was successfully deduced (Wank *et al.*, 1992a).

Another important and powerful technique is expression cloning by which cDNAs, prepared from mRNA from supposed target tissues for the peptides, are transfected into suitable cells. These cells are subsequently screened for expression of the receptor by hormone binding or other measures. The structure of the gastrin receptor was deduced in this way (Kopin *et al.*, 1992) and, in as much as the gastrin and CCK peptides are related, so were the gastrin and CCK receptors; both bind CCK with high affinity, but only the gastrin receptor (also called the CCK-B receptor) binds gastrin with high affinity.

As more and more receptor structures were identified, it became apparent that they all belong to the so-called seven-transmembrane-spanning, G-protein-coupled receptor superfamily (Laburthe *et al.*, 1994). Many of the receptors, including the CCK receptors, show a high degree of structural and functional homology with the rhodopsin subfamily of these receptors. The receptors for the secretin/glucagon family of peptides constitute a distinct subfamily that also includes the receptors for calcitonin and parathyroid hormone (Lok *et al.*, 1994). For these receptors, structural and functional information is much more scanty; characteristically, they couple to adenylate cyclase.

The fact that all of the gut peptide receptors belong to the same superfamily is the background for the homology cloning techniques widely employed since, 1989 (Libert *et al.*, 1989). With this approach, short nucleotide primers, constructed to correspond to receptor domains that show a high degree of homology, are used to amplify DNA sequences from relevant tissues using polymerase chain reaction (PCR) techniques. Receptor-like sequences are subsequently isolated and subjected to further investigation. By this extremely powerful technique, it is evident that many peptides may bind to several receptors. Thus, at least six different receptor genes seem to exist for NPY and the related peptides (Widdowson *et al.*, 1997). Five receptors are known for somatostatin (Møller *et al.*, 2000). Although it is difficult to understand the physiological significance of all these subtypes, it seems clear that different subtypes are often expressed in different tissues, and that some of them show characteristic differences with respect to binding and activation by synthetic analogues. These observations may have therapeutic applications, because the differences will allow pharmaceutical targeting of a specific receptor subtype in a specific tissue. Moreover, the cloned receptors, introduced into suitable reporter systems, may be used for drug screening in a search for non-peptide agonists and antagonists that may eventually be used to treat disorders in which the parent peptides are suspected to play a pathophysiological or regulatory role, or in which a regulation of organ function may be expedient.

The techniques of gene targeting (Wei, 1997) presently attract great interest among physiologists. With such techniques it is possible to amplify (knock in) or obliterate (knock out) the gene of a peptide ligand or its receptor. The functions of the ligand/receptor couple in the adult and the developing animal can then be studied by analysing the phenotype of the homozygous or heterozygous offspring of the mutated animals. Frequently, the outcome of some of these experiments has been predicted, e.g. development of severe diabetes in animals with insulin receptor knockout, or hypoacidity and mucosal atrophy in gastrin knockouts. In other cases, the mutations have had surprising consequences, such as the finding that mutations or knockout of the endothelin 3 gene or endothelin receptor B gene causes Hirschprung's disease (Wartiovaara *et al.*, 1998). This particular ligand/receptor couple, therefore, seems to play an important role in the maturation and expression of certain neural-crest-derived cell lineages. It is important to recognize the difference between experiments involving receptor antagonists and receptor knockout. The use of an efficacious receptor antagonist can reveal the acute effects of the lack of a certain signal, whereas the knockout phenotype reflects the consequences of the lifelong lack of the signal. Apart from the developmental implications the latter might have, there is also the possibility that compensatory mechanisms have developed, with the consequence that a physiologically important function of a peptide may be concealed by the substituting functions of redundant or compensatory mechanisms. The inconspicuous effects on body weight or appetite of a knockout of the neuropeptide NPY (Erickson *et al.*, 1996) are probably due to the actions of such compensatory mechanisms; a host of other experimental data support the idea that NPY is probably the most important cerebral promoter of food intake.

METABOLISM OF GUT PEPTIDES

It seems to be a general rule pertaining to all the regulatory peptides of the gut that they circulate in low concentrations in the plasma, that they do not exhibit protein binding and that they are eliminated rapidly, i.e. with half-lives of a few minutes. Being peptides that cannot cross cell membranes in the absence of specific transport proteins, their apparent volume of distribution generally corresponds to the volume of the extracellular space. Some of the peptides may be subjected to receptor-mediated elimination in their target organs, others may be eliminated by, largely unknown, enzymatic mechanisms in specific organs like the lungs and the liver, but it applies to all that the kidneys are a main site of elimination (Henriksen, 1991). The peptides are freely filtered and metabolized by brush-border enzymes of the proximal tubules and the resulting amino acids are reabsorbed. For many of the peptides, however, renal extraction exceeds the filtered amount, suggesting the presence of peritubular uptake, perhaps in agreement with the fact that the kidneys often express receptors for the peptides. Some peptides (somatostatin, GLP-1, GIP, PYY) may be degraded by aminopeptidases while circulating, which may significantly limit their biological effect. On the other hand, this renders the enzymes responsible as potential drug targets (Holst and Deacon, 1998). The neuropeptides are usually eliminated locally with remarkable efficiency, and a large local release of a neuropeptide is rarely reflected in measurable changes in the concentration of the peptide in peripheral plasma. This is likely to be essential. In patients with neuroendocrine tumours, the plasma levels of the neuropeptides may reach 'endocrine' levels, perhaps because of the absence of local elimination, with sometimes dramatic consequences. Thus, life-threatening diarrhoea may result in patients with VIP-producing tumours when the plasma levels increase above 90 pmol/L. More or less specific enzymatic mechanisms may be responsible for the local elimination. For the hormonal peptides, their rapid elimination is in keeping with the notion that they are fast acting, regulating cell function within seconds or minutes, as would be expected of hormones that function to adjust metabolism to the rapidly changing conditions of feeding and fasting.

GASTROINTESTINAL HORMONES

Gastrin

Gastrin, a 17-amino-acid polypeptide secreted from the antral G-cells, is essential for gastric secretion and growth (Sawada and Dickinson, 1997).

Gastric acid secretion is regulated in a complex interplay between endocrine, neural and paracrine factors. Elegant physiological experiments by Walsh and co-workers have established the important role of gastrin in acid secretion. In these experiments, neutralizing antibodies against gastrin were employed to gauge the relative importance of this hormone in meal-induced acid secretion (Kovacs *et al.*, 1989). In dogs stimulated with intragastric peptone (protein hydrolysate) instillation, antibody infusion almost abolished acid secretion and, in rats, a 40 per cent reduction was observed. Thus, species differences may exist, but the results are in concert with previous studies comparing the plasma gastrin responses to meal ingestion in humans and the secretory results of infusions of gastrin to similar plasma levels (the so-called *mimicry* method to evaluate the functional significance of hormone secretion), which also indicated that gastrin is reponsible for a large part of the secretory response to meal ingestion (Walsh, 1993).

Both gastrin gene knockout experiments and CCK-B receptor (gastrin receptor) knockouts confirm the importance of gastrin for acid secretion (Friis-Hansen *et al.*, 1998) and its functions as a trophic factor for parietal and enterochromaffin-like cells (ECL cells; see below). Other regulatory functions of the gastrins were not apparent in mice whose phenotype, apart from the gastric changes, was unremarkable. The importance of gastrin for the secretion of pepsinogen has been less rigorously studied, but it is clear that the chief cells express a different set of receptors compared to the parietal cells and that their rate of secretion is regulated differently. The CCK-B receptor (the gastrin receptor) was cloned from a canine parietal cell library (Kopin *et al.*, 1992), confirming its expected expression in this particular cell type, where receptor activation leads to increased intracellular calcium and inositoltriphosphate (IP_3) concentrations. However, to date there is general agreement that, in most species, the primary target for gastrin is likely to be the histamine-producing ECL cells (Håkanson *et al.*, 1994). Thus, gastrin activates the parietal cells indirectly via histamine release from the ECL cells (Gantz *et al.*, 1991), a finding which explains the extreme efficiency of histamine H_2 receptor antagonists to inhibit acid secretion. The trophic effects of gastrin are evident in the transgenic mice as mentioned (Nagata *et al.*, 1996; Wang *et al.*, 1996; Koh *et al.*, 1997) and also appear in patients with gastrin-producing tumours, in whom the gastric mucosa shows gross hyperplasia. It has been contended that gastrin also might act as a trophic factor for the intestinal epithelium, and a role in the development of colon cancers has been suggested (Baldwin and Whitehead, 1994), but the latter is a matter of considerable controversy (Joshi and Gardner, 1996).

Pathogenetically, gastrin is considered as one of the key hormones in the development of duodenal ulcers, where, apparently, the infection with *Helicobacter pylori* causes hypersecretion of gastrin (Calam *et al.*, 1997). Its key role in the pathogenesis of the Zollinger–Ellison syndrome has been clearly established (Vinayek *et al.*, 1990). It has been discussed whether or to what extent gastrin influences pancreatic exocrine and endocrine secretion. The original identification of the CCK-A receptors (cholecystokinin preferring) in the pancreas would seem incompatible with a major role for gastrin in this respect, but subsequent research has shown that the pattern of receptor expression may vary between species. Thus, in humans (Monstein *et al.*, 1996) and pigs (Morriset *et al.*, 1996; Philippe *et al.*, 1997) the CCK-B receptor is also expressed in the pancreas, possibly explaining the significant secretory effects of gastrin in these species.

Cholecystokinin

Cholecystokinin, secreted from the I-cells of the small intestinal mucosa (Reeve and Eysselein, 1994; Liddle, 1997), like gastrin, shows a pronounced molecular heterogeneity, and there has been considerable disagreement about which molecular form is the most abundant or important. As in the case of gastrin, the different molecular forms arise by more or less extensive proteolytic cleavage of a large precursor molecule (Takahashi *et al.*, 1985). All of the biological activity apparently resides in a sulphated and amidated C-terminal octapeptide, localized near the C-terminus of the precursor, and this fragment is also the most potent. The N-terminally elongated form CCK-33 (of 33 amino acids), which was isolated first (Mutt and Jorpes, 1968), is also highly active and the two constitute, perhaps together with another elongated form consisting of 22 amino acids, the predominating circulating forms (Rehfeld, 1998). Plasma also contains a very large form, CCK-58, which has been claimed to be the most abundant form in canine plasma, but not in human plasma. CCK is produced both in the I-cells and in numerous neurons, particularly in the central nervous system, where the peptide (mainly the octapeptide) seems to function as transmitter in a variety of circuits. Some of the peripheral actions also seem to involve neural mechanisms and this has made the precise elucidation of its physiological actions difficult (Liddle, 1997). It is secreted from the intestinal mucosa in response to the luminal presence of micellar fat and protein digests, particularly during acidic conditions. Because luminal administration of trypsin inhibitors may increase CCK secretion, it is assumed that secretion may be regulated in a local feedback circuit. Further research along these lines led to the discovery of two CCK-releasing peptides (the 'monitor peptide' and the 'luminal CCK-releasing factor' (Miyasaka and Funakoshi, 1998)). At present, their physiological significance remains uncertain, particularly in humans, who respond with pancreatic enzyme secretion after administration of trypsin inhibitors but not with CCK secretion.

CCK shares its receptors with gastrin as discussed above, but interacts with the so-called CCK-A receptor with a 1000 times higher potency than gastrin (Wank *et al.*, 1992a,b). The development of specific agonists and antagonists for the CCK-A and B receptors (Jensen, 1996) has helped identify the physiological functions of these receptors, and recent studies involving targeted disruptions of the receptors have also provided important information (Samuelson *et al.*, 1996). In addition, it seems that the so-called Otsukyu Long-Evans Tokushima Fatty rats (OLETF rats) may constitute a useful rat model for CCK-A receptor deficiency, harbouring a nonsense mutation of the receptor gene (Takiguchi *et al.*, 1997).

The knockout and antagonist studies all point to a major role for CCK in the regulation of gallbladder and bile duct motility (Schmidt *et al.*, 1991; Cantor *et al.*, 1992; Kopin *et al.*, 1996). Thus, potent CCK-A receptor antagonists can completely block meal-induced gallbladder emptying (Liddle *et al.*, 1989), and the knockout mice develop gallstones. The gallbladder smooth muscles are equipped with CCK-A receptors, which may account for this endocrine effect of CCK. However, gallbladder function is also neurally regulated, and some actions may depend on neural interactions.

With respect to the pancreas, intravenous infusions of CCK stimulate the secretion of proteins, i.e. enzymes. The pancreatic secretory response to meal stimulation (duodenal instillation of nutrient solutions), on the other hand, is only partially or weakly antagonized by specific CCK-A antagonists, whereas muscarinic antagonists may completely inhibit the response (Adler *et al.*, 1991, 1995). Thus, physiologically, the actions of CCK may depend on interaction with autonomic cholinergic neurones. Recent studies suggest that CCK interacts with afferent nerve fibres localized both in the duodenal mucosa and elsewhere, which in turn reflexly activate efferent neurones whose fibres innervate the pancreas. As mentioned, however, the human pancreas possesses both CCK-A and CCK-B receptors (Monstein *et al.*, 1996), a fact that may explain in part the inefficiency of the CCK-A receptor antagonists to inhibit meal-induced secretory responses (Adler *et al.*, 1991; Cantor *et al.*, 1992).

Another important action of CCK, which is counteracted by the antagonists, is pancreatic growth. This action aroused an interest in the possible use of CCK-A antagonists to treat pancreatic cancer, but so far successful treatment has not been reported. Antagonist studies also suggest that CCK plays a role in the regulation of gastric motility, which is enhanced by CCK-A antagonists, and the antagonists have also shed some light on the role of CCK in the regulation of acid secretion. CCK would be expected to interact equally with gastrin on the CCK-B receptors of parietal and ECL cells of the gastric mucosa and, therefore, to act as a full agonist for acid secretion. However, it has long been known that CCK is a weak and partial agonist for acid secretion, particularly in higher doses. It now turns out that CCK activates CCK-A receptors on D-cells located in the vicinity of the parietal cells, and that somatostatin released from these cells inhibits parietal cell secretion; because of the extreme inhibitory potency of somatostatin on acid secretion, inhibition predominates (Schmidt *et al.*, 1994).

Finally, CCK seems to play an important role in the regulation of food intake, acting as a meal-related satiety signal to terminate ingestion (Read *et al.*, 1994). This concept was not supported by studies on knockout mice that develop normally and do not become obese. However, it is generally conceded that knockout of one of the many factors regulating food intake cannot be expected to result in a striking phenotype as the regulatory function of the deficient factor is taken over by other mechanisms, as discussed above. CCK administration reliably inhibits food intake, and in certain studies antagonist administration has resulted in increased food intake (Rose *et al.*, 1996). Moreover, the OLETF rats do develop obesity (Moran *et al.*, 1998). Again, the inhibitory mechanism seems to involve afferent sensory nerve fibres. CCK has been included among the incretin hormones because it stimulates insulin secretion in rodents. In humans, however, it is without effect (Fieseler *et al.*, 1995).

Secretin

The physiological importance of secretin is demonstrated by studies involving the mimicry technique (Schaffalitzky de Muckadell *et al.*, 1979) and immunoneutralization studies (Chey *et al.*, 1979). The secretin receptor has been cloned and its localization conforms with the expected targets of secretin action (Ulrich *et al.*, 1998). Like CCK, secretin circulates in extremely low concentrations (a few pmol/L); the physiological variations are sufficient to influence pancreatic bicarbonate secretion. For a while there was confusion because the plasma secretin concentrations do not exhibit a clear relation to meal ingestion, but subsequent studies showed that secretion closely follows the most important physiological stimulus: the concentration of hydrogen ions in the chyme that enters the duodenum (Schaffalitzky de Muckadell *et al.*, 1981). During ingestion of meals with a high buffering capacity, the gastric pH increases and the chyme that enters the duodenum may have a pH that is too high to stimulate secretin secretion, for which a pH around 2–3 is required. In contrast, in the fasting state, the boluses of chyme that enter the duodenum may have a low pH, and may cause secretion of short pulses of secretin. On the other hand, if the frequency of chyme expulsion from the stomach is low, a low average secretin concentration in plasma will be the result. As the postprandial gastric chyme eventually becomes acidified, a more frequent (because of the meal) emptying of acidic chyme may cause a more sustained increase in plasma secretin (Schaffalitzky de Muckadell *et al.*, 1981). The cellular mechanism whereby the low pH of the duodenal contents stimulates secretin secretion is not known; a high tension of CO_2 has no influence on secretion, indicating that the hydrogen ions themselves, rather than changes in intracellular pH, trigger secretion.

Recent experimental evidence points to the existence of secretin-releasing peptides analogous to the CCK-releasing peptides (Herzig, 1998), but their physiological significance is not established. Secretin acts on the ductular epithelium of the pancreas to increase secretion of bicarbonate and water, and, although progress has been made, for instance, with regard to the involvement of the cystic fibrosis transmembrane conductance regulator (CFTR) protein, which plays an important role for the exchange of chloride and bicarbonate between the lumen and the interstitium, the secretory mechanism is still far from elucidated (Argent and Case, 1994). Secretin has no effect on pancreatic protein secretion. The secretory actions of secretin, on the one hand, and cholinergic agonists and CCK on the other, exhibit strong potentiating synergism (Park *et al.*, 1998). Thus, combinations of small or even subthreshold amounts of the three factors may cause considerable pancreatic secretion of fluid as well as protein and bicarbonate, illustrating the importance of neuroendocrine regulation of the pancreas (Holst *et al.*, 1979). In addition to its pancreatic actions, secretin is thought to play a role as a choleretic agent (Erlinger, 1996; Marinelli *et al.*, 1997). Early immunoneutralization studies suggested that secretin may be a physiological inhibitor of gastric acid secretion in dogs, but this could not be reproduced in humans using a mimicry approach (Kleibeuker *et al.*, 1984). On the other hand, physiological elevations of plasma secretin inhibit gastric emptying and this effect, which was also evident from the immunoneutralization studies, may therefore be physiologically relevant. However, as an enterogastrone (intestinal hormonal inhibitor of gastric functions), secretin may be much more potent in dogs (Chey *et al.*, 1981; Lloyd *et al.*, 1997) than in humans.

A clear, secretin-related pathology does not seem to exist. Recently, a family of hypocretins, hypothalamus-specific peptides with neuroexcitatory activity and strong amino-acid homology with secretin, were uncovered (deLecea *et al.*, 1998). These peptides cause an increased food intake when administered into the cerebral ventricles, and were therefore designated orexins (Sakurai *et al.*, 1998). This discovery may provide an explanation for the episodic detections of immunoreactive secretin in neurons of the brain. Surprisingly, however, injection of secretin into the cerebral ventricles influences pancreatic secretion (Conter *et al.*, 1996).

Motilin

Motilin is a 22-amino-acid peptide produced in endocrine cells of the upper intestinal mucosa (Itoh, 1997). Motilin is also produced in certain regions of the brain, and motilin binding sites are also present there, but little is known about its functional importance as a brain peptide (Depoortere *et al.*, 1997a,b). Motilin is encoded by a gene from the sixth chromosome and its precursor is a peptide of 114 amino acids (Seino *et al.*, 1987). Nothing is known about the possible functions of the non-motilin parts of the precursor. It is secreted in response to intraluminal changes in pH and the presence of bile (Goll *et al.*, 1996). However, important differences between species seem to exist in this respect. In humans, its secretion parallels the occurrence of the migrating myoelectric complexes (MMCs) in the fasting state. Its functions seem to be related to the regulation of gastrointestinal motility. Thus, infusion of motilin can induce premature MMCs and, in immunoneutralization studies (Poitras, 1984), infusion of motilin antiserum disrupted the spontaneous (fasting) motility pattern in the upper gut. However, the cyclic variations in the secretion of motilin could also reflect the cyclic neural interdigestive activity, which is reflected also in the periodic bursts of gastrointestinal secretion and emptying of the gallbladder (Qvist *et al.*, 1995).

So far, motilin receptors have not been cloned. Binding studies have revealed different pharmacological characteristics for receptors (binding sites) occurring in the antrum and the duodenum (Poitras *et al.*, 1996). It is generally assumed that motilin may activate smooth muscles directly in high concentrations. In lower concentrations, motilin seems to activate cholinergic neural networks and it appears that the cyclic changes in plasma motilin can initiate cyclic changes in parasympathetic efferent activity (Boivin *et al.*, 1997). Potent motilin receptor antagonists that might help clarify its physiological functions have not yet been developed. However, erythromycin and related macrolide antibiotics are potent agonists, and the stimulation of gastrointestinal motor activity that can be elicited with erythromycin is thought to reflect its interaction with motilin receptors (Peeters, 1993; Peeters and Depoortere, 1994; Itoh, 1997). Moreover, infusions of motilin (as norLeu-13-motilin, which is more stable) and erythromycin and related substances have been demonstrated to have beneficial effects in patients with impaired gastrointestinal motility, such as diabetic gastroparesis (Ishii *et al.*, 1997). Disturbed secretion of motilin has, so far, not been implicated in the pathogenesis of states of disease.

Gastric inhibitory polypeptide or glucose-dependent insulinotropic peptide

GIP is a peptide composed of 42 amino acids and belongs to the glucagon–secretin family of peptides. The sequence homology is particularly strong in the N-terminal part. It is processed from a precursor of 153 amino acids (Takeda *et al.*, 1987), but specific functions for other fragments of the precursor have not been identified. Most antisera raised against GIP cross-react to some extent with a larger molecule, designated GIP 8000, but its relation to GIP is not established (Krarup, 1988). It does not seem to be a product of the GIP precursor. In some instances, 'GIP 8000' may have been due to the presence of the related peptide glicentin, which may cross-react with some antisera. Preferably GIP assays should not show a cross-reaction with GIP 8000. The GIP receptor has been cloned and is related to the receptors for the other members of the glucagon–secretin family of peptides. It is expressed in the pancreatic islets and also in the gut, adipose tissue, heart, pituitary, in the adrenal cortex and in several regions of the brain (Usdin *et al.*, 1993).

GIP is secreted from specific endocrine cells, the so-called K-cells, which exhibit the highest density in the duodenum, but actually GIP cells are found in the entire small intestinal mucosa. Their secretion is stimulated by absorbable carbohydrates and by lipids. GIP secretion is, therefore, greatly increased in response to meal ingestion, resulting in 10–20-fold elevations of the plasma concentration (Pederson, 1994).

Interaction of GIP with its receptor on the pancreatic β-cells causes an elevation of cAMP levels, which in turn increases the intracellular calcium concentration and enhances the exocytosis of insulin-containing granules by a mechanism distal to the elevation of calcium (Gromada *et al.*, 1998). In agreement with this, GIP is considered one of the incretin hormones, the insulinotropic hormones, which enhance and potentiate meal-related, substrate-induced insulin secretion. The incretin function of GIP has been probed in immunoneutralization studies (Lauritsen *et al.*, 1981) and, more recently, in studies employing a fragment, GIP 7–30 amide, which turns out to be a GIP receptor antagonist (Tseng *et al.*, 1996). Both treatments reduced insulin responses to oral glucose and impaired glucose tolerance. GIP receptor tolerance is associated with glucose intolerance.

GIP influences lipid metabolism (Morgan, 1997). In particular, the hormone enhances lipoprotein lipase activity, inhibits lipolysis and promotes synthesis of triglycerides, all of which promote the postprandial clearance of dietary lipids.

As suggested from the name, GIP was isolated as an inhibitor of acid secretion. In humans, however, its activity in this respect is weak and the peptide also seems to have little effect on gastrointestinal motility (Walsh, 1994).

Pathophysiologically, GIP is implicated in two diseases. One is the recently described postprandial Cushing syndrome (DeHerder *et al.*, 1996), which seems to be due to adrenal overexpression and/or sensitivity of adrenal GIP receptors, with subseqent hypersecretion of adrenal corticosteroids in relation to meal ingestion, when GIP levels are high. The other, quantitatively more important, disease is type II (non-insulin-dependent) diabetes mellitus. These patients have been reported to hypersecrete GIP, but this is noted only with certain assays and may reflect different specificities of the assays. However, it has been demonstrated that the patients have a weak or absent incretin function, and that exogenous GIP has little or no insulinotropic effect (Holst *et al.*, 1997a). Thus, type II diabetes seems to be characterized by a defective function of the pancreatic GIP receptor, a finding which could be of great pathophysiological significance. Detected polymorphisms in the coding region of the GIP receptor gene were not associated with diabetes, however (Kubota *et al.*, 1996). Disturbances of GIP secretion or action in other metabolic diseases, notably in obesity, have not been established, but the deranged lipid metabolism in type II diabetes and other dyslipidaemic disorders could represent another target (Gama *et al.*, 1997).

Somatostatin

Somatostatin is a 14-amino-acid peptide (SS 14) originally isolated as the growth-hormone release-inhibiting factor from the hypothalamus. The single somatostatin gene is expressed in numerous endocrine cells in the gastrointestinal system, including the gastric mucosa and the pancreatic islets. In addition, it is expressed in many neurones of the enteric nervous system (*see* Chapter 1). In the intestinal mucosa, however, the 92-amino-acid precursor is processed to release a 28-amino-acid peptide (SS 28), of which SS 14 occupies the C-terminal 14 positions (Chiba and Yamada, 1994; Walsh, 1994). Thus, upon appropriate stimulation, it is SS 28 rather than the tetradecapeptide that is released from the gut (Baldissera *et al.*, 1985). Its halflife in the circulation is considerably longer than that of the tetradecapeptide, in keeping with the notion that SS 28 functions as a circulating hormone, whereas the SS 14 functions in local regulation, as a neurotransmitter or in paracrine systems. The somatostatins act on a total of five different but related receptor molecules (Bell and Reisine, 1993; Møller *et al.*, 2000). The fifth receptor (sst 5) seems to prefer SS 28, whereas the others have similar affinitites for SS 14 and SS 28. The receptor subtype composition varies characteristically between the different somatostatin responsive tissues. Generally, in the gastrointestinal tract, expression of the sst 2 and sst 3 isoforms predominate. All receptors seem to inhibit cell function, most through inhibition of adenylate cyclase via an inhibitory G-protein, but other signalling pathways may also be activated, e.g. activation of tyrosine phosphatases, which could transmit the inhibitory effects on growth exerted by somatostatin in certain tissues.

Somatostatin 28 is released in relation to meal ingestion. A low pH in the upper intestine may be the stimulus proper. The increases are small, however. Somatostatin released from nerves or paracrine cells (SS 14) is usually not detectable in peripheral blood, and therefore probably does not play a role in the endocrine regulation of the organs.

If the arterial concentration of somatostatin reaches sufficient levels, the hormone could affect the functions of virtually any organ. This is because somatostatin is capable of inhibiting the secretion of most hormones including the gastrointestinal hormones. It may also inhibit exocrine secretion from the entire gastrointestinal tract and has effects on blood flow, absorption and growth. Finally, it has variable but highly significant effects on gastrointestinal motility. It has been shown that somatostatin 28, as a hormone, has at least the potential to inhibit, for instance, pancreatic exocrine secretion (Hildebrand *et al.*, 1992). However, the extent to which SS 28 exerts such regulatory functions is generally not known. Clearly, the diversity of its receptors and functions makes it extremely complicated to analyse the effects of any gene knockouts; potent and selective antagonists have generally not been available. Immunoneutralization studies have suggested, however, that circulating somatostatin may play a role as an enterogastrone hormone mediating inhibition of upper gastrointestinal functions elicited by the presence of lipids or acid in the small intestine (Orloff *et al.*, 1992). Possibly, somatostatin also participates in the regulation of absorption, but whether this is a local effect or is due to circulating SS 28 is not known (Schusdziarra *et al.*, 1980).

Clinical conditions associated with a deficiency of somatostatin secretion have not been described, but several patients have been discovered to suffer from somatostatin-secreting tumours (Service, 1997). Some of these have been located in the pancreas, others may be duodenal. These patients exhibit, to a variable degree, disturbances related to the actions of somatostatin. Impaired biliary function with gallstone formation seems to be a frequent feature, and most patients have some degree of diabetes mellitus. A metabolically stable form of somatostatin, octreotide (Arnold, 1996), is commonly used to treat endocrine tumours (gastrointestinal and pituitary), and patients on constant therapy with this compound may develop diarrhoea and steatorrhoea. It deserves mentioning that scintigraphy after injection of radioactively labelled octreotide is the most useful tool in the diagnosis of neuroendocrine tumours, which often express a high density of somatostatin receptors (Reubi, 1997).

Distal gut hormones

PRO-GLUCAGON-DERIVED PEPTIDES

The glucagon gene is expressed not only in the pancreatic A-cells but also in the endocrine, so-called L-cells, of the intestinal mucosa, which show the highest density in the lower small intestine. Here the primary translation product, pro-glucagon (a peptide of 160 amino acids) is cleaved, not to release glucagon and the major pro-glucagon fragment (MPGF; corresponding to the pro-glucagon (PG) sequences 33–61 and 78–158, respectively) as in the pancreas (Holst *et al.*, 1994), but to release glicentin (or 'enteroglucagon', corresponding to PG 1–69) and the two glucagon-like peptides contained in the major pro-glucagon fragment: glucagon-like peptide 1 (PG 78–107 amide) and 2 (PG 126–158), or GLP-1 and 2 (Ørskov *et al.*, 1986; Holst *et al.*, 1997b). Both the major pro-glucagon fragment from the pancreas and glicentin seem to be biologically inactive. Thus, in the pancreas, the two specific gut products (GLP-1 and 2) are inactivated by being incorporated in the MPGF, while, in the gut, the glucagon sequence is inactivated by incorporation in glicentin. Minor amounts of glicentin may be cleaved *in vivo* to release oxyntomodulin (PG 33–69), which shares some of the activities of glucagon (because of their common N-terminus), but generally with low potency (Holst, 1997). Glicentin and GLP-1 and 2 are secreted in relation to meal ingestion. The presence of carbohydrates and fat in the gut lumen seems to be the appropriate stimulus for the L-cells, which are of the open type, but, because the meal response is rapid, it has been speculated that neuroendocrine regulation may also play a role. As already mentioned, glicentin seems to be inactive, but a considerable literature about glicentin (enteroglucagon) secretion has accumulated over the years (Holst, 1997). Because the three peptides are secreted in parallel, the results of these older studies do, to some extent, apply to the glucagon-like peptides.

GLP-1, a 30-amino-acid peptide with 50 per cent homology with glucagon, interacts with a single receptor, which belongs to the receptors of the glucagon–secretin family (Thorens *et al.*, 1993). The main site of expression is in the pancreatic islets, but receptors are also present in the lungs, the stomach and in the brain. Activation of the β-cell receptor causes a stimulation of insulin secretion with similar characteristics to the secretion elicited by GIP (see above) (Gromada *et al.*, 1998). GLP-1 is, therefore, considered to be the more distal incretin hormone (Nauck *et al.*, 1993), playing a role when not only the upper but also the lower small intestine is exposed to nutrients, mainly carbohydrates but also lipids. Unlike GIP secretion, which is either 'on' or 'off', GLP-1 secretion, and therefore plasma levels, reflect the size of the meal and/or the rate of gastric emptying. Its function as an incretin hormone has been probed with both receptor antagonists and in receptor knockout studies. A truncated form of exendin-4, a lizard peptide, has been shown to interact rather specifically with the GLP-1 receptor (Thorens *et al.*, 1993), and administration of the antagonist together with (oral) glucose impairs insulin responses as well as glucose tolerance (Kolligs *et al.*, 1995). Mice with a targeted disruption of the GLP-1 receptor gene are glucose intolerant and the males have fasting hyperglycaemia (Schrocchi *et al.*, 1996). Unlike GIP, the incretin effect of GLP-1 is completely preserved in patients with type II diabetes mellitus, and infusions of small amounts of GLP-1 have been shown to be able to normalize the blood glucose levels completely of patients with even long-standing diabetes (Nauck *et al.*, 1993). Part of the efficacy of GLP-1 in this respect is due to its inhibitory effect on glucagon secretion (which is not shared by GIP). Thereby, GLP-1 efficiently lowers the hepatic glucose production, which is elevated in these patients.

At present, considerable efforts are being made to convert this metabolically unstable peptide into a clinically useful therapeutic agent (Holst, 1998). Physiologically, the gastrointestinal actions of GLP-1 may be more important (Holst, 1997). GLP-1 strongly inhibits upper gastrointestinal secretion and motility (Wettergren *et al.*, 1993), and, if it is infused together with a meal, the meal-induced insulin secretion actually decreases (Nauck *et al.*, 1997). This is because GLP-1 slows motility and absorption so that the nutrient-induced insulin secretion (and thereby the response that is potentiated by GLP-1) decreases. This inhibitory mechanism, which constitutes a part of the so-called ileal brake mechanism (MacFarlane *et al.*, 1983) seems to involve activation of afferent sensory nerve fibres that reflexly inhibit the cephalic parasympathetic outflow and thereby functions that are regulated by the vagus nerves (Wettergren *et al.*, 1996, 1997). Surprisingly, GLP-1 is rapidly inactivated by a local enzyme (dipeptidyl peptidase IV; DPP-IV), so that about half of the GLP-1 that leaves the gut is already inactive (Holst and

Deacon, 1998). This may suggest that, physiologically, GLP-1 interacts with local afferent nerve fibres immediately upon its release before it is degraded. GLP-1 also also inhibits appetite and food intake (Flint *et al.*, 1998) and may represent one of the meal-related intestinal satiety signals that terminate food intake (Read *et al.*, 1994). Another signal may, as noted above, be CCK released from the upper intestine. GLP-1 receptors are also expressed in the brain, particularly in the hypothalamus (Wei and Mojsov, 1995), where they seem to be targets for GLP-1 produced in neurons with cell bodies located in the brainstem. GLP-1 strongly inhibits food intake if injected into the cerebral ventricles (Turton *et al.*, 1996), but this mechanism seems to be unrelated to the satiating effects of peripheral GLP-1.

Glucagon-like peptide 2 is released in parallel with GLP-1, in relation to meal ingestion. It shares with GLP-1 the inhibitory effects on upper gastrointestinal motility and secretion, but has attracted more interest because of its growth-promoting effects. Although its physiological role in this respect is not yet known precisely, infusions or injections of GLP-2 to rodents cause a marked growth of the entire intestine with most marked effects on the small intestine (Drucker *et al.*, 1996). Both the length and the weight of the gut increase as well as crypt depth and villus height. GLP-2 has, therefore, been proposed to be the endocrine factor that induces adaptive growth, e.g. in relation to intestinal transposition or resection studies. For a decade, enteroglucagon was thought to be involved in this mechanism because of the striking relationship between plasma levels of enteroglucagon and adaptive growth (Bloom, 1987). As mentioned, GLP-2 secretion is likely to show the same correlation because they are secreted in parallel. Of clinical interest is the demonstration that the intestinal atrophy that accompanies total parenteral nutrition can be completely prevented by GLP-2 infusion (Chance *et al.*, 1997). A receptor mediating the actions of GLP-2 has recently been identified.

NEUROTENSIN

Neurotensin (NT) is a 13-amino-acid peptide produced in the so-called N-cells, the distribution of which resembles that of the L-cell (Shulkes, 1994). The neurotensin gene encodes a precursor of 170 amino acids, in which neurotensin is located near the C-terminus (Dobner *et al.*, 1987). Immediately N-terminally to neurotensin resides the sequence of neuromedin N, another biologically active peptide. Neuromedin N, however, is not released from the precursor in the N-cells, but is released from the many neurons in the peripheral and particularly in the central nervous system that express the NT gene. There is little doubt that neurotensin plays an important role as a transmitter in the central nervous system, e.g. in nociceptive and neuroendocrine systems (Rostene and Alexander, 1997), whereas as a hormone, its function is less clear.

Neurotensin may interact with two receptors, a high-affinity (Tanaka *et al.*, 1990) and a low-affinity (Yamada *et al.*, 1998) receptor, both of which are expressed in numerous neural tissues. In the periphery, receptors (high affinity) are mainly localized in the colon, followed by the liver, and then the duodenum and the pancreas in that order (Mendez *et al.*, 1997). Neurotensin secretion is stimulated particularly by the luminal presence of lipids, but the plasma concentration rises by only a few picomoles per litre. The peptide seems to be cleaved almost immediately upon secretion into the inactive (peripherally) 1–8 fragment. When reproduced by infusion, the low circulating concentrations of NT have little effect (Mogard *et al.*, 1987), whereas higher concentrations have marked inhibitory effects on gastric function and stimulatory effects on pancreatic secretion (Gullo *et al.*, 1992). Its effects seem to depend on an intact vagal innervation, and it seems possible that NT, like GLP-1, could act locally on sensory afferent nerve fibres before it is degraded. A similar mechanism may apply to PYY (see below) and may thus characterize the entire ileal-brake mechanism. Neurotensin's functions have not yet been probed in gene-targeting studies; such studies would be expected to mainly reflect its functions in the nervous system. High-affinity receptor antagonists are now available (Gully *et al.*, 1996) but do not seem to have been applied in studies of its functions as a gastrointestinal hormone.

PEPTIDE YY

Peptide YY is a peptide of 36 amino acids that belongs to a family of peptides (the PP-fold family, signifying a common, characteristic molecular configuration) comprising, in addition, neuropeptide Y and pancreatic polypeptide (PP). All contain 36 amino acids, exhibit a high degree of sequence homology, and have one or two terminal tyrosine residues (hence the Ys). Whereas neuropeptide Y (phylogenetically the oldest) is an obligatory neuropeptide, PYY and PP are hormones, and PP is secreted from certain cells of the pancreatic islets and PYY from endocrine cells of the distal intestinal mucosa (Larhammar, 1996a). At least some of the latter also produce the pro-glucagon-derived peptides discussed above, and under some, but apparently not all, experimental conditions the secretion of PYY and GLP-1 is parallel. Like GLP-1, PYY is attacked by the enzyme DPP-IV, but whereas all stored GLP-1 is intact, part of PYY is stored and secreted as the metabolite PYY 3–36. PYY is secreted in relation to meal ingestion, but lipids seem to be particularly effective as stimulants (Maas *et al.*, 1998). A stimulatory loop from the upper to the distal gut may exist with CCK or gastrin stimulating PYY secretion, which in turn may inhibit gastrin and CCK secretion (Liu *et al.*, 1996).

The PP family operates via a family of receptors comprising six members, the Y_{1-6} receptors, all of which have been cloned (Larhammar, 1996b; Widdowson *et al.*, 1997). Of these, the Y_4 has the highest affinity for PP, whereas the others can be distinguished, not only on the basis of structural differences, but also by their interactions with various analogues and fragments of the PP family of peptides. With NPY being the most widely distributed member, it is perhaps not surprising that the receptors are also expressed in neural tissues, central as well as peripheral. NPY and PYY both activate the Y_1 and Y_2 receptors equally well, whereas C-terminal fragments of PYY, including PYY 3–36, interact only with the Y_2 receptor. Since the tissue distribution of the two receptor types is markedly distinct, it follows that the conversion of PYY by the enzyme DPP-IV has important functional consequences. PYY does not immediately cross the blood–brain barrier and is therefore not capable of interacting with the Y receptors of the central nervous system. Whereas NPY at the various neuroeffector junctions may reach high local concentrations upon activation of the nerves, the plasma concentrations of PYY are in the low picomolar range, and circulating PYY, therefore, activates only accessible, high-affinity receptors. This probably limits the physiological actions of PYY. In functional studies, PYY has been shown to operate as an inhibitor of many gastrointestinal functions, including upper gastrointestinal secretion and motility, but it also inhibits intestinal secretion and promotes absorption (Nakanishi *et al.*, 1996). It seems possible that its effect on, for example, intestinal secretion may be exerted locally, i.e. it acts as a paracrine regulator. As was the case for GLP-1, its inhibitory effects on gastric and pancreatic function seem to involve the parasympathetic nervous system (Chen and Rogers, 1995), and the two peptides may act in very similar ways (Wettergren *et al.*, 1994). As inhibitors of gastric secretion, the two peptides have additive effects, and strongly inhibit acid secretion at very low concentrations (Wettergren *et al., 1996).* In dogs, PYY may be the most important peptide of the ileal-brake mechanism (Lloyd *et al.*, 1997), whereas in humans GLP-1 may be more prominent. PYY has been reported to be secreted in response to the luminal presence of fibre and short-chain fatty acids, but in humans, both GLP-1 and PYY remained unaffected by colonic carbohydrate fermentation (Ropert *et al.*, 1996). Both are released in response to the luminal presence of bile and bile salts. So far there have been no reported knockouts of the Y-receptors or PYY (whereas a knockout of NPY had mainly cerebral effects (Erickson *et al.*, 1996)). Selective agonist and antagonist studies have shed little light on the physiology of PYY, but an immunoneutralization study (Lin *et al.*, 1996) confirmed that the fat-induced ileal-brake effects in dogs depend on the actions of PYY. A pathology specifically related to PYY secretion has not been identified. The endocrine functions of PP are largely unknown, but it may act as an inhibitor of the motility and secretion of the biliary system (Adrian *et al.*, 1982).

Hormones of the colon

All of the hormones from the distal small intestine are also produced in the numerous endocrine cells of the colon and rectal mucosa. However, very little is known about the functional role of these endocrine cells (Christiansen *et al.*, 1990), nor is it known if regulation of the secretion from the colon differs from that of the ileum. Resection studies have not been informative.

PARACRINE REGULATION OF THE GASTROINTESTINAL TRACT

The most prominent examples of paracrine regulation are both related to gastric secretion, although it appears likely that paracrine mechanisms regulate function throughout the gastrointestinal tract. One paracrine regulator is histamine secreted from the ECL cells of the gastric mucosa. Recent studies have suggested that a local histamine release from these cells, with histamine subsequently diffusing towards the parietal cell for interaction with its stimulatory histamine H_2-receptors, represents one of the most important stimulatory pathways for acid secretion. Histamine release from the ECL cell, in turn, is regulated by gastrin secretion and by neural or paracrine mechanisms. The other prominent paracrine transmitter is somatostatin. Somatostatin as a gastrointestinal hormone was discussed previously. In the gastric mucosa, somatostatin is produced in the D-cells, which, in the corpus and fundus, are mainly endocrine cells of the closed type (no luminal contact), whereas in the antral glands they appear characteristically open. The somatostatin cells may send out dendrite-like cytoplasmic processes, which seem to establish close contact with neighbouring cells, and it was this characteristic feature that led to the hypothesis that gastric somatostatin might act as a paracrine rather than an endocrine transmitter (Larsson *et al.*, 1979).

The activity of paracrine cells is not likely to be reflected in the concentrations of the transmitter in the peripheral plasma, but a spillover of the transmitter after activation of the paracrine cells may be detected in the local veins draining the region. For somatostatin in the antrum, the main target seems to be the gastrin cells, and the main stimulus to the D-cells seems to be luminal pH. Thus a high acidity in the antral lumen stimulates paracrine somatostatin release, which in turn inhibits gastrin secretion, thus creating a negative feedback loop (Holst *et al.*, 1992a,b). Antral somatostatin secretion is also regulated by neural factors and

CCK (see below). In the corpus region, the parietal and/or the ECL cells are the targets for D-cell secretion and somatostatin has been demonstrated to be an exceedingly potent inhibitor of acid secretion, acting via receptors located on the the parietal (or ECL) cells. Neural stimuli seem to regulate D-cell secretion, with inhibitory cholinergic influences probably being the most important (Holst *et al.*, 1992c). Activation of vagal cholinergic fibres may, therefore, stimulate acid secretion, partly by interacting with stimulatory cholinergic receptors on the parietal cells, and partly by inhibiting tonically inhibitory paracrine D-cells. The D-cells possess CCK-A receptors, which may be activated by CCK from the duodenum (Park *et al.*, 1987; Beglinger *et al.*, 1992). As discussed above, this probably explains why CCK (which is a full agonist for the CCK-B receptors on ECL cells and parietal cells, and therefore should be a full agonist for acid secretion) is in fact a partial agonist and may actually inhibit gastrin-stimulated secretion, by stimulation of the paracrine, inhibitory D-cells (Schmidt *et al.*, 1994). It is of interest that the antral paracrine regulation of gastrin secretion seems to be one of the targets of *Helicobacter pylori* infection that causes the hypersecretion of gastrin in duodenal ulcer patients (Calam *et al.*, 1997).

NEUROPEPTIDES OF THE GUT

The innervation of the gut may be divided into intrinsic and extrinsic systems (Furness and Costa, 1987). The extrinsic system comprises efferent and afferent sympathetic and parasympathetic pathways. The cell bodies from which the fibres emerge are located outside the gut. The intrinsic system contains the numerous (more than 10^8 cell bodies) neurons of the enteric nervous system (*see* Chapter 1) that remain intact after extrinsic denervation. These cell bodies are mainly located in the plexuses of the gut, the myenteric and the submucous plexuses. The enteric nervous system (the ENS) comprises sensory neurons, and a large number of interneurons and effector neurons. It is thus able to create full reflex loops without involving the spinal cord. Both the intrinsic and the extrinsic systems are sources of numerous neuropeptides (Daniel, 1990; Furness *et al.*, 1992). The neuropeptides may coexist with each other and with non-peptide transmitters, such as acetylcholine, noradrenaline and serotonin. The system is incredibly diverse and it is extremely difficult to dissect out the particular functions of the individual peptides. An indication of the importance of the neuropeptides for gut function is provided by hypersecretion of the peptides in neuroendocrine tumours. Thus, hyperproduction of vasoactive intestinal polypeptide is the pathogenetic mechanism behind the watery diarrhoea and hypokalaemia syndrome or Werner–Morrison syndrome, with its dramatic secretory diarrhoea. The somatinoma syndrome has been alluded to above. It should be emphasized that the intestinal neuropeptides, although in many cases isolated from and identified for the first time in the gut, are widely distributed in the entire organism, and have numerous important functions beyond the gut, which are outside the focus of this presentation.

With respect to the occurrence and distribution of the neuropeptides in the gut, certain differences between species have been noted. This means that information gathered from experimental animals cannot immediately be applied to humans. However, in higher mammals, many features are similar.

VIP is one of the most abundant neuropeptides, and regulates both motility and secretion. It is a peptide of 27 amino acids and belongs to the glucagon–secretin family. Upstream in the VIP precursor is the homologous peptide PHI or PHM (peptide histidine isoleucine in pigs and methionine in humans), which is released in parallel with VIP during the processing of the precursor (Itoh *et al.*, 1983). It shares many of the actions of VIP and seems to be an example of amplification of a neural signal by duplication of the transmitter in the precursor. Closely related to VIP is the peptide pituitary adenylate cyclase-activating polypeptide (PACAP), a peptide of 38 amino acids, originally isolated from the hypothalamus. VIP/PACAP operate via at least three receptors that are structurally related to the other receptors of this peptide family. However, one receptor is PACAP preferring (has the highest affinity for PACAP), while the remaining receptors may be activated equally by both peptides (Forsmann, 1998). Again, because of the complexity of the peptide and receptor distribution patterns, the precise functions of these peptides are difficult to unravel, and antagonist studies so far have not provided much information. It seems well established, however, that at least VIP functions in the descending relaxation of the circular muscles of the gut that constitutes part of peristalsis. All three receptors typically activate adenylate cyclase, which is known, via cAMP, to cause relaxation of the smooth muscles, but activation of NO synthase, leading to a production of the inhibitory transmitter nitric oxide (which activates the guanylate cyclase of the smooth muscles), also seems to play a role. As already alluded to, stimulation of intestinal secretion of electrolytes and water may be another important effect of the VIPergic neurones, and it is well established that the VIPergic fibres, by their relaxing effect on the smooth muscles of the vascular walls, play an important role in the regulation of blood flow in the intestine as well as elsewhere in the body.

Neuropeptide Y, discussed above, is another abundant neuropeptide in the gut. It is present both in intrinsic neurones and in extrinsic sympathetic nerve fibres where it coexists with noradrenaline, whose actions it seems to potentiate. The intrinsic NPY neurones may funtion mainly in the regulation of secretion and absorption.

Another important group of peptides is the tachykinins, the most important of which are substance P and neurokinin A. They emerge by differential processing of the mRNA as well as the peptide precursors resulting from expression of the preprotachykinin gene (Nakanishi, 1987), which explains why they coexist in most tissues and nerve fibres. They activate a group of receptors, designated NK_{1-3} (Nakanishi, 1991), which are expressed in several structures of the gut, including smooth muscles and other neurones. Importantly, the tachykinins seem to coexist with acetylcholine in excitatory motor neurones. The function of the tachykinins has been probed with specific receptor antagonists and, although the cholinergic activation of the muscles predominates, there is little doubt that the tachykinins act to support or enhance intestinal contractions stimulated by reflex, and may therefore play an important role in generating the ascending contractions of peristalsis (Schmidt and Holst, 1997). Substance P is also found in extrinsic sensory nerve fibres, thought to transmit nociceptive information to the dorsal horns of the spinal cord. The importance of the tachykinins for nociception and inflammation was clearly demonstrated in mice with deletion of either the preprotachykinin or the NK_1-receptor genes (Cao *et al.*, 1998; De Filipe *et al.*, 1998). In these sensory fibres, substance P coexists with the calcitonin-gene related polypetide, a product of calcitonin gene expression. When expressed in neural tissue, the calcitonin part is excised as an intron, while the neuropeptide sequence is transcribed, another example of differential RNA precursor splicing (Rosenfeld *et al.*, 1983). CGRP, however, is also found in intrinsic neurones, presumably interneurones that seem to activate cholinergic motor neurones. CGRP-containing fibres are often associated with blood vessels and may help regulate blood flow, causing pronounced vasodilatation. The tachykinins are often produced in large amounts in carcinoids (Mertz and Walsh, 1994), the neuroendocrine tumours of the gut, where excessive concentrations of tachykinins together with an overproduction of serotonin may cause flushing and diarrhoea, particularly when metastases are present in the liver, which otherwise efficiently clears the plasma of the substances that cause the syndrome.

Opioid peptides (enkephalins, dynorphin and related products) are also widely distributed in the ENS. Acting via opioid receptors, it has been possible to evaluate their specific functions using specific agonists and antagonists of these receptors, but the results have been confusing. Possibly, their main effect is to modulate neural transmission via presynaptic inhibition, as is observed in other parts of the nervous system. Gastrin-releasing peptide (GRP; mammalian bombesin) and the truncated form, neuromedin C, constituting the C-terminal decapeptide of GRP, are best known for their effects on gastrin secretion, but GRP fibres are scattered throughout the gastrointestinal tract, and, in general, GRP has a stimulatory or excitatory effect on motility as well as exocrine or endocrine secretion. Four receptors have been cloned and effective antagonists are available (Milusheva *et al.*, 1998; Pradhan *et al.*, 1998). The recent development of mice with a knockout of the high-affinity GRP receptor gene should prove helpful (Wada *et al.*, 1997). In addition, it is of considerable interest that mice with a null mutation of the low-affinity GRP receptor (bombesin receptor subtype-3) develop obesity, hypertension and impaired glucose metabolism, which characterize the ‘metabolic syndrome’ or ‘syndrome x’, one of the scourges of modern civilization (Okhi-Hamasaki *et al.*, 1997). GRP is also considered to be an autocrine growth factor for, for example, small cell lung cancers (Cuttitta *et al.*, 1985).

Galanin and somatostatin are also widespread neuropeptides (Harling *et al.*, 1991; Skak Nielsen *et al.*, 1987). Both peptides may affect gut motility, galanin being predominantly inhibitory (Rattan, 1991) and somatostatin mostly excitatory. The latter was surprising in view of the generally inhibitory responses elicited by this peptide in other tissues. In agreement with this, somatostatin is known to profoundly inhibit neural transmission in the ganglia, and it is thought that its motor effects may be due to inhibition of an inhibitory neurone.

REFERENCES

Adler, G., Beglinger, C., Braun, U. *et al.* 1991: Interaction of the cholinergic system and cholecystokinin in the regulation of endogenous and exogenous stimulation of pancreatic secretion in humans. *Gastroenterology* 100, 537–43.

Adler, G., Nelson, D.K., Katschinski, M., Beglinger, C. 1995: Neurohormonal control of human pancreatic exocrine secretion. *Pancreas* 10, 1–13.

Adrian, T.E., Mitchenere. P., Sagor, G., Bloom, S.R. 1982: Effect of pancreatic polypeptide on gall bladder pressure and hepatic bile secretion. *American Journal of Physiology* 243, G204–7.

Argent, B.E., Case, R.M. 1994: Pancreatic ducts. Cellular mechanism and control of bicarbonate secretion. In Johnson, L.R. (ed.), *Physiology of the gastrointestinal tract*. New York: Raven Press, 1473–97.

Arnold, R. (ed.) 1996: Somatostatin analogues. Basic and clinical perspectives. *Digestion* 57, S1–120.

Baldissera, F.G.A., Nielsen, O.V., Holst, J.J. 1985: The intestinal mucosa preferentially releases somatostatin-28 in pigs. *Regulatory Peptides* 11, 251–62.

Baldwin, G.S., Whitehead, R.H. 1994: Gut hormones, growth and malignancy. In Fuller, P., Shulkes, A. (eds), *Bailliere's clinical endocrinology and metabolism*. London: Bailliere Tindall, 185–214.

Bayliss, W.M., Starling, E.H. 1902: The mechanism of pancreatic secretion. *Journal of Physiology (London)* 28, 330–2.

Beglinger, C., Hildebrand, P., Meier, R. *et al.* 1992: A physiological role for cholecystokinin as a regulator of gastrin secretion. *Gastroenterology* 103, 490–5.

Bell, G.I. 1986: The glucagon superfamily: precursor structure and gene organization. *Peptides* 7(Suppl. 1), 27–36.

Bell, G.I., Reisine, T. 1993: Molecular biology of somatostatin receptors. *Trends in Neuroscience* 16, 34–8.

Berson, S.A., Yalow, R.S. 1967: Radioimmunoassays of peptide hormones in plasma. *New England Journal of Medicine* 277, 640–7.

Bishop, E.A., Bloom, S.R., Polak, J.M. 1988: Cytochemical techniques in work with gastrointestinal hormones. In Mutt, V. (ed.), *Gastrointestinal hormones*. San Diego: Academic Press, 11–44.

Bloom, S.R. 1987: Gut hormones in adaptation. *Gut* 28 (Suppl. 1), 31–5.

Boivin, M., Pinelo, L.R., St Pierre, S., Poitras, P. 1997: Neural mediation of the motilin motor effect on the human antrum. *American Journal of Physiology* 272, G71–6.

Brand, S.J., Babyatsky, M., Bachwich, D., Tillotson, L., Wang, T. 1994: Molecular approaches to the study of gut peptides. In Walsh, J.H., Dockray, G.J. (eds), *Gut peptides*. New York: Raven Press, 11–32.

Calam, J., Gibbons, A., Healey, Z.V., Bliss, P., Arebi, N. 1997: How does Helicobacter pylori cause mucosal damage? Its effect on acid and gastrin physiology. *Gastroenterology* 113, S43–9.

Cantor, P., Mortensen, P.E., Myhre, J. *et al.* 1992: The effect of the cholecystokinin receptor antagonists MK-329 on meal-stimulated pancreaticobiliary output in humans. *Gastroenterology* 102, 1742–51.

Cao, Y.Q., Mantyh, P.W., Carlson, E.J., Gillespie, A.-M., Epstein C.J., Basbaum, A.I., 1998: Primary afferent tachykinins are required to experience moderate to intense pain. *Nature* 392, 390–4.

Chance, W.T., Foley-Nelson, T., Thomas, I., Balasubramaniam, A. 1997: Prevention of nutrition-induced gut hypoplasia by co-infusion of glucagon-like peptide-2. *American Journal of Physiology* 273, G559–63.

Chen, C.H., Rogers, R.C. 1995: Central inhibitory action of peptide YY on gastric motility in rats. *American Journal of Physiology* 169, R787–92.

Chey, W.Y., Kim, M.S., Lee, K.Y., Chang, T.M. 1979: Effect of rabbit antiserum on postprandial pancreatic secretion in dogs. *Gastroenterology* 77, 1266–75.

Chey, W.Y., Kim, M.S., Lee, KY., Chang, T.M. 1981: Secretin is an enterogastrone in the dog. *American Journal of Physiology* 240, G239–44.

Chiba, T., Yamada, T. 1994: Gut somatostatin. In Walsh, J.H., Dockray, G.J. (eds), *Gut peptides*. New York: Raven Press, 123–46.

Christiansen, J., Lorentzen, M., Holst, J. 1990: Influence of peptides on anorectal function. *Annals of Medicine* 22, 413–18.

Conter, R.L., Hughes, M.T., Kauffmann, G.L. 1996: Intracerebroventricular secretin enhances pancreatic volume and bicarbonate response in rats. *Surgery* 119, 208–13.

Cuttita, F., Carney, D.N., Mulshine, J. *et al.* 1985: Bombesin-like peptides can function as autocrine growth factors in human small-cell lung cancer. *Nature* 316, 823–6.

Daniel, E.E. 1990: *Neuropeptide function in the gastrointestinal tract*. Boca Raton: CRC Press, 1–510.

De Felipe, C., Herreo, J.F., O'Brien, J.A. *et al.* 1998: Altered nociception, analgesia and aggression in mice lacking the receptor for substance P. *Nature* 392, 394–7.

DeHerder, W.W., Hofland, L.J., Usdin, T.B. *et al.* 1996: Food-dependent Cushing's syndrome resulting from abundant expression of gastric inhibitory polypeptide receptors in adrenal adenoma cells. *Journal of Clinical Endocrinology and Metabolism* 81, 3168–72.

deLecea, L., Kilduff, T.S., Peyron, C. *et al.* 1998: The hypocretins: hypothalamus specific peptides with neuroexcitatory activity. *Proceedings of the National Academy of Sciences USA* 95, 322–7.

Depoortere, I., DeClercq, P., Svoboda, M., Bare, L., Peeters, T.L. 1997a: Identification of motilin mRNA in the brain of man and rabbit. Conservation of polymorphisms of the motilin gene across species. *Peptides* 18, 1497–503.

Depoortere, I., Van Assche, G., Peeters, T.L. 1997b: Distribution and subcellular localization of motilin binding sites in the rabbit brain. *Brain Research* 777, 103–9.

Dobner, P.R., Barber, D.L., Villa-Komaroff, L., McKiernan, C. 1987: Cloning and sequence analysis of cDNA for the canine neurotensin/neuromedin N precursor. *Proceedings of the National Academy of Sciences USA* 84, 3516–20.

Drucker, D.J., Ehrlich P., Asa, L., Brubaker, P.L. 1996: Induction of intestinal epithelial proliferation by glucagon-like-peptide-2. *Proceedings of the National Academy of Sciences USA* 93, 7911–16.

Edkins, J.S. 1905: On the chemical mechanism of gastric secretion. *Proceedings of the Royal Society of London (Biology)* 76, 376–80.

Erickson, J.C., Clegg, K.E., Palmiter, R.D. 1996: Sensitivity to leptin and susceptibility to seizures of mice lacking neuropeptide Y. *Nature* 381, 415–21.

Erlinger, S. 1996: Review article: new insights into the mechanisms of hepatic transport and bile secretion. *Journal of Gastroenterology and Hepatology* 11, 575–9.

Fahrenkrug, J., Galbo, H., Holst, J.J., Schaffalitzky de Muckadell, O.B. 1978: Influence of the autonomic nervous system on the release of vasoactive intestinal polypeptide, from the gastrointestinal tract. *Journal of Physiology* 280, 405–22.

Feyrter, F. 1938: *Über diffuse endokrine epitheliale Organe*. Leipzig: Barth.

Fieseler, P., Bridenbaugh, S., Nustede, R., Martell, R., Ørskov, C., Holst, J.J., Nauck, M.A. 1995: Physiological augmentation of amino-acid induced insulin secretion by gastric inhibitory polypeptide and glucagon-like peptide-1 (GLP-1), but not cholecystokinin (CCK-8) in normal man. *American Journal of Physiology* 268, E949–55.

Flint, A., Raben, A., Astrup, A., Holst, J.J. 1998: Glucagon-like peptide-1 promotes satiety and suppresses energy intake in humans. *Journal of Clinical Investigation* 101, 515–20.

Forssmann, W.G. (ed.) 1998: VIP, PACAP and related peptides. Proceedings of the Third International Symposium. *Annals of the New York Academy of Science* 865, 1–611.

Friis-Hansen, L., Sundler, F., Li, Y., *et al.* 1998: Impaired gastric acid secretion in gastrin-deficient mice. *American Journal of Physiology* 274, G561–8.

Furness, J., Costa, M. 1987: *The enteric nervous system.* Edinburgh: Churchill Livingstone, 1–290.

Furness, J.B., Bornstein, J.C., Murphy, R., Pompolo, S. 1992: Role of peptides in transmission in the enteric nervous system. *Trends in Neurosciences* 15, 66–71.

Furuta, M., Yano, H., Zhou, A. *et al.* 1997: Defective prohormone processing and altered pancreatic islet morphology in mice lacking active SPC2. *Proceedings of the National Academy of Sciences USA* 94, 6646–51.

Gama, R., Norris, F., Morgan, L., Hampton, S., Wright, J., Marks, V. 1997: Elevated post-prandial gastric inhibitory polypeptide concentrations in hypertriglyceridemic subjects. *Clinical Science* 93, 343–7.

Gantz, I., Schaffer, M., DelValle, J. *et al.* 1991: Molecular cloning of a gene encoding the histamine H2 receptor. *Proceedings of the National Academy of Sciences USA* 88, 429–33.

Goll, R., Haagen Nielsen, S., Holst, J.J. 1996: Regulation of motilin release from isolated perfused duodenum. *Digestion* 57, 341–8.

Gromada, J., Holst, J.J., Rorsman, P. 1998: Cellular regulation of islet hormone secretion by the incretin hormone, glucagon-like peptide 1. *European Journal of Physiology* 435, 583–94.

Gubler, U., Seeburg, P., Hoffman, B.J., Gage, L.P., Udenfriend, S. 1982: Molecular cloning establishes proenkephalin as precursor of enkephalin-containing peptides. *Nature* 295, 206–9.

Gullo, L., De Giorgio, R., Corinaldesi, R., Barbara, L. 1992: Neurotensin: a physiological regulator of exocrine pancreatic secretion? *Italian Journal of Gastroenterology* 24, 347–51.

Gully, D., Lespy, L., Canton, M. *et al.* 1996: Effect of the neurotensin receptor antagonist SR48692 on rat blood pressure modulation by neurotensin. *Life Sciences* 58, 665–74.

Håkanson, R., Chen, D., Sundler, F. 1994: The ECL cells. In Johnson, L.R. (ed.), *Physiology of the gastrointestinal tract*, 3rd edn. New York: Raven Press, 1171–84.

Harling, H., Messell, T., Poulsen, S.S., Rasmussen, T.N., Holst, J.J. 1991: Galanin and vasoactive intestinal polypeptide: coexistence and corelease from the vascularly perfused pig ileum during distension and chemical stimulation of the mucosa. *Digestion* 50, 61–71.

Harper, A.A., Raper, H.S. 1943: Pancreozymin, a stimulant of secretion of pancreatic enzymes in extracts of the small intestine. *Journal of Physiology* 102, 115–25.

Henriksen, J.H. (ed.) 1991: Degradation of bioactive substances. *Physiology and Pathophysiology*. Boca Raton: CRC Press.

Herzig, K.H. 1998: Cholecystokinin- and secretin-releasing peptides in the intestine – a new regulatory interendocrine mechanism in the gastrointestinal tract. *Regulatory Peptides* 73, 89–94.

Hildebrand, P., Ensinck, J.W., Gyr, K. *et al.* 1992: Evidence for hormonal inhibition of exocrine pancreatic functions by somatostatin 28 in humans. *Gastroenterology* 103: 240–7.

Holst, J.J. 1997: Enteroglucagon. *Annual Review of Physiology* 59, 257–72.

Holst, J.J. 1998: Treatment of type 2 diabetes with glucagon-like peptide 1 (GLP-1). *Current Opinion in Endocrinology and Diabetes* 5, 108–15.

Holst, J.J., Deacon, C.F. 1998: Inhibition of the activity of dipeptidyl-peptidase IV as a treatment for type II diabetes mellitus. Perspectives in Diabetes. *Diabetes* 47, 1663–70.

Holst, J.J., Schaffalitzky de Muckadell, O.B., Fahrenkrug, J. 1979: Vagal control of pancreatic exocrine secretion in pigs. *Acta Physiologica Scandinavica* 105, 33–51.

Holst, J.J., Fahrenkrug, J., Knuhtsen, S., Jensen, S.L., Nielsen, O.V., Lundberg, J. 1987: VIP and PHI in the pig pancreas: co-existence, co-release and co-operative effects. *American Journal of Physiology* 252, G182–90.

Holst, J.J., Jørgensen, P.N., Rasmussen, T.N., Schmidt, P. 1992a: Somatostatin restraint of gastrin secretion in porcine antrum revealed by monoclonal antibody immunoneutralization. *American Journal of Physiology* 263, G908–12.

Holst, J.J., Ørskov, C., Seier Poulsen, S. 1992b: Somatostatin is an essential paracrine link in acid inhibition of gastrin secretion. *Digestion* 51, 95–102.

Holst, J.J., Skak-Nielsen, T., Øskov, C., Poulsen, S.S. 1992c: Vagal control of the release of somatostatin, vasoactive intestinal polypeptide, gastrin-releasing peptide and HCl from porcine non-antral stomach. *Scandinavian Journal of Gastroenterology* 27, 677–85.

Holst, J.J., Bersani, M., Johnsen, A.H., Kofod, H., Hartmann, B., Ørskov, C. 1994: Proglucagon processing in porcine and human pancreas. *Journal of Biological Chemistry* 269, 18827–33.

Holst, J.J., Gromada, J., Nauck, M.A. 1997a: The pathogenesis of non-insulin dependent diabetes mellitus involves a defective expression of the GIP receptor. *Diabetologia* 40, 984–6.

Holst, J.J., Ørskov, C., Hartmann, B., Deacon, C.F. 1997b: Posttranslational processing of proglucagon and postsecretory fate of proglucagon products. In Fehmann, H.C., Göke, B. (eds), *The insulinotropic gut hormone glucagon-like peptide-1. Frontiers in diabetes,* Vol. 1. Basel: Karger, 24–48.

Ishii, M., Nakamura, T., Kasai, F., Baba, T., Takebe, K. 1997: Erythromycin derivative improves gastric emptying and insulin requirement in diabetic patients with gastroparesis. *Diabetes Care* 20, 1134–7.

Itoh, N., Obata, K., Yanaihara, N., Okamoto, H. 1983: Human preprovasoactive intestinal polypeptide contains a novel PHI-like peptide, PHM-27. *Nature* 304, 547–9.

Itoh, Z. 1997: Motilin and clinical application. *Peptides* 18, 593–608.

Ivy, A.C., Olberg, E. 1928: A hormone mechanism for gallbladder contraction and evacuation. *American Journal of Physiology* 65, 599–613.

Jackson, R.S., Creemers, J.W., Ohagi, S. *et al.* 1997: Obesity and impaired prohormone processing associated with mutations in the human prohormone convertase 1 gene. *Nature Genetics* 16, 303–6.

Jensen, R.T. 1996: CCK B/gastrin receptor antagonists: recent advances and potential uses in gastric secretory disorders. *Yale Journal of Biology and Medicine* 69, 245–59.

Joshi, S., Gardner, J.D. 1996: Gastrin and colon cancer: a unifying hypothesis. *Digestive Diseases* 14, 334–44.

Kleibeuker, J.H., Weysselein, V.E., Maxwell, V.E., Walsh, J.H. 1984: Role of endogenous secretin in acid-induced inhibition of human gastric function. *Journal of Clinical Investigation* 73, 526–32.

Koh, T.J., Goldenring, Jl.R., Ito, S. *et al.* 1997: Gastrin deficiency results in altered gastric differentiation and decreased colonic proliferation in mice. *Gastroenterology* 113, 1015–25.

Kolligs, F., Fehmann, H.C., Göke, R., Göke, B. 1995: Reduction of the incretin effect in rats by the glucagon-like peptide-1 receptor antagonist exendin (9–39)amide. *Diabetes* 44, 16–19.

Kopin, A.S., Lee, Y.-M., McBride, E.W. *et al.* 1992: Expression cloning and characterization of the canine parietal cell gastrin receptor. *Proceedings of the National Academy of Sciences USA* 89, 3605–9.

Kopin, A.S., Nguyen, M., Chui, M. *et al.* 1996: CCK-A receptor deficient mice develop gallstones and lack of CCK mediated inhibition of food intake. *Regulatory Peptides* 64, 97.

Kovacs, T.O.G., Walsh, J.H., Maxwell, V., Wong, H.C., Azuma, T., Katt, E. 1989: Gastrin is a major mediator of the gastric phase of acid secretion in dogs: proof by monoclonal antibody neutralization. *Gastroenterology* 97, 1406–13.

Krarup, T. 1988: Immunoreactive gastric inhibitory polypeptide. *Endocrine Reviews* 9, 122–34.

Kubota, A., Yamada, Y., Hayami, T. *et al.* 1996: Identification of two missense mutations in the GIP receptor gene: a functional study and association analysis with NIDDM: no evidence of association with Japanese NIDDM subjects. *Diabetes* 45, 1701–5.

Labarre, J. 1932: Sur les possibilités d'un traitement due diabète par l'incretine. *Bulletin d'Academie Royale de Médicine Belgique* 12, 620–34.

Laburthe, M., Couvineau, A., Amiranoff, B., Voisin, T. 1994: Receptors for gut regulatory peptides. *Bailliere's Clinical Endocrinology and Metabolism* 8, 77–110.

Larhammar, D. 1996a: Evolution of neuropeptide Y, peptide YY and pancreatic polypeptide. *Regulatory Peptides* 62, 1–11.

Larhammar, D. 1996b: Structural diversity of receptors for neuropeptide Y, peptide YY and pancreatic polypeptide. *Regulatory Peptides* 65, 165–74.

Larsson, L.I., Fahrenkrug, J.F., Schaffalitzky de Muckadell, O.B., Sundler, F., Håkanson, R., Rehfeld, J.F. 1976: Localization of vasoactive intestinal polypeptide (VIP) to central and peripheral neurons. *Proceedings of the National Academy of Sciences USA* 73, 3197–200.

Larsson, L.I., Goltermann, N., De Magistris, L., Rehfeld, J.F., Schwartz, T.W. 1979: Somatostatin cell processes as pathways for paracrine secretion. *Science* 205, 1393–5.

Lauritsen, K.B., Holst, J.J., Moody, A.J. 1981: GIP antiserum depression of insulin release and glucose tolerance in rats. *Scandinavian Journal of Gastroenterology* 16, 417–20.

Leiter, E.H. 1997: Carboxypeptidase E and obesity in the mouse. *Journal of Endocrinology* 155, 211–14.

Libert, F., Parmentier, M., Lefort, A. *et al.* 1989: Selective amplification and cloning of four new members of the G protein-coupled receptor family. *Science* 244, 569–72.

Liddle, R.A. 1997: Cholecystokinin cells. *Annual Review of Physiology* 59, 221–42.

Liddle, R.A., Gertz, B.J.K., Kanayama, S. *et al.* 1989: Effects of a novel cholecystokinin receptor antagonist, MK-329 on gall bladder contraction and gastric emptying in humans. *Journal of Clinical Investigation* 84, 1220–5.

Lin, H.C., Zhao, X.T., Wang, L., Wong, H. 1996: Fat-induced ileal brake in the dog depends on peptide YY. *Gastroenterology* 110, 1491–5.

Liu, C.D., Hines, O.J., Newton, T.R. *et al.* 1996: Cholecystokinin mediation of colonic absorption via peptide YY: foregut-hindgut axis. *World Journal of Surgery* 20, 221–7.

Lloyd, K.C., Amirmoazzami, S., Friedik, F., Heynio, A., Solomon, T.E., Walsh, J.H. 1997: Candidate canine enterogastrones: acid inhibition before and after vagotomy. *American Journal of Physiology* 272, G1236–42.

Lok, S., Kuijper, J.L., Jelinek, L.J. *et al.* 1994: The human glucagon receptor encoding gene: structure, cDNA sequence and chromosomal localization. *Gene* 140, 203–9.

Maas, M.I., Hopman, W.P., Kartan, M.B., Jansen, J.B. 1998: Release of peptide YY and inhibition of gastric acid secretion by long-chain and medium-chain triglycerides but not by sucrose polyester in man. *European Journal of Clinical Investigation* 28, 123–30.

MacFarlane, A., Kinsman, R., Read, N.W. 1983: The ileal brake: ileal fat slows small bowel transit and gastric emptying in man. *Gut* 24, 471–2.

Mannon, P., Taylor, I.L. 1994: The pancreatic polypeptide family. In Walsh, J.H., Dockray, G.J. (eds), *Gut peptides, biochemistry and physiology*. New York: Raven Press, 341–70.

Marinelli, R.A., Pham, L., Agre, P., LaRusso, N.F. 1997: Secretin promotes osmotic water transport in rat cholangiocytes by increasing aquaporin-1 water channels in plasma membrane. Evidence for a secretin-induced vesicular translocation of aquaporin-1. *Journal of Biological Chemistry* 272, 12984–8.

Mendez, M., Souaze, F., Nagano, M., Kelly, P.A., Rostene, W., Forgez, P. 1997: High affinity neurotensin receptor mRNA distribution in the rat brain and peripheral tissues. *Journal of Molecular Neuroscience* 9, 983–1102.

Mertz, H.R., Walsh, J.H. 1994: Gastrointestinal neuroendocrine tumours. In Walsh, J.H., Dockray, G.J. (eds), *Gut peptides*. New York: Raven Press, 785–801.

Meunier, J.C., Mollereaud, C., Toll, L. *et al*. 1995: Isolation and structure of the endogenous agonist of opioid receptor-like ORL_1 receptor. *Nature* 377, 532–5.

Milusheva, E.A., Kortezova, N.I., Mizhorkova, Z.N. *et al*. 1998: Role of different bombesin receptor subtypes mediating contractile activity in cat upper gastrointestinal tract. *Peptides* 19, 549–56.

Miyasaka, K., Funakoshi, A. 1998: Luminal feed-back regulation, monitor peptide, CCK-releasing peptide, and CCK receptors. *Pancreas* 16, 2877–83.

Mogard, M.H., Maxwell, V., Sytnik, B., Walsh, J.H. 1987: Regulation of gastric acid secretion by neurotensin in man. Evidence against a hormonal role. *Journal of Clinical Investigation* 80, 1064–7.

Møller, L.N., Stidsen, C., Holst J.J. 2000: Somatostatin receptors. *Physiological Reviews* (in press).

Monstein, H.J., Nylander, A.G., Salehi, A., Chen, D., Lundquist, I., Håkanson, R. 1996: Cholecystokinin-A and cholecystokinin-B/gastrin receptor mRNA expression in the gastrointestinal tract and pancreas of the rat and man. *Scandinavian Journal of Gastroenterology* 31, 383–90.

Moran, T.H., Katz, L.F., Plata-Salaman, C.R., Schwartz, G.J. 1998: Disordered food intake and obesity in rats lacking cholecystokinin A receptors. *American Journal of Physiology* 274, R618–25.

Morgan, L.M. 1997: The metabolic role of GIP: physiology and pathology. *Biochemical Society Transactions* 24, 585–91.

Morriset, J., Levenez, F., Corring, T., Benrezzak, O., Pelletier, G., Calvo, E. 1996: Pig pancreatic acinar cells possess predominantly the CCK-B receptor subtype. *American Journal of Physiology* 271, E397–402.

Mutt, V., Jorpes, J.E. 1968: Structure of porcine cholecysto-kinin-pancreozymin. Cleavage with thrombin and with trypsin. *European Journal of Biochemistry* 6, 156–62.

Mutt, V., Jorpes, J.E., Magnusson, S. 1970: Structure of porcine secretin: the amino acid sequence. *European Journal of Biochemistry* 15, 513–20.

Nagata, A., Ito, M., Iwata, N. *et al*. 1996: G protein-coupled cholecystokinin-B/gastrin receptors are responsible for physiological cell growth of the stomach mucosa in vivo. *Proceedings of the National Academy of Sciences USA* 93, 11825–30.

Nakanishi, S. 1987: Substance P precursor and kininogen: their structures, gene organization, and regulation. *Physiological Reviews* 67, 1117–42.

Nakanishi, S. 1991: Mammalian tachykinin receptors. *Annual Review of Neuroscience* 14, 123–36.

Nakanishi, T., Kanayama, S., Kiyohara, T., Okuino, M., Shinomura, Y., Matsusawa, Y. 1996: Peptide YY induced alteration of colonic electrolyte transport in the rat. *Regulatory Peptides* 61, 149–54.

Nauck, M.A., Bartels, E., Ørskov, C., Ebert, R., Creutzfeldt, W. 1993: Additive insulinotropic effects of exogenous synthetic human gastric inhibitory polypeptide and glucagon-like peptide 1 (7–36) amide infused at near-physiological insulinotropic and glucose concentrations. *Journal of Clinical Endocrinology and Metabolism* 76, 912–17.

Nauck, M.A., Niedereichholz, V., Ettler, R. *et al*. 1997: Glucagon-like peptide 1 inhibition of gastric emptying outweighs its insulinotrophic effects in healthy humans. *American Journal of Physiology* 273, E981–8.

Ohki-Hamazaki, H., Watase, K., Yamamoto, K. *et al*. 1997: Mice lacking bombesin receptor subtype-3 develop metabolic defects and obesity. *Nature* 390, 165–9.

Orloff, S.L., Bunnet, N.W., Walsh, J.H., Debas, H.T. 1992: Intestinal acid inhibits gastric acid secretion by neural and hormonal mechanisms in rats. *American Journal of Physiology* 262, G165–70.

Ørskov, C., Holst, J.J., Knuhtsen, S., Baldissera, F.G.A., Poulsen, S.S., Nielsen, O.V. 1986: Glucagon-like peptides GLP-1 and GLP-2, predicted products of the glucagon gene, are secreted separately from the pig small intestine, but not pancreas. *Endocrinology* 119, 1467–75.

Park, H.S., Lee, Y.L., Kwon, H.Y., Chey, W.Y., Park, H.J. 1998: Significant cholinergic role in secretin-stimulated exocrine secretion in isolated rat pancreas. *American Journal of Physiology* 274, G413–18.

Park, J., Chiba, T., Yakabi, K., Yamada, T. 1987: Cholecystokinin (CCK) stimulates somatostatin release from isolated canine D-cells via both gastrin and CCK-selective receptors. *Gastroenterology* 92, 1566–72.

Pederson, R.A. 1994: Gastric inhibitory polypeptide. In Walsh, J.H., Dockray, G.J. (eds), *Gut peptides*. New York: Raven Press, 217–60.

Peeters, T.L. 1993: Erythromycin and other macrolides as prokinetic agents. *Gastroenterology* 105, 1886–99.

Peeters, T.L., Depoortere, I. 1994: Motilin receptor: a model for development of prokinetics. *Digestive Diseases and Sciences* 39(Suppl. 12), 76–8S.

Philippe, C., Lhoste, E.F., Dufresne, M., Moroder, L., Corring, T., Fourmy, D. 1997: Pharmacological and biochemical evidence for the simultaneous expression of CCKB/gastrin and CCKA receptors in the pig pancreas. *British Journal of Pharmacology* 120, 447–54.

Poitras, P. 1984: Motilin is a digestive hormone in the dog. *Gastroenterology* 87, 909–13.

Poitras, P., Miller, P., Dickner, M., Mao, Y.K., Daniel, E.E., St Pierre, S., Trudel, L. 1996: Heterogeneity of motilin receptors in the gastrointestinal tract of the rabbit. *Peptides* 17, 701–7.

Polak, J.M., Bloom, S.R. 1979: The diffuse neuroendocrine system. *Journal of Histochemistry and Cytochemistry* 27, 1398–400.

Pradhan, T.K., Katsuno, T., Taylor, J.E. *et al.* 1998: Identification of a unique ligand which has high affinity for all four bombesin receptor subtypes. *European Journal of Pharmacology* 343, 275–87.

Qvist, N., Øster-Jørgensen, E., Pedersen, S.A., Rasmussen, L., Hovendal, C., Holst, J.J. 1995: Increases in plasma motilin follow each episode of gallbladder emptying during the interdigestive period and changes in serum bile acid concentration correlate to plasma motilin. *Scandinavian Journal of Gastroenterology* 30: 122–7.

Rattan, S. 1991: Role of galanin in the gut. *Gastroenterology* 100, 1762–8.

Read, N., French, S., Cunningham, K. 1994: The role of the gut in regulating food intake in man. *Nutrition Reviews* 52, 1–10.

Reeve, J., Eysselein, V. (eds) 1994: Cholecystokinin. *Annals of the New York Academy of Science* 713, 1–450.

Rehfeld, J.F. 1998: Accurate measurement of cholecystokinin in plasma. *Clinical Chemistry* 44, 991–1001.

Reubi, J.C. 1997: Regulatory peptide receptors as molecular targets for cancer diagnosis and therapy. *Quarterly Journal of Nuclear Medicine* 41, 63–70.

Ropert, A., Cherbut, C., Roze, C. *et al.* 1996: Colonic fermentation and proximal gastric tone in humans. *Gastroenterology* 111, 289–96.

Rose, C., Vargas, F., Facchinetti, P. *et al.* 1996: Characterization and inhibition of a cholecystokinin-inactivating serine peptidase. *Nature* 380, 403–9.

Rosenfeld, M.G., Mermod, J.J., Amara, S.G. *et al.* 1983: Production of a novel neuropeptide encoded by the calcitonin gene via tissue-specific RNA processing. *Nature* 304, 129–35.

Rosetene, W.H., Alexander, M.J. 1997: Neurotensin and neuroendocrine regulation. *Frontiers in Neuroendocrinology* 18, 115–73.

Sakurai, T., Amemiya, A., Ishii, M. 1998: Orexins and orexin receptors: a family of hypothalamic neuropeptides and G protein-coupled receptors that regulate feeding behaviour. *Cell* 92, 573–5.

Samuelson, L.C., Gillespie, P.J., May, J.M., Swanberg, L.J., Seasholtz, A.F., Saunders, T.L. 1996: Generation of a CCK loss of function mutation in the mouse by homologous recombination in ES cells. *Regulatory Peptides* 64, 166.

Sawada, M., Dickinson, C.J. 1997: The G cell. *Annual Review of Physiology* 59, 273–98.

Schaffalitzky de Muckadell, O.B., Fahrenkrug, J., Matzen, P., Rune, S.J., Worning, H. 1979: Physiological significance of secretin in the pancreatic bicarbonate response to a physiological increase in plasma concentration. *Scandinavian Journal of Gastroenterology* 14, 85–90.

Schaffalitzky de Muckadell, O.B., Fahrenkrug, J., Nielsen, J., Westphall, I., Worning, H. 1981: Meal-stimulated secretin release in man: effect of acid and bile. *Scandinavian Journal of Gastroenterology* 1, 981–8.

Schmidt, P., Holst, J.J. 1997: Use of antagonists to define tachykininergic control of intestinal motility in pigs. *Peptides* 18, 373–9.

Schmidt, W.E., Creutzfeldt, W., Schleser, A. *et al.* 1991: Role of CCK in regulation of pancreaticobiliary functions and GI motility in humans: effects of loxiglumide. *American Journal of Physiology* 260: G197–206.

Schmidt, W.E., Schenck, S., Nustede, R., Rovati, L.C., Holst, J.J., Fölsch, U., Creutzfeldt, W. 1994: Cholecystokinin is a negative regulator of gastric acid secretion and postprandial release of gastrin in humans. *Gastroenterology* 107, 1610–20.

Schusdziarra, V., Zyznar, E., Rouiller, D., Boden, G., Brown, J.C., Arimura, A., Unger, R.H. 1980: Splanchnic somatostatin: a hormonal regulator of nutrient homeostasis. *Science* 207, 530–2.

Scrocchi, L., Brown, T.J., MacLusky, N., Brubaker, P.L., Auerbach, A.B., Joyner, A.L., Drucker, D.J. 1996: Glucose intolerance but normal satiety in mice with a null mutation in the glucagon-like peptide 1 receptor gene. *Nature Medicine* 2, 1254–8.

Seino, Y., Tanaka, K., Takeda, J. 1987: Sequence of an intestinal cDNA encoding human motilin precursor. *FEBS Letters* 223, 74–6.

Service, F.J. 1997: Insulinoma and other islet-cell tumors. *Cancer Treatment and Research* 89, 335–46.

Shulkes, A. 1994: Neurotensin. In Walsh, J.H., Dockray, G.J. (eds), *Gut peptides: biochemistry and physiology*. New York: Raven Press, 371–88.

Skak Nielsen, T., Holst, J.J., Baldissera, F.G.A., Seier Poulsen, S. 1987: Localization in the gastrointestinal tract of immunoreactive prosomatostatin. *Regulatory Peptides* 19, 183–96.

Solcia, E., Polak, J.M., Larsson, L.I., Buchan, A.M.J., Capella, C. 1981: Update on Lausanne classification of endocrine cells. In Bloom, S.R., Polak, J.M. (eds), *Gut hormones*. Edinburgh: Churchill Livingstone, 96–100.

Tager, H., Steiner, D.F. 1974: Peptide hormones. *Annual Review of Biochemistry* 43, 509–38.

Takahashi, Y., Kato, K., Hayashizaki, Y. *et al.* 1985: Molecular cloning of the human cholecystokinin gene by use of a synthetic probe containing deoxyinosine. *Proceedings of the National Academy of Sciences USA* 82, 1931–5.

Takeda, J., Seino, Yl., Tanaka, K. *et al.* 1987: Sequence of an intestinal cDNA encoding human gastric inhibitory polypeptide precursor. *Proceedings of the National Academy of Sciences USA* 84, 7005–8.

Takiguchi, S., Takata, Y., Funakoshi, A. *et al.* 1997: Disrupted cholecystokinin type-A receptor (CCKAR) gene in OLETF rats. *Gene* 197, 169–75.

Tanaka, K., Masu, M., Nakanishi, S. 1990: Structure and functional expression of the cloned rat neurotensin receptor. *Neuron* 4, 847–54.

Tatemoto, K., Mutt, V. 1982: Isolation of two novel candidate hormones using a chemical method for finding naturally occurring hormones. *Nature* 285, 417–18.

Thorens, B., Porret, A., Bühler, L., Deng, S.H., Morel, P., Widmann, C. 1993: Cloning and functional expression of the human islet GLP-1 receptor. Demonstration that exendin 4 is an agonist and exendin 9–39 an antagonist of the receptor. *Diabetes* 42, 1678–82.

Tseng, C.C., Kieffer, T.J., Jarboe, L.A., Usdin, T.B., Wolfe, M.M. 1996: Postprandial stimulation of insulin release by glucose-dependent insulinotropic polypeptide (GIP). Effect of a specific glucose dependent insulinotropic polypeptide receptor antagonist in the rat. *Journal of Clinical Investigation* 98, 2440–5.

Turton, M.D., O'Shea, D., Gunn, I. *et al.* 1996: A role for glucagon-like peptide-1 in the regulation of feeding. *Nature* 379, 69–72.

Ulrich, C.D., Holtmann, M., Miler, L.J. 1998: Secretin and vasoactive intestinal peptide receptors: members of a unique family of G protein-coupled receptors. *Gastroenterology* 114, 328–97.

Usdin, T.B., Mezey, E., Button, D.C., Brownstein, M.J., Bonner, T.I. 1993: Gastric inhibitory polypeptide receptor, a member of the secretin-vasoactive intestinal peptide receptor family, is widely distributed in peripheral organs and the brain. *Endocrinology* 133, 2861–70.

Vinayek, K.J., Frucht, H., Chiang, H.-C.V. *et al.* 1990: Zollinger–Ellison syndrome: recent advances in the management of gastrinoma. *Gastroenterology Clinics of North America* 19, 197–218.

Wada, E., Watase, K., Yamada, K. *et. al.* 1997: Generation and characterization of mice lacking gastrin-releasing peptide receptor. *Biochemical and Biophysical Research Communications* 239, 28–33.

Walsh, J.H. (ed.) 1993: *Gastrin*. New York: Raven Press, 1–432.

Walsh, J.H. 1994: Gastrointestinal hormones. In Johnson, L.R. (ed.), *Physiology of the gastrointestinal tract*, 3rd edn. New York: Raven Press, 1–128.

Wang, T.C., Koh, T.J., Varro, A. *et al.* 1996: Processing and proliferative effects of human progastrin in transgenic mice. *Journal of Clinical Investigation* 98, 1918–29.

Wank, S.A., Harkins, R., Jensen, R.T., Shapira, H., De Weerth, A., Slattery, T. 1992a: Purification, molecular cloning, and functional expression of the cholecystokinin receptor from rat pancreas. *Proceedings of the National Academy of Sciences USA* 89, 3125–9.

Wank, S.A., Pisegna, J.R., De Weerth, A. 1992b: Brain and gastrointestinal cholecystokinin receptor family: structure and functional expression. *Proceedings of the Nattional Academy of Sciences USA* 89, 8691–5.

Wartiovaara, K., Salo, M., Sariola, H. 1998: Hirschsprung's disease genes and the development of the enteric nervous system. *Annals of Medicine* 30, 66–74.

Wei, L.-N. 1997: Transgenic animals as new approaches in pharmacological studies. *Annual Review of Pharmacology and Toxicology* 37, 119–41.

Wei, Y., Mojsov, S. 1995: Tissue specific expression of the human receptor for glucagon-like peptide-1: brain, heart and pancreatic forms have the same deduced amino acid sequence. *FEBS Letters* 358, 219–24.

Wettergren, A., Schjoldager, B., Mortensen, P.E., Myhre, J., Christiansen, J., Holst, J.J. 1993: Truncated GLP-1 (proglucagon 72–107amide) inhibits gastric and pancreatic function in man. *Digestive Diseases* 38, 665–73.

Wettergren, A., Petersen, H., Ørskov, C., Christiansen, J., Holst, J.J. 1994: Glucagon-like peptide-1 (GLP-1) 7–36amide and peptide YY from the L-cell of the ileal mucosa are potent inhibitors of vagally induced acid secretion in man. *Scandinavian Journal of Gastroenterology* 29, 501–5.

Wettergren, A., Maina, P., Boesby, S., Holst, J.J. 1996: The effect of GLP-1 and PYY on acid secretion in man. *Regulatory Peptides* 64, 208.

Wettergren, A., Wøjdemann, M., Meisner, S., Stadil, F., Holst, J.J. 1997: The inhibitory effect of glucagon-like peptide-1 (GLP-1) 7–36 amide on gastric acid secretion in humans depends on an intact vagal innervation. *Gut* 40, 597–601.

Wiborg, O., Berglund, L., Boel, E. *et al.* 1981: Structure of a human gastrin gene. *Proceedings of the National Academy of Sciences USA* 26, 1067–9.

Widdowson, P.S., Buckingham, R., Williams, G. 1997: Distribution of (Leu31, Pro34)NPY-sensitive, BIBP3226-insensitive (125I)PYY (3–36) binding sites in rat brain: possible relationship to Y5 NPY receptors. *Brain Research* 778, 242–50.

Yamada, M., Yamada, M., Lombet, A.W., Forgez, P., Rostene, W. 1998: Distinct functional characteristics of levocabastine sensitive rat neurotensin NT2 receptor expressed in Chinese hamster ovary cells. *Life Sciences* 62, PL375–80.

FURTHER READING

In addition to the specific references listed below, the reader is referred to the following more comprehensive presentations on the subject.

Daniel, E.E. 1990: *Neuropeptide function in the gastrointestinal tract*. Boca Raton, FL: CRC Press, 1–510.

Dockray, G.J., Walsh, J.H. 1994: Regulatory peptide systems of the gut. In Walsh, J.H., Dockray, G.J. (eds) *Gut peptides*. New York: Raven Press, 1–10.

Holst, J.J., Schmidt, P. 1994: Gut hormones and intestinal function. In Fuller, P., Shulkes, A. (eds) *Bailliere's clinical endocrinology and metabolism. The gut as an endocrine organ*. London: Bailliere Tindall, 137–64.

Walsh, J.H., Dockray, G.J. 1994: *Gut peptides*. New York: Raven Press, 1–884.

8

Absorption and secretion of water and electrolytes

MRINALINI C RAO

OVERVIEW

The intestine is constantly faced with the predicament of keeping its luminal contents fluid while having to reabsorb the >7 L of liquid that reach its lumen daily. The intestine, in turn, adds 1.5–2 L of fluid to this volume. In a healthy individual, the small intestine reabsorbs >80 per cent of these 9 L of fluid. The structural and functional design of the intestine is conducive both to optimal nutrient absorption and this demand of fluid transport. Structural features, such as the folds of Kerckring, villi and crypts amplify the surface area to create a three-dimensional geometry that allows for effective movement of fluid. The bases of net fluid movement are specific electrolyte transport mechanisms in the enterocytes, with a spatial separation of absorption occurring chiefly in the villi and secretion in the crypts. In addition to fluid, mucous glycoproteins secreted by the goblet cells provide necessary lubrication and protection. Protection is also achieved by secretion of immunoglobulin A (IgA), secretion of paracrine modulators such as defensins from the Paneth cells and the physical barrier provided by the epithelium *per se*. Coordination of absorption as well as secretion demands a tight regulation, which is achieved by a plethora of regulatory factors. These factors could be locally released from endocrine cells in the epithelium, from neural or immune elements in the underlying mesenchyme or systemically transported by the rich vasculature in the submucosa. Finally, the overall transit of intestinal contents is influenced by the motility function of the smooth muscle layers. The challenges of coordinating function in a complex tissue like the intestine are underscored by the discovery, especially in the past two decades, of multiple transporters, each regulated by multiple signals and with extensive cross-talk between the various signaling pathways. An important corollary is that there is species- and cell-type variability.

There are a number of excellent reviews on the concepts of small intestinal fluid and electrolyte transport (Armstrong, 1987; Chang and Rao, 1991, 1994; Sullivan and Field, 1991), and this chapter provides a broad overview of ion transport and its regulation with an emphasis on recent insights.*

DESIGN OF THE INTESTINE AND MODELS USED TO STUDY ION TRANSPORT

In examining the dynamics of fluid transport in the intestine, both the overall, long, tube-like structure of the intestine as well as the compartmentalization created by the villi and the crypts need to be considered. Details of the architecture of the mucosa are provided in Chapters 1–3. Clearly there is no simple model in

*For the sake of brevity, the bibliography is chiefly composed of recent reviews and is not comprehensive. Any omissions from the vast volume of excellent work are unintentional and regretted.

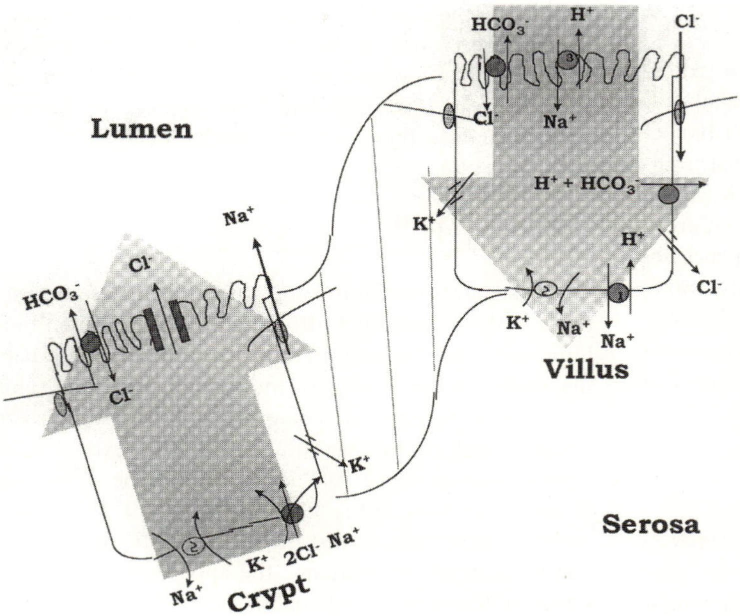

Figure 8.1 *Model of small intestinal ion transport processes. There is a morphological and functional separation of absorptive and secretory enterocytes in the villus and crypt regions, respectively. The driving force for net ion and fluid transport is the Na^+/K^+-ATPase located on the basolateral membrane. In the crypt cells, Cl^- enters via the Na^+–K^+–$2Cl^-$ co-transporter on the basolateral membrane and exits via Cl^- channels on the apical membrane. The basolateral membrane has an essential K^+ leak pathway. The apical membrane has Cl^-/HCO_3^- exchangers that could be involved in net HCO_3^- secretion. Movement of Na^+ from serosa to the lumen is paracellular. In the villus cells, the apical membrane has the NHE-3 and NHE-2 (not shown) isoforms of the Na^+/H^+ exchanger, which are responsible for vectorial Na^+ transport. In ileal (shown here) and not jejunal cells, there is also an apical Cl^-/HCO_3^- exchanger. In jejunal cells, HCO_3^- exits via the basolateral membrane. The basolateral membrane also has the NHE-1 isoform, which is quiescent in an actively absorbing epithelium. The movement of Cl^- is paracellular in the villar epithelium.*

which all these parameters can be studied effectively. Our current understanding of ion transport in the normal human intestine stems from *in vivo* perfusion studies, studies conducted *in vitro* on human intestinal explants, membrane vesicle preparations and from extrapolation of studies on cell lines and animal models. While *in vivo* perfusion studies in the human are the most physiological, they at best represent a composite picture of net transport. To delineate the individual ionic components of transport, intact intestinal epithelial sheets and/or biopsies have been studied *ex vivo*. However, even when stripped of underlying muscle layers, these tissues are heterogeneous, being composed of the epithelium, lamina propria and submucosal layers. Apical and basolateral membrane vesicle preparations are good models for delineating events at the membrane level but are not amenable to studying neurohumoral signaling cascades. Extensive information has been extrapolated from studies using animal models and immortalized cell lines of animal (e.g. rat IEC cells) and human (Caco-2, T-84 and HT-29 from the colon) origin. The Caco-2 cell line has been invaluable because it possesses a number of features akin to the human small intestine, despite its colonic origin. However, the increasing evidence for species-, segment- and cell-specific differences in a variety of ion transport mechanisms and their regulation lend a note of caution to making sweeping generalizations based on other models.

Mucosal epithelium

The small intestinal epithelium is essentially a barrier separating two iso-osmotic compartments, that of the lumen and that of the blood. In effect it acts as a semipermeable sheet, exhibits a transepithelial electrical potential difference and a transepithelial resistance (TER), and can serve as an osmotic barrier. The small intestine is a 'leaky' epithelium with the TER increasing from the duodenum ($\leq 25\ \Omega{\cdot}cm^2$ in some species) to the jejunum to the ileum ($\approx 90\ \Omega{\cdot}cm^2$ in the human). Tissue resistance increases to $\approx 200\ \Omega{\cdot}cm^2$ in the colon (Armstrong, 1987). Despite the low TER, the small intestinal epithelial cells are polarized with distinct tight junctions and a well-defined apical brush-border membrane (BBM) and basolateral membranes (BLM). The geometry of the lateral space between the enterocytes may be contorted by the presence of intercellular connections like gap junctions and desmosomes, and can influence transepithelial fluid flow. All four major cell types of the small intestinal epithelium – enterocytes, goblet, endocrine and Paneth cells – contribute directly or indirectly to fluid transport. The spatial organization of the mucosal epithelium into villi and crypts is accompanied by a functional differentiation, with the villi being the major sites of ion and nutrient absorption and the crypts being the sites of IgA and fluid secretion (Fig. 8.1).

ENTEROCYTES

Enterocytes are the 'workhorses' of electrolyte transport. The villar enterocytes are columnar epithelial cells with a highly differentiated apical brush-border microvillar membrane that is supported by a well-organized cytoskeletal scaffold. In contrast, the crypt enterocytes have a less pronounced BBM. The differentiation of nutrient transporters and metabolic processes along the crypt–villus axis has been well documented. This is paralleled by biochemical and functional differences in the nature of the electrolyte transport processes in the two cell types as described in 'Cellular basis of electrolyte and water transport'.

OTHER EPITHELIAL CELLS

These include Paneth cells at the base of the crypts of Lieberkuhn, endocrine cells chiefly in the lower two-thirds of the crypts and goblet cells distributed throughout the mucosa. The pyramidal Paneth cells, which are most abundant in the ileum, have received significant attention in recent years as the site of production of antimicrobial proteins. These include lysozyme, secretory phospholipase A_2 and defensins. Defensins, a family of small molecular weight antimicrobial peptides, with three intramolecular S–S bonds are also secreted by other epithelia and cells of myeloid origin. They can kill pathogens including viruses, bacteria, mycobacteria and protozoa, and exhibit cytolytic activity against mammalian cells. Intestinal defensins, termed cryptidins, are secreted into the crypt lumen, where they can achieve high local concentrations. Paneth cells secrete cryptidins either in response to serosal cholinergic activation and/or to the luminal presence of bacteria and lipopolysaccharides. The appearance of cryptidins increases with age (Lehrer *et al.*, 1998). The generally cationic defensins appear to attack their target cell membrane by binding to anionic sites and forming voltage-regulated channels. Recently, cryptidin was shown to transport Cl^- (Lencer *et al.*, 1997), and its release may be a local flushing defense mechanism in the crypt lumen.

Endocrine cells are scattered throughout the intestinal mucosa, and the peptides and biogenic amines elaborated by these cells are known to alter down the cephalocaudal axis. A large number of these modulators are released basolaterally into the subepithelial compartment from where they can be transported as classical endocrine substances or elicit paracrine effects. There is increasing evidence that some modulators are released from the apical membrane into the lumen where they can have local, paracrine/juxtacrine effects. For example, the peptide modulator guanylin is found both in the lumen, where it can activate surface receptors on the enterocytes, and in the serum (*see* 'Activators of cGMP'). The goblet cells secrete a variety of mucins copiously by classic exocrine mechanisms. Mucins are crucial in the maintenance of the glycocalyx, in lubrication and in protection. Lastly, immune cells such as intraepithelial lymphocytes are gaining prominence for their role in epithelial defence.

Support system

The basement membrane and underlying mesenchyme provide the structural scaffolding on which the epithelium rests, and the latter plays a pivotal role in modulating epithelial ion transport and barrier functions. This has been demonstrated using cell cultures, where the separate and combined influences of the extracellular matrix and mesenchymal elements can be examined (Chang and Rao, 1991, 1994; Barrett, 1997). Interestingly, in these reductionist models, a paucity of cell–cell contact appears to influence the appearance of certain types of transport mechanisms. The rich network of vasculature, neural elements and the entire gut-associated lymphoid tissue (GALT) in the wall of the intestine provide myriads of modulators that have a tremendous influence on epithelial function (Castro and Powell, 1994). The musculature contributes to net fluid movement both in terms of bulk motility and in releasing tissue metabolites in the intestinal wall. These metabolites, like adenosine and histamine, have profound effects on epithelial cell function.

CELLULAR BASIS OF ELECTROLYTE AND WATER TRANSPORT

Net transport of fluid and electrolytes across leaky epithelia can occur by both passive and active transport processes. Active transport is cellular (Fig. 8.1), whereas the bulk of passive transport is paracellular in the small intestine.

Paracellular transport

Passive forces, such as chemical, electrical,* osmotic and hydrostatic gradients, can drive ion and fluid transport; for example, in the small intestine, movement of K^+ out of the lumen primarily occurs via solvent drag. As discussed earlier in the section on the mucosal epithelium, the geometry of the paracellular space could influence net flow in response to these gradients. In the last decade much has been learned about the molecular

*The luminal surface of the mammalian small intestine is generally negative (approx. –10 mV) with respect to the serosal aspect.

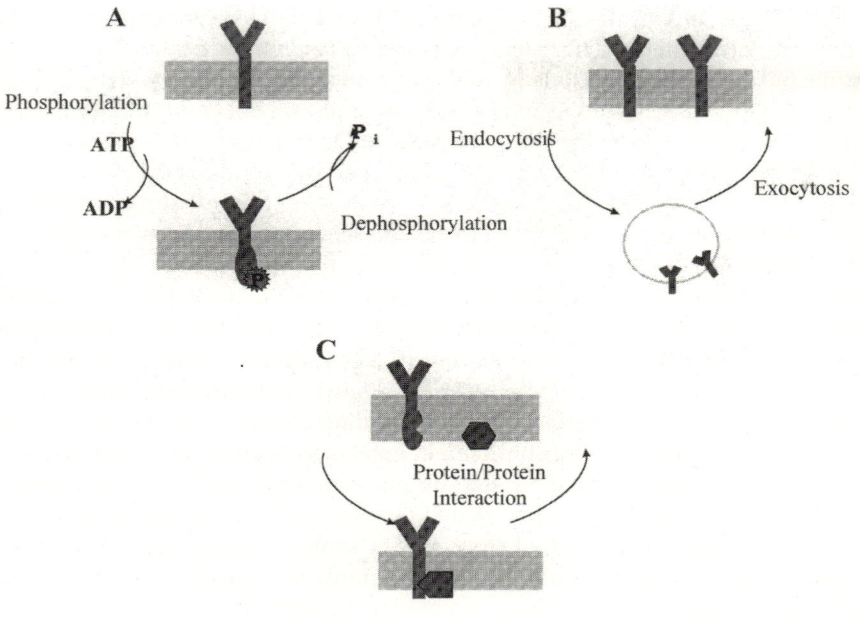

Figure 8.2 *Mechanisms for regulating ion transport. (a) Phosphorylation/dephosphorylation events can alter the activity of a transporter. Multiple phosphorylations may be required for sustained activation. (b) Stimulation of transport can be achieved by recruiting new transporters into the membrane and inhibition by sequestration of transporters into vesicles. Post-translational modifications such as phosphorylation can regulate these processes. (c) Activity of a transporter can be stimulated or inhibited by association with another protein. The modulator protein could be the site of second messenger-directed phosphorylation.*

nature of the proteins that line the paracellular route. A transmembrane protein, occludin, is the major protein associated with the tight junction, and various cadherins (proteins that mediate Ca^{2+}-dependent intercellular adhesion) form the zonula adherens subadjacent to this. However, these proteins do not function in isolation, but are part of a complex lattice of membrane, cytosolic and cytoskeletal proteins (Anderson and van Itallie, 1995). Thus, junctional proteins, and consequently the paracellular conduit, are subject to regulation by cellular mediators. Equally important is the contractility of the perijunctional actomyosin ring that collars the apical end of the enterocyte. This plays an active role in paracellular permeability as demonstrated in association with nutrient transport (Madara, 1989). Bacterial toxins, such as the zonula occludens toxin (ZOT) of *Vibrio cholera*, can also alter paracellular permeability (Fasano, 1998).

General principles of cellular transport

The *sine qua non* of all transepithelial active transport processes is the Na^+/K^+ ATPase (reviewed in Pressley, 1996) located on the BLM of most epithelial cells. The inherent gradient generated by the pump provides the driving force for the majority of electrolyte and solute transport mechanisms, making most of them secondary active transport processes. Blocking the pump with the cardiac glycoside, ouabain, inhibits net ion and solute transport. The pump is a P-type (or E1–E2) ATPase, which undergoes phosphorylation during the catalytic cycle and contributes to the membrane potential as it extrudes three Na^+ ions in exchange for two K^+. The Na^+/K^+ ATPase protein is heteromeric with an α subunit, the site of catalytic activity and a β-subunit; multiple isoforms of each subunit exist. The pump is a target site for regulation, especially by modulators, such as steroids, invoking transcriptional control. As detailed in the section on regulation of electrolyte transport, regulation of this and other transporters can occur either via post-translational modifications such as phosphorylation of the transporter molecule, via protein–protein interactions, and by sequestration to or release from subplasmalemmal vesicles (Fig. 8.2). While the pump is present in all cells of the intestinal epithelium, ion absorptive and secretory processes are not. An impressive body of work led to the dogma that crypt regions are the major sites of Cl^- and fluid secretion in the intestine, whereas absorptive processes are restricted to the villar or surface regions (Sullivan and Field, 1991). Recent evidence suggests that this division of function may not be an all or none phenomenon but that crypts are predominantly secretory and villi predominantly absorptive (Greger *et al.*, 1996). The molecular identity of many of these transporters has become available only in the past decade but a number remain to be identified.*

Transport pathways leading to fluid absorption

Net fluid absorption is inexorably linked to the movement of Na^+, either in conjunction with solutes or

*The molecular identification of ion transporters poses a number of challenges, e.g. an intact membrane system is required for assay. Since most transporters are widely distributed, cells lacking them need to be developed and/or identified. A number of innovative strategies have been used.

with parallel anion movement. The major anions absorbed are Cl^- and HCO_3^- (Fig. 8.1). Little fluid absorption occurs in the duodenum, the bulk occurring in the jejunum and ileum.

Na^+ SOLUTE TRANSPORTERS

A variety of solutes, including sugars, amino acids and bile acids, utilize the Na^+ gradient to be transported across the BBM against their concentration gradient. Within the enterocyte, the transported solutes could be partially utilized for the cell's own metabolism, but generally the bulk of them exit across the BLM, down their concentration gradient, via facilitated diffusion carriers (*see* Chapter 9). Many nutrient co-transporters, their isoforms and variants have been cloned. Indeed the Na^+-dependent glucose symporter was the first co-transporter to be cloned, and these studies revolutionized the field of transport biology by introducing the strategy of expression cloning using *Xenopus* oocytes.

Na^+/H^+ EXCHANGERS

In addition to solute-coupled transport, the bulk of Na^+ transport in the small intestine is achieved via Na^+/H^+ antiport.* While this antiport is relatively new in the pantheon of ion transporters, with the first detailed report appearing just over two decades ago (reviewed in Orlowski and Grinstein, 1997; Wakabayashi *et al.*, 1997; Donowitz *et al.*, 1998), there has been an explosion of information on this process. In cells, Na^+/H^+ antiport utilizes the Na^+ gradient to transport Na^+ into the cell, in a 1:1 exchange for H^+, resulting in a net alkalinization of the cell. The transport mechanism is driven by relative Na^+ and H^+ gradients and therefore is bidirectional. This fundamental transport process is ubiquitously distributed in all vertebrate cells where it functions to maintain cell pH and volume, and plays a role in growth regulation. Despite the 1:1 stoichiometry and a hyperbolic dependence on extracellular Na^+, the transporter activity exhibits a sigmoidal relationship with respect to intracellular H^+ concentration. This led to the demonstration that the exchanger has an internal H^+-sensitive allosteric site; thus as the intracellular pH falls below a threshold set point, the exchanger is rapidly activated. Is this widely distributed 'housekeeping' exchanger also responsible for vectorial Na^+ transport across epithelia? The answer is 'no', but it is carried out by processes which share some similarity with the 'housekeeping' exchanger. Earlier pharmacological studies and more recent cloning studies demonstrate the existence of these related transporters.

Molecular identification of the Na^+/H^+ exchanger was achieved by an ingenious approach: the bidirectional property of the antiporter was used to acid-kill a fibroblast population and the few survivors were clonally isolated, demonstrated to be NHE-deficient and so provided an ideal expression system. Cloning of the ubiquitous Na^+/H^+ exchanger (NHE) led rapidly to the discovery that there is a family of NHEs (reviewed in Orlowski and Grinstein, 1997; Wakabayashi *et al.*, 1997; Donowitz *et al.*, 1998). In mammalian systems at least five isoforms (NHE 1–5) have been identified and an NHE-6 isoform has been isolated. There is ≥ 34 per cent identity between NHE 1 to 5 isoforms at the amino acid level, whereas NHE-6 shows ≈ 20 per cent identity. These proteins are coded for by distinct genes, and the proteins exhibit distinct kinetic, tissue and cellular distribution and regulation profiles. They are all inhibited by the diuretic amiloride and its analogs with a potency that is isoform-specific. All members of the NHE family have a similar topology with two major regions: an NH_2-terminal hydrophobic domain with 12 membrane-spanning segments (M1–12) and a COOH-terminal cytoplasmic domain. Most of the isoforms have potential glycosylation sites on the extracellular loops. The transmembrane domain is conserved between the isoforms, is responsible for transport activity and bears the site of amiloride interaction (M4). The C-terminal domain is less conserved, and each isoform has distinct regulatory regions, which impart specificity to the role of the isoform. Regulators act to alter the sensitivity of the H^+-modifier site and/or the V_{max} value of the transporter.

In the intestine, NHE-1, the ubiquitous isoform, has been localized to the BLM and is responsible for the 'housekeeping' functions. In the differentiated enterocyte, NHE-1 is largely quiescent, since it would be counterproductive to move Na^+ into a vectorially transporting cell across the same membrane where it is being pumped out of the cell. Vectorial transport across the intestine is achieved by the NHE-2 and NHE-3 isoforms located on the BBM. They exhibit a descending villus–crypt gradient and are more abundant in the jejunum than in the ileum (Wakabayashi *et al.*, 1997; Donowitz *et al.*, 1998). Highly specific primers detected abundant NHE-2, but not NHE-4, in the rat intestine, whereas NHE-4, but not NHE-2, was localized to the rat kidney (Bookstein *et al.*, 1997). The distribution of the isoforms even within a membrane is not uniform. Immunolocalization and biochemical studies suggest that NHE-1 and the apical isoforms may be sequestered at specific sites associated with distinctive cytoskeletal proteins. Studies in cell lines transfected with the different NHE isoforms and in intact intestinal tissues demonstrate that NHE-2 and NHE-3 have distinct kinetics and patterns of regulation. Thus, while both NHE-2 and NHE-3 are involved in vectorial transport of Na^+, they may be differentially regulated under conditions of short-term or long-term alterations in Na^+ load. For example, up-regulation of Na^+ absorption

*Electrogenic Na^+ transport via Na^+ channels is present in the colon but is not a major mechanism in the small intestine.

in the small intestine by glucocorticoids correlates well with up-regulation of NHE-3 but not NHE-2 levels and activity, although both are present in abundance. Finally targeted gene disruption of these NHEs reveals that NHE-3-deficient, but not NHE-2-deficient, mice show impaired fluid absorption (Schultheis *et al.*, 1998a,b). These results suggest that NHE-3 is the major isoform underlying Na^+ absorption.

ANION ABSORPTION AND Cl^-/HCO_3^- EXCHANGERS

The major anions to consider are Cl^- and HCO_3^-, although transporters for other anions such as SO_4^{2-} and PO_4^{3-} are known to be present (reviewed in Armstrong, 1987; Sullivan and Field, 1991). In the jejunum, the movement of Cl^- is largely paracellular, passively following the electrical gradient. Technical difficulties in studying net HCO_3^- transport have made it hard to elucidate the underlying cellular processes. In the jejunum the intracellular HCO_3^-, generated by carbonic anhydrase to 'fuel' the Na^+/H^+ antiporter, generally exits the BLM by mechanisms that remain to be characterized. In contrast, the ileum has transporter(s) in its apical membrane for Cl^--dependent HCO_3^- transport. The latter has long been implicated as a major mechanism for HCO_3^- extrusion into the intestinal lumen using both *in vivo* and *in vitro* techniques. The prototype for all eukaryotic anion antiporters is the extensively characterized red blood cell anion exchanger (AE). This protein, originally termed Band 3, because of its migration on sodium dodecyl sulfate (SDS)-polyacrylamide gels, is now referred to as AE-1 and belongs to a family of proteins coded for by distinct genes, but with structural and functional similarities (reviewed in Alper, 1994). There are at least two other isoforms, AE-2 and AE-3; AE-3 has two subtypes, the brain (bAE-3) and cardiac (cAE-3) forms, which differ in their amino-terminal sequence. Recently, human intestine has been shown to have only AE-2 and bAE-3, but not AE-1 or cAE-3 (Alrefai *et al.*, 2000). The AEs are integral membrane proteins with 12 membrane-spanning helices in the C-terminal half of the molecule and a long cytoplasmic NH_2–terminal domain. The latter bears the major regulatory domain and at least in AE-1 interacts with a number of cytoskeletal proteins. The AEs transport Cl^- and HCO_3^- with a 1:1 stoichiometry and are sensitive to a variety of stilbene derivatives, such as 4,4'-diisothiocyanatostilbene-2,2'-disulfonic acid (DIDS) and 4-acetamido-4'-isothiocyanatostilbene-2,2'-disulfonic acid (SITS), and their potency is isoform-specific, being less effective against AE-2 and AE-3. While functional studies with isolated BBM vesicles clearly demonstrate the presence of Cl^-/HCO_3^- activity, with the exception of one study (Chow *et al.*, 1996), most immunolocalization studies detect AE-2 and AE-3 only on the BLM (Alrefai *et al.*, 2000). This has led to the suggestion that another AE isoform and/or exchanger may be responsible for apical Cl^-/HCO_3^- activity. A possible candidate is the product (DRA) of the *dra* (down-regulated in adenoma) gene, which encodes a SO_4^{2-}/anion exchange protein. A study of patients with the rare congenital chloride diarrhea (CLD) correlated mutations in *dra* with the disease. It remains to be determined if DRA itself is the BBM Cl^-/HCO_3^- exchanger or if it is a modulator thereof (Hoglund *et al.*, 1996).

Electrolyte transport pathways leading to secretion

Most, if not all, fluid-secreting epithelia utilize cellular Cl^- secretory mechanisms in concert with the Na^+/K^+-ATPase to drive water and electrolytes from the serosal to the luminal compartments. At least three transporters other than the pump are needed: Cl^- entry and exit steps, and a K^+ leak pathway (Fig. 8.1).

THE ENTRY STEP, $Na^+/K^+/2Cl^-$ CO-TRANSPORT

Chloride is above its electrochemical equilibrium in the cell and therefore entry into the cell has to be uphill. A cardinal component of the secretory process is a complex secondary active symporter that transports $1Na^+:1K^+:2Cl^-$ ions simultaneously. The Na^+ gradient is sufficient to drive Cl^- entry across the BLM, by this symporter, allowing the cell to gain two Cl^- ions for the expenditure of one Na^+ ion; Cl^- can accumulate up to levels as much as five-fold above its electrochemical equilibrium (reviewed in Armstrong, 1987; Kaplan *et al.*, 1996; Sullivan and Field, 1991; Begenisich and Melvin, 1998; Haas and Forbush, 1998). While the $Na^+/K^+/2Cl^-$ (NKCC) co-transport proteins were cloned recently, much has been known about the unique characteristics and regulation of these co-transporters before their molecular sequence was identified (reviewed in Kaplan *et al.*, 1996; Haas and Forbush, 1998). There are at least two known isoforms of the NKCC co-transporter: NKCC-1, the secretory form that is chiefly localized to the BLM of secretory epithelia; and the NKCC-2 isoform, which appears restricted to the apical membrane of absorptive epithelia. Although a major route of absorption in the intestine of euryhaline fish such as flounder (Suvitayavat *et al.*, 1994), NKCC is not a conduit for salt absorption in mammalian intestines but occurs in mammalian kidney (Kaplan *et al.*, 1996; Haas and Forbush, 1998). While NKCC-1 and -2 differ in their location and regulation, they share some fundamental properties such as their high degree of ion specificity. Thus, while Rb^+ can substitute for K^+, and Li^+ can substitute for Na^+, only Br^-, but not the other halides, I^- and F^-, can partially substitute for Cl^-. Another hallmark of NKCCs is their inhibition by the 5-sulfamoyl benzoic acid derivatives with a rank order of potency of furosemide < piretanide < bumetanide < benzmatinide. The NKCCs are large (≈ 150–180 kDa), integral membrane glycoproteins with 12 transmembrane helices, sandwiched between two very large NH_2–terminal and COOH-terminal cytoplasmic domains. The proteins contain consensus sequences for a variety of protein kinases, and it is known that their phosphorylation state often correlates with the activity of the transporter. Intracellular Cl^- concentration, the cytoskeleton, other transmembrane regulatory proteins and transcriptional control are also known to regulate NKCC. In keeping with the postulate that the crypts are the major sites of Cl^- secretion, the transcripts of NKCC-1 show a dramatic decline along the crypt–villus axis and in cell lines made to undergo crypt to villus differentiation (Matthews *et al.*, 1998).

K^+ CHANNELS

A leak mechanism for K^+ to return to the extracellular compartment is essential for maintaining Cl^- secretion. This enables the cell to move its electrical potential closer to the K^+ equilibrium potential and helps maintain the electrical driving force for Cl^- exit across the apical membrane. Conversely, exit of Cl^- depolarizes the cell and therefore can activate K^+ efflux. There are multiple classes of K^+ channels in the BLM, at least one of which is modulated by cAMP and another by Ca^{2+} (Barrett, 1993, 1997). The molecular identity of the intestinal isoforms remain to be established, although they are most likely related to the well-characterized K^+ channels of other tissues (reviewed in Durell *et al.*, 1998). These are multimeric transmembrane proteins with cytoplasmic regulatory domains which are believed to occlude the ion conductance pore in the resting cell. Stimulation causes a conformational change releasing the block and activating the channel. This 'ball and chain' model of regulation is gaining credence for a number of transporters including CFTR (*see* 'What is CFTR?').

EXIT STEP, Cl^- CHANNELS

Unraveling the molecular basis of two major diseases has revolutionized our understanding of the importance and the role of Cl^- secretion (reviewed in Field and Semrad, 1993). First came the discovery of how cholera toxin acted at the cellular level to stimulate Cl^- secretion. The seminal finding that the toxin affected electrolyte but not solute transport mechanisms led to the important therapeutic strategy of oral rehydration therapy (Reviewed in Field and Semrad, 1993). The second and more recent discovery was the cloning of the gene responsible for cystic fibrosis (CF) (reviewed in Welsh *et al.*, 1995; Jilling and Kirk, 1997). The protein product of the CF gene, termed cystic fibrosis transmembrane conductance regulator (CFTR), is the prominent, Cl^- channel in the apical membrane of an array of secretory epithelia, including the intestinal mucosa. Studying aberrations in epithelial ion transport both in human CF subjects and in the CF mouse model has revealed basic differences in how various tissues regulate Cl^- transport and therefore their secretory function. As described above and in Fig. 8.1, exit of Cl^- across the BBM is downhill and occurs via channels. Since 1989, although much attention has been focused on CFTR as *the* intestinal Cl^- channel, there is evidence that other Cl^- channels may also be present (Begenisich and Melvin, 1998). The role(s) of these in the human small intestine needs to be substantiated.

What is CFTR?

As its name suggests, CFTR was first thought to be a regulator of Cl^- transport rather than the channel *per se*. Numerous elegant studies, including the conclusive demonstration that purified CFTR incorporated into a planar lipid bilayer can transport Cl^- (Bear *et al.*, 1992) proved that CFTR is a Cl^- channel. Structurally CFTR falls under the rubric of the large family of ABC (ATP binding cassette) proteins, so named because they contain ≥ 1 domain(s) that have the signature ATP-binding sequence called the Walker motif. CFTR has 1480 amino acids and, depending on its state of glycosylation, exhibits a molecular weight of 160 000–180 000, with the latter being the mature form. The molecule can be roughly designated into two topologically similar, but not identical, halves separated by a large cytoplasmic region termed the regulatory or 'R' domain. The similar halves each comprise a transmembrane region (TM1 and TM2) with six α helices, immediately followed by a cytoplasmic nucleotide binding domain (NBD1 and NBD2). The unique R domain bears consensus sequences for a number of protein kinases and is not found in other ABC proteins. Functionally, CFTR is a low-conductance (G_t: 5–10 pS) linear channel with a permselectivity of $Br^- \geq Cl^- \geq I^- \geq F^-$. Although over 550 mutations of CFTR have been mapped, nearly two-thirds of all CF patients bear a deletion mutation of phe 508 (ΔF508). This is in NBD1, and the deletion results in improper protein folding, earmarking it for degradation rather than allowing it to be trafficked to its site on the apical membrane (Jilling and Kirk, 1997). Other mutations affect ion selectivity, nucleotide processing and translation. Current models suggest a two-step process for activation of CFTR as an ion channel. First, the R domain needs to be phosphorylated to induce a conformational change that will expose the ion pore formed by the transmembrane domains (TMs) but keeps it in a closed state. This is similar to the 'ball and chain' model proposed for the K^+ channels. Opening is rendered by ATP binding to NBD1 and its hydrolysis, whereas the duration of opening is regulated by ATP binding to NBD2. Since CF pathology is complex, it is no surprise that, with the discovery of the underlying defect, CFTR was assigned multiple roles. These have ranged from being a transporter for HCO_3^-, ATP and water to being a regulator of other ion channels, such as the outwardly rectifying large conductance Cl^- channel and the epithelial Na^+ channel (Greger *et al.*, 1996). Intracellularly, CFTR has been proposed to have a role(s) in acidification of endosomes, vesicular trafficking and endosome fusion. As CFTR is in low abundance, most of these studies have been carried out in other cell types transfected with CFTR. There is some evidence for these role(s) of CFTR in the small intestine (Welsh *et al.*, 1995; Jilling and Kirk, 1997; Grubb and Gabriel, 1998), and their physiological relevance is only beginning to be understood. In the small intestine CFTR is distributed largely in the crypts, although there is some evidence for its presence in villus enterocytes and goblet cells.

Other types of Cl^- channels

The intestine may possess at least three other classes of Cl^- channels, and their molecular identity and extent of their involvement in net fluid transport remains to be determined (reviewed in Begenisich and Melvin, 1998). These include the following:

1. The voltage-gated ClC family. The ClC-2 isoform is an inwardly rectifying, 3–5 pS G_t channel expressed in secretory tissues such as the rat small intestinal BBM. It is activated by an increase in cell volume and regulated by second messengers.
2. Volume-activated channels, which are widely distributed and have a G_t of 15–50 pS.
3. Ca^{2+}-activated Cl^- channels. The issue of a Ca^{2+}-dependent Cl^- channel in the intestine is interesting. It has long been suggested, based in part on the refractoriness of CF intestine to Ca^{2+}-dependent secretagogues, that all Ca^{2+}-regulated transport occurs via activation of BLM K^+ channels (reviewed in Barrett, 1993, 1997; Welsh *et al.*, 1995). However, recent evidence in T-84 cells, the archetype of intestinal Cl^- secretion, suggests that there is a Cl^- conductance, activated by Ca–CaM PK II and inhibited by inositol 3,4,5,6-tetrakisphosphate (IP_4) and the Ca^{2+}-binding protein annexin IV (Xie *et al.*, 1996).

HCO_3^- SECRETION

Bicarbonate secretion is needed for maintaining pH in the luminal membrane microenvironment throughout the length of the intestine. Recent investigations have focused on the duodenum as the major intestinal site of HCO_3^- secretion and the key role it plays in neutralizing acidic chyme. A number of transport mechanisms, including electrogenic secretion through channels and $Na^+/(HCO_3^-)_n$ symporters as well as electroneutral Na^+-independent (i.e. AEs, *see* 'Anion absorption and Cl^-/HCO_3^- exchangers') and Na^+-dependent Cl^-/HCO_3^- ($1Na^+:2HCO_3^-/1Cl^-$) exchangers, have been implicated in contributing to net HCO_3^- secretion (Sullivan and Field, 1991). The molecular identity of these transporters in the human intestines is not known. The relative contribution of the various pathways is not clear but exciting insights have been provided recently by comparing HCO_3^- secretion and its regulation in CFTR-deficient mice (CF-mice) and their normal littermates (Seidler *et al.*, 1997). Since CFTR is known to conduct HCO_3^-, albeit less so than Cl^-, this also addressed the question of whether there were separate HCO_3^- channels. A major portion of net duodenal HCO_3^- secretion is electrogenic, and the absence of CFTR caused a reduction in this response to cAMP, cGMP and Ca^{2+}-dependent secretagogues, without altering the Cl^-/HCO_3^- antiport capacity of the BBM. This study demonstrates that there are no separate 'HCO_3^- channels' and shows the central role of CFTR in HCO_3^- secretion. It remains to be determined whether HCO_3^- secretion occurs primarily through CFTR or through the Cl^-/HCO_3^- antiporter, which in turn is functionally linked to Cl^-. Such a mechanism has long been suggested for pancreatic and distal intestinal HCO_3^- secretion. In the ileum, Cl^-/HCO_3^- antiport plays a major role in electroneutral HCO_3^- secretion.

Water transport including water channels

The permeability of plasma membranes to water varies greatly with cell types. Water can move across the plasma membrane either by a slow diffusion across the lipid bilayer or by traversing through aqueous pores. Although Koefoed-Johnsen and Ussing (1953) predicted the existence of 'water pores', it was not until the early 1990s that a water-channel protein was cloned. A family of at least nine water-channel proteins, termed aquaporins (AQP),* not surprisingly, are distributed throughout the plant, animal and bacterial kingdom (Zeidel, 1998). Aquaporin isoforms were rapidly identified in tissues such as red blood cells, and renal and lens epithelia. Structurally, the AQPs are intrinsic proteins, with six predicted transmembrane helices and cytoplasmic NH_2- and COOH-terminal domains. AQPs probably function as tetramers, and they all have two characteristic asp-pro-ala motifs that may be involved in forming the aqueous pore.

*As in most 'new' families, the nomenclature has been confusing. Aquaporins have been classed as CHIP28, MIWC, AQP-CD and MIP. The latest classification of AQP 0–8 is used in this text.

Table 8.1 *Major neurohumoral substances and toxins that modulate intestinal fluid transport*

Intracellular mediators				
Cyclic AMP	**Cyclic GMP**	**PKC and/or Ca2+**	**Tyrosine kinase**	**Others**
Promoters of secretion[a]				
VIP	Guanylin	Bradykinin	EGF	Vasopressin
Prostaglandins	Uroguanylin	Acetylcholine		Histamine
Bradykinin	STa	Prostaglandins		Adenosine
Adenosine		Gastrin-releasing peptide		*C. difficile* enterotoxin
Histamine		Neurotensin		
Cholera toxin		Substance P		
LT		Serotonin		
Promoters of absorption				
α_2-Adrenergic agonists[b]				Dopamine
Somatostatin[b]				Aldosterone
Neuropeptide Y[b]				Glucocorticoid

[a]These agents stimulate second messenger systems.
[b]These agents attenuate second messenger systems.
LT, *E. coli* heat-labile enterotoxin; EGF, epidermal growth factor.

As the water permeabilities of the BBM and BLM *per se* are low, the intestines were thought to be a major location for AQPs. However, to date, AQPs have been detected only in the colon (AQPs 1, 3, 4 and 8) but not in the small intestine (e.g. Ma *et al.*, 1997; Zeidel, 1998). How then, does the human small intestine absorb up to 8–10 L of water a day in the absence of any overt hydrostatic or osmotic gradients? Recent studies reveal an intriguing alternate route for water transport, the Na^+-solute transporters. The well-established observation that water movement is coupled to Na^+-solute absorption in the small intestine was presumed to occur due to the generation of local osmotic gradients. However, the presence of such a gradient has not been demonstrated in the small intestine. Using the *Xenopus* oocyte expression system, it was demonstrated that the Na^+-glucose co-transporter transports Na^+:glucose: water with a stoichiometry of 2:1:>205–260 molecules across the membrane. The movement of water can occur uphill and therefore is via secondary active transport (Loo *et al.*, 1996; Meinild *et al.*, 1998). It is postulated that a variety of co-transporters, such as the H^+/amino acid and K^+/Cl^- co-transporters, are capable of transporting water molecules and may be responsible for water transport across the BLM. It has been calculated that, based on the absorption of 1 mole of glucose/day, the Na^+-glucose co-transporter could account for the absorption of as much as 5 L of water a day. Thus the small intestine could be a highly water-permeable epithelium without an apparent presence of classic AQP water channels. In contrast, the colon, where reabsorption of water from the stool occurs, may require a separate molecule such as AQP8 for transport. The conduit for water secretion remains to be identified.

REGULATION OF ELECTROLYTE TRANSPORT IN HEALTH AND DISEASE

The intestinal epithelium is bathed with a plethora of hormones, neurotransmitters, immunomodulators and autocoids (autocrine regulators such as arachidonic acid metabolites) on the serosal aspect, and a profusion of 'foreign' dietary substances and the local physiological factors released in response to luminal stimulation on the mucosal aspect. Clearly not all the luminal stimuli are beneficial, and the epithelium also has to respond to deleterious substances. Provided in Table 8.1 is a list, by no means exhaustive, of the major neurohumoral substances and toxins that modulate intestinal fluid transport.* It is teleologically sound that agents that promote net fluid secretion generally inhibit Na^+ absorption and stimulate Cl^- secretion, whereas agents that promote net fluid absorption increase Na^+ uptake and attenuate Cl^- secretion. In a healthy individual, net absorption prevails, and, when this balance is disrupted, diarrhea can ensue.

Signal transduction cascades – drives and brakes

The burgeoning literature on signaling cascades is an index of the challenges in understanding complex

*The distinction between the various classes of regulatory molecules, e.g. classic endocrine versus neural versus paracrine substances, is becoming murkier, reinforcing the high degree of plasticity and redundancy in nature. Thus most classifications are arbitrary.

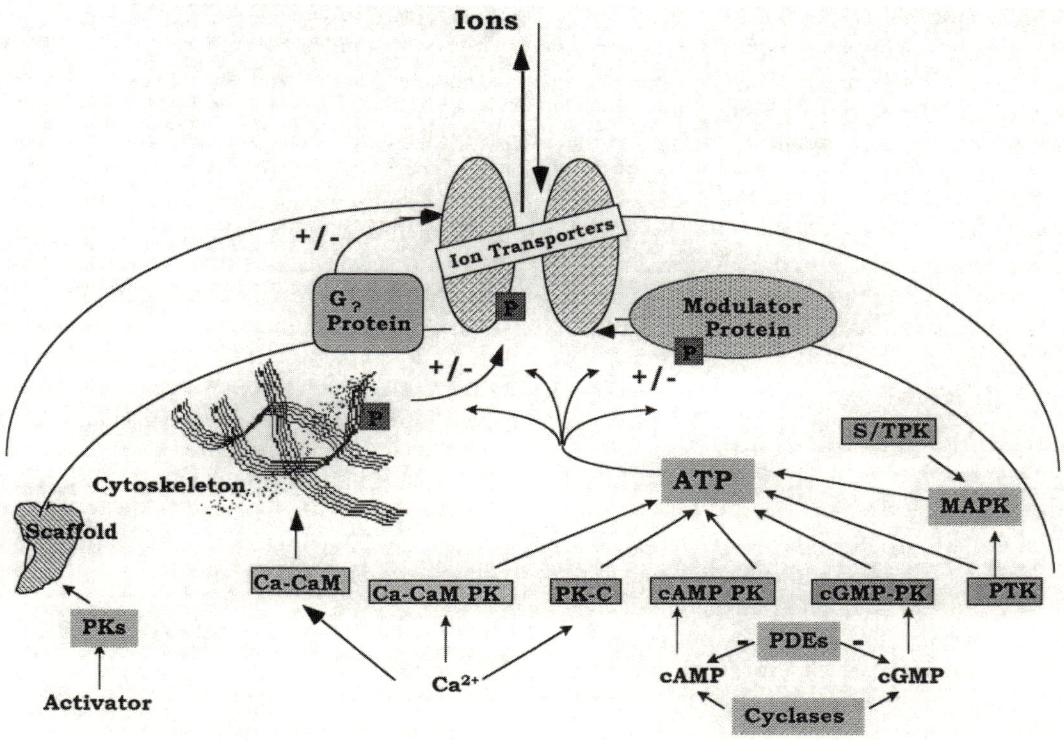

Figure 8.3 *Protein kinase cascades that could regulate intestinal ion transport. Activation of a variety of protein kinases (PKs) by specific second messengers could phosphorylate (P) one or more targets. These could be the ion transporter itself, modulator proteins and/or cytoskeletal proteins. The phosphorylation event could either activate (+) or inhibit (–) the transport process. All these events are reversed by the action of protein phosphatases (not shown here). The second messengers could be cyclic AMP (cAMP) or cyclic GMP (cGMP) whose levels are increased by the activation of cyclases and decreased by phosphodiesterases (PDEs). Other regulators could increase intracellular calcium (Ca^{2+}), which can act via binding proteins such as calmodulin (CaM) or via protein kinase C (PKC). Ca^{2+}-calmodulin can activate various processes directly or via PKs. Cyclic nucleotide and Ca^{2+}-dependent kinases are serine–threonine kinases (S/TPK). The protein tyrosine kinases (PTK) and dual-specificity kinases (MAPK) can also influence ion transport. All the S/TPKs, PTKs and MAPKs can cross-talk at multiple steps in their respective signaling cascades (not shown). Compartmentalization can be achieved by anchoring PKs, phosphatases and/or substrates to scaffolding proteins.*

phenomena such as net epithelial ion and fluid transport. The necessity for having rapid response cascades in place is offset by the equally important need to have rapid turn-off mechanisms. For example, while cyclases are poised to synthesize cyclic nucleotides, there are phosphodiesterases set to degrade them (Fig. 8.3). The net biological response will be governed by the relative contributions of the accentuating and attenuating processes. How is this achieved and what are the compounding variables? First, the molecules at almost every step in the signal transduction cascade, beginning with the activating hormone to the receptor, to the cyclase, the kinases/phosphatases and, finally, the transporters exist as multiple isoforms and/or variants (Fig. 8.3). These isoforms exhibit species, tissue, cell type and subcellular distribution differences, and are subject to regulation in response to routine physiological demands as well as during development. Second, the cannonical cascade of a stimulus → a second messenger → a kinase → a response is a gross oversimplification. There is extensive cross-talk between different signaling pathways at multiple steps. Within a signaling cascade, there are critical feedforward and feedback regulatory steps. Equally important is the recognition that there is no universal 'dogma' in signaling, e.g. protein phosphorylation is not synonymous with activation. Third, the pivotal role of compartmentalization* of specific components of the signaling cascade as a means of regulation is especially germane to the polarized enterocyte (Fig. 8.2). In this context, specific protein–protein interaction to promote docking of various enzymes and substrates has gained much importance (Fig. 8.3). Fourth, new signaling molecules and pathways are continuously being discovered, and their role in regulating epithelial ion transport remains to be elucidated. Finally, all signal transduction mechanisms need to be

*It is no longer true that 'compartmentalization' is a default explanation of data that does not fit conventional wisdom.

assessed with respect to their physiological relevance in the intact intestine. While reductionist models are a necessity for unraveling molecular mechanisms, they do not provide the complete picture. With these caveats, some common themes have emerged. Thus agents that elevate intracellular cAMP, cGMP or Ca^{2+} increase fluid secretion (Table 8.1). Fluid absorption is associated with a decrease in these messengers and/or an activation of some tyrosine kinase pathways. This section provides a brief description of how these signaling cascades, in particular those of cAMP, cGMP or Ca^{2+}, regulate intestinal ion transport.*

Post-translational modifications

Post-translational protein modifications ranging from glycosylation to myristylation (covalent linkage of a fatty acid to a soluble protein to help membrane localization of the protein) and phosphorylation/dephosphorylation are critical for delivering transporters to their correct location as well as for regulating their function. Phosphorylation and dephosphorylation, which utilize protein kinases (PKs) and protein phosphatases (PPases), respectively, have received tremendous attention as a rapid control system (reviewed in Hanks and Hunter, 1995; Barford, 1996; Fauman and Saper, 1996). The PKs catalyse the transfer of the terminal PO_4^{3-} of Mg-ATP to the –OH on a serine (ser), threonine (thr) or tyrosine (tyr) residue of a protein to form a phosphomonoester bond. At physiological pH, this adds two negative charges to the protein, which are sufficient to cause significant conformational change(s) in the substrate. This may result in altered function and/or interaction with other proteins, thereby initiating a variety of biological responses. PKs exhibit specificity both in terms of their activators and their substrates, and their action is essentially irreversible in living cells. Phosphoproteins can only be dephosphorylated by the action of separate enzymes, the PPases. The phosphoproteins could be the transporter itself and/or modulator proteins that are located in the membrane or cytosol (Fig. 8.3).

Both PKs and PPases are extensively regulated by cell signals. Based on whether they alter ser/thr or tyr, these enzymes are classified as ser/thr PKs (or PPases) or tyr PKs (or PPases) (reviewed in Hanks and Hunter, 1995; Barford, 1996; Fauman and Saper, 1996). The tyr-specific and ser/thr-specific PKs/PPases can act at different sites on the same substrate but generally cannot substitute for each other, although exceptions are known. The basic topology of a kinase involves a fairly well-conserved catalytic domain bearing ATP binding, phosphoryl transferase and peptide recognition sites and a highly divergent (between classes of PKs) regulatory domain. The peptide recognition site generally binds to a specific consensus sequence on the substrate that includes the phosphorylatable amino acid. The enzymes often possess a pseudosubstrate site, which holds the catalytic domain in an inactive state; when the regulator binds to the PK, this 'inhibition' is released, and the enzyme is activated. The PKs/PPases can themselves be phosphorylated. Various classes of Ca^{2+} and cyclic nucleotide-specific PKs are ser/thr PKs, whereas tyr-specific PKs are associated with receptors of a number of hormones involved in growth. Until the early 1990s it was thought that these two signaling pathways were distinct. Furthermore, the discovery of dual-specificity PKs (Cobb and Goldsmith, 1995), which can phosphorylate a specific sequence containing tyr and thr, opened up the entire field of cross-talk in signaling pathways. Similarly there are dual-specificity PPases.

cAMP cascade

The pioneering work of Field and others (Field and Semrad, 1993) identified cAMP as a key signal in the action of cholera toxin (CT), elaborated by *Vibrio cholera* and humoral secretagogues such as secretin, vasoactive intestinal peptide and prostaglandins. All of them activate, albeit by different types of receptors, the integral membrane protein, adenylate cyclase, which hydrolyzes ATP to form cAMP. Indeed, elucidation of the action of CT was seminal in our comprehension of adenylate cyclase signaling. Adenylate cyclases are integral membrane proteins similar in topology to ABC transporters like CFTR (*see* 'What is CFTR?') and require both of their cytoplasmic domains for activity (Taussig and Gilman, 1995). Receptors linked to adenylate cyclase activation are members of a superfamily of heptahelical transmembrane proteins that are located on the BLM in intestinal epithelia. Binding of hormones changes the receptor conformation, which is transduced to adenylate cyclases via heterotrimeric GTP-binding proteins (G proteins) in the membrane.

The seminal prediction, nearly 30 years ago, that there has to be a transducer that connects multifarious receptors to the cyclase, led to the discovery of G proteins (Rodbell, 1980). Heterotrimeric G proteins, composed of α, β and γ subunits, are a subgroup of a larger family of G proteins. The α subunit has a receptor interacting domain and, in the quiescent state, is associated with $\beta\gamma$ and GDP. Receptor activation increases affinity for GTP and a dissociation of α from $\beta\gamma$. There is heterogeneity in G_α, and $G_{\alpha s}$ stimulates adenylate cyclase and the production of cAMP. G proteins have nascent GTPase activity, which hydrolyses GTP to GDP, resulting in the reassociation of G_α with $\beta\gamma$. The receptor signaling cascade is different for CT

*Space restrictions preclude doing justice to all the signaling pathways examined in the intestine and therefore general concepts and a few highlights are provided.

and other enterotoxins, such as *Escherichia coli* heat-labile toxin (Sears and Kaper, 1996; Fasano, 1998). The receptors for CT are the ubiquitous GM_1 gangliosides. In the intestine, the pentameric B subunit of CT binds to GM_1 ganglioside on the BBM. This allows for the insertion and translocation of the A subunit into the membrane where its S–S bonds are reduced to release the active A_1 fragment. A_1 has enzymatic activity, which causes the ADP ribosylation of arginine residues on $G_{\alpha s}$. This irreversibly inactivates the nascent GTPase and renders $G_{\alpha s}$ constitutively active. Thus, as long as the cell has activated $G_{\alpha s}$, the adenylate cyclase remains activated, accounting for the large amounts of cAMP generated and the consequent copious fluid secretion. The puzzling issue of how cholera toxin entering apically can affect basolateral adenylate cyclase has recently been demonstrated to involve transcellular cytosis through endocytic vesicles (reviewed in Sears and Kaper, 1996; Fasano, 1998). The intestine also has important modulators that decrease cAMP content, including somatostatin and epinephrine, the latter acting through α_2 receptors. Binding of these receptors activates $G_{\alpha i}$, another subset of G_α proteins. Activation of $G_{\alpha i}$ also dissociates it from $\beta\gamma$ and results in GTP displacing GDP. The mechanism(s) by which this leads to decreased cyclase activity appears to depend on the cyclase isoform and the cell type, e.g. myristylated $G_{\alpha i}$ inhibits Type V, whereas $\beta\gamma$ inhibits Type 1 cyclase (Taussig and Gilman, 1995). The distribution of the G_α proteins in the enterocyte is polarized with the BBM having abundant $G_{\alpha s}$, and $G_{\alpha i}$ being localized to the BLM.

Cyclic AMP causes many of its actions by activating cAMP-specific PKs (de Jonge and Rao, 1990). These tetrameric enzymes have two regulatory subunits, each with two cAMP binding sites and two catalytic subunits. Binding of cAMP releases the catalytic subunits from the regulatory dimer and renders them active. CFTR has a number of consensus sequences for cAMP-PK, and phosphorylation of five specific sequences is necessary for the activation of the R domain (reviewed in Welsh *et al.*, 1995; Jilling and Kirk, 1997). The ser/thr PPases, PP2a and PP2c, dephosphorylate and thereby inactivate CFTR. Cyclic AMP-specific phosphorylation also plays a role in the sequestration and release of CFTR-containing endosomal vesicles from and to the apical membrane. Cyclic AMP stimulates NKCC-1 and inhibits NHE-3 activity. The regulation of NHE-3 appears to occur either by direct phosphorylation of the transporter, and/or by interaction with specific cAMP-modulated binding protein(s) and/or by sequestration into vesicles (Orlowski and Grinstein, 1997; Wakabayashi *et al.*, 1997).

Activators of cGMP

Unlike those of cAMP, the signaling systems utilizing cGMP are more restricted in their distribution and regulate more specialized functions. With the exception of the phototransduction system, investigations on the role of cGMP have generally lagged behind those on cAMP. The discovery that the heat-stable enterotoxin of *E. coli*, STa, causes rapid secretory diarrhea by increasing cGMP content opened a new area of investigation (Rao, 1985; Field and Semrad, 1993; Sears and Kaper, 1996). Although the final outcome is the stimulation of Cl^- secretion and the inhibition of Na^+ absorption (Chang and Rao, 1991), a number of features set the STa-cGMP cascade apart from the CT-cAMP cascade. These include the locus of action, the STa receptor, the endogenous ligands for STa and the cGMP-PK cascades (de Jonge and Rao, 1990; Lohmann *et al.*, 1997).

STa action, unlike that of CT, is highly tissue-specific, eliciting biological effects only in defined intestinal segments (Rao, 1985). STa acts only luminally and exhibits a decreasing villus to crypt gradation in activation of BBM guanylate cyclase. The STa receptor was identified in 1990 as a membrane form of guanylate cyclase, GC-C (Schulz *et al.*, 1990). The tissue-specific localization of STa receptors/action led to the prediction and discovery of a family of endogenous STa homologs, guanylin (reviewed in Forte and Hamra, 1996). Guanylin and uroguanylin are synthesized in precursor form and are structurally similar to STa, but have four rather than six cysteine residues. They presumably bind to GC-C on the BBM and are less potent than STa. Guanylins are secreted luminally, where they have a paracrine effect, and basolaterally into the serum. With some species differences, uroguanylin appears to be produced largely by the enterochromaffin cells of the proximal small intestine, whereas proguanylin appears to be localized more frequently to ileal and colonic goblet cells. In keeping with this distribution, uroguanylin has a more acidic pH optimum for its action than guanylin.

In contrast to the triumvirate of membrane receptor–G protein–cyclase of the cAMP cascade, there are membrane and cytosolic isoforms of guanylate cyclases in which the recognition and catalytic sites reside on the same protein (Schulz *et al.*, 1990; Wedel and Garbers, 1997). In intestinal epithelia, the bulk of GC is membrane-localized, with little, if any, being detected in the cytosol. This is unusual since in other tissues such as intestinal smooth muscle, the major GC isoforms are cytosolic and are involved in nitric oxide signaling. While nitric oxide can influence fluid transport in the intestine, it is thought to occur indirectly via submucosal elements. The STa receptor, GC-C, and a recently identified orphan receptor, GC-G, are the only representatives of the particulate GC family (GC-A to GC-G) detected in enterocytes. Although atrial natriuretic peptides regulate

*Small molecular weight peptides, high in S–S bonds like these and cryptidin (*see* 'Other epithelial cells') tend to be protease resistant and may be a motif of luminally active secretagogues.

renal fluid homeostasis via GC-A and GC-B, they have no effect on the enterocyte. GC-C acts as a dimer, and each monomer is a single-pass transmembrane glycoprotein (140–160 kDa) with an NH_2-terminal extracellular domain bearing the ligand recognition site, a 21-amino-acid transmembrane domain, and a > 550-amino-acid cytoplasmic tail. The cytoplasmic region immediately adjacent to the membrane has a protein kinase-like domain, followed by a catalytic domain and finally a 70-amino-acid COOH-terminal, which is the site of cytoskeletal interaction. GC-C appears to be the sole STa receptor since the only defect in GC-C-deficient mice was an insensitivity to STa-induced secretion (Mann *et al.*, 1997; Schulz *et al.*, 1997). This brings into question what, if any, are the other roles of GC-C and why has it survived natural selection?

The intestine is also unique with respect to the cGMP-PKs in that, rather than the ubiquitous PKG-I isoforms, it possesses a tissue-restricted isoform, PKG-II. In contrast to GC-C, PKG-II shows an increase in activity from villus to crypt in keeping with the distribution of CFTR. Like all cGMP-PKs, PKG-II has the regulatory and catalytic domains on the same molecule and requires dimerization for activity. Activation occurs as a result of two cGMPs binding to the regulatory domain. In addition, PKG-II has an NH_2–terminal myristylation site that allows it to anchor to the membrane (reviewed in (de Jonge and Rao, 1990; Lohmann *et al.*, 1997). In an elegant series of studies, de Jonge and collaborators have demonstrated that the docking of PKG-II at a site on the BBM close to CFTR, allows phosphorylation and activation of the latter (French *et al.*, 1995). The system provides an interesting example of complexity in signaling: both PKG-I and PKG-II can phosphorylate CFTR in membranes, but only PKG-II can activate Cl^- conductance, emphasizing the importance of the membrane milieu. Thus GC-C, PKG-II and CFTR are in close proximity in the BBM and poised for activation by luminal peptides, perhaps to provide a local flushing response. The mechanism by which cGMP inhibits Na^+ absorption is not known (Chang and Rao, 1991). PKG-II knockout mice not only show refractoriness to STa stimulation but were also defective in endochondrial ossification (Pfiefer *et al.*, 1996). Other features that make the cGMP cascade distinct from the cAMP cascade include: its responsiveness to cGMP is segment and development specific; the intestine is one of the few secretory epithelia that possesses the GC-C→PKG-II→CFTR cascade; and STa is a potent stimulator of duodenal HCO_3^- secretion. All these lend credence to the suggestion that this cascade perhaps has a highly specialized role(s) in intestinal function.

*PKG-II is also found in brain, kidney and bone.

Phosphodiesterases

Phosphodiesterases (PDE) are relatively new contenders in the assortment of pathways that affect electrolyte transport and are subject to hormonal regulation. They are a family of dimeric enzymes that hydrolyse 3',5'-cyclic nucleotides to their 5'-congeners and thereby modulate the levels of available cyclic nucleotides. The 11 isoforms have different allosteric sites and active sites (Beavo, 1995). For example, PDE II is activated by cGMP, whereas PDE III is inhibited by cGMP, and both prefer cAMP as a substrate. PDE V is cGMP-sensitive and acts on cGMP. While PDEs play a crucial role in signal amplification in visual transduction, until recently it was assumed that they had only a constitutive role in epithelia and were not subject to regulation. However, studies on cGMP signaling suggest that PDEs can be regulated. For example, in rat colon, cGMP activates secretion by inhibiting a cAMP PDE (PDE III?) and thereby increasing cAMP (Lohmann *et al.*, 1997). In T84 cells, desensitization to STa stimulation is due to an activation of PDE V (Bakre and Visweswariah, 1997) and may contribute to the transient nature of the STa response.

Calcium and DAG signaling

Hormones and neurotransmitters such as substance P, neurotensin and acetylcholine activate secretion by increasing intracellular Ca^{2+} (reviewed in Rao and de Jonge, 1990; Berridge, 1997; Holda *et al.*, 1998). The well-recognized pathway is via activation of membrane receptors that are coupled to the heterotrimeric G protein, in particular $G_{\alpha q}$, cascade. Activated $G_{\alpha q}$ in turn stimulates phospholipase C-β to hydrolyze phosphatidyl inositol to release diacylglycerol (DAG) and inositol 1,4,5–trisphosphate (IP_3). DAG can also be produced indirectly by the activation of phospholipase D by tyrosine kinase receptors, via the release of phosphatidic acid. The rise in DAG is generally transient as it is rapidly metabolized, and its major action is by stimulating protein kinase C (PKC). DAG *per se* does not increase intracellular Ca^{2+}.

The profile of intracellular Ca^{2+} in response to a secretagogue is biphasic with an initial rapid and transient peak which declines to a plateau that is higher than basal values. The peak could be either due to release from intracellular stores and/or influx through plasma membrane Ca^{2+} channels. The plateau phase is generally dependent on the presence of extracellular Ca^{2+} (see below). The IP_3 acts on specific receptors to release Ca^{2+} from intracellular stores and increases free cytosolic Ca^{2+} concentrations. The increase in cytosolic Ca^{2+} is transient, with the Ca^{2+} being resequestered by Ca^{2+}-dependent ATPases on the endoplasmic reticulum or effluxed by Na^+/Ca^{2+} exchange on the plasma membrane. Recent studies demonstrate that epithelia also possess ryanodine receptors, which are well characterized in muscle cells as the sites of Ca^{2+}-induced Ca^{2+} release. Cyclic ADP ribose, not IP_3, is the putative signaling molecule for the ryanodine-sensitive receptor (Holda *et al.*, 1998). The kinetics of the IP_3 receptor channel and the ryanodine receptors are distinct, and the two mechanisms may help the cell distinguish between different types of signals. Undoubtedly, the intracellular Ca^{2+} stores are not limitless and need to be replenished from extracellular Ca^{2+}. This mechanism has been termed 'capacitative calcium entry' and represents the plateau phase of the Ca^{2+} profile. The molecular basis of these capacitance channels and the process by which the intracellular stores signal to the plasma membrane to replenish the stores is being actively investigated. While the IP_3 cascade has been characterized in the small intestine, the presence of the other Ca^{2+} pathways remains to be demonstrated.

The transience of Ca^{2+} signaling and desensitization to Ca^{2+}-dependent secretagogues have been well documented in intestinal epithelia. The underlying mechanisms, however, are not defined. One possibility is the concomitant release of signals that dampen the response. Thus, phospholipase C (PLC) activation releases other polyinositol phosphates, such as IP_4, which function as ileal brakes and attenuate Ca^{2+}-induced Cl^- secretion (Xie *et al.*, 1996; Barrett, 1997). How the increase in intracellular Ca^{2+} causes an activation or inhibition of specific ion transport mechanisms is a complex and at times controversial issue. Activation of Ca^{2+}-binding proteins and/or Ca^{2+}-sensitive PKs are the major mechanisms.

Protein kinase C

The common feature of this class of ser/thr PKs is their requirement for phosphatidylserine, although they were originally described as Ca^{2+}- and phospholipid-dependent. In addition to phosphatidylserine, depending on the isoform, PKCs can be activated by DAG, Ca^{2+} and other lipid second messengers (reviewed in Rao and de Jonge, 1990; Newton, 1995). The early observations, that the tumor-promoting phorbol esters are potent activators of PKC by virtue of their similar conformation to DAG but are not easily metabolized, have been extensively exploited in elucidating the actions of PKC. In contrast to the cyclic nucleotide PKs, PKCs have less stringent requirements for substrate stereospecificity, which may account for their wide range of functions. Currently there are at least 11 members of this family, which are divided into three groups: the traditional DAG- and Ca^{2+}-dependent or 'conventional isoforms' (cPKCs), α, β I and II and γ; the Ca^{2+}-independent, DAG-dependent or 'novel' isoforms (nPKCs), δ, ϵ, η, θ and the related μ (also known as PKD); and the atypical forms (aPKCs), ζ and λ, which require neither Ca^{2+} nor DAG. In all PKCs but μ, the pseudosubstrate domain resides in the extreme NH_2–terminal region. This is followed by two major 'conserved' regions (C1 and C2) comprising the regulatory domain of the enzyme, a hinge region and the C-terminal catalytic domain which bears the ATP- (C3) and substrate-binding (C4) regions. The C1 region is the site of DAG or phorbol ester binding in cPKCs and nPKCs. The C2 region bears the phosphatidylserine and, in cPKCs, also the Ca^{2+} binding sites.

There are two key components to PKC regulation. First, the enzyme itself has to be made catalytically functional and second it has to be activated by its regulators. PKC is synthesized as an inactive precursor, which is associated with a cytoskeletal fraction. Three important phosphorylations occur in series at the C-terminal end of PKC, which properly aligns the activation loop of the enzyme and releases it into the cytosol in a catalytically competent but inactive form. Phorbol esters or DAG increase affinity of PKC for the membrane and for phosphatidylserine, and stabilize its active conformation. In cPKCs, Ca^{2+} also has this role. These events result in the translocation of PKC to the membrane, with the C1 and C2 domains being the sites of association. The active conformation leads to the release of the pseudosubstrate domain from the substrate binding site and thereby renders the latter to be available for specific substrates (Newton, 1995). Despite the multiple isoforms, there is considerable overlap in the substrate specificity and activator sensitivity between the different isoforms. Another mechanism by which specificity of action is ensured is by the anchoring of isoforms to specific sites within the cell (see 'Cross-talk and the role of other kinase pathways' Mochly-Rosen and Gordon, 1998).

Studies, largely using phorbol esters, have indicated that PKC has multifarious effects on ion transport in intestinal epithelia. For example, it increases paracellular permeability (Tai *et al.*, 1996), stimulates NHE-1 but inhibits NHE-3 (Orlowski and Grinstein, 1997; Wakabayashi *et al.*, 1997) and stimulates Cl^- secretion (Chang and Rao, 1991, 1994). There has been some debate as to whether PKC is an activator of Cl^- transport (Sahi *et al.*, 1994) or if it is chiefly involved in the down-regulation of cAMP-stimulated pathways (Barrett, 1997). Recent evidence indicates that PKC-specific phosphorylation is required for continued activation of CFTR by PKA (Jia *et al.*, 1997).

Calcium-calmodulin (Ca-CaM) PKs and PPs

Calcium signals are also transduced by its binding to small molecular weight proteins, such as the ubiquitous calmodulin, which has four Ca^{2+} binding sites. When bound to Ca^{2+}, CaM undergoes a conformational change that allows it to modulate both structural proteins, like actin, and classes of phosphodiesterases, PKs and PPases. Calmodulin modulates NHE-1 function by PK-independent binding to specific sites (Wakabayashi *et al.*, 1997).

Annexins, another group of Ca^{2+}-binding proteins, also modulate CFTR function (Xie *et al.*, 1996). Calcineurin or PP-2B is the only ser/thr PPase to be activated by Ca-CaM and affects a wide assortment of cell functions (Klee *et al.*, 1998). The identification of calcineurin as the target for the immunosuppressive drugs, FK506 and cyclosporin, emphasized not only the pleiotropic role of calcineurin but also the overall significance of dephosphorylation mechanisms in cell function. Calcineurin is present in the enterocyte BBM, and inhibitor studies imply a role in ion transport that needs to be analyzed (Rao and de Jonge, 1990).

The family of Ca^{2+}-CaM PKs comprises at least seven members, three of which have narrow substrate specificity and the rest phosphorylate a broader range of substrates (reviewed in Rao and de Jonge, 1990; Braun and Schulman, 1995; Soderling, 1996; Heist and Schulman, 1998). The former are myosin light-chain kinase (MLCK), Ca-CaM PK III and phosphorylase kinase, which phosphorylate MLC, elongation factor 2 (EF-2) and phosphorylase. While all three enzymes and their substrates are present in the intestine, their role in ion transport is best defined for MLCK. The terminal web is rich in myosin, and MLCK activity alters brush-border motility, paracellular permeability and NHE activity (Rao, M.C., unpublished observations). While increases in Ca^{2+} increase EF-2 phosphorylation in the intestine, the implications for ion transport are not clear. The broad range Ca^{2+}-CaM PKs include the multifunctional CaM-PK II, Ca-CaM PK I, IV and CaM-kinase kinase. The last three form an interesting signaling cascade: activation of CaM by Ca^{2+} directly activates Ca-CaM PK I and IV and also triggers CaM kinase kinase to phosphorylate and further activate these enzymes. Ca-CaM PK IV has a number of nuclear substrates. The CaM-PK II is the best characterized and perhaps the largest of the ser/thr PKs with 10–12 subunits (approx. 650 kDa) in a 'floral' configuration. Each 'petal' bears the catalytic domain, which is inhibited by a pseudosubstrate domain in the basal state. Upon activation, the enzyme undergoes autophosphorylation by intersubunit catalysis, a process that renders it constitutively active and Ca^{2+}-independent. Thus, this PK can remain active in the absence of the signal and returns to the basal state by the action of PPases. CaM-PK I and II are in high abundance in the BBM, and the latter activates the Ca^{2+}-dependent Cl^- channel. In addition, roles for CaM-PK II in inhibiting basal NHE activity and stimulating BLM K^+ channels have been suggested (Donowitz *et al.*, 1998).

Cross-talk and the role of other kinase pathways

There is extensive cross-talk not only amongst the ser/thr PKs and PPases, but also between them and the tyr PKs and PPases (reviewed in Hanks and Hunter, 1995; Fauman and Saper, 1996) (Fig. 8.3). Some of this is direct interaction between the pathways and others through the intervention of the dual-specificity kinase cascades as exemplified by the MEK family (mitogen and extracellular receptor kinase) (Cobb and Goldsmith, 1995). While the roles of tyrosine PKs and PPases are well defined in growth regulation, their influence on ion transport is only beginning to be explored. The tyr PPases are in far greater excess than the PKs and are subject to multiple regulatory pathways. In general, activation of tyrosine kinases appears to promote absorption and inhibit secretion. For example, epidermal growth factor (EGF), which activates a tyrosine kinase receptor on the BLM, stimulates NHE-3 activity on the BBM via the activation of both a tyr PK, the PI 3-kinase and PKCζ. In contrast, muscarinic cholinergic stimulation causes inhibition of NHE-3 by activation of a tyr PK to modulate PLCγ and by PKC. Similarly, tyrosine PK inhibitors are known to activate CFTR and, as mentioned above, both PKA and PKC phosphorylation are needed for sustained CFTR activation (Jia *et al.*, 1997; Jilling and Kirk, 1997). The intricacies of the complex circuitry between these cascades are just beginning to be explored (Donowitz *et al.*, 1998).

Compartmentalization – cytoskeletal runners, anchoring proteins and vesicular traffic

Localization of transporters and the components of their signaling systems into specific subcellular domains is becoming the norm rather than the exception. This is a dynamic and thereby a highly regulatable process. Compartmentalization can be achieved by specific domains on the protein tethering to the cytoskeleton and/or membrane, e.g. GC-C and PKG-II have cytoskeletal- and membrane-interacting domains, respectively, which allow them to be in close proximity to CFTR in the BBM. A new class of molecules that has gained attention as a mechanism for ensuring specificity of location is the anchoring or scaffolding proteins (Fig. 8.3). These proteins act as docking sites for kinases, making them available for substrates in their proximity. PPases, in particular PP-1, associated with glycogen particles, are a classic example of targeted distribution. More recently, docking proteins, such as RACK, RICK, PICK and AKAP,* which target PKC and PKA, have been characterized (reviewed in Faux and Scott, 1996; Mochly-Rosen and Gordon, 1998). An interesting example of multienzyme signaling complexes is

*RACK: receptor for activated C kinase; RICK: receptor for inactive C kinase; PICK: proteins that interact with C kinase; AKAP: A kinase anchoring proteins.

provided by AKAP-79, a protein which has separate docking domains for PKA, PKC and PP-2B, thereby serving as an anchor for three separate second messengers – cAMP, Ca^{2+}-phospholipid and Ca^{2+}-calmodulin (Faux and Scott, 1996). A physiological role for AKAP-79 is proposed in postsynaptic densities and similar roles for proteins like it can be conceived in regulating BBM ion transport. Finally, trafficking of transporters into and out of the membrane via endosomal vesicles is an effective way of rapidly altering the V_{max} of the transporter (Fig. 8.2). For example, cAMP increases CFTR translocation to the membrane and NHE-3 retrieval from the membrane, resulting in an increase in Cl^- secretion and a decrease in Na^+ absorption.

PERSPECTIVES

The intestine efficiently handles 9 L of fluid a day by orchestrating an intricate series of ion transport processes. In the past decade, great progress has been made towards our understanding of the molecular nature of intestinal ion transporters and the mechanisms by which they are regulated. The research has raised as many or more exciting questions than it has answered. Finally, the cell type, tissue- and species-specificity leading to complex signaling circuitry only underscore the necessity to translate findings in the test-tube to the intact human intestine.

Acknowledgments The author is especially appreciative of Dr J. Venkatasubramanian's assistance with the illustrations and for the critical comments of Dr J. Venkatasubramanian, Ms R. Prasad and N. Selvaraj. The author thanks all her laboratory colleagues for their suggestions. This work is supported by grants from the National Institutes of Health.

REFERENCES

Alper, S.L. 1994: The band 3-related AE anion exchanger gene family. *Cellular Physiology and Biochemistry* 4, 265–81.

Alrefai, W.A., Tyagi, S., Nazir, T.M. *et al.* 2000: Human intestinal anion exchanger isoforms: expression, distribution and membrane localization. *American Journal of Physiology* (submitted).

Anderson, J.M., van Itallie, C.M. 1995: Tight junctions and the molecular basis for regulation of paracellular permeability. *American Journal of Physiology* 269, G467–75.

Armstrong, W.M. 1987: Cellular mechanisms of ion transport in the small intestine. In Johnson L.R. (ed.), *Physiology of the gastrointestinal tract*, 2nd edn. New York: Raven Press, 1251–65.

Bakre, M.M., Visweswariah, S.S. 1997: Dual regulation of heat-stable enterotoxin mediated cGMP accumulation in T84 cells by receptor desensitization and increased phosphodiesterase activity. *FEBS Letters* 408, 345–9.

Barford, D. 1996: Molecular mechanisms of the protein serine/threonine phosphatases. *Trends in Biochemical Sciences* 21, 407–12.

Barrett, K.E. 1993: Positive and negative regulation of chloride secretion in T84 cells. *American Journal of Physiology* 265, C859–69.

Barrett, K.E. 1997: Integrated regulation of intestinal epithelial transport: intercellular and intracellular pathways. *American Journal of Physiology* 272, C1069–76.

Bear, C.E., Li, C., Kartner, N., Bridges, R.J., Jensen, T.J., Ramjeesingh M., Riordan, J.R. 1992: Purification and functional reconstitution of the cystic fibrosis transmembrane conductance regulator (CFTR). *Cell* 68, 809–18.

Beavo, J.A. 1995: Cyclic nucleotide phosphodiesterases: functional implications of multiple isoforms. *Physiological Reviews* 75, 725–48.

Begenisich, T., Melvin, J.E. 1998: Regulation of chloride channels in secretory epithelia. *Journal of Membrane Biology* 163, 77–85.

Berridge, M. 1997: Elementary and global aspects of calcium signaling. *Journal of Physiology* 499, 291–306.

Bookstein, C., Rabenau, K., Xie, Y., Musch, M.W., McSwine, R., Rao, M.C., Chang, E.B. 1997: Tissue distribution of Na^+/H^+ exchanger isoforms NHE-2 and NHE-4 in rat intestine and kidney. *American Journal of Physiology* 273, C1496–505.

Braun, A.P., Schulman, H. 1995: The multifunctional calcium/calmodulin-dependent protein kinase: from form to function. *Annual Reviews of Physiology* 57, 417–45.

Castro, G.A., Powell, D.W. 1994: The physiology of the mucosal immune system and immune-mediated responses in the gastrointestinal tract. In Johnson, L.R. (ed.), *Physiology of the gastrointestinal tract*, 3rd edn. New York: Raven Press, 709–50.

Chang, E.B., Rao, M.C. 1991: Intracellular mediators of intestinal electrolyte transport. In Field, M. (ed.), *Diarrheal diseases* (Current Topics in Gastroenterology). New York: Elsevier, 49–72.

Chang, E.B., Rao, M.C. 1994: Intestinal electrolyte and water transport. In Johnson, L.R. (ed.), *Physiology of the gastrointestinal tract*, 3rd edn. New York: Raven Press, 2028–81.

Chow, A., Zhou, W., Jacobson, R. 1996: Regulation of AE2 Cl^-/HCO_3^-exchanger during intestinal development. *American Journal of Physiology* 271, G330–7.

Cobb, M.H., Goldsmith, E.J. 1995: How MAP kinases are regulated. *Journal of Biological Chemistry* 270, 14843–6.

de Jonge, H.R., Rao, M.C. 1990: Cyclic nucleotide-dependent kinases. In Lebenthal, E., Duffey, M. (eds), *Textbook of secretory diarrhea*. New York: Raven Press, 191–207.

Donowitz, M., Khurana, S., Tse, C.M., Yun, C.H.C. 1998: G

protein-coupled receptors in gastrointestinal physiology III. Asymmetry in plasma membrane signal transduction: lessons from brush-border Na^+/H^+ exchangers. *American Journal of Physiology* 274, G971–7.

Durell, S.R., Hao, J., Guy, H.R. 1998: Structural models of the transmembrane region of voltage-gated and other K^+ channels in open, closed, and inactivated conformations. *Journal of Structural Biology* 121, 263–84.

Fasano, A. 1998: Cellular microbiology: how enteric pathogens socialize with their intestinal host. *Journal of Pediatric Gastroenterology and Nutrition* 26, 520–32.

Fauman, E.B., Saper, M.A. 1996: Structure and function of the protein tyrosine phosphatases. *Trends in Biochemical Science* 21, 413–17.

Faux, M.C., Scott, J.D. 1996: More on target with protein phosphorylation: conferring specificity by location. *Trends in Biochemical Sciences* 21, 312–15.

Field, M., Semrad, C.E. 1993: Toxigenic diarrheas, congenital diarrheas, and cystic fibrosis: disorders of intestinal transport. *Annual Reviews in Physiology* 55, 631–55.

Forte, L.R., Hamra, F.K. 1996: Guanylin and uroguanylin: intestinal peptide hormones that regulate epithelial transport. *News in Physiological Sciences* 11, 17–24.

French, P.J., Bijman, J., Edixhoven, M. *et al.* 1995: Isotype-specific activation of cystic fibrosis transmembrane conductance regulator-chloride channels by cGMP-dependent protein kinase II. *Journal of Biological Chemistry* 270, 26626–31.

Greger, R., Mall, M., Bleich, J., Ecke, D., Warth, R., Riedemann, N., Kunzelmann, K. 1996: Regulation of epithelial ion channels by the cystic fibrosis transmembrane conductance regulator (CFTR). *Journal of Molecular Medicine* 74, 527–34.

Grubb, B.R., Gabriel, S.E. 1998: Intestinal physiology and pathology in gene-targeted mouse models of cystic fibrosis. *American Journal of Physiology* 273, G258–66.

Haas, M., Forbush B. III. 1998: The Na-K-Cl cotransporters. *Journal of Bioenergetics and Biomembranes* 30, 161–72.

Hanks, S.K., Hunter, T. 1995: The eukaryotic protein kinase superfamily: kinase (catalytic) domain structure and classification. *FASEB Journal* 9, 576–96.

Heist, E.K., Schulman, H. 1998: The role of Ca^{2+}/calmodulin-dependent protein kinases within the nucleus. *Cell Calcium* 23, 103–14.

Hoglund, P., Haila S., Socha J. *et al.* 1996: Mutations of the down regulated in adenoma (DRA) gene causing congenital chloride diarrhoea. *Nature Genetics* 14, 316–19.

Holda, J.R., Klishin, A., Sedova, M., Huser, J., Blatter, L.A. 1998: Capacitative calcium entry. *News in Physiological Sciences* 13, 157–63.

Jia, J., Mathews, C.J., Hanrahan, J.W. 1997: Phosphorylation by protein kinase C is required for acute activation of cystic fibrosis transmembrane conductance regulator by protein kinase A. *Journal of Biological Chemistry* 272, 4978–84.

Jilling, T., Kirk, K.L. 1997: The biogenesis, traffic and function of the cystic fibrosis transmembrane conductance regulator. *International Review of Cytology* 172, 193–241.

Kaplan, M.R., Mount, D.B., Delpire, E., Gamba, G., Hebert, S.C. 1996: Molecular mechanisms of NaCl cotransport. *Annual Reviews in Physiology* 58, 649–68.

Klee, C.B., Ren, H., Wang, X. 1998: Regulation of the calmodulin-stimulated protein phosphatase, calcineurin. *Journal of Biological Chemistry* 273, 13367–70.

Koefoed-Johnsen, V., Ussing, H.H. 1953: The contributions of diffusion and flow to the passage of D2O through living membranes: effect of neurohypophyseal hormone on isolated anuran skin. *Acta Physiologica Scandinavica* 28, 60–7.

Lehrer, R.I., Bevins, C.L., Ganz, T. 1998: Defensins and other antimicrobial peptides. In Ogra, P.L., Mestecky, J., Lamm, M.E., Strober, W.M., Bienstock, J. (eds), *Mucosal immunology*. New York: Academic Press, 89–99.

Lencer, W.I., Cheung, G., Strohmeier, G.R., Currie, M.G., Ouellette, A.J., Selsted, M.E., Madara, J.L. 1997: Induction of epithelial chloride secretion by channel forming cryptidins 2 and 3. *Proceedings of the National Academy of Sciences USA* 94, 8585–9.

Lohmann, S.M., Vaandrager, A.B., Smolenski, A., Walter, U., de Jonge, H.R. 1997: Distinct and specific functions of cGMP-dependent protein kinases. *Trends in Biochemical Sciences* 22, 307–12.

Loo, D.D.F., Zeuthen, T., Chandy, G., Wright, E.M. 1996: Cotransport of water by the Na^+/glucose cotransporter. *Proceedings in National Academy of Sciences USA* 2, 13367–70.

Ma, T., Yang, B., Verkman, A.S. 1997: Cloning of a novel water and urea-permeable aquaporin from mouse expressed strongly in colon, placenta, liver and heart. *Biochemical and Biophysical Research Communications* 240, 324–8.

Madara, J.L. 1989: Loosening tight junctions– lessons from the intestine. *Journal of Clinical Investigation* 83: 1089–94.

Mann, E.A., Jump, M.L., Wu, J., Yee, E., Giannella, R.A. 1997: Mice lacking the guanylyl cyclase C receptor are resistant to STa-induced intestinal secretion. *Biochemical and Biophysical Research Communications* 239: 463–6.

Matthews, J.B., Hassan, I., Meng, S., Archer, S.Y., Hrnjez, B.J., Hodin, R.A. 1998: Na-K-2Cl cotransporter gene expression and function during enterocyte differentiation. *Journal of Clinical Investigation* 101, 2072–9.

Meinild, A.-K., Klaerke, D.A., Loo, D.D.F., Wright, E.M., Zeuthen, T. 1998: The human Na^+-glucose cotransporter is a molecular water pump. *Journal of Physiology* 508, 15–21.

Mochly-Rosen, D., Gordon, A.S. 1998: Anchoring proteins for protein kinase C: a means for isozyme selectivity. *FASEB Journal* 12, 35–42.

Newton, A.C. 1995: Protein kinase C: structure, function

and regulation. *Journal of Biological Chemistry* 270: 28495–8.

Orlowski, J., Grinstein, S. 1997: Na^+/H^+ exchangers of mammalian cells. *Journal of Biological Chemistry* 272, 22373–6.

Pfeifer, A., Aszodi, A., Seidler, U., Ruth, P., Hofmann, F., Fassler, R. 1996: Intestinal secretory defects and dwarfism in mice lacking cGMP-dependent protein kinase II. *Science* 274, 2082–6.

Pressley, T.A. 1996: Structure and function of the Na, K pump: ten years of molecular biology. *Minerals and Electrolyte Metabolism* 22: 264–71.

Rao, M.C. 1985: Toxins which activate guanylate cyclase: heat-stable enterotoxins. In *Microbial toxins and diarrhoeal disease*. Ciba Foundation Symposium, no. 112, 74–93.

Rao, M.C., de Jonge, H.R. 1990: Ca and phospholipid-dependent protein kinases. In Lebenthal, E., Duffey, M. (eds), *Textbook of secretory diarrhea*. New York: Raven Press, 209–32.

Rodbell, M. 1980: The role of hormone receptors and GTP-regulatory proteins in membrane transduction. *Nature* 284, 17–22.

Sahi, J., Goldstein, J.L., Layden T.J., Rao, M.C. 1994: Cyclic AMP and phorbol ester regulated chloride permeabilities in primary cultures of human and rabbit colonocytes. *American Journal of Physiology* 266, G846–55.

Schultheis, P.J., Clarke, L.L., Meneton, P. *et al.* 1998a: Targeted disruption of the murine Na^+/H^+ exchanger isoform 2 gene causes reduced viability of gastric parietal cells and loss of net acid secretion. *Journal of Clinical Investigation* 101, 1243–53.

Schultheis, P.J., Clarke, L.L., Meneton, P. *et al.* 1998b: Renal and intestinal absorptive defects in mice lacking the NHE3 Na^+/H^+ exchanger. *Nature Genetics* 19, 282–5.

Schulz, S., Green, C.K., Yuen, P.S.T., Garbers, D.L. 1990: Guanylyl cyclase is a heat-stable enterotoxin receptor. *Cell* 63, 941–8.

Schulz, S., Lopez, M.J., Kuhn, M., Garbers, D.L. 1997: Disruption of the guanylyl cyclase-c gene leads to a paradoxical phenotype of viable but heat-stable enterotoxin-resistant mice. *Journal of Clinical Investigation* 100, 1590–5.

Sears, C.L., Kaper, J.B. 1996: Enteric bacterial toxins: mechanisms of action and linkage to intestinal secretion. *Microbiological Reviews* 60, 167–215.

Seidler, U., Blumenstein, I., Kretz, A. *et al.* 1997: A functional CFTR protein is required for mouse intestinal cAMP-, cGMP- and Ca^{2+}-dependent HCO_3^- secretion. *Journal of Physiology* 505, 411–23.

Soderling, T.R. 1996: Structure and regulation of calcium/calmodulin-dependent protein kinases II and IV. *Biochimica et Biophysica Acta* 1297, 131–8.

Sullivan, S.K., Field, M. 1991: Ion transport across mammalian small intestine. In Schultz, S.G. (ed.), *Handbook of physiology. Section 6: The gastrointestinal system, Volume IV. Intestinal absorption and secretion*. Bethesda, MD: American Physiology Society, 287–301.

Suvitayavat, W., Haas, M., Dunham, P.B., Rao, M.C. 1994: Molecular characterization of the intestinal brush border Na^+-K^+-$2Cl^-$ cotransporter. *American Journal of Physiology* 267, C375–84.

Tai, Y.-H., Flick, J., Levine, S.A., Madara, J.L., Sharp, G.W.G., Donowitz, M. 1996: Regulation of tight junction resistance in T84 monolayers by elevation in intracellular Ca^{2+}: a protein kinase C effect. *Journal of Membrane Biology* 149, 71–9.

Taussig, R., Gilman, A.G. 1995: Mammalian membrane-bound adenylyl cyclases. *Journal of Biological Chemistry* 270, 1–4.

Wakabayashi, S., Shigekawa, M., Pouyssegur, J. 1997: Molecular physiology of vertebrate Na^+/H^+ exchangers. *Physiological Reviews* 77, 51–74.

Wedel, B.J., Garbers, D.L. 1997: New insights on the functions of guanylyl cyclase receptors. *FEBS Letters* 410, 29–33.

Welsh, M.J., Tsui, L.-C., Boat, T.F., Beaudet, A.L. 1995: Cystic fibrosis. In Scriver, C.R, Beaudet, A.L., Sly, W.S., Valle, D. (eds), *The metabolic and molecular basis of inherited disease*, Vol. 7. New York: McGraw-Hill, 3799–876.

Xie, W., Kaetzel, M.A., Bruzik, K.S., Dedman, J.R., Shears, S.B., Nelson, D.J. 1996: Inositol 3,4,5,6-tetrakisphosphate inhibits the calmodulin-dependent protein kinase II-activated chloride conductance in T84 colonic epithelial cells. *Journal of Biological Chemistry* 271, 14092–7.

Zeidel, M.L. 1998: Recent advances in water transport. *Seminars in Nephrology* 18, 167–77.

9

Absorption of vitamins and minerals

RANJIT N RATNAIKE, PETER D ZALEWSKI

INTRODUCTION

Vitamins are a group of organic substances present in food in minute quantities that are essential to normal functioning of the body. Insufficient quantities in the diet can lead to deficiency diseases. In addition to the deficiency disorders, there is now increasing evidence that the lack of vitamins is implicated in a wider spectrum of conditions involving physical and mental well-being. The activities of the 13 vitamins listed in Table 9.1 are relevant to humans for a variety of metabolic functions. There is accumulating evidence that a number of these compounds are important as antitumour agents (Taylor *et al.*, 1994). The vitamins that are antioxidants are widely recommended for their role in the prevention of atherosclerosis.

Some vitamins are designated by their chemical name while others have the prefix vitamin. Vitamins containing one chemical substance are designated by their chemical name and those with more than one substance are termed vitamins.

In the USA, there is a view that, especially in older persons, the recommended dietary allowances (RDAs) be increased for riboflavin, vitamin B_6, folic acid, vitamin B_{12} and vitamin D (and calcium), and reduced for vitamin A (Russell, 1997). A British study on a cohort of elderly 'free-living' subjects, carried out before and after a 2-year period, found that a small proportion were at risk of deficiency of folate (7 per cent and 3 per cent), thiamine (12 per cent and 3 per cent), vitamin C (15 per cent and 17 per cent), vitamin B_6 (42 per cent

Table 9.1 *Vitamins necessary for human metabolism*

Group	Name	Alternative name
Fat soluble	Vitamin A	
	Vitamin D	
	Vitamin E	
	Vitamin K	
Water soluble	Thiamin	Vitamin B_1
	Riboflavin	Vitamin B_2
	Biotin	
	Pyridoxine	Vitamin B_6
	Ascorbic acid	Vitamin C
	Niacin	
	Pantothenic acid	
	Folate	
	Cyanocobalamin	Vitamin B_{12}

and 47 per cent) and riboflavin (77 per cent and 79 per cent); it was concluded that the requirements of the elderly for vitamins be reviewed (Bailey *et al.*, 1997).

The recommended daily intake of vitamins and minerals given in this chapter is based on the guidelines of the National Health and Medical Research Council of Australia. These values may differ in other countries and, for example, in situations of increased requirements, such as during pregnancy and lactation, in children, and in other special circumstances.

FAT-SOLUBLE VITAMINS

The fat-soluble vitamins are not water soluble and therefore need a mechanism to cross the unstirred water layer of the small intestine to reach the mucosal surface for absorption to occur. Food fats serve as a vehicle for the absorption of vitamins A, D, E and K. Bile salts play an important role, enabling these vitamins to be transported to the mucosa within micelles (*see* Chapter 16). Prolonged cholestasis or other conditions that deplete bile salt production or availability within the intestinal lumen will compromise the formation of the micelles that are necessary for the absorption of these vitamins.

Absorption of fat-soluble vitamins occurs in the proximal small intestine by passive diffusion. All fat-soluble vitamins are absorbed more effectively in an acid environment (Hollander, 1981). After absorption, vitamin A is transported as a non-polar lipid, vitamin D is transported in the blood by binding proteins, vitamin E by low-density lipoproteins and vitamin K by intestinal lymph into the circulation. The fat-soluble vitamins (as with vitamin B_{12}) are stored in the liver. The body has large stores of vitamin A, vitamin D and vitamin B_{12}, in contrast to vitamin K and vitamin E. All the fat-soluble vitamins cause toxicity if excessive amounts are ingested.

VITAMIN A

There is now increasing interest in vitamin A owing to evidence that it influences an increasing range of beneficial processes. Vitamin A may have a specific role in the immune system, and is an antioxidant that prevents the effects of oxidative free radicals (Bates, 1995).

The basic molecule of vitamin A is retinol. This is present in food and tissues as an ester combined with long-chain fatty acids. The main food source of preformed vitamin A is liver; other sources include fish, oils, eggs and margarine. Plant-derived carotenoids (compounds with yellow to red pigments that are precursors of vitamin A) are present in dark-green leafy vegetables, carrots, mango and pumpkin. Carotenoids are classified as alpha- and beta-carotene, beta-cryptoxanthin and lutein; all of these are absorbed from the ileum. They are transported mainly as non-polar lipids and do not combine with transport proteins. Alpha- and beta-carotene and beta-cryptoxanthin can be converted to vitamin A by oxygenase present in the intestine and elsewhere at a variable conversion efficiency (Bates, 1995). Lutein cannot be converted to vitamin A, but possesses antioxidant properties. After absorption, retinol is transported from the enterocyte to the liver by chylomicrons where it is stored as retinyl esters. A retinol-binding protein transports the retinol from the liver to the tissues.

Vitamin A maintains the integrity of mucosal surfaces, retinal and immune function, and the production of mucus.

The clinical features of vitamin A deficiency are night blindness (the earliest symptom) and a variety of ocular manifestations due to structural abnormalities. These ocular changes are termed xerophthalmia (Plate 9.1). The non-ocular consequences of vitamin A deficiency are dryness of the skin (xerosis), keratinization of the hair follicles and atrophy of sebaceous glands.

Toxicity

Toxicity can occur through excessive ingestion of foods high in vitamin A, such as liver, or as a side-effect of inappropriate therapy. Acute hypervitaminosis can result within hours from a single toxic dose. Headache is a dominant feature. Generalized desquamation of the skin occurs after a few days but rapid recovery occurs. Nausea and vomiting, abdominal pain, blurred vision, papilloedema, dizziness and sluggishness are other clinical features. The symptoms and signs of *chronic* toxicity are anorexia, dry lips, weight loss, hepatosplenomegaly, bone and joint pain, hyperostosis, hair loss, benign intracranial hypertension, low-grade fever and pruritus.

Treatment

Owing to its teratogenic effect, vitamin A should not be prescribed during pregnancy. The synthetic vitamin A is more teratogenic than the natural vitamin A. In patients with xerophthalmia, vitamin A may be administered as retinol palmitate intramuscularly, 100 000 IU. Xerophthalmia can be prevented with oral vitamin A, 100 000 IU every 4 months. Attention is now focused on the treatment of measles with vitamin A. The demand for the vitamin is increased in measles and vitamin A supplementation (a high dose, e.g. 120 g) results in significant clinical improvement and survival (Hussey and Klein, 1990). A beneficial link between vitamin A therapy and respiratory and diarrhoeal diseases is inconclusive (Bates, 1995), but needs further study.

VITAMIN E

Vitamin E, first detected in 1922, is present as eight naturally occurring compounds, each with different biological activities. There are two classes, tocopherols and tocotrienols. Each class has four isomers: alpha, beta, gamma and delta. The most biologically active and widely available form in food is D-alpha-tocopherol. The important food sources are vegetable oils, butter, margarine, nuts, eggs and meat. Vitamin E is available pharmaceutically as an equal mixture of the eight stereoisomers of alpha-tocopherol (Meydani, 1995). Vitamin E acts as a major antioxidant in the body by preventing the oxidation of polyunsaturated fatty acids by free radicals and thus has a potential role in the prevention of coronary artery disease.

The recommended daily intake is 7–10 mg a day for adults. Vitamin E is transported by low-density lipoprotein (LDL). In abetalipoproteinaemia (*see* Chapter 16), vitamin E concentrations are decreased and this deficiency is responsible for the neurological abnormalities. Owing to the importance of vitamin E in normal neurological function, it is recommended that vitamin E concentrations be measured in all patients with spinocerebellar disorders, whatever the aetiology (Muller, 1986). Vitamin E deficiency is associated with free radical damage to membranes on nerve cells resulting in neurological abnormalities and haemolytic anaemia due to red blood cell membrane damage (Anonymous, 1986).

In patients on total parental nutrition (*see* Chapter 29), inadequate vitamin supplements can cause vitamin E deficiency. In the rare condition, the brown bowel syndrome (*see* Chapter 27), vitamin E deficiency is significant, although other fat-soluble vitamins are also malabsorbed (Drake *et al.*, 1996). Isolated vitamin E deficiency has been reported.

In chronic disorders of fat malabsorption and other conditions associated with vitamin E deficiency, such as abetalipoproteinaemia, chronic liver disease and cystic fibrosis, the replacement of vitamin E is essential at a dose of 200 mg a day.

Toxicity

Vitamin E toxicity may cause malaise, vague gastrointestinal tract symptoms, headaches and possibly hypertension. Vitamin E in massive doses can antagonize vitamin K and therefore prolong the prothrombin time. Premature infants given vitamin E have developed hepatosplenomegaly with ascites, cholestatic jaundice, azotemia and thrombocytopenia.

VITAMIN K

Vitamin K occurs naturally as a single plant form phylloquinone (vitamin K_1) and as a family of bacterially synthesized menaquinones (vitamin K_2). The primary dietary source is green leafy vegetables and to a lesser extent other plant sources such as soya bean oil, olive oil and rape seed oils. While the major source of menaquinones is by bacterial synthesis, moderate concentrations are present in cheese (Shearer *et al.*, 1996). Bacterial synthesis occurs both in the terminal ileum and the colon. Major intestinal forms are MK-10 (menaquinone 10) and MK-11, produced by Bacterioides, MK-8 produced by enterobacteria, MK-7 by *Veillonella* species and MK-6 by *Eubacterium lentum* (Shearer, 1995).

The bulk of menaquinones are synthesized by the conversion of chorismate to isochorismate by the enzyme isochorismate synthase by the *menF* gene (Daruwala *et al.*, 1997).

The daily dietary requirement is 100–200 mg a day.

Vitamin K is absorbed predominantly in the terminal ileum. The body stores of vitamin K are not large. In the absence of daily supplementation, the storage pool may be exhausted in 7 days. A total of 60–70 per cent of the dietary intake is lost by excretion and therefore the tissue reserves should be maintained continuously (Shearer *et al.*, 1996). Clinical consequences may not be manifest if the gut bacteria continue to synthesize vitamin K_2. However, this view is now being increasingly challenged, as the contribution of menaquinones may be much less relevant than presumed (Suttie, 1995). In the liver, the vitamin K stores last for 30 days but in acutely ill patients deficiency can occur within 7–10 days.

Vitamin K is essential for normal homeostatic and antithrombotic mechanisms of the body. Vitamin K is a co-factor in the synthesis of carboxyglutamic acid (Gla), which is an integral part of the protein molecule, and necessary for the manufacture of several blood coagulation factors (II, VII, IX and X) and coagulation inhibitors (proteins C and S) in the liver, and other extrahepatic proteins such as the bone protein osteocalcin (Shearer, 1992).

Deficiency results from diseases in which there is fat malabsorption or with the use of oral antibiotics that eliminate the bacterial source for vitamin K when the dietary intake is limited. Vitamin K deficiency is also associated with primary biliary cirrhosis and cholestatic liver disease. In the MELAS syndrome (mitochondrial myopathy, encephalopathy, lactic acidosis and stroke-like episodes) vitamin K is an important therapeutic agent (Barak *et al.*, 1995). Vitamin K-dependent blood-clotting proteins should be administered in conjunction with vitamin K.

Vitamin K can also be administered orally or subcutaneously. Replacement therapy consists of vitamin K by injection, 10 mg a day. In instances of significantly prolonged prothrombin time, intramuscular injections of vitamin K should be avoided. Intravenous vitamin K results in a rapid action but allergic reactions may occur. If bleeding is serious, fresh-frozen plasma that contains vitamin K will restore the vitamin K level and normalize prothrombin time in 8–10 hours. As a rule, 1 μg/kg of body weight per day is probably adequate, based on coagulation function as a marker.

Vitamin K in large amounts can block the effect of oral anticoagulants and, when given to pregnant women, can cause jaundice in the newborn.

VITAMIN D

Vitamin D was first described as a fat-soluble vitamin, but is now regarded as a hormone and not a vitamin. Its classification as a nutrient has persisted because it is administered orally.

The subscripts D_1, D_2 and D_3 attached to vitamin D reflect the chronological sequence of their isolation. The term vitamin D_1 is no longer used, as it is a mixture of vitamin D_2 and vitamin D_3. At present, the term 'vitamin D' denotes both vitamin D_2 and vitamin D_3. Vitamin D_2 (ergocalciferol) and vitamin D_3 (cholecalciferol) differ in their chemical structure, but they are similar in their metabolism and biological activity.

Sources

The body obtains vitamin D from two sources. Vitamin D_2 is the plant-derived compound and vitamin D_3 is the form produced in the skin. Vitamin D_2 (ergocalciferol) is not found naturally in large quantities, but is available in pharmaceutical preparations. It is produced by ultraviolet irradiation of steroid ergosterol found in yeast and fungi. This naturally occurring vitamin D_2 from food is of far less importance than vitamin D_3 produced in the skin, but contributes to much of the vitamin D requirements in some pathological states. Foods with a high content of vitamin D are fish liver oils, fatty fish (herring, mackerel, pilchards, salmon, sardines and tuna), and eggs. Most dairy products are fortified with vitamin D. The recommended daily intake for adults is 2.5 μg. For children under the age of five and for women who are pregnant or lactating the dose is 10 μg.

The main source of vitamin D is produced by ultraviolet activation (photoactivation) of 7-dehydrocholesterol (the immediate precursor of cholesterol), which is present in the skin. Ultraviolet light converts the 7-dehydrocholesterol to *previtamin* D_3, which is then spontaneously converted to vitamin D_3 (cholecalciferol) by a temperature-dependent molecular rearrangement of its conjugated triene system (triple bond). At body temperature, it takes approximately 24 hours for the previtamin to be completely converted to the vitamin. This process occurs in actively growing areas of the epidermis where the temperature is relatively constant. The quantity of vitamin D_3 produced by this mechanism is normally sufficient to meet daily requirements. However, for a variety of reasons, shown in Table 9.2, the activation of the precursor 7-dehydrocholesterol by ultraviolet light may be suboptimal.

Table 9.2 *Causes of decreased activation of 7-dehydrocholesterol*

Inadequate exposure of the body to sunlight
Increased melanin pigmentation of the skin
Hyperkeratosis
Sunscreen lotions

Absorption and metabolism

Absorption and metabolism of vitamin D are regulated by parathyroid hormone (PTH). Dietary vitamin D is absorbed in the jejunum (Hollander and Muralidhara, 1978), and, being fat-soluble, requires micellar solubilization for absorption into the enterocyte. Thus, those factors that decrease in micelle formation (*see* Chapter 16) affect vitamin D absorption. Most of the vitamin appears in the lymph in the chylomicron fraction.

Vitamin D is bound to a vitamin D-binding protein (DBP) and transported to the liver. Here vitamin D is hydroxylated in the '25' position of the sterol to 25-hydroxycholecalciferol, 25(OH)D. In hepatocellular disease, this activity is decreased. The 25(OH)D is then bound to a DBP and transported to the kidney. In the proximal renal tubular cells of the kidney, 25(OH)D-1-alpha-hydroxylase converts 25(OH)D to form the active metabolite 1,25-dihydroxycholecalciferol, $1,25(OH)_2D$. The causes of increased and decreased $1,25(OH)_2D$ synthesis are shown in Tables 9.3 and 9.4, respectively.

Table 9.3 *Causes of increased synthesis of* $1,25(OH)_2D$

Hyperparathyroidism
Low-phosphate concentration
Hypocalcaemia
Growth hormone excess
Hyperprolactinaemia
Oestrogen excess

Table 9.4 *Causes of decreased synthesis of 1,25(OH)$_2$D*

Deficiency of vitamin D
Chronic renal disease
Liver disease
Hypoparathyroidism

Action

Vitamin D enhances calcium and phosphate absorption from the small intestine, and calcium efflux from bone, to maintain normal calcium and phosphate concentrations in the blood. Vitamin D interacts with specific receptors in the nuclei of a variety cells, increasing the production of hormone-specific messenger RNA (mRNA), which regulates the transcription of various proteins. These receptors are present in the intestine, bone, kidney, skin, breast, pituitary, parathyroid glands, beta cells of the pancreatic islets, gonads, brain, skeletal muscle, circulating monocytes and activated T and B lymphocytes.

In bone, vitamin D acts on the receptors of immature osteoclast precursors to become mature osteoclasts. Osteoblasts produce cytokines, which stimulate the activity of mature osteoclasts that mobilize calcium stores from bone (Holick, 1996). In the enterocyte of the small intestine, vitamin D binds with receptors to form a specific protein that increases calcium absorption. The active renal metabolite 1,25(OH)$_2$D and its immediate precursor 25(OH)D, which is synthesized in the liver, stimulate the active intestinal absorption of calcium and phosphate.

Vitamin D deficiency

Vitamin D deficiency results in decreased osteoblastic activity in the synthesis and mineralization of the matrix of bone. The aetiology of decreased vitamin D availability is shown in Table 9.5. The consequence in children is rickets (Plate 9.2), and osteomalacia in adults. In most children with rickets, skeletal growth is stunted and with advanced disease they appear apathetic, irritable and hypokinetic. The initial symptoms of osteomalacia include fatigue, malaise or bone pain. In advanced disease there is proximal muscle weakness.

The major cause of vitamin D deficiency is decreased cutaneous production of vitamin D$_3$ owing to the conditions previously described in Table 9.2. Osteomalacia may also occur with malabsorption, liver disease, resistance to the action of vitamin D, hypophosphataemia, hypocalcaemia or toxic effects on osteoblastic function (Francis and Selby, 1997). Twelve per cent of upper femoral fractures are reportedly due to osteomalacia (Rush, 1977).

Table 9.5 *Causes of decreased vitamin D*

Decreased vitamin D$_3$ synthesis in skin (*see* Table 9.2)
Decreased (dietary) intake
Decreased absorption
Small intestinal mucosal disease (*see* Chapter 16)
Small intestinal resection (*see* Chapters 28 and 29)
Small intestinal revision
Jejuno–ileal bypass
Liver and biliary disease
Decreased bile salt production
Obstruction of bile flow to the intestine resulting in decreased micelle formation
Chronic pancreatic disease
Drugs
Cholestyramine
Corticosteroids
Phenobarbitone
Phenytoin
Decreased metabolism
Parenchymal liver disease
Chronic renal failure
Hypothyroidism

Diagnosis

The diagnosis of rickets and osteomalacia is confirmed by bone X-rays, where there is generalized osteopenia. In rickets, the undermineralized osteoid within the zone of provisional calcification leads to increased lucency, widening, elongation, irregularity and cupping of the metaphyses. The most common complication is skeletal deformity, resulting in bowing of the long bones in arms and legs, scoliosis, basilar invagination of the skull and slipped capital femoral epiphyses.

In adult osteomalacia, the radiological findings are non-specific (Fig. 9.1). There is generalized osteopenia, and the bony trabeculae are coarse and indistinct. Looser's zone or pseudofracture is a more specific sign, appearing as linear areas of undermineralized osteoid that occur in a symmetrical distribution. The characteristic sites are the margins of the femoral neck, proximal ulna, axillary margin of the scapula, pubic rami and ribs. Other skeletal abnormalities include end-plate deformities and fractures of vertebral bodies, bowing and fractures of long bones and basilar invagination of the skull.

The major laboratory finding in osteomalacia is a raised serum alkaline phosphatase due to increased bone turnover. The concentrations of 25-hydroxycholecalciferol and 1,25-dihydroxycholecalciferol will be decreased.

Treatment

The treatment of vitamin D deficiency is determined by the cause. Treatment may involve adequate exposure to

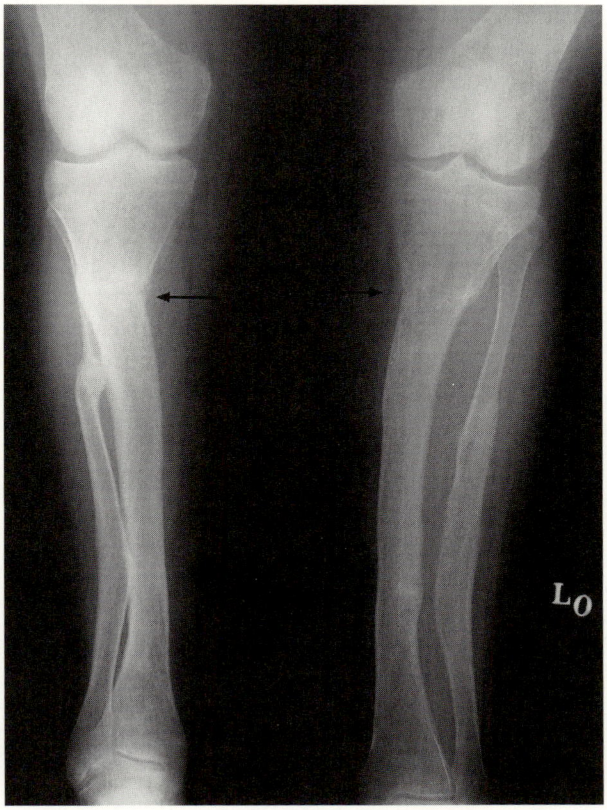

Figure 9.1 *Osteomalacia (both lower legs). The bones are osteopenic. Narrow 2–3 mm wide lucencies are present in both upper tibiae (Looser's zones). These are pseudofractures which are in the healing phase. Note healing fractures of the fibula bilaterally. The long bones are bowed medially due to softening. (Courtesy of Dr Anil B. Utturkar, Radiology Department, The Queen Elizabeth Hospital, Woodville, South Australia.)*

sunlight and counselling regarding diet. Vitamin D_2 supplements can be given orally (4000 units a day) to patients with inadequate dietary intake. Patients with malabsorption and evidence of vitamin D deficiency are treated with vitamin D (25 000–50 000 units, three times per week) and the cause of malabsorption addressed. Vitamin D deficiency in gastrointestinal disease appears to be due to the malabsorption of calcium that raises the vitamin D demand, consequently depleting the vitamin D reserves. Therefore, in treating vitamin D deficiency due to gastrointestinal tract causes, a more rational approach to management would be to increase the supply of dietary calcium (Fraser, 1995).

Both calcium and vitamin D must be given to patients with renal failure. The dose is usually 0.25–1 μg of alfacalcidol per 24 hours, given orally. In renal disease it is important to decrease the amount of phosphate to reduce the risk of metastatic calcification.

Hypervitaminosis D

Toxicity occurs only with large amounts of synthetic vitamin D, 50 000–100 000 IU a day, administered for weeks or months. This results in hypercalcaemia, the many associated manifestations and even death.

The symptoms of hypercalcaemia are abdominal pain, nausea, vomiting, constipation, polyuria, polydipsia, depression, anorexia, weight loss, tiredness, weakness, reduced blood pressure, clouding of consciousness, pyrexia, sudden cardiac arrest, renal calculi, renal failure, corneal calcification and reduced Q-T interval on electrocardiogram. Coma may eventually develop. The reason for this toxicity is not known. The upper limit of normal intake is thought to be 2.5 g of vitamin D per 100 kcal (Chesney, 1989).

Studies of domestic animals suggest that persistent feeding of dietary vitamin D may be associated with the development of chronic vascular disease.

Treatment

Treatment is directed towards reducing serum calcium levels and withholding the vitamin D.

WATER-SOLUBLE VITAMINS

The water-soluble vitamins are:

- thiamine (vitamin B_1)
- riboflavin (vitamin B_2)
- biotin
- pyridoxine (vitamin B_6)
- ascorbic acid (vitamin C)
- niacin
- pantothenic acid
- folate
- cyanocobalamin (vitamin B_{12})

These vitamins are available in food sources in the normal diet, usually as complex coenzyme forms. Their breakdown into simpler forms is necessary to ensure absorption. Digestion may occur intraluminally or at the brush border of the small intestinal enterocyte.

The duodenum and proximal jejunum are the site of absorption of the water-soluble vitamins except vitamin B_{12}, which is absorbed in the terminal ileum. A variety of mechanisms are involved in the transport of these vitamins or their active form across the brush-border membrane of the enterocyte.

The water-soluble vitamins act, after they are metabolized, as coenzymes to facilitate a variety of biochemical reactions. Vitamin C serves primarily as a water-soluble antioxidant.

At higher luminal concentrations of vitamins, absorption occurs by a separate passive process of diffusion transcellularly or using a paracellular pathway. Toxicity occurs most often with excessive intake of vitamin A and vitamin B_6 (pyridoxine).

The B group of vitamins comprises:

- thiamine (vitamin B_1)
- riboflavin (vitamin B_2)
- pyridoxine (vitamin B_6).

All three vitamins are absorbed in the upper small intestine.

THIAMINE (VITAMIN B_1)

Thiamine is involved in a number of reactions in the glycolytic and pentose phosphate pathways of glucose metabolism. The metabolic consequences of thiamine deficiency are the inability to metabolize glucose aerobically with subsequent glucose deprivation of the central nervous system. Tissues that are dependent on carbohydrate metabolism are most adversely affected. Demyelination is a feature because the pentose pathway is involved in lipid metabolism. Thiamine deficiency also leads to the accumulation of pyruvic acid and then lactic acid, which causes vasodilatation leading to cardiac failure.

The food sources are in the husk and germ of grains, yeast and milk. The hydrolysis of dietary phosphoesters results in free thiamine in the intestinal lumen, where absorption occurs by active transport. The recommended daily dose is 0.7–1.1 mg.

Thiamine deficiency now occurs in the more industrialized countries and most often in chronic alcoholics. In some developing countries, infants may suffer from thiamine deficiency owing to low concentrations in maternal milk, reflecting low dietary intake. Alcoholics with a poor nutritional status are most susceptible to Wernicke's encephalopathy, with the features of confusion, ataxia and ophthalmoplegia, and Korsakoff's psychosis, a memory disorder in which confabulation is a prominent feature.

The clinical diagnosis is confirmed by a low red blood cell transketolase activity. Red blood cell transketolase is an enzyme active in the pentose phosphate pathway and requires thiamine as a co-factor. The treatment should be immediate, initially with an intravenous injection of 50 mg of thiamine and then a once daily dose of 50 mg of thiamine for 1 week.

Beriberi

In the East, especially in South Asia and East Asia, although now no longer common, severe nutritional depletion of thiamine caused beriberi. In these countries, rice is the dietary staple. At the end of the nineteenth century, machinery was introduced to mill rice. This resulted in 'polished' rice with vitamins such as thiamine, riboflavin, niacin, pantothenic acid and pyridoxine, and other components of the outer covering of the grain of rice, calcium, iodine and iron, being removed in the milling process. The word is derived from Sinhalese spoken in Sri Lanka, corrupted phonetically from the word 'bari' that means 'cannot'. This reflected the severity of the illness with the patient saying: 'bari, bari', 'cannot, cannot'.

This form of ('wet') beriberi can manifest two clinical presentations. Owing to severe dilatation of the blood vessels, fluid loss into the tissue causes significant oedema (Plate 9.3). Cardiac failure due to cardiac dilatation may occur.

Transketolase concentration in the red blood cells is low. Treatment is with thiamine, initially intravenously (50 mg), followed by oral thiamine 10 mg three times a day until full recovery is achieved. The response to the initial dose of thiamine is rapid with a dramatic improvement in symptoms.

DRY BERIBERI

Dry beriberi is a chronic form of thiamine deficiency in which the major features are a peripheral neuropathy and, with time, muscle wasting may occur.

RIBOFLAVIN (VITAMIN B_2)

Riboflavin is important in cellular oxidation, serving as a coenzyme to the flavodehydrogenases. These are riboflavin-linked dehydrogenases involved in electron transport in or to the respiratory chain. The food sources are dairy products, liver, kidney, muscle meat, fish and pulses, such as beans, peas and lentils. The requirement is 1.2–1.7 mg/day. Riboflavin is absorbed in the proximal small intestine by a carrier-mediated process that is sodium independent and electroneutral (Rose, 1996). Riboflavin deficiency is often associated in conjunction with other deficiency states. Deficiency occurs as a result of a diet inadequate in riboflavin, especially during pregnancy owing to increased demand, and in chronic alcoholism.

The clinical features of deficiency are non-specific, and are angular stomatitis, cheilosis (Plate 9.4) and sore throat. A typical finding is nasolabial dyssebacea, which is an enlargement of the follicles around the sides of the nose owing to excess sebaceous material, leading to seborrhoeic dermatitis. The characteristic seborrhoeic dermatitis around the mouth, ears and eyelids may also extend to the genital area, perineal and perianal areas. A normochromic normocytic anaemia may occur, which responds to riboflavin. The diagnosis is clinical but may be confirmed by decreased glutathione activity in red blood cells. The replacement therapy is 5 mg of riboflavin three times a day.

BIOTIN

Biotin functions as a coenzyme for four carboxylase enzymes in the metabolism of carbohydrates, fatty acids and amino acids. The food sources are ubiquitous. The daily requirement of biotin is 30–100 μg. Biotin is absorbed in the proximal or mid-small intestine (Said *et al.*, 1988) by an electrochemical process (Said and Redha, 1988). Biotin deficiency occurs with excessive consumption of raw egg white, which contains a glycoprotein called avidin that binds to biotin and prevents its absorption. Biotin deficiency may also occur from a lack of holocarboxylase synthetase (biotinidase), which is necessary to hydrolyse the protein-bound biotin in the diet.

The clinical features of deficiency are dermatitis, conjunctivitis, alopecia and ataxia. The treatment is with biotin 100 μg daily.

PYRIDOXINE (VITAMIN B_6)

This vitamin serves as a co-factor in amino-acid metabolism. The food sources are muscle meat, liver, bananas, peanuts and whole-grain cereals. The biologically active form is pyridoxal phosphate, which is absorbed in the proximal small intestine. The daily requirement of vitamin B_6 is 1.1–2.0 mg. The requirements are increased in pregnancy, chronic renal dialysis and in patients with chronic alcoholism, those on oestrogen therapy, and on penicillamine and isoniazid. Deficiency is rarely due to inadequate dietary intake. The clinical picture is that of glossitis (Plate 9.5), dry skin, a peripheral neuropathy, irritability and mental confusion. Vitamin B_6 has been used in treating both congenital and acquired sideroblastic anaemia (May and Fitzsimmons, 1994). The daily replacement dose is 5–20 mg. Excess vitamin B_6 may lead to neurotoxicity.

ASCORBIC ACID (VITAMIN C)

Ascorbic acid maintains connective tissue integrity and enhances iron absorption. Ascorbic acid is essential in the crucial step of proline hydroxylation to hydroxyproline, the essential amino acid in the formation of collagen necessary for the integrity of connective tissue.

The importance of ascorbic acid is being recognized owing to its antioxidant function, serving as a scavenger 'mopping up' free oxygen radicals, which may react with and damage tissues (Rose, 1996).

The food sources are fresh green vegetables and fruit. Foods extremely high in ascorbic acid are tomatoes, citrus fruits, blackberries and guavas. Ascorbic acid is easily destroyed by heat, and cooking therefore significantly reduces its content. Ascorbic acid is absorbed in the ileum against a concentration gradient. The recommended daily intake varies in different countries and ranges from 30 mg to 75 mg. The body stores last for about 3 months.

The classic deficiency is scurvy manifested by swollen spongy gums that bleed easily. Other features are perifollicular haemorrhages, petechial haemorrhages and ecchymoses, and delayed wound healing.

Ascorbic acid deficiency is established by low plasma or leucocyte concentrations of the vitamin. A dietary history, especially in the elderly, is useful.

Treatment consists of ascorbic acid 100 mg three times a day.

NIACIN (NICOTINIC ACID, NICOTINAMIDE)

Niacin refers to both nicotinic acid and nicotinamide. Nicotinic acid is converted in the body to nicotinamide. Both compounds have equal biological activity. Niacin is an integral part of the two pyridine nucleotides, NAD and NADP, which are an integral part of the cellular respiratory cycle. The dietary sources are liver, kidney, meat, fish, beans, peas, peanuts and yeast extract. In the body niacin is manufactured from tryptophan. The two sources of tryptophan are high-protein foods such as eggs and cheese. The recommended daily intake of niacin is 10–20 mg.

Niacin is absorbed by both active and passive transport in the small intestine. Pellagra is the nutritional consequence of niacin deficiency. Maize, in contrast to other cereals, has a low concentration of tryptophan, and diets heavily reliant on maize may cause niacin deficiency. In Hartnup disease (*see* Chapter 10), tryptophan malabsorption occurs and the symptoms are due in part to the resulting niacin deficiency. The other causes of niacin deficiency are therapy with isoniazid, low-protein diets and protein loss in, for example, the nephrotic syndrome. In the carcinoid syndrome, large quantities of dietary tryptophan are converted to serotonin, thus depleting tryptophan necessary for niacin production.

Pellagra is characterized by the 'three Ds': dermatitis, diarrhoea and dementia, but this triad may not be present except in severe cases. Patients may present initially with glossitis, cheilosis and angular stomatitis, mild diarrhoea and confusion. Severe niacin deficiency leads to encephalopathy and spasticity. The dermatitis is well demarcated, symmetrical and the initially erythematous lesions progress to thickening and cracking, which is prominent in areas exposed to the sun. A classic sign is 'Casal's necklace' around the neck (Plate 9.6). The perineum, perianal area and vulva are also affected. The diarrhoea is possibly due to inflammation of the gastrointestinal tract and perhaps villous atrophy is described. Dementia is a late manifestation.

The treatment of niacin deficiency is with a daily dose of 500 mg of nicotinic acid. Niacin is effective as a lipid-lowering agent, and in combination with gemfibrozil is reported to lower cholesterol and LDL by 14 per cent, elevate high-density lipoprotein (HDL) by 24 per cent, lower the ratio of total cholesterol to HDL by 30 per cent and decrease triglycerides by 52 per cent (Spencer *et al.*, 1996).

FOLIC ACID

Folic acid is a collective term for pteroylglutamic acids and their oligoglutamic conjugates. Folic acid is essential for the normal production of red cells by the pteroylpolyglutamates participating in the transfer of 1-carbon moieties required for the synthesis of purine and pyrimidine bases necessary for DNA synthesis.

Food sources

In food, the major forms of folic acid exist as conjugates of glutamyl peptides (polyglutamates). Foods rich in folate are yeast, liver, kidney, nuts, legumes, green leafy vegetables and mushrooms. The dietary forms are thermolabile and are destroyed by cooking for over 15 minutes and by canning. On a normal Western diet, 700–1500 μg of folate is ingested daily, 80 per cent as polyglutamates (Rosenberg and Godwin, 1971). The minimum daily requirement of folate is about 200 μg, and significantly increases with increased demand when cell division occurs, as in pregnancy, when the recommended daily intake is 500 μg. It is advisable to increase the folate intake in advance of pregnancy. During lactation the recommended daily intake is 350 μg.

Chemical composition

The major portions of the molecule include a pteridine ring linked by a methylene bridge to para-aminobenzoic acid, which is joined by an amide linkage to glutamic acid.

Body stores

The body stores of folate are 5–20 mg. Folate deficiency occurs rapidly if dietary folate intake is inadequate or in conditions of small bowel malabsorption. The other causes of folate deficiency are listed in Table 9.6. The body stores of folate last for about 4 months (Herbert, 1985). Folate is stored primarily in the liver.

Absorption

The major site of folate absorption is the jejunum, although absorption occurs to some extent more distally in the small intestine. Folate ingested in the pteroylpolyglutamate form is not readily absorbed owing to the presence of the highly 'polar' side chain. The polyglutamates are therefore hydrolysed to pteroylmonoglutamates on the brush border of the jejunum by the enzyme pteroylpolyglutamate hydrolase, which is an endopeptide (Chandler *et al.*, 1986; Halstead, 1989).

Inhibition of folate absorption occurs with a variety of drugs listed in Table 9.6. In the plasma, about two-thirds of the absorbed folate is bound to serum proteins. Folate is in the form of a monoglutamate, N^5–methyltetrahydrofolate. Within the cell the N^5–methyl group is removed in a reaction that requires vitamin B_{12}.

Metabolic role

Folic acid is essential for the biosynthesis of DNA. Folic acid transfers 1-carbon moieties from 'donor compounds' to a pool. Examples of these carbon moieties are methyl, methylene, formyl and formimino. From this pool they are donated to 'acceptor compounds'. These 'acceptor compounds' form metabolic intermediates necessary for the synthesis of DNA. An obligatory first step is the conversion of folic acid to the tetrahydrofolate for this activity to occur.

Folic acid deficiency

Folic acid deficiency is associated with a variety of causes listed in Table 9.6. Serum folate levels are rapidly normalized by even a single hospital meal, even if folate deficiency is present, and false elevation can also occur

Table 9.6 *Aetiology of folic acid deficiency*

Congenital	
Deficiency of folate-metabolising enzymes	
Decreased intake	
Alcoholics	
Malnutrition	
Increased utilization	
Pregnancy	
Lactation	
Children	
Chronic haemolytic anaemia	
Chronic haemodialysis	
Decreased absorption	
Proximal small bowel mucosal damage (*see* Chapter 16)	
Drug interference	
DNA synthesis inhibitors	
	Azathioprine
	Mercaptopurine
	Thioguanine
	5-Fluorouracil
	Cytosine arabinose (cytarabine)
	Zidovudine (AZT)
Folate antagonists	
	Methotrexate
	Pyrimethamine
	Triamterene
	Trimethoprim
	Pentamidine
Miscellaneous	
	Oral contraceptives
	Phenytoin
	Phenobarbitone
	Primidone
	Sulphasalazine

with mild haemolysis. The diagnosis of folate deficiency is based on macrocytosis and an abnormally low serum folate concentration. Red cell folate concentrations are a more accurate indicator of folate deficiency because serum folate fluctuates with dietary folate intake (Antony, 1991) (*see* Chapter 13).

The primary cause should be addressed. Folate supplementation is 5–15 mg/day. If folate deficiency and vitamin B_{12} deficiency are both present, treatment of *only* folate deficiency can precipitate subacute combined degeneration of the spinal cord.

CYANOCOBALAMIN (VITAMIN B_{12})

Vitamin B_{12} malabsorption (as with folic acid deficiency) is a prominent cause of megaloblastic anaemia. Owing to a lack of vitamin B_{12} (or of folic acid), DNA replication is arrested, thwarting normal cell division. However, the synthesis of cytoplasmic RNA and protein are unaffected and continue. The consequence is a megaloblast. Indeed, the most diagnostic finding (as in folate deficiency) is evidence of megaloblastosis in the bone marrow and peripheral blood. Precursor cells die within the bone marrow and mature functional cells are greatly decreased in number. The consequence is one of ineffective erythropoiesis.

Food sources

Vitamin B_{12} cannot be synthesized in the human body (except for small quantities synthesized in the colon but not absorbed) nor by plant sources. Animals obtain vitamin B_{12} manufactured by bacteria in their food. The main source is therefore animal products, such as meat and dairy products, and egg yolk. High concentrations are present in liver, kidney, oysters and clams, and moderate concentrations in ocean fish, lobsters and crabs (Antony, 1991).

The average Western diet contains 5–7 μg/day of vitamin B_{12}. About 2 μg is absorbed per day (Corcino *et al.*, 1970). Vitamin B_{12} deficiency due to a nutritional cause occurs in vegans who do not eat animal or dairy products, and in chronic alcoholics.

The minimum daily requirement is 2.5 μg.

Terminology

Vitamin B_{12} is the generic term for compounds with the biological activity of cyanocobalamin. The therapeutic preparation is cyanocobalamin. Vitamin B complex is a pharmaceutical term for compounds that usually contain vitamins B_1 and B_2.

Chemical composition

Vitamin B_{12} is chemically cyanocobalamin, which must be converted to an active form, cobalamin. Structurally, cyanocobalamin is a tetrapyrrole molecule with a cobalt atom within a corrin ring bound to a 5'-deoxyadenosyl moiety and a benzimidole moiety. In food, vitamin B_{12} is in the form of two coenzymes, methylcobalamin (Me-cbl) and 5'-deoxyadenosyl cobalamin (Ado-cbl).

Body stores

The total body stores of vitamin B_{12} are 2–5 mg distributed between the liver (1 mg) and other tissues. If the daily requirements are not exceeded, the body stores last up to 3–6 years in the absence of any vitamin B_{12} absorption. This is in contrast to the much shorter duration of folate body stores where the 5–20 mg of stored folate is depleted in 4 months.

Functions

Vitamin B_{12} regulates DNA synthesis by serving as a co-factor in folate metabolism in the transfer of one carbon moiety from one compound to another. The two coenzyme forms of cobalamin, methylcobalamin (Me-cbl) and 5'-deoxyadenosyl cobalamin (Ado-cbl) participate in the following. The conversion of N^5-methyltetrahydrofolate to tetrahydrofolate is necessary for the conversion of homocysteine to methionine. This pathway provides both methionine and tetrahydrofolate, which contributes a one carbon atom unit to deoxyuridylate, to form thymidylate and DNA. This is catalysed by methionine synthetase, and methyl cobalamin (Me-cbl) is a co-factor.

The second key function of vitamin B_{12} is in the conversion of L-methylmalonyl CoA to succinyl CoA. 5'-Deoxyadenosyl cobalamin (Ado-cbl) is the co-factor for the enzyme methylmalonyl-CoA mutase.

Absorption

In the stomach vitamin B_{12} from the ingested food is released and binds to a glycoprotein, the R protein binder. The release of vitamin B_{12} from food requires a low gastric pH (Cooper and Castle, 1960). There is evidence that decreased gastric acidity due to H-2 receptor antagonists interferes with this process (Steinbert *et al.*, 1980). The R protein binder is termed haptocorrin (Markle, 1996). The vitamin B_{12}–R protein binder complex is digested in the duodenum and vitamin B_{12} is released by the action of pancreatic proteases. This may, however, not be an essential requirement for the release of the R protein binder because total pancreatectomy does not result in vitamin B_{12} malabsorption (Kano *et al.*, 1985).

Binding between vitamin B_{12} and intrinsic factor (IF) then occurs, forming a vitamin B_{12}–IF complex that is resistant to digestion by proteolytic enzymes (Allen *et al.*, 1978a). Intrinsic factor is a 50 000–60 000 molecular weight glycoprotein secreted from the gastric parietal cells (Fischer and Taylor, 1969). Although gastric parietal cells (also) secrete gastric acid, compounds that decrease gastric acid secretion (H-2 receptor blockers; proton pump inhibitors; the hormone, secretin) do not affect IF secretion. Two molecules of IF aggregate to form a dimer within the stomach to which two molecules of vitamin B_{12} bind in the duodenum. IF serves as a carrier protein conveying the vitamin B_{12} to the terminal ileum, where the complex is taken up by endocytosis (Kapadia *et al.*, 1983) by way of specific brush-border receptors (Donaldson *et al.*, 1967). These receptors in the terminal ileum have been isolated and consist of two subunits (Seetharam *et al.*, 1981). Calcium ions form a 'salt bridge' between the receptor and IF. Optimal binding requires a neutral pH and bile salts.

In the enterocyte, IF in the vitamin B_{12}–IF complex is degraded and proteolysis occurs (a process that may assist in subsequent vitamin B_{12} binding for transport) and the vitamin B_{12} is released. The vitamin B_{12} then forms a complex with transcobalamin (TC) II, a polypeptide of molecular weight 38 000 synthesized in the liver, macrophages and ileum. TC II is essential for the transfer of vitamin B_{12} to cell surface receptors and across cell membranes. The transfer of vitamin B_{12} to TC II and release to the portal circulation takes 6–8 hours. TC II is rapidly cleared from the blood and vitamin B_{12} is now transported by another carrier protein, TC I, a glycoprotein which is cleared at a much lower rate than TC II. TC I is the primary carrier protein of vitamin B_{12}. Most vitamin B_{12} is taken up by the liver and bone marrow.

Clinical features

Anaemia is the most prominent feature and may be of sufficient severity to lead to cardiac failure. This complication is not restricted to the elderly patient. Mild scleral icterus (due to haemolysis), a beefy, red sore tongue and a palpable spleen are common findings. The neurological signs due to demyelination, degeneration and cell death should be sought. This occurs in the posterior and lateral columns, the cerebrum and the peripheral nerves. Other features are dementia, optic atrophy, peripheral neuropathy and subacute combined degeneration of the spinal cord, characterized by lower limb loss of vibration sense (more so than position sense) and upper motor neurone signs of hyper-reflexia and clonus.

Small bowel pathology

In patients with vitamin B_{12} deficiency, small intestinal villi are shortened and these changes reverse with treatment (Foroozan and Trier, 1967). The morphological changes of the mucosa of the small intestine may reflect the adverse impact of vitamin B_{12} on DNA synthesis and cell division. In a group of 28 patients with vitamin B_{12} deficiency, a significant number were unable to absorb orally administered vitamin B_{12} with intrinsic factor and a few had abnormal D-xylose absorption (Lindenbaum *et al.*, 1974). These abnormalities reversed within 2–3 weeks on vitamin B_{12} therapy, suggesting that malabsorption may be a feature of pernicious anaemia.

Vitamin B_{12} deficiency

CONGENITAL CAUSES

Conditions affecting vitamin B_{12} status associated with transcobalamin II deficiency (Cooper and Rosenblatt,

1987) and defective transcobalamin II (Haurani *et al.*, 1979; Seligman *et al.*, 1980) are documented. Transcobalamin II deficiency is an autosomal recessive condition. Although transcobalamin II transports only small quantities of vitamin B_{12}, its role is crucial as it is the only carrier that conveys vitamin B_{12} to tissues. The disorder is manifest soon after birth and the features are of severe megaloblastic anaemia.

DIETARY DEFICIENCY

Dietary causes of vitamin B_{12} deficiency are extremely rare and occur only in vegans who consume no animal or dairy products for prolonged amounts of time. In a study of 138 vegetarians in India who only consumed the animal products milk and yoghurt, vitamin B_{12} deficiency was present in 95 (69 per cent) of the subjects (Chanarin *et al.*, 1985).

DECREASED GASTRIC ACIDITY

In conditions of hypochlorhydria or achlorhydria, the release of vitamin B_{12} from food sources is impaired (Carmel, 1978) from lack of gastric acid. In states of reduced gastric mucosal surface – for example, partial or total gastrectomy – vitamin B_{12} absorption is decreased due to lack of gastric acid, decreased IF secretion and bacterial overgrowth. This problem occurs most often in Bilroth II and in subtotal and total gastrectomy.

INTRINSIC FACTOR DEFICIENCY

An absence or lack of intrinsic factor production by the gastric parietal cells occurs in pernicious anaemia. Pernicious anaemia is an autoimmune condition associated with gastritis, lack of IF production and achlorhydria, and in conditions of reduced gastric surface area as with gastric resections. Other autoimmune diseases associated with pernicious anaemia are diabetes mellitus, Crohn's disease, Hashimoto's thyroiditis, Addison's disease and vitiligo. Juvenile pernicious anaemia, an autosomal recessive condition, is a heterogeneous group of disorders due to: (1) inadequate synthesis of IF; (2) a block in IF secretion; (3) the secretion of an abnormal IF that does not bind to cobalamin; or (4) the secretion of other abnormal IFs with other functional defects (Levine and Allen, 1985). These patients have IF concentrations that are absent or subnormal, but, unlike older patients, have neither gastric atrophy nor achlorhydria.

ILEAL MUCOSAL CAUSES

In disorders of malabsorption (Chapter 16), the most common cause of megaloblastic anaemia is folate deficiency; however, terminal ileal involvement and vitamin B_{12} deficiency occurs in a variety of diseases discussed in detail in subsequent chapters. In tropical sprue (Chapter 21), ileal involvement and cobalamin malabsorption are a more common feature (Baker, 1972). Severe coeliac disease (*see* Chapter 23), owing to the extension of the mucosal lesion to the ileum, may cause vitamin B_{12} malabsorption, although this is uncommon. The drugs listed in Table 9.7 interfere with the transepithelial transport of vitamin B_{12}, most probably through mucosal damage. In Crohn's disease (*see* Chapter 25) vitamin B_{12} malabsorption due to terminal ileal disease occurs in severe ileal involvement. In patients with resection of the distal ileum greater than 50 cm, cobalamin malabsorption is inevitable (Alcock, 1961), and also occurs when the ileum is surgically bypassed (Coyle *et al.*, 1977).

Table 9.7 *Causes of vitamin B_{12} malabsorption*

Congenital
Transcobalamin II deficiency
R-protein binder deficiency

Dietary deficiency

Decreased gastric acidity
Atrophic gastritis
Hypochlorhydria
Omeprazole

Intrinsic factor deficiency
Pernicious anaemia
- Adult pernicious anaemia
- Juvenile pernicious anaemia
- Gastric surgery (partial or total gastrectomy)

Ileal mucosal causes
Mucosal diseases
- Inflammatory bowel disease (Crohn's disease)
- Tropical sprue
- Severe coeliac disease
- Tuberculosis
- Whipple's disease
- Lymphoma

Drugs
- Neomycin
- Colchicine
- Biguanides
- Potassium supplements
- Para-amino salicylic acid

Ileal resection
Immerslund–Gräsbeck syndrome (familial selective vitamin B_{12} absorption)

Intraluminal causes
Bacterial overgrowth
Parasitic causes
- *Diphyllobothrium latum*

Pancreatic disease
- Inactivation of pancreatic proteins
- Zollinger–Ellison syndrome

In the Immerslund–Gräsbeck syndrome (familial selective vitamin B_{12} malabsorption), malabsorption of the intrinsic factor-bound vitamin B_{12} complex occurs at the site of the terminal ileal receptors owing to a congenital defect in the transcellular transport of cobalamin. The clinical features are megaloblastic anaemia and albuminuria due to a renal tubular defect (Immerslund, 1960; Gräsbeck *et al.*, 1960). The anaemia responds to vitamin B_{12} therapy.

INTRAMURAL CAUSES

Several mechanisms are implicated in the malabsorption of vitamin B_{12} in states of small intestinal bacterial overgrowth. The range of bacteria that are able to bind vitamin B_{12} is extensive. Anaerobic species, especially Bacteroides, have a high capacity to bind both cobalamin and the intrinsic factor vitamin B_{12} combination (Giannella *et al.*, 1972; Welkos *et al.*, 1981). Clostridium, *E. coli* and Propionibacterium metabolize cobalamin to cobamides, which are metabolically inactive substances (Brandt *et al.*, 1977). These substances may combine with intrinsic factor and block ileal receptors (Mathan *et al.*, 1974). Vitamin B_{12} may be consumed by the fish tapeworm *Diphyllobothrium latum*. This parasite (*see* Chapter 19) is commonly found in freshwater fish, such as pike in the lakes of north central USA and in Scandinavia, the Baltic states and Russia. Infection occurs by eating raw or undercooked fish. *Diphyllobothrium latum* absorbs significant quantities of vitamin B_{12}. The worms are located in jejunum, where vitamin B_{12} is consumed before the vitamin reaches the terminal ileum. It is interesting that megaloblastic anaemia occurs most often in Finland. The diagnosis is made by identifying the ova in stools. Treatment consists of vitamin B_{12} supplements and eradication of the worm, with praziquantel, one dose of 5–10 mg per kg body weight.

MISCELLANEOUS CAUSES

Pancreatic protease enzymes degrade the R proteins in the vitamin B_{12}–R protein binder complex to prevent competition with intrinsic factor. In chronic pancreatic disease, megaloblastic anaemia occurs due to the lack of pancreatic proteases (Allen *et al.*, 1978b; Marcoullis *et al.*, 1980). Among the drugs that cause vitamin B_{12} malabsorption are neomycin (Jacobsen, 1960), colchicine (Webb *et al.*, 1968), omeprazole (Bellou *et al.*, 1966) and potassium chloride (Palva *et al.*, 1972). Vitamin B_{12} malabsorption is reported as a side-effect of para-amino salicylic acid and the mechanism is not due to mucosal atrophy or related to intrinsic factor (Palva *et al.*, 1966).

Tests of vitamin B_{12} absorption (*see* Chapter 13)

Deficiency of vitamin B_{12} is established by low serum concentrations. The tests of vitamin B_{12} absorption are discussed in detail in Chapter 13. The Schilling test serves to establish if vitamin B_{12} deficiency is due to the absence of intrinsic factor. If pernicious anaemia is not the cause of low vitamin B_{12} concentrations, other possibilities related to the causes as discussed above and listed in Table 9.7 should be considered. If bacterial contamination of the gut is suspected, the use of antibiotics in conjunction with the Schilling test will enable a diagnosis to be established.

Management

The use of cyanocobalamin is no longer advocated for the treatment of vitamin B_{12} deficiency. Hydroxocobalamin is the preferred form, since it is retained longer and is also biologically more available than cyanocobalamin. The principle is to replenish body stores, and maintain regular therapy depending upon the underlying cause. A variety of treatment regimes abound for the treatment of vitamin B_{12} deficiency (Lee, 1999). Body stores would be replenished by six 1000 μg doses administered intramuscularly at 3–7 day intervals; and for maintenance therapy, the same dose is given intramuscularly every 3 months (Hoffbrand, 1999). A reticulocyte response occurs about 5–10 days after treatment. The rapid formation of new cells may be associated with significant hypokalaemia.

MINERALS

Transition metals (e.g. iron, copper and zinc) and alkaline earth metals (e.g. calcium and magnesium) are essential dietary components required for numerous functions within cells and tissues. Inadequate intake of any of these is accompanied by a number of clinical manifestations, which may prove fatal unless treated. In addition, excess of the metals interferes with macromolecular synthesis and function and is toxic to cells. To maintain appropriate and safe concentrations of metals in the body, elaborate homeostatic regulatory processes exist. One level of this regulation is at the point of entry of metals in the body, the small intestine. The efficiency by which a specific metal is absorbed depends very much on several intraluminal environmental factors: the luminal pH, the redox state of the mineral, and the formation of chelates and other complexes that impede if not prevent absorption. Although the mechanisms that underlie metal absorption and homeostasis are still being defined and remain key questions in current research, some of the critical regulatory proteins have now been identified and cloned. This section integrates older information pertaining to the absorption and function of these metals with recent findings at the molecular front.

IRON

An adult male contains about 4 g of iron, comprising haem iron in haemoglobin and myoglobin as well as non-haem iron, either as ferric or ferrous iron in complex with various ligands. Haem iron serves as a carrier of oxygen from the lungs to the tissues, while non-haem iron is found in cytochromes and other proteins, where it participates in redox reactions required for oxidative metabolism and macromolecular synthesis (reviewed in Lombard *et al.*, 1997). Like the other biologically important transition metals, iron has to be continually absorbed from the diet, delivered to tissues and organs, and then utilized in physiological processes. At the same time, it is important that the body stores of iron do not exceed critical tissue concentrations or toxic effects will ensue. This section describes our current knowledge of the absorption and homeostatic regulation of iron in the body, with particular emphasis on the role of the small intestine.

Dietary sources and bioavailability

The recommended daily allowances (USA) for iron are 6–10 mg/day for infants, 10 mg/day for children, 12 mg/day for teenagers, 15 mg/day for adults and lactating women, and 30 mg/day for pregnant women (Table 9.8). A typical diet contains 10–14 mg of iron per day, which is provided by meat, cereals, vegetables and fruit (Passmore and Eastwood, 1986). Pregnant women need iron tablet supplementation to achieve 30 mg/day. The infant obtains most of its iron from stores in the liver, formed during gestation. Dietary iron can be present as haem or non-haem iron. Between 10 per cent and 20 per cent of iron in the Western diet is ferrous haem iron, largely derived from animal food products. This iron is readily absorbed by the intestine, and may constitute 30 per cent of the absorbed iron. Non-haem ferric iron constitutes the bulk of dietary iron and is abundant in vegetable-derived foods, where it is bound to a variety of ligands that may interfere with absorption, thereby limiting its bioavailability (Passmore and Eastwood, 1986). Bioavailability is an index of the level at which a nutrient is absorbed by the intestine. Thus, iron in cereal is poorly absorbed due to being complexed with phytates (Lombard *et al.*, 1997).

Absorption of iron

The bulk of iron is absorbed in the first portion of the duodenum, in which the action of acidic gastric juices promotes solubilization and membrane transport of iron (Raja *et al.*, 1992). Iron may also be absorbed in the jejunum and, to a lesser extent, in more distal regions. Both energy-dependent and passive transport mechanisms are implicated and homeostatic mechanisms ensure that uptake of iron is promoted in iron deficiency. Another factor thought to be involved in iron absorption is gastric mucin, which binds and solubilizes iron at acidic pH and facilitates its absorption in the duodenum, where the pH is more alkaline (Conrad and Umbreit, 1993).

Molecules involved in iron absorption and transport

The well-known effects of iron deficiency in anaemia have led to numerous studies of the mechanisms and

Table 9.8 *USA recommended daily allowances for minerals*

Minerals	Infants (0–1 years)	Children (1–10 years)	Teenagers (15–18 years)	Adults	Pregnant women	Lactating women
Calcium (mg)	400–600	800	1200	800	1200	1200
Magnesium (mg)	40–60	80–170	270–400	350	320	355,[a] 340[b]
Iron (mg)	6–10	10	12	15	30	15
Zinc (mg)	5	10	15	15	15	19,[a] 16[b]
Copper (mg)	0.6–0.7	1–2	1.5–3	1.5–3	1.5–3	1.5–3
Manganese (mg)	0.3–1.0	2–3	2–5	2–5	2–5	2–5
Iodine (μg)	40–50	70–120	150	150	175	200
Chromium (μg)	10–60	50–200	50–200	50–200	50–200	50–200
Selenium (μg)	10–15	20–30	40–50	70	65	75

[a]First 6 months of lactation.
[b]Second 6 months of lactation.
Adapted from Recommended Dietary Allowances: National Academy of Sciences, published on web page: http://www.nal.usda.gov/fnic/Dietary/rda.html.

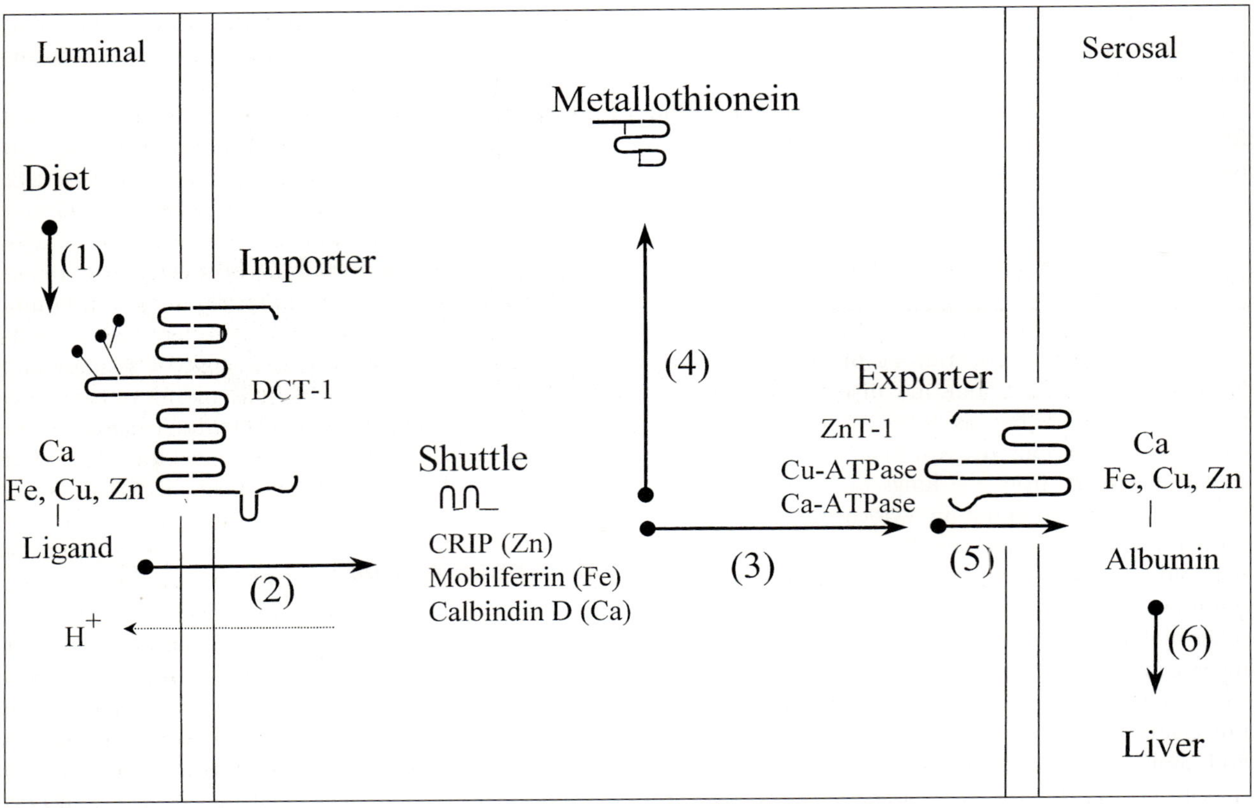

Figure 9.2 *Model of transcellular metal transport across the intestine. Essential metals (iron, copper, zinc and calcium) obtained in the diet appear in the lumen (1) complexed to small molecular weight ligands (e.g. histidine for zinc). The metals are taken up across the brush border by specific transporters, including the multispecific importer DCT-1, which involves exchange of H^+ (2). Once internalized, metal ions are transported through the cytosol of the enterocyte by shuttle proteins, CRIP for zinc (and possibly copper), mobilferrin for iron and calbindin D for calcium (3). Excess zinc and copper are trapped by metallothionein (4), and either diverted to excretory routes or utilized by the intestinal cells. Metals destined for the body are exported across the basolateral membrane via specific or non-specific transporters (5), e.g. via the recently cloned zinc efflux protein ZnT-1, the copper efflux protein Cu-ATPase and the Ca-ATPase. Metals released into the portal circulation are transported to the liver, probably in complex with plasma proteins such as albumin (6), and then to other tissues.*

molecules that control intestinal absorption, excretion and homeostasis of this metal. These are discussed below and a model is shown in Fig. 9.2. Although transferrin promotes iron uptake across cell membranes, it is not thought to be important in luminal absorption of this metal, although it may mediate reabsorption (see below) (Conrad *et al.*, 1996). Conrad and Umbreit (1993) have proposed a model of iron transport across the enterocyte in which integrins at the luminal end of enterocytes bind iron and facilitate its transit through the brush border. In addition, the putative high-affinity copper uptake transporter hCRT-1 (discussed later) has been found to rescue yeast defective in both copper and iron uptake. Its possible role in small intestinal absorption of iron now needs investigation. However, the most exciting clues to intestinal absorption of iron have followed the cloning of DCT-1.

The recent discovery of the role of DCT-1 in cellular uptake of iron and certain other metals had its origins in genetic studies to map the gene whose mutation is responsible for an iron deficiency-like microcytic anaemia in mice. This gene was mapped to a locus known to contain the *Nramp2* gene, which confers susceptibility to some intracellular pathogens but with no obvious role in iron uptake (Fleming *et al.*, 1997). Gunshin and colleagues in 1997 made the exciting link to iron transport by showing that expression of the rat homologue of the *Nramp2* gene, in a *Xenopus* oocyte functional-expression cloning model, stimulated cellular iron uptake by about 200-fold. Since this gene product was also able to transport zinc and copper, at least *in vitro*, it was given the more general term of divalent cation transporter (DCT-1). A model of the structure of DCT-1 is depicted in Fig. 9.3a. It is a 561-amino-acid protein with 12 putative membrane-spanning domains. The N- and C-termini are on the cytoplasmic side, while the extracellular portion features a large loop with putative glycosylation sites. DCT-1 mediates active

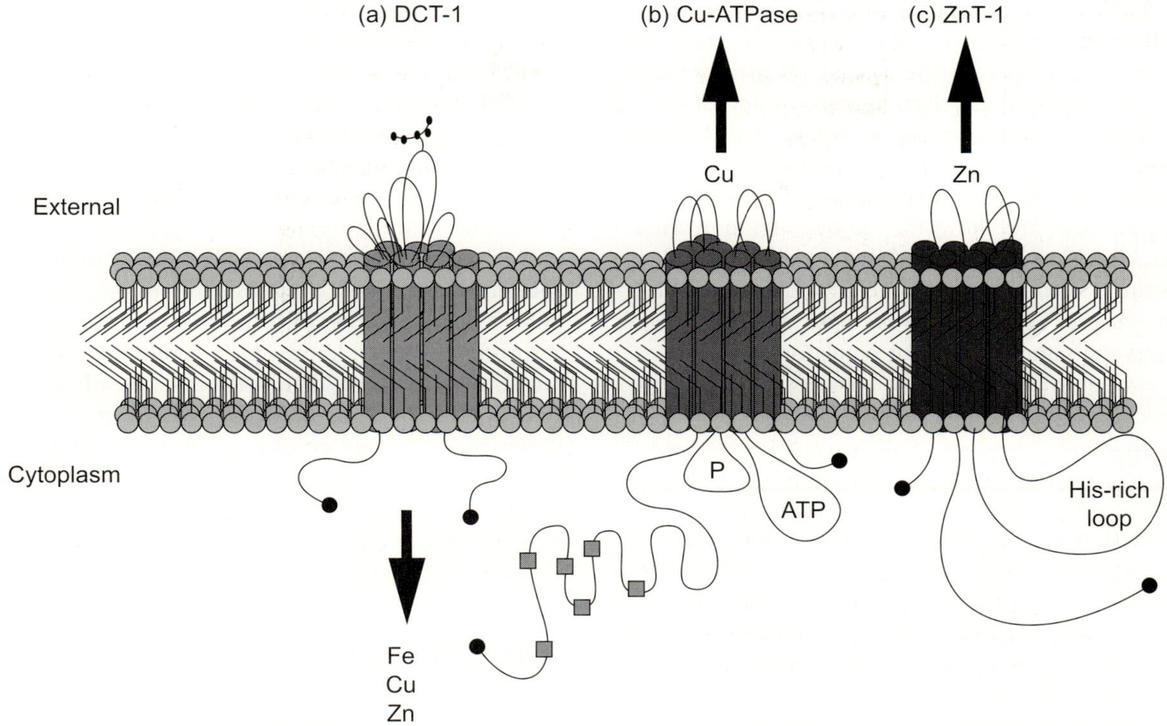

Figure 9.3 *Plasma membrane metal ion transporters. A schema of the structures of three different types of metal ion transporters with their predicted orientation across the plasma membrane. (a) The structure of the multispecific divalent cation transporter DCT-1 with its 12 putative transmembrane domains is shown. Between domains 7 and 8 on the extracellular side, the polypeptide contains a predicted glycosylation site (sugars are indicated by black circles). DCT-1 is enriched in the enterocyte luminal plasma membrane where it mediates influx of metal ions in a process linked to proton transport. (b) The copper-transporting ATPase is shown. At the N-terminal end of the polypeptide, within the cytoplasm, are the putative copper-binding sites. The structure is thought to have eight transmembrane domains. Loops containing phosphatase (P) and the ATP-binding site are shown. (c) ZnT-1 is a plasma membrane Zn transporter involved in efflux of Zn out of many types of cell, including the enterocyte where it mediates serosal transport. ZnT-1 has six putative transmembrane domains. On the cytoplasmic side, there is a large loop rich in histidine, which may bind zinc ions.*

influx of metal ions by a mechanism coupled to proton-transport and dependent on the cell membrane potential (Gunshin *et al.*, 1997). Its preferential expression at the apical membranes of the enterocytes lining the small intestinal lumen, as well as its up-regulation in dietary iron deficiency, strongly implicates DCT-1 in iron absorption. It is particularly enriched in the proximal duodenum, especially in the crypts and in the lower segments of the villi, and levels decrease towards the colon. The current thinking is that DCT-1 serves as a multispecific metal ion transporter mediating iron absorption at the luminal surface of enterocytes (Fig. 9.2), although this has yet to be substantiated.

Once iron is absorbed across the brush border, how is it transported to the basolateral surface and excreted into the portal circulation? One study has pointed towards a cytosolic iron binding protein called mobilferrin, which may act to shuttle iron across the enterocyte (Fig. 9.2). Part of the homeostatic regulation of iron uptake may be at the level of iron binding sites on mobilferrin (Conrad *et al.*, 1996). An efflux mechanism at the serosal end, which may mediate the release of iron from the enterocyte into the portal blood, has not yet been identified. One candidate for the iron efflux transporter has emerged from a study of hereditary haemochromatosis, an autosomal recessive disorder resulting in excessive iron overload of the body and multiple organ dysfunction. This phenotype implies that a defect exists in the capacity of the intestine to regulate homeostasis of iron. The gene responsible for this disease, *Hfe*, is closely related to the major histocompatibility complex class I family, and missense mutations in *Hfe* account for more than 80 per cent of the patients (Feder *et al.*, 1996). Another factor may also operate because, in an X-linked form of microcytic anaemia in mice, there is normal intestinal uptake of iron but defective export into the portal circulation – *see* Vulpe and Gitschier (1997) for further discussion and references. Identification of the normal function of this gene product, sla, as well as that of *Hfe*, and the relationship of these proteins to the pathways of export of iron from the intestinal epithelium should provide new insights into the mechanisms of iron homeostasis. Finally, there are homeostatic mechanisms involving transferrin receptors on the basolateral membranes of enterocytes that are involved in reabsorption of iron in conditions of iron overload (Conrad and Umbreit, 1993).

Elucidation of the individual roles of these various gene products and how they cooperate to maintain normal levels of iron in the body presents a challenge for future research. It will be equally important to determine whether homeostasis of other essential metals involves the same or different regulatory proteins.

COPPER

This section reviews the physiology, absorption and transport of copper in the body. For more information, the reader is referred to an excellent series of review articles on copper in a supplement to volume 67 (1998) of the *American Journal for Clinical Nutrition*. The most exciting new finding in copper research has been the identification of at least two structurally related copper-transporting ATPases, which mediate efflux of copper from cells and which are defective in diseases of abnormal copper homeostasis, one in Menkes' disease (see below) and the other in Wilson's disease (see below).

Copper and physiology

Copper is far less abundant than iron; adult humans contain 70–100 mg of copper, which exists in two oxidation states, cuprous (I) and cupric (II). Copper is not distributed uniformly throughout the body but is most abundant in skeletal muscle (25 per cent of body copper), bone (19 per cent), skin (15 per cent), bone marrow (15 per cent), liver (8–15 per cent), and brain (8 per cent). When expressed as a concentration in wet tissues, it is highest in brain and liver (5–6 μg/g) (Solomons, 1988). In the body, the only function of copper is in copper metalloenzymes, all of which are involved in redox reactions, which commonly consume oxygen or oxyradicals and generate hydrogen peroxide or water. Examples are cytochrome c oxidase, which is involved in mitochondrial oxidative phosphorylation, and lysyl oxidase, which catalyses oxidative deamination reactions needed for cross-linking of collagen and elastin (Solomons, 1988).

Copper and diet

The recommended daily allowances (USA) for copper are 0.6–0.7 mg/day for infants, 1–2 mg/day for children, and 1.5–3 mg/day for teenagers, adults, lactating and pregnant women (Table 9.8). Legumes are the major source of copper in the diet, while animal proteins supply much less. Copper in vegetables is complexed to a variety of ligands (including lectins and glycoproteins), which may interfere with absorption, although phytates may not be important (Lonnerdal, 1996; Wapnir, 1998). Food processing (such as milling of grains and canning of vegetables) can result in significant losses of copper (Clydesdale, 1988). Copper is also abundant in shellfish, but very low in rice and cow's milk. Of the dietary factors that influence copper absorption, the best known are a component of human breast milk, yet to be identified, which greatly facilitates absorption, and ascorbic acid (Milne *et al.*, 1981). Prolonged consumption of high levels of dietary ascorbic acid has been found to lower serum copper and ceruloplasmin levels in monkeys, and thereby interfere with the role of copper in regulating cholesterol metabolism.

Copper deficiency

Copper deficiency was not identified in humans until 1964 in severely malnourished infants on milk-based diets, which were low in copper (Cordano *et al.*, 1964). Subsequently, copper deficiency was found in patients on total parenteral nutrition without appropriate supplementation (Solomons, 1988). Typical features of copper deficiency are microcytic hypochromic anaemia and neutropenia; there may also be skeletal changes (especially in growing children), loss of pigmentation of integumentary tissues (owing to the lack of the copper metalloenzyme tyrosinase), and defective elastin formation and decreased collagen deposition (owing to the lack of the copper-dependent enzyme lysyl oxidase) (Beshgetoor and Hambridge, 1998; Solomons, 1988).

One inherited form of copper deficiency is Menkes' disease, although it might also be considered as an abnormality of copper homeostasis because some organs have little copper (e.g. liver), while others (e.g. kidney) actually accumulate copper. Menkes' disease is an X-linked disease of male infants characterized by growth retardation, cerebral degeneration leading to coma and mental retardation, depigmentation of skin and hair, and bone demineralization. It is usually fatal in early childhood. This disease is also known as kinky hair syndrome because the hair has the appearance of steel wool (Fig. 9.4). Its resemblance to the abnormalities of wool seen in copper-deficient sheep in Australia led to the realization that Menkes' disease was due to copper deficiency. The pathogenesis of Menkes' disease is a consequence both of impaired intestinal absorption of copper and defective incorporation into copper proteins. Recently, the Menkes' gene was cloned and identified as a copper-transporting P-type ATPase that is thought to regulate the efflux of copper from cells,

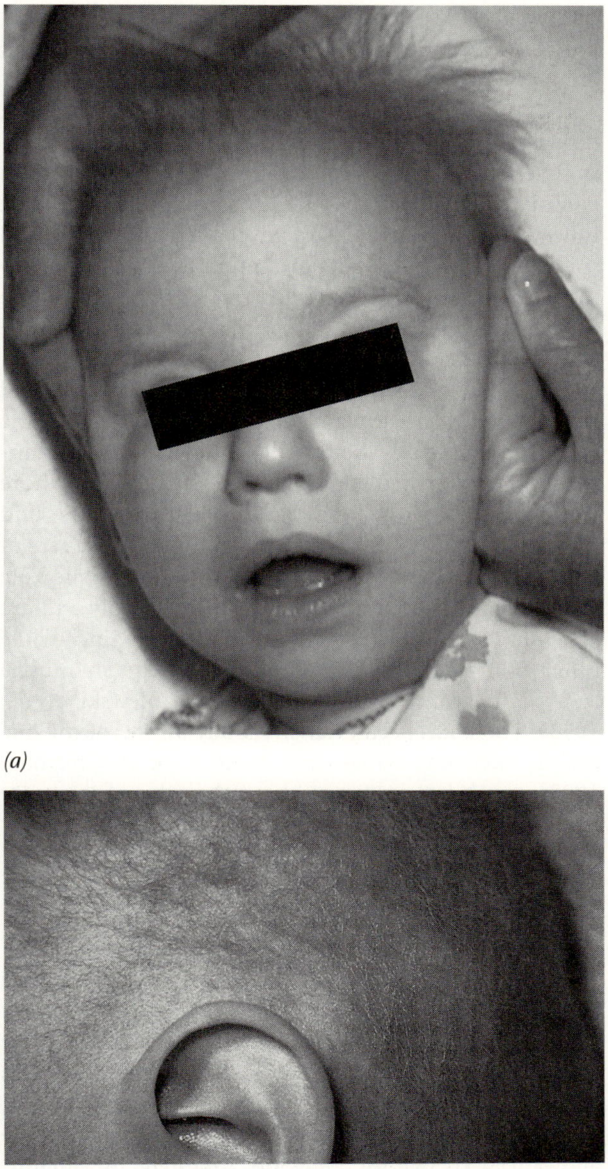

(a)

(b)

Figure 9.4 *(a) A child with Menkes' disease. (b) Note the typical, short, kinky hair in close up.*

driven by the hydrolysis of ATP (see below) (reviewed in Mercer, 1998).

Another disease of altered copper homeostasis is Wilson's disease. In this autosomal recessive disorder, the affected locus also encodes a P-type ATPase, which is 57 per cent homologous to the Menkes' ATPase (Dameron and Harrison, 1998). Since the Wilson's ATPase is highly expressed in the liver and thought to be important in the excretion of copper in the bile, there is accumulation of copper in the liver, kidney and basal ganglia, to toxic levels. Wilson's disease is associated with abnormally low levels of ceruloplasmin and with impairment of biliary excretion (Harris *et al.*, 1998). It can be treated by copper chelation therapy (e.g. with penicillamine) or by excessive zinc intake to induce intestinal metallothionein, thereby interfering with copper absorption (see later).

Absorption of copper

In adult humans, the net absorption of dietary copper is approximately 1 mg/day (30–40 per cent of ingested copper). Soluble copper is absorbed in the stomach and upper duodenum in man. However, since digestion is required for the liberation of free ionic copper from foods, the major sites of copper absorption are thought to be beyond the duodenum (Solomons, 1988). Factors considered important in the absorption of copper are pH of the lumen, presence of histidine and other facilitatory ligands and competition for uptake by iron. Although long-term supplementation of zinc may result in copper-deficient anaemia, this is more likely the consequence of induction of metallothionein by zinc, resulting in trapping of the copper in the intestinal mucosa, rather than direct competition between zinc and copper for absorption (Fischer *et al.*, 1983). As for the other metals, the fractional absorption of copper is decreased when copper intake is excessive, thereby restricting intake of copper in the body in conditions of overload (Wapnir, 1998). Malabsorption of copper may occur in coeliac disease (*see* Chapter 23), short bowel syndrome (*see* Chapter 29) and chronic diarrhoea (especially in infants) (*see* Chapter 14); deficiencies in copper uptake in the elderly have not been reported.

Copper is taken up across the intestinal mucosa largely by a carrier-mediated diffusion, although some copper may enter enterocytes by the active transport of histidine-bound copper (Wapnir, 1998). It is not yet clear whether DCT-1 is a major participant in uptake of copper but its uptake *in vitro* was stimulated by this metal ion transporter (Gunshin *et al.*, 1997). Another protein that may also participate in mammalian copper absorption was identified by Zhou and Gitschier in 1997 at the University of California in San Francisco. Their strategy was to screen for human genes that were able to rescue mutant yeast defective in copper uptake. In yeast, three copper uptake genes, CTR1–3, have been identified. Two of these, CTR1 and CTR3, encode high-affinity copper-transport proteins while the other encodes a low-affinity receptor. The human gene hCTR1 was able to complement yeast defective in CTR1 and, when overexpressed in yeast, made them vulnerable to excessive copper concentrations in the medium. Although hCTR1 is expressed in the small intestine, there is little known about its distribution within the intestinal epithelium (e.g. apical versus basolateral) and we must await proof that it mediates intestinal copper absorption *in vivo*.

Once copper is absorbed, a fraction remains within the enterocyte, owing to tight binding to metallothionein. At the basolateral end, copper is released from the enterocyte by an efflux mechanism that is thought to be mediated by the copper-transporting ATPase (Cu-ATPase). The recognition of the role of this enzyme in copper transport followed its identification as the affected locus in Menkes' disease (see earlier). Patients with Menkes' disease are able to absorb copper into the enterocytes, since these cells are rich in copper, but apparently cannot efflux it efficiently into the portal blood, resulting in severe copper deficiency (Mercer, 1998). The structure of this form of Cu-ATPase is shown in Fig. 9.3 as item (b). It is a very large protein (exactly 1500 amino acids) with P-type ATPase activity; the P refers to the phosphorylation on a conserved aspartic acid residue during the ATP hydrolysis reaction. There are six putative copper-binding regions in the N-terminal cysteine-rich region that lies under the plasma membrane (Mercer, 1998). It has been suggested that conformational changes induced by binding of copper result in the exposure of the aspartic acid and its phosphorylation, events required for the translocation of copper across the cell membrane. Menkes'-type Cu-ATPase is also found in the membranes of vesicles of the trans-Golgi network in some other types of cell, and may play roles in sequestration and secretion of copper.

Copper released into the portal blood supply is transported via albumin to the liver where it is coupled to ceruloplasmin, which can bind up to six atoms of copper per molecule of protein. Liver copper is then transported to other organs or, when in excess, it is returned to the gastrointestinal tract via bile. There is little excretion of copper in the urine.

ZINC

This section reviews the physiology, absorption and transport of zinc in the body. For more information, the reader is referred to a series of review articles on zinc in a forthcoming supplement (2000) in the *Journal of Nutrition*. This series was based on a workshop 'Zinc and Health: Current Status and Future Directions' sponsored by the National Institutes of Health Office of Dietary Supplements in November 1998.

Physiology

Zinc is a group IIb metal, and is required for the healthy functioning of the body. The importance of zinc for the functional integrity of many organ tissues systems and as a structural component of hundreds of metalloenzymes and zinc finger transcription factors has emerged only in the last four decades. Zinc is also required for growth, development and tissue repair in humans and animals (Solomons, 1988).

The total zinc content in the human body is 2–3 g distributed non-uniformly throughout all organs, secretions, fluids and tissues of the body. Most tissues contain about 20–200 μg of zinc per gram of tissue; however, the retina, prostate, pancreatic islets and sperm contain much higher amounts (800–3000 μg/g) (Vallee and Falchuk, 1993). The majority of zinc in the body is in two distinct intracellular pools. Firstly, the bulk of cellular zinc exists tightly bound to metalloenzymes, where it serves both catalytic and structural functions. This pool of zinc is largely non-exchangeable and little affected by dietary intake of zinc. The remaining 5–10 per cent of the body's zinc exists in a more dynamic pool, which is rapidly exchangeable and readily depleted in zinc deficiency. Therefore the rate of zinc turnover in the body is tissue-specific; labile zinc pools (e.g. in liver and bone) turn over rapidly and are very susceptible to alterations in dietary zinc, while other non-readily exchangeable pools (e.g. in muscle and brain) turn over more slowly (Zalewski *et al.*, 1993). There has been extensive study of the role of zinc within metalloenzymes and zinc fingers (Coleman, 1992); much less is known about the roles of the more labile pools in cellular function.

Dietary sources and bioavailability

The foods from which copper is acquired differ to a large extent from those providing zinc. Zinc is normally obtained in foods such as red meat, seafoods, dairy foods, grains and nuts (Dreosti, 1993). Green vegetables and fruits also contain adequate levels of zinc; however, this zinc is less bioavailable. The recommended daily allowances (USA) for zinc are 5 mg/day for infants, 10 mg/day for children, 15 mg/day for teenagers, adults and pregnant women, and 16–19 mg/day for lactating women (Table 9.8). In an Australian national random survey in 1991, 67 per cent of men and 85 per cent of women consumed diets with zinc content below 12 mg/day. In this study (Baghurst *et al.*, 1991), the major individual food sources for zinc in men were steak (11 per cent of total Zn intake), bread (9 per cent), milk (8 per cent), cheese (6 per cent), minced meat (4 per cent) and breakfast cereals (3 per cent).

The bioavailability of zinc is dependent on a variety of factors. These include the presence of ligands (phosphates and oxalates), which decrease absorption, as well as ligands (carboxylic acids, glucose and amino acids, such as histidine and methionine), which increase uptake. Some of the latter have been utilized in zinc supplements. The amount of protein in a meal can promote zinc absorption, although each protein affects zinc absorptivity differently. Certain factors, including lactoferrin and whey factor in human milk, have been shown to promote zinc absorption. Solomons (1988) reported that, although the concentration of zinc in cow's milk exceeded that in human milk, zinc was more readily absorbed across an infant's intestine from human milk.

One important dietary factor that negatively influences zinc absorption is phytate, commonly present in staple foods such as cereals, corn and rice. Some of the common forms of phytate responsible for zinc chelation include inositol hexaphosphate and pentaphosphate. Studies performed by Freeland-Graves and colleagues in 1980 found that, although vegetarian diets, which are high in legumes and green vegetables, did contain adequate amounts of zinc, the metal was largely chelated to fibre and phytic acid, which decreased its absorptivity. Vegetarians can increase their intake of zinc by consuming seeds, nuts and wholegrain breads. Similarly, the lowering of phytate levels via the enzymic activity of phytase (commonly found in fermented soy bean meals) can also increase zinc bioavailability as it results in the degradation of phytic acid (Hirabayashi *et al.*, 1998). Resistant starch may also promote zinc absorption by meals rich in phytic acid.

Zinc deficiency

The classic features of zinc deficiency include retardation of growth, severe immunodeficiency, characteristic skin lesions, delayed sexual maturation and gastrointestinal problems; this reflects the extreme sensitivity of the tissues and organs in which there is rapid turnover of cells (e.g. bone, thymus, epidermis, testis, intestinal crypts). Even in severe zinc deficiency, the total cellular zinc (as measured by atomic absorption spectroscopy) is decreased only slightly or not at all. Therefore, the zinc that is most susceptible to depletion resides in the minor, readily exchangeable labile pools (Zalewski *et al.*, 1993). Other than in plasma, tissue zinc levels of adult animals fed a zinc-deficient diet generally do not fall unless the deficiency extends for considerable periods of time.

Severe primary zinc deficiency is relatively rare. Zinc is limiting in the diet of some indigenous peoples including Australian aborigines (Cheek *et al.*, 1984). Others (such as the sexually immature male dwarves of Egypt and Iran studied in the 1960s) consumed a staple diet adequate in zinc but also rich in phytate. Zinc deficiency may also follow parenteral nutrition lacking extra zinc supplementation, and occurs in anorexia nervosa and protein-energy malnutrition. Other metals such as iron and copper can compete for zinc transporters, hence having a negative effect on zinc absorption; this is particularly important in infants and pregnant women on iron-fortified diet formulas (Dreosti, 1993; Lonnerdal, 1996). Other causes of zinc deficiency result from decreased absorption across the intestinal brush border (e.g. in acrodermatitis enteropathica) and/or increased loss of zinc in the urine (e.g. in diabetes mellitus and alcoholic cirrhosis).

One of the major pathophysiological abnormalities contributing to secondary zinc deficiency is zinc malabsorption. An important factor is the functional integrity of the intestinal mucosa, which is compromised in a number of disorders, including alcoholism and gastrointestinal disorders (Solomons, 1988). The autosomal recessive disease acrodermatitis enteropathica is an inherited abnormality of zinc absorption, characterized by hyperpigmented skin lesions (especially over the acral surfaces of elbows and knees), severe immunodeficiency and stunted growth. Oral zinc sulphate therapy produces complete clinical remission. The efficiency of zinc absorption is reduced in this disease, but the precise abnormalities have yet to be identified.

It remains controversial whether mild zinc deficiency is common in the Western population. Recent information on zinc intake in Australian men and women is scanty. However, according to the 1983 National Dietary Survey of Adults in Australia, 27 per cent of men and 54 per cent of women had zinc intakes that were less than 70 per cent of the recommended daily intake. Similar studies in the USA and Canada suggest that a significant proportion of Western people are at risk of zinc deficiency, especially children, the elderly and pregnant women (Sandstead, 1991).

Absorption

Zinc homeostasis is regulated largely at the level of the gastrointestinal tract, by absorption and excretion. There are no stores of zinc in the body (unlike iron), although bone and liver zinc may act as reservoirs. Both stable isotopes and ^{65}Zn radioisotope have been utilized in tracer studies to provide information on efficiency of zinc uptake across the intestine (Hambidge *et al.*, 1998). Fractional absorption of zinc decreases as the intraluminal concentration of zinc is increased, while zinc deficiency has the opposite effect. Increased fractional absorption of zinc occurs in pregnancy, lactation and infancy, where zinc demands are high (Krebs *et al.*, 1998).

It is generally believed that the primary site of zinc absorption is the distal duodenum or proximal jejunum. However, at least one recent study in mice has also indicated significant absorption in the ileum (Sorensen *et al.*, 1998). The kinetics of absorption are slower in the jejunum than the rest of the small intestine. Overall, the transit time for zinc is very short, as large quantities of zinc were found to pass through the small intestine within 1 hour. In mice, the stomach, caecum and colon appeared to be insignificant sites of zinc absorption (Sorensen *et al.*, 1998). The effect of ageing on zinc absorption is unclear but a recent study of nine young and eight elderly healthy men showed no significant effect of ageing on zinc absorption, even up to the age of 80 years (Couzy *et al.*, 1993).

Molecular mechanisms

The mechanisms involved in transport of zinc across the intestinal membranes are still poorly defined. Absorption across the intestinal mucosa may be both carrier-mediated and by simple diffusion of either ionic zinc or zinc complexed to various ligands, including histidine, citric acid and picolinic acid (Vallee and Falchuk, 1993). One candidate for the membrane transporter is DCT-1, which probably serves as a multispecific metal ion transporter mediating zinc, copper and iron absorption at the luminal surface of enterocytes (Fig. 9.2), although this has yet to be substantiated.

After absorption across the brush border, zinc is thought to be coupled to either of two intracellular transporters, cysteine-rich intestinal protein (CRIP) and metallothionein. CRIP is a 77-amino-acid protein in mucosal cytosol. It contains two cysteine- and/or histidine-rich zinc-finger motifs, which bind zinc and which may participate in protein–protein interactions (Fernandes *et al.*, 1997; Khoo *et al.*, 1997). It is thought that CRIP may serve as a shuttle for zinc transport from apical to basolateral surfaces, analogous to mobilferrin for iron. In rats fed a moderate amount of zinc, CRIP was reported to bind a large proportion of the zinc entering the intestinal cells, whereas when zinc intake was excessive, the bulk of intestinal zinc was associated with another cysteine-rich protein, metallothionein. Metallothionein retains zinc in the enterocyte either for local use or to prevent zinc overload during periods of high zinc intake (Davis *et al.*, 1998). Zinc can have a number of functions in the intestine including enzymatic regulation (e.g. brush-border zinc-dependent ATPase) and gene regulation (e.g. up-regulation of the uroguanylin precursor) (Blanchard and Cousins, 1997). An abundant pool of intestinal zinc also resides in the granules of the Paneth cells, pyramidal cells of unknown function at the bases of small intestinal crypts (Sawada *et al.*, 1993). How zinc gets to these cells and for what purpose is not known.

At the basolateral surface, export of zinc is likely to be mediated by the zinc efflux protein ZnT-1 (Fig. 9.2c), analogous to the role of Cu-ATPase in the export of copper, although quite different in structure. These transporters have been likened to sensors that control the intracellular levels of copper and zinc and prevent them from reaching toxic levels. ZnT-1 was the first Zn-specific transporter cloned and is associated with zinc efflux out of cells rather than zinc influx (McMahon and Cousins, 1998a). It is a member of a larger family of Zn transporters, all of which encode proteins with predicted multiple membrane-spanning regions, and most have a histidine-rich intracellular loop, which may be the site of binding of zinc (Fig. 9.3c). Consistent with a role in serosal zinc efflux, ZnT-1 is localized to the basolateral membrane of villous enterocytes lining the duodenum and jejunum, although it is absent from the ileum. Curiously, intestinal ZnT-1 mRNA (but not ZnT-1 protein) was found to be up-regulated by dietary zinc intake (McMahon and Cousins, 1998b). The significance of this finding is unclear.

The remaining absorbed zinc continues its passage through the enterocytes into the blood by an active transport process and is carried by proteins, especially albumin, to the liver and other tissues. The rapid uptake of ^{65}Zn into the nuclei of liver, kidney and spleen cells, shortly after ingestion, argues for a direct pathway of exchangeable zinc from dietary to intracellular labile pools (Cousins and Lee-Ambrose, 1992). A substantial proportion (70–80 per cent) of the ingested zinc is excreted in faeces, while only a small amount of zinc is normally lost in the urine, except in diseases such as diabetes mellitus (Vallee and Falchuk, 1993). Excreted zinc originates from either unabsorbed zinc, or the absorbed zinc which is largely returned via the pancreatic and biliary secretions, as well as sloughing of mucosal cells. That the loss of zinc by these processes may be important in homeostatic regulation of body zinc status is suggested by the finding that the amounts of zinc excreted increase with zinc intake (Krebs *et al.*, 1998).

CALCIUM

Two major functions of calcium in the body are in bone and tooth formation and as an intracellular second messenger in many cellular processes (e.g. protein phosphorylation, cell division, fertilization and even cell death). Other functions include blood clotting and muscle, nerve and cardiac function. More than 99 per cent of the 1 kg of calcium in humans is within the skeleton. Bone calcium not only has structural function but can serve as a reservoir to maintain plasma calcium concentrations in the 2–3 mM range, since resorption of bone is triggered in response to low plasma calcium, a process that is mediated by release of parathyroid hormone. Understanding the mechanism of calcium absorption and utilization has important implications for prevention and treatment of osteoporosis, a disabling condition with increasing public health ramifications in modern society.

Dietary sources

The recommended daily allowances (USA) for calcium are 400–600 mg/day for infants, 800 mg/day for children, 1200 mg/day for teenagers and 800 mg/day for adults (Table 9.8). A higher intake of 1200 mg/day is recommended for pregnant and lactating women, as well as to help prevent osteoporosis in postmenopausal women. The tolerable upper limit for calcium has been put at 2500 mg/day. Like most other minerals, calcium is absorbed from the diet and excreted in the faeces. The major food sources of calcium are dairy products, leafy green vegetables, dried legumes, nuts and grains.

Intestinal absorption

About 20–30 per cent of dietary calcium is absorbed by the intestine, and this may increase during growth, lactation and pregnancy. Most of the calcium is absorbed in the ileum (Marcus and Lengemann, 1962), but absorption can take place in the jejunum, duodenum and, to a limited extent, in the caecum and the ascending colon (Petith and Schedl, 1976). The latter is particularly important in calcium absorption after small bowel resection, but may also account for about 10 per cent of calcium absorbed by the healthy individual, at least in rodents (Bronner and Pansu, 1999). Amongst the factors that hinder calcium absorption is insolubility due to the alkalinity of the small bowel (Duflos *et al.*, 1995). In order to be absorbed by the small intestine, calcium should exist in the ionized form (Ca^{2+}), and this is promoted by an acidic environment. Other factors include chelation by dietary ligands (e.g. fibre) and formation of soaps with excess saturated fats. Although vegetables are rich in calcium, the metal is bound to a variety of organic ions, which reduces bioavailability, and extensive digestion is required before this calcium can be absorbed. Some substances (e.g. casein phosphopeptides and lactose in milk) promote calcium absorption (Bronner and Pansu, 1999).

Differences in mechanisms of calcium uptake occur in different regions of the intestine. An energy-requiring transcellular transport is localized to the upper duodenum and is totally dependent on vitamin D (Pansu *et al.*, 1983), while a passive paracellular absorption, mediated by diffusion from intestinal lumen to lymph and blood down an electrochemical gradient, occurs in the jejunum and ileum. Both processes are found in the colon. Passive uptake predominates in the intestine when calcium intake is high because active transport is inhibited (Buckley and Bronner, 1980). When calcium uptake is low, active transport in the duodenum is up-regulated and may account for up to 50 per cent of the total absorbed (Bronner *et al.*, 1986).

Paracellular absorption is intercellular via tight junctions between neighbouring enterocytes. Transcellular absorption, on the other hand, is intracellular and involves uptake via calcium channels and shuttling across the cell to the basolateral pole (Bronner, 1997). This process occurs down a favourable electrochemical gradient and therefore does not require energy. A series of papers by Kowarski and colleagues described a calcium binding protein IMCAL, which may serve as a calcium carrier at the brush border (Schachter and Kowarski, 1982), but there has been little new information on this protein in the last decade, and its role in calcium absorption still remains unclear. Shuttling of calcium through the enterocyte cytosol requires a cytosolic protein calbindin D. The levels of calbindin D are directly regulated by vitamin D metabolites and therefore calcium absorption is linked to vitamin D levels (Stein, 1992; Wasserman and Fullmer, 1995). In this process, vitamin D_3 (cholecalciferol) is first hydroxylated to 25-hydroxycholecalciferol in the liver, and then metabolized in the kidney to 1,25-dihydroxycholecalciferol, which is the active form. This metabolite then enters the nucleus and stimulates the transcription of calbindin D. Decreased synthesis of the vitamin D metabolites causes impaired calcium absorption. In addition to transporting calcium ions across the intestinal cell, calbindin ensures that the free cytosolic calcium ion concentration remains tightly controlled.

From the enterocyte, calcium is extruded in a process mediated by membrane Ca/Mg-ATPase (Carafoli, 1994). Calcium is transferred from calbindin D to the cytoplasmic end of this enzyme, which then undergoes a phosphorylation-induced conformational change leading to the opening of a calcium channel. Calcium is extruded against an electrochemical gradient, thus making transcellular calcium uptake energy-requiring. The released calbindin D relocates to the brush-border region where it picks up another calcium ion.

In addition to this process, evidence has also been presented for a more rapid calcium absorption involving cytosolic vesicles, which bud off from the brush-border membrane, picking up calcium ions in the process. These then pass through the cell and fuse with the basolateral membrane, resulting in release of calcium ions and thereby net transport through the intestine (Nemere and Norman, 1990). This rapid calcium absorption, occurring within minutes, has been named transcaltachia.

Disorders of absorption

Factors that decrease calcium absorption include: vitamin D deficiency; chronic renal failure; hypochlorhydria or achlorhydria, which are common in the elderly; increased small intestinal motility and other abnormalities; and certain medications and drugs (e.g. anticonvulsants: phenobarbitone and phenytoin, glucocorticoids and ethanol (Krawitt *et al.*, 1975; Recker, 1985; Bronner, 1997).

MAGNESIUM

About half of the total magnesium in the body is present in bone, where it is important for bone and tooth formation. The remaining magnesium is largely within soft tissues and is critical for heart, nervous tissue and muscle function. Less than 1 per cent of body magnesium is present in plasma. Magnesium is a component of more than 300 enzymes, many involving ATP, and is essential for protein synthesis and anaerobic phosphorylation. As for calcium, maintaining body supplies of magnesium is especially important in prevention of osteoporosis, but it may also be beneficial in a number of other common disorders including chronic fatigue syndrome and attention deficit hyperactivity disorder. In a recent study in Belgium, 45 per cent of patients suffering from chronic fatigue had low magnesium status (Moorkens *et al.*, 1997). Low levels of magnesium may also result in hardening of the arteries. Symptoms of magnesium deficiency are growth retardation, muscle weakness and cramps, heart failure and hypertension. Amongst the causes of magnesium deficiency are ageing, diabetes, chronic laxative abuse, excess purified fibre intake and poor absorption. Diuretics can also lower body magnesium levels. Hypomagnesemia is frequently encountered in patients admitted to intensive care units.

Dietary sources

The recommended daily allowances (USA) for magnesium are 40–60 mg/day for infants, 80–170 mg/day for children, 270–400 mg/day for teenagers, 350 mg/day for adults, and 320–355 mg/day for pregnant and lactating women (Table 9.8). In a national random survey of Australian adults in 1991, the diets of 50 per cent of men and 39 per cent of women were below these levels (Baghurst *et al.*, 1991). In this study, the major individual food sources of magnesium for men were bread (14 per cent), milk (10 per cent), breakfast cereals (5 per cent), beer (5 per cent) and bananas (5 per cent). Green vegetables are also rich in magnesium, since it is a component of chlorophyll. Magnesium absorption is facilitated by dietary protein and fructose in humans, and decreased by dietary cellulose and phytate. However, as pointed out by Brink and Beynen (1992), the fall in apparent magnesium absorption caused by phytate and cellulose is, to some extent, compensated by the generally higher contents of magnesium that is present in foods rich in these chelators. An additional complexing factor is that, as part of homeostatic mechanisms, changes in magnesium absorption are accompanied by opposite changes in urinary excretion of this metal.

Intestinal absorption

The predominant site of magnesium absorption is the ileum, but it can also occur in the colon (Hardwick *et al.*, 1991; Kayne and Lee, 1993). In humans, peak levels of magnesium in the blood occur 4–7 hours after ingestion. As for calcium, both transcellular and paracellular absorption routes of absorption exist. The mechanisms involved are less certain than for the other metals, although evidence for specific magnesium transporters has been inferred (Bijvelds *et al.*, 1998). These may be especially important for absorption at low dietary magnesium intakes. The most important factor in absorption of magnesium is its luminal concentration. Although high doses of vitamin D increase magnesium absorption in both vitamin D-deficient and vitamin D-replete animals, generally magnesium absorption is independent of vitamin D; the latter, in fact, may reduce net intake of magnesium by increasing urinary magnesium excretion (Hardwick *et al.*, 1991).

Interactions between magnesium and either calcium or phosphate have been demonstrated. Increasing dietary calcium decreases magnesium absorption in humans and animals. This may be due to competition for transporter sites or interactions at other sites on these molecules, with resultant effects on conformation and/or function. To what extent interactions may also occur at the level of dietary chelators and enhancing factors is not known. Increasing dietary phosphate also depresses magnesium absorption, attributed to the formation of an insoluble complex between the two ions (Hardwick *et al.*, 1991). Poor magnesium absorption may arise from protein-calorie malnutrition, chronic watery diarrhoea and steatorrhoea, short bowel syndrome, bowel fistula and, rarely, primary familial magnesium malabsorption (al-Ghamdi *et al.*, 1994). Failure of magnesium absorption occurs in children with a rare inborn error of magnesium transport, primary hypomagnesemia.

ABSORPTION OF OTHER METALS: SELENIUM, IODINE, MANGANESE, COBALT AND CHROMIUM

Much less is known about the absorption of other metals. Selenium is an antioxidant, deficiency of which can lead to anaemia, enlargement of cardiac muscle and arrythmias (Thomson, 1998). The recommended daily allowances (USA) for selenium are 10–15 μg/day for infants, 20–30 μg/day for children, 40–50 μg/day for teenagers, 70 μg/day for adults, 75 μg/day for lactating women and 65 μg/day for pregnant women (Table 9.8). Absorption of selenium is relatively efficient, 60 per cent of dietary selenium being absorbed across the intestine. Selenium is rapidly absorbed as a complex with amino acids (e.g. selenomethionine). It has been suggested that absorption of selenium is primarily by active transport via specific amino-acid carriers (Reasbeck *et al.*, 1985). Coffee and excess Zn or Cu decrease selenium absorption. Whether this implies that the Zn/Cu transporters also participate in selenium transport is unclear. Selenium deficiency is common in patients with severe gastrointestinal disorders (Rannem *et al.*, 1998).

Iodine is absorbed as inorganic iodide and concentrated in the thyroid, where it is incorporated into thyroid hormones, tri-iodothyronine (T_3) and throxine (T_4) (Passmore and Eastwood, 1986; Saller *et al.*, 1998). It is therefore an essential element and iodine deficiency leads to thyroid gland enlargement (goitre). The recommended daily allowances (USA) for iodine are 40–50 μg/day for infants, 70–120 μg/day for children, 150 μg/day for teenagers and adults, 175 μg/day for pregnant women and 200 μg/day for lactating women (Table 9.8). The major food source of iodine is seafood, although small amounts are also found in fruits, vegetables, cereals and meat (Passmore and Eastwood, 1986).

Other essential metals include manganese, cobalt and chromium. Manganese is essential for bone formation and as a cofactor in many enzymes, especially phosphohydrolases and phosphotransferases. Typical diets provide about 1–8 mg/day. Deficiencies in manganese can cause deformities of bone, growth retardation, hypertension, joint problems and heart conditions. Cobalt is a cofactor for vitamin B_{12} and this vitamin is the only food source of cobalt for man, although bacteria in the stomachs of ruminants are able to incorporate cobalt into vitamin B_{12}. Chromium, which exists in a trivalent state (Cr^{3+}), is present in humans at about 5–10 mg. Its functions and mechanisms of absorption are poorly understood. Dietary chromium is found both in the inorganic form and as organic complexes. Chromium is only poorly absorbed (0.5–2 per cent of dietary intake). Absorbed chromium is transported bound to transferrin or other plasma proteins, or as a complex with glucose tolerance factor (Ducros, 1992). While little is known about uptake of these metals by the intestine, the recently cloned mammalian metal ion transporter DCT-1 not only has specificity for Fe, Cu and Zn, but also binds Co and Mn (Gunshin *et al.*, 1997). Further characterization of DCT-1 and related transporters may open up new lines of investigation into absorption of some of the trace metals.

FUTURE PRIORITIES

In the last three decades since the recognition that deficiencies in the transition, alkaline earth and ultratrace metals can occur in man, a wealth of literature has been acquired on the roles of these metals in normal physiology. However, we are still far from answering one of the fundamental questions of metal biochemistry: how are metals absorbed across the intestine and across cell membranes? Recent advances in the identification and cloning of the first groups of mammalian metal ion transporters should open up new avenues of research and begin to address the following questions. What are the metal ion specificities of these transporters? What mechanisms up-regulate and down-regulate their expression on enterocytes and other types of cell? What abnormalities occur in their expression in disease? What is the molecular lesion in acrodermatitis enteropathica and why is there a specific deficiency of zinc but not copper or iron? Is there is a defect, in this disease, in a specific zinc transporter regulating the import of zinc from the lumen or is the defect in export from the intestinal epithelium? Evidence that integrins, major cell adhesion molecules of cells, influence iron absorption prompts the question of whether metal transport across membranes involves cooperation between the transporters and other membrane molecules.

One of the evolutionary pressures for ancestral life was the utilization of readily available, but potentially toxic, metals in their environment for the catalysis of a wide range of biochemical processes. Learning how the mechanisms evolved for absorbing these metals presents an exciting challenge for future research.

REFERENCES

Alcock, E. 1961: Absorption of vitamin B_{12} in man following extensive resection of the jejunum, ileum and colon. *Gastroenterology* 40, 81–4.

al-Ghamdi, S.M., Cameron, E.C., Sutton, R.A. 1994: Magnesium deficiency: pathophysiologic and clinical overview. *American Journal of Kidney Disease* 24, 737–52.

Allen, R.H., Seetharam, B., Allen, N.C., Podell, E.R., Alpers, D.H. 1978a: Correlation of cobalamin malabsorption in pancreatic insufficiency with a cobalamin analogue that binds with high affinity to R protein but not to intrinsic factor. In vivo evidence that a failure to partially degrade R protein is responsible for cobalamin malabsorption in pancreatic insufficiency. *Journal of Clinical Investigation* 61, 1628–34.

Allen, R.H., Seetharam, B., Podell, E.R., Alpers, D.H. 1978b: Effect of proteolytic enzymes on the binding of cobalamin to R protein and intrinsic factor. In vitro evidence that a failure to partially degrade R protein is responsible for cobalamin malabsorption in pancreatic deficiency. *Journal of Clinical Investigation* 61, 47–54.

Anonymous 1986: Vitamin E deficiency (editorial). *Lancet* 1, 423–4.

Antony, A.C. 1991: Megaloblastic anaemias. In Hoffman, R., Benz, E.J., Jr, Shattil, S.J., Furie, B., Cohen, H.J. (eds), *Haematology basic principles and practice*. New York: Churchill Livingstone, 392–422.

Baghurst, K.I., Dreosti, I.E., Syrette, J.A., Record, S.J., Baghurst, P.A., Buckley, R.A., Chem, H.C. 1991: Zinc and magnesium status of Australian adults. *Nutrition Research* 11, 23–32.

Bailey, A.L., Maisey, S., Southon, S., Wright, A.J., Finglas, P.M., Fulcher, R.A. 1997: Relationships between micronutrient intake and biochemical indicators of nutrient adequacy in a 'free-living' elderly UK population. *British Journal of Nutrition* 77, 225–42.

Baker, S.J. 1972: Vitamin B_{12} and tropical sprue. *British Journal of Haematology* 23(Suppl), 135–46.

Barak, Y., Arnon, S., Wolach, B., Raz, Y., Ashkenasi, A., Glick, B., Shapira, Y. 1995: MELAS syndrome: peripheral neuropathy and cytochrome C-oxidase deficiency: a case report and review of the literature. *Israel Journal of Medical Sciences* 31, 224–9.

Bates, C.J. 1995: Vitamin A. *Lancet* 345, 31–5.

Bellou, A., Aimone-Gastin, I., De Korwin, J.D. *et al.* 1966: Cobalamin deficiency with megaloblastic anaemia in one patient under long-term omeprazole therapy. *Journal of Internal Medicine* 240, 161–4.

Beshgetoor, D., Hambridge, M. 1998: Clinical conditions altering copper metabolism in humans. *American Journal of Clinical Nutrition* 67(Suppl), 1017–21S.

Bijvelds, M.J., Flik, G., Kolar, Z.I. 1998: Cellular magnesium transport in the vertebrate intestine. *Magnesium Research* 11, 315–22.

Blanchard, R.K., Cousins, R.J. 1997: Upregulation of rat intestinal uroguanylin mRNA by dietary zinc restriction. *American Journal of Physiology* 272, G972–8.

Brandt, L.J., Bernstein, L.H., Wagle, A. 1977: Production of vitamin B_{12} analogues in patients with small bowel overgrowth. *Annals of Internal Medicine* 87, 546–51.

Brink, E.J., Beynen, A.C. 1992: Nutrition and magnesium absorption: a review. *Progress in Food and Nutrition Science* 16, 125–62.

Bronner, F. 1997: Calcium. In O'Dell, B.L., Sunde, R.A. (eds), *Handbook of nutritionally essential mineral elements.* New York: Marcel Dekker, 13–61.

Bronner, F., Pansu, D. 1999: Nutritional aspects of calcium absorption. *Journal of Nutrition* 129, 9–12.

Bronner, F., Pansu, D., Stein, W.D. 1986: An analysis of intestinal calcium transport across the rat intestine. *American Journal of Physiology 250: Gastrointestinal and Liver Physiology* 13, G561–9.

Buckley, M., Bronner, F. 1980: Calcium-binding protein biosynthesis in the rat: regulation by calcium and 1,25-dihydroxyvitamin D_3. *Archives of Biochemistry and Biophysics* 202, 235–41.

Carafoli, E. 1994: Biogenesis: plasma membrane Ca ATPase: 15 years of work on the purified enzyme. *FASEB Journal* 8, 993–1002.

Carmel, R. 1978: Nutritional vitamin B_{12} deficiency: possible contributory role of subtle vitamin B_{12} malabsorption. *Annals of Internal Medicine* 88, 647.

Chanarin, I., Malkowska, V., O'Hea, A.M., Rinsler, M.G., Price, A.B. 1985: Megaloblastic anaemia in the vegetarian Hindu community. *Lancet* 2, 1168–72.

Chandler, C.J., Wang, T.T., Halstead, C.H. 1986: Pteroylpolyglutamate hydrolase from human jejunal brush borders. Purification and characterization. *Journal of Biological Chemistry* 261, 928–33.

Cheek, D.B., Hay, H.J., Lattanzio, L., Ness, D., Ludwigsen, N., Spargo, R. 1984: Zinc content of red and white blood cells in aboriginal children. *Australian and New Zealand Journal of Medicine* 14, 638–42.

Chesney, R.W. 1989: Vitamin D: can an upper limit be defined? *Journal of Nutrition* 119, 1825–8.

Clydesdale, F.M. 1988: Minerals: their chemistry and fate in food. In Smith, K.T. (ed.), *Trace minerals in foods.* New York: Marcel Dekker, 57–94.

Coleman, J.E. 1992: Zinc proteins: enzymes, storage proteins, transcription factors and replication proteins. *Annual Review of Biochemistry* 61, 897–946.

Conrad, M.E., Umbreit, J.N. 1993: A concise review: iron absorption – the mucin-mobilferrin-integrin pathway. A competitive pathway for metal absorption. *American Journal of Hematology* 42, 67–73.

Conrad, M.E., Umbreit, J.N., Moore, E.G., Heiman, D. 1996: Mobilferrin is an intermediate in iron transport between transferrin and hemoglobin in K562 cells. *Journal of Clinical Investigation* 98, 1449–54.

Cooper, B.A., Castle, W.B. 1960: Sequential mechanisms in the enhanced absorption of vitamin B_{12} by intrinsic factor in the rat. *Journal of Clinical Investigation* 39, 199.

Cooper, B.A., Rosenblatt, D.S. 1987: Inherited defects of vitamin B12 metabolism. *Annual Review of Nutrition* 7, 291–320.

Corcino, J.J., Waxman, S., Herbert, V. 1970: Absorption and malabsorption of vitamin B_{12}. *American Journal of Medicine* 48, 562–9.

Cordano, A., Baertl, J.M., Graham, G.G. 1964: Copper deficiency in infancy. *Pediatrics* 34, 324–36.

Cousins, R.J., Lee-Ambrose, L.M. 1992: Nuclear zinc uptake and interactions with metallothionein gene expression are influenced by dietary zinc in rats. *Journal of Nutrition* 122, 56–64.

Couzy, F., Kastenmayer, P., Mansourian, R., Guinchard, S., Munoz-Box, R., Dirren, H. 1993: Zinc absorption in healthy elderly humans and the effect of diet. *American Journal of Clinical Nutrition* 58, 690–4.

Coyle, J.J., Varco, R.L., Buchwald, H. 1977: Vitamin B_{12} absorption following human intestinal bypass surgery. *American Journal of Digestive Diseases* 22, 1069–71.

Dameron, C.T., Harrison, M.D. 1998: Mechanisms for protection against copper toxicity. *American Journal of Clinical Nutrition* 67(Suppl), 1091–7S.

Daruwala, R., Bhattacharyya, D.K., Kwon, O., Meganathan, R. 1997: Menaquinone (vitamin K2) biosynthesis: overexpression, purification, and characterization of a new isochorismate synthase from Escherichia coli. *Journal of Bacteriology* 179, 3133–8.

Davis, S.R., McMahon, R.J., Cousins, R.J. 1998: Metallothionein knockout and transgenic mice exhibit altered intestinal processing of zinc with uniform zinc-dependent zinc transporter-1 expression. *Journal of Nutrition* 128, 825–31.

Donaldson, R.M., Jr, Mackenzie, I.L., Trier, J.S. 1967: Intrinsic factor-mediated attachment of vitamin B_{12} to brush borders and microvillous membranes of hamster intestine. *Journal of Clinical Investigation* 46, 1215–28.

Drake, W.M., Winter, T.A., Price, S.K., O'Keefe, S.J. 1996: Small bowel intussusception and brown bowel syndrome in association with severe malnutrition. *American Journal of Gastroenterology* 91, 1450–2.

Dreosti, I.E. 1993: Recommended dietary intakes of iron, zinc, and other inorganic nutrients and their chemical form and bioavailability. *Nutrition* 9, 542–5.

Ducros, V. 1992: Chromium metabolism. A literature review. *Biological Trace Element Research* 32, 65–77.

Duflos, C., Bellaton, C., Pansu, D., Bronner, F. 1995: Calcium solubility, intestinal sojourn time and paracellular permeability codetermine passive Ca absorption in rats. *Journal of Nutrition* 125, 2348–55.

Feder, J.N., Gnirke, A., Thomas, W. *et al.* 1996: A novel MHC class I-like gene is mutated in patients with hereditary haemochromatosis. *Nature Genetics* 13, 399–408.

Fernandes, P.R., Samuelson, D.A., Clark, W.R., Cousins, R.J. 1997: Immunohistochemical localization of cysteine-rich intestinal protein in rat small intestine. *American Journal of Physiology* 272, G751–9.

Fischer, J.M., Taylor, K.B. 1969: The intracellular localization of Castele's intrinsic factor by an immunofluorescent technique using auto antibodies. *Immunology* 16, 779–84.

Fischer, P.W., Giroux, A., L'Abbe, M.R. 1983: Effects of zinc on mucosal copper binding and on the kinetics of copper absorption. *Journal of Nutrition* 113, 462–9.

Fleming, M.D., Trenor, C.C., Su, M.A., Foernzler, D., Beier, D.R., Dietrich, W.F., Andrews, N.C. 1997: Microcytic anaemia mice have a mutation in Nramp2, a candidate iron transporter gene. *Nature Genetics* 16, 383–6.

Foroozan, P., Trier, J.S. 1967: Mucosa of the small intestine in pernicious anemia. *New England Journal of Medicine* 277, 553–9.

Francis, R.M., Selby, P.L. 1997: Osteomalacia. *Baillieres Clinical Endocrinology and Metabolism* 11, 145–63.

Fraser, D.R. 1995: Vitamin D. *Lancet* 345, 104–7.

Freeland-Graves, J.H., Bodzy, P.W., Eppright, M.A. 1980: Zinc status of vegetarians. *Journal of the American Dietetic Association* 77, 655–61.

Giannella, R.A., Broitman, S.A., Zamcheck, N. 1972: Competition between bacteria and intrinsic factor for vitamin B_{12}: implications for vitamin B_{12} malabsorption in intestinal bacterial overgrowth. *Gastroenterology* 62, 255–60.

Gräsbeck, R., Gordin, R., Kangero, I., Kuhlback, B. 1960: Selective vitamin B_{12} malabsorption and proteinuria in young people: a syndrome. *Acta Medica Scandinavica* 167, 289–96.

Gunshin, H., Mackenzie, B., Berger, U.V. *et al.* 1997: Cloning and characterization of a mammalian proton-coupled metal-ion transporter. *Nature* 388, 482–8.

Halstead, C.H. 1989: The intestinal absorption of dietary folate in health and disease. *Journal of the American College of Nutrition* 8, 650–8.

Hambidge, K.M., Krebs, N.F., Miller, L. 1998: Evaluation of zinc metabolism with use of stable-isotope techniques: implications for the assessment of zinc status. *American Journal of Clinical Nutrition* 68(Suppl), 410–13S.

Hardwick, L.L., Jones, M.R., Brautbar, N., Lee, D.B. 1991: Magnesium absorption: mechanisms and the influence of vitamin D, calcium and phosphate. *Journal of Nutrition* 121, 13–23.

Harris, E.D., Qian, Y., Reddy, M.C. 1998: Genes regulating copper metabolism. *Molecular and Cellular Biochemistry* 188, 57–62.

Haurani, F.I., Hall, C.A., Rubin, R. 1979: Megaloblastic anaemia as a result of an abnormal transcobalamin II (Cardeza). *Journal of Clinical Investigation* 64, 1253–9.

Herbert, V. 1985: Biology of disease. Megaloblastic anaemias. *Laboratory Investigations* 52, 3.

Hirabayashi, M., Matsui, T., Yano, H. 1998: Fermentation of soybean meal with Aspergillus usamii improves zinc availability in rats. *Biological Trace Element Research* 61, 227–34.

Hoffbrand, A.V. 1999: Megaloblastic anaemia. In Hoffbrand, A.V., Lewis, S.M., Tuddenham, E.G.D. (eds), *Postgraduate haematology*, 4th edn. Oxford: Butterworth-Heinemann, 47–67.

Holick, M.F. 1996: Vitamin D and bone health. *Journal of Nutrition* 126, 1159–64S.

Hollander, D. 1981: Intestinal absorption of vitamins A, E, D and K. *Journal of Laboratory and Clinical Medicine* 97, 449–61.

Hollander, D., Muralidhara, K.S. 1978: Vitamin D3 intestinal absorption in vivo: influence of fatty acids, bile salts, and perfusate pH on absorption. *Gut* 19, 267–72.

Hussey, G.D., Klein, M. 1990: A randomised controlled trial of vitamin A in children with severe measles. *New England Journal of Medicine* 323, 160–4.

Immerslund, O. 1960: Idiopathic chronic megaloblastic anemia in children. *Acta Paediatrica* 119, 1–6.

Jacobsen, E.D. 1960: An experimental malabsorption syndrome induced by neomycin. *American Journal of Medicine* 28, 524–6.

Kano, Y., Sakamoto, S., Miura, Y., Takaku, F. 1985: Disorders of cobalamin metabolism. *CRC Critical Reviews in Oncology and Hematology* 3, 1–34.

Kapadia, C.R., Serfilippi, D., Voloshin, D., Donaldson, R.M., Jr. 1983: Intrinsic factor-mediated absorption of cobalamin by guinea pig ileal cells. *Journal of Clinical Investigation* 71, 440–8.

Kayne, L.H., Lee, D.B. 1993: Intestinal magnesium absorption. *Mineral and Electrolyte Metabolism* 19, 210–17.

Khoo, C., Blanchard, R.K., Sullivan, V.K., Cousins, R.J. 1997: Human cysteine-rich intestinal protein: cDNA cloning and expression of recombinant protein and identification in human peripheral blood mononuclear cells. *Protein Expression and Purification* 9, 379–87.

Krawitt, E.L., Sampson, H.W., Katagini, C.A. 1975: Effect of 1,25-dihydroxycholecalciferol on ethanol mediated suppression of calcium absorption. *Calcified Tissue Research* 18, 119–24.

Krebs, N.F., Westcott, J.E., Miller, L.V., Huffer, J.W. 1998: Absorption of exogenous zinc and secretion of endogenous zinc in the human small intestine. *Federation of American Society for Experimental Biology Journal* 12, A345.

Lee, G.R. 1999: Pernicious anaemia and other causes of vitamin B12 (cobalamin) deficiency. In Lee, G.R. *et al.* (eds), *Wintrobe's clinical haematology*, 10th edn. Baltimore: Williams and Wilkins, 941–64.

Levine, J.S., Allen, R.H. 1985: Intrinsic factor within parietal cells of patients with juvenile pernicious anaemia. A retrospective immunohistochemical study. *Gastroenterology* 88, 1132–6.

Lindenbaum, J., Pezzementi, J.F., Shea, N. 1974: Small-intestinal function in vitamin B12 deficiency. *Annals of Internal Medicine* 80, 326–31.

Lombard, M., Chua, E., O'Toole, P. 1997: Regulation of intestinal non-haem iron absorption. *Gut* 40, 435–9.

Lonnerdal, B. 1996: Bioavailability of copper. *American Journal of Clinical Nutrition* 63, 821–9S.

Marcoullis, G., Parmentier, Y., Nicolas, J.P., Jimenez, M., Gerard, P. 1980: Cobalamin malabsorption due to nondegradation of R proteins in the human intestine. *Journal of Clinical Investigation* 66, 430–40.

Marcus, C.S., Lengemann, F.W. 1962: Absorption of Ca^{45} and Sr^{85} from solid and liquid food at various levels of the alimentary tract of the rat. *Journal of Nutrition* 77, 155–60.

Markle, H.V. 1996: Cobalamin. *Critical Reviews in Clinical and Laboratory Science* 33, 247–356.

Mathan, V.I., Babior, B.M., Donaldson, R.M. 1974: Kinetics of the attachment of intrinsic factor-bound cobamides to ileal receptors. *Journal of Clinical Investigation* 54, 598–608.

May, A., Fitzsimmons, R. 1994: Sideroblastic anaemia. *Baillieres Clinical Haematology* 7, 851–79.

McMahon, R.J., Cousins, R.J. 1998a: Mammalian zinc transporters. *Journal of Nutrition* 128, 667–70.

McMahon, R.J., Cousins, R.J. 1998b: Regulation of the zinc transporter zincT-1 by dietary zinc. *Proceedings of the National Academy of Sciences USA* 95, 4841–6.

Mercer, J.F. 1998: Menkes syndrome and animal models. *American Journal of Clinical Nutrition* 67(Suppl), 1022–8S.

Meydani, M. 1995: Vitamin E. *Lancet* 345, 170–5.

Milne, D.B., Omaye, S.T., Amos, W.H., Jr. 1981: Effect of ascorbic acid on copper and cholesterol in adult cynomolgus monkeys fed a diet marginal in copper. *American Journal of Clinical Nutrition* 34, 2389–93.

Moorkens, G., Manuel, Y., Keenoy, B., Vertommen, J., Meludu, S., Noe, M., De Leeuw, I. 1997: Magnesium deficit in a sample of the Belgian population presenting with chronic fatigue. *Magnesium Research* 10, 329–37.

Muller, D.P. 1986: Vitamin-E: its role in neurological function. *Postgraduate Medical Journal* 62, 107–12.

Nemere, I., Norman, A.W. 1990: Transcaltachia, vesicular calcium transport and microtubule-associated calbindin-D28K: emerging views of 1,25-dihydroxyvitamin D3-mediated intestinal calcium absorption. *Mineral and Electrolyte Metabolism* 16, 109–14.

Palva, I.P., Heinivaara, O., Mattila, M. 1966: Drug-induced malabsorption of vitamin B-12. 3. Interference of PAS and folic acid in the absorption of vitamin B-12. *Scandinavian Journal of Haematology* 3, 149–53.

Palva, I.P., Salokannel, S.J., Timonen, T., Palva, H.L. 1972: Drug-induced malabsorption of vitamin B_{12}. Malabsorption and deficiency of B_{12} during treatment with slow-release potassium chloride. *Acta Medica Scandinavica* 191, 335–7.

Pansu, D., Bellaton, C., Roche, C., Bronner, F. 1983: Duodenal and ileal calcium absorption in the rat and effects of vitamin D. *American Journal of Physiology 244: Gastrointestinal and Liver Physiology* 7, G695–700.

Passmore, R., Eastwood, M.A. 1986: Iron, zinc and other trace minerals. In Davidson, S., Passmore, R. (eds), *Human nutrition and dietetics.* Edinburgh: Churchill Livingstone, 115–20.

Petith, M.M., Schedl, H.P. 1976: Intestinal adaptation to dietary calcium restriction: in vivo cecal and colonic calcium transport in the rat. *Gastroenterology* 71, 1039–42.

Raja, K.B., Simpson, R.J., Peters, T.J. 1992: Investigation of a role for reduction in ferric iron uptake by mouse duodenum. *Biochimica et Biophysica Acta* 1135, 141–6.

Rannem, T., Ladefoged, K., Hylander, E., Hegnhoj, J., Staun, M. 1998: Selenium depletion in patients with gastrointestinal diseases: are there any predictive factors? *Scandinavian Journal of Gastroenterology* 33, 1057–61.

Reasbeck, P.G., Barbezat, G.O., Weber, F.L., Robinson, M.F., Thomson, C.D. 1985: Selenium absorption by canine jejunum. *Digestive Diseases and Sciences* 30, 489–94.

Recker, R.R. 1985: Calcium absorption and achlorhydria. *New England Journal of Medicine* 313, 70–3.

Rose, R.C. 1996: Intestinal absorption of water-soluble vitamins. *Proceedings of the Society for Experimental Biology and Medicine* 212, 191–8.

Rosenberg, I.H., Godwin, H.A. 1971: The digestion and absorption of dietary folate. *Gastroenterology* 60, 445–63.

Rush, J.H. 1977: Osteomalacia in the elderly. *Australian and New Zealand Journal of Surgery* 47, 186–8.

Russell, R.M. 1997: New views on the RDAs for older adults. *Journal of the American Dietetic Association* 97, 515–18.

Said, H.M., Redha, R. 1988: Biotin transport in rat intestinal brush border membranes vesicles. *Biochimica et Biophysica Acta* 945, 195–201.

Said, H.M., Redha, R., Nylander, W. 1988: Biotin transport in the human intestine: site of maximal transport and effect of pH. *Gastroenterology* 95, 1312–17.

Saller, B., Fink, H., Mann, K. 1998: Kinetics of acute and chronic iodine excess. *Experimental and Clinical Endocrinology and Diabetes* 106(Suppl 3), S34–8.

Sandstead, H.H. 1991: Zinc deficiency. A public health problem. *American Journal of the Diseases of Children* 145, 853–9.

Sawada, M., Nishikawa, M., Adachi, T., Midorikawa, O., Hiai, H. 1993: A Paneth cell specific zinc-binding protein in the rat. Purification and immunohistochemical localization. *European Journal of Biochemistry* 211, 377–80.

Schachter, D., Kowarski, S. 1982: Isolation of the protein IMCal, a vitamin D-dependent membrane component of the intestinal transport mechanism for calcium. *Federation Proceedings* 41, 84–7.

Seetharam, B., Alpers, D.H., Allen, R.H. 1981: Isolation and characterization of the ileal receptor for intrinsic factor. *Journal of Biological Chemistry* 256, 3785–90.

Seligman, P.A., Steiner, L.L., Allens, R.H. 1980: Studies of a patient with megaloblastic anaemia and an abnormal transcobalamin II. *New England Journal of Medicine* 303, 1209–12.

Shearer, M.J. 1992: Vitamin K metabolism and nutrition. *Blood Reviews* 6, 92–104.

Shearer, M.J. 1995: Vitamin K. *Lancet* 345, 229–34.

Shearer, M.J., Bach, A., Kohlmeier, M. 1996: Chemistry, nutritional sources, tissue distribution and metabolism of vitamin K with special reference to bone health. *Journal of Nutrition* 126, 1181–6S.

Solomons, N.W. 1988: Zinc and copper. In Shils, M.E., Young, V.R. (eds), *Modern nutrition in health and disease*, 7th edn. Philadelphia: Lea and Febiger, 238–62.

Sorensen, J.A., Andersen, O., Nielsen, J.B. 1998: An in vivo study of the gastrointestinal absorption site for zinc chloride in mice. *Journal of Trace Elements in Medicine and Biology* 12, 16–22.

Spencer, G.A., Wirebaugh, S., Whitney, E.J. 1996: Effect of a combination of genfibrozil and niacin on lipid levels. *Journal of Clinical Pharmacology* 36, 696–700.

Stein, W.D. 1992: Facilitated diffusion of calcium across the intestinal epithelial cell. *Journal of Nutrition* 122(3S), 651–6.

Steinbert, W., King, C.E., Toskes, P.P. 1980: Malabsorption of protein bound cobalamin but not unbound cobalamin during cimetidine administration. *Digestive Diseases and Sciences* 25, 188–91.

Suttie, J.W. 1995: The importance of menaquinones in human nutrition. *Annual Review of Nutrition* 15, 399–417.

Taylor, P.R., Li, B., Dawsey, S.M., Li, J.Y., Yang, C.S., Guo, W., Blot, W.J. 1994: Prevention of esophageal cancer: the nutrition intervention trials in Linxian, China. Linxian Nutrition Intervention Trials Study Group. *Cancer Research* 54(7 Suppl), 2029–31s.

Thomson, C.D. 1998: Selenium speciation in human body fluids. *Analyst* 123, 827–31.

Vallee, B.L., Falchuk, K.H. 1993: The biochemical basis of zinc physiology. *Physiological Reviews* 73, 79–118.

Vulpe, C., Gitschier, J. 1997: Ironing out anaemia. *Nature Genetics* 16, 319–20.

Wapnir, R.A. 1998: Copper absorption and bioavailability. *American Journal of Clinical Nutrition* 67(Suppl), 1054–60S.

Wasserman, R.H., Fullmer, C.S. 1995: Vitamin D and intestinal calcium transport: facts, speculations and hypotheses. *Journal of Nutrition* 125, 1971–9S.

Webb, D.I., Chodos, R.B., Mahar, C.Q., Faloon, W.W. 1968: Mechanism of vitamin B12 malabsorption in patients receiving colchicine. *New England Journal of Medicine* 279, 845–50.

Welkos, S.L., Toskes, P.P., Baer, H. 1981: Importance of anaerobic bacteria in the cobalamin malabsorption of the experimental rat blind loop syndrome. *Gastroenterology* 70, 249–58.

Zalewski, P.D., Forbes, I.J., Betts, W.H. 1993: Correlation of apoptosis with change in intracellular labile Zn, using Zinquin, a new specific fluorescent probe for zinc. *Biochemical Journal* 296, 403–8.

Zhou, B., Gitschier, J. 1997: hCRT1: a human gene for copper uptake identified by complementation in yeast. *Proceedings of the National Academy of Sciences USA* 94, 7481–6.

10

Digestion and absorption of carbohydrates, fat and proteins

EMILE LEVY

INTRODUCTION

Normal digestion and absorption of macronutrients in the gastrointestinal tract are essential for adequate growth and development in the newborn as well as good health throughout life. Most ingested carbohydrates, lipids and proteins are efficiently assimilated via the intestine with less than 5 per cent being excreted in the stool. Malabsorption of these major nutrients may lead to steatorrhoea and various other disorders, including malnutrition. Overall health may even be threatened. This chapter provides an overview of the complex interactions involved in digestive and absorptive mechanisms, while emphasizing their relevance to conditions commonly encountered in clinical practice. An increased understanding of how dietary components are optimally handled by the gastrointestinal tract will help towards evaluating patients, establishing correct diagnoses and recommending appropriate treatment.

DIGESTION AND ABSORPTION OF CARBOHYDRATES

DIETARY CARBOHYDRATES

In the West, carbohydrates provide 45–60 per cent of total daily energy requirements. Sixty per cent of this dietary source comes from plant starch (potatoes, rice, wheat, legumes, tubers, some vegetables and fruit). Carbohydrates consist of amylose, a very large and straight glucose polymer linked by $\alpha(1\text{–}4)$ bonds, and amylopectin, containing $\alpha(1\text{–}6)$ glucosidic bonds

Table 10.1 *Carbohydrates and their corresponding digestive enzymes*

Carbohydrate	Substrate properties	Enzyme	Source	Products
Amylose	Linear polymer of glucose (α-1,4), MW 10^5–10^6	α-Amylase	Mouth Pancreas	Maltose Maltotriose
		Sucrase-isomaltase Maltase-glucoamylase	Small intestine	Glucose
Amylipectin (starch)	Branched polymer of glucose (α-14, α-1,6) MW 10^7–10^8	α-Amylase	Mouth Pancreas	α-Limit dextrins Maltotriose Maltose
		Sucrase-isomaltase Maltase-glucoamylase	Small intestine	Glucose
Sucrose	Disaccharide (α-1,4-linked glu-fru) MW 360	Sucrase-isomaltase	Small intestine	Glucose, fructose
Lactose	Disaccharide (β-1,4-linked gal-glu) MW 360	Lactase	Small intestine	Glucose, galactose
Maltose	Disaccharide (α-1,4-linked glu-glu) MW 360	Maltase-glucoamylase Sucrase-isomaltase	Small intestine	Glucose
Trehalose	Disaccharide (glucosyl-α, α-glucose)	Trehalase	Small intestine	Glucose

MW, molecular weight.

branching off from the main chain of α(1–4)-linked glucose residues. Limited amounts of polysaccharides are present in animal foods, such as meat, fish and poultry, except for small amounts of glycogen with a branched structure similar to that of amylopectin. Carbohydrates ingested during the neonatal period are usually in the form of disaccharides, especially lactose, which is found exclusively in mammalian milk. This molecule consists of a galactose and glucose residue, joined by a β(1–4) glycosidic bond. The other disaccharides are: (1) sucrose (fruit and vegetables), composed of a glucose and fructose residue joined by an α(1–4) glucosidic bond; (2) maltose (produced during digestion of starches) composed of two glucose residues α(1–4) linked; and (3) trehalose (mushrooms) consisting of a non-reducing dimer of glucose-bound α(1–4)α′. Three monosaccharides (glucose, galactose and fructose) also occur in the diet. They are principally derived from fruit and to a lesser extent from honey.

ORAL AND INTRALUMINAL DIGESTION

The digestion of polysaccharides, oligosaccharides and disaccharides is crucial for the transport of these products across the plasma membranes of enterocytes (Table 10.1).

Salivary and pancreatic amylase

The hydrolysis of carbohydrates with a high molecular weight is initiated by salivary α-amylase (McMichael, 1976). In view of the fact that only a limited amount of chewing usually takes place and the amylase is inactivated by the acidic pH of the stomach, salivary amylase plays but a minor role in the intraluminal degration of starch (McMichael, 1976). Careful, slow chewing may, however, provide optimal salivary action. Most ingested starch reaches the duodenum and the cleavage continues in the duodenum by means of α-amylase released through the exocrine pancreas (Alpers, 1994). Both amylases or endoglucosidases, with nearly identical structures, act on the internal α(1–4) bonds of amylose and amylopectin, leading to short oligosaccharides (or α-limit dextrins), maltose and maltotriose. Free glucose is minimally released under the action of both salivary and pancreatic α-amylase. The bulk of starch breakdown occurs within the lumen. The branches of α(1–6) glycosidic side chains located in amylopectin are fully resistant to the action of α-amylases and are further hydrolysed by sucrase-isomaltase.

Brush-border hydrolases

The continued breakdown of newly formed glycosyl oligosaccharides occurs by surface enzymes along the enterocytes' brush border of the duodenum and jejunum. At this site, maltase-glucoamylase acts on α(1–4)-linked oligomers containing 5–9 glucose residues, releasing glucose monomers. Hydrolysis of α(1–6) glucosidic bonds also occurs to some extent. It should be noted that human maltase-glucoamylase (335 kDa), isolated from brush-border membrane, exists solely as a single molecular form. It is first synthesized as a 285 kDa, high-mannose *N*-glycan-containing precursor, which is then converted into the 335 kDa, *N*-glycosylated brush-border form. It is fully functional as maltase and glucoamylase without being cleaved proteolytically (Naim *et al.*, 1988a). Similarly, sucrase-isomaltase (sucrase-α-dextrinase) removes glucose molecules from the non-reducing end of α-limit dextrins. Of note is the ability of isomaltase to split the 1–6 glycosidic linkage into α-limit dextrins.

Disaccharides are also too large to cross the brush-border membrane and must, therefore, be hydrolysed before absorption. They are hydrolysed by disaccharidases, physically close to the monosaccharide co-transporter systems in the membrane, thus maintaining efficient absorption.

SUCRASE-ISOMALTASE

The digestion of sucrose and maltose is assigned to this enzymatic complex, which represents 10 per cent of total brush-border membrane proteins. Sucrase-isomaltase is a dimeric enzyme consisting of two peptide chains, each with an active site. One is specific for sucrose and maltose and the other for isomaltose and maltose (Semenza, 1986). The two polypeptides are almost identical in size and are linked by non-convalent bonds. Exoglucosidase is synthesized in the endoplasmic reticulum as a single polypeptide precursor: pro-sucrase-isomaltase, which displays a high molecular weight (260 kDa). *N*-Glycosylation with mannose allows proper folding and transport of sucrase-isomaltase from the endoplasmic reticulum compartment to the Golgi. There, it acquires additional *N*- and *O*-glycosylation before being inserted into the apical brush-border membrane. The N-terminal end of isomaltase acts as a hydrophobic anchor segment incorporated into the lipid bilayer (Frank *et al.*, 1978; Montgomery *et al.*, 1981), where it is cleft into two subunits by pancreatic proteinases. The subunits remain associated and continue to have independent activities (Dahlqvist *et al.*, 1963), although they are complementary to each other regarding the cleavage of oligosaccharides (Gray, 1981). Naturally occurring mutations in human sucrase-isomaltase often lead to the transport of incompetent enzyme molecules (Naim *et al.*, 1988b). Whereas intact sucrase-isomaltase is efficiently transported to the apical membrane through vectorial transport (polarized migration toward the tip of the villus), defective sucrase-isomaltase is rapidly transcytosed to the apical membrane (LeBivic *et al.*, 1990). Furthermore, the absence of proteinases prohibits conversion to mature sucrase (Fransen *et al.*, 1991; Shapiro *et al.*, 1991).

LACTASE

The enzymatic hydrolysis of lactose into equimolar amounts of glucose and galactose is carried out by means of small intestinal lactase. This purified enzyme also splits phlorizin and other β-glucosides. Classically, this enzyme complex carries a double name, lactase-phlorizin hydrolase. Previously, substrate specificity was studied using a series of chemically defined lactose-like components that are either hydrophilic (lactose and cellulose) or hydrophobic (phlorizin and β-glycosylceramides). The mature enzyme was found to contain only one polypeptide with two active sites for lactose and phlorizin. Available data indicate that apical brush-border lactase is the product of an intracellularly larger glycoprotein (pro-lactase), the precursor form located in the endoplasmic reticulum. Pro-lactase is synthesized, *N*-glycosylated (200–220 kDa), folded in the rough endoplasmic reticulum, and subsequently converted into an *O*-glycosylated form (220–240 kDa) in the Golgi. Intrinsic proteolysis of the lactase precursor occurs during transport to the brush-border membrane and prior to insertion in the lipid bilayer. The large 'pro' portion and a short signal sequence do not appear in the mature membrane-spanning enzyme. The preparation of lactase isolation consists of two components: a minor polypeptide of 200–240 kDa (representing lactase precursor) and a predominant polypeptide of 130–160 kDa (mature lactase). Both are tightly membrane associated.

TREHALASE

This enzyme hydrolyses non-reducing disaccharide trehalose, a storage disaccharide in many fungi, and is not abundant in the small intestinal epithelium (less than 0.1 per cent of total brush-border protein). It is tightly linked to the brush-border membrane by a glycosyl phosphatidylinositol anchor (Ruf *et al.*, 1990), which also serves as a specific targeting signal for apical transport. It contains a cleavable hydrophobic signal sequence for translocation into the rough endoplasmic reticulum (Ruf *et al.*, 1990). In addition, the extreme C-terminus contains a hydrophobic sequence, which could function in membrane-anchoring. This region is most likely transient and is replaced in the rough endoplasmic reticulum by the glycosyl phosphatidylinositol (Ruf *et al.*, 1990). Trehalase contains many *N*-glycosylation sites and there is no evidence of *O*-glycosylation.

ABSORPTION OF CARBOHYDRATES

Glucose (galactose) transport across the mucosa

Monosaccharides (glucose, galactose and fructose) resulting from enzymatic hydrolysis are transported through the brush-border membrane. Their cellular uptake requires specific transport processes, which are rate-limiting steps in carbohydrate absorption. The absorption of D-glucose and D-galactose occurs by means of an energy-dependent process involving the Na^+ extracellular to intracellular chemical gradient. The sodium pump (Na^+, K^+-ATPase), located at the basolateral membrane of the enterocyte, generates a low intra-

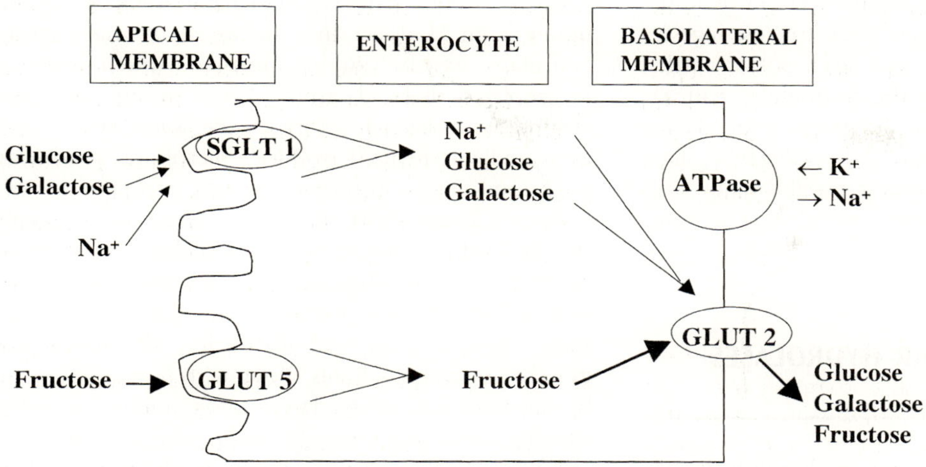

Figure 10.1 *Illustration of intracellular hexose transport. Both SGLT1 and GLUT5 carriers are localized in the apical membrane of the enterocyte, whereas GLUT2 is found in the basolateral membrane allowing the facilitated movement of hexose out of the cell. The Na^+/K^+-ATPase pumps the Na^+ outside.*

cellular Na^+ concentration, allowing the entrance of Na^+ from the apical membrane down its gradient. The consumption of adenosine triphosphate provides energy for the extrusion of Na^+ into the intercellular space. Thus, the uphill transport of glucose (or galactose), coupled with Na^+, is mediated by the Na^+ glucose co-transporter protein (SGLT1) (Fig. 10.1). On the other hand, hexoses exit across the basolateral membrane, down their concentration gradients into the systemic system via a facilitated sugar transporter, GLUT 2 (Thorens, 1993). The transport capacity of the latter has been shown to exceed apical SGLT1 (Kimmich and Carter-Su, 1978). The presence of either luminal D-glucose or D-galactose induces SGLT1 (Dyer *et al.*, 1994), and this regulation seems to be post-transcriptional (Freeman *et al.*, 1993; Lescale-Matys *et al.*, 1993). Similarly, non-metabolizable substrates, such as methyl-α, D-glucopyranoside or 3-0-methyl-α, D-glucopyranoside, increase SGLT1 protein amounts, suggesting there is no prerequisite for the substrate to be metabolized by the enterocytes in SGLT1 induction. Even inappropriate substrates result in the induction of functional SGLT1, indicating the presence of a sugar-sensing system located on the external face of the luminal membrane (Hopfer, 1987; Wright *et al.*, 1994).

The human SGLT1 gene is located on chromosome 22 at q11.2→qter. The SGLT1 clone was isolated and codes for a protein of 664 amino acid residues (Hediger *et al.*, 19891a), which share a high degree of similarity (86 per cent) to rabbit SGLT1 (Hediger *et al.*, 1989b). SGLT1's three-dimensional structure in the membrane remains unknown, but the model secondary structure displays 12 membrane-spanning domains in a helical conformation with the amino- and carboxyl-termini in the cytoplasm (Wright *et al.*, 1991). The molecular weight is about 75 kDa, including 15 kDa glycosylation mass (Shirazi-Beechey *et al.*, 1991; Wright *et al.*, 1991).

It has also been suggested that facilitated and passive diffusion transports hexoses (monosaccharides with six carbons). However, the studies were performed only on rodents and the experimental evidence for such movement is weak. The first process appears to be mediated by both a saturable, electrogenic, phlorizin-sensitive mechanism (Debnam and Levin, 1975) and a non-saturating, phlorizin-insensitive non-electrogenic mechanism. The second process implies that glucose and galactose, present in higher concentrations in the intestinal rather than the intracellular compartment, will be passively transported (Gray, 1981). When this hexose concentration gradient is dissipated, glucose and galactose can then be transported by means of the active transport process.

Fructose absorption

The absorption of fructose is distinct from the glucose-Na^+ co-transporter (Schultz and Strecker, 1970), since its transport takes place (1) even in sufferers from glucose-galactose malabsorption, and (2) despite the presence of phlorizin, which completely inhibits the active movement of glucose. Although a few reports propose a mode of carrier-mediated facilitated diffusion for fructose, other studies suggest an energy- and Na^+-dependent process that follows saturation kinetics (Gracey *et al.*, 1972). Fructose absorption and its facilitated transport may be mediated by another glucose transporter isoform known as GLUT5 (Burant *et al.*, 1992), located in the brush-border membrane (Davidson *et al.*, 1992). The latter is abundant in the jejunum and does not display any homology with SGLT1. Fructose utilizes the glucose transporter GLUT2, located on the enterocyte basolateral membrane, to exit the absorptive epithelial cells (Thorens, 1992; Cheeseman, 1993). Fructose absorption from sucrose or in the presence of glucose appears to be more efficient than the uptake of dietary fructose alone (Riby and Fujisawa, 1993). In order to explain the enhancement of fructose absorption by the presence of glucose, some investigators propose rapid glucose-dependent and slow glucose-independent systems. When glucose and fructose are ingested together, they can use the efficient disaccharidase-related transport system, whereas fructose ingested alone cannot follow this route. Another hypothesis is that fructose is absorbed through the paracellular pathway when tight junctions open in the presence of glucose (Madara *et al.*, 1992). Recently, Shi *et al.* (1997) have shown that fructose is transported transcellularly by facilitated diffusion and paracellularly via glucose-activated solution drag.

DEVELOPMENT OF SUGAR HYDROLASES AND TRANSPORTERS

α-Amylase in human infants is not developed during the first 6 months of life (Auricchio *et al.*, 1968; Danielsen *et al.*, 1981). On the other hand, disaccharidases are first detectable during week 10 of gestation (Dahlqvist and Lindberg, 1965). In human infants, sucrase activity is high by week 20 of gestation, being nearly 50–75 per cent full-term infant and adult levels. Its activity reaches adult human intestine levels for the rest of foetal life, with a marked increase noted at term (Antonowicz *et al.*, 1974; Antonowicz and Lebenthal, 1977). Similarly, glucoamylase activity develops early in gestation and contributes to the digestion of starch after birth (Auricchio *et al.*, 1968). In human neonates, it represents 50–100 per cent that of adults (Lebenthal and Lee, 1980). In contrast, lactase activity is low before the 24th week of gestation (Antonowicz *et al.*, 1974; Antonowicz and Lebenthal, 1977). At this stage, it begins to increase, especially in the third trimester, and peaks in full-term neonates, finally decreasing 3–4 times in infants 2–11 months of age (Antonowicz *et al.*, 1974; Antonowicz and Lebenthal, 1977).

Early studies have demonstrated that active intestinal uptake is detectable in 11-week-old foetuses, increasing fourfold by 19 weeks of gestation, steadily rising during the first months of life to reach maturational glucose transport (Koldovsky *et al.*, 1965; Younoszai, 1974). The basolateral Na^+, K^+-ATPase is present early in gestation in all polar epithelial cells. In view of the sequential development of intraluminal hydrolases, premature infants born between 26 and 30 weeks of gestation, in particular, can experience abnormal digestion and absorption of lactose. Mucosal monosaccharide transporters follow a similar development. By week 11 of gestation, the small intestine expresses specific mRNA of SGLT1, GLUT5 and GLUT2 (Davidson *et al.*, 1992).

CARBOHYDRATE MALABSORPTION

Under healthy conditions, the major digestive processes occur within the duodenum, whereas the absorption of ingested carbohydrates is completed in the jejunum and upper ileum. However, in some disorders, brush-border hydrolase activity can be impaired, which leads to incompletely digested carbohydrates. In this case, non-absorbable carbohydrates reach the colon, where they are rapidly fermented by local microflora, producing gases and acids, primarily acetate, propionate and butyrate. These short-chain fatty acids are normally metabolized by colonocytes. Nevertheless, the overproduction of carbon dioxide, hydrogen and methane, as well as short-chain fatty acids, causes abdominal distension, cramps, pain and flatulence. Moreover, the presence of carbohydrates, along with lactate generated by fermentation in the large bowel lumen, provokes osmotic pressure, thereby increasing the flow of water, and leading to diarrhoea. Obviously, the fermentation of monosaccharides and disaccharides is faster than the handling of polysaccharides, owing to their rapid transit and their suitable form for microflora. Different defects in carbohydrate digestion lead to malabsorption.

Congenital sucrase-isomaltase deficiency

The hydrolysis of sucrose can be defective, as was first reported by Weijers *et al.* in 1960. The inability to digest sucrose is detectable mainly in infants and children, although it can also be present at different ages.

Primary sucrase-isomaltase deficiency follows an autosomal recessive trait of inheritance, with heterozygotes having intermediate enzymatic activity (Kerry and Townley, 1965; Gray, 1981). The frequency of congenital sucrase-isomaltase deficiency in North Americans is about 0.2–0.8 per cent (Kerry and Townley, 1965; Welsh *et al.*, 1978) and in Danes less than 0.1 per cent (Gudmand-Høyer *et al.*, 1987), whereas the incidence appears to be much higher in Native Alaskans (3 per cent), Canadian native peoples (3.6–7.1 per cent) and Greenland Eskimos (2–10 per cent) (Gudmand-Høyer *et al.*, 1987; Bell *et al.*, 1973; Ellestad-Sayad *et al.*, 1978).

Most patients have a double defect, lacking both sucrase and isomaltase. Others lack sucrase activity but have residual isomaltase activity, suggesting genotypic heterogeneity. Studies on this enzyme deficiency reveal different phenotypes: the lack of enzyme production (McMichael, 1976); intracellular accumulation in the endoplasmic reticulum as a membrane-associated high-mannose precursor (Alpers, 1994); failure to be integrated in the brush-border membrane, given retention and degradation in the Golgi apparatus (Naim *et al.*, 1988a); transport of catalytically altered sucrase to the cell surface (Semenza, 1986); partial missorting to the basolateral membrane (Montgomery *et al.*, 1981); and intracellular loss of sucrase subunits and expression of isomaltase subunits at the brush-border membrane (Hauri *et al.*, 1986; Louvard *et al.*, 1992).

Sucrase-isomaltase deficiency is frequently misdiagnosed because the patients have no family history or are presumed to have cow's milk or soy protein allergy. The initial onset of symptoms usually occurs in the first months of life with the introduction of sucrose into the diet. Diarrhoea is the main symptom in association with other non-specific findings, including abdominal distension, flatulence, excoriated buttocks, diaper rash, colic and sporadic vomiting. Patients are clinically malnourished and show growth retardation, particularly in individuals diagnosed after the age of 5, with long episodes of chronic diarrhoea and abdominal pain. The administration of a sucrose-free diet results in the normalization of bowel movements, and sick patients who fail to thrive can gain weight and height. Striking differences as to the severity of diarrhoea and the incidence of malnutrition are clearly noted in the published series. The varying clinical presentations depend on infant feeding practices. In fact, diarrhoea is more severe in patients experiencing precocious administration of sucrose, whereas simultaneous delayed introduction and decreased quantity modify the course and symptoms of the disease. Similarly, reducing sucrose load in the diet through the avoidance of fruits, vegetables (peas, beans and lentils), fruit juices and soft drinks in children diagnosed late will ameliorate symptoms.

The determination of stool pH 5.5, the detection of reducing substances before and after hydrolysis of stools by HCl, and a clear rise in breath hydrogen after a sucrose load are the clues to diagnosis. In view of false negatives reported in the literature, the measurement of intestinal disaccharidases remains the key to diagnosis of sucrase-isomaltase deficiency. In addition to lifelong adherence to a strict sucrose-free diet, liquid yeast sucrase as an enzyme substitution therapy may prevent and ameliorate symptoms. The rigid exclusion of sucrose from the diet and treatment with liquid yeast sucrase may also be beneficial for secondary sucrase deficiency.

Congenital lactase deficiency

This is a very rare disorder in infancy, which displays a complete absence of both enzymatic activity and protein immunoreactivity. It is inherited as an autosomal recessive trait and studies are needed to determine the defect at the molecular level. A pattern of decrease is observed in lactase activity after weaning and the residual activity represents 10 per cent of birth values. Maximal lactase activity, observed in the perinatal period, is maintained throughout life only in Northern Europeans, North Americans, Aboriginal subjects of Australia and Oceania, and in various people in South-East Asia. However, half the adult population in most parts of the world experiences symptoms of lactose intolerance, probably due to genetically controlled 'switching off' lactase synthesis by intestinal cells. Recent work has attempted to characterize the molecular basis of human adult-onset lactase decline (Harvey *et al.*, 1995). The findings have suggested that each allele is independently regulated and that a *cis*-acting control mechanism may determine human adult-onset lactase decline. These conclusions were reached when individuals with high lactase activity showed equal expression from both alleles, whereas those with intermediate lactase activity revealed a preferential expression of only one of the alleles.

The symptoms of lactose maldigestion include bloating, borborygmia, colics, flatulence and diarrhoea (Büller and Grand, 1990). However, these manifestations vary among subjects owing to differences in the rates of gastric emptying, intestinal transit and colonic flora. Primary lactase deficiency can be diagnosed on the basis of acid pH in stools (less than 3.8), high reducing substances in stool, lack of increase in blood sugar after a lactose load with accompanying uncharacteristic abdominal complaints and diarrhoea, and enhanced excretion of hydrogen in exhaled air. The assessment of lactase deficiency on small-bowel biopsy in the absence of mucosal damage allows secondary lactase deficiency to be excluded. Thus, dietary lactose restriction can be advised in patients with lactose intolerance. Commercial yogurt, ice cream, sherbets, cheese, milk chocolate, desserts prepared with milk, etc., should be avoided. Furthermore, many enzymatic preparations (i.e. lactase from *Kluyveromyces lactis*) can be added to dairy products to predigest lactose.

Calcium supplements are often necessary in view of the decreased calcium intake resulting from self-imposed restriction of dairy products or from the interference of undigested lactose with calcium absorption. Calcium supplements are particularly recommended for postmenopausal women and the elderly because of the risk factor for developing osteoporosis.

Congenital maltase-glucoamylase deficiency

Many patients with decreased maltase-glucoamylase were defined as having secondary deficiencies in view of their abnormal mucosal morphology. However, recent studies were able to determine primary maltase-glucoamylase deficiency in patients with normal intestinal morphology and appropriate activity of lactase, sucrase, maltase, isomaltase and pancreatic α-amylase (Lebenthal *et al.*, 1994). Suppression of starch or short glucose polymers in their diet improves their condition. This congenital disease is very rare, and necessitates further investigation in order to assess its impact on carbohydrate digestion and nutrition.

Congenital trehalase deficiency

Trehalose maldigestion has also been reported. Decreased trehalase activity was found in Greenlandic individuals and confirmed by a low trehalose tolerance test (Gudmand-Høyer *et al.*, 1988). The prevalence in Greenland Inuits is about 10 per cent, but this primary disorder is very rare among adult White Americans. Additional investigation is necessary to define this disorder further.

Congenital glucose–galactose malabsorption

As mentioned earlier, glucose and galactose are both absorbed in the small intestine by the same active transport system. Theoretically, any defect in the specific carrier is able to impair the absorption of both of these sugars. Patients with glucose–galactose malabsorption cannot accumulate hexoses, probably due to a specific defect in Na^+-dependent absorption of glucose in the brush border as noted with the incubation of intestinal biopsies with various monosaccharides (Elsas *et al.*, 1970; Stirling *et al.*, 1972; Booth *et al.*, 1988). In the congenital disorder, known as glucose–galactose malabsorption, a mutation of Na^+-dependent glucose transporter SGLT1 was detected (Turk *et al.*, 1991; Wright *et al.*, 1991). A single nucleotide base change (guanine to adenine) was discovered at position 92 of the cloned and sequenced cDNA from two sisters presenting with this disorder (Turk *et al.*, 1991; Wright *et al.*, 1991). The parents were also investigated and were found to carry the mutation. The inheritance of this form of malabsorption seems to occur by an autosomal recessive mode. At present, it appears that practically all glucose absorption is by SGLT1 and the malfunction of this transporter is lethal. The patients develop profuse watery diarrhoea within a few days after birth, and occasionally later, resulting in severe dehydration and metabolic acidosis. Among the gastrointestinal signs and symptoms are abdomen distension, flatulence and vomiting. The findings of glycosuria, despite low blood sugar, and the presence of reducing substances in faeces, are suggestive of glucose–galactose malabsorption. An oral glucose/galactose tolerance test yields flat blood response curves. As with disaccharide malabsorption, the breath hydrogen test proves to be sensitive in the syndrome. Breath hydrogen can exceed 20 ppm within 3 hours of glucose or galactose loading. Once again, jejunal biopsies can offer better diagnosis by measuring glucose or galactose uptake and accumulation. Treatment is offered through a glucose–galactose-free diet. Fructose can be added to the alimentary regimen.

Fructose malabsorption

Various studies have reported cases of malabsorption related to the ingestion of foods containing significant quantities of fructose (Andersson and Nygren, 1978). Malabsorption is particularly common in children who consume large amounts of fruit juice or high-fructose syrup. The mechanisms have not been elucidated. However, the ingestion of small amounts of fructose in the presence of glucose prevents discomfort. The reduction in the severity of fructose malabsorption when glucose is ingested simultaneously confirms: (1) the need for two subsites of the disaccharidase-related transport system to be occupied by both monosaccharides; and (2) increased frucose absorption occurs through the paracellular pathway when tight junctions open in the presence of glucose.

Secondary carbohydrate malabsorption

In addition to severe pancreatic insufficiency or congenital disaccharidase deficiency, insult to the intestinal mucosa or impairment of the gastrointestinal tract function may result in carbohydrate malabsorption. Examples of these disorders associated with carbohydrate malassimilation are listed in Table 10.2, and also include toxic infectious and pharmacologic agents. In some cases, secondary enzyme deficiencies have been considered to complicate an already existing gastrointestinal disease. For example, lactase deficiency provokes diarrhoea and abdominal discomfort in patients with ulcerative colitis, Crohn's disease and irritable bowel syndrome (Gudmand-Høyer and Jarnum, 1970; Gudmand-Høyer and Busk, 1975). In

Table 10.2 *Conditions associated with secondary glycohydrolase deficiency*

Pancreatic insufficiency (e.g. cystic fibrosis)
Gastric or intestinal surgery
Blind loop syndrome
Inflammatory bowel disease (e.g. Crohn's disease) (Jönsson and Bodemar, 1990; Saavedra, 1994)
Radiation enteritis and drug-induced enteritis
Severe malnutrition
Bacterial gastroenteritis (e.g. acute diarrhoea caused by rotaviral infection) (Saavedra, 1994; Collins *et al.*, 1990)
Giardiasis and ascariasis (Tolboom *et al.*, 1987)
Immune defects (e.g. sensitivity to cow's milk, soy protein and gluten; AIDS) (Montes and Perman, 1980; Saavedra and Perman, 1989; Beeken, 1973)
Drugs (e.g. laxative abuse commonly seen in anorexia nervosa (McMichael, 1976); neomycin; colchicine; sufasazine; dephenylhydantoin; disaccharidase-inhibitory drugs (Puls *et al.*, 1977)

general, the severity and duration of secondary carbohydrate deficiency are determined by the primary aetiology. Treatment includes the elimination of the offending carbohydrate from the diet and therapy of the underlying mucosal injury.

DIAGNOSTIC EVALUATION

As discussed before, malabsorbed carbohydrates are fermented by colonic bacteria into gases and organic acids. Thus, the presence of organic acids in the stool decreases the pH to below 6 and suggests carbohydrate malabsorption. Intraluminal H_2 is absorbed into the circulation and exhaled as a function of the amount of ingested carbohydrate. Therefore, the hydrogen breath test is a useful tool to evaluate carbohydrate malabsorption. Furthermore, a defect in carbohydrate absorption following the oral disaccharide tolerance test will result in a flat serum glucose curve. Finally, the determination of disaccharidase mucosal activity will complete the laboratory investigation.

CONCLUDING REMARKS

Advances in cellular and molecular biology provide efficient tools to investigate the luminal and cellular processes controlling intestinal sugar absorption. Intensive efforts are still needed to delineate the possible causative mechanisms associated with primary and secondary disorders of carbohydrate malabsorption. Hopefully, the combination of present and future knowledge of basic concepts will improve the general diagnostic approach, thereby making it possible to offer more appropriate treatment.

DIGESTION AND ABSORPTION OF LIPIDS

DIETARY LIPIDS

The daily diet of the average Western adult contains 120–150 g triglycerides, 4–8 g phospholipids and 300–500 mg cholesterol. These fats are derived mainly from meat, eggs and dairy products. Bile provides an additional source of intraluminal cholesterol (800–1200 mg/day) and phospholipids (10–20 g/day), with phosphatidylcholine (lecithin) as the major class. The turnover of intestinal mucosal epithelium is estimated to contribute 250–400 mg of cholesterol per day (Cheng and Stanley, 1959). Dietary lipids also include plant and shellfish sterols, waxes, lipovitamins and commercial synthetic fat.

DIGESTIVE AND MICELLAR PHASE

Prepyloric digestion

Fat digestion is a complex process given the particular physicochemical properties of lipids. Coordinated events are required in order to ensure the efficient digestion of dietary hydrophobic fat. In fact, fat digestion begins with mastication and mixing with saliva in the mouth. The mechanical crude emulsification continues with peristalsis in the stomach that leads to dispersing fat into unstable droplets. The emulsion becomes more stable when dietary phospholipids and protein proteolytic products coat the triglyceride core. At this stage, a considerable proportion (20–30 per cent) of alimentary triglycerides are digested locally without being disturbed by the low gastric pH (Hamosh *et al.*, 1981). Prepyloric lipases are fully active in the acidic environment and are not dependent on the presence of co-lipase or bile salts. The acid-stable lipases are secreted by the serous glands of Ebner at the base of the tongue and gastric mucosal cells.

If lingual lipase, originating from Von Ebner glands beneath the circumvallate papillae, is dominant in many animal species (Hamosh *et al.*, 1981; Levy *et al.*, 1981), true gastric lipase of fundic origin represents the major lipolytic enzyme at work in the stomach of humans (Moreau *et al.*, 1988). It hydrolyses the medium-chain triglycerides more rapidly than long-chain triglycerides, and acts mostly on fatty acids on the primary positions of the triglyceride backbone. This gastric lipase plays a significant role when pancreatic function is impaired, as in cystic fibrosis or premature birth (Smith *et al.*, 1986). The digestion of triglycerides in the stomach also appears to be a prerequisite for efficient intestinal lipolysis: (1) milk lipid globules are resistant to intestinal lipolysis by pancreatic lipase unless first exposed to gastric lipase (Bernback *et al.*, 1990); (2) gastric and intestinal emulsification is assisted by the small amount of fatty acids liberated by intragastric lipolysis (Armand *et al.*, 1994); and (3) these fatty acids release cholecystokinin, a messenger transmitting signal, which triggers pancreatobiliary secretions essential for integrated and coordinated intestinal events conducting to remarkably efficient absorption (Liddle *et al.*, 1985).

Solubilization and absorption of lipolytic products

Following gastric peristalsis and intermittent relaxation of the pyloric musculature, gastric lipid content is delivered to the duodenum. As mentioned earlier, the fatty acids in the gastric chyme stimulate the release of cholecystokinin from the duodenal mucosa, thereby provoking the release of exocrine pancreatic enzymes and sustained gallbladder excretion of bile containing bile acids, phospholipids and cholesterol. Furthermore, cholecystokinin promotes pancreatic bicarbonate secretion that ensures a persistent alkalization of acid chyme in the duodenum, which is optimal for enzymatic activity (You *et al.*, 1983). These active constituents bring about the chemical hydrolysis of lipids and physical dispersion of their lipolytic products. Pancreatic lipase is of major importance for the digestion of dietary lipids in the small intestine lumen. It contains 420 amino-acid residues with six disulphide bridges ending in a molecular weight of 46 000 Da (Winkler *et al.*, 1990).

Pancreatic lipase, which is responsible for most hydrolysis in adults, cannot act on the triglyceride emulsion covered at the oil and aqueous interface by amphiphilic proteins and lipids (Lowe, 1994). Although bile salts remove these substances from the interface, they inhibit pancreatic lipase by sequestering the substrate from lipolytic attack (Donner *et al.*, 1976). Co-lipase, a coenzyme for lipase also secreted in the pancreatic juice, enables pancreatic lipase to reach its substrate interface in the presence of bile salts and restores lipolytic activity (Donner *et al.*, 1976). The hypothesis was put forward that lipase–co-lipase complex, in a 1:1 ratio favouring a new pancreatic lipase conformation, supplants bile salts and allows binding to the surface of triglyceride droplets (Lowe, 1994). The mixed micelles present in bile (consisting of bile salts, phospholipids and cholesterol), adsorb to this complex, remove the lipolytic products (2-monoglycerides and fatty acids) and promote binding of the lipase–co-lipase complex to the emulsion surface (Carey and Small, 1970, 1972; Lowe, 1994; Björkhem and Boberg, 1995). Pancreatic phospholipase A_2 is catalytically active against phospholipids (e.g. phosphatidylcholine), producing fatty acids and lysophosphatidylcholine, which has an important role in solubilizing other lipid digestion products (VanDeenen *et al.*, 1963). Cholesterol esterase (carboxyl ester hydrolase) is a further pancreatic enzyme that hydrolyses both lipid-soluble and water-soluble esters (cholesterol esters, lipophilic vitamin esters, triolein) (Lombardo and Guy, 1980). Bile salts are required for the optimal activity of the last two enzymes (Ihse and Arnesjö, 1973; Jacobson *et al*, 1990). The absorption of cholesterol is absolutely dependent on the presence of bile (Westergaard and Dietschy, 1976).

After digestion, the micelles convey the non-polar lipid molecules to the epithelial cell surface. These lipolytic products have to be transported across the diffusion barrier because of the unstirred water layer bordering the enterocyte membrane (Westergaard and Dietschy, 1974, 1976). Since the microclimate at this location is slightly acidic (because of the activity of the Na^+/H^+ exchanger in the brush-border membrane), the solubility of fatty acids in micelles decreases. Thus, the fatty acids dissociate from micelles, become protonated and diffuse into the lipophilic cell membrane where they become trapped (Ahrens, 1957). Furthermore, 2-monoglycerides lysophosphatidylcholine and free cholesterol are also transferred to the mucosa. Then, the majority of bile acids reach the terminal ileum where they are absorbed by active transport and carried in the portal venous blood to the liver.

Related disorders of maldigestion

Abnormalities in lipid hydrolysis and micelle formation impair the normal processes of digestion and absorption. Specific disorders are addressed in order to document the mechanisms, which can be encountered in various diseases.

CYSTIC FIBROSIS AS AN EXOCRINE PANCREATIC INSUFFICIENCY

Cystic fibrosis (CF) is the most common fatal genetic disorder of the Caucasian population. It is inherited in an autosomal recessive manner and affects 1 in 2000 live births, while the carrier frequency has been estimated to be about 1 in 20. The disease is characterized by progressive lung disease, pancreatic dysfunction, elevated sweat electrolytes and male infertility (Koch and Hoiby, 1993; Shalon and Adelson, 1996). The gene is located on the long arm of chromosome 7 at position 7q31, which encodes a cyclic AMP-regulated chloride channel protein of 1480 amino acids (Riordan *et al.*, 1989). This CF gene product, named cystic fibrosis transmembrane conductance regulator (CFTR), is located on the apical membrane of many types of epithelial cells, including pancreatic, intestinal, salivary, sweat, airway, vas deferens and biliary duct (Morris *et al.*, 1993). The most common mutation is referred to as ΔF 508, indicating a 3-nucleotide base-pair deletion that results in a missing phenylalanine at position 508 in the amino-acid sequence (Lucotte and Loirat, 1993). All mutations lead to the failure of Cl^- transport limiting fluid secretion, which predisposes the ducts to obstruction (Lucotte and Loirat, 1993). CFTR dysfunction in the pancreas does not allow the delivery of alkaline fluid containing HCO_3^- and pancreatic enzymes in exchange of lumenal Cl^- (Shalon and Adelson, 1996). Plugging and obstruction of the pancreatic ducts occur, and the organ is destroyed (Oppenheimer and Esterly, 1975). Both impaired pancreatic enzyme secretion and defective delivery of alkalinizing pancreatic fluid necessary for gastric acid neutralization contribute to malabsorption.

Maldigestion of fat is also due to the reduction in the total bile acid pool in view of the decreased ileal reabsorption and hepatic disorders predisposing to the formation of lithogenic bile (Roy *et al.*, 1977, 1982; Roy *et al.*, 1982; Gaskin *et al.*, 1988). Approximately 85 per cent of patients have steatorrhoea at the time of diagnosis. This is accompanied by abnormal tests of secretin-pancreozymin, fat load, faecal chymotrypsin and impaired ultrasound examination. It has been shown that the degree of pancreatic insufficiency is determined by the nature of the CF mutation (Hamosh and Corey, 1993). Young CF patients very often show failure-to-thrive and malnutrition. Aggressive nutritional therapy is necessary to cope with steatorrhoea, increased energy requirements and poor intake. A deficiency of essential fatty acids is very often observed (Levy *et al.*, 1987b; Roy *et al.*, 1987) and fat-soluble vitamin decrease (A, D, E and K) is present unless persistently liberal fat intake with proportional pancreatic enzyme replacement, along with supplementation of essential fatty acids and vitamins, contribute to normalizing the precarious nutritional state. Taurine may be supplied in view of the excess of glycoconjugates versus tauroconjugates that tend to precipitate at an acid pH and are, therefore, not available for micelle formation (Belli *et al.*, 1987).

Conjunctival xerosis, and eventually xerophthalmia with corneal ulceration, night blindness and conjunctival abnormalities have been reported in both children and adults with CF. Vitamin A intake (8000 IU daily for adults) may limit these abnormalities. Neurologic problems in CF patients due to long-standing severe deficiency of vitamin E may be resolved with an intake of 200–400 mg daily (adult recommendation). Furthermore, low levels of bone mineralization may be helped through the recommended intake of vitamin D (800 IU daily for adults). Of note is a deficiency in vitamin K reported in CF patients with liver disease or long-term antibiotic therapy. Attempts to influence essential fatty acid deficiency must be undertaken.

OTHER EXOCRINE PANCREATIC INSUFFICIENCIES

Pancreatitis

Fat malabsorption, although not severe, can occur in chronic pancreatitis. Obstruction may be produced by a stone, oedema, spasm, or from an acquired or congenital anomaly. The obstructed duct provokes the activation of pancreatic enzymes, resulting in pancreatic autodigestion (Lott, 1982; Balart and Ferrante, 1982). Exocrine pancreatic dysfunction can be diagnosed through the direct analysis of pancreatic secretion, a 3-day stool fat collection or the bentiromide test (BT-PABA). Pain and fat malabsorption may be relieved by enzyme replacement therapy.

Shwachman–Diamond syndrome

This is a very common condition of pancreatic insufficiency in children (Shwachman *et al.*, 1964). Steatorrhoea and growth failure are important clinical features. In contrast to cystic fibrosis, patients with this syndrome have normal sweat electrolytes and bicarbonate secretion is less severely affected. However, the enzyme response to pancreatic stimulation is markedly reduced.

Zollinger–Ellison syndrome

Large amounts of gastrin in Zollinger–Ellison syndrome increase the capacity of the stomach to secrete hydrochloric acid via the expansion of the gastric parietal cell mass. Acid hypersecretion in the lumen of the small intestine may cause morphologic abnormalities and diarrhoea (Isenberg *et al.*, 1973). Steatorrhoea is probably the consequence of inactivated pancreatic lipase and insoluble primary bile salts, which impair the hydrolysis of intraluminal triglycerides and the formation of micelles. The surgical removal of the gastrinoma eliminates the source of excessive gastrin secretion, which induces gastric acid secretion, and provides help in reducing steatorrhoea. Among the powerful antisecretory agents, H-2 receptor antagonists omeprazole, ranitidine and famotidine proved effective in producing symptom relief and reducing acid secretion. The use of omeprazole, an inhibitor of the proton pump potassium ATPase, is preferable in view of the development of resistance to H-2 blockers (McGuigan, 1993).

Other disorders are characterized by hypergastrinaemia and gastric acid hypersecretion. They include: antral G hyperplasia, protracted pyloric obstruction, chronic renal failure, short bowel syndrome, duodenal ulcer and hyperparathyroidism.

DISORDERS ASSOCIATED WITH BILE ACID ABNORMALITIES

Brief overall physiology

As mentioned before, bile is necessary for the efficient digestion and absorption of dietary fat. Primary or hepatocellular bile is elaborated by the hepatocytes at the level of the canaliculus by a process of osmotic filtration. Bile flows in the canalicular system, enters biliary ductules and ducts, is concentrated by the gallbladder mucosa and finally is released into the duodenum. Bile is composed of water, inorganic electrolytes and organic solutes, such as bile acids, cholesterol, phospholipids and bilirubin. Bile acids are the principal metabolites of cholesterol in the liver and the major solutes in bile. They induce bile flow by their osmotic effects and biliary lipid secretion. Once in the intestinal lumen, they take part in the emulsification and hydrolysis of fat. More than 90 per cent of bile acids are efficiently recovered from the small bowel, reabsorbed predominantly by the distal ileum through active transport, returned to the liver via the portal superior mesenteric vein and promptly resecreted into bile (Hofmann, 1989). Bile acids, not absorbed from the ileum by a process requiring energy and specific carriers, are taken up by passive diffusion by the large bowel. In this organ, they first undergo further metabolism by local, abundant bacteria: removal of the conjugating group (amino acid, glucuronide, glucoside, sulphate) and modification of the steroid nucleus (dehydroxylation and oxidation reduction). They are then absorbed into the inferior (left colon) and superior (right colon) mesenteric veins, thus completing the minor branch of the enterohepatic circulation. Numerous liver diseases affect small bowel functions and lead to malabsorption. A number of factors may be responsible for fat malabsorption in patients with liver diseases.

Defective bile acid biosynthesis

More than 15 enzymatic steps are involved in bile acid biosynthesis from cholesterol as a precursor in the liver. An inborn error affecting bile acid biogenesis will alter the enterohepatic circulation with repercussions on micelle-forming bile acids and fat absorption (Björkhem and Boberg, 1995). Unfortunately, diagnosing these errors of bile acid formation is not easy and requires sophisticated determinations such as the isotope dilution technique (using radioactive or stable isotopes) or molecular biology methodology. The identification of enzymatic step defects will help optimize treatment through the administration of specific exogenous bile acids.

Cholestasis resulting in abnormal bile secretion

Cholestasis results from many different forms of liver injury that impair bile secretion. It is characterized by pruritus, jaundice and elevation of the serum alkaline phosphatase. The initiation of cholestasis in humans often remains ill-defined because bile formation is a complex multistep process. More than one abnormality may disturb the overall mechanism comprising liver perfusion, hepatocyte uptake, transcellular transport system, bile acid excretion, canalicular contraction involving canalicular microfilaments, tight junctions, etc. Patients with chronic cholestasis develop the inability to digest alimentary fat, resulting from impaired intestinal bile-acid delivery. Pancreatic enzyme deficiency, small bowel disease and cholestyramine may be also contributing factors (Gleeson and Boyer, 1991). Steatorrhoea and weight loss are therefore common in patients with advanced chronic cholestasis. As a consequence of lipid malabsorption, a deficiency of fat-soluble vitamins and calcium is frequently observed. The low levels of vitamin A lead to the impairment of dark adaptation. Decreased blood concentrations result in hyporeflexia, ataxia, loss of vibration and position sensation, peripheral neuropathy, gaze palsies and quadriplegia. Vitamin K deficiency causes the prolongation of the prothrombin time (due to the impaired activity of factors II, VII and X). Impaired calcium absorption due to the formation of insoluble calcium–fatty acid complexes may cause bone diseases with decreased vitamin D as a contributory factor. Administration of these vitamins and calcium is necessary to correct their deficiency in long-standing cholestasis. However, the effective treatment of the primary liver disorder that causes cholestasis will improve fat absorption, and both calcium and vitamin deficiencies. In addition, a low-fat diet and medium-chain triglyceride supplementation correct the steatorrhoea of chronic cholestasis. In some refractory cases, cystic fibrosis or coeliac disease may be the causes of steatorrhoea, and, in this case, pancreatic enzyme replacement or withdrawal of gluten may be beneficial.

Bile acid malabsorption

The defective function of ileal absorption occurs in patients with small intestinal resection or inflammatory bowel disease. In such cases, increased bile acid synthesis compensates for the considerable bile acid malabsorption. The bile acids, which pass into the colon, undergo dehydroxylation by colonic bacteria and this leads to diarrhoea. However, patients with large ileal resections cannot compensate for the important loss of bile acids (Hofmann, 1993). There is, therefore, diminished bile acid secretion into the duodenum. Bile acids may precipitate and their reduced concentrations are not sufficient to potentialize fat digestion. It is recommended that patients limit fat consumption and these are given supplements of medium-chain triglycerides and fat-soluble vitamins.

Other disturbances in the bile enterohepatic circulation of bile associated with fat malabsorption

The latter can occur in patients with the following conditions:

1 Cholelithiasis, where ileal dysfunction causes bile acid malabsorption and a high prevalence of gallstones.
2 Enhanced bile acid deconjugation in the stagnant loop syndrome, resulting in intraluminal bile acid deficiency. This augmented deconjugation can be measured by measuring $^{14}CO_2$ after the administration of 1-^{14}C-cholylglycine or by detecting an increased concentration of unconjugated bile acids in plasma.
3 Defective gallbladder contraction because of the diminished cholecystokinin characteristic of coeliac sprue.
4 Cirrhosis, which is often accompanied with numerous abnormalities in the portal systemic

shunting, hepatic uptake, 12-hydroxylation of newly synthesized bile acids and reconjugation. Thus, there is a fall in intraduodenal bile-acid concentrations, thereby limiting adequate solubilization and micellar incorporation of dietary lipid and fat-soluble vitamins.

Primary bile acid malabsorption

Primary bile acid malabsorption is an idiopathic intestinal disorder associated with chronic diarrhoea beginning in early infancy, interruption of the enterohepatic circulation of bile acids and reduced plasma cholesterol (Heubi *et al.*, 1982; Balistreri *et al.*, 1983). Several conflicting mechanisms have been postulated. However, impaired ileal uptake of bile acids has been documented in several patients (Heubi *et al.*, 1982; Jonas *et al.*, 1986), thus reducing the solubilization of dietary lipids. Recent studies have established that molecular defects in the human ileal Na^+/bile acid co-transporter gene can cause primary bile acid malabsorption (Wong *et al.*, 1995).

The enterohepatic circulation of bile acids is an extremely efficient process and only 10 per cent of the intestinal bile acids escape reabsorption to be eliminated in the faeces. The first stage in the active uptake of bile acids from the intestine is mediated by a Na^+-gradient-driven transporter located on the apical membrane of the ileal enterocyte (Hofmann, 1994). Inherited mutations in the ileal Na^+/bile acid co-transporter gene, localized to chromosome 13q33, abolished the transport of taurocholate and other bile acids (Oelkers *et al.*, 1997).

MUCOSAL UPTAKE AND INTRACELLULAR PROCESSING

Lipolytic products are absorbed in the proximal intestine. The transfer process does not seem to require energy. Passive diffusion apparently takes place, initiated by a gradient across the brush-border membrane resulting from the abundant lipid content in the lumen and poor concentration in the cytosol of enterocytes. However, suggestions have been advanced that fatty-acid uptake is mediated by microvillus membrane fatty acid-binding (40 kDa), since the process is saturable, heat sensitive, trypsin inactivated and competitive (Stremmel *et al.*, 1985). Additional microvillous membrane carrier proteins may be involved in the uptake of the other lipolytic products (Stremmel, 1988). The majority of absorbed lipolytic products migrate to the endoplasmic reticulum following binding to low molecular weight cytosolic proteins (Fig. 10.2).

It has been postulated that the intracellular transport of fatty acids is facilitated or promoted by cytosolic fatty-acid binding protein (FABP). Two different FABPs

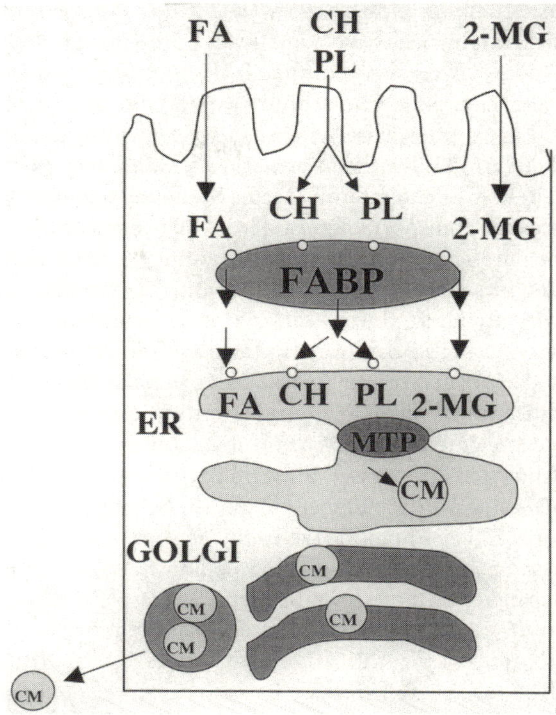

Figure 10.2 *Intracellular lipid transport and chylomicron formation. FA, fatty acids; CH, cholesterol; PL, phospholipid; 2-MG, 2-microsomal transfer protein; CM, chlyomicron; ERR, endoplasmic reticulum.*

are expressed along the small intestine. The first, termed intestinal FABP (I-FABP), is strictly confined to this organ, whereas the second, liver FABP (L-FABP), is also found in the liver and kidneys (Gordon and Lowe, 1985). These two proteins may exert different physiological functions intracellularly.

After interiorization into the endoplasmic reticulum, fatty acids are re-esterified into triglycerides via the monoacylglycerol pathway or, alternatively, via the α-glycerophosphate pathway. Most triglycerides are synthesized by the monoacylglycerol pathway, which involves sequential direct acylation of absorbed exogenous 2-monoglycerides to form the diglycerides and ultimately triglycerides in the smooth endoplasmic reticulum (Senior and Isselbacher, 1962; Tso, 1994). The α-glycerophosphate pathway becomes active when alimentary monoglycerides are not available or during fasting. In this case, the enzymes are predominantly located in the smooth endoplasmic reticulum, and the substrates, glycerol-3-phosphate and lysolecithin, are derived from glucose metabolism and bile, respectively (Parthasarathy *et al.*, 1974; Popper *et al.*, 1985).

It is also through the monoacylglycerol pathway that absorbed lysophosphatidylcholine is reacylated to form phosphatidylcholine (or lecithin) with the enzymatic cooperation of lysophatidylcholine acyl transferase (Parthasarathy *et al.*, 1974). Another important route of phosphololipid synthesis is via the phosphatidic acid–phosphorylcholine pathway involving the substrates glycerol-3-phosphate, derived from glucose metabolism and lysolecithin hydrolysis, and CDP (cytidine diphosphate)-choline, derived from biliary and dietary choline (Scow *et al.*, 1967; Mansbach, 1977).

The rate of cholesterol esterification may regulate the lymphatic transport of this sterol. Two enzymes have been implicated in the esterification of cholesterol within intestinal mucosal cells: cholesterol esterase (also commonly referred to as carboxyl ester lipase) and acyl coenzyme A:cholesterol acyltransferase (ACAT). There is a controversy as to which enzyme plays the more significant role in cholesterol esterification and other aspects of intestinal cholesterol metabolism.

Cholesterol esterase is secreted by the exocrine pancreas and by a number of species in milk, where it ensures efficient lipid uptake in the newborn (Wang and Hartsuck, 1993). cDNA cloning demonstrates that milk and pancreatic forms of cholesterol esterase are derived from the same gene (Nilsson *et al.*, 1990). Not only has it been proposed that this enzyme hydrolyses lipid nutrients in the intestinal lumen, but it has also been suggested that cholesterol esterase facilitates the movement of lipids into the enterocyte, directing them into functional intracellular sites (Lopez-Candales *et al.*, 1993). Its role in the uptake of dietary cholesteryl ester has been established by studying gene knockout mice (Howles *et al.*, 1996). The interaction of cholesterol esterase with micellar bile salt seems to be required for cholesterol esterification (Wang and Hartsuck, 1993). Diet manipulations may alter the expression at the molecular level of this lipid-metabolizing enzyme, thereby modulating the absorption of cholesterol (Lopez-Candales *et al.*, 1996).

There is also evidence suggesting that ACAT is the key enzyme that regulates intestinal cholesterol transport. Inhibiting ACAT activity results in the decreased secretion of cholesteryl esters in lymph chylomicrons and very-low-density lipoprotein (VLDL) (Bennett Clark and Tercyak, 1984). On the other hand, the ingestion of cholesterol leads to a stimulation of ACAT activity (Bennett Clark and Tercyak, 1984). The use of Caco-2 cells, a human intestinal epithelial cell line, has uncovered much information about the function of this enzyme in cholesterol transport: (1) changes in ACAT activity affect lipoprotein assembly or secretion of triglyceride-enriched lipoproteins; (2) inhibition of ACAT activity provokes triglyceride accumulation intracellularly (Field *et al.*, 1987; Kam *et al.*, 1989, 1990; Levy *et al.*, 1995); and (3) arrest of cholesterol synthesis, and esterification by neutralizing both 3-hydroxy-3-methylglutanyl-Coenzyme A (HMG-CoA) reductase (key enzyme in cholesterol synthesis) and ACAT by lovastatin leads to a decrease in the secretion of newly synthesized triglycerides and cholesteryl esters.

It is likely that a form of cooperation exists between ACAT and cholesterol esterase as was suggested many years ago. Cholesterol esterase may catalyse the esterification of cholesterol on the cell surface and its hydrolysis in the inner leaflet of the plasma membrane, thereby allowing intracellularly liberated free cholesterol to be re-esterified by ACAT.

The aforementioned lipid molecule types migrate through the cisternae of the smooth endoplasmic reticulum to the rough endoplasmic reticulum. The transfer of triglycerides, mainly, but also of phospholipids and cholesteryl esters to apo B-48 by microsomal transfer protein (MTP) is essential for the formation of triglyceride-rich lipoproteins (Wetterau *et al.*, 1997). Other apolipoproteins (A-I, A-IV and C-III) are added to these nascent particles, which are then transported to the Golgi apparatus for final assembly (Havel, 1987; Davidson, 1994; Tso, 1994; Black, 1995). Glycosylation of apolipoproteins, initiated in the rough endoplasmic reticulum, is completed in the Golgi apparatus. Finally, extrusion of the completed prechylomicrons into intercellular space occurs subsequent to the fusion of Golgi vesicles containing well-individualized prechylomicrons with the lateral plasma membrane. Chylomicrons are secreted into the intestinal lymphatics for ultimate entry into the systemic circulation for metabolism.

CHYLOMICRON STRUCTURE AND METABOLISM

Circulating chylomicrons (80–500 nm) consisting of more than 87 per cent triglycerides and about 1–2 per cent cholesteryl esters together with liposoluble vitamins are enclosed in a thin, stabilizing coat of 9 per cent phospholipids, 1 per cent free cholesterol and 2 per cent apolipoproteins. Apoprotein B-48 (Apo B-48) is the major protein and apo C-III the minor protein on the chylomicron surface, whereas apo A-I and apo A-IV are abundant components of the particle coat. Other apolipoproteins, such as apo E and apo C-II, join chylomicrons in the circulation. The major function of chylomicrons is to deliver triglyceride-fatty acids to peripheral tissues. As they circulate, they transiently adhere to glycoaminoglycan molecules on endothelial cells, where they encounter lipoprotein lipase. Chylomicron triglycerides are then hydrolysed after the activation of lipoprotein lipase by apo C-II. Fatty acids released during lipolysis are utilized by muscles for energy production or are stored in adipose tissue. Chylomicron remnants are removed rapidly by the liver through the mediation of apo E receptor.

SYNTHESIS AND SECRETION OF OTHER INTESTINAL LIPOPROTEINS

With only limited dietary lipids in the lumen or during fasting, 'small chylomicrons' or intestinal VLDL

(25–80 nm) are formed by the small intestine. They transport mainly endogenous lipids and their chemical composition resembles chylomicrons more than plasma VLDL of liver origin. Although chylomicrons and VLDL may follow the same biosynthetic pathway (Mahley *et al.*, 1971), the utilization of Pluronic L-81 (a hydrophobic surfactant) suggests different pathways for their formation. Pluronic L-81 reduces chylomicron secretion by enterocytes without affecting the transport of VLDL-sized particles. Nevertheless, both lipoproteins share a similar catabolism.

In addition to the production of triglyceride-rich particles, the intestine produces nascent spherical or disc-shaped particles (6–13 nm). They are enriched in phospholipids and cholesteryl esters and contain apo A-I and apo A-IV at their surface (Magun *et al.*, 1985). However, another high-density lipoprotein (HDL) population has been characterized and shows the presence of apo B-48 (Magun *et al.*, 1985). This lipoprotein fraction may constitute chylomicron precursors. Additional investigation is needed to determine the metabolism of intestinal HDL.

APOLIPOPROTEIN B AND RELATED DISORDERS

Over the two last decades, the mechanistic aspects of the assembly and secretion of triglyceride-rich lipoproteins have been explored by focusing on the biogenesis of apo B. Genetic disorders of this molecule have afforded new insights into the mechanisms involved in intestinal lipid handling and lipoprotein metabolism. Additional studies using conventional transgenic mice and gene-targeted mice help in the understanding of apo B structure and function relationships, the regulation of apo B gene expression in the intestine and the mechanisms involved in apo B deficiency syndrome (familial hypobetalipoproteinaemia).

Apo B and mRNA editing

The small gut elaborates the apo B-48 short form, consisting of the N-terminal 2152 amino acids of apo B-100 (Kane, 1983). Apo B-48 is synthesized by a novel post-transcriptional modification of the mRNA, referred to as mRNA editing (Chen *et al.*, 1987; Powell *et al.*, 1987; Teng *et al.*, 1993). This molecular mechanism deaminates a specific cytidine (nucleotide nt 6666) to form a uridine, resulting in the conversion of glutamine (CAA) into a premature stop codon (UAA) at codon 2153. APOBEC-1 (apo B mRNA-editing enzyme catalytic polypeptide 1) is the catalytic subunit of the apo B mRNA editing complex (Teng *et al.*, 1993). The mRNA editing occurs in the small intestine of mammals. It is also present in the livers of rats, mice, dogs and horses, where it is regulated by growth hormone, thyroxine, cortisol, fasting and diet (Baun *et al.*, 1990; Leighton *et al.*, 1990; Sjöberg *et al.*, 1992; Funahashi *et al.*, 1995). Overexpression of APOBEC-1 in the liver of transgenic animals lowers apo B-100 and LDL concentrations, and concomitantly results in liver dysplasia and hepatocellular carcinomas (Teng *et al.*, 1994). The latter observation severely compromises its potential use in gene therapy in order to reduce plasma LDL levels, thereby preventing atherosclerosis. Interestingly, both apo B-48 and apo B-100 have been revealed in subcellular compartments of human enterocytes of normal children (Levy *et al.*, 1990). It is not clear whether a substantial amount of apo B-100 escapes apo B mRNA editing.

Translational and translocational control of apo B expression

The transport of triglycerides in the form of chylomicrons by the intestine appears to be a very complex process similar to VLDL formation by the liver. Apo B-48 synthesis is an important prerequisite for the assembly and exocytosis of triglyceride-rich lipoproteins. Most acute stimuli of apolipoprotein production do not involve changes in transcription (Adeli *et al.*, 1995). Increasing evidence has been accumulating that apo B production is regulated translationally. For example, hepatic apo B production was shown to be reduced primarily in diabetic animals as a result of the impaired ribosome transit of apo B mRNA elongation or translation (Yamanaka *et al.*, 1995b). The regulation of apo B secretion may also be achieved by controlling the rate of translocation across the endoplasmic reticulum. A pause-transfer mechanism translocates apo B across the endoplasmic membrane, and protein chains blocked in the endoplasmic reticulum membrane increase intracellular degradation of apo B (Yamanaka *et al.*, 1995a). The intracellular degradative pathway regulates the proportion of apo B, which enters the secretory pathway.

Among a variety of factors modulating apo B secretion efficiency, the availability of lipids is the most important factor. In fact, the assembly of triglyceride-rich lipoproteins is likely to be achieved through two discrete steps (Boren *et al.*, 1994; Rustaeus *et al.*, 1995). During the first step of assembly, apo B is lipidated co-translationally and translocated across the endoplasmic reticulum membrane. The lipid content of the primordial lipoproteins is directly related to the length of apo B polypeptides (Boren *et al.*, 1992; Yao *et al.*, 1991). MTP plays an obligatory role in this initial stage of apo B lipidation (Wetterau *et al.*, 1997). Incorrect lipidation leads to increased degradation, probably because a protease cleavage site becomes exposed, resulting in a loss of the N-terminal globular domain of apo B (Adeli, 1994; Du *et al.*, 1994). In the second step, primordial lipoprotein particles acquire additional neutralipids to form mature lipoproteins (Yao *et al.*, 1991; Boren *et al.*, 1992). The recruitment of lipids at this stage does not seem to require MTP and is not governed by the length of apo B (Innerarity *et al.*, 1996).

Genetic abnormalities in apo B

Numerous and various mutations in the apo B gene affect plasma cholesterol levels and the phenotype segregates as an autosomal co-dominant trait (Table 10.3). Homozygotes display low-density lipoprotein (LDL) cholesterol in the lowest tenth percentile and heterozygotes present with their LDL cholesterol in the lowest fifth percentile. The homozygous form of familial hypocholesterolaemia shows excessive lipid retention in small-intestinal enterocytes and complete absence of the postprandial delivery of chylomicrons and VLDLs to the circulation (Farese *et al.*, 1992; Schonfeld, 1995).

Fat malabsorption is accompanied by steatorrhoea, red cell acanthocytosis, bleeding diathesis due to a vitamin K deficiency, atypical retinitis pigmentosa and progressive neurologic disease. The neurologic deficits appear to be related to vitamin E deficiency and may respond favourably to vitamin E therapy. Essential fatty acid deficiency is very often acquired and supplementation is recommended. Although most heterozygous patients have no symptoms, they can also present with signs of fat malabsorption and neurologic abnormalities. Sometimes young symptomatic heterozygous hypobetalipoproteinaemia patients have a transient inability to form apo B (Levy *et al.*, 1994).

Today, more than 25 different truncations of apo B have been identified (Young and Linton, 1991). They produce nonsense or frameshift mutations, resulting in the formation of a premature stop codon. Techniques of molecular genetics have helped define apo B defects that range from apo B-2 to apo B-89 (2–89 per cent of apo B-100 length). Truncations shorter than apo B-48 are likely to be produced in the intestine. However, the molecular defects and genetic aetiologies of many patients with hypolipoproteinaemia are unknown. Potential mechanisms are that truncated apo B may be synthesized at very low rates or removed rapidly from the plasma.

The development of transgenic mice and gene-targeted mice has provided new insights into the role of apo B-48 and apo B-100 in lipoprotein metabolism and familial hypobetalipoproteinaemia. An apo B-70 mouse was obtained by insertion of a large stretch of foreign DNA into exon 26 of the apo B gene (Kim and Young, 1998). The resulting lipoprotein profile was similar to that observed in human homozygotes with familial hypocholesterolaemia. Another mouse heterozygous for apo B was generated by inserting an apo B-83 mutation (Leu 3798 Stop) into the apo B gene. In addition to the Leu 3798 Stop mutation, the apo B-83-only allele contained a CTA-missense mutation and codon 2153, which abrogates apo B-48 formation (Kim and Young, 1998). Traces of apo B-83 were noted in the plasma, a profile very similar to the pattern observed in human familial hypocholesterolaemia heterozygotes with apo B-83 mutation (Kim and Young, 1998). Only the VLDL fraction contained apo B-83, which was virtually absent in LDL particles. A reduction of apo B-83 mRNA (76 per cent) and apo B-83 secretion (72 per cent) was found in hepatocytes of these mice. This mechanism may apply to familial hypocholesterolaemia.

It is noteworthy that the homozygosity for the apo B-83 caused lethal developmental abnormalities, including exencephalus, haemorrhaging from the brain into the amniotic fluid, growth retardation and herniation of the liver into the umbilical cord. Possibly a certain amount of apo B synthesis is required for normal mouse development.

MTP AND GENETIC DISORDERS

Physiological role of MTP

MTP is a heterodimeric protein composed of the multifunctional enzyme protein disulphide isomerase (PDI) of low molecular weight (58 kDa), and a unique 97-kDa large subunit (Wetterau *et al.*, 1997). While PDI has been revealed to be a ubiquitous protein, the large subunit confers lipid transfer activity to the complex (Wetterau *et al.*, 1997). Although PDI seems to maintain the large subunit in a soluble form and dissociation of the complex abolishes MTP activity (Wetterau *et al.*, 1997), its contribution to the transfer function is not known. MTP resides in the lumen of the endoplasmic reticulum of the intestine and liver (Gordon *et al.*, 1995) and functions in the loading of apo B with lipid. Evidence has been accumulating that the genetic loss of functioning MTP constitutes the basis of the human autosomal recessive abetalipoproteinaemia. MTP mutation of the gene localized on chromosome 4q22–24 was identified in both alleles of all individuals with abetalipoproteinaemia (Wetterau *et al.*, 1992). Confirmation was obtained with genetically engineered cell mutants. Coexpression of the large subunit of MTP with apo B in non-lipoprotein-producing cell lines (Hela, COS cells) was essential and sufficient for the assembly and secretion of apo B-containing lipoproteins in these cells (Gordon *et al.*, 1994; Lin *et al.*, 1995). The level of MTP influences lipoprotein production. Insulin and ethanol inhibit MTP gene transcription in HepG2 cells (Lin *et al.*, 1995) and an MTP inhibitor decreases apo B secretion in a dose-dependent manner (Jamil *et al.*, 1996). In contrast, high fat and sucrose diets increase hepatic MTP large subunit mRNA levels in the

Table 10.3 *Similarities and differences characterizing genetic disorders of intestinal fat transport*

Features	Abetalipoproteinaemia	Hypobetalipoproteinaemia	Chylomicron retention disease
Mandelian condition	Recessive	Dominant	Recessive
Molecular defect	MTP	Apo B	Unknown
Intestinal malabsorption	Severe	Severe	Severe
Failure to thrive (in early childhood)	Severe	Severe	Severe
Neuro-ophthalmic complications	Present	Present	Present
Deficiency of fat-soluble vitamins	Present	Present	Present
Deficiency of essential fatty acids	Present	Present	Present
Triglyceride	Very low	Very low	N
Cholesterol	Very low	Very low	Low
LDL-cholesterol	ND	ND	Low
HDL-cholesterol	Low	Low	Low
Apo A-I	Low	Low	Low
Apo B	ND	ND	Low
Triglyceride-rich lipoproteins			
CM	ND	ND	ND
VLDL	ND	ND	N

MTP, microsomal transfer protein; Apo, apolipoprotein; LDL, low-density lipoprotein; HDL, high-density lipoprotein; CM, chylomicron; VLDL, very-low-density lipoprotein; ND, not detectable; N, normal.

liver (55 per cent) and intestine (126 per cent) with a positive correlation with VLDL + LDL cholesterol or triglyceride concentrations in hamsters (Lin *et al.*, 1994). Saturated fat increased mRNA levels more than diets enriched in polyunsaturates in parallel with the rise of VLDL, LDL or HDL-cholesterol (Bennett *et al.*, 1995).

If these studies clearly indicate how essential MTP is in the processing of triglyceride-rich lipoproteins, the precise steps in lipoprotein assembly that are mediated by MTP remain less obvious. More investigation is necessary to determine whether MTP is actually involved in the first basal lipidation step in which apo B-48 undergoes an MTP-dependent co-translational lipidation to form a lipoprotein with HDL size. In a second step, these small particles are converted to large triglyceride-rich lipoproteins containing apo B-48 (chylomicrons/VLDL).

Abetalipoproteinaemia

The hallmark of this disease is the absence of apo B-containing lipoproteins, including chylomicrons from the small intestine and VLDL from the liver (Gordon *et al.*, 1995). Similarly, the LDL fraction that is derived from the catabolism of VLDL is virtually absent. As a result, plasma triglycerides are often unmeasurable, and practically all the plasma cholesterol is contained in HDL. Fat malabsorption is common and begins in infancy with steatorrhoea and poor weight gain. No increase in triglycerides over fasting levels is registered in response to a fat load (Levy *et al.*, 1988). Morphologic studies of the intestinal mucosa depict engorgement of enterocytes by large lipid droplets and the absence of chylomicrons from the cisternae of the Golgi apparatus.

Impaired absorption of fat-soluble vitamins (due to the inability to secrete chylomicrons) is responsible for several clinical features of abetalipoproteinaemia. Deficiencies of vitamins A and E and essential fatty acids account for the retinal and neurologic complications (Table 10.3). Indeed, the patients develop atypical retinitis pigmentosa and the loss of deep-tendon reflexes. This is followed by decreased distal lower extremity vibratory and proprioceptive senses and cerebellar signs, including dysmetria, ataxia and spastic gait. The high ratio of free cholesterol to phospholipids and the altered qualitative pattern of membrane phospholipids lead to acanthocytes of circulating red blood cells.

The intake of large doses of vitamin E, vitamin A and vitamin K may prevent, delay or stop the progression of neurologic and retinal lesions (Levy *et al.*, 1987b; Gordon *et al.*, 1995). The restriction of dietary triglycerides containing saturated long-chain fatty acids is recommended. Whereas the supplementation of essential fatty acids is encouraged (if tolerated), caution should be taken with medium-chain triglycerides in view of hepatic complications.

CHYLOMICRON RETENTION DISEASE

The examination of plasma of this disorder, also known as Anderson's disease, reveals apo B-100 containing particles of hepatic origin (Levy *et al.*, 1987a; Roy *et al.*, 1987; Pessah *et al.*, 1991). However, plasma levels of apo B, apo A-IV, LDL and HDL are all decreased in contrast to the normal plasma concentration of fasting triglycerides. Similarly, fat-soluble vitamins, especially A and E, are extremely low (Table 10.3).

Morphologic studies show fat particles vesiculating the endoplasmic reticulum and well-individualized chylomicron-size lipid structures within dilated vesicles in the Golgi complex. Absence of fat in the intercellular spaces and lacteals is consistent with the inability to secrete chylomicrons after oral fat load characteristic of this syndrome. The molecular defect does not appear to be related to apo B, since: (1) immunoperoxidase localization of apo B on fasting biopsies illustrates normal to elevated staining; (2) jejunal explants demonstrate the ability to synthesize apo B-48; and (3) the intestinal transcription of apo B-100 mRNA and its editing to apo B-48 mRNA seems to proceed at normal rates. Whether the defect in chylomicron retention disease involves the final assembly, modification or delivery of chylomicrons needs to be clarified.

As with abetalipoproteinaemia and homozygous hypobetalipoproteinaemia, chylomicron retention disease is rare. It appears to follow a recessive pattern of inheritance. However, this condition needs to be recognized early in view of its adverse effects on growth and neuro-ophthalmic complications. Deficiency of vitamin E and essential fatty acids is probably behind these abnormalities. In fact, patients treated with essential and medium-chain fats and fat-soluble vitamins normalize their symptoms.

DIAGNOSTIC EVALUATION

Following the clinical suspicion of fat malabsorption, laboratory tests are necessary to confirm the diagnosis, assess the severity and determine the underlying cause. One should establish whether malassimilation is due to abnormalities of intraluminal digestion or intramural absorption. Steatorrhoea will reveal the presence of a disorder involving the pancreas, biliary system or the small intestinal mucosa. An indication of possible steatorrhoea is obtained with a qualitative sudan stain. Quantitative faecal fat determination remains the most accurate method of evaluating fat absorption and providing a definitive diagnosis. Stools must be collected for 72 hours from the patient consuming 60–100 g fat/day. The ^{13}C-triolein breath test can also be used as a measure of fat absorption. Patients with altered lipid hydrolysis and absorption will develop altered carbon dioxide. This technique, however, may provide erroneous results in the presence of various diseases (diabetes, lung dysfunction, etc.).

D-Xylose test and small bowel radiographs may help distinguish between intraluminal and intramural disorders. Although high specificity and sensitivity have been reported, false-positive results may occur with the D-xylose test.

Pancreatic function is assessed by the secretin stimulation. The secretory capacity of the exocrine pancreas, bicarbonate concentration and enzyme output can be measured after a tube is placed in the duodenum adjacent to the ampullae of Vater.

The rapid deconjugation of bile acids by bacterial overgrowth limiting micellar solubilization and failed bile acid reabsorption is determined by the Schilling test for vitamin B_{12} or by the ^{13}C-labelled bile acid breath test. Finally, a small intestinal biopsy represents the key to clarifying unexplained malabsorption.

CONCLUSIONS

Tremendous progress has been made in understanding the complex series of events governing the processes of digestion and absorption. The resulting huge knowledge allows us to establish whether steatorrhoea is associated with defects in luminal or intracellular processes. Tools are available for laboratory diagnosis and efficient treatment.

DIGESTION AND ABSORPTION OF PROTEINS

SOURCE OF PROTEINS

Dietary proteins are the major source of amino acids, some of which are essential because they cannot be synthesized in the body. This group of essential amino acids includes histidine, isoleucine, leucine, lysine, methionine, phenylalanine, threonine, tryptophan and valine. For infants, histidine is also indispensable for growth and recent studies report its requirement for total parental nutrition.

Western diets provide about 10–15 per cent of energy intake in the form of proteins and the WHO/FAO/UNO (1995) set the daily adult protein requirement as 0.75 g/kg body weight. However, the requirement is much greater for infants, children and pregnant women, since a nitrogen balance is positive in view of tissue growth. In general, protein quality is determined by its amino-acid composition, capacity to support growth and digestibility. Plant proteins are less digestible than animal proteins (Linder, 1991). Proteins consumed in the diet are enzymatically hydrolysed in the alimentary

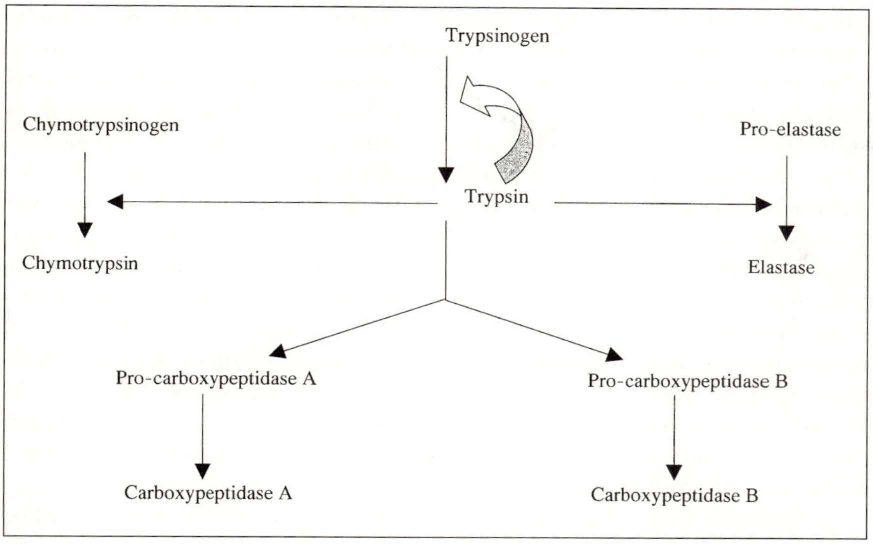

Figure 10.3 *Activation of pancreatic proteolytic enzymes.*

tract. A series of complex interactive and complementary steps, beginning in the stomach and ending with the transport of digestive products from the small intestine epithelium, assures the assimilation of dietary proteins.

Gastric phase of digestion

Digestion of proteins begins in the stomach, where chief cells secrete pepsin as pepsinogen, an inactive precursor form. Effectors, such as gastrin, histamine, and cholinergic excitation stimulate pepsinogen release (Samloff, 1981). The conversion of pepsinogen to pepsin is initiated in an acidic milieu and completed by autoactivation with the formation of the first, active pepsin molecules.

Pepsins are, in fact, a family of proteolytic enzymes presenting distinct electrophoretic and immunologic properties. The acid pH is necessary not only for the activation of their analogous pepsinogens, but also for their optimal gastric activity. Even if activated pepsins hydrolyse proteins into polypeptides of diverse size, their involvement in protein digestion does not appear essential. Subjects with total gastrectomy, decreased gastric emptying, pyloroplasty or pernicious anaemia with achlorhydria assimilate protein normally.

Small intestine: intraluminal phase of digestion

On entering the small bowel, gastric protein content is attacked by proteolytic enzymes from the pancreas and the intestinal mucosa. Pancreatic enzymes are also secreted in an inactivated precursor form (zymogen or pro-enzyme), which becomes activated after the loss of a small part of their peptide chains. The removal of the N-terminal hexapeptide from trypsinogen is catalysed by the enterokinase, a brush-border membrane enteropeptidase located in the duodenum and proximal jejunum (Nordstrom, 1972). This process in turn is followed by a cascade of activation of the other pancreatic proenzymes, initiated by the action of trypsin (Fig. 10.3). Among these proteases, there are endopeptidases and exopeptidases. The endopeptidases include trypsin, chymotrypsin and elastase, and act inside the protein molecule to produce oligopeptides (2–6 amino acid residues in length). On the other hand, exopeptidases include carboxypeptidases A and B. They cleave the terminal bond of the protein, releasing a single amino acid. The enzymes have an optimum pH of 8.0. All the proteolytic enzymes successively split peptide bonds selected on their amino-acid affinity. The whole cooperative activity yields polypeptides of six or fewer amino-acid residues together with neutral and basic amino acids. Overall, luminal protein digestion produces 70 per cent oligopeptides and 30 per cent amino acids (Nixon and Mawer, 1970).

Mucosal phase of digestion

Peptidases located in the small bowel epithelium are capable of continuing the hydrolysis of small peptides. They are composed of two groups, brush border and cytosol enzymes, differing in their physicochemical and immunochemical features (Kim *et al.*, 1972; Noren *et al.*, 1977; Tobey *et al.*, 1985).

BRUSH-BORDER PEPTIDASES

These enzymes are associated with villus but not crypt epithelial cells, and are attached to the outer surface of the microvillous membrane of the enterocyte. There are at least seven brush-border peptidases, which appear to be unique to the human small bowel: three aminopeptidases displaying a specificity for peptides or amino acids at the amino terminus; two carboxypeptidases releasing peptides or amino acids from the carboxy terminus; γ-glutamyl transpeptidase splitting γ-glutamyl peptide bonds, with the transfer of the γ-glutamyl group to another amino acid to form a γ-glutamyl amino acid or peptide derivative, and finally one or two endopeptidases (Alpers, 1987). As much as 90 per cent of the total mucosal peptidehydrolase activity for peptides with four amino acids and more is found in the brush border, which contained only 10 per cent dipeptidases. The brush-border membrane hydrolysis rate is most rapid for tripeptides, slowest for dipeptides and intermediate for tetrapeptides and pentapeptides. Each specific peptidase is synthesized in the rough endoplasmic reticulum (100 000 Da), transferred to the Golgi apparatus and transported to the brush-border membrane, where it is inserted by exocytic fusion (Ahnen *et al.*, 1983; Danielsen *et al.*, 1984). After post-translational processing, it remains linked to the brush-border membrane by short hydrophobic pieces (3000–4500 Da).

CYTOSOLIC PEPTIDASES

Many dietary dipeptides and tripeptides are absorbed intact and are split within the enterocyte by cytosolic peptide hydrolases, which do not make direct contact with the luminal content. These enzymes are not specific for the intestine since they have been found in various tissues. About 90 per cent of the dipeptidases are found in the cytoplasm with only a limited proportion of peptidases capable of hydrolysing oligopeptides with a chain length greater than three amino acids. Cytoplasmic dipeptidases are optimally active at alkaline pH 7.5–8.0. They depend on Mn^{2+} or Zn^{2+}, and are much more heat labile than brush-border membrane hydrolases. Three types of cytoplasmic peptidases have been reported: dipeptidases, aminopeptidase and proline dipeptidase. The complementarity of proteolytic steps on the brush border and within the cytosol of the surface epithelial cell is evident regarding the peptide length. Brush-border hydrolases split the oligopeptides of six or fewer amino acids produced by pancreatic digestion, and cytosolic hydrolases hydrolyse tripeptides and dipeptides into amino acids, which ultimately enter the portal circulation. The complementary action of these enzymes is striking, as well, with respect to the peptide site at which hydrolysis occurs.

Absorption

AMINO ACIDS

The end products of protein digestion are absorbed through the mucosal cells of the small intestine. As mentioned before, hydrolysis of a small proportion of dietary peptides into free amino acids occurs prior to absorption. The transport of these amino acids into the mucosa involves energy-dependent carrier proteins sited on villous enterocytes. In this process, absorption is initiated by coupling the amino acid and Na^+ to the protein carrier at the luminal surface, transferring them across the microvillus membrane and releasing them within the enterocyte. An active Na^+ pump at the basolateral membrane maintains a low intracellular Na^+ concentration and, thereby, provides an electrochemical gradient for Na^+, which maintains the Na^+-amino acid coupled transport. The transporters remain ill-defined in view of their overlapping specificities. For example, four active processes for the transport of neutral amino acids across the apical cell membrane have been identified (Hopfer, 1987). There are at least three group-specific membrane carrier systems for neutral, basic and acidic amino acids. There is also some evidence to suggest that other sodium-independent, facilitated amino-acid transport systems are present in the enterocyte on both the microvillus and basolateral membrane.

PEPTIDES

Specific protein carriers transport dipeptides and tripeptides, which are further hydrolysed by cytosolic enzymes before transport of the amino acids into the portal circulation. The absorption appears to occur by active transport, which is mediated by specific carrier proteins. Tripeptides as well as dipeptides can be transported intact across the small intestinal wall and their transport is generally more efficient than the absorption of individual amino acids. Nevertheless, some tripeptides have to be hydrolysed at the brush border before absorption. In the human intestine, the uptake of GlyLeu (glycine-leucine peptide) has been shown to be competitively inhibited by a large variety of dipeptides *in vitro*, suggesting that there is only one peptide carrier that accepts a wide variety of peptides (Das and Radhakrishnan, 1975). The presence of luminal glucose, acidification of the D-isomers of amino acids, and the short length of amino-acid side chains lower the affinity for the transport system. Furthermore, single amino-acid absorption is able to inhibit dipeptide and tripeptide uptake, which indicates a separate transporter system for amino acids and tripeptides.

PROTEIN MALABSORPTION

Protein malabsorption may have severe consequences, such as oedema and diminished muscle mass. Evidently, impaired protein synthesis from liver diseases and excessive protein loss in renal disease will further aggravate protein deficiencies. The immune system, which depends upon adequate protein supply, will weaken, resulting in recurrent infections.

Trypsin

Absent trypsin, chymotrypsin and carboxypeptidase activity were found in two unrelated children who presented in infancy with severe growth failure, hypoproteinaemia, and oedema (Townes *et al.*, 1967). With the addition of exogenous trypsin, the activity of these enzymes reverted to normal, emphasizing the deficiency of trypsin alone and the requirement of active trypsin for the conversion of chymotrypsinogen and carboxypeptidase into full active forms. Growth failure and oedema were corrected with the introduction of predigested proteins.

Congenital enterokinase deficiency

Primary enterokinase absence is a very rare disease. It results in marked malabsorption of protein with generalized oedema, vomiting and loose stools. These clinical features occur shortly after birth and include impaired development and growth (Lebenthal *et al.*, 1976; Ghishan *et al.*, 1983). Given the inability of trypsinogen to be converted into active trypsin, which in turn activates other pro-enzymes, hypoproteinaemia and anaemia develop. Vitamin B_{12} malabsorption is probably due to the lack of proteolytic enzymes needed for the hydrolysis of vitamin B_{12} from R proteins, enabling its attachment to intrinsic factor (Mann *et al.*, 1984). It is possible to improve vitamin B_{12} concentrations after pancreatic replacement therapy.

Congenital defects in the absorption of amino acids

Specific congenital defects in peptide digestion and absorption have not been observed, probably because more than one transport system is available for these molecules. Thus, people with abnormal peptide transporters may remain undiagnosed. In contrast, specific absorption defects affect amino acids.

CYSTINURIA

This heritable autosomal disorder of cystine, lysine, arginine and ornithine affects the epithelial cells of the gastrointestinal tract and renal tubules. The prevalence of the disorder is variable. It is estimated at 1 in 100 000 in Sweden, 1 in 20 000 in England and 1 in 2500 in Israeli Jews of Libyan origin (McCutcheon and Race, 1962). The disease is characterized by the formation of calculi in the urinary tract, sometimes accompanied by obstruction infections and renal insufficiency. Heterozygous and homozygous subjects excrete the dibasic amino acids in higher quantities than normal. Cystic and uric acid stones form readily and a simple diagnostic procedure involves the microscopy of urinary sediment and typical cystine crystals. Improvement is obtained with dietary restriction, decreasing cystine production and excretion, increased cystine solubility, and conversion of cystine to a more soluble compound.

HARTNUP DISORDER

Hartnup disorder is a genetic defect in neutral amino acid (*see* Table 10.4) transport across the intestinal and renal epithelium. The disorder is transmitted as an autosomal recessive trait. The disease is characterized by renal neutral hyperaminoaciduria and a defect in the intestinal absorption of free amino acids (not linked by a peptide bond) (Newman *et al.*, 1988). Some individuals with Hartnup disorder develop an unusual combination of a photosensitive rash and neuropsychiatric manifestations. There is an amelioration of the rash, ataxia and psychotic-type behaviour with nicotinic acid or nitotinamide treatment. Furthermore, a high-protein diet is beneficial for patients with low plasma amino-acid values.

LYSINURIC PROTEIN INTOLERANCE

Inheritance follows a pattern of autosomal recessive disease, such as 1 in 60 000 in Finland (Simell, 1995).

Table 10.4 *Types of amino acids*

Acidic	
Aspartic acid	Side chains negatively charged at physiological pH
Glutamic acid	
Basic	
Lysine	Side chains positively charged at physiological pH
Arginine	
Neutral	
Essential	
e.g. tryptophan, leucine, methionine	Cannot be synthesized by the body and must be ingested. (No charge on their side chains)
Non-essential	
e.g. serine, glycine, alanine	Normally synthesized by the body
Dibasic	
Arginine	Contains two amino groups

The defect has been localized to the basolateral membranes of the intestine and kidney for the transport of basic and dibasic amino acids, such as arginine, ornithine and lysine (*see* Table 10.4). As a direct consequence, ornithine deficiency and increased turnaround of the urea cycle occur. Hyperammonaemia has also been reported. Nausea, vomiting and mild diarrhoea appear at birth or shortly after weaning. Then, infants develop failure to thrive, marked muscular hypotonia and hepatosplenomegaly. Later, osteoporosis becomes evident and patients experience fractures. Since lysine is an integral part of most proteins in the body, its defective intestinal absorption and increased renal excretion result in the aforementioned disorders and organ abnormalities. Urinary excretion of lysine is massively increased, whereas that of arginine and ornithine is moderately increased. Very often, plasma concentrations of lysine, arginine and ornithine are decreased, while the levels of serine, glycine, citrulline, proline, alanine and glutamine are elevated. Blood ammonium is also elevated after regular meals.

Treatment of lysinuric protein intolerance consists of protein restriction and supplementation with oral citrulline, a third urea cycle intermediate that is efficiently absorbed by the intestine and metabolized into arginine. Thus it is able to abolish hyperammonaemia in patients with lysinuria.

OTHER CONGENITAL AMINO-ACID DEFECTS

These disorders include iminoglycinuria (Chesney, 1985), blue diaper syndrome (Drummond *et al.*, 1964), oasthouse syndrome (Hooft *et al.*, 1965) and Lowe's oculocerebrorenal syndrome (Wadelius *et al.*, 1989). All are characterized by the impairment of the intestinal transport of specific amino acids: proline, hydroxyproline and glycine in iminoglycinuria; tryptophan in blue diaper syndrome; methionine in oasthouse syndrome (methionine malabsorption syndrome, in which the urine has a characteristic odour resembling that of the interior of an oasthouse due to the formation of α-hydroxybutyric acid by bacterial action on the unabsorbed methionine); and lysine and arginine in Lowe's oculocerebrorenal syndrome.

SECONDARY MALDIGESTION AND MALABSORPTION OF PROTEINS

In diffuse diseases of the small bowel, acquired enterokinase deficiency may be responsible for functional pancreatic insufficiency, resulting in maldigestion and malabsorption. Patients with coeliac sprue develop pancreatic insufficiency and need pancreatic replacement therapy in addition to a gluten-free diet (Wadelius *et al.*, 1989). Since bile acids are important in the activation of trypsinogen by enterokinase, conditions leading to abnormal biliary output disturb enterokinase activity. Examples of this category are impaired release of secretin and cholecystokinin, chronic cholestasis and gastrectomy. Furthermore, protein malabsorption results from pancreatic insufficiency (chronic pancreatitis, cystic fibrosis, pancreatic cancer and pancreatectomy). The treatment includes dietary management and pancreatic enzyme supplementation.

CONCLUSIONS

In this section, the digestion of proteins and the intestinal transport of amino acids have been reviewed. Several issues have been addressed, including the mechanisms behind protein malabsorption, the clinical assessment of patients with impaired absorption, the description of the tests available for investigation and the general principles of management. It should be emphasized that relatively few inherited defects have been reported because of the redundant processes of protein assimilation. As with carbohydrate malabsorption, specific diseases cause acquired disorders that occur at different steps of protein assimilation, such as exocrine pancreatic insufficiency (cystic fibrosis, pancreatitis malignancy), small intestine mucosa damage (coeliac disease), and defects in portal and lymphatic flow. Tests of protein absorption are rarely used to confirm the diagnosis of protein malabsorption, and are reserved only for the patients with protein-losing enteropathy.

REFERENCES

Adeli, K. 1994: Regulated intracellular degradation of apolipoprotein B in semipermeable HepG2 cells. *Journal of Biological Chemistry* 269, 9166–75.

Adeli, K., Mohammadi, A., Macri, J. 1995: Regulation of apolipoprotein B biogenesis in human hepatocytes: posttranscriptional control mechanisms that determine the hepatic production of apolipoprotein B-containing lipoproteins. *Clin Biochim* 28, 123–30.

Ahnen, D.J., Mircheff, A.K., Santiago, N.A. *et al.* 1983: Intestinal surface amino-oligopeptidase. Distinct molecular forms during assembly in intracellular membranes in vivo. *Journal of Biological Chemistry* 258, 5960–6.

Ahrens, E.H., Jr 1957: Nutritional factors and serum lipid levels. *American Journal of Medicine* 23, 928–52.

Alpers, D.H. 1987: Digestion and absorption of carbohydrates and proteins. In Johnson, L.R. (ed.) *Physiology of the gastrointestinal tract*, 2nd edn. New York: Raven Press, 1469.

Alpers, D.H. 1994: Digestion and absorption of

carbohydrates and proteins. In Johnson, L.R. (ed.) *Physiology of the gastrointestinal tract*, 3rd edn. New York: Raven Press, 1723–46.

Andersson, D.E.H., Nygren, A. 1978: Four cases of long-standing diarrhea and colic pains cured by fructose free diet. *Acta Medica Scandinavica* 203, 87–92.

Antonowicz, I., Lebenthal, E. 1977: Developmental pattern of small intestinal enterokinase and disaccharidase activity in the human fetus. *Gastroenterology* 72, 1299–303.

Antonowicz, I., Chang, S.K., Grand, R.J. 1974: Development and distribution of lysosomal enzymes and disaccharidases in human fetal intestine. *Gastroenterology* 67, 51–8.

Armand, M., Borel, P., Dubois, C. *et al.* 1994: Characterization of emulsions and lipolysis of dietary lipids in the human stomach. *American Journal of Physiology* 226 (*Gastrointestinal and Liver Physiology* 29), G372–81.

Auricchio, S., Ciccimara, F., Rubino, A. *et al.* 1968: Studies on intestinal digestion of starch in man. III. The absorption coefficient of starch in infants and children. *Enzymol Biol Clin* 9, 321–7.

Balart, L.A., Ferrante, W.A. 1982: Pathophysiology of acute and chronic pancreatitis. *Archives of Internal Medicine* 42, 113–17.

Balistreri, W.F., Heubi, J.E., Suchy, F.J. 1983: Bile acid metabolism: relationship of bile acid malabsorption and diarrhea. *Journal of Pediatric Gastroenterology and Nutrition* 2, 105–21.

Baun, C.L., Teng, B.-B., Davidson, N.O. 1990: Apolipoprotein B messenger RNA editing in the rat liver. Modulation by fasting and refeeding a high carbohydrate diet. *Journal of Biological Chemistry* 265, 19263–70.

Beeken, W. 1973: Absorptive defects in young people with regional enteritis. *Pediatrics* 52, 69–74.

Bell, R.R., Draper, H.H., Bergan, J.G. 1973: Sucrose, lactose, and glucose tolerance in northern Alaskan Eskimos. *American Journal of Clinical Nutrition* 26, 1185–90.

Belli, D.C., Levy, E., Darling, P. *et al.* 1987: Taurine improves the absorption of a fat meal in cystic fibrosis patients. *Pediatrics* 80, 517–23.

Bennett, A.J., Billett, M.A., Salter, A.M. *et al.* 1995: Regulation of hamster hepatic MTP mRNA levels by dietary fats. *Biochemical and Biophysical Research Communications* 212, 473–8.

Bennett Clark, S., Tercyak, A.M. 1984: Reduced cholesterol transmucosal transport in rats inhibited mucosal acyl CoA:cholesterol acyltransferase and normal pancreatic function. *Journal of Lipid Resarch* 25, 148–59.

Bernback, S., Blackberg, L., Hernell, O. 1990: The complete digestion of human milk triacylglycerol in vitro requires gastric lipase, pancreatic colipase-dependent lipase, and bile salt-stimulated lipase. *Journal of Clinical Investigation* 85, 1221–6.

Björkhem, I., Boberg, K.M. 1995: Inborn errors in bile acid biosynthesis and storage of sterols other than cholesterol. In Scriven, G.R., Beaudet, A.L., Sly, W.S., Valle, D. (eds) *The Metabolic and Molecular Bases of Inherited Disease,* 7th edn. New York: McGraw-Hill, 2073–99.

Black, D.D. 1995: Intestinal lipoprotein metabolism. *Journal of Pediatric Gastroenterology and Nutrition* 20, 125–47.

Booth, I.W., Patel, P.B., Sule, D. *et al.* 1988: Glucose-galactose malabsorption: demonstration of specific jejunal brush border membrane defect. *Gut* 29, 1661–5.

Boren, J., Graham, L., Wettesten, M. *et al.* 1992: The assembly and secretion of apo B 100-containing lipoproteins in Hep G2 cells. Apo B 100 is cotranslationally integrated into lipoproteins. *Journal of Biological Chemistry* 267, 9858–67.

Boren, J., Rustaeus, S., Olofsson, S.-O. 1994: Studies on the assembly of apolipoprotein B-100 and B-48 containing very low density lipoproteins in McA-RH7777 cells. *Journal of Biological Chemistry* 269, 25879–88.

Borgström, B. 1980: Importance of phospholipids, pancreatic phospholipase A_2 and fatty acid for the digestion of dietary fat. *Gastroenterology* 78, 954–62.

Büller, H.A., Grand, R.J. 1990: Lactose intolerance. *Annual Review of Medicine* 41, 141–8.

Burant, C.F., Takeda, J., Brot-Laroche, E. *et al.* 1992: Fructose transporter in human spermatozoa and small intestine is GLUT 5. *Journal of Biological Chemistry* 267, 14523–6.

Carey, M.C., Small, D.M. 1970: The characteristics of mixed micellar solutions with particular reference to man. *American Journal of Medicine* 49, 590–608.

Carey, M.C., Small, D.M. 1972: Micelle formation by bile salts. *Archives of Internal Medicine* 130, 506–27.

Cheeseman, C.I. 1993: GLUT2 is the transporter for fructose across the rat intestinal basolateral membrane. *Gastroenterology* 105, 1050–6.

Chen, S.-H., Habib, G., Yang, C.-Y. *et al.* 1987: Apolipoprotein B-48 is the product of a messenger RNA with an organ-specific in-frame stop codon. *Science* 238, 363–6.

Cheng, S.H., Stanley, M.M. 1959: Secretion of cholesterol by intestinal mucosa in patients with complete common bile duct obstruction. *Proceedings of the Society for Experimental Biology and Medicine* 48, 223–5.

Chesney, R.W. 1985: Iminoglycinuria. In Scriver, C.R., Beaudet, A.L., Sly, W.S., Valle, D. (eds) *The metabolic basis of inherited disease*, 7th edn. New York: McGraw-Hill, 3643–53.

Collins, J., Candy, D.C.A., Starkey, W.G., Spencer, A.J., Osborne, M.P., Stephen, J. 1990: Disaccharidase activities in small intestine of rotavirus-infected suckling mice: a histochemical study. *Journal of Pediatric Gastroenterology and Nutrition* 11, 395–403.

Dahlqvist, A., Lindberg, T. 1965: Fetal development of the small intestinal disaccharidase and alkaline phosphatase in the human. *Biology of the Neonate* 9, 24–32.

Dahlqvist, A., Auricchio, S., Semenza, G. *et al.* 1963: Human intestinal disaccharidases and hereditary disaccharide intolerance: the hydrolysis of sucrose, isomaltose, palatinose (isomaltulose), and a 1,6-α-oligosaccharide (isomalto-oligosaccharide) preparation. *Journal of Clinical Investigation* 42, 556–62.

Danielsen, E.M., Skovbjerg, H., Noren, O. *et al.* 1981: Biosynthesis of intestinal proteins. Nature of precursor forms of microvillar enzymes from Na^{2+}-precipitated enterocyte membranes. *FEBS Letters* 132, 197–200.

Danielsen, E.M., Cowell, G.M., Noren, O. *et al.* 1984: Biosynthesis of microvillar proteins. *Biochemical Journal* 221, 1–14.

Das, M., Radhakrishnan, A.N. 1975: Studies on a wide-spectrum intestinal dipeptide uptake system in the monkey and in the human. *Biochemical Journal* 146, 133–9.

Davidson, N.O. 1994: Cellular and molecular mechanisms of small intestinal lipid transport. In Johnson, L.R. (ed.) *Physiology of the gastrointestinal tract*, 3rd edn. New York: Raven Press, 1909–34.

Davidson, N.O., Hausman, A.M.L., Ifkovits, C.A. *et al.* 1992: Human intestinal transporter expression and localization of GLUT 5. *American Journal of Physiology* 262, C795–800.

Debnam, E.S., Levin, R.J. 1975: An experimental method of identifying and quantifying the active transfer of electrogenic component from the diffuse component during sugar absorption measured in vivo. *Journal of Physiology (London)* 246, 181–96.

Donner, J., Spink, C.H., Borgström, B. *et al.* 1976: Interactions between pancreatic lipase, colipase and taurodeoxycholate in the absence of triglyceride substrate. *Biochemistry* 15, 5413–17.

Drummond, K., Michael, A.F., Ulstrom, R.A. 1964: The blue diaper syndrome: familial hypercalcemia with nephrocalcinosis and indicanuria. *American Journal of Medicine* 37, 928–48.

Du, E.Z., Kurth, J., Wang, S.-L. *et al.* 1994: Proteolysis-coupled secretion of the N-terminus of apolipoprotein B: characterization of a transient, translocation-arrested intermediate. *Journal of Biological Chemistry* 269, 24169–76.

Dyer, J., Scott, D., Beechey, R.B. *et al.* 1994: Dietary regulation of intestinal glucose transport. In Lentze, M.J., Grand, R.J., Naim, H.Y. (eds) *Mammalian brush-border membrane proteins*, Part 2. Stuttgart, New York: Thieme Verlag, 65–72.

Ellestad-Sayad, J.J., Haworth, J.C., Hildes, J.A. 1978: Disaccharide malabsorption and dietary pattern in two Canadian Eskimo communities. *American Journal of Clinical Nutrition* 31, 1473–8.

Elsas, L.J., Hillman, R.E., Patterson, J.H. *et al.* 1970: Renal and intestinal hexose transport in familial glucose-galactose malabsorption. *Journal of Clinical Investigation* 49, 576–85.

Farese, R.V., Jr, Linton, M.F., Young, S.G. 1992: Apolipoprotein B gene mutations affecting cholesterol levels. *Journal of International Medicine* 231, 643–52.

Field, F.J., Albright, E., Mathur, S.N. 1987: Regulation of cholesterol esterification by micellar cholesterol in Caco-2 cells. *Journal of Lipid Research* 28, 1057–66.

Frank, G., Brunner, J., Hauser, H. *et al.* 1978: The hydrophobic anchor of small-intestinal sucrase-isomaltase. *FEBS Letters* 96, 183–8.

Fransen, J.A.M., Hauri, H.P., Ginsel, L.A. *et al.* 1991: Naturally occurring mutations in intestinal sucrase-isomaltase provide evidence for the existence of an intracellular sorting signal in the isomaltase subunit. *Journal of Cell Biology* 115, 45–57.

Freeman, T.C., Wood, I.S., Sirinathsinghji, D.J.S. *et al.* 1993: The expression of Na^+ glucose co-transporter (SGLT1) gene in lamb small intestine during postnatal development. *Biochimica et Biophysica Acta* 1146, 203–12.

Funahashi, T., Giannoni, F., DePaoli, A.M. *et al.* 1995: Tissue-specific, developmental and nutritional regulation of the gene encoding the catalytic subunit of the rat apolipoprotein B mRNA editing enzyme: functional role in the modulation of apo B mRNA editing. *Journal of Lipid Research* 36, 414–28.

Gaskin, K.J., Waters, D., Dorney, S. *et al.* 1988: Liver disease and common-bile-duct stenosis in cystic fibrosis. *New England Journal of Medicine* 318, 340–6.

Ghishan, F.K., Lee, P.C., Lebenthal, E. *et al.* 1983: Isolated congenital enterokinase deficiency. *Gastroenterology* 85, 727–31.

Gleeson, D., Boyer, J.L. 1991: Intrahepatic cholestasis. In McIntyre, N., Benhamou, J.-P., Bircher, J., Rizzette, M., Rodes, J. (eds) *Oxford textbook of clinical hepatology*. 1087–107.

Gordon, D.A., Jamil, H., Sharp, D. *et al.* 1994: Secretion of apolipoprotein B-containing lipoproteins from HeLa cells is dependent on expression of the microsomal triglyceride transfer protein and is regulated by lipid availability. *Proceedings of the National Academy of Sciences USA* 91, 7628–32.

Gordon, D.A., Wetterau, J., Gregg, R.E. 1995: Microsomal triglyceride transfer protein: a protein complex required for the assembly of lipoprotein particles. *Trends in Cell Biology* 268, 22794–801.

Gordon, J.I., Lowe, J.B. 1985: Analyzing the structures, functions and evolution of two abundant gastrointestinal fatty acid-binding proteins with recombinant DNA and computational techniques. *Chemistry and Physics of Lipids* 38, 137.

Gracey, M., Burke, V., Oshin, A. 1972: Active intestinal transport of D-fructose. *Biochimica et Biophysica Acta* 266, 397–406.

Gray, G.M. 1981: Carbohydrate absorption and malabsorption. In Johnson, L.R. (ed.) *Physiology of the gastrointestinal tract*. New York: Raven Press, 1063–72.

Gudmand-Høyer, E., Busk, H.E. 1975: Laktose malabsorption hos fremmedarbejdere. *Ugeskr Laeger* 137, 1584–5.

Gudmand-Høyer, E., Jarnum, S. 1970: Incidence and clinical significance of lactose malabsorption in ulcerative colitis and Crohn's disease. *Gut* 11, 338–43.

Gudmand-Høyer, E., Fenger, H.J., Kern-Hansen, P. *et al.* 1987: Sucrase deficiency in Greenland. *Scandinavian Journal of Gastroenterology* 22, 24–8.

Gudmand-Høyer, E., Fenger, H.J., Skovbjerg, H. *et al.* 1988: Trehalase deficiency in Greenland. *Scandinavian Journal of Gastroenterology* 23, 775–8.

Hamosh, A., Corey, M. 1993: Correlation between genotype and phenotype in patients with cystic fibrosis. *New England Journal of Medicine* 329, 1308–15.

Hamosh, M., Scanlon, J.W., Ganot, D. *et al.* 1981: Fat digestion in the newborn: characterization of lipid gastric aspirates of premature and term infants. *Journal of Clinical Investigation* 67, 838–46.

Harvey, C.B., Pratt, W.S., Islam, I. *et al.* 1995: DNA polymorphisms in the lactase gene: linkage disequilibrium across the 70-kb region. *European Journal of Human Genetics* 3, 27–41.

Hauri, H.P., Sterchi, E.E., Bienz, D. *et al.* 1986: Expression and intracellular transport of microvillus membrane hydrolases in human intestinal epithelial cell. *Journal of Cell Biology* 101, 838–51.

Havel, R.J. 1987: Lipid transport function of lipoproteins in blood plasma. *American Journal of Physiology* 253, E1–5.

Hediger, M.A., Turk, E., Wright, E. 1989a: Homology of the human intestinal Na^+ glucose and E. coli Na^+/proline cotransporters. *Proceedings of the National Academy of Sciences USA* 86, 5748–52.

Hediger, M.A., Budarf, M., Emanuel, B. *et al.* 1989b: Assignment of the human intestinal Na^+ glucose cotransporter gene SGLT1 of the q11.2 $\rightarrow$ qter region of chromosome 22. *Genomics* 4, 297–300.

Heubi, J.E., Balistreri, W.F., Fondacaro, J.D. *et al.* 1982: Primary bile acid malabsorption: defective *in vitro* ileal active bile acid transport. *Gastroenterology* 83, 804–11.

Hofmann, A.F. 1989: Enterohepatic circulation of bile acids. In Schul, S.G. (ed.) *Handbook of physiology. Section on the gastrointestinal system*. Bethesda, MD: American Physiological Society, 567–96.

Hofmann, A.F. 1993: The enterohepatic circulation of bile acids in health and disease. In Steisenger, M.H., Fordtran, J.S. (eds) *Gastrointestinal disease: pathophysiology, diagnosis, management*, 5th edn. Philadelphia: WB Saunders, 127–50.

Hofmann, A.F. 1994: Intestinal absorption of bile acids and biliary constituents: the intestinal component of the enterohepatic circulation and the integrated system. In Johnson, L.R. (ed.) *Physiology of the gastrointestinal tract.* New York: Raven Press, 1845–65.

Hooft, C., Timmermans, J., Snoeck, J., Antener, I., Oyaert, W., Van den Hende, C. 1965: Methionine malabsorption syndrome. *Annals of Paediatrics and International Review of Pediatrics* 205, 73–104.

Hopfer, U. 1987: Membrane transport mechanisms for hexose and amino acids in the small intestine. In Johnson, L.R. (ed.) *Physiology of the gastrointestinal tract*, 2nd edn. New York: Raven Press, 1499–526.

Howles, P.N., Carter, C.P., Hui, D.Y. 1996: Dietary free and esterified cholesterol absorption in cholesterol esterase (bile salt-stimulated lipase) gene-targeted mice. *Journal of Biological Chemistry* 271, 7196–7202.

Ihse, I., Arnesjö, B. 1973: The phospholipase A_2 activity of human small intestinal contents. *Acta Chemica Scandinavica* 27, 2749–56.

Innerarity, T.L., Boren, J., Yamanaka, S. *et al.* 1996: Biosynthesis of apolipoprotein B48-containing lipoproteins. Regulation by novel post-transcriptional mechanisms. *Journal of Biological Chemistry* 271, 2353–6.

Isenberg, J.I., Walsh, J.H., Grossman, M.I. 1973: Zollinger–Ellison syndrome. *Gastroenterology* 65, 140–65.

Jacobson, P.W., Wiesenfeld, P.W., Gallo, L.L. 1990: Sodium cholate-induced changes in the conformation of activity of rat pancreatic cholesterol esterase. *Journal of Biological Chemistry* 265, 515–21.

Jamil, H., Gordon, D.A., Eustice, D.C. *et al.* 1996: An inhibitor of the microsomal triglyceride transfer protein inhibits apo B secretion from HepG2 cells. *Proceedings of the National Academy of Sciences USA* 93, 11991–5.

Jonas, A., Diver-Haber, A., Avigad, S. 1986: Well-compensated primary bile acid malabsorption presenting as chronic nonspecific diarrhea. *Journal of Pediatric Gasteroenterology and Nutrition* 5, 143–6.

Jönsson, K.A., Bodemar, G. 1990: Low activities of disaccharidases associated with inflamed duodenal bulb mucosa. *Hepatogastroenterology* 37, 217–22.

Kam, N.T.P., Albright, E., Mathur, S.N. *et al.* 1989: Inhibition of acylcoenzyme A:cholesterol acyltransferase activity in Caco-2 cells results in intracellular triglyceride accumulation. *Journal of Lipid Research* 30, 371–7.

Kam, N.T.P., Albright, E., Mathus, S. *et al.* 1990: Effect of lovastatin on acyl-CoA:cholesterol O-acyltransferase (ACAT) activity and the basolateral-membrane secretion of newly synthesized lipids by Caco-2 cells. *Biochemical Journal* 272, 427–33.

Kane, J.P. 1983: Apolipoprotein B: structural and metabolic heterogeneity. *Annual Review of Physiology* 45, 637–50.

Kerry, K.R., Townley, R.R.W. 1965: Genetic aspects of intestinal sucrase-isomaltase deficiency. *Australian Paediatric Journal* 1(4): 223–35.

Kim, E., Young, S.G. 1998: Genetically modified mice for the study of apolipoprotein B. *Journal of Lipid Research* 39, 703–23.

Kim, Y.S., Birthwhistle, W., Kim, Y.W. 1972: Peptide hydrolases in the brush border and soluble fractions of small intestinal mucosa of rat and man. *Journal of Clinical Investigation* 51, 1419–30.

Kimmich, G.A., Carter-Su, C. 1978: Membrane potentials and the energetics of intestinal Na^+-dependent transport systems. *American Journal of Physiology* 235, C78–81.

Koch, C., Hoiby, N. 1993: Pathogenesis of cystic fibrosis. *Lancet* 341, 1065–70.

Koldovsky, O., Heringova, A., Jirsova, V. *et al.* 1965: Transport of glucose against a concentration gradient in everted sacs of jejunum and ileum of human fetuses. *Gastroenterology* 48, 185–7.

Lebenthal, E., Lee, P.C. 1980: Glucoamylase and disaccharidase activities in normal subjects and in patients with musocal injury of the small intestine. *Journal of Pediatrics* 97, 389–93.

Lebenthal, E., Antonowicz, I., Shwachman, H. 1976: Enterokinase and trypsin activities in pancreatic insufficiency and diseases of the small intestine. *Gastroenterology* 70, 508–12.

Lebenthal, E., Khin-Maung, U., Zheng, B.Y. *et al.* 1994: Small intestinal glucoamylase deficiency and starch malabsorption: a newly recognized alpha-glucosidase deficiency in children. *Journal of Pediatrics* 124, 541–6.

LeBivic, A., Quaroni, A., Nichols, B. 1990: Biogenic pathways of plasma membrane proteins in Caco-2, a human intestinal cell line. *Journal of Cell Biology* 111, 1351–61.

Lescale-Matys, L., Dyer, J., Scott, D. *et al.* 1993: Regulation of the ovine intestinal Na^+ glucose co-transporter (SGLT1) is dissociated from mRNA abundance. *Biochemical Journal* 291, 435–40.

Leighton, J.K., Joyner, J., Zamarripa, J. *et al.* 1990: Fasting decreases apolipoprotein B mRNA editing and the secretion of small molecular weight apo B by rat hepatocytes: evidence that the total amount of apo B secreted is regulated post-transcriptionally. *Journal of Lipid Research* 31, 1663–8.

Levy, E., Goldstein, R., Freier, S. *et al.* 1981: Characterization of gastric lipolytic activity. *Biochimica et Biophysica Acta* 664, 316–26.

Levy, E., Marcel, Y., Deckelbaum, R.J. *et al.* 1987a: Intestinal apo B synthesis, lipids, and lipoproteins in chylomicron retention disease. *Journal of Lipid Research* 28, 1263–74.

Levy, E., Marcel, Y., Milne, R.W. *et al.* 1987b: Absence of intestinal synthesis of apoprotein B-48 in two cases of abetalipoproteinemia. *Gastroenterology* 93, 1119–26.

Levy, E., Chouraqui, J.P., Roy, C.C. 1988: Steatorrhea and disorders of chylomicron synthesis and secretion. *Pediatric Clinics of North America* 35, 53–67.

Levy, E., Rochette, C., Londono, I. *et al.* 1990: Apolipoprotein B-100: immunolocalization and synthesis in human intestinal mucosa. *Journal of Lipid Research* 31, 1937–46.

Levy, E., Roy, C.C., Thibault, L., Bonin, A., Brochu, P., Seidman, E.G. 1994: Variable expression of familial heterozygous hypobetalipoproteinemia: transient malabsorption during infancy. *Journal of Lipid Research* 35, 2170–7.

Levy, E., Mehran, M., Seidman, E. 1995: Caco-2 cells as a model for intestinal lipoprotein synthesis and secretion. *FASEB Journal* 9, 626–35.

Liddle, R.A., Goldfine, I.D., Rosen, M.S. *et al.* 1985: Cholecystokinin bioactivity in human plasma. Molecular forms, responses to feeding, and relationship to gallbladder contraction. *Journal of Clinical Investigation* 75, 114–52.

Lin, M.C.M., Arbeeny, C., Bergquist, K. *et al.* 1994: Cloning and regulation of hamster microsomal triglyceride transfer protein: the regulation is independent from that of other hepatic and intestinal proteins which participate in the transport of fatty acids and triglycerides. *Journal of Biological Chemistry* 269, 29138–45.

Lin, M.C.M., Gordon, D., Wetterau, J.R. 1995: Microsomal triglyceride transfer protein (MTP) regulation in HepG2 cells: insulin negatively regulates MTP gene expression. *Journal of Lipid Research* 36, 1073–81.

Linder, M.C. 1991: Nutritional biochemistry and metabolism. In Linder, M.C. (ed.) *Nutritional biochemistry and metabolism*, 2nd edn. New York: Elsevier, 87–109.

Lombardo, D., Guy, O. 1980: Studies on the substrate specificity of a carboxyl ester hydrolase from pancreatic juice. Action on cholesterol esters and lipid-soluble vitamin esters. *Biochimica et Biophysica Acta* 611, 147–55.

Lopez-Candales, A., Bosner, M.S., Spilburg, C.A. *et al.* 1993: Cholesterol transport function of pancreatic cholesterol esterase: directed sterol uptake and esterification in enterocytes. *Biochemistry* 32, 12085–9.

Lopez-Candales, A., Grosjlos, J., Sasser, T. *et al.* 1996: Dietary induction of pancreatic cholesterol esterase: a regulatory cycle for the intestinal absorption of cholesterol. *Biochem Cell Biology* 74, 257–64.

Lott, J.A. 1982: Inflammatory disease of the pancreas. *CRC Critical Reviews of Clinical Laboratory Science* 17, 201–28.

Louvard, D., Kedinger, M., Hauri, H.P. 1992: The differentiating intestinal epithelial cell. *Annual Review of Cell Biology* 8, 157–95.

Lowe, M.E. 1994: The structure and function of pancreatic enzymes. In Johnson, L.R. (ed.) *Physiology of the gastrointestinal tract*. New York: Raven Press, 1531–42.

Lucotte, G., Loirat, F. 1993: A more detailed map of the cystic fibrosis mutation delta F508 frequencies in Europe. *Human Biology* 65, 503.

Madara, J.L., Parkos, C., Colgan, S. *et al.* 1992: The movement of solutes and cells across tight junctions. *Annals of the New York Academy of Sciences* 664, 47–60.

Magun, A.M., Brasitis, T.A., Glickman, R.M. 1985: Isolation of high density lipoproteins from rat intestinal epithelial cells. *Journal of Clinical Investigation* 75, 209–18.

Mahley, R.W., Bennett, B.D., Moore, D.J. *et al.* 1971: Lipoproteins associated with Golgi apparatus isolated from epithelial cells of rat small intestine. *Laboratory Investigation* 25, 435–44.

Mann, N.S., Nair, P.K., Russman, H.B. *et al.* 1984: Enterokinase deficiency and vitamin B12 absorption. *Gastroenterology* 86, 384–5.

Mansbach, C.M., II 1977: The origin of chylomicron phosphatidylcholine in the rat. *Journal of Clinical Investigation* 60, 411–20.

McCutcheon, A.D., Race, D. 1962: Experimental pancreatitis: a possible etiology of postoperative pancreatitis. *Annals of Surgery* 155, 523–31.

McGuigan, J.E. 1993: Zollinger–Ellison syndrome and other hypersecretory states. In Sleisenger, M.H., Fordtran, J.S. (eds) *Gastrointestinal diseases: pathophysiology, diagnosis, management*, 5th edn. Philadelphia: WB Saunders, 679–97.

McMichael, H.B. 1976: Disorders of carbohydrate digestion and absorption. *Clinical Endocrinology and Metabolism* 5, 627–43.

Montes, R.G., Perman, J.A. 1990: Disorders of carbohydrate absorption in clinical practice. *Maryland Medical Journal* 39, 383–8.

Montgomery, R.K., Sybicki, M.A., Forcier, A.G. *et al.* 1981: Rat intestinal microvillus membrane sucrase-isomaltase is a single high molecular weight protein and fully active enzyme in the absence of luminal factors. *Biochimica et Biophysica Acta* 661, 346–9.

Moreau, H., Laugier, R., Gargouri, Y. *et al.* 1988: Human preduodenal lipase is entirely of gastric fundic origin. *Gastroenterology* 95, 1221–6.

Morris, A.P., Cunningham, S.A., Frizzell, R.A. 1993: CFTR targeting in epithelial cells. *Journal of Bioenergics and Biomembranes* 25, 21–6.

Naim, H.Y., Sterchi, E.E., Lentze, M.J. 1988a: Structure, biosynthesis, and glucosylation of human small intestinal maltase-glucoamylase. *Journal of Biological Chemistry* 263, 19709–17.

Naim, H.Y., Roth, J., Sterchi, E.E. *et al.* 1988b: Sucrase-isomaltase deficiency in humans. Different mutations disrupt intracellular transport, processing, and function of an intestinal brush border enzyme. *Journal of Clinical Investigation* 82, 667–9.

Newman, B.M., Brooks, S., Tajiri, H. *et al.* 1988: Long-term pancreatic-biliary diversion in the rat. *Digestion* 41, 172–9.

Nilsson, J., Blackberg, P., Carlsson, S. *et al.* 1990: cDNA cloning of human-milk bile-salt-stimulated lipase and evidence for its identity to pancreatic carboxylic ester hydrolase. *European Journal of Biochemistry* 192, 543–50.

Nixon, S.E., Mawer, G.E. 1970: The digestion and absorption of proteins in man. II. The form in which digested protein is absorbed. *British Journal of Nutrition* 24, 241–58.

Nordstrom, C. 1972: Release of enteropeptidase and other brush border enzymes from the small intestinal wall in the rat. *Biochimica et Biophysica Acta* 289, 367–77.

Noren, O., Dabelsteen, W., Sjöström, H. *et al.* 1977: Histological localization of two dipeptidases in the pig small intestine and liver, using immunofluorescence. *Gastroenterology* 72, 8792.

Oelkers, P., Kirby, L.C., Heubi, J.E. *et al.* 1997: Primary bile acid malabsorption caused by mutations in the ileal sodium-dependent bile acid transporter gene (SLC10A2). *Journal of Clinical Investigation* 99, 1880–7.

Oppenheimer, E.H., Esterly, J.F. 1975: Pathology of cystic fibrosis, review of the literature and comparison with 146 autopsied cases. In *Perspectives in pediatric pathology*, Vol. 2. Chicago: Year Book Publishers, 2451.

Parthasarathy, S., Papasani, S.V., Ganguly, J. 1974: The mechanism of intestinal absorption of phosphatidylcholine in rats. *Biochemical Journal* 140, 503–8.

Pessah, M., Benlian, P., Beucler, I. *et al.* 1991: Anderson's disease: genetic exclusion of the apolipoprotein-B gene in two families. *Journal of Clinical Investigation* 87, 367–70.

Popper, D.A., Shiau, Y.F., Reed, M. 1985: Role of small intestine in pathogenesis of hyperlipidemia in diabetic rats. *American Journal of Physiology* 249, G161–7.

Powell, L.M., Wallis, S.C., Pease, R.J. *et al.* 1987: A novel form of tissue-specific RNA processing produces apolipoprotein B-48 in intestine. *Cell* 50, 831–40.

Puls, W., Kemp, U., Krause, H.P., Thomas, G., Hoffmeister, F. 1977: Glucosidase inhibition: a new approach to the treatment of diabetes, obesity and hypolipoproteinemia. *Naturwissenshaften* 65, 536–7.

Riby, J.E., Fujisawa, T. 1993: Fructose absorption. *American Journal of Clinical Nutrition* 58(Suppl), 748–53S.

Riordan, J.R., Rommens, J.M., Kerem, B. *et al.* 1989: Identification of the cystic fibrosis gene: cloning and characterization of complementary DNA. *Science* 245, 1066–73.

Roy, C.C., Weber, A.M., Morin, C.L. *et al.* 1977: Abnormal biliary lipid composition in cystic fibrosis: effect of pancreatic enzymes. *New England Journal of Medicine* 297, 1301–5.

Roy, C.C., Weber, A.M., Morin, C.L. *et al.* 1982: Hepatobiliary disease in cystic fibrosis: a survey of current issues and concepts. *Journal of Pediatric Gastroenterology and Nutrition* 1, 469–78.

Roy, C.C., Levy, E., Green, P.H.R. *et al.* 1987: Malabsorption, hypocholesterolemia, and fat-filled enterocytes with increased intestinal apoprotein B. Chylomicron retention disease. *Gastroenterology* 92, 390–9.

Ruf, J., Wacker, H., James, P. *et al.* 1990: Rabbit small intestinal trehalase. Purification, cDNA cloning, expression, and verification of glycosylphosphatidylinositol anchoring. *Journal of Biological Chemistry* 265, 15034–9.

Rustaeus, S., Boren, J., Wettesten, M. *et al.* 1995: In Woodford, F.P., Davignon, J., Sniderman, A. (eds) *Atherosclerosis X*. Amsterdam: Elsevier Science Publishers BV, 958–65.

Saavedra, J.M., Perman, J.A. 1989: Current concepts in lactose malabsorption and intolerance. *Annual Review of Nutrition* 9, 475–502.

Saavedra, J.M., Bauman, N.A., Dung, I., Perman, J.A., Yolker, R.H. 1994: Feeding of bifidobacterium bifidum and Streptococcus thermophilus to infants in hospital for prevention of diarrhoea and shedding of rotavirus. *Lancet* 344, 1046–9.

Samloff, I.M. 1981: Pepsins, peptic activity and peptic inhibitors. *Journal of Clinical Gastroenterology* 3, 91–4.

Schonfeld, G. 1995: The hypobetalipoproteinemias. *Annual Review of Nutrition* 15, 23–34.

Schultz, S.G., Strecker, C.K. 1970: Fructose influx across the brush border of rabbit ileum. *Biophysica et Biochimica Acta* 211, 586–8.

Scow, R.O., Stein, Y., Stein, O. 1967: Incorporation of dietary lecithin and lysolecithin into lymph chylomicrons in the rat. *Journal of Biological Chemistry* 242, 4919–24.

Semenza, G. 1986: Anchoring and biosynthesis of stalked brush border membrane proteins. *Annual Review of Cell Biology* 2, 255–313.

Senior, J.R., Isselbacher, K.J. 1962: Direct esterification of monoglycerides with palmityl coenzyme A by intestinal epithelial subcellular fractions. *Journal of Biological Chemistry* 237, 1454–9.

Shalon, L.B., Adelson, J.W. 1996: Cystic fibrosis. Gastrointestinal complications and gene therapy. *Pediatric Gastroenterology* 43, 157–96.

Shapiro, G.L., Bulow, S.D., Conklin, K.A. *et al.* 1991: Postinsertional processing of sucrase-α-dextrinase precursor to authentic subunits: multiple step cleavage by trypsin. *American Journal of Physiology* 261, G847–57.

Shi, X., Scheld, H.P., Summers, R.M. *et al.* 1997: Fructose transport mechanisms in human. *Gastroenterology* 113, 1171–9.

Shirazi-Beechey, S.P., Hirayama, B.A., Wang, Y. *et al.* 1991: Ontogenic development of lamb intestinal sodium-glucose cotransporter is regulated by diet. *Journal of Physiology* 437, 699–708.

Shwachman, H., Diamond, L.K., Oski, F.A. *et al.* 1964: The syndrome of pancreatic insufficiency and bone marrow dysfunction. *Journal of Pediatrics* 65, 645–63.

Simell, O. 1995: Lysinuric protein intolerance and other cationic aminoacidurias. In Scriver, C.R., Beaudet, A.L., Sly, W.S., Valle, D. (eds) *The metabolic basis of inherited disease*, 7th edn. New York: McGraw-Hill, 3603–27.

Sjöberg, A., Oscarsson, J., Boström, K. *et al.* 1992: Effects of growth hormone on apolipoprotein-B (apo B) messenger ribonucleic acid editing, and apo B 48 and apo B 100 synthesis and secretion in the rat liver. *Endocrinology* 130, 3356–64.

Smith, L.J., Kamisky, S., D'Souza, S.W. 1986: Neonatal fat digestion and lingual lipase. *Acta Paediatrica Scandinavica* 175, 313–18.

Stirling, C.E., Schneider, A.J., Wong, M.D. *et al.* 1972: Quantitative radioautography of sugar transport in intestinal biopsies from normal humans and a patient with glucose-galactose malabsorption. *Journal of Clinical Investigation* 51, 438–51.

Stremmel, W. 1988: Uptake of fatty acids by jejunal mucosal cells is mediated by a fatty acid-binding membrane protein. *Journal of Clinical Investigation* 82, 2001.

Stremmel, W., Strohmeyer, G., Borchard, F. *et al.* 1985: Identification, isolation and partial characterization of a fatty acid-binding protein from rat jejunal microvillous membrane. *Journal of Clinical Investigation* 75, 1068–76.

Teng, B.B., Burant, C.F., Davidson, N.O. 1993: Molecular cloning of an apolipoprotein B messenger RNA editing protein. *Science* 264, 1816–19.

Teng, B., Blumenthal, S., Forte, T. *et al.* 1994: Adenovirus-mediated gene transfer of rat apolipoprotein B mRNA-editing protein in mice virtually eliminates apolipoprotein B-100 and normal low density lipoprotein production. *Journal of Biological Chemistry* 269, 29395–404.

Thorens, B. 1992: Molecular and cellular physiology of GLUT-2, a high-Km facilitated diffusion glucose transporter. *International Review of Cytology* 137A, 209–38.

Thorens, B. 1993: Facilitated glucose transporters in epithelial cells. *Annual Review of Physiology* 55, 591–608.

Tobey, N., Yeh, R., Huang, T.I. *et al.* 1985: Human intestinal brush border peptidases. *Gastroenterology* 88, 913–26.

Tolboom, J.J., Kabin, H., Molasteli, P. *et al.* 1987: Lactose malabsorption and giardiasis in Basoto school children. *Acta Pediatrica Scandinavica* 76, 60–5.

Townes, P.L., Bryson, M.F., Miller, G. 1967: Further observation on trypsinogen deficiency disease: report of a second case. *Journal of Pediatrics* 71, 220.

Tso, P. 1994: Intestinal lipid absorption. In Johnson, L.R. (ed.) *Physiology of the gastrointestinal tract*. New York: Raven Press, 1867–907.

Turk, E., Zabel, B., Muindlos, S. *et al.* 1991: Glucose-galactose malabsorption caused by a defect in the Na^+/glucose cotransporter. *Nature* 350, 354–6.

VanDeenen, L.L.M., DeHass, G.H., Heemskerk, C.H.Th. 1963: Hydrolysis of synthetic mixed acid phosphatides by phospholipase A from human pancreas. *Biochimica et Biophysica Acta* 67, 411–17.

Wadelius, C., Faguholm, P., Petterson, U. 1989: Lowe oculocerebrorenal syndrome: DNA-based linkage of the gene to Xq24–q26, using tightly linked flanking markers and the correlation to lens examination in carrier diagnosis. *American Journal of Human Genetics* 44, 241–7.

Wang, C.-S., Hartsuck, J.A. 1993: Bile salt-activated lipase, a multiple function lipolytic enzyme. *Biochimica et Biophysica Acta* 1166, 1–19.

Weijers, H.A., Van de Kamer, J.H., Mossel, D.D.A. *et al.* 1960: Diarrhoea caused by deficiency of sugar splitting enzymes. *Lancet* 2, 296–7.

Welsh, J.D., Poley, J.R., Bhatia, M. *et al.* 1978: Intestinal disaccharidase activities in relation to age, race, and mucosal damage. *Gastroenterology* 75, 847–55.

Westergaard, H., Dietschy, J.M. 1974: Delineation of the dimensions and permeability characteristics of the two major diffusion barriers to passive mucosal uptake in the rabbit intestine. *Journal of Clinical Investigation* 54, 718–32.

Westergaard, H., Dietschy, J.M. 1976: The mechanism whereby bile acid micelles increase the rate of fatty acid and cholesterol uptake into the intestinal mucosal cell. *Journal of Clinical Investigation* 58, 97–108.

Wetterau, J.R., Aggerbeck, L.P., Bouma, M.-E. *et al.* 1992: Absence of microsomal triglyceride transfer protein in individuals with abetalipoproteinemia. *Science* 258, 999–1001.

Wetterau, J.R., Lin, M.C.M., Jamil, H. 1997: Microsomal triglyceride transfer protein. *Biochimica et Biophysica Acta* 1345, 136–50.

WHO/FAO/UNO (World Health Organization/Food Agriculture Organization/United Nations Office) 1995: *Energy and protein requirements*. WHO Technical Report Series no. 724. Geneva: WHO.

Winkler, F.K., D'Arcy, A., Hunziker, W. 1990: Structure of human pancreatic lipase. *Nature* 343, 771–4.

Wong, M.H., Oelkers, P., Dawson, P.A. 1995: Identification of a mutation in the ileal sodium-dependent bile acid transporter gene that abolishes transport activity. *Journal of Biological Chemistry* 270, 27228–34.

Wright, E.M., Turk, E., Zabel, B. *et al.* 1991: Molecular genetics of intestinal glucose transport. *Journal of Clinical Investigation* 88, 1435–40.

Wright, E.M., Hirayama, B.A., Loo, D.D.F. *et al.* 1994: Intestinal sugar transport. In Johnson, L.R. (ed.) *Physiology of the gastrointestinal tract*, 2nd edn. New York: Raven Press, 1751–72.

Yamanaka, S., Balestra, M.E., Ferrell, L.D. *et al.* 1995a: Apolipoprotein B mRNA-editing protein induces hepatocellular carcinoma and dysplasia in transgenic animals. *Proceedings of the National Academy of Sciences USA* 92, 8483–7.

Yamanaka, S., Poksay, K.S., Balestra, M.E. *et al.* 1995b: Protein–protein interaction in apolipoprotein B mRNA editing complex. *Circulation* 92(Suppl 1), 1–165.

Yao, Z., Blackhart, B.D., Linton, M.F. *et al.* 1991: Expression of carboxyl-terminally truncated forms of human apolipoprotein B in rat hepatoma cells. Evidence that the length of apolipoprotein B has a major effect on the buoyant density of the secreted lipoproteins. *Journal of Biological Chemistry* 266, 3300–8.

You, C.H., Rominger, J.M., Chey, W.Y. 1983: Potentiation effect of cholecystokinin-octapeptide on pancreatic bicarbonate secretion stimulated by a physiological dose of secretin in humans. *Gastroenterology* 85, 40–5.

Young, S.G., Linton, M.R.F. 1991: Genetic abnormalities in apolipoprotein B. *Trends in Cardiovascular Medicine* 1, 59–65.

Younoszai, M.K. 1974: Jejunal absorption of hexose in infants and adults. *Journal of Pediatrics* 85, 446–8.

11

Small intestinal motility

WEI MING SUN

Our knowledge of small intestinal motility has increased enormously in the past three decades, but the characteristics of small bowel motor dysfunction in localized or systemic diseases are still poorly understood. Nevertheless, some small intestinal motor problems have been demonstrated. This chapter summarizes the normal motor functions of the small intestine and their control mechanisms, and discusses the current understanding of abnormal small intestinal motility in disease.

NORMAL SMALL INTESTINAL MOTOR FUNCTION

Anatomy of the small intestine (*see* Chapter 1)

The small intestine is a long muscular tube that extends from the stomach to the cecum. The muscular wall of the small intestine has three layers: a longitudinal and a circular muscle layer, and a thin layer of muscularis mucosa that sends fibers up into the villi. The longitudinal and circular layers of smooth muscle are mainly responsible for the movement of intestinal contents. Phasic contraction of the muscularis mucosae may shorten the villi and stir the microclimate adjacent to the mucosa; tonic contraction of this layer may act as a barrier to fluid absorption. Smooth muscle cells are connected to one another by nexuses or gap junctions. The cells in the circular muscle layer are considered to be linked electrically to those in the longitudinal layer via the interstitial cells of Cajal (ICC) (Cajal, 1893). There is evidence now that the interstitial cells of Cajal generate electrical control activity (Sanders, 1996), the most basic control mechanism for small intestinal motor activity (see below). It has been hypothesized that the c-*kit* pathway is a major signal for interstitial cell differentiation. The proto-oncogene c-*kit* encodes a receptor tyrosine kinase. The gene product of c-*kit* is a 160-kilodalton protein (c-Kit). Antibodies directed against c-Kit protein are used to detect the c-*kit* activity. Cells that express c-Kit-like immunoreactivity are found in the same anatomical positions within the gastrointestinal tract as ICC (Torihashi *et al.*, 1995). Interstitial cells adjacent to neural tissue and exposed to c-Kit differentiate into interstitial cells, while those not exposed become smooth muscle.

An extensive network of enteric nervous system, connected to ganglion cells, lies between the circular and longitudinal layers of smooth muscle. Another nerve plexus lies in the submucosa. These enteric nerve nets are linked to sensory receptors in the epithelium, the submucosa and muscular layers, and supply motor nerve fibers to the smooth muscle.

Electrical basis of small intestinal contraction

ELECTRIC CONTROL ACTIVITY

The timing, maximum frequency and rate of propagation of contractions in the small intestine are all determined by the regular oscillations in the membrane potential of the smooth muscle cells. These rhythmic oscillations are termed electrical control activity (ECA), slow waves or pacesetter potentials. These signals can be recorded, *in vitro*, by intracellular microelectrodes within individual cells or by extracellular electrodes from a group of muscles.

In humans, the *in vivo* recordings are usually done by serosal surface electrodes placed during laparotomy, with the leads passing through the drainage hole. The electrodes are removed when the drainage is extracted, hence the recording time is limited. Furthermore, the conditions under which the recordings are made are hardly physiological. Intraluminal electrodes attached to oro-intestinal catheters have also been used. However, it is difficult to keep the electrodes in position and the mucosa is not the closest or most direct approach to the muscles.

The frequency of the slow waves declines from the duodenum (12/min) to the distal small intestine (8/min in the ileum). The slow wave is propagated rapidly in a circumferential direction, creating the condition for the development of a ring constriction. Propagation in an aboral direction is slow.

ELECTRIC RESPONSE ACTIVITY

Unlike in cardiac muscle, not all slow waves are associated with smooth muscle contractions, but each contraction is coupled with a slow wave. Contraction of intestinal smooth muscle only occurs when membrane depolarization exceeds a given threshold. This is associated with a burst of spike potentials, an action potential or an electric response activity (ERA), which are superimposed on the slow waves. Although the slow wave determines the timing and frequency of contractions, the actual occurrence of contractions depends on the presence or absence of spikes, and the strength of the contractions is determined by the number of spikes associated with the slow waves.

Pattern of contractile activity

MIGRATING MOTOR COMPLEX

Under fasting conditions, a regular cycle of motility in the small intestine is observed in most mammalian species. This recurrent pattern of different phases is known as migrating motor complex (MMC) (Szurszewski, 1969). Since the MMC only occurs during fasting, it is more appropriate to call it interdigestive motor complex (Kellow *et al.*, 1986). The cycle of 90–120 min is then divided into three parts: phase I, a period of quiescence when spikes are absent; phase II, during which intermittent contractile activity resembles the activity that normally occurs after a meal; and phase III, a short period of intense contractile activity when contractions and spike bursts are superimposed upon every slow wave (Code and Marlett, 1975). Phase III usually starts in the upper small intestine or the stomach but may start lower in the intestine; it migrates at a slow rate (~ 8 cm/min) towards the ileum.

The MMC is thought to clear the small intestine of bacteria and food residues between meals. For this reason, it has been called the intestinal housekeeper, sweeping away the debris of the last meal. Absence of MMCs are associated with evidence of bacterial overgrowth both in man and in the rat (Vantrappen *et al.*, 1977; Scott and Cahall, 1982). There is also evidence to suggest that phase III of the MMC is associated with a burst of intestinal secretion (Read, 1980).

FED PATTERN OF MOTOR ACTIVITY

Eating disrupts the interdigestive cycle, leading to a prolonged period of apparently irregular activity. The duration directly correlates with the size of the meal (DeWever *et al.*, 1978). Food contents also influence the pattern of postprandial motor activity. A meal rich in fat disrupts the MMC pattern longer than isocaloric meals in the form of protein and carbohydrate (DeWever *et al.*, 1978). This is associated with more contractions after a carbohydrate meal and less contractions after a fatty meal. Infusion of fats into the small intestine, particularly the distal part of the small intestine, reduces the postprandial contraction rate, amplitude and degree of propagation (Welch *et al.*, 1985).

The conversion of the fasting to fed pattern and the length of the fed pattern can be inhibited by vagotomy or vagal freezing, suggesting that vagal activity suppresses the interdigestive pattern. The return of the MMC after a meal occurs sooner if the meal is conveyed rapidly down the small intestine.

OTHER PATTERNS

Migrating clusters of contraction

Migrating clustered contractions occur during both phase II of the MMC and postprandially in animals (Schemann and Ehrlein, 1986) and humans (Fleckenstein and Oigaard, 1978; Summers *et al.*, 1983). Unlike the MMC, migrating clustered contractions do not have a regular frequency, are less than 1 minute in duration and have a velocity of up to 20 cm/s. This pattern is often associated with diarrhea, intestinal obstruction or pseudo-obstruction and the irritable bowel syndrome (Kellow and Phillips, 1987).

Retrograde propulsive contractions

In the dog, retrograde propulsive contractions are frequently seen during vomiting (Lang *et al.*, 1986) and are believed to lead to rapid orad propulsion of intestinal contents. These are recorded mainly in the mid or distal small intestine, and are associated with relaxation of the proximal stomach and lower esophageal sphincter. This is also observed in diabetic patients with cardiac autonomic neuropathy (Hackelsberger *et al.*, 1997) and in children with vomiting and abdominal pain (Hyman *et al.*, 1990).

Giant migrating contractions

Giant migrating contractions are isolated, high-amplitude (60 mmHg), long duration (20–40 s) contractions, which occur mainly in the jejunum or ileum, and migrate distally to the colon in the dog at about 1 cm/s (Quigley *et al.*, 1984a; Sarna, 1987). This pattern of small intestinal motor activity has been characteristically observed in response to injury, particularly inflammation due to infection (Cowles and Sarna, 1990), radiation enteritis (Otterson and Sarna, 1992) or noxious substances (Kruis *et al.*, 1985) in animals. They are believed to cause rapid movement of small intestinal contents distally (Kruis *et al.*, 1985). Similar characteristics of giant migrating contraction have been described in patients with irritable bowel syndrome, associated with abdominal cramps and discomfort (Kellow and Phillips, 1987).

Control of motor patterns

Despite much research, the mechanisms of regulation of intestinal contractile activity remain poorly understood. Factors that influence gastrointestinal motility include smooth muscle cells (see above), enteric nervous system and the extrinsic sympathetic and parasympathetic nervous systems, and the effects of various chemicals that reach the nerves and muscles of the gut.

ENTERIC NERVOUS SYSTEM (*see* Chapter 7)

Patterns of contractile activity are largely coordinated by the intrinsic nerves of the gut – the gut brain – and generated by reflexes triggered by the interaction of intraluminal contents with receptors in the bowel wall. Most studies have been carried out by inhibiting and activating those nerves. The enteric nervous system is programmed to regulate motor patterns when certain stimuli are present in the gut lumen. Acetylcholine is the major excitatory postganglionic neurotransmitter. Inhibitory neurotransmitters such as nitric oxide (NO) and vasoactive intestinal polypeptide (VIP) are important in providing tonic neural inhibition of the small intestine (Sanders and Ward, 1992).

EXTRINSIC NERVES

The small intestine receives an extrinsic innervation from parasympathetic nerves from the vagus and sympathetic nerves from the thoracicolumbar outflow. Most of these nerves end at the level of the enteric nervous system. Basic patterns of motor activity are regulated in the enteric nervous system, and the extrinsic nervous system is not essential but may modulate the activity of the intrinsic system in response to extra-enteric influences. The role of extrinsic nerves as modulators of gut motor activity is supported by the fact that there are approximately 108 ganglion cells in the enteric nervous system and only 104–105 efferent fibers in the vagus or splanchnic nerves (Furness and Costa, 1980).

PEPTIDES (*see* Chapter 7)

Studies on the effects of peptides on the contractility of the small intestine indicate that gastrin, motilin and cholecystokinin (CCK) increase contractility, whereas VIP, glucagon and secretin decrease contractility. Some of these agents may be present in enteric neurones and function as neurosecretors or neurotransmitters.

Ileocolonic junction

A high resting pressure zone exists at the end of the ileum where it projects into the cecum (Quigley *et al.*, 1983). It relaxes in response to proximal distension and contracts when the proximal colon is distended, supporting the concept of a true ileocolonic sphincter. Two types of motor activity are recorded; discrete clusters of contractions and prolonged propagated contractions. However, phase III of the MMC often does not reach the terminal ileum (Quigley *et al.*, 1984a,b).

Small intestinal transit

It takes 2–12 hours for a solid meal to travel down the small intestine to the ileum. Most material is absorbed by the time the chyme reaches the ileocecal junction. In humans, up to 1–2 L are emptied every day into the colon. The small intestinal transit is closely regulated. Under normal postprandial conditions, there is a balanced relationship between the patterns of small intestinal motor activity, food composition, transit and absorption. Most of this is achieved by the enteric nervous system. A meal consisting of more unabsorbable carbohydrate will accelerate small bowel transit time, probably by absorbing water, causing distension and inducing propagation (Read *et al.*, 1980), while a meal rich in fat will delay small bowel transit (Read *et al.*, 1984).

Adequate absorption depends on the time of exposure to the small intestinal epithelium. The absorption of foods that are either more slowly digested or transported across the epithelium will be limited by transit time. Nutrient reaching the distal small intestine inhibits gastric emptying and small bowel transit. This effect may last for hours and influence the emptying and absorption of the subsequent meal. The degree of absorption is also influenced by the area of the intestine exposed to luminal contents. Motor patterns that increase the contact area include propulsion, rhythmic movements of the longitudinal muscle, ring-like contraction of circular smooth muscle and rhythmic contractions of muscularis mucosae, and piston-like movements of the intestinal villi (Sessions *et al.*, 1968; Melville *et al.*, 1975; Lee, 1983). Mixing enhances absorption by increasing the interactions between food and enzymes, and between products of digestion and the epithelium.

SMALL INTESTINAL MOTILITY IN DISEASE

The small intestinal motor abnormalities described below are not disease specific but rather quantitative measures, which are crude because of the complexity of motor dysfunctions. Different motor patterns occur in one abnormality, or several disease entities share the same motor abnormalities. Most studies have focused on the pattern of the MMC activity. Recently, attempts have made to study the temporal and spatial relationships among small intestinal pressure waves in different segments of the small intestine.

Diarrhea

Abnormal intestinal secretion, absorption and motility are contributory mechanisms (*see* Chapter 15) for diarrhoea to occur. Theoretically, increased intestinal motility may shorten the transit time, and hence decrease absorption. However, the nature of the relationship between disturbed motility and diarrhea is not always clear. In some instances it is possible that the abnormal motility may be the consequence rather than the cause of diarrhea. For example, impaired epithelial absorption of fluid or stimulation of secretion increases the net amount of fluid in the intestinal lumen. This will increase the rate of flow and decrease the transit time by the passive influence of the increased volume in the lumen as well as by stimulating propulsive movements. Because these factors interplay, studies of the motor function alone may not be enough, but certainly give some insight as to the pathogenesis of diarrhea. More information can be gained by combined study of the motor activity, measurement of flow and transit.

The interdigestive motor complex is a highly efficient mechanism for cleaning up the remnants of the preceding meal. The absence of this may result in the accumulation of food remnants, desquamated cells and secretions, thus creating a medium favorable to bacterial colonization of the small intestine (Vantrappen *et al.*, 1977), leading to diarrhea (*see* Chapter 15). In contrast, if nutrients entering the small intestine do not interrupt the MMC, and therefore fail to produce a postprandial motor pattern, the phase III of the MMC will swipe the bowel contents through the lumen in a much shorter period of time. This has been indicated as one of the mechanisms for functional diarrhea in toddlers (Fenton, 1983).

Short bowel syndrome (*see* Chapter 29)

Such a condition is caused by intestinal volvulus, strangulated hernia and mesenteric infarction, and Crohn's disease is the most common underlying diagnosis presently. These patients often have a jejunostomy. Two types of short-bowel patients can be distinguished: those with a jejunostomy, and those with their jejunum anastomosed to a functioning colon. Both types of patients have problems with macronutrient absorption. The underlying motility abnormality is still not clear. In a group of patients who had distal small bowel resections of greater than 100 cm, the duration of the MMC was shorter, particularly the phase II activity, but the postprandial motor activity was unchanged when compared to controls. Interestingly, loperamide increased the postprandial motor activity in the residual small intestine but shortened the period of postprandial motor activity (Remington, 1983). In a more recent study (Schmidt *et al.*, 1996a), seven patients with short bowel syndrome after total ileal and partial jejunal resection (residual jejunal segments between 60 and 100 cm) and six patients with limited distal ileal resection (resected segment between 30 and 70 cm) underwent ambulatory 24-hour jejunal manometry 6–24 months after the operation. Limited ileal resection did not result in changed jejunal motility.

After extensive distal resection, patients had a significantly shorter MMC cycle and a significantly shorter duration of the postprandial motor response compared with controls. On the other hand, intestinal resection had no influence on jejunal contraction frequency and amplitude, and did not lead to any abnormal motor pattern. The shortening of digestive motility and the increased frequency of MMC cycling probably explains the mechanism of malabsorption and diarrhea in the short bowel syndrome (Schmidt *et al.*, 1996b). In dogs, the crucial length of resection to develop abnormal intestinal motor patterns and short bowel syndrome is resection of 75 per cent of the distal small intestine (Quigley and Thompson, 1993). However, there are no clear-cut conclusions in humans.

The severity of symptoms can be reduced by a nipple valve construction at the distal end of the remnant in patients, but hypoalbuminemia, motor activity and transit are similar in those without the valve construction. This suggests that a simple low-grade mechanical obstruction may enhance absorption (Quigley and Thompson, 1994). Similar results of prolongation of small bowel transit have been achieved by various methods of valve construction (Waddell *et al.*, 1970; Vinograd *et al.*, 1984).

Ileal pouch

An ileal pouch with different fashions of construction is used widely after total colectomy for ulcerative colitis. The electrical and motor patterns of the undistended ileum are similar in ileal pouch and Brooke ileostomy (Akwari *et al.*, 1980), but the anatomical and motor properties of the pouch allow it to accept far larger intraluminal volumes both during fasting and after feeding (Akwari *et al.*, 1980). One of the adverse effects, after an ileal pouch–anal anastomosis, from the motility point of view, is multiple bowel actions and incontinence. The duration, velocity of propagation and periodicity of the MMC are usually similar between patients and normal controls. Discrete bursts of clustered contractions are recorded in both groups, which are confined to the terminal ileum in normal controls, but are also present in the jejunoileum in patients, up to 125 cm proximal to the ileal pouch. These large-amplitude, rapidly propagating waves in the proximal jejunoileum may be a response to increased storage within and distension of the distal bowel (Stryker *et al.*, 1985), and also responsible for frequent bowel actions (Levitt *et al.*, 1994). These abnormal motor functions are associated with inflammation in the pouch, since both substance P, which may play a role in mediating inflammatory processes, and VIP, which may contribute to the regulation of intestinal motility, are increased in the pouch (Keranen *et al.*, 1996).

Some patients become incontinent after the procedure. The internal anal sphincter is unstable, characterized by a spontaneous reduction in pressure (Sun *et al.*, 1994), and may or may not be associated with a simultaneous rise in pouch pressure (Levitt *et al.*, 1994). All patients lose discriminative rectal sensation during pouch ('neo-rectum') balloon distension and usually cannot perceive a normal desire to defecate (Sun *et al.*, 1994). These pathophysiological features after ileal pouch–anal anastomosis are probably due to damage to the autonomic and enteric nerve supplies (Sun *et al.*, 1994). Loperamide may be useful in treating those patients as it increases resting anal pressure by approximately 20 per cent, with reduced bowel frequency, an improved night-time continence, and less soiling thus reducing the need to wear a protective pad (Hallgren *et al.*, 1994).

Chronic intestinal pseudo-obstruction

Chronic pseudo-obstruction is a rare syndrome characterized by recurrent episodes of symptoms and signs of intestinal obstruction without mechanical obstruction. Symptoms include nausea, vomiting and abdominal pain, which are sometimes severe enough to result in nutritional disturbances which require nutritional support. Chronic pseudo-obstruction may be 'primary', with the disorder intrinsic to the small intestine, or 'secondary', as part of a systemic disease such as diabetes or progressive systemic sclerosis. Patients may be relatively well between attacks. However, when a patient first presents, the diagnosis is usually difficult because of the lack of specificity of the clinical features and the absence of diagnostic radiological characteristics. Overlap with the symptoms and signs of other 'functional syndromes', such as irritable bowel syndromes and chronic constipation, is common.

Chronic pseudo-obstruction results from dysfunction of the neuromuscular control mechanism of the gut, which may be either myopathic or neuropathic in nature (Camilleri *et al.*, 1993). Motor disturbances in chronic pseudo-obstruction are not restricted to the small intestine, the clinical manifestations may also include dysphagia, heartburn, distension and constipation. For example, gastric emptying of solids is delayed and mouth-to-cecum transit of solids and liquids is significantly prolonged (Camilleri *et al.*, 1986; Mayer *et al.*, 1988). Extraintestinal smooth muscle organs, such as the urinary bladder, particularly in patients with myopathic processes, such as scleroderma, may sometimes be associated with chronic pseudo-obstruction.

Manometric studies in the human small intestine show a variety of motor dysfunctions, which are likely to reflect, at least in part, differences in the underlying pathophysiology (Summers *et al.*, 1983; Stanghellini *et al.*, 1987; Colemont and Camilleri, 1989). Reported abnormalities include a reduction in the frequency and amplitude of pressure waves, clustered migrating contractions (Vantrappen *et al.*, 1977), and a reduction or absence of phase III activity (Summers *et al.*, 1983). Abnormal propagation of interdigestive motor complexes, non-propagating bursts of phasic pressure activity, and failure to convert to fed patterns have also been reported (Camilleri *et al.*, 1986). It has not been established which of these abnormalities contributes to a delay in small intestinal transit. Furthermore, there is no consensus on the criteria of diagnosis of chronic pseudo-obstruction of the small intestine.

A recent workshop reports the view that the diagnosis of chronic intestinal pseudo-obstruction is frequently made without adequate proof and that this leads to both inappropriate and overaggressive therapies (Rudolph *et al.*, 1997). A more rigid definition of pseudo-obstruction is advocated based on the demonstration of radiographic evidence of obstruction in the absence of a fixed lumen-occluding lesion. However, it has been pointed out that there is a practical difficulty drawing a line between the definition of intestinal dysmotility and pseudo-obstruction (Camilleri, 1997). There is a need for diagnostic criteria that are objective and well validated, and that can be relied upon by all clinicians managing these patients. There is evidence to suggest that small intestinal manometry is also valuable in assessing the prognosis of patients with intestinal pseudo-obstruction. In children, a manometric pattern of low-amplitude phase III activity or very reduced motor activity might predict an unfavorable outcome or a requirement for parenteral nutrition, while children with higher-amplitude pressure waves do significantly better (Di Lorenzo *et al.*, 1995; Fell *et al.*, 1996).

Functional gastrointestinal disorders

A functional gastrointestinal disorder is a disorder with symptoms attributable to the gastrointestinal tract without evidence of organic diseases (Drossman, 1990). The symptoms include nausea, heartburn, early satiety, abdominal pain, bloating or distension, and various symptoms of disordered defecation. The pathophysiologies of these symptoms are unknown. Diagnosis depends principally on the history. Management requires an early confident diagnosis, together with attention to abnormal illness behavior or psychosocial abnormalities, which, along with the somatic symptoms, may account for the consultation. In this section, only the pathophysiological aspect of functional bowel disorder is discussed.

IRRITABLE BOWEL SYNDROME

Irritable bowel syndrome (IBS) is a functional bowel disorder characterized by abdominal pain or discomfort associated with features of disordered defecation and with distension. These symptoms should last for at least 3 months as the diagnostic criteria (Thompson, 1989; Drossman, 1990). IBS is common in the general population, particularly in urban inhabitants in industrialized countries.

Many have sought to identify a physiological abnormality that is unique to IBS patients. Dysmotility of the small intestine has been reported in patients with IBS (Kellow and Phillips, 1987; Kellow *et al.*, 1990). While IBS patients as a group show an exaggerated or altered response in the small and large intestines to various stimuli, which include diet, fatty acids, bile salts, hormones, and physical and psychological stress (Kellow *et al.*, 1992), no test has been established as a diagnostic standard for the individual with IBS, although the majority of studies have been done in the colon and anorectum because of their easier accessibility (Snape *et al.*, 1977; Swarbrick *et al.*, 1980; Whitehead *et al.* 1980; Sun *et al.*, 1990; Prior *et al.*, 1993).

Gorard *et al.* (1994) recorded fasting ambulatory motility in the jejunum and ileum in the diarrhea-predominant IBS patients and controls. During the day, periodicity of migrating motor complexes did not differ between patients and controls. In both groups, aboral progression of phase III fronts was associated with a slowing of propagation velocity and maximum contractile rate, but an increase in mean amplitude of contraction. Discrete clustered contractions were also similar between the two groups during daytime phase II activity. Pain episodes were not associated with any specific motility patterns. Despite the lack of motility differences between the two groups, orocecal transit time in the IBS patients was shorter than in the controls. This ambulant study failed to show any abnormalities of fasting small intestinal motility that might distinguish diarrhea-predominant IBS patients from healthy controls (Gorard *et al.*, 1994). In contrast, an ambulatory jejunal motility recording in IBS patients with predominant diarrhea showed heterogeneous pressure patterns in the small bowel but the preponderance of patients demonstrated a longer duration of phase II with higher amplitudes during both fasting and postprandial status (Schmidt *et al.*, 1996a).

In another ambulatory jejunal motility study, the differences in the amplitudes and frequency of pressure waves were minor between patients and controls, and there was no difference in the number of discrete cluster contractions between the two groups (Small *et al.*, 1997). Therefore, the discrete cluster contractions do not appear to be a useful marker for IBS (Gorard *et al.*, 1994; Small *et al.*, 1997). Further studies are required to clarify this discrepancy with previous data. However, there are data to suggest that motilin and cholecystokinin secretion in response to water and fat ingestion is abnormal in patients with IBS (Sjolund *et al.*, 1996). The possible motor abnormality associated with peptide change remains unclear.

The human MMC and sleep cycle have a similar periodicity, and there is some contention as to whether these biorhythms are linked in the irritable bowel syndromes, where episodes of intestinal dysmotility have been described during sleep (Kumar *et al.*, 1992). These patients often complain of poor sleep, which is associated with a remarkable increase in rapid eye movement (REM) sleep (Kumar *et al.*, 1992). A study using non-invasive indirect measurement of gastric function, the electrogastrogram (EGG), which measures the electrical control activity of the stomach, showed that the amplitude of the dominant EGG frequency did not decrease from waking to non-REM sleep and that there was a subsequent increase in the amplitude from non-REM to REM sleep in IBS patients compared to the control group. These data suggest that there is an intrinsic alteration in autonomic and central nervous system functioning in patients with IBS (Orr *et al.*, 1997). However, another study using direct measurement of gut motility showed that, despite increased depression in the IBS patients, the proportions of time awake, in non-REM and REM sleep, and nocturnal motility were similar in controls and IBS patients (Gorard *et al.*, 1995).

A recent study also indicates that there may be specific associations between the autonomic nervous system, predominant physical symptoms, bowel transit time and psychological factors in patients with irritable bowel syndrome. Aggarwal *et al.* (1994) showed that a diarrhea-predominant subgroup had a prolonged postural adjustment ratio (a sympathetic adrenergic test), while a constipation-predominant subgroup showed a shorter R-R interval (a vagal cholinergic test) when compared with normals (Aggarwal *et al.*, 1994). This area needs further investigation as the evidence is scarce at the moment.

HELICOBACTER PYLORI INFECTION

H. pylori infection has been suspected to be associated with functional dyspepsia because gastric and duodenal afferents partly project to the same anatomic areas. The dyspeptic symptoms suggest that the gastric and/or duodenal motility is impaired in these patients.

A possible etiological role for *H. pylori* in dyspepsia has been sought in three major types of study (Armstrong, 1996). Epidemiological studies have suggested that *H. pylori* is not a major cause of non-ulcerative dyspepsia. However, both dyspepsia and *H. pylori* are common. Pathophysiological studies have commonly reported a variety of motor and sensory 'abnormalities' in association with *H. pylori*, but none has been confirmed or reproduced. In eradication studies, there is continuing debate as to whether dyspeptic symptoms diminish with treatment. This is partly because of the high placebo-response rate and partly because many treatment regimens have not cured the infection. Suppression of bacterial growth may not affect symptoms significantly, if they are due to mucosal inflammation, and symptom resolution may take many weeks or months after curing *H. pylori* and the associated gastritis.

Recent findings have shown that symptom reduction is more evident 1 year after eradication of *H. pylori* than after 4 weeks. Therefore, to confirm or disprove an association between *H. pylori*-induced gastritis and non-ulcerative dyspepsia is difficult. The reasons include: current definitions of dyspepsia reflect a number of underlying pathophysiological processes, rather than a specific disease entity (Talley, 1991); little is known about variations in host susceptibility and *H. pylori* virulence, or their potential effect on symptomatology; and the mechanisms responsible for dyspeptic symptoms are unknown, regardless of whether or not there is concomitant *H. pylori*-induced inflammation (Armstrong, 1996).

In a recent study, patients with functional dyspepsia for more than 6 months had heightened small intestinal sensory thresholds and lower tolerance of duodenal balloon distension compared to controls. However, there was no difference in the threshold for first perception and maximum tolerance between *H. pylori*-positive and *H. pylori*-negative patients. During duodenal nutrient infusion, the duodenal motility index increased in all subjects, and was not significantly different in patients and controls or in *H. pylori*-negative or *H. pylori*-positive subjects (Holtmann *et al.*, 1996). There is a continuing and urgent need for well-designed studies to assess the long-term effect of *H. pylori* and its cure on both gastrointestinal function and dyspeptic symptoms (Armstrong, 1996).

Diabetes mellitus

There is substantial evidence that the prevalence of gastrointestinal symptoms is high in patients with diabetes mellitus (Kassander, 1958; Feldman and Schiller, 1983; Janatuinen *et al.*, 1993; Schvarcz *et al.*, 1996). These are associated with abnormal gastrointestinal motility that leads to potential sequelae of malnutrition, poor glycemic control and impaired absorption of orally administered drugs (Horowitz and Fraser, 1994; Camilleri, 1996).

Small intestinal motility is frequently disordered in diabetes and the motor dysfunction is heterogeneous (Camilleri and Malagelada, 1984; Kim *et al.*, 1991; Fraser *et al.*, 1993). Both normal, slow and rapid small intestinal transit have been reported, probably partly reflecting differences in subject selection and the methodology used to evaluate small intestinal transit (Keshavarzian *et al.*, 1987; Wegener *et al.*, 1990; Kawagishi *et al.*, 1992; Werth *et al.*, 1992). Diarrhea occurs in up to 20 per cent of diabetic patients (Feldman and Schiller, 1983) and is considered to result primarily from small intestinal motor dysfunction. The diarrhea classically is nocturnal, but can occur at any time of the day, and is often associated with fecal incontinence. Diarrhea may be intermittent and be precipitated by enteral nutrients introduced for nutritional support. More rapid small intestinal transit is likely to contribute to diarrhea by reducing the time available for absorption of nutrients, electrolytes and bile salts. Animal models of diabetes suggest that impaired adrenergic control of intestinal secretion may also be important (Chang *et al.*, 1986). In a review article (Valdovinos *et al.*, 1993), diabetic diarrhea examined at the Mayo Clinic is frequently due to celiac sprue, bacterial overgrowth in the small bowel or fecal incontinence in conjunction with anorectal dysfunction. However, in almost 50 per cent of the patients, these causes are excluded, and abnormal intestinal motility or secretion is postulated to be one of the likely causes of the diarrhea. Therapeutic trials with opioids, clonidine hydrochloride and, rarely, cholestyramine resin or octreotide acetate (or both methods) are effective in many patients (Valdovinos *et al.*, 1993).

In type I diabetic patients with dyspeptic symptoms, the frequency and duration of the MMC are affected in both the antrum and duodenum when compared to control subjects. After a meal, the duration of the fed state was shorter in diabetic patients with symptoms during the study than in diabetic patients without symptoms and in control subjects. In diabetic patients with the clinical diagnosis of gastroparesis, either duodeno-jejunal phasic pressure activity was reduced or there were non-propagated long bursts of powerful contractions (Camilleri and Malagelada, 1984). Prolonged recording of gastrointestinal motility in type II diabetics with diarrhea revealed abnormal MMC that commenced in the distal duodenum or jejunum with short duration, or even absence of phase III activity of MMC. The velocity of propagation was increased between recording sites (Dooley *et al.*, 1988). However, there is no correlation between manometric parameters and the degree of cardiac autonomic neuropathy (Jebbink *et al.*, 1993). Currently, there is no specific test to evaluate gastrointestinal autonomic neuropathy. The commonly performed autonomic nervous system tests can be divided into three groups: sympathetic adrenergic tests, sympathetic cholinergic tests and vagal tests.

Orthostatic changes in blood pressure in response to head-up tilt are dependent on sympathetic adrenergic function. The drop in blood pressure is normally less than 25 mmHg for systolic and 15 mmHg for diastolic when the subject is tilted from horizontal to 80°. The postural adjustment ratio is also commonly used and tests a reflex barostatic response. Doppler flow measurements of the superior mesenteric artery have been tried as an indicator of abdominal sympathetic adrenergic function (Chaudhuri *et al.*, 1992).

Postganglionic sympathetic adrenergic function is assessed by the response of the plasma norepinephrine response to intravenous edrophonium, which is a short-acting anticholinesterase (Leveston *et al.*, 1979). The plasma level of norepinephrine is measured by sampling blood every 1 or 2 minutes over a period of 10 minutes. This test is not a pure gastrointestinal sympathetic test because the norepinephrine is also released from skin, lung and kidneys.

Sympathetic cholinergic activity is measured by thermoregulatory sweat test or quantitative sudomotor axon reflex test, involving iontophoresing acetylcholine into one area of the skin and measuring the sweat output into an adjacent but physically separated area.

For testing vagal function, cardiovagal tests are the most commonly used, in which R-R interval response to deep breathing is measured. It is based on an assumption that abdominal branches of the vagus are affected before the cardiac braches. In a longitudinal study, among the five cardiovascular autonomic measures, only the R-R response to the Valsalva maneuver deteriorated after 9-year follow-ups (Levitt *et al.*, 1996).

The abdominal vagus function can be tested by stimulating the vagal nuclei in the brainstem by insulin-induced hypoglycemia or modified sham-feeding using a chew-and-spit technique (Schwartz *et al.*, 1978; Taylor *et al.*, 1978). This causes secretion of gastric acid and pancreatic polypeptide. The latter technique is safer, easier to perform and is therefore more acceptable to patients.

There is a strong body of data suggesting that acute changes in the blood glucose concentration have significant but potentially reversible effect on gastrointestinal motility (MacGregor *et al.*, 1976; Fraser *et al.*, 1991; De Boer *et al.*, 1992a,b; Oster-Jorgensen *et al.*, 1992; Chey *et al.*, 1995; Hasler *et al.*, 1995; Boeckxstaens *et al.*, 1996; Hebbard *et al.*, 1996; Russo *et al.*, 1996, 1997). The postprandial blood glucose control may be manipulated by altering the dietary fibers, which affect small intestinal motility. For example, sugar beet or ispaghula fibers have been shown to inhibit stationary contractile activity and increase the propagation length and velocity of propagated activity, and hence delay glucose absorption (Cherbut *et al.*, 1994). Further studies are required to define the pathways mediating the effects of the blood glucose concentration on gastrointestinal motor function and the perception of signals arising from the gastrointestinal tract, and to carry out clinical trials to determine whether or not the impact of modulation of gastric emptying on long-term glycemic controls in both type I and type II diabetes is beneficial. The mechanisms mediating the effects of the blood glucose concentration on gastrointestinal motor function are likely to be indirect and related, at least in part, to changes in cholinergic activity (De Boer *et al.*, 1992a; Horowitz and Fraser, 1994; Yeap *et al.*, 1996). A direct effect on smooth muscle appears unlikely as both smooth muscle stimulation and inhibition occur during hyperglycemia (Horowitz *et al.*, 1997). A central nervous system effect is supported by animal studies (Hirano and Niijima, 1980). There is debate as to whether insulin affects gastrointestinal motor function; however, the effect of insulin on changes in the blood glucose concentration is likely to be minor in type I diabetes. Hyperglycemia is associated with changes in the secretion of a number of hormones, including pancreatic polypeptide and motilin (Barnett and Owyang, 1988; De Boer *et al.*, 1992a; Schvarcz *et al.*, 1997). There is no information about factors which may mediate the effects of hyperglycemia on gastrointestinal sensation.

SUMMARY

More motor abnormalities have been identified recently because of the increasing awareness of their existence and partly due to the available diagnostic methods. New technology, in particular non-invasive methods, will advance our understanding of small intestinal motor abnormalities, which will in turn improve the diagnosis and management of these problems.

REFERENCES

Aggarwal, A., Cutts, T.F., Abell, T.L. *et al.* 1994: Predominant symptoms in irritable bowel syndrome correlate with specific autonomic nervous system abnormalities. *Gastroenterology* 106, 945–50.

Akwari, O.E., Kelly, K.A., Phillips, S.F. 1980: Myoelectric and motor patterns of continent pouch and conventional ileostomy. *Surgical Gynecology and Obstetrics* 150, 363–71.

Armstrong, D. 1996: Helicobacter pylori infection and dyspepsia. *Scandinavian Journal of Gastroenterology* 215, 38–47.

Barnett, J.L., Owyang, C. 1988: Serum glucose concentration as a modulator of interdigestive gastric motility. *Gastroenterology* 94, 739–44.

Boeckxstaens, G., Horowitz, M., Bermingham, H. *et al.* 1996: Physiological variations in blood glucose concentration affect oesophageal motility and sensation in normal subjects. *Gastroenterology* 110, A636.

Cajal, S.R. 1893: Sur les ganglions et plexus nerveus de l'intestin. *Comptes rendus de séances de la Société de Biologie, Paris* 45, 217–23.

Camilleri, M. 1996: Gastrointestinal problems in diabetes. *Endocrinolology and Metabolism Clinics of North America* 25, 361–78.

Camilleri, M. 1997: Intestinal dysmotility: does the x-ray resolve the real dilemma? *Journal of Pediatric Gastroenterology and Nutrition* 24, 100–1.

Camilleri, M., Malagelada, J.R. 1984: Abnormal intestinal motility in diabetics with the gastroparesis syndrome. *European Journal of Clinical Investigation* 14, 420–7.

Camilleri, M., Brown, M.L., Malagelada, J.R. 1986: Impaired transit of chyme in chronic intestinal pseudo-obstruction: correction by cisapride. *Gastroenterology* 91, 619–26.

Camilleri, M., Balm, R.K., Low, P.A. 1993: Autonomic dysfunction in patients with chronic intestinal pseudo-obstruction. *Clinical Autonomic Research* 3, 95–100.

Chang, E.B., Fedorak, R.N., Field, M. 1986: Experimental diabetic diarrhea in rats. Intestinal mucosal denervation, hypersensitivity and treatment with clonidine. *Gastroenterology* 91, 564–9.

Chaudhuri, K.R., Thomaides, T., Mathias, C.J. 1992: Abnormality of superior mesenteric artery blood flow responses in human sympathetic failure. *Journal of Physiology* (*London*) 457, 477–89.

Cherbut, C., Bruley-des-Varannes, S., Schnee, M. *et al.* 1994: Involvement of small intestinal motility in blood glucose response to dietary fibre in man. *British Journal of Nutrition* 71, 675–85.

Chey, W.D., Kim, M., Hasler, W. *et al.* 1995: Hyperglycemia alters perception of rectal distention and blunts the rectoanal inhibitory reflex in healthy volunteers. *Gastroenterology* 105, 1700–8.

Code, C.F., Marlett, J.A. 1975: The interdigestive myoelectric complex of the stomach and small bowel of dogs. *Journal of Physiology* (*London*) 246, 289–309.

Colemont, L., Camilleri, M. 1989: Chronic intestinal pseudoobstruction: diagnosis and treatment. *Mayo Clinic Proceedings* 64, 60–70.

Cowles, V.E., Sarna, S.K. 1990: Effect of cholera toxin on small intestinal motor activity in the fed state. *Digestive Diseases and Sciences* 35, 353–9.

De Boer, S.Y., Masclee, A.A., Lamers, C.B. 1992a: Effect of hyperglycemia on gastrointestinal and gallbladder motility. *Scandinavian Journal of Gastroenterology* 194, 13–18.

De Boer, S.Y., Masclee, A.A.M., Lam, W.F. *et al.* 1992b: Effect of acute hyperglycemia on esophageal motility and lower esophageal sphincter pressure in humans. *Gastroenterology* 103, 775–80.

DeWever, I., Eeckhout, C., Vantrappen, G. *et al.* 1978: Disruptive effect of test meals on interdigestive motor complex in dogs. *American Journal of Physiology* 235, G661–5.

Di Lorenzo, C., Flores, A.F., Buie, T. *et al.* 1995: Intestinal motility and jejunal bleeding in children with chronic intestinal pseudo-obstruction. *Gastroenterology* 108, 1379–85.

Dooley, C.P., El-Newihi, H.M., Zeidler, A. *et al.* 1988: Abnormalities of the migrating motor complex in diabetics with autonomic neuropathy and diarrhea. *Scandinavian Journal of Gastroenterology* 23, 217–23.

Drossman, D.A. 1990: Identification of subgroups of functional bowel disorders. *Gastroenterology International* 3, 159–72.

Feldman, M., Schiller, L.R. 1983: Disorders of gastrointestinal motility associated with diabetes mellitus. *Annals of Internal Medicine* 98, 378–84.

Fell, J., Smith, V., Milla, P. 1996: Infantile chronic idiopathic intestinal pseudo-obstruction: the role of intestinal manometry as a diagnostic tool and prognostic indicator. *Gut* 39, 303–11.

Fenton, T.R. 1983: Disordered small intestinal motility: a rational basis for toddlers diarrhoea. *Gut* 24, 897–903.

Fleckenstein, P., Oigaard, A. 1978: Electrical spike activity in the human small intestine. A multiple electrode study of fasting diurnal variations. *American Journal of Digestive Diseases* 23, 776–80.

Fraser, R., Horowitz, M., Dent, J. 1991: Hyperglycaemia stimulates pyloric motility in normal subjects. *Gut* 32, 475–8.

Fraser, R., Horowitz, M., Maddox, A. *et al.* 1993: Organization of antral pyloric and duodenal motility in patients with gastroparesis. *Journal of Gastrointestinal Motility* 5, 167–75.

Furness, J.B., Costa, M. 1980: Types of nerves in the enteric nervous system. *Neuroscience* 5, 1–20.

Gorard, D.A., Libby, G.W., Farthing, M.J. 1994: Ambulatory small intestinal motility in 'diarrhoea' predominant irritable bowel syndrome. *Gut* 35, 203–10.

Gorard, D.A., Vesselinova-Jenkins, C.K., Libby, G.W. *et al.* 1995: Migrating motor complex and sleep in health and irritable bowel syndrome. *Digestive Diseases and Sciences* 40, 2383–9.

Hackelsberger, N., Schmidt, T., Renner, R. *et al.* 1997: Ambulatory long-term jejunal manometry in diabetic patients with cardiac autonomic neuropathy. *Neurogastroenterology and Motility* 9, 77–83.

Hallgren, T., Fasth, S., Delbro, D.S. *et al.* 1994: Loperamide improves anal sphincter function and continence after restorative proctocolectomy. *Digestive Diseases and Sciences* 39, 2612–18.

Hasler, W.L., Soudah, H.C., Dulai, G. *et al.* 1995: Mediation of hyperglycemia-evoked gastric slow-wave dysrhythmias by endogenous prostaglandins. *Gastroenterology* 108, 727–36.

Hebbard, G.S., Samsom, M., Sun, W.M. *et al.* 1996: Hyperglycemia affects proximal gastric motor and sensory function during small intestinal triglyceride infusion. *American Journal of Physiology* 271, G814–19.

Hirano, T., Niijima, A. 1980: Effects of 2-deoxy-D-glucose, glucose and insulin on efferent activity in gastric vagus nerve. *Experientia* 36, 1197–8.

Holtmann, G., Talley, N.J., Goebell, H. 1996: Association between H. pylori, duodenal mechanosensory thresholds, and small intestinal motility in chronic unexplained dyspepsia. *Digestive Diseases and Sciences* 41, 1285–91.

Horowitz, M., Fraser, R. 1994: Disordered gastric motor function in diabetes mellitus. *Diabetologia* 37, 543–51.

Horowitz, M., Fraser, R.J.L., Hebbard, G.S. *et al.* 1997: Effects of diabetes mellitus on gastrointestinal motor function. *Neuroscience Research Communications* 21, 75–82.

Hyman, P.E., Napolitano, J.A., Diego, A. *et al.* 1990: Antroduodenal manometry in the evaluation of chronic functional gastrointestinal symptoms. *Pediatrics* 86, 39–44.

Janatuinen, E., Pikkarainen, P., Laakso, M. *et al.* 1993: Gastrointestinal symptoms in middle-aged diabetic patients. *Scandinavian Journal of Gastroenterology* 28, 427–32.

Jebbink, H.J., Bravenboer, B., Akkermans, L.M. *et al.* 1993: Relationships between dyspeptic symptoms and gastrointestinal motility in patients with type 1 (insulin-dependent) diabetes mellitus. *Diabetologia* 36, 948–54.

Kassander, P. 1958: Asymptomatic gastric retention in diabetics (gastroparesis diabeticorum). *Annals of Internal Medicine* 48, 797–812.

Kawagishi, T., Nishizawa, Y., Okuno, Y. *et al.* 1992: Segmental gut transit in diabetes mellitus: effect of cisapride. *Diabetes Research and Clinical Practice* 17, 137–44.

Kellow, J.E., Phillips, S.E. 1987: Altered small bowel motility in irritable bowel syndrome is correlated with symptoms. *Gastroenterology* 92, 1885–93.

Kellow, J.E., Borody, T.J., Phillips, S.F. *et al.* 1986: Human interdigestive motility: variations in patterns from esophagus to colon. *Gastroenterology* 91, 386–95.

Kellow, J.E., Gill, R.C., Wingate, D. 1990: Prolonged ambulant recordings of small bowel motility demonstrate abnormalities in the irritable bowel syndrome. *Gastroenterology* 98, 1208–18.

Kellow, J.E., Langeluddecke, P.M., Eckersley, G.M. *et al.* 1992: Effects of acute psychologic stress on small-intestinal motility in health and the irritable bowel syndrome. *Scandinavian Journal of Gastroenterology* 27, 53–8.

Keranen, U., Jarvinen, H., Kiviluoto, T. *et al.* 1996: Substance P- and vasoactive intestinal polypeptide-immunoreactive innervation in normal and inflamed pouches after restorative proctocolectomy for ulcerative colitis. *Digestive Diseases and Sciences* 41, 1658–64.

Keshavarzian, A., Iber, F.L., Vaeth, J. 1987: Gastric emptying in patients with insulin-requiring diabetes mellitus. *American Journal of Gastroenterology* 82, 29–35.

Kim, C.H., Kennedy, F.P., Camilleri, M. *et al.* 1991: The relationship between clinical factors and gastrointestinal dysmotility in diabetes mellitus. *Journal of Gastrointestinal Motility* 3, 268–72.

Kruis, W., Azpiroz, F., Phillips, S.F. 1985: Contractile patterns and transit of fluid in canine terminal ileum. *American Journal of Physiology* 249, G264–70.

Kumar, D., Thompson, P.D., Wingate, D.L., *et al.* 1992: Abnormal REM sleep in the irritable bowel syndrome. *Gastroenterology* 103, 12–17.

Lang, I., Marvig, J., Sarna, S. *et al.* 1986: Gastrointestinal myoelectric correlates of vomiting in the dog. *American Journal of Physiology* 251, G830–6.

Lee, J.S. 1983: Effect of stretching and stirring on water and glucose absorption by canine mucosal membrane. *Journal of Physiology* (*London*) 345, 335–43.

Leveston, S.A., Shah, S.D., Cryer, P.E. 1979: Cholinergic stimulation of norepinephrine release in man. *Journal of Clinical Investigation* 64, 374–80.

Levitt, M.D., Kamm, M.A., van-der-Sijp, J.R. *et al.* 1994: Ambulatory pouch and anal motility in patients with ileo-anal reservoirs. *International Journal of Colorectal Disease* 9, 40–4.

Levitt, N.S., Stansberry, K.B., Wynchank, S. *et al.* 1996: The natural progression of autonomic neuropathy and autonomic function tests in a cohort of people with IDDM. *Diabetes Care* 19, 751–4.

MacGregor, I.L., Gueller, R., Watts, H.D. *et al.* 1976: The effect of acute hyperglycaemia on gastric emptying in man. *Gastroenterology* 70, 190–6.

Mayer, E.A., Elashoff, J., Hawkins, R. *et al.* 1988: Gastric emptying of mixed solid-liquid meal in patients with intestinal pseudoobstruction. *Digestive Diseases and Sciences* 33, 10–18.

Melville, J., Macagno, E., Christensen, J. 1975: Longitudinal contractions in the duodenum, their fluid mechanical function. *American Journal of Physiology* 228, 1887–92.

Orr, W.C., Crowell, M.D., Lin, B. *et al.* 1997: Sleep and gastric function in irritable bowel syndrome: derailing the brain–gut axis. *Gut* 41, 390–3.

Oster-Jorgensen, E., Qvist, N., Pedersen, S.A. *et al.* 1992: The influence of induced hyperglycaemia on the characteristics of intestinal motility and bile kinetics in healthy men. *Scandinavian Journal of Gastroenterology* 27, 285–8.

Otterson, M.F., Sarna, S.K. 1992: Fractionated doses of ionizing radiation alter postprandial small intestinal motor activity. *Digestive Diseases and Sciences* 37, 709–15.

Prior, A., Sorial, E., Sun, W.M. *et al.* 1993: Irritable bowel syndrome: differences between patients who show rectal sensitivity and those who do not. *European Journal of Gastroenterology and Hepatology* 5, 343–9.

Quigley, E.M., Thompson, J.S. 1993: The motor response to intestinal resection: motor activity in the canine small intestine following distal resection. *Gastroenterology* 105, 791–8.

Quigley, E.M., Thompson, J.S. 1994: Effects of artificial ileocolonic sphincter on motility in intestinal remnant following subtotal small intestinal resection in the dog. *Digestive Diseases and Sciences* 39, 1222–9.

Quigley, E.M.M., Phillips, E.S., Dent, J. *et al.* 1983: Myoelectric activity and intraluminal pressure of the canine ileocolonic sphincter. *Gastroenterology* 85, 1054–62.

Quigley, E.M.M., Phillips, S., Dent, J. 1984a: Distinctive patterns of interdigestive motility at the canine ileocolonic junction. *Gastroenterology* 87, 836–44.

Quigley, E.M.M., Borody, T.J., Phillips, S.F. *et al.* 1984b: Motility of the terminal ileum and ileocecal sphincter in healthy humans. *Gastroenterology* 87, 857–66.

Read, N.W. 1980: The migrating motor complex and spontaneous fluctuations of transmural potential difference in the human small intestine. In International Symposium on Gastrointestinal Motility *Gastrointestinal motility*. New York: Raven Press, 299–306.

Read, N.W., Miles, C.A., Fisher, D. 1980: Transit of a meal through the small intestine and colon in normal subjects and its role in the pathogenesis of diarrhoea. *Gastroenterology* 79, 1276–82.

Read, N.W., McFarlane, A., Kinsman, R.I. *et al.* 1984: Effect of infusion of nutrient solutions into the ileum on gastrointestinal transit and plasma levels of neurotensin and enteroglucagon. *Gastroenterology* 86, 274–80.

Remington, M. 1983: Abnormalities in gastrointestinal motor activity in patients with short bowels: effects of a synthetic opiate. *Gastroenterology* 85, 629–36.

Rudolph, C., Hyman, P., Altschuler, S. *et al.* 1997: Diagnosis and treatment of chronic intestinal pseudo-obstruction in children: report of consensus workshop. *Journal of Pediatric Gastroenterology and Nutrition* 24, 102–12.

Russo, A., Fraser, R., Horowitz, M. 1996: The effect of acute hyperglycaemia on small intestinal motility in normal subjects. *Diabetologia* 39, 984–9.

Russo, A., Sun, W.M., Sattawatthamrong, Y. *et al.* 1997: Acute hyperglycaemia affects anorectal motor and sensory function in normal subjects. *Gut* 41, 494–9.

Sanders, K. 1996: A case for interstitial cells of Cajal as pacemakers and mediators of neurotransmission in the gastrointestinal tract. *Gastroenterology* 111, 492–515.

Sanders, K.M., Ward, S.M. 1992: Nitric oxide as a mediator of nonadrenergic noncholinergic neurotransmission. *American Journal of Physiology* 262, G379–92.

Sarna, S.K. 1987: Giant migrating contractions and their myoelectric correlates in the small intestine. *American Journal of Physiology* 253, G687–705.

Schemann, M., Ehrlein, H.J. 1986: Postprandial patterns of canine jejunal motility and transit of luminal content. *Gastroenterology* 90, 991–1000.

Schmidt, T., Hackelsberger, N., Widmer, R. *et al.* 1996a: Ambulatory 24-hour jejunal motility in diarrhea-predominant irritable bowel syndrome. *Scandinavian Journal of Gastroenterology* 31, 581–9.

Schmidt, T., Pfeiffer, A., Hackelsberger, N. *et al.* 1996b: Effect of intestinal resection on human small bowel motility. *Gut* 38, 859–63.

Schvarcz, E., Palmer, M., Ingberg, C. *et al.* 1996: Increased prevalence of upper gastrointestinal symptoms in long-term Type 1 diabetes mellitus. *Diabetic Medicine* 13, 478–81.

Schvarcz, E., Palmer, M., Aman, J. *et al.* 1997: Changes in blood glucose within the physiological range affect gastric emptying in normal subjects and patients with insulin dependent diabetes mellitus. *Gastroenterology* 113, 60–6.

Schwartz, T.W., Holst, J.J., Fahenhrug, J. *et al.* 1978: Vagal, cholinergic regulation of pancreatic polypeptide secretion. *Journal of Clinical Investigation* 61, 781–9.

Scott, L.D., Cahall, D.L. 1982: Influence of the interdigestive myoelectric complex on enteric flora in the rat. *Gastroenterology* 82, 737–45.

Sessions, J.T., Viegas de Indrade, S.R., Kokas, E. 1968: Intestinal villi. Forward motility in relation to function. In Glass, G.B.J. (ed.) *Progress in gastroenterology*. New York: Grune & Stratton, 248–60.

Sjolund, K., Ekman, R., Lindgren, S. *et al.* 1996: Disturbed motilin and cholecystokinin release in the irritable bowel syndrome. *Scandinavian Journal of Gastroenterology* 31, 1110–14.

Small, P., Loudon, M., Hau, C. *et al.* 1997: Large-scale ambulatory study of postprandial jejunal motility in irritable bowel syndrome. *Scandinavian Journal of Gastroenterology* 32, 39–47.

Snape, W.J., Jr, Carlson, G.M., Matarazzo, S.A. *et al.* 1977: Evidence that abnormal myoelectrical activity produces colonic motor dysfunction in the irritable bowel syndrome. *Gastroenterology* 72, 383–7.

Stanghellini, V., Camilleri, M., Malagelada, J.R. 1987: Chronic idiopathic intestinal pseudo-obstruction: clinical and intestinal manometric findings. *Gut* 28, 5–12.

Stryker, S.J., Borody, T.J., Phillips, S.F. *et al.* 1985: Motility of the small intestine after proctocolectomy and ileal pouch-anal anastomosis. *Annals of Surgery* 201, 351–6.

Summers, R.W., Anuras, S., Green, J. 1983: Jejunal manometry patterns in health, partial intestinal obstruction and pseudo-obstruction. *Gastroenterology* 85, 1290–300.

Sun, W.M., Edwards, C.A., Prior, A. *et al.* 1990: The effect of oral nicardipine on anorectal function in human volunteers and patients with irritable bowel syndrome. *Digestive Diseases and Sciences* 35, 885–90.

Sun, W.M., Read, N.W., Katsinelos, P. *et al.* 1994: Anorectal function after restorative proctocolectomy and low anterior resection with coloanal anastomosis. *British Journal of Surgery* 81, 280–4.

Swarbrick, E.T., Bat, L., Hegarty, J.E. *et al.* 1980: Site of pain from the iritable bowel syndrome. *Lancet* 2, 443–6.

Szurszewski, J.H. 1969: A migrating electrical complex in canine small intestine. *American Journal of Physiology* 217, 1757–63.

Talley, N.J. 1991: Non-ulcer dyspepsia: myths and realities. *Alimentary Pharmacology and Therapeutics* 1, 145–62.

Taylor, I., Feldman, M., Richardson, C. *et al.* 1978: Gastric and cephalic stimulation of human pancreatic polypeptide release. *Gastroenterology* 75, 432–7.

Thompson, W.G. 1989: Irritable bowel syndrome: guidelines for the diagnosis. *Gastroenterology International* 2, 92–5.

Torihashi, S., Ward, S.M., Nishikawa, S.I. *et al.* 1995: c-kit-dependent development of interstitial cells and electrical activity in the murine gastrointestinal tract. *Cell and Tissue Research* 280, 97–111.

Valdovinos, M.A., Camilleri, M., Zimmerman, B.R. 1993: Chronic diarrhea in diabetes mellitus: mechanisms and an approach to diagnosis and treatment. *Mayo Clinic Proceedings* 68, 691–702.

Vantrappen, G., Janssens, J., Hellemans, J., Ghoos, Y. 1977: The interdigestive motor complex of normal subjects and patients with bacterial overgrowth of the small intestine. *Journal of Clinical Investigation* 59, 1158–66.

Vinograd, I., Merguerian, P., Udassin, R. *et al.* 1984: An experimental model of a submucosally tunnelled valve for the replacement of the ileo-cecal valve. *Journal of Pediatric Surgery* 19, 726–31.

Waddell, W.R., Kern, F., Jr, Halgrimson, C.G. *et al.* 1970: A simple jejunocolic 'valve'. For relief of rapid transit and the short bowel syndrome. *Archives of Surgery* 100, 438–44.

Wegener, M., Borsch, G., Schaffstein, J. *et al.* 1990: Gastrointestinal transit disorders in patients with insulin-treated diabetes mellitus. *Digestive Disease* 8, 23–36.

Welch, I., Saunders, K., Read, N.W. 1985: Effect of ileal and intravenous infusions of fat emulsions on feeding and satiety in human volunteers. *Gastroenterology* 89, 1293–7.

Werth, B., Meyer-Wyss, B., Spinas, G.A. *et al.* 1992: Non-invasive assessment of gastrointestinal motility disorders in diabetic patients with and without cardiovascular signs of autonomic neuropathy. *Gut* 33, 1199–203.

Whitehead, W.E., Engel, B.T., Schuster, M. 1980: Irritable bowel syndrome. *Digestive Diseases and Sciences* 25, 404–13.

Yeap, B., Russo, A., Fraser, R. *et al.*, 1996: Hyperglycaemia affects autonomic nerve function in healthy volunteers. *Diabetic Care* 19, 880–2.

12

Ecology of the small intestine

ADRIAN G CUMMINS

ESTABLISHMENT OF POSTNATAL BACTERIAL FLORA IN THE SMALL INTESTINE

The gastrointestinal tract of the neonate becomes colonized with bacteria within 24 hours of birth (Simon and Gorbach, 1984; Gracey, 1993). There is initially less bacterial colonization in neonates during the first 48 hours after Caesarean section than after vaginal delivery. Gram-positive organisms tend to predominate in breast-fed infants and Gram-negative organisms predominate in bottle-fed infants, with a microflora that is stable by 3–4 weeks after birth and remains so for a lifetime (Toskes and Donaldson, 1993). It has been claimed that maternal transfer of anaerobic bacteria to the neonatal gastrointestinal tract is reduced in Western countries owing to excessive hygiene (Bengmark, 1998). Colonization occurs sequentially from an oral to anal direction. Initially, *Escherichia coli* and *Streptococcus* colonize on the first day (within hours), coliforms, lactobacilli and enterococci on the second day, *Bacteroides* species and other anaerobes on the third day, and *Bifidobacter* species on the tenth day, especially in breast-fed infants (Simon and Gorbach, 1984). The progressive colonization of the gastrointestinal tract with different species of bacteria changes the redox potential and prepares the environment for later anaerobic organisms, especially in the colon. The initial luminal environment has a positive redox potential (+175 to +200 mV), which changes to a negative redox potential (–100 to –110 mV) and encourages growth of anaerobic organisms.

In the small intestine, breast milk promotes Gram-positive bacteria (mostly lactobacilli) but this changes to a mixed Gram-positive and Gram-negative flora during weaning, at least in the laboratory rat (Cummins *et al.*, 1988). In humans, about 90 per cent of faecal bacteria are Gram-positive in breast-fed infants, whereas *Bacteroides* and enterobacteria predominate in the faeces of formula-fed infants. Thus, the ratio of bifidobacteria:enterobacteria in faeces from breast-fed infants is 1000:1 but from formula-fed infants is 1:10. This is the basis of the bifidus effect in which Bifidobacteria colonization is promoted by breast milk, which also reduces colonization with *Bacteroides* and enterobacteria. Weaning removes the differences in bacterial flora between breast-fed and formula-fed infants. It is also claimed that modern human diets are too hygienic, with low bacteria numbers, which contrasts with the heavy bacterial (mainly *Lactobacillus* species) colonization of food that would have characterized prehistoric human diets (Bengmark, 1998).

DISTRIBUTION OF BACTERIAL FLORA ALONG THE GASTROINTESTINAL TRACT

The normal bacterial flora of the gastrointestinal tract has been reviewed (Simon and Gorbach 1984). This is summarized in Table 12.1. The stomach has $< 10^3$ colony-forming units (CFU)/ml in gastric juice with luminal flora consisting of predominantly Gram-positive aerobic organisms. This does not include

Table 12.1 *Bacterial flora of the gastrointestinal tract expressed as colony-forming units per gram of intestinal content*

	Stomach	Jejunum	Ileum	Caecum
Total bacterial counts	$0–10^3$	$0–10^4$	$10^5–10^8$	$10^{10}–10^{12}$
Predominant species	Gram-positive aerobic	Gram-positive aerobic	Mixed Gram aerobic/anaerobic	Gram-negative/ anaerobic
Anaerobes	0	0	$10^3–10^7$	$10^9–10^{12}$
Enterobacteria	Few	$< 10^3$	$10^2–10^6$	$10^4–10^{10}$
Luminal pH	3.0	6.0–7.0	7.5	6.8–7.3

Data taken from Toskes and Donaldson (1993).

Helicobacter pylori (Gram-negative) bacteria, which reside in the mucus layer of the stomach (Marshall, 1983; Warren, 1983). The bacterial flora of the proximal small intestine is similar to that of the stomach, i.e. mainly Gram-positive aerobic organisms. Typical species of bacteria are streptococci, lactobacilli, and lesser numbers of staphylococci, enterobacteria and bifidobacteria. In the distal ileum, Gram-negative organisms begin to outnumber Gram-positive organisms. Enterobacteria and anaerobes are also present (Simon and Gorbach, 1984). Bacteria in the colon are mainly Gram-negative anaerobic organisms. About one-third to one-half of the dry weight of faeces is bacteria.

FACTORS AFFECTING BACTERIAL FLORA IN THE GASTROINTESTINAL TRACT

Stability of bacterial flora in the gastrointestinal tract

Once bacterial flora are established postnatally, there is very little change in composition over a lifetime, at least in the colon. However, the bacterial flora of the stomach and proximal small intestine may change under certain situations, such as changes in gastric acid acidity or intestinal motility (Table 12.2). Colonization of the stomach with *Helicobacter pylori* is lifelong and is unusual in that not many bacterial infections of man are chronic replicating organisms. This affects the luminal bacterial flora if gastric atrophy and achlorhydria result. This leads to bacterial overgrowth both within the stomach and in the proximal small intestine. Gastric acid is an important protective mechanism in maintaining only sparse bacterial numbers in the upper gastrointestinal tract (*see* Chapter 5). Only acid-resistant organisms such as lactobacilli, streptococci and fungi survive transit through the stomach. Similarly, treatment with omeprazole and other proton pump inhibitors leads to bacterial overgrowth from loss of the gastric acid barrier. Decreased intestinal motility leads to bacterial overgrowth of the proximal gastrointestinal tract. This is classically seen in surgical blind loops in which there is considerable stasis. Lesser degrees of bacterial overgrowth with impaired intestinal motility are seen in various medical conditions, such as cirrhosis of the liver, chronic renal failure and generally with ageing (Roberts *et al.*, 1977; Husebye, 1995; Morencos *et al.*, 1995). Incontinence of the ileo-caecal valve (or surgical resection) can result in contamination of the ileum with colonic organisms. Immunodeficiency may also lead to bacterial overgrowth of the small intestine (Pignata *et al.*, 1990). This occurs in both congenital and acquired syndromes, including the acquired immunodeficiency syndrome (AIDS) and common variable immunodeficiency. Antibiotics for 4 days reduce breath H_2 and CH_4 fourfold after lactulose (Bjorneklett and Midtvedt, 1981).

Probiotics

Diet does not tend to have a major effect in altering the composition of the bacterial flora, except for the postnatal effect of breast milk. The difficulty is that changes in bacterial flora of the small intestine either have to be studied from proximal intestinal sampling or inferred from faecal cultures. A high meat diet also causes a small increase in faecal anaerobes, whereas a meatless diet is associated with a small increase in faecal coliforms (Hentges, 1978). Perhaps the main controversy regarding diet is the effect of supplementation of

Table 12.2 *Factors affecting bacterial flora of the gastrointestinal tract*

Factor	Effect
Breast feeding versus formula feeding	Favours Gram-positive bacteria
Achlorhydria	Bacterial overgrowth in stomach and small intestine
Decreased motility	Bacterial overgrowth in stomach and small intestine
Antibiotics	Reduce Gram-negative organisms but anaerobes persist
Immunodeficiency	Bacterial overgrowth of Gram-positive organisms

lactobacilli (probiotics) on the small and large intestines (Bengmark, 1998). Metchnikoff (1908) attributed the longevity of Bulgarian peasants to their consumption of yoghurt.

Probiotics such as yoghurt are being promoted for a variety of gastrointestinal conditions, to ameliorate gastroenteritis, to prevent antibiotic-associated diarrhoea, to prevent traveller's diarrhoea, to improve small bowel overgrowth, to ameliorate mucositis after radiotherapy or chemotherapy, and in the long term to prevent bowel cancer and promote better general health (Salminen *et al.*, 1996; Simenhoff *et al.*, 1996). The evidence for most of these claims is poor and circumstantial. A small study has shown that probiotics decrease intestinal permeability of the small bowel (Southcott *et al.*, 1997). Probiotics did not improve bacterial overgrowth when *Lactobacillus* was given to 17 patients for 4 weeks in a double-blind cross-over study (Stotzer *et al.*, 1996); *Lactobacillus* could only be recovered in the faeces of two of the subjects. There is evidence that *Lactobacillus* reduces colon cancers in rats given the cancer-inducing agent, dimethylhydrazine (Goldin *et al.*, 1996). There is better evidence that *Lactobacillus* will ameliorate rotavirus gastroenteritis in children (Rautanen *et al.*, 1998). This study has found that administration of two 1.25 g sachets of *Lactobacillus* GG (a strain thought to be adhesive on to enterocytes) early on the day of admission for diarrhoea will reduce the duration of diarrhoea from 30 to 18 hours. Infants were also given a glucose electrolyte mixture for rehydration.

EFFECT OF BACTERIAL FLORA ON INTESTINAL MORPHOLOGY AND FUNCTION

The effect of bacterial flora on the small intestine comes from studies of germ-free animals in which the small intestine is relatively immature (Abrams *et al.*, 1963). The intestine has small finger-like villi, small crypts and low proliferation. Exposure to a conventional environment results in 'physiological inflammation' and maturation of the small intestine. This process is similar to that during postnatal growth and weaning (Thompson *et al.*, 1998). Bacteria, especially Gram-negative organisms with lipopolysaccharide, are likely to prime the gut-associated immune system, and expand and activate dendritic (antigen-presenting) cells that assist food antigens to activate specific immune cells (Cummins and Thompson, 1997).

Luminal bacteria metabolize certain substrates in the small intestine, which is perhaps more important for animals than humans, e.g. rats utilize vitamin K from bacteria either absorbed directly or through coprophagy. Nevertheless, luminal bacteria in humans deconjugate sex hormones, which are subject to enterohepatic circulation. Hence, antibiotics can reduce circulating levels of androgens and oestrogens (Boxenbaum *et al.*, 1979). Similarly, the biliary excreted conjugate of digoxin can be degraded to an inactive form. Other actions of luminal bacteria occur but these are located in the colon rather than the small intestine (e.g. conversion of sulphasalazine to 5-aminosalicylic acid and sulphapyridine, and conversion of urea to ammonia). In small bowel bacterial overgrowth, various metabolic actions of the increased numbers of bacteria on specific ingested substrates are used to investigate this condition. Thus luminal breakdown of xylose occurs to CO_2, glucose or lactulose to H_2 or CH_4, or deconjugation of bile acids to CO_2, and these are detected in expired air. Some patients with bacterial overgrowth have changes in liver function tests and evidence of non-alcoholic steatohepatitis, which could be due to absorption of bacterial products (Lichtman *et al.*, 1990).

BACTERIAL OVERGROWTH

Bacterial overgrowth varies from asymptomatic to a severe malabsorption syndrome. Up to one-third of patients with bacterial overgrowth lose weight. In bacterial overgrowth, the flora of the proximal small intestine resembles that of the colon. It may cause diarrhoea, which is probably multifactorial but includes a component of steatorrhoea as well as mucosal damage, and patients may develop vitamin B_{12} deficiency if the condition is prolonged. The vitamin B_{12} deficiency is not corrected by intrinsic factor but by antibiotics. Competitive uptake of vitamin B_{12} is particularly characteristic of Gram-negative aerobes and certain anaerobes (*Bacteroides*).

Bacterial overgrowth is difficult to diagnose and is probably underdiagnosed. Apart from its association with classical structural abnormalities (jejunal diverticula, surgical blind loops), it may be associated with cirrhosis of the liver, chronic pancreatitis, chronic renal failure, and human immunodeficiency virus (HIV) enteropathy and it generally increases with ageing (Roberts *et al.*, 1977; McEvoy, 1983; Lembeke *et al.*, 1985; Montogomery, 1986; Pignata *et al.*, 1990; Morencos *et al.*, 1995). Bacterial overgrowth also occurs in immunodeficiency syndromes but tends to be of Gram-positive oral organisms (e.g. *Streptococcus* and *Staphylococcus*) (Pignata *et al.*, 1990), as compared to other causes of bacterial overgrowth in which Gram-negative organisms occur. Thus, bacterial overgrowth may be present in a variety of general medical conditions, which may obscure or distract from its diagnosis. Its presence is suggested by high folate levels in blood and perhaps by false-positive antigliadin antibodies. Bacterial overgrowth may explain why many patients, especially the elderly with chronic diarrhoea or just weight loss, improve after an empirical course of antibiotic, and presumably explains why serum vitamin B_{12} levels tend to decline with age.

The traditional test for bacterial overgrowth is quantitative culture of duodenal or jejunal fluid, but this may underestimate the condition, as it is always difficult to intubate far enough along the gastrointestinal tract to where it is presumed the bacterial overgrowth is maximally located, i.e. the mid and distal small intestine. Nevertheless, quantitative culture of intestinal fluid remains the gold standard, although it is realized that it may miss some bacterial overgrowth (Tillman *et al.*, 1981). Bacterial overgrowth is diagnosed if quantitative culture yields total bacteria counts of $> 10^5$ CFU/ml (g), or counts of aerobic bacteria $> 10^4$ CFU/ml (g), or counts of Gram-negative bacteria $> 10^3$ CFU/ml (g) or counts of anaerobes $> 10^2$ CFU/ml (g) (Table 12.1). Probably the first or second criterion is sufficient in routine practice. Although it is commonly advocated that strict anaerobic collection and culture be used, the benefit of this is dubious, as overgrowth usually consists of aerobic Gram-negative (coliform) bacteria despite the fact that anaerobes may be variably present.

If endoscopy is used for collection of intestinal fluid, then a lubricant without antiseptic should be employed on the instrument. Modern routine endoscopes are certainly easier to pass into the third and sometimes the fourth part of the duodenum. It is also advocated that a sealed outer tube (that is later broken *in situ*) be used and passed down the biopsy channel for fluid collection, although once again the importance of this outside of research studies is not proven. In fact, there is a high correlation between an open-ended and closed-ended tube for collection (Tillman *et al.*, 1981). In spite of the limitation of quantitative intestinal culture in diagnosing bacterial overgrowth, studies have shown that repeated sampling a few days apart still yields concordant results, as does sampling of the intestine from the ligament of Treitz as compared to more distally in the jejunum (Kalser *et al.*, 1966; Tillman *et al.*, 1981). As with many studies of bacterial overgrowth, the results probably depend on the patient population and severity of bacterial overgrowth under study. A very practical difficulty sometimes is the sparseness of fluid present that can be successfully aspirated. A recent technique has cultured endoscopic biopsies of the duodenum and is attractive because of simplicity and because it samples adherent bacteria in mucus (Riordan *et al.*, 1995). The authors found that the weight (4.0–84 mg) of the biopsy did not influence the bacteria count, which was highly correlated with the luminal aerobic bacteria count.

The mainstay of treatment for bacterial overgrowth consists of low-dose antibiotics (e.g. tetracycline, augmentin, cephalexin), which can be given either once only, cyclically (1 week every 4 weeks), or continuously in severe cases. Occasionally a patient may respond to cisapride on the presumption that the bacterial overgrowth is due to impaired intestinal motility or where the patient refuses to take antibiotics. Gastrointestinal lavage and probiotics have also been used in a few patients with short bowel syndrome and bacterial overgrowth with success (Vanderhoof *et al.*, 1998). The theory is that lactic acid bacteria inhibit Gram-negative bacteria, especially live lactobacilli, which adhere to the mucosal surface. They thereby compete with facultative anaerobic bacteria that adhere to the mucosal surface and injure by the production of enterotoxins.

Table 12.3 *Tests for bacterial overgrowth of the small intestine*

Test	Sensitivity	Specificity
Culture	High	High
^{14}C-Cholylglycine	Fair	Poor
^{14}C-D-Xylose	High	Medium–high
H_2 + CH_4/glucose or lactulose	Low	Medium

A variety of indirect tests have been developed that have the advantage of being non-invasive but perhaps more efficacious in testing bacterial flora in the mid and distal small intestine (Table 12.3). They rely on administering an ingested substrate (e.g. xylose, lactulose, bile acids) and following its transit through the small intestine over 4–6 hours. Catabolism of the substrate is assessed by breath $H_2 + CH_4$ or $^{13}CO_2$ or $^{14}CO_2$. The main disadvantage of these tests is differentiating between catabolism in the small bowel and large bowel (King and Toskes, 1986). This is especially difficult in short bowel syndrome.

The first indirect breath test was ^{14}C-cholylglycine and relied on deconjugation of the labelled bile acid by luminal bacteria. Its disadvantage is that it will be abnormal if the substrate is not fully absorbed in the ileum because of ileal resection or Crohn's disease. The labelled bile acid enters the colon and is deconjugated giving a false-positive result. Equivocal or false-positive results also occur if there is rapid transit into the colon.

Toskes and co-workers introduced the ^{14}C-D-xylose breath test in 1979 (King *et al.*, 1979). A non-radioactive version using ^{13}C-D-xylose has also been described (Dellert *et al.*, 1997). D-Xylose was believed to be better than labelled bile acid because xylose is metabolized by luminal Gram-negative aerobic bacteria, it is not metabolized by mammalian cells, and it is absorbed in the jejunum. The sensitivity for detecting bacterial overgrowth was initially reported as 95 per cent compared with 60–70 per cent for the ^{14}C-cholylglycine breath test. These values probably overestimate the sensitivity of both tests. In practice, there is also some spillover into the colon with false-positive results. This has led to combined tests of ^{14}C-D-xylose with a transit marker such as breath $H_2 + CH_4$ and lactulose or ^{99m}Tc-labelled colloid (Lewis *et al.*, 1997), which increased the specificity from 85 per cent

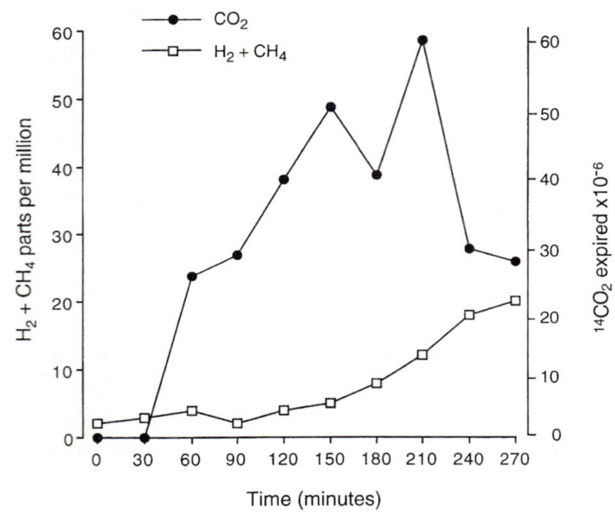

Figure 12.1 *Combined ^{14}C-D-xylose and H_2 + CH_4 breath test after lactulose ingestion. An example of a positive ^{14}C-D-xylose breath test for bacterial overgrowth that was nevertheless relatively mild and associated with an irritable bowel syndrome. The ^{14}C-D-xylose breath test was combined with measurement of breath H_2 and CH_4 after lactulose ingestion. The rise in breath H_2 and CH_4 from 180 minutes indicates that the substrate bolus has reached the distal ileum and/or caecum. Therefore any $^{14}CO_2$ rise prior to that time represents small bowel catabolism of xylose.*

to 94 per cent. An example of a combined ^{14}C-D-xylose and breath H_2 + CH_4 after lactulose is given in Fig. 12.1.

Recently, ^{13}C-sorbitol has been evaluated as a test for bacterial overgrowth, with 89 per cent sensitivity compared to 56 per cent and 67 per cent sensitivity for ^{14}C-xylose or ^{13}C-xylose (Somogyi *et al.*, 1998). Another simple breath test is to give a carbohydrate substrate, such as lactulose or glucose, and measure breath H_2 + CH_4. The major disadvantage is the low sensitivity (40–70 per cent) even when CH_4 is measured to overcome the problem of non-hydrogen-producing individuals. The considerable variation sometimes in reported sensitivity and specificity values of all breath tests presumably relates to the patient population and the spectrum of severity of bacterial overgrowth. Often patients are selected on the basis of jejunal culture, which overlooks some false-negative individuals. A true sensitivity rate for jejunal culture could be only 74 per cent but this is often considered as the gold standard of tests (Corazza *et al.*, 1990).

TROPICAL SPRUE AND ENTEROPATHY

Tropical sprue (*see* Chapter 21) comes from the Dutch term '*Indische spouw*' and describes a syndrome that was identified by military surgeons of the European maritime powers from the 1700s onwards. This syndrome consisted of chronic diarrhoea, followed by anorexia and weight loss, glossitis, and profound weakness with emaciation. Later malabsorption was associated with steatorrhoea and megaloblastic anaemia. Although originally described in European expatriates, it was later appreciated that it occurs in indigenous inhabitants. The small intestine of inhabitants of the tropics shows changes in structure and function as compared to those living in temperate zones. It is apparently acquired after birth, as stillborn foetuses in India have normal finger-like villi (Baker *et al.*, 1962). Usually this enteropathy is asymptomatic and is termed 'tropical enteropathy', but is designated 'tropical sprue' when symptomatic.

Tropical enteropathy has been reported in apparently healthy subjects in Thailand (Sprinz *et al.*, 1962), Malaysia (England and O'Brein, 1966), India (Baker and Mathan, 1972), Pakistan (Lindenbaum *et al.*, 1966) and Burma (Aung-Than-BaTu *et al.*, 1970). Tropical sprue may lead to significant malabsorption of carbohydrate. For example, malabsorption of rice is common in 80–90 per cent of infants less than 2 years old, 74 per cent of children from 3 to 5 years old, and 60 per cent of 5-year-old children, as well as 60 per cent of adults (Bolin *et al.*, 1996), which is presumably due to tropical enteropathy. Tropical enteropathy arises from small intestinal bacterial overgrowth perhaps predisposed by loss of the gastric acid barrier (Dale *et al.*, 1998), decreased motility and impaired intraluminal killing of coliform bacteria (Donaldson, 1968; Gracey, 1982). The major factor may be loss of the gastric acid barrier, perhaps through early acquisition of *Helicobacter pylori* infection (Dale *et al.*, 1998); it has been shown that even well-nourished Bangladeshi children do not have sufficient gastric acid to kill enteropathogenic bacteria (Gilman *et al.*, 1988). The other major reason could be slow intestinal transit, but orocaecal transit time, as measured by lactulose-breath hydrogen, seems to be in the same range of 60–90 minutes and is independent of country of origin, age or socioeconomic condition (Solomons *et al.*, 1977; Vreugdenhil *et al.*, 1986; Vajro *et al.*, 1988). It differs subtly from intestinal bacterial overgrowth in that there is only one or at most a few species of Gram-negative bacteria (e.g. *Klebsiella*) in the proximal small intestine, and folate deficiency may be associated in contrast to most cases of bacterial overgrowth in which there is folate excess.

Folic acid (usually with vitamin B_{12}) supplementation improves the glossitis, megaloblastic anaemia, lethargy and loss of appetite, whereas antibiotics improve the gastrointestinal symptoms. It has also been considered that other factors are involved such as environmental toxins, but these have never been confirmed as an additional aetiological agent.

REFERENCES

Abrams, G.D., Bauer, H., Sprinz, H. 1963: Influence of the normal flora on mucosal morphology and cellular renewal in the ileum. A comparison of germ-free and conventional mice. *Laboratory Investigations* 12, 355–64.

Aung-Than-BaTu, Marlar-Than, Hla-Pe 1970: Small intestinal morphology on healthy Burmese adults. *Union of Burma Journal of Life Science* 3, 365–70.

Baker, S.J., Mathan, V.I. 1972: Tropical enteropathy and tropical sprue. *American Journal of Clinical Nutrition* 25, 1047–55.

Baker, S.J., Ignatius, M., Mathan, V.I., Vasih, S.K., Chacko, C.C. 1962: Intestinal biopsy. In Wolstenholme, G.E.W., Cameron, M.P. (eds), *Intestinal biopsy*. Boston: Little, Brown and Co., 84.

Bengmark, S. 1998: Ecological control of the gastro-intestinal tract. The role of probiotic flora. *Gut* 42, 2–7.

Bjorneklett, A., Midtvedt, T. 1981: Influence of three antimicrobial agents – penicillin, metronidazole, and doxycyclin – on the intestinal microflora of healthy humans. *Scandinavian Journal of Gastroenterology* 16, 473–80.

Bolin, T.D., Myo-Kin, Soe-Aung, Genge, J.R., Duncombe, V.M. 1996: Correlation of hydrogen and methane production to rice carbohydrate malabsorption in Burmese (Myanmar) children. *Journal of Pediatric Gastroenterology and Nutrition* 22, 144–7.

Boxenbaum, H.G., Bejersky, I., Jack, M.L., Kaplan, S.A. 1979: Influence of gut microflora on bioavailability. *Drug Metabolism and Review* 9, 259–79.

Corazza, G.R., Menozzi, M.G., Strocchi, A. *et al.* 1990: The diagnosis of small bowel bacterial overgrowth. Reliability of jejunal culture and inadequacy of breath hydrogen testing. *Gastroenterology* 98, 302–9.

Cummins, A.G., Thompson, F.M. 1997: Postnatal changes in mucosal immune response: a physiological perspective of breast feeding and weaning. *Immunology and Cell Biology* 75, 419–29.

Cummins, A.G., Steele, T.W., LaBrooy, J.T., Shearman, D.J.C. 1988: Maturation of the rat small intestine at weaning: changes in epithelial cell kinetics, bacterial flora and mucosal immune activity. *Gut* 29, 1672–9.

Dale, A., Thomas, J.E., Darboe, M.K., Coward, W.A., Harding, M., Weaver, L.T. 1998: *Helicobacter pylori* infection, gastric acid secretion and infant growth. *Journal of Pediatric Gastroenterology and Nutrition* 26, 393–7.

Dellert, S.F., Nowicki, M.J., Farrell, M.K., Delente, J., Heubi, J.E. 1997: The ^{13}C-xylose breath test for the diagnosis of small bowel overgrowth in children. *Journal of Pediatric Gastroenterology and Nutrition* 25, 153–8.

Donaldson, R.M. 1968: Significance of small bowel bacteria. *American Journal of Clinical Nutrition* 21, 1088–96.

England, N.W., O'Brein, W. 1966: Appearances of the jejunal mucosa in acute tropical sprue in Singapore. *Gut* 7, 128–39.

Gilman, R.H., Partanen, R., Brown, K.H. *et al.* 1988: Decreased gastric acid secretion and bacterial colonization of the stomach in severely malnourished Bangladeshi children. *Gastroenterology* 94, 1308–14.

Goldin, B.R., Gualtieri, L.J., Moore, R.P. 1996: The effect of *Lactobacillus GG* on the initiation and promotion of DMH-induced intestinal tumors in the rat. *Nutrition and Cancer* 25, 197–204.

Gracey, M. 1982: Intestinal microflora and bacterial overgrowth in early life. *Journal of Pediatric Gastroenterology and Nutrition* 1, 13–22.

Gracey, M. 1993: Intestinal microflora. In Gracey, M., Burke, V. (eds), *Pediatric gastroenterology and hepatology.* Boston: Blackwell Scientific Publications, 200–8.

Hentges, D.J. 1978: Faecal flora of volunteers on controlled diets. *American Journal of Clinical Nutrition* 31, S123–4.

Husebye, E. 1995: Gastrointestinal motility disorders and bacterial overgrowth. *Journal of Internal Medicine* 237, 419–27.

Kalser, M.H., Cohen, R., Arteaga, I., Yawn, E., Maydral, L., Hoffert, W.R., Frazier, D. 1966: Normal viral and bacterial flora of the human small and large intestine. *New England Journal of Medicine* 274, 500–5.

King, C., Toskes, P. 1986: Comparison of the 1-gram [^{14}C]xylose, 10-gram lactulose-H_2 and 80-gram glucose breath tests in patients with small intestine bacterial overgrowth. *Gastroenterology* 91, 1447–51.

King, C.E., Toskes, P.P., Spivey, J.C., Lorenz, E., Welkos, S. 1979: Detection of small intestinal bacterial overgrowth by means of a ^{14}C-D-xylose breath test. *Gastroenterology* 77, 75–82.

Lembeke, B., Kraus, B., Lankisch, P.G. 1985: Small intestinal function in chronic relapsing pancreatitis. *Hepatogastroenterology* 32, 149–51.

Lewis, S.J., Young, G., Mann, M., Franco, S., O'Keefe, S.J.S. 1997: Improvement in specificity of [^{14}C]D-xylose breath test for bacterial overgrowth. *Digestive Diseases and Sciences* 42, 1587–92.

Lichtman, S.N., Sartor, R.B., Keku, J., Schwab, J.H. 1990: Hepatic inflammation in rats with experimental small intestinal bacterial overgrowth. *Gastroenterology* 98, 414–23.

Lindenbaum, J., Alam, J.A.K., Kent, T.H. 1966: Subclinical small-intestinal disease in East Pakistan. *British Medical Journal* 2, 1616–19.

Marshall, B. 1983: Unidentified curved bacilli on gastric epithelium in active chronic gastritis. *Lancet* 1, 1273–5.

McEvoy, A. 1983: Bacterial contamination of the small intestine is an important cause of occult malabsorption in the elderly. *British Medical Journal* 287, 789–93.

Metchnikoff, E. 1908: *The prolongation of life.* New York: Putnam.

Montogomery, R.D. 1986: Causes of malabsorption in the elderly. *Age and Ageing* 15, 235–40.

Morencos, F., De Las Castano, G., Martin Ramos, L., Lopez Arias, M.J., Ledesma, F., Pons Romero, F. 1995: Small bowel bacterial overgrowth in patients with alcoholic cirrhosis. *Digestive Diseases and Sciences* 40, 1252–6.

Pignata, C., Budillon, G., Monaco, G., Nani, E., Cuomo, R., Parill, G., Ciccimarra, F. 1990: Jejunal bacterial overgrowth and intestinal permeability in children with immunodeficiency syndromes. *Gut* 31, 879–82.

Rautanen, T., Isolauri, E., Salo, E., Vesikari, T. 1998: Management of acute diarrhoea with low osmolarity oral rehydration solutions and *Lactobacillus* strain GG. *Archives of Disease of Childhood* 79, 157–60.

Riordan, S., Mciver, C., Duncombe, V., Bolin, T. 1995: Bacteriologic analysis of mucosal biopsy specimens for detecting small-intestinal bacterial overgrowth. *Scandinavian Journal of Gastroenterology* 30, 681–5.

Roberts, S.H., James, O., Jarvis, E.H. 1977: Bacterial overgrowth without 'blind loop': a cause for malnutrition in the elderly. *Lancet* 2, 1193–5.

Salminen, S., Isolauri, E., Salminen, E. 1996: Clinical uses of probiotics of stabilizing the gut mucosal barrier: successful strains and future challenges. *Antonie Van Leeuwenhoek* 70, 347–58.

Simenhoff, M.L., Dunn, S.R., Zollner, G.P., Fitzpatrick, M.E., Emery, S.M., Sandine, S.M., Ayres, J.W. 1996: Biomodulation of the toxic and nutritional effects of small bowel bacterial overgrowth in end stage kidney disease using freeze-dried *Lactobacillus acidophilus*. *Mineral and Electrolyte Metabolism* 22, 92–6.

Simon, G.L., Gorbach, S.L. 1984: Intestinal flora in health and disease. *Gastroenterology* 86, 174–93.

Solomons, N., Vásquez, L., Torún, B., Viteri, F. 1977: A non-invasive methology for mouth-to-colon transit time in pre-school children using hydrogen (H2) breath analysis. *Gastroenterology* 32, A112/1135.

Somogyi, L., Amann, S., Wagner, D.A., Toskes, P.P. 1998: Preliminary evaluation of ^{13}C-sorbitol breath test in diagnosis of small bowel bacterial overgrowth. *Gastroenterology* 114, A417.

Southcott, E.K., Butler, R.N., Davidson, G.P. 1997: Probiotics decrease small intestinal permeability in children. *Journal of Gastroenterology and Hepatology* 12, A104.

Sprinz, H., Sribhibhadh, R., Gangarosa, E.J., Benyajsti, C., Kundel, D., Halstead, S. 1962: Biopsy of the small bowel of Thai people with special reference to recovery from Asiatic cholera and to an intestinal malabsorption syndrome. *American Journal of Clinical Pathology* 38, 43–51.

Stotzer, P.O., Blomberg, L., Conway, P.L., Henriksson, A., Abrahamsson, H. 1996: Probiotics treatment of small intestinal bacterial overgrowth by *Lactobacillus fermentum KLD. Scandinavian Journal of Infectious Disease* 28, 615–19.

Thompson, F.M., Catto-Smith, A.G., Moore, D., Davidson, G., Cummins, A. 1998: Epithelial growth of the small intestine in human infants. *Journal of Pediatric Gastroenterology and Nutrition* 26, 506–12.

Tillman, R., King, C., Toskes, P. 1981: Continued experience with xylose breath test: evidence that the small bowel culture as the gold standard for bacterial overgrowth may be tarnished. *Gastroenterology* 80, 1304.

Toskes, P.P., Donaldson, R.M. 1993: Enteric bacterial flora and bacterial overgrowth syndrome. In Sleisenger, M.H., Fordtran, J.S. (eds), *Gastrointestinal disease. Pathophysiology, diagnosis and management.* Philadelphia: W.B. Saunders, 1106–18.

Vajro, P., Silano, G., Longo, D., Staiano, A., Fontanella, A. 1988: Orocaecal transit time in healthy and constipated children. *Acta Paediatrica Scandinavica* 77, 583–6.

Vanderhoof, J.A., Young, R.J., Murray, N., Kaufman, S.S. 1998: Treatment strategies for small bowel bacterial overgrowth in short bowel syndrome. *Journal of Pediatric Gastroenterology and Nutrition* 27, 155–60.

Vreugdenhil, C., Sinaasappel, M., Bouquet, J. 1986: A comparative study of the mouth to caecum transit time in children and adults using a weighted adapted lactulose dose. *Acta Paediatrica Scandinavica* 75, 483–8.

Warren, J.R. 1983: Unidentified curved bacilli on gastric epithelium in active chronic gastritis. *Lancet* 1, 1273.

13

Diagnostic tests of small intestinal function

13.1

Endoscopy

IAN C ROBERTS-THOMSON

INTRODUCTION

Endoscopy, sometimes combined with small bowel biopsy, is an early investigation for most patients with suspected small bowel disorders. The most common approach is the use of upper gastrointestinal endoscopy for intubation of the duodenum. The terminal ileum can also be visualized at the time of colonoscopy, although success rates among endoscopists for intubation of the ileum vary widely from about 10 per cent to 90 per cent. Intubation of the ileum is easier after a colonic resection (usually a hemicolectomy) and is readily performed after an ileostomy.

There is only limited experience with endoscopic procedures for visualization of the small bowel between the third part of the duodenum and the terminal ileum. The first prototype endoscopes were enteroscopic probes, which advanced along the small bowel by peristalsis (Lewis and Waye, 1987; D'Agostino *et al.*, 1997). A major disadvantage was the duration of the procedure, often several hours. More recently, 'push-type' enteroscopes have been developed that can be used either through the upper gastrointestinal tract or through the colon (Barkin *et al.*, 1992; Landi *et al.*, 1998). When introduced through the upper gastrointestinal tract, entry into the lower small bowel can be facilitated by the use of a gastric overtube (Barkin *et al.*, 1994). Nevertheless, 'push-type' enteroscopes rarely permit visualization of the entire small bowel.

Under certain circumstances, previous operative procedures can facilitate visualization of the jejunum with routine endoscopes. These procedures include a gastroenterostomy, Billroth II (Polya) gastrectomy and an operative jejunostomy.

NORMAL SMALL BOWEL

The duodenum is the most proximal portion of small bowel and forms a C-shaped loop that is moulded around the head of the pancreas. The adult duodenum is about 30 cm long and has been subdivided into four parts on the basis of angular changes in its course. The first part is approximately 5 cm long and incorporates the duodenal bulb or cap, a proximal region about 4 cm long and 2 cm wide. The second part of the duodenum courses inferiorly for 7–10 cm and almost always incorporates the ampulla of Vater and the accessory ampulla. The third part of the duodenum is about 10 cm in length and courses transversely to the aorta and inferior vena cava, while the fourth part courses upwards and to the left to the duodeno-jejunal flexure, which is fixed posteriorly by the ligament of Treitz.

The relationship between the endoscopic appearance and the site of lesions in the duodenal bulb may be of importance. This can be assisted by the relationship of duodenal structures to antral structures but, in general, posterior lesions are seen at the 3 o'clock position, inferior lesions at 6 o'clock, anterior lesions at 9 o'clock and superior lesions at 12 o'clock. When compared to the antrum of the stomach, the mucosa of the bulb is somewhat pale and yellow–grey (Plate 13.1.1). With close inspection, the villous architecture has a finely granular appearance with tiny dots of reflected light.

Small-calibre endoscopes can sometimes be retroflexed within the duodenal bulb to examine the pylorobulbar junction and the fornices.

The second part of the duodenum is characterized by the presence of bile and by numerous circular folds known as valvulae conniventes, plicae circulares or Kerckring's folds (Plate 13.1.2). The ampullae can be seen with end-viewing endoscopes but are better examined with side-viewing duodenoscopes. The minor ampulla is located about 2 cm above and anterior to the major ampulla. The second part of the duodenum has a yellow–orange colour when compared to the duller appearance of the duodenal bulb. The presence of small white spots is usually due to lipid in lacteals in the lamina propria and may reflect a recent meal or slow gastric emptying.

The terminal ileum is similar to the duodenum but has fewer circular folds and often has more vigorous motor activity (Plate 13.1.3). In addition, small nodules, 1–5 mm in size, may be seen and are usually lymphoid nodules covered by normal mucosa. With suction, the lumen of the terminal ileum tends to collapse more readily than the lumen of the ascending colon.

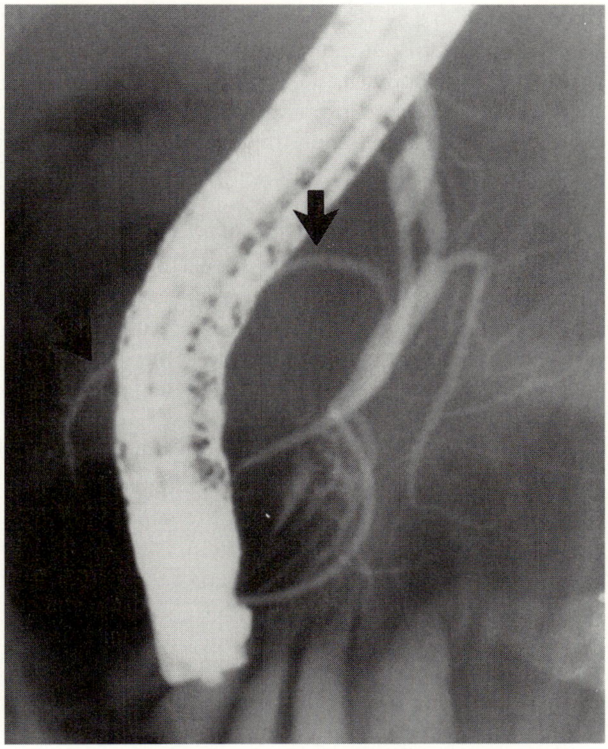

Figure 13.1.1 *A retrograde pancreatogram in a patient with annular pancreas showing an anomalous pancreatic duct encircling the duodenum (arrows).*

DEVELOPMENTAL ANOMALIES

Congenital anomalies

It is unusual for congenital anomalies of the small bowel to be recognized by endoscopists. This reflects the low incidence of anomalies in most populations as well as the likelihood that some anomalies will be diagnosed and treated early in life, usually without endoscopy.

The most common anomaly is a Meckel's diverticulum, which, based on autopsy studies, occurs in about 1–3 per cent of the population. Only a minority of diverticula, however, contain gastric tissue with the potential for ulceration and bleeding, either within the diverticulum or in the adjacent ileum (Turgeon and Barnett, 1990). Furthermore, the orifice of the diverticulum is usually outside the reach of the colonoscope and reports of ileal ulceration identified by endoscopy are rare.

Annular pancreas occurs in about 1:10 000 live births and often results in narrowing or obstruction of the second part of the duodenum (Urayama *et al.*, 1995). While the majority of patients are diagnosed in infancy, some present with obstructive symptoms as teenagers or adults. Endoscopy reveals focal narrowing of the second part of the duodenum. If the stricture can be negotiated with a duodenoscope, the papilla is normally located below the stricture, while pancreatography reveals an anomalous duct encircling the duodenum (Fig. 13.1.1).

Congenital anomalies of intestinal rotation are rare and most present with symptoms of intestinal obstruction within the first 2 months of life (Yanez and Spitz, 1986). Occasionally, however, endoscopy for abdominal pain will suggest a partial rotation. If this involves the duodenum, one clue may be difficulty with orientation of the papilla at the time of endoscopic retrograde cholangiopancreatography (ERCP).

Duplication cysts of the intestine are also rare and, again, usually present within the first year of life with obstruction or a palpable mass (Ildstad *et al.*, 1988). The majority of cysts do not communicate with the intestinal lumen and, therefore, would only be suspected because of duodenal distortion. In addition, duplication cysts of the small intestine are less common in the duodenum than in the jejunum or ileum. Finally, rare patients may present later in life with obstructive symptoms owing to a congenital diaphragm of the small bowel. These are usually located within the duodenum and are probably due to incomplete intestinal atresia.

Acquired anomalies

The major acquired anomaly is that of small bowel diverticula. These are more common in the duodenum than in other regions and are usually associated with the ampulla of Vater (major ampulla). Additional diverticula can be associated with the minor ampulla or can occur in other regions of the small bowel distal to the major ampulla. The relationship of the ampulla to the diverticulum varies but, in the majority of patients, the orifice of the ampulla is adjacent to or just below the orifice of the diverticulum and is readily cannulated at the time of ERCP. In about 10 per cent of patients, the orifice of the papilla is on the margin of the diverticulum, within the diverticulum or in a ridge of tissue which separates two diverticula (Plate 13.1.4).

Periampullary duodenal diverticula are rare before the age of 50 years but, thereafter, increase in frequency to a prevalence of about 20 per cent at the age of 80 years. Higher frequencies are observed in patients with bile duct stones, perhaps because diverticula predispose to stone formation through bile stasis and bacterial contamination of bile (Chandy *et al.*, 1997). The lumen of large diverticula may be filled with food debris. Rarely, diverticula extend into the lumen of the duodenum and can be seen as sacular structures, often with an opening that is adjacent to the lumen of the second part of the duodenum (Karoll *et al.*, 1983). These intraluminal duodenal diverticula or 'windsock' diverticula vary in size and may be filled with food debris if there is an inadequate opening in the distal portion of the diverticulum. Jejunal diverticula are rarely seen at endoscopy but can be identified by barium follow-through x-rays in about 1:400 adults (Tsiotos *et al.*, 1994).

Another disorder, which may be identified by duodenal endoscopy at the time of ERCP, is that of a choledochocoele (Venu *et al.*, 1984). This is seen as a cystic structure in the hood of the papilla and represents dilatation of the intraduodenal portion of the lower bile duct (Fig. 13.1.2). Whether this is a congenital or acquired anomaly remains unclear; some authors classify choledochocoeles as one of a number of manifestations of choledochal cysts.

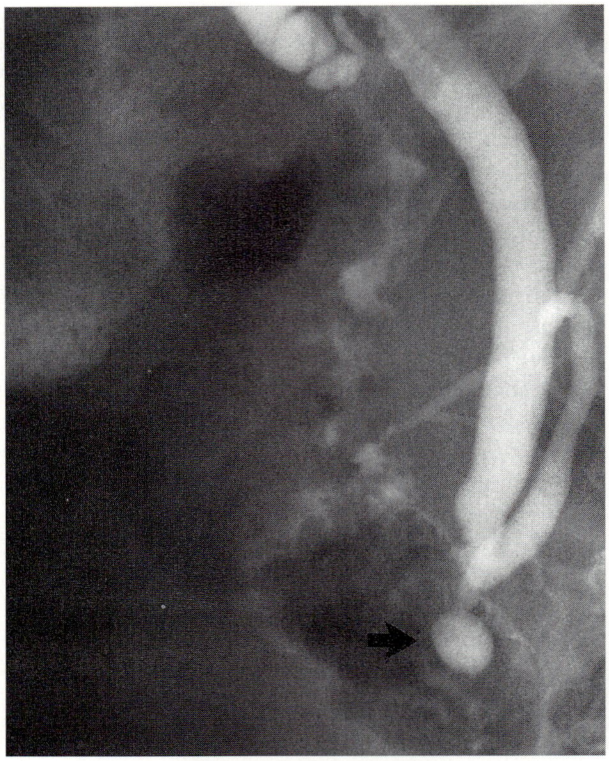

Figure 13.1.2 *Retrograde cholangiogram and pancreatogram showing contrast within a choledochocoele (arrow) in the intraduodenal portion of the lower bile duct.*

SMALL BOWEL ULCERATION

Peptic ulceration of the bulb and duodenum

Duodenal ulceration and duodenitis are two of the most common abnormalities recognized at the time of upper gastrointestinal endoscopy. Although the relationship of duodenitis to chronic duodenal ulceration is still debated, a consensus view is that duodenitis is part of the spectrum of ulcer disease, and can occur either prior to ulcer development or as a manifestation of the healing phase. Some patients, however, appear to have recurrent symptomatic duodenitis without the development of a definite chronic ulcer.

Most endoscopists recognize two forms of ulceration, a typical chronic ulcer (Plate 13.1.5) and duodenal erosions (Plate 13.1.6), the latter being small (1–5 mm in diameter), superficial and often multiple. Erosions are more likely to be associated with non-steroidal anti-inflammatory drugs and usually heal within 1–4 days, either spontaneously or after treatment with H-2 receptor antagonist drugs.

Most chronic ulcers are located on the anterior (50 per cent) or posterior walls (30 per cent) of the proximal duodenal bulb (within 2 cm of the pylorobulbar junction). About 15 per cent of patients have two or more ulcers, the most common being ulcers on both the anterior and posterior walls ('kissing ulcers'). Most ulcers are roughly spherical in shape with a diameter of between 5 and 10 mm and a depth of 1–2 mm. However, ulcers that are substantially larger and deeper can occur. About 20 per cent of patients have ulcers that are either linear or markedly irregular, probably largely because of previous scar formation. Pseudodiverticula are common in recurrent ulcer disease and may reflect the effects of scar formation, perhaps aggravated by stretching of the uninvolved duodenal wall. Pseudodiverticula can be single or multiple, and typically occur at the fornices and the mid-portion of the bulb.

Atypical peptic ulceration

Multiple ulcers of the duodenal bulb and second part of the duodenum should raise the strong possibility of a gastrinoma (Zollinger–Ellison syndrome). This is often associated with diffuse duodenal erythema, which, on biopsy, reveals duodenal inflammation with partial villous atrophy.

Peptic ulceration of the jejunum may occur in patients who have previously been treated with a gastroenterostomy or a Billroth II gastrectomy. After a gastroenterostomy, ulceration usually occurs in the efferent (jejunal) loop and within 3 cm of the gastroenterostomy stoma (Plate 13.1.7). After a Billroth II gastrectomy, ulceration may occur either in the efferent loop or in the region of the stoma. These jejunal ulcers have a similar appearance to chronic ulcers in the duodenal bulb but appear to be associated with a higher risk for perforation. A minority of patients with jejunal ulceration will have a gastrinoma or, after Billroth II gastrectomy, hypergastrinaemia due to retained antrum in the closed duodenal stump.

Ulceration associated with non-steroidal anti-inflammatory drugs

The use of non-steroidal anti-inflammatory drugs (NSAIDs) is associated with an increased risk for duodenal erosions and chronic duodenal ulcers (Soll, 1991). Furthermore, ulceration can also occur more distally in the small bowel. For example, small bowel enteroscopy revealed jejunal or ileal erosions or chronic ulcers in 40 per cent of a selected group of patients treated with NSAIDs who had rheumatoid arthritis and unexplained iron-deficiency anaemia (Morris *et al.*, 1991). Furthermore, a postmortem study by Allison *et al.* (1992) revealed that the frequency of non-specific small bowel ulceration was higher in users of NSAIDs (8 per cent) than in non-users (1 per cent). Three of the patients who were long-term users of NSAIDs died from perforated chronic ulcers of the small bowel.

SMALL BOWEL INFLAMMATION

While peptic inflammation can be readily identified in the duodenal bulb, the endoscopic features of other chronic inflammatory disorders are much more subtle unless inflammation is associated with ulceration as in Crohn's disease. For example, duodenal endoscopy in giardiasis is normal despite widespread inflammation on small bowel biopsies. Similarly, duodenal endoscopy is normal in most patients infected with *Strongyloides stercoralis*, although a minority have mild or more severe duodenal inflammation (Bone *et al.*, 1982).

Whipple's disease is extremely rare but has been associated with a number of endoscopic abnormalities, including patchy yellow–white discoloration of the duodenal mucosa, sometimes associated with an irregular mosaic pattern (Geboes *et al.*, 1990). These pale patches have been attributed to lipid accumulation in cells and lymphatic vessels, perhaps because of a degree of lymphatic obstruction associated with enlarged mesenteric lymph nodes. Similar endoscopic abnormalities have been observed in patients with acquired immunodeficiency syndrome (AIDS) who are infected with *Mycobacterium avium-intracellulare*.

The small bowel may also be affected by eosinophilic gastroenteritis, another rare inflammatory disorder characterized histologically by a predominant infiltrate of eosinophils. At endoscopy, a variety of abnormalities have been described ranging from thickened duodenal folds to small or larger nodules, usually covered by normal or reddened mucosa (Kalantar *et al.*, 1997). More recently, Croese *et al.* (1994) highlighted a form of eosinophilic enteritis, which was attributed to the canine hookworm, *Ankylostoma caninum*. Colonoscopy with intubation of the terminal ileum revealed abnormalities in a minority of patients, usually ileal ulceration. In a second study by Croese *et al.* (1996), patients with ileal ulceration identified at colonoscopy often had biopsy evidence of eosinophilic enteritis (33 per cent), elevated serum levels of immunoglobulin E (IgE) (55 per cent) and elevated antibody titres to *A. caninum* (47 per cent).

Although a variety of endoscopic abnormalities have been described in coeliac disease, some of these changes are relatively minor and only rarely lead to small bowel biopsy in the absence of other clinical indications. However, both loss of valvulae conniventes in the second part of the duodenum and scalloping of valvulae conniventes were predictive of coeliac disease in two prospective studies (Brocchi *et al.*, 1988; Jabbari *et al.*, 1988). Brocchi *et al.* (1996) also described an association between duodenal bulb micronodules and coeliac disease, although this endoscopic feature appears to be unusual. More recently, Niveloni *et al.* (1998) reported a larger prospective study of the endoscopic features of coeliac disease, including the use of methylene blue to highlight mucosal changes. Endoscopic procedures were recorded on videotape and reviewed by five experienced endoscopists in a blinded and random protocol. Videoendoscopic inspection alone correctly identified 75 of 80 subjects with total villous atrophy and 86 of 87 with normal mucosa. The presence of a mosaic pattern (89 per cent) and scalloped folds (86 per cent) were the most useful endoscopic signs. The use of methylene blue highlighted mucosal changes but did not provide additional information to the experienced endoscopist. Interobserver agreement was high for the mosaic pattern and scalloped folds but was only fair for loss of duodenal folds. An example of a mosaic pattern is shown in Plate 13.1.8. The optimal site of biopsy for the diagnosis of coeliac disease has also been debated, although it is now established that results from histological evaluation of endoscopic biopsies from the second part of the duodenum are similar to that of specimens taken by a suction capsule from the fourth part of the duodenum (Mee *et al.*, 1985).

The endoscopic features of Crohn's disease are more likely to involve the terminal ileum (about 60 per cent of cases) than the duodenum (about 2 per cent of cases). Indeed, almost all patients with duodenal Crohn's disease have other small bowel lesions and/or involvement of the antrum of the stomach. The sequence of endoscopic changes in Crohn's disease is still poorly understood but the first lesions appear to be small, shallow 'aphthous' ulcers with a surrounding rim of erythema (Plate 13.1.9). These aphthous ulcers may coalesce to form large shallow ulcers and may subsequently erode into the bowel wall causing areas of deep ulceration or long 'serpiginous' ulcers. In some patients, the major endoscopic feature is patchy or diffuse inflammation with mucosal oedema and friability, sometimes creating a nodular or 'cobblestone' appearance (Plate 13.1.10). Extension of inflammation through the bowel wall may result in fistula formation but it is uncommon to identify the opening of a fistulous tract in the small bowel at the time of duodenal or ileal endoscopy. Pseudopolyps in Crohn's disease appear to be less common in the small bowel than in the large bowel. In contrast, the small bowel is the more likely site of a symptomatic stricture, which, in active disease, is usually associated with marked inflammation and a small or larger chronic ulcer.

Thus far, activity indices for Crohn's disease have not been based on the site or severity of endoscopic changes. This reflects the difficulty of comparing the overall effect of inflammation that may be localized and severe, with inflammation that may be mild but is more widespread.

VASCULAR DISEASES OF THE SMALL BOWEL

Fortunately, vascular abnormalities of the small bowel are an uncommon cause for recurrent or occult bleeding from the gastrointestinal tract. Although a large number of syndromes have been described, most vascular abnormalities can be categorized as vascular ectasia (angiodysplasia), arteriovenous malformations, haemangiomas or hereditary haemorrhagic telangiectasiae (Osler–Weber–Rendu syndrome) (Moretó *et al.*, 1986). In addition, vascular changes in the small bowel may be secondary to irradiation, vasculitis, renal failure and portal hypertension.

Vascular ectasia is the most common abnormality and is probably a degenerative lesion associated with ageing. The endoscopic appearance varies from a red tuft of small blood vessels to a small or larger red area associated with dilated and tortuous larger vessels. True arteriovenous malformations of the small bowel are rare but may appear as red and raised lesions of variable size at the time of endoscopy. Haemangiomas vary in appearance from a red and nodular mass, which can be confused with a tumour, to a diffuse abnormality of small blood vessels, which may extend over a distance of several centimetres. In hereditary haemorrhagic telangiectasiae, vascular abnormalities can be seen throughout the small bowel but are most likely to be identified as cherry red spots in the duodenum, usually about 1–3 mm in diameter.

Endoscopic changes due to irradiation or vasculitis are less likely to be recognized in the small bowel than in the colon. However, the delayed effects of irradiation include mucosal pallor, largely due to fibrosis and oedema, and fragile small and irregular blood vessels, which have been attributed to neovascularization. Vasculitis of the small bowel usually appears as small red spots (petechiae) but other changes have been recorded, including pale areas with central erythema and superficial (aphthous) ulceration. Duodenal varices are an uncommon manifestation of portal hypertension but may be identified as undulating and tortuous protuberances, often on the posterior wall of the apex of the duodenal bulb. Identification is sometimes facilitated by a faint blue or grey–blue colour.

TUMOURS OF THE SMALL BOWEL

Tumours of the small bowel are uncommon when compared to the frequency of tumours in the colon and stomach (Lowenfels, 1973). Furthermore, the pathological nature of nodules in the duodenal bulb differs from that in other regions of the small bowel.

Multiple polypoid lesions in the duodenal bulb

Small nodules (2–4 mm in diameter) are a common finding at endoscopy and are usually due to small inflammatory polyps or to ectopic (heterotopic) gastric mucosa. The former are often associated with duodenitis and deformity, while the latter have a pale pink or red colour and are typically located in the proximal portion of the bulb (Plate 13.1.11). Another entity, hyperplasia of Brunner's glands, may cause larger nodules (5 mm) in the duodenal bulb as well as nodules in the second part of the duodenum (Plate 13.1.12). These nodules are covered by normal duodenal mucosa and may be difficult to distinguish from nodular lymphoid hyperplasia, a rare condition which is usually associated with common variable hypogammaglobulinaemia.

Single polypoid lesion of the duodenal bulb

Single polypoid lesions may be due to inflammatory polyps, but can also be due to a variety of benign neoplasms including a leiomyoma, lipoma, carcinoid, hamartoma or adenoma. These may be difficult to differentiate at the time of endoscopy, although a minority of leiomyomas have central ulceration and some lipomas become pedunculated.

Benign neoplasms of the small bowel

The most common benign neoplasms are stromal tumours, adenomas and lipomas. Stromal tumours are evenly distributed throughout the small bowel, adenomas are somewhat more common in the duodenum and ileum, while lipomas are more common in the ileum.

The most common endoscopic appearance of stromal tumours is a nodule projecting into the intestinal lumen. Small nodules are smooth and are covered by normal mucosa, while larger nodules may be lobulated or somewhat irregular in shape with a surface which is red, friable and sometimes ulcerated. Superficial biopsies are often unhelpful but deep biopsies reveal spindle-cell neoplasms, sometimes with features of smooth muscle (leiomyoma) or neural (neurofibroma, schwannoma) differentiation. Apical ulceration may be more common in leiomyomas than in other stromal tumours.

The endoscopic appearances of small bowel adenomas are similar to those of colonic adenomas. Small adenomas (< 5 mm) are usually covered by mucosa, which appears either normal or near-normal. Larger adenomas are often pedunculated with a clearly-defined 'tuft' with a red or speckled appearance (Plate 13.1.13). Sessile adenomas are more likely to be classified histologically as villous adenomas and are more likely to undergo malignant change (Plate 13.1.14).

Multiple adenomas of the duodenum should raise the possibility of familial adenomatous polyposis (FAP). Duodenal polyps occur in 70–80 per cent of FAP patients and are largely located in the second and third parts of the duodenum (Plate 13.1.15). In addition, the majority of these patients have endoscopic or histological abnormalities in the periampullary region, which seem likely to account for a higher than expected frequency of cancer of the ampulla of Vater (Jagelman *et al.*, 1988; Offerhaus *et al.*, 1992).

Malignant neoplasms of the small bowel

The ratio of malignant to benign neoplasms of the small bowel is probably of the order of 2:1. The most common malignant tumours are adenocarcinomas (40 per cent), followed by carcinoid tumours (30 per cent), lymphomas (17 per cent) and sarcomas (13 per cent). Adenocarcinomas are more common in the duodenum, while lymphomas and carcinoid tumours are more common in the ileum. Sarcomas are more evenly distributed with a slight predilection for the jejunum (Weiss and Yang, 1987).

The endoscopic appearances of adenocarcinomas of the small bowel are similar to adenocarcinomas of the stomach and colon. The typical appearance is that of a nodular and ulcerated mass, often extending circumferentially in the duodenum, with duodenal narrowing and prominent contact bleeding. Adenocarcinomas that are identified at an earlier stage can appear as ulcers with raised and irregular margins, or as irregular exophytic or polypoid masses. Biopsies are more reliable when taken from the margins of ulcerated or nodular lesions.

Cancers of the ampulla of Vater are identified in about 5 per cent of patients with obstructive jaundice due to malignant disease (Plate 13.1.16). These cancers are best identified with duodenoscopes at the time of ERCP and can be broadly categorized into ulcerative or polypoid lesions with about equal frequency. In addition, the orifice of the ampulla can usually be identified within the tumour mass, while retrograde cholangiograms and pancreatograms reveal duct obstruction in the region of the ampulla. If the orifice of the ampulla is not within the tumour mass, the more likely diagnosis is that of malignant infiltration of the periampullary area by cancer of the head of the pancreas. Indeed, extension of pancreatic cancer into the duodenum is more common than primary duodenal cancer and cancer of the ampulla of Vater.

The small bowel is the most common site for carcinoid tumours of clinical significance. Furthermore, carcinoids in the small bowel may be more likely to metastasize than carcinoids in the rectum or appendix, although there is a relationship between the size of the tumour and the probability of spread in all regions. Endoscopically, most carcinoid tumours appear as regular or slightly irregular nodules projecting into the lumen of the intestine (Plate 13.1.17). Small nodules are usually covered by normal mucosa, but larger nodules may have a red or mottled appearance, sometimes with small areas of ulceration and prominent contact bleeding. Endoscopic biopsies are usually inconclusive when smaller nodules are covered by normal mucosa, but histological confirmation is possible in the presence of ulceration.

Lymphomatous involvement of the small bowel can be either primary or secondary. The latter is more common than the former, although the origin of some lymphomas remains unclear. Lymphomas complicating coeliac disease are more common in the jejunum and may be multifocal. Other primary lymphomas are more common in the ileum. Primary lymphoma of the duodenum is extremely rare but duodenal lesions may be seen when gastric lymphoma extends through the pylorus. The endoscopic appearance of lymphoma is highly variable but includes polypoid lesions (sometimes with central ulceration), multiple nodules or plaques, diffuse thickening of the bowel wall and large polypoid or fungating masses (Halphen *et al.*, 1986). One example is shown in Plate 13.1.18. Immunoproliferative small intestinal disease (heavy-chain disease) is a low-grade B-cell lymphoma, which usually involves the duodenum and may be recognized because of the presence of thick and mildly irregular duodenal folds.

Sarcomas of the small bowel are rare and, at endoscopy, have a similar appearance to adenocarcinomas. Kaposi's sarcoma appears as reddish brown lesions of variable size, which can be identified in both the stomach and proximal duodenum. Metastases in the small bowel are rare in most patients with advanced cancer, with the exception of malignant melanoma where metastases appear as elevated, pigmented nodules of variable size, sometimes associated with central ulceration.

REFERENCES

Allison, M.C., Howatson A.G., Torrance, C.J., Lee, F.D., Russell, R.I. 1992: Gastrointestinal damage associated with the use of nonsteroidal antiinflammatory drugs. *New England Journal of Medicine* 327, 749–54.

Barkin, J.S., Lewis, B.S., Reiner, D.K., Waye, J.D., Goldberg, R.I., Phillips, R.S. 1992: Diagnostic and therapeutic jejunoscopy with a new, longer enteroscope. *Gastrointestinal Endoscopy* 38, 55–8.

Barkin, J.S., Chong, J., Reiner, D.K. 1994: First-generation video enteroscope: fourth-generation push-type small bowel enteroscopy utilizing an overtube. *Gastrointestinal Endoscopy* 40, 743–7.

Bone, M.F., Chesner, I.M., Oliver, R., Asquith, P. 1982: Endoscopic appearances of duodenitis due to strongyloidiasis. *Gastrointestinal Endoscopy* 28, 190–1.

Brocchi, E., Corazza, G.R., Caletti, G., Treggiari, E.A., Barbara, L., Gasbarrini, G. 1988: Endoscopic demonstration of loss of duodenal folds in the diagnosis of celiac disease. *The New England Journal of Medicine* 319, 741–4.

Brocchi, E., Corazza, G.R., Brusco, G., Mangia, L., Gasbarrini, G. 1996: Unsuspected celiac disease diagnosed by endoscopic visualization of duodenal bulb micronodules. *Gastrointestinal Endoscopy* 44, 610–11.

Chandy, G., Hart, W.J., Roberts-Thomson, I.C. 1997: An analysis of the relationship between bile duct stones and periampullary duodenal diverticula. *Journal of Gastroenterology and Hepatology* 12, 29–33.

Croese, J., Loukas, A., Opdebeeck, J., Prociv, P. 1994: Occult enteric infection by *Ancylostoma caninum*: a previously unrecognized zoonosis. *Gastroenterology* 106, 3–12.

Croese, J., Fairley, S., Loukas, A., Hack, J., Stronach, P. 1996: A distinctive aphthous ileitis linked to *Ancylostoma caninum*. *Journal of Gastroenterology and Hepatology* 11, 524–31.

D'Agostino, J.A., Petros, J.G., Semegran, A.B., Cave, D.R., Lopez, M.J. 1997: Complete intraoperative Sonde enteroscopy in the evaluation of recurrent partial small-bowel obstruction. *Gastrointestinal Endoscopy* 46, 577–8.

Geboes, K., Ectors, N., Heidbuchel, H., Rutgeerts, P., Desmet, V., Vantrappen, G. 1990: Whipple's disease: endoscopic aspects before and after therapy. *Gastrointestinal Endoscopy* 36, 247–52.

Halphen, M., Najjar, T., Jaafoura, H., Cammoun, M., Tufrali, G. 1986: Diagnostic value of upper intestinal fiber endoscopy in primary small intestinal lymphoma. *Cancer* 58, 2140–5.

Ildstad, S.T., Tollerud, D.J., Weiss, R.G., Ryan, D.P., McGowan, M.A., Martin, L.W. 1988: Duplications of the alimentary tract. Clinical characteristics, preferred treatment, and associated malformations. *Annals of Surgery* 208, 184–9.

Jabbari, M., Wild, G., Goresky, C.A., Daly, D.S., Lough, J.O., Cleland, D.P., Kinnear, D.G. 1988: Scalloped valvulae conniventes: an endoscopic marker of celiac sprue. *Gastroenterology* 95, 1518–22.

Jagelman, D.G., DeCosse, J.J., Bussey, H.J.R. 1988: Upper gastrointestinal cancer in familial adenomatous polyposis. *Lancet* i, 1149–51.

Kalantar, S.J., Marks, R., Lambert, J.R., Badov, D., Talley, N.J. 1997: Dyspepsia due to eosinophilic gastroenteritis. *Digestive Diseases and Sciences* 42, 2327–32.

Karoll, M.P., Ghahremani, G.G., Port, R.B., Rosenberg, J.L. 1983: Diagnosis and management of intraluminal duodenal diverticulum. *Digestive Diseases and Sciences* 28, 411–16.

Landi, B., Tkoub, M., Gaudric, M. *et al.* 1998: Diagnostic yield of push-type enteroscopy in relation to indication. *Gut* 42, 421–5.

Lewis, B.S., Waye, J.D. 1987: Total small bowel enteroscopy. *Gastrointestinal Endoscopy* 33, 435–8.

Lowenfels, A.B. 1973: Why are small-bowel tumours so rare? *Lancet* 1, 24–6.

Mee, A.S., Burke, M., Vallon, A.G., Newman, J., Cotton, P.B. 1985: Small bowel biopsy for malabsorption: comparison of the diagnostic adequacy of endoscopic forceps and capsule biopsy specimens. *British Medical Journal* 291, 769–72.

Moretó, M., Figa, M., Ojembarrena, E., Zabella, M. 1986: Vascular malformations of the stomach and duodenum: an endoscopic classification. *Endoscopy* 18, 227–9.

Morris, A.J., Madhok, R., Sturrock, R.D., Capeld, H.A., Mackenzie, J.F. 1991: Enteroscopic diagnosis of small bowel ulceration in patients receiving non-steroidal anti-inflammatory drugs. *Lancet* 337, 520.

Niveloni, S., Fiorini, A., Dezi, R. *et al.* 1998: Usefulness of videoduodenoscopy and vital dye staining as indicators of mucosal atrophy of celiac disease: assessment of interobserver agreement. *Gastrointestinal Endoscopy* 47, 223–9.

Offerhaus, G.J.A., Giardiello, F.M., Krush, A.J., Booker, S.V., Tersmette, A.C., Kelley, N.C., Hamilton, S.R. 1992: The risk of upper gastrointestinal cancer in familial adenomatous polyposis. *Gastroenterology* 102, 1980–2.

Soll, A.H. (moderator) 1991: Nonsteroidal anti-inflammatory drugs and peptic ulcer disease. *Annals of Intestinal Medicine* 114, 307–19.

Tsiotos, G.G., Farnell, M.B., Ilstrup, D.M. 1994: Nonmechelian jejunal or ileal diverticulosis. An analysis of 112 cases. *Surgery* 116, 726–32.

Turgeon, D.K., Barnett, J.L. 1990: Meckel's diverticulum. *American Journal of Gastroenterology* 85, 777–81.

Urayama, S., Korazek, R., Ball, T. 1995: Presentation and treatment of annular pancreas in an adult population. *American Journal of Gastroenterology* 90, 995–9.

Venu, R.P., Geenen, J.E., Hogan, W.J., Dodds, W.J., Wilson, S.W., Stewart, E.T., Soergel, K.H. 1984: Role of endoscopic retrograde cholangiopancreatography in the diagnosis and treatment of choledochocele. *Gastroenterology* 87, 1144–6.

Weiss, N.S., Yang, C.-P. 1987: Incidence of histologic types of cancer of the small intestine. *Journal of National Cancer Institute* 78, 653–6.

Yanez, R., Spitz, L. 1986: Intestinal malrotation presenting outside the neonatal period. *Archives of Disease in Childhood* 61, 682–5.

13.2

Small intestinal mucosal biopsy

MINNIE M MATHAN

The mucosal lining of the small intestine, a primary barrier between the external environment in the lumen of the bowel and the internal environment of the body, was only accessible for biopsy at laparotomy or autopsy till the mid-1950s. In the late 1950s and early 1960s, a series of elegant peroral biopsy instruments were designed by investigators interested in studying small intestinal physiology or pathophysiology, especially the malabsorption syndromes (Shiner, 1956; Crosby and Kugler, 1957; Brandborg *et al*., 1959; Baker and Hughes, 1960; Flick *et al*., 1961; McCarthy *et al*., 1964). With the advent of flexible fibreoptic upper gastrointestinal endoscopes and flexible biopsy forceps, targeted biopsies of the mucosa of the second and third part of the duodenum are now performed frequently. An enteroscope to visualize the entire small intestine and to obtain targeted mucosal biopsies at any level is also available, though not yet extensively used. The wide availability of fibreoptic endoscopy has made the use of the earlier intestinal biopsy instruments relatively rare except for research purposes.

PERORAL SMALL INTESTINAL MUCOSAL BIOPSY INSTRUMENTS

Three types of peroral biopsy instruments: wire-operated, multiple-retrieving hydraulic tubes, and capsules on thin flexible tubes, are available.

Wire-operated biopsy tubes

These instruments modified the principle of the Wood's gastric biopsy tube (Wood *et al*., 1949) with a hollow cylindrical knife mounted on a wire, fitted into a cylindrical capsule with one or more round holes on the side for sucking in knuckles of mucosa, attached to a flexible coated spring tube through which the wire passes. By applying suction to the top of the tube, a knuckle of mucosa is sucked in. Pulling sharply on the wire cuts the knuckle of mucosa. The entire tube has to be removed to retrieve the biopsy (Shiner, 1956; Brandborg *et al*., 1959). These tubes are seldom used now.

Hydraulic multiple-retrieving biopsy tubes

These tubes are particularly useful for obtaining biopsies from multiple sites or several specimens from the same area to reduce sampling error (Baker and Hughes, 1960; Flick *et al*., 1961). A cylindrical knife with a one-way fluid valve is placed in a cylindrical capsule with side holes for sucking in a small knuckle of mucosa. The knife and capsule are attached to a double tube: one for the hydraulic fluid, usually normal saline, and the other for negative suction to suck in the mucosal knucle and to wash out the biopsy specimen. The knife is kept in the open position by applying negative suction through the hydraulic tube. Once a knuckle of mucosa is sucked in, the pressure in the hydraulic system is rapidly reversed, pushing the knife forward and cutting off the biopsy. The fluid flushes the biopsy out through the coated spring tube. The knife and cylinder can be repositioned and made ready for the next biopsy by applying negative pressure to the hydraulic tube to open the knife.

These tubes are relatively large and uncomfortable for the patient, and positioning involves fluoroscopy. They are now seldom used except for research purposes.

Biopsy capsules

These are cylindrical capsules, 1 cm × 0.5 cm, with rounded ends, containing a spring-loaded knife block assembly, which can be triggered by suction and a lateral hole (3 mm diameter for adults, 2 mm for children) into which a knuckle of mucosa can be sucked (Crosby and Kugler, 1957; McCarthy *et al.*, 1964). The distal one-third of the capsule is separated by a rubber diaphragm from the rest of the capsule containing the knife block, creating a small chamber with air when the capsule is assembled. The capsule with the cocked knife block is attached to a long thin flexible and preferably radio-opaque plastic tube to which suction can be applied to sample the mucosa. When the knuckle of mucosa is sucked in, continuing negative pressure causes the rubber diaphragm to bulge and push the knife block off the stop against which it is cocked. The spring-loaded knife swirls around cutting the knuckle of mucosa. The entire capsule is pulled back and the distal end opened to retrieve the biopsy. The capsule is best positioned under fluoroscopy.

All these biopsy instruments have the advantage of obtaining relatively large pieces of tissue with intact muscularis mucosa, enabling precise orientation of the tissue for fixation and embedding. The biopsy specimen can be examined with a hand lens and mounted flat on monofilament mesh with the villus surface up, before immersion in fixatives. However, biopsy skills have to be developed and the procedure requires good cooperation from the patient and is time consuming. Deep sedation or anaesthesia may be necessary in children. There is also exposure of the patient and the doctor to ionizing radiation while positioning the capsule.

ENDOSCOPIC DUODENAL BIOPSIES

Small intestinal mucosal biopsies using pinch biopsy forceps are easily obtained from the second part of the duodenum at endoscopy. This does not require fluoroscopy for positioning and, with more recent endoscopes, larger biopsy forceps can be used. Although the cups of the forceps have holes for mucosa to bulge through, the mucosal samples may show artefacts, especially if there are central fixing pins on the jaws. It is difficult to orient the 1–2 mm size bits, thereby multiple step sections are required to ensure that adequate interpretation is possible. Several biopsy bits can be obtained at one endoscopy session, reducing sampling errors. Comparisons of the diagnostic utility of endoscopic biopsies with capsule biopsies (Achkar *et al.*, 1986) and of biopsies from the proximal jejunum to proximal duodenum (Gear and Dobbins, 1969; Dandalides *et al.*, 1989) have validated the utility of endoscopic biopsies. This technique is now most widely used to sample proximal small intestinal mucosa (Karn and Foroozan, 1974; Kreuning *et al.*, 1978; Goldman and Antonioli, 1982; Rotterdam, 1983; Lawson, 1989).

INDICATIONS FOR SMALL INTESTINAL MUCOSAL BIOPSY

A small intestinal mucosal biopsy is of diagnostic value in pathology diffusely involving the upper small intestinal mucosa (Table 13.2.1). The best examples are untreated coeliac disease (gluten-sensitive enteropathy),

Table 13.2.1 *Conditions in which upper small bowel mucosal biopsy will help in diagnosis*

Diffuse mucosal lesions with diagnostic features
Coeliac sprue (gluten-sensitive enteropathy)
Whipple's disease
Abetalipoproteinaemia
Hypogammaglobulinaemia
Graft versus host disease
Diffuse mucosal lesions with malabsorption but changes are not diagnostic
Tropical sprue
Folate and vitamin B_{12} deficiency
Radiation enteritis
Zollinger–Ellison syndrome
HIV infection of the gut
Patchy mucosal lesion with diagnostic features, which may be missed due to sampling error
Amyloidosis
Capillariasis, strongyloidiasis, cryptosporidiosis, giardiasis and coccidial parasites
Crohn's disease
Eosinophilic enteritis
Lymphangiectasia
Lymphoma
Mastocytosis
Mycobacterium avium-intercellulare
Immunoproliferative small intestinal disease (IPSID)
Malabsorption present but biopsy is normal
Pancreatic disease
Primary disaccharidase deficiency
Liver disease

abetalipoproteinaemia, Whipple's disease and certain immunodeficiency syndromes. When the mucosal lesion is patchy as in amyloidosis, cryptosporidiosis, other coccidiosis, parasitic infections and intestinal lymphangiectasia, while the histological features may be diagnostic, a single apparently normal biopsy does not rule out the diagnosis.

The appearance of the biopsy is abnormal but not diagnostic in several conditions associated with a malabsorbption syndrome (Rubin and Dobbins, 1965; Trier, 1971; Brandborg, 1979; Goldman and Antonioli, 1982). Before the availability of endoscopic biopsies, algorithms were developed to minimize the need for small bowel mucosal biopsies. However, the relative ease and safety of endoscopic biopsies has changed the situation and an upper small intestinal (duodenal) biopsy would be considered a mandatory diagnostic test in patients with a malabsorption syndrome.

COMPLICATIONS OF SMALL INTESTINAL MUCOSAL BIOPSIES

Tethering of the biopsy tube or capsule to the mucosa, owing to an incomplete cut during triggering of the knife and detachment of the biopsy capsule, are relatively minor complications. The former problem is solved by leaving the capsule tethered for about 6 hours, after which it can easily be pulled out, as autolysis of the partially biopsied piece of mucosa releases the capsule. The latter problem requires collection of all faecal matter to retrieve the capsule. Perforation of the small intestine and bleeding from the site of biopsy are major complications. In over 10 000 biopsies of the upper small intestinal mucosa with multiple-retrieving instruments and the Crosby capsule, only two perforations were encountered, both in patients with suspected intestinal lymphoma who had been scheduled for laparotomy. If care is taken to ensure normal coagulation parameters before biopsy, bleeding is seldom encountered. None of these complications have been encountered in endoscopic upper small intestinal biopsies.

HANDLING AND PROCESSING OF SMALL INTESTINAL MUCOSAL BIOPSIES

The biopsied mucosal sample should be expeditiously processed to minimize autolytic changes. It is also essential to orient the tissue appropriately, with the muscularis spread over a monofilament mesh with villi projecting upward, before fixation in 10 per cent neutral or buffered formaldehyde or any other fixative (Perera *et al.*, 1975; Petras, 1989; Morson *et al.*, 1990). This is relatively easy, especially using a hand lens, with capsule biopsies, but more difficult in endoscopic biopsies even with large biopsy forceps, and step sectioning is usually advisable. Facilities for rapidly placing the biopsies in fixative or quench freezing in liquid nitrogen should be available in the room where the biopsies are performed. Further processing is according to standard techniques depending upon the type of work planned: histology, frozen sections, histochemistry or electron microscopy (Lee and Toner, 1980; Morson *et al.*, 1990; Rotterdam *et al.*, 1993). For routine histopathological evaluation, in addition to haematoxylin and eosin stains, the periodic acid–Schiff stain (for Whipple's disease and *Mycobacterium avium-intercellulare*) and a trichrome stain for collagen, which also stains *Giardia*, are useful.

EVALUATION OF SMALL INTESTINAL MUCOSAL BIOPSIES

Adequate interpretation of small intestinal pathology is possible only if the normal structure and histology is well understood (Segal and Petras, 1992). In addition, there are geographic variations in the morphology of the small bowel mucosa (Baker, 1973) and this must be kept in mind when biopsies have to be interpreted. Ideally slides with 5–7 serial sections (5–6 μm thick) should be evaluated. The villus architecture, surface and crypt epithelial cells, the lamina propria constituents, any submucosal tissue and any parasite, microbe or exudate adherent to the surface of the epithelium should be systematically evaluated. Ideally at least four well-oriented villi must be identified (Perera *et al.*, 1975). Variations in length, shape and orientation of the villi can occur, especially if there is tangential sectioning or if the muscularis mucosa is not included in the biopsy.

Descriptions of the more commonly encountered small intestinal pathologies are presented in Chapter 2. More detailed reviews of the pathological changes can be found in Fenoglio *et al.* (1989), Mathan and Mathan (1990), Mathan (1995) and Rotterdam *et al.* (1993).

Acknowledgements The ICDDR,B Centre for Health and Population Research is supported by countries and agencies that share its concern for the health problems of developing countries. Current donors providing unrestricted support include: the aid agencies of the Governments of Australia, Bangladesh, Belgium, Canada, Saudi Arabia, Sweden, Switzerland, the United Kingdom and the United States of America; international organizations include the United Nations Children's Fund (UNICEF).

The secretarial assistance of Mrs Saleha Chowdhury is gratefully acknowledged.

REFERENCES

Achkar, E., Carey, W.D., Petras, R., Sivak, M.V., Revta, R. 1986: Comparison of suction capsule and endoscopic biopsy of small bowel mucosa. *Gastrointestinal Endoscopy* 32, 278–81.

Baker, S.J. 1973: Geographical variations in the morphology of the small intestinal mucosa in apparently healthy individuals. *Pathology and Microbiology* 39, 222–34.

Baker, S.J., Hughes, A. 1960: A multiple retrieving small intestinal biopsy tube. *Lancet* ii, 686–7.

Brandborg, L.L. 1979: Histologic diagnosis of diseases of malabsorption. *American Journal of Medicine* 67, 999–1006.

Brandborg, L.L., Rubin, C.E., Quinton, W.E. 1959: A multipurpose instrument for suction biopsy of the esophagus, stomach, small bowel and colon. *Gastroenterology* 37, 1–16.

Crosby, W.H., Kugler, H.W. 1957: Intraluminal biopsy of the small intestine: the intestinal biopsy capsule. *American Journal of Digestive Diseases* 2, 236–41.

Dandalides, S.M., Carey, W.D., Petras, R., Achkar, E. 1989: Endoscopic small bowel mucosal biopsy: a controlled trial evaluating forceps size and biopsy location in the diagnosis of normal and abnormal mucosal architecture. *Gastrointestinal Endoscopy* 35, 197–200.

Fenoglio, P.C.M., Lantz, P.E., Listrom, M.D., Davis, M., Rillae, F.O. 1989: *Gastrointestinal pathology: an atlas and text.* New York: Raven Press, 262–357.

Flick, A.L., Quinton, W.E., Rubin, C.E. 1961: A peroral hydraulic biopsy tube for multiple sampling at any site of the gastrointestinal tract. *Gastroenterology* 40, 120–6.

Gear, E.V., Dobbins, W.O., III 1969: The histologic spectrum of proximal duodenal biopsy in adult males. *American Journal of Medical Sciences* 257, 90–9.

Goldman, H., Antonioli, D.A. 1982: Mucosal biopsy of the esophagus, stomach and proximal duodenum. *Human Pathology* 13, 423–48.

Karn, E.R., Foroozan, P. 1974: Endoscopic biopsies of normal duodenal mucosa. *Gastrointestinal Endoscopy* 21, 51–4.

Kreuning, J., Bosman, F.T., Kuiper, G., Van der Wal, A.M., Lindeman, J. 1978: Gastric and duodenal mucosa in 'healthy' individuals: an endoscopic and histopathologic study in 50 volunteers. *Journal of Clinical Pathology* 31, 69–77.

Lawson, H.H. 1989: The duodenal mucosa in health and diseases: a clinical and experimental study. *Surgery Annual* 21, 157–80.

Lee, F.D., Toner, P.G. 1980: The handling of biopsy. In Lee, F.D., Toner, P.G. (eds) *Biopsy pathology of the small intestine.* London: Chapman and Hall, 6–16.

Mathan, M.M. 1995: Specific infections and tropical sprue. In Whitehead, R. (ed.) *Gastrointestinal and oesophageal pathology.* London: Churchill Livingstone, 525–47.

Mathan, M.M., Mathan, V.I. 1990: Gastrointestinal biopsy diagnosis. In William, G.T. (ed.) *Current topics in pathology, 81. Gastrointestinal pathology.* London: Springer Verlag, 104–31.

McCarthy, C.F., Gough, K.R., Rodriguez, M., Read, A.E. 1964: Peroral intestinal mucosal biopsy with a small Crosby capsule. *British Medical Journal* 1, 1620.

Morson, B.C., Dawson, I.M.P., Day, D.W., Jans, J.R., Price, A.G., Williams, G.T. (eds) 1990: Reception and examination of biopsy and surgical specimens and special investigation. In *Morson and Dawson's gastrointestinal pathology.* Oxford: Blackwell Scientific Publications, 3–17.

Perera, D.R., Weinstein, W.M., Rubin, C.E. 1975: Small intestinal biopsy. *Human Pathology* 6, 157–217.

Petras, R.E. 1989: Non-neoplastic intestinal diseases. In Sternberg, S.S. (ed.) *Diagnostic surgical pathology*, Vol. 2. New York: Raven Press, 967–1014.

Rotterdam, H. 1983: Contributions of gastrointestinal biopsy to an understanding of gastrointestinal disease. *American Journal of Gastroenterology* 78, 140–8.

Rotterdam, H., Sheahan, D.G., Sommers, S.C. 1993: *Biopsy diagnosis of the digestive tract.* New York: Raven Press, 315–575.

Rubin, C.E., Dobbins, W.O. 1965: Peroral biopsy of the small intestine. A review of its diagnostic usefulness. *Gastroenterology* 49, 676–97.

Segal, G.H., Petras, R.E. 1992: Small intestine. In Sternberg, S.S. (ed.) *Histology for pathologists.* New York: Raven Press, 547–71.

Shiner, M. 1956: Duodenal biopsy. *Lancet* i, 17–19.

Trier, J.S. 1971: Diagnostic value of peroral biopsy of the proximal small intestine. *New England Journal of Medicine* 285, 1470–3.

Wood, I.J., Doig, R.K., Motteram, R., Hughes, A. 1949: Gastric biopsy: report on fifty five biopsies using new flexible biopsy tubes. *Lancet* 1, 18–21.

13.3

Biochemical tests of small intestinal function

ROSS BUTLER

INTRODUCTION

The small intestine is an organ with a large functional residual capacity. Even with impaired function or loss of a substantial percentage of the absorptive area, adequate, but not necessarily optimal, nutrition may be maintained (*see* Chapter 29). It is not surprising then that the development of sensitive and specific tests of dysfunction has been a relatively difficult task. To compound this, the dual role of maintaining an efficient absorptive surface and an effective barrier to environmental hazards contained in food and other ingested substances needs to be considered when tests are being established. In addition, being aware of the potential for impairment of both absorption and secretion creates further hurdles in developing adequately standardized tests of small intestinal function. A third factor that can contribute significantly to the variability of biochemical tests in the small intestine is variable transit times (Wutzke *et al.*, 1997).

This chapter concentrates on non-invasive biochemical tests of gastrointestinal function that are directly related to the small intestinal mucosa or that can affect its functional efficiency.

Four areas of gut function will be addressed:

1 absorption and malabsorption of macronutrients
2 bacterial overgrowth
3 small intestinal integrity – barrier function
4 motility and transit time.

ABSORPTION AND MALABSORPTION OF MACRONUTRIENTS

Normal intestinal absorption requires adequate digestion in the stomach, adequate pancreatic function and enough absorptive area, i.e. patent and metabolically active mature epithelial cells. Of the three major macronutrients, fats depend on both bile acids and pancreatic lipases for absorption; carbohydrates need salivary and pancreatic amylases, but the most likely rate-limiting factors are the brush-border disaccharides, primarily lactase and also sucrase-isomaltase; and proteins are firstly broken down in the stomach by pepsins and thence the pancreatic peptidases followed by brush-border peptidases.

Fats

Fat malabsorption can occur because any one of several components necessary for full absorption may be impaired (*see* Chapters 10 and 16).

Tests for fat malabsorption include 3-day faecal fat – a test that is not well tolerated and hard to complete in a standardized manner (see below), and microscopic detection of fat in stool, which is not quantitative. For a totally reliable faecal fat balance to be obtained, a 5-day hospital stay is required (Thorsgaard Pederson, 1987). More recently, breath tests have been described

(Newcomer *et al.*, 1979; Butler *et al.*, 1984), particularly ^{13}C-labelled fat tests (Ghoos *et al.*, 1981; Lembcke *et al.*, 1996). These have been used for both overall fat absorption and as a specific test designed to detect changes in lipase activity to assess pancreatic function. An alternative test that also holds promise is the use of faecal elastase (Loser *et al.*, 1996). This test depends on the observation that human pancreatic elastase remains undegraded during intestinal transit, thus its concentration in faeces reflects exocrine pancreatic function. Briefly, an enzyme-linked immunosorption assay plate is coated with monoclonal antibody against human pancreatic elastase 1 (E1). When the samples are incubated in the plates, the antigen binds to the immobilized antibody. A second biotinylated antibody against E1 is then added, which binds to elastase 1 and is measured photometrically after addition of peroxidase, streptavidin and ABTS (2,2′-azino-bis-(3-ethylbenzothiazolin-6-sulphonic acid) diammonium salt), which when it is oxidized turns dark green. It has a high sensitivity and specificity (> 90 per cent in both cases) and, in contrast to the chymotrypsin assay, can detect moderate pancreatic insufficiency (Loser *et al.*, 1995). Nonetheless, the assay still suffers from an inability to provide a quantitative result.

Principle of breath tests

Because a number of different breath tests will be described in this section, the principle of these tests is provided. Figure 13.3.1 shows the principle of a ^{13}C-labelled breath test to detect a metabolic difference, such as altered fat absorption and also the presence of bacteria in the stomach or small bowel as a bacterial overgrowth.

Various reports have suggested that the triolein breath test, using the radioactive ^{14}C label, has been useful and is able to detect fat malabsorption due to both pancreatic insufficiency as well as mucosal disease, although discrimination of moderate pancreatic disease from normal function is still difficult (Butler *et al.*, 1984; Vantrappen *et al.*, 1989). The stable isotope ^{13}C mixed triglyceride test has been in use for less time but appears to be a useful test for determining pancreatic dysfunction and is likely to be particularly useful in patients with cystic fibrosis (Amarri *et al.*, 1997; Swart *et al.*, 1997). One reason why these tests have not yet been widely accepted is the radioactivity associated with ^{14}C and, in the case of the stable isotope ^{13}C, the cost, although it is likely that this will decrease dramatically with the increased availability of instruments to measure $^{13}CO_2$ (e.g. isotope ratio mass spectrometers and infrared spectrometers). While full quantitative analysis using breath testing techniques is not possible, they are acceptable to patients, easily carried out and user friendly for laboratory staff. In addition, the technique offers a dynamic and integrated result of the overall fat absorption process.

Some caveats associated with these methods are that the patient must be sedentary, as exercise alters the output of CO_2, and that as yet no truly standardized amount of fat, type of fat and stable isotopes required have been universally accepted. Considering the alternatives, the fat breath tests, once validated and standardized in a number of laboratories, are likely to be of enormous benefit for clinical diagnosis and monitoring of fat malabsorption syndromes both in adults and in

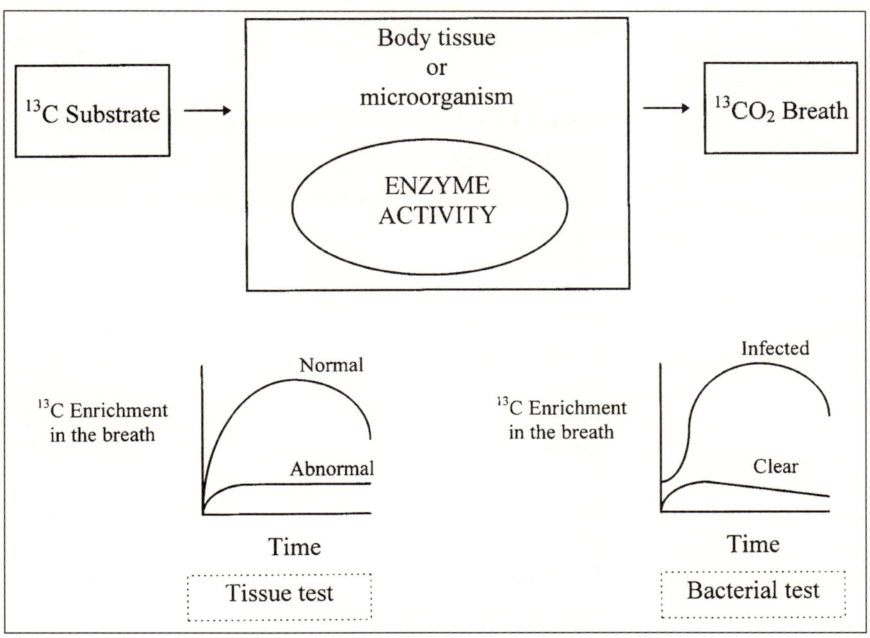

Figure 13.3.1 *Principles of $^{13}CO_2$ breath tests. Theoretical enrichment curves are presented for $^{13}CO_2$ enrichment in breath for ^{13}C stable isotope breath tests. Patients are given a single oral dose of ^{13}C-labelled substrate, which is labelled at a target bond. Breath samples are collected at timed intervals and ^{13}C enrichment is measured by an isotope ratio mass spectrometer (IRMS). Ideal excretion curves are illustrated for tissue test (assessment of small gastrointestinal function) and bacterial test (assessment of infection or overgrowth) analyses.*

particular in children. Most other pancreatic function tests (excepting faecal elastase, which is not quantitative) are highly invasive, e.g. the collection of pancreatic juice, and measurement of lipase activity and bicarbonate output after administration of a secretagogue such as secretin-caerulein.

Three-day faecal fat test

The quantitative estimation of fat (the 3-day faecal fat estimation) was invariably ordered in the past to establish steatorrhoea, but has now been replaced by tests less challenging for both patients and laboratory staff. The procedure to carry out the 3-day faecal fat estimation is to collect stools over a period of 3 days, ensuring that urine contamination is excluded. The faecal samples are stored below 10°C until the collection is complete. These are then homogenized and a weighed sample is hydrolysed at 100°C for 30 minutes with 36 per cent hydrochloric acid to release fatty acids. The sample is then extracted overnight into diethyl ether. A measured aliquot of the ether layer is evaporated in a preweighed dish and the weight of the residual solids, the fatty residue, is determined.

The weight of residue is related back to the original proportions of the sample to multiply the extracted fat weight in grams by the dilution factor. This is multiplied by 3.52 to convert grams of fat into millimoles of fat (as stearate), then divided by 3 (the number of days over which the sample is collected) to obtain the faecal fat excreted in millimoles each day. The normal range should be from zero to 20 mmol faecal fat per day.

The D-xylose absorption test

The test is listed under tests of carbohydrate malabsorption in some texts. Its essential purpose is to establish the integrity of the small intestinal mucosa in terms of absorptive function and to determine whether steatorrhoea is of small intestinal mucosal origin. However, the D-xylose absorption test reflects the capacity of the small bowel to absorb luminal contents, not specifically carbohydrates.

Xylose is a pentose sugar that is absorbed, unchanged, in the upper small intestine, mainly by passive diffusion, not via a specific sugar-transport mechanism. The measurement of blood xylose and urine xylose after an oral dose is a measure of the absorptive capacity of the small intestine as a whole, and reflects its surface area and overall permeability. An abnormal D-xylose test suggests a small bowel mucosal lesion which is impairing its absorptive capacity. The D-xylose absorption test has a number of drawbacks as it is influenced by:

- the rate of gastric emptying;
- impaired renal function;
- small bowel bacterial overgrowth;
- the state of hydration;
- the presence of ascites;
- portal hypertension;
- therapy with aspirin, indomethacin, neomycin or glypizide (Riley and Marsh, 1993).

Since the D-xylose absorption test specifically reflects small intestinal pathology, some practitioners prefer to perform an endoscopic small bowel biopsy to seek evidence of morphological abnormalities of the mucosa, rather than requesting a D-xylose absorption test.

Carbohydrates

These are presented to the small bowel in a variety of forms, as monosaccharides, disaccharides and oligosaccharides, and also as polymers of glucose (starches) that are broken down by amylases (salivary and pancreatic), as resistant starches that resist this action and reach the colon where they and other dietary fibres are fermented (*see* Chapter 10).

However, from a clinical perspective, the most important carbohydrates, particularly in children, are those ingested as disaccharides, lactose and sucrose, and the monosaccharide fructose. Over 70 per cent of the world's population of adults are lactase deficient with differing degrees of deficiency (Table 13.3.1; *see* Chapter 24).

Children, on the other hand, are not usually lactase deficient in early life but, with variation in different cultures and geographic areas, proceed to develop some malabsorption of this milk sugar as they mature (Davidson, 1991). The role lactose malabsorption plays in adult disease is controversial (e.g. irritable bowel syndrome); however, the best test for defining

Table 13.3.1 *Prevalence of primary lactase deficiency for different populations*

Population	Incidence within the population (%)
Australian	
White	10
Indigenous	80–90
Mediterranean	36
North American	
White	5–20
Black	70–75
Asian	
Indian	55
Japanese	90
Thai	97
Greek	60–80

Modified from Davidson (1984).

this problem is the lactose breath H_2 test (Cuatrecasas *et al.*, 1965).

Principle of the breath hydrogen test

When a physiological dose of lactose is ingested (up to 20 g lactose depending on age and body weight) in individuals who are lactase sufficient, all of the lactose will be efficiently absorbed in the small intestine. However, in those who are either partially or totally unable to break down the lactose because they lack the brush-border enzyme lactase or have a damaged mucosa with diminished lactase activity, the lactose will reach the large intestine, where some of the 400 species of bacteria will metabolize the unabsorbed lactose and produce H_2. It has been shown that the amount of H_2 in the breath is proportional to that produced in the large bowel. On this basis, the breath H_2 test was established (Davidson *et al.*, 1984).

It has been reported that only 10 per cent of individuals do not produce H_2. In fact probably everybody possesses the bacteria to produce H_2. It is just that some also have other organisms that utilize the H_2, such as methanogens (Levitt and Bond, 1970). This may reduce the number of patients who can use this test, although measurement of other gases, e.g. methane, may increase the diagnostic sensitivity of the test (Corazza *et al.*, 1994; Rumessen *et al.*, 1994). At present more than 85 per cent of all patients can be tested effectively using the H_2 breath test alone.

Expiration of $^{13}CO_2$ from labelled lactose has not yet been adequately evaluated to assess whether all who are lactose intolerant can be detected and whether a quantitative index of the degree of lactose deficiency can be established, although the early studies are promising (Hiele *et al.*, 1988). Alternative tests such as detection of reducing sugars in stool or the measurement of glucose in serum after administration of lactose are less useful (Newcomer *et al.*, 1975).

Other sugars are also malabsorbed. Sucrose malabsorption occurs in a small number of individuals and, in infants, fructose malabsorption can be a major problem (Strocchi and Levitt, 1993; Gudmand-Hoyer and Skovbjerg, 1996). These sugars and indeed others, including monosaccharides such as galactose and other complex carbohydrates, can be assessed for malabsorption using breath H_2 analysis. This is a particularly useful test in young infants who may have an immature gastrointestinal tract.

Protein

Protein malabsorption has been a difficult entity to detect and monitor and, although a variety of tests, including α1-antitrypsin (see below), have been used, none are universally accepted (Evenpoel *et al.*, 1997). Nevertheless, an experimental stable isotope breath test holds great hope for a simple and rapid method to follow these malfunctions dynamically (Evenpoel *et al.*, 1997).

α1-Antitrypsin clearance

α1-Antitrypsin is produced by the liver, and small amounts are normally found in stools. This glycoprotein is very resistant to enzymatic degradation and is therefore considered to be a good indicator of loss of protein into the gastrointestinal tract. A 3-day faecal sample is collected, along with a single serum sample. Quantitative determination of α1-antitrypsin in the serum is done by laser nephelometry, where the rate of increase of light scattering due to complexes formed between antibodies to human α1-antitrypsin and α1-antitrypsin in a sample is determined and related back to standard concentrations. The faecal sample is too heavily contaminated to use the same measurement technique. A small sample is taken from the 3-day faecal collection and suspended in buffer and centrifuged to remove solids. A radial immunodiffusion technique is used to determine the concentration of α1-antitrypsin in this sample.

In this radial immunodiffusion technique, an agar gel contains antibody to human α1-antitrypsin. The faecal sample is placed in a central well and allowed to diffuse into the gel where the resultant antigen–antibody precipitation appears as a ring with a radius proportional to the concentration of the antigen (α1-antitrypsin). The clearance rate is then determined from the values of the serum sample and the faecal sample.

BACTERIAL OVERGROWTH

Bacterial overgrowth in the small intestine is defined as an increase in number or alteration in the type of enteric flora of sufficient magnitude to have clinical significance ($> 10^6$ per gram of contents of the gastrointestinal tract). Clinical significance is usually defined as the presence of pain, or signs such as malabsorption indicated by weight loss or dietary deficiency. Amelioration of these symptoms or signs by administration of antibiotics indicates that bacterial overgrowth was responsible (Toskes and Kumar, 1998) (*see* also Chapter 12).

The upper gastrointestinal tract is relatively free of bacteria. The discovery in 1984 by Marshall and Warren of *Helicobacter pylori* changed this view markedly and ushered in the use of breath tests with the use of ^{13}C urea to detect this organism (Graham *et al.*, 1986). Thus a specific probe for a particular bacterial overgrowth (*Helicobacter pylori*) in the stomach and the duodenum was developed. *Helicobacter pylori* is now the accepted causative agent for duodenal ulcers and is found in association with approximately 70 per cent of gastric ulcers (Peura and Graham, 1994).

The test is remarkably robust and is being constantly modified both in terms of the sensitivity (by lowering the cut-off point for positive detection) and in terms of other information that might be gleaned from it, such as the density of bacterial load and the depth of inflammation (Perri *et al.*, 1998). This test has also heralded a wider application of breath tests in gastroenterology, in particular to assess regional differences in the upper bowel and to assess gastric and small intestinal motility (Swart and Van Den Berg, 1998).

Bacterial overgrowth in different parts of the small intestine, i.e. proximal versus distal, occurs when one or more of the following mechanisms are perturbed.

1 Gastric acidity is diminished (*see* Chapter 5).
2 Intestinal propulsive activity is altered (slowed) (*see* Chapters 5 and 11).
3 Loss of competency of the ileo-caecal valve allows reflux of colonic bacteria (*see* Chapter 5).
4 There is impaired secretion of antibacterial agents such as immunoglobulin A (IgA), bile acids (in bile) and defensins (*see* Chapter 4).

Defects in propulsion are the most frequent cause of bacterial overgrowth and these may be caused by surgery, inborn neuropathic or myogenic defects, or acquired in conditions such as scleroderma or diabetes (*see* Chapter 12).

A number of different breath tests have been suggested for assessing bacterial overgrowth but with little regard for the region of overgrowth. The first test to be proposed, which also indirectly assessed bile acid malabsorption, was the bile acid breath test (Fromm and Hofmann, 1971). An alternative test for assessing bile acid malabsorption, which is relatively simple and non-invasive, is the ^{75}Se-23-homocholic acid taurine (SeHCAT) retention test (Merrick *et al.*, 1985). The disadvantage of this test is the radioactivity and inconvenience involving determinations at days 0 and 7 of the retained radioactivity, with the results being expressed as a percentage of the SeHCAT retained at 7 days. It does, however, provide a reliable measure of bile acid malabsorption.

The bile acid breath test has fallen out of favour because of its low sensitivity and specificity (Fromm *et al.*, 1973; Lauterberg *et al.*, 1978). This is not surprising given that it is designed to test for bacterial overgrowth in an area, the ileum, where hugely variable bacterial colonization would be expected, and the bacteria need to be able to hydrolyse the amide bond between glycine and the steroid moiety of glycocholic acid. The labelled CO_2 exhaled in the breath, after administration of glycocholic acid labelled in the amino-acid glycine portion of the molecule, indicates the presence of bacteria in the small bowel if a rise of greater than 1 per cent of the dose is seen within 3 hours of ingestion of the probe molecule.

The other three breath tests that have been used are a glucose breath test for a proximal bacterial overgrowth (Onderdonk, 1991) and the lactulose breath test (Metz *et al.*, 1976), both of which have given variable results when compared to the gold standard of intubation and culture. The third and probably most reliable is the ^{13}C/^{14}C-xylose breath test developed by King *et al.* (1980). This test is gaining in stature and can be claimed for a medical rebate in the USA. This test relies on the same principle as the other tests, the ability of bacteria to metabolize a 1-g dose of ^{14}C-xylose after ingestion within a 4-hour time frame, detected as a peak level of $^{14}CO_2$ in the breath.

SMALL INTESTINAL INTEGRITY: BARRIER FUNCTION

This area of study is probably the most exciting to emerge over the last two decades but has yet to be widely accepted. There are many situations where small intestinal integrity is altered and there are several variants of the method of detection. The dual sugar permeability test (Fig. 13.3.2), using either lactulose with rhamnose or lactulose with mannitol, was first devised by Menzies and the sugar measurement was originally performed using high-performance thin-layer chromatography (Menzies, 1974).

The measurement of urinary excretion of non-metabolized sugars as a marker of intestinal integrity is based on the fact that clear differences in uptake of monosaccharides or disaccharides in the pathological mucosa have been demonstrated. Monosaccharides such as mannitol and L-rhamnose pass via transcellular routes, whereas disaccharides such as lactulose will only follow a paracellular pathway, reflecting loss of integrity of tight junctions between epithelial cells (Travis and Menzies, 1992).

More recently, a number of different high-performance liquid chromatography techniques have been described (Miki *et al.*, 1996; Ryan *et al.*, 1996) which allow better resolution of the sugars both in urine and in serum samples. This test measures changes in permeability that may occur as a consequence of infection (e.g. rotavirus), of effects of non-steroidal anti-inflammatory drugs, after chemotherapy and in Crohn's disease and coeliac disease. While the test is non-specific, it is an important marker of severity, and in some cases can be used to monitor disease activity and likelihood of relapse (in Crohn's disease; *see* Chapter 25) (Sanderson *et al.*, 1987), and the adherence to diet (in coeliac disease; *see* Chapter 23) (Cummins *et al.*,

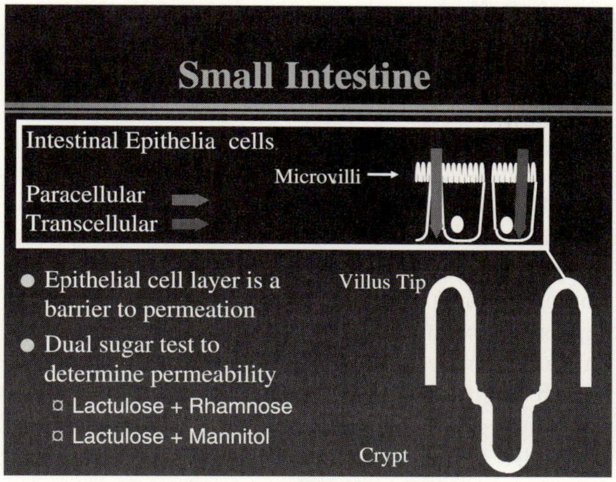

Figure 13.3.2 *The principle of the dual-sugar permeability tests using either lactulose/rhamnose or lactulose/mannitol. The synthetic disaccharide lactulose is not absorbed in the small intestine but if loss of barrier function has occurred, with loosening of tight junctions between epithelial cells, this sugar will cross the mucosa between the cells (paracellular movement) and be excreted in the urine. In the case of the monosaccharides, such as rhamnose or mannitol, the sugars permeate the epithelium transcellularly and appear in increased concentrations in the urine, where the cell mass is decreased due to damage. The ratio between the two sugars is a measure of the permeability and thus the integrity of the small intestine.*

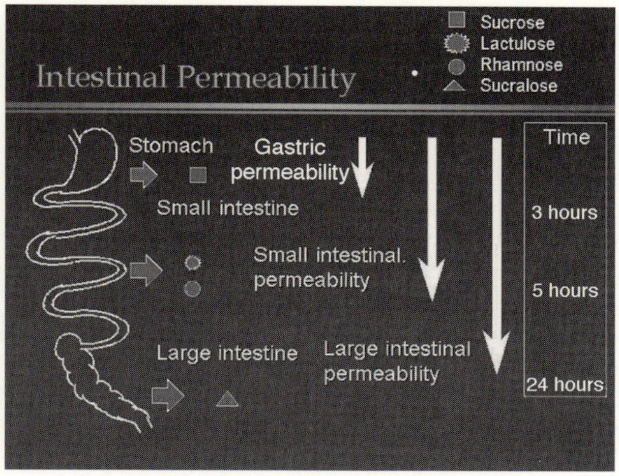

Figure 13.3.3 *The use of four sugars to ascertain the integrity of the intestine from the gastric mucosa, small intestine and the large bowel by measuring urinary ratios of sucrose to lactulose, lactulose to rhamnose and sucralose to lactulose, respectively. (Adapted from Meddings and Gibbons, 1998.)*

1991). In the case of chemotherapy, it is an early side-effect in the course of chemotherapy and may in the future be used to select patients who are particularly susceptible to gut mucositis.

On a broader front, considering the relationship of gut permeability to absorption and to small intestinal function, from the standpoint of the mucosal immune system, relatively little has been done. It is in this area that the understanding of the interactive role of regional permeability and absorptive processes will be very fruitful. The use of the sucrose permeability test to detect gastric and upper small bowel permeability combined with lactulose and rhamnose have been shown in the rat to detect regional damage that is not yet detectable by histology. Similarly, in the distal small bowel, the use of a sucralose to lactulose ratio is likely to prove very important and provide understanding for the region affected and the extent of that dysfunction (Meddings and Gibbons, 1998).

Principle of the sugar permeability tests

As shown in Fig. 13.3.3, the four sugars are sucrose, lactulose, rhamnose and sucralose (Meddings and Gibbons, 1998). Sucralose is a synthetic disaccharide used as an artificial sweetener that is non-absorbable and also resists degradation by colonic bacteria, making it an ideal probe for both small and large bowel permeability.

These tests have great potential utility and, while they lack specificity, they can confer significant diagnostic sensitivity. For example, in coeliac disease the detection of both antigliadin and antiendomysial antibodies as diagnostic tools has increased our awareness of a higher incidence of this disease than previously believed (Catassi *et al.*, 1996). Evidence has now emerged suggesting that the addition of a small intestinal permeability measurement may reveal an even higher occurrence of coeliac disease (Rostami *et al.*, 1998).

MOTILITY AND TRANSIT TIME

While small intestinal function can be partially described in health and disease by some of the aforementioned tests, one of the major rate-limiting factors that will determine its function is the transit time, or the time of contact of any nutrient with the small intestinal mucosa. One of the controlling processes in this is the rate of gastric emptying. Until recently, this has only been measurable by using highly invasive techniques requiring radioisotopes or by using ultrasound, with the necessity of trained individuals and high-level interpretative skills.

Stable isotope breath testing has the potential to change this. Using either ^{13}C-labelled octanoic acid or ^{13}C-labelled acetic acid, liquid gastric emptying rates can be measured and compared in health and disease before and after therapy.

While these breath tests are similar to those previously described, they require a significant mathematical input, usually in the form of curve-fitting algorithms or integration of areas under curves generated. A series of differing patterns can arise from altered gastric emptying that are usually more complex for the emptying of solids (which generally take longer) than liquids and, at this point, there is controversy over the best technique to use (Ghoos *et al.*, 1993; Choi *et al.*, 1997; Maes *et al.*, 1998).

This technology is still evolving but, even so, the advantages of the method are likely to outweigh the disadvantages. These assays can be done in free-living, ambulatory individuals, and can be performed in remote areas and analysed at a central laboratory after sending the samples via the mail. Clinically, patients with reflux disease, diabetes and a variety of other conditions, e.g. premature infants, can now be easily and rapidly assessed for gastric emptying abnormalities. The effect of alterations in gastric emptying and small intestinal function can now also be assessed, including their role in modifying absorptive efficiency. The capacity to absorb various nutrients can be markedly altered by the transit time of these nutrients through the small intestine. We have only been able to assess this transit time by using lactulose and measuring breath hydrogen up until now (Read *et al.*, 1980). While this tells us how long this laxative synthetic disaccharide takes to traverse the small intestine, it may not give us a true index of transit time. Indeed, the very fact that lactulose has laxative properties probably renders it less than ideal for this measurement. In our laboratory in over 1000 individuals, both adults and children, the mean oro-caecal transit time is 77 ± 12 minutes (mean ± SD). This relatively fast transit time probably depends partly on the dose of lactulose, and a new stable isotope breath test is being developed that may be the solution for the simple measurement of small intestinal transit.

The lactose ^{13}C-labelled ureide test is still in its infancy but early indications suggest that it will become a very useful tool in estimating small intestinal transit time (Wutzke *et al.*, 1997). Combining this with gastric emptying will give the clinician an unprecedented grasp on the dynamics of small intestinal function without having to resort to highly invasive and costly nuclear medicine and other imaging procedures in the first instance.

As inaccessible as they are, the different regions of the small intestine can now be probed with a variety of simple biochemical tests. These tests do not provide a pictorial view of the disease processes but they will allow decision trees for clinical management to be constructed on a more objective basis, and should help to avoid invasive and costly procedures unless they are necessary. Indeed, in children, where these studies are ideal, the decision to perform elaborate tests that are uncomfortable, sometimes unwarranted and costly to both the patient and the community is taken less readily compared with diagnosis in adults. The only limits to our diagnostic and prognostic probes for the small intestine are the innovativeness of those researchers involved in this area. The classical tests for malabsorption or malfunction in the small intestine are now being superseded by studies that describe the patency of the barrier function and the ability of different regions to absorb specific agents and foodstuffs. Tests such as the Schilling test are still useful but this test, as do many of the older tests, unfortunately requires a significant exposure to radioactivity. The D-xylose test was probably the forerunner to the newer permeability tests and has now largely been discarded (see below).

No simple objective index of small intestinal function or gut well-being has yet been devised analagous to, for example, blood pressure measurement for heart and vascular health, and respiratory function in the lung. This is partly due to the complexity of the gastrointestinal tract, which is an interlinked network of interactive, but at the same time, independent organs. If we view it in this way, then the most likely differences between individuals that could confer an increased risk of disease and manifest illness are differences in gastrointestinal motility and the extent to which different parts of the gastrointestinal tract are colonized by microorganisms. The interaction of these two factors and their effects on absorptive function and physiological well-being can now begin to be probed using the techniques described in this chapter. Furthermore, the role these factors play in disease processes can now be more accurately ascertained using a wide variety of non-invasive breath tests combined with tests of mucosal barrier function in patients and subjects of all ages, from premature infants to the elderly. As these tests become standardized and validated in different clinical settings, their utility as diagnostic tools in clinical management will increase. We are at the beginning of a reawakening of the potential of the measurement of substances (labelled with non-radioactive isotopes and naturally occurring compounds) in breath as well as other effluents (e.g. urine, saliva and faeces) to give meaningful data on small intestinal function that may be useful in clinical management.

OTHER TESTS OF INTESTINAL FUNCTION

Assessment of intestinal permeability

The patient fasts overnight, but drinking water is allowed. Then a drink containing 5 g of lactulose, 1 g of rhamnose and 22.6 g of glucose is consumed. Urine output is collected over the next 5 hours, the volume recorded, and an aliquot taken for later analysis by high-performance thin-layer chromatography (Cummins *et al.*, 1991).

Glucose is present as an osmotic filler in preference to lactose, or lactose and sucrose, because these are likely to be malabsorbed in villous atrophy. Intestinal permeability is expressed as the ratio of urinary lactulose to rhamnose, with each expressed as a percentage of the ingested dose (Cummins *et al.*, 1991).

REFERENCES

Amarri, S., Harding, M., Coward, W.A., Evans, T.J., Weaver, L.T. 1997: ^{13}Carbon mixed triglyceride breath test and pancreatic enzyme supplementation in cystic fibrosis. *Archives of Disease in Childhood* 76, 349–51.

Butler, R.N., Gehling, N.J., Lawson, M.J., Grant, A.K. 1984: Clinical evaluation of the ^{14}C triolein breath test: a critical analysis. *Australia and New Zealand Journal of Medicine* 14, 111–13.

Catassi, C., Fabiani, E., Ratsch, I.M. *et al.* 1996: The coeliac iceberg in Italy. A multicenter antigliadin antibodies screening for coeliac disease in school-age subjects. *Acta Paediatrica Supplement* 412, 29–35.

Choi, M.G., Camilleri, M., Burton, D.D., Zinsmeister, A.R., Forstrom, L.A., Nair, K.S. 1997: [^{13}C]Octanoic acid breath test for gastric emptying of solids: accuracy, reproducibility and comparison with scintigraphy. *Gastroenterology* 112, 1155–62.

Corazza, G.R., Benati, G., Strocchi, A., Malservisi, S., Gasbarrini, G. 1994: The possible role of breath methane measurement in detecting carbohydrate malabsorption. *Journal of Laboratory and Clinical Medicine* 124, 695–700.

Cuatrecasas, P., Lockwood, D.H., Caldwell, J.R. 1965: Lactase deficiency in the adult: a common occurrence. *Lancet* 1, 14–18.

Cummins, A.G., Penttila, I.A., Labrooy, J.T., Robb, T.A., Davidson, G.P. 1991: Recovery of the small intestine in coeliac disease on a gluten-free diet: changes in intestinal permeability, small bowel morphology and T-cell activity. *Journal of Gastroenterology and Hepatology* 6, 53–7.

Davidson, G.P. 1984: Lactase deficiency–diagnosis and management. *Medical Journal of Australia* 141, 442–4.

Davidson, G.P. 1991: The physiology and pathology of carbohydrate absorption in children. *Current Opinion in Paediatrics* 3, 999–1003.

Davidson, G.P., Goodwin, D., Robb, T.A. 1984: Incidence and duration of lactose malabsorption in children hospitalized with acute enteritis: a study in a well nourished urban population. *Journal of Paediatrics* 105, 620–2.

Evenpoel, P., Hiele, M., Luypaerts, A. *et al.* 1997: Production of egg proteins, enriched with L-leucine ^{13}Cl, for the study of protein assimilation in humans using the breath test techniques. *Journal of Nutrition* 127, 327–31.

Fromm, H., Hofmann, A.F. 1971: Breath test for altered bile acid metabolism. *Lancet* 2, 621–5.

Fromm, H., Thomas, P.J., Hofmann, A.F. 1973: Sensitivity and specificity in tests of distal ileal function: prospective comparisons of bile acid and vitamin B12 absorption in ileal resection patients. *Gastroenterology* 64, 1077–90.

Ghoos, Y.F., Vantrappen, G.R., Rutgeerts, P.J., Schurmans, P.C. 1981: A mixed-triglyceride breath test for intraluminal fat digestive activity. *Digestion* 22, 239–47.

Ghoos, Y.F., Maes, B.D., Geypens, B.J., Mys, G., Hiele, M.I., Rutgeerts, P.J., Vantrappen, G. 1993: Measurement of gastric emptying rate of solids by means of a carbon-labelled octanoic acid breath test. *Gastroenterology* 104, 1640–7.

Graham, D.Y., Klein, P.D., Evans, D.G. *et al.* 1986: Rapid non-invasive diagnostic of gastric Camylobacter by a ^{13}C urea breath test. *Gastroenterology* 90, 1435.

Gudmand-Hoyer, E., Skovbjerg, H. 1996: Disaccharide digestion and maldigestion. *Scandinavian Journal of Gastroenterology* 31, 111–21.

Hiele, M., Ghoos, Y.F., Rutgeerts, P., Vantrappen, G., Carchon, H., Eggermont, E. 1988: $^{13}CO_2$ breath test using naturally ^{13}C-enriched lactose for detection of lactase deficiency in patients with gastrointestinal symptoms. *Journal of Laboratory and Clinical Medicine* 112, 193–200.

King, C.E., Toskes, P.P., Guilarte, T.R., Lorenz, E., Welkos, S.L. 1980: Comparison of the one gram ^{14}C-xylose breath test to the ^{14}C-bile acid breath test in patients with small intestine bacterial overgrowth. *Digestive Diseases Science* 25, 53–8.

Lauterberg, B.H, Newcomer, A.D., Hofmann, A.F. 1978: Clinical value of the bile acid breath test: evaluation of Mayo Clinic experience. *Mayo Clinic Proceedings* 53, 227–33.

Lembcke, B., Braden, B., Caspary, W.F. 1996: Exocrine pancreatic insufficiency: accuracy and clinical value of the uniformly labelled ^{13}C-triolein breath test. *Gut* 39, 668–74.

Levitt, M.D., Bond, J.H. 1970: Volume, composition and source of intestinal gas. *Gastroenterology* 59, 1058.

Loser, C., Molgaard, A., Folsch, U.R. 1995: Elastase 1 in faeces: a novel, highly sensitive, and specific pancreatic function test for easy and inexpensive routine application. *Digestion* 56, 301.

Loser, C., Molgaard, A., Folsch, U.R. 1996: Faecal elastase 1: a novel, highly sensitive, and specific pancreatic function test. *Gut* 39, 580–6.

Maes, B.D., Mys, G., Geypens, B.J., Evenepoel, P., Ghoos, Y.F., Rutgeerts, P.J. 1998: Gastric emptying flow curves separated from carbon-labelled octanoic acid breath test results. *American Journal of Physiology* 275, G169–75.

Marshall, B.J., Warren, J.R. 1984: Unidentified curved bacilli in the stomach of patients with gastritis and peptic ulceration. *Lancet* 1, 1311–15.

Meddings, J., Gibbons, I. 1998: Discrimination of site-specific alterations in gastrointestinal permeability in the rat. *Gastroenterology* 114, 83–92.

Menzies, I.S. 1974: Absorption of intact oligosaccharide in health and disease. *Biochemical Society Transcripts* 2, 1040–6.

Merrick, M.V., Eastwood, M.A., Ford, M.J. 1985: Is bile acid malabsorption underdiagnosed? An evaluation of accuracy of diagnosis by measurement of SeHCAT retention. *British Medical Journal* 290, 665–86.

Metz, G., Gassull, M.A., Drasar, B.S., Jenkins, D.J., Blendis, L.M. 1976: Breath-hydrogen test for small intestinal bacterial colonization. *Lancet* 1, 668–9.

Miki, K., Butler, R.N., Moore, D., Davidson, G. 1996: Rapid simultaneous quantification of rhamnose, mannitol and lactulose in urine by HPLC for estimating intestinal permeability in paediatric practice. *Clinical Chemistry* 42, 71–5.

Newcomer, A.D., McGill, B.D., Thomas, P.J., Hofmann, A.F. 1975: Prospective comparison of indirect methods for detecting lactase deficiency. *New England Journal of Medicine* 293, 1232–36.

Newcomer, A.D., Hofmann, A.F., DiMagno, E.P., Thomas, P.J., Carlson, G.L. 1979: Triolein breath test: a sensitive and specific test for fat malabsorption. *Gastroenterology* 76, 6–13.

Onderdonk, A.B. 1991: Intestinal microflora: control and overgrowth. In Blum, H.E., Bode, C., Bode, J.C., Sartor, R.B. (eds) *Gut and the liver*. Dordrecht: Kluwer Academic Publishers, 3–11.

Perri, F., Clemente, R., Pastore, M. *et al.* 1998: The ^{13}C urea breath test as a predictor of intragastric bacterial load and severity of Helicobacter pylori gastritis. *Scandinavian Journal of Clinical Laboratory Investigation* 58, 19–28.

Peura, D.A., Graham, D.Y. 1994: Helicobacter pylori: consensus reached: peptic ulcer disease is on the way to becoming an historic disease. *American Journal of Gastroenterology* 89, 1137–9.

Read, N.W., Mils, C.A., Fisher, D. *et al.* 1980: Transit of a meal through the stomach, small intestine, and colon in normal subjects and its role in the pathogenesis of diarrhoea. *Gastroenterology* 79, 1276–82.

Riley, S.A., Marsh, M.N. 1993: Maldigestion and malabsorption. In Feldman, M., Scharschmidt, B.F., Sleisenger, M.H. (eds) *Sleisenger and Fordtran's gastrointestinal and liver disease*, Vol. I. Philadelphia: W.B. Saunders, 1501–22.

Rostami, K., Kerckhaert, J., von Blomberg, B.M.E., Meijer, J.W.R., Wahab, P., Mulder, C.J.J. 1998: SAT and serology in adult coeliacs; seronegative coeliac disease seems a reality. *Netherlands Journal of Medicine* 53, 15–19.

Rumessen, J.J., Nordgaard-Andersen, I., Gudmand-Hoyer, E. 1994: Carbohydrate malabsorption: quantification by methane and hydrogen breath tests. *Scandinavian Journal of Gastroenterology* 29, 826–32.

Ryan, A.J., Chang, R.J., Gisolfi, C.V. 1996: Gastrointestinal permeability following aspirin intake and prolonged running. *Medicine and Science in Sports Exercise* 28, 698–705.

Sanderson, I.R., Boulton, P., Menzies, I., Walker-Smith, J.A. 1987: Improvement of abnormal lactulose/rhamnose permeability in active Crohn's disease of the small bowel by an elemental diet. *Gut* 28, 1073–6.

Strocchi, A., Levitt, M.D. 1993: Intestinal gas. In Sleisinger, M.H., Fordtran, J.S. (eds) *Gastrointestinal disease*. Philadelphia: W.B. Saunders, 1035–42.

Swart, G.R., Van Den Berg, J.W.O. 1998: ^{13}C breath tests in gastroenterological practice. *Scandinavian Journal of Gastroenterology* 33(Suppl 225), 13–18.

Swart, G.R., Baartman, E.A., Wattimena, J.L., Rietvald, T., Overbeek, S.E., Van Den Berg, J.W. 1997: Evaluation studies of the ^{13}C mixed triglyceride breath test in healthy controls and adult cystic fibrosis patients with exocrine pancreatic insufficiency. *Digestion* 58, 415–20.

Thorsgaard Pederson, N. 1987: Fat digestion tests. *Digestion* 37(Suppl 1), 25–34.

Toskes, P.P., Kumar, A. 1998: Enteric bacterial flora and bacterial overgrowth syndrome. In Sleisinger, M.H., Fordtran, J.S. (eds) *Gastrointestinal and liver disease*, 6th edn, Vol. 2. Philadelphia: W.B. Saunders, 1523–35.

Travis, S., Menzies, I. 1992: Intestinal permeability: functional assessment and significance. *Clinical Science* 82, 471–88.

Vantrappen, G.R., Rutgeerts, P.J., Ghoos, Y.F., Hiele, M.I. 1989: Mixed triglyceride breath tests: a non-invasive test of pancreatic lipase activity in the duodenum. *Gastroenterology* 96, 1126–34.

Wutzke, K.D., Heine, W.E., Plath, C. *et al.* 1997: Evaluation of oro-caecal transmit time: a comparison of the lactose-[^{13}C,^{15}N] ureide $^{13}CO_2$ and the H_2 breath test in humans. *European Journal of Clinical Nutrition* 51, 11–19.

13.4

Microbiological tests

PETER LAWSON, AUSTIN G MILTON

SPECIMEN

Ideally, a fresh sample of 20–40 g of stool should be examined within 30 minutes of collection. While some organisms responsible for diarrhoea are quite hardy, others succumb to the fall in pH, drying and the accumulation of products of bacterial metabolism. Similarly, leucocytes and amoebic trophozoites are rapidly disrupted after passage of the stool.

Microbiologists are often amused to receive a request form with diarrhoea listed as the reason for sending a pellet of faeces so hard that it rattles when the container is shaken. It is important that the specimen submitted is consistent with clinical expectations before accepting a negative microscopy and culture result.

Most laboratories will provide a macroscopic description of the specimen as part of their report. The stool appearance, along with presence of pus and blood, is a guide to whether the diarrhoea, if bacterial, is of a penetrating inflammatory type, as in shigellosis, or the watery toxin-mediated type like cholera. Microbiology laboratories tend to 'tailor' their examination of a stool specimen subject to the macroscopic appearance, clinical information provided and local knowledge, such as the requesting specialty and current epidemiology. For example, a history of recent seafood ingestion is a valuable pointer to inoculate *Vibrio* isolation media. A history of immune deficiency warrants a workup that includes examination for *Cryptosporidium* and other parasites.

BASIC LABORATORY PROCEDURES

Pathogens detectable on microscopy

In the laboratory, areas of the stool that appear mucoid or bloody are emulsified into a drop of saline on a slide, and examined for white and red blood cells and parasites. Stains such as methylene blue, phloxine, iodine or eosin are used to visualize cells, trophozoites and cysts.

A rigorous examination for parasites includes a stool concentration method using salt or sugar flotation, or more often a formol–ether centrifugation process. Trophozoite and cyst identification is based on size and fine structure using high-power microscopy on fixed smears stained with an iron-haematoxylin stain.

The presence of many leucocytes in the stool suggests large intestinal pathology of inflammatory origin. Leucocytes are detected in the faeces by microscopy on a wet preparation stained with Loeffler's methylene blue.

Some microscopic features used to identify protozoa are given in the following section (Table 13.4.1).

PARASITES

Giardia lamblia

Cysts of the protozoan parasite *Giardia* excyst in the duodenum and infect the duodenum and jejunum.

Table 13.4.1 *Major protozoal parasites of the human gastrointestinal tract*

Species	Detection method
Flagellates	
Giardia lamblia	Oocysts, or flagellated trophozoites in stools
Amoebae	
Entamoeba histolytica	Red blood cells containing parasite in stools
Ciliates	
Balantidium coli	Large ciliated protozoa in stools
Spore-formers	
Cryptosporidium parvum	4–6 μm oocysts in stools
Cyclospora cayetanensis	8–9 μm oocysts in stools
Isospora belli	15 × 24 μm elliptical oocysts in stools
Sarcocystis species	Oocysts similar to *Isospora*, but more regularly ovoid in shape
Microsporidia:	
Enterocytozoon bieneusi	1–2 μm spores in stools, but difficult to see
Encephalitozoon intestinalis	1–2 μm spores in stools, but difficult to see

Motile *Giardia* are detected in a saline wet mount of a liquid stool or duodenal aspirate by their vigorous activity, and identified by the overall leaf-like shape and distinctive internal features. In formed stools, the cysts can be concentrated by the formol–ether or flotation techniques, and are identifiable by their axostyle and other internal features (Ash and Orihel, 1994).

Balantidium coli

This large ciliate protozoan is a relatively uncommon parasite of humans. It is easily identified in saline wet mounts by its size (50–200 μm) and peripheral cilia (Ash and Orihel, 1994). Ingested cysts of the parasite excyst in the small intestine and are swept into the colon. Here they penetrate the epithelium, occasionally also affecting the terminal ileum.

Cryptosporidium species

Ingested oocyts excyst in the small intestine, where they attach to the epithelium of both the small and large intestine, destroying the microvilli. This organism is detected by making a smear of the specimen on a slide, which is then heat fixed and stained with a modified Kinyoun acid-fast stain similar to that used for *Mycobacterium tuberculosis* (Owen, 1989). The parasites are stained with sufficient contrast so that they are relatively easily recognized against the background of faecal bacteria and debris. With a size of 3–6 μm, they may be confused with yeast cells; mature oocysts contain four sausage-shaped naked sporozoites (Ash and Orihel, 1994).

Isospora belli and *Sarcocystis hominis*

Ingested oocyts excyst in the small intestine, where the sporozoites invade the epithelium. *Isospora belli* is best detected and identified in modified acid-fast (Kinyoun) stained preparations (Isenberg, 1992). The oocyst is an elliptical acid-fast structure 22–33 by 10–15 μm, often showing two internal sporocysts. *S. hominis* is similar in appearance, but the oocyst is more regularly ovoid in shape (Ash and Orihel, 1994).

Microsporidia

Microsporidia, for example, species from the genuses Enterocytozoon and Encephalitozoon, are obligate intracellular protozoa. Spores from faeces, or contained in muscle and other tissues eaten by carnivores, transmit the infection. Infections of the small intestine are seen frequently in patients with the acquired immunodeficiency syndrome (AIDS), and healthy adults in tropical areas are also prone to infection. The infections are hard to detect, since the spores in stool are very small (about 1–2 μm). There are no current tests to diagnose infection, but biopsy specimens of small intestinal epithelium will allow demonstration of small inclusions in the apical cytoplasm of enterocytes (Owen, 1989; Garcia and Shimizu, 1993).

Roundworms (nematodes)

Most roundworm infections are detected by examination of stools for eggs, most of which are fairly characteristic in size and shape to enable identification of the parasite (Table 13.4.2). However, *Strongyloides stercoralis*

Table 13.4.2 *Major helminthic parasites of the human gastrointestinal tract*

Species	Detection method
Roundworms	
Ancylostoma duodenale	40 × 60 μm eggs in stools
Angiostrongylus costaricensis	Undetectable in stools
Anisakis species	Undetectable in stools
Ascaris lumbricoides	Large numbers of eggs in stools; fertilized: ovoid 50 × 70 μm double-walled; unfertilized: oval 40 × 90 μm with a single wall; distinct mammillated external layer
Capillaria philippinensis	Eggs and larvae detectable, usually in large numbers
Necator americanus	40 × 60 μm eggs in stools
Strongyloides stercoralis	Stage 1 larvae in stools or duodenal aspirates
Trichinella spiralis	Worms in muscle biopsy, undetectable in stools
Trichuris trichiura	3–10 days in small intestine, then relocates to colon; barrel-shaped ova in stools, 50 μm long
Flukes	
Echinostoma species	Eggs in stools
Fasciolopsis buski	Eggs in stools: 140 μm long ovals
Heterophyes heterophyes	Eggs in stools: 30 μm long ovals
Metagonimus yokogawai	Eggs in stools: 25 μm long ovals
Schistosoma japonicum	Eggs in stools: 90 μm long ovoid, almost round
Schistosoma mansoni	Eggs in stools: 150 μm long, pointed ovals with double walls
Tapeworms	
Diphyllobothrium latum	40 × 60 μm eggs in stools
Hymenolepis nana	30 × 50 μm eggs in stools; distinct separate outer wall
Hymenolepis diminuta	80 μm round eggs in stools; distinct separate outer wall
Taenia saginata/Taenia solium	30 × 40 μm eggs in stools, but proglottids need to be seen to distinguish *Taenia saginata* from *T. solium*

is usually detected by identifying stage 1 larval forms in stools or duodenal aspirates, since eggs are rarely found in stools other than during severe diarrhoea. *Trichinella spiralis* is rarely detected in stools, but requires biopsy of infected muscle tissue to detect the presence of worms. Serological tests are available (Nishiyama *et al.*, 1992).

Angiostrongylus costaricensis does not pass eggs detectable in stools because the eggs stay in the tissues in which they are laid (Pearson and Guerrant, 1995). Similarly, eggs from infecting *Anisakis* organisms are undetectable in stools; the worms partially embed themselves into the stomach wall and larvae may be found in the walls of the intestines (Pearson and Guerrant, 1995).

Ascaris infection is detected by the presence of large numbers of eggs, which are large and may be of two sizes. Fertilized eggs are large and ovoid, while unfertilized eggs are narrower and longer. Most eggs have a distinctive mammillated external layer, which is a characteristic marker of *Ascaris* species (Ash and Orihel, 1994). If the infection is by male worms, no eggs will be found and detection of the adult worm will usually require radiographic demonstration. Sputum and vomitus may demonstrate adult worms and, during the pneumonitis that accompanies the initial phase of the infection, larvae can be found in sputum.

Capillaria philippinensis and *Strongyloides stercoralis* are two parasites of humans where a mechanism known as autoinfection occurs. In this process, the parasite multiplies inside the gut of an infected person, rather than merely growing and passing eggs, which may infect another person or species. This often produces an overwhelming infection. Eggs and larvae may be detected in stools, and protein-losing enteropathy is a typical laboratory finding, with fat, mineral and vitamin malabsorption and electrolyte loss (Pearson and Guerrant, 1995). Major nematode parasites of the gastrointestinal tract are listed in Table 13.4.2.

Flukes (trematodes)

Schistosomiasis is caused by trematodes, which are commonly found in contaminated water in the tropics and subtropics, and which have a life cycle that requires a specific snail as an intermediate host. *Fasciolopsis buski* is the giant intestinal fluke of Asia that has a similar requirement for an intermediate host snail. Both may be detected by the presence of eggs in stools. Other flukes that are found to parasitize humans are listed in Table 13.4.2 and are considered in detail in Chapter 19 (Ash and Orihel, 1994; Nash, 1995).

Tapeworms (cestodes)

While a number of species of adult tapeworms can be found in human gastrointestinal systems, only a few involve parasitization of the small intestine. These include the fish tapeworm *Diphyllobothrium latum*, which is ingested from infected raw fish, *Taenia saginata* and *Taenia solium*, owing to ingestion of infected meat that is raw or inadequately cooked, from cattle or pigs, respectively, and *Hymenolepis nana*, which has no intermediate host but directly infects via embryonated eggs from another infected person, often a family member or from contact with fellow institutionalized members. The eggs of the *Hymenolepis* species possess a characteristically distinguishable double-layered cell wall, which has a distinct inner membrane separated by a large space from the thick outer shell (Ash and Orihel, 1995).

The larval form of tapeworms attaches to the small intestine wall, where they cause irritation of the host intestine due to metabolic wastes produced by the parasite. Sufficiently large numbers of the parasite can cause intestinal obstruction, especially in the beef tapeworm, *Taenia saginata*, which grows to a great length. The fish tapeworm can cause vitamin B_{12} deficiency, by competing with the host for this dietary resource.

These parasites can be detected by the presence in the faeces of eggs, which are often produced in great number. Differential diagnosis of which *Taenia* species, *T. saginata* or *T. solium*, is present requires the examination of proglottids (egg-producing body segments shed by adult worms), which are also passed into stools, or even the recovery of an evacuated scolex (the head part of the worm, which anchors the parasite to the host intestinal mucosa) (Ash and Orihel, 1995).

BACTERIA

Most laboratories choose their basic media to recover *Salmonella*, *Shigella* and *Campylobacter*. In the hospital setting particularly, an attempt will be made to check for *Clostridium difficile* by culture, toxin detection or both. Less common pathogens such as *Aeromonas*, *Yersinia* and *Vibrio* can be detected by experienced microbiologists on the basic *Salmonella–Shigella* media set, although more specific media yield a better chance of isolation. It is the minor differences in nutritional activity and resistance to toxic compounds of these organisms that are exploited in the complex culture media used to isolate them.

The wide choice of differential–selective agar media currently popular in laboratories for the isolation of *Salmonella* species and *Shigella* species include xylose–lysine–desoxycholate (XLD), *Salmonella–Shigella* (SS) and MacConkey medium. A laboratory will commonly use two of these to increase isolation rates. The media contain a variety of compounds, such as bile salts, that selectively suppress growth of some normal bowel flora, for example, *Escherichia* and *Enterococcus*, while allowing a minority population of *Salmonella* or *Shigella* to grow (Isenberg, 1992).

The media are also rendered 'differential' by including a nutrient substrate, such as lactose, along with a pH indicator. Organisms that ferment lactose produce lactic acid, resulting in a red-coloured colony. More complex and elegant biochemical differentiators of nutritional activity can be used, such as are present in XLD medium to show the fermentation of xylose, the decarboxylation of lysine and indicate the production of hydrogen sulphide to differentiate *Salmonella* and *Shigella* from other bacteria (Isenberg, 1992).

One or more types of enrichment broth will be inoculated. For example, selenite broth and Rappaport's medium are formulated to support preferentially the growth of some pathogenic species of interest while suppressing or holding static the numbers of the normal bowel flora.

The agar plates are inoculated with the specimen, streaked and incubated for 18–24 hours. After incubation, plates are examined for 'suspect' colonies. Growth from a faecal inoculum on selective–differential media is rarely pure, even in the case of a florid salmonellosis, and colonies are not easily distinguishable from *Proteus* by their pale colour on a medium containing lactose, since both organisms are non-lactose fermenters. Therefore, several of each morphological type of suspect colony are 'picked off' and subcultured into a range of differential broth media. *Proteus*, for instance, are rapidly screened out by their ability to split urea to ammonia. The colour change occurs within an hour or two of inoculation of the detection broth (Isenberg, 1992).

Various commercially prepared differential sugar identification systems for Enterobacteriaceae are now employed widely. These consist of plastic strips or plates containing moulded wells or bubbles into which sugar or substrate mixtures, along with indicator agents, have been freeze-dried.

A suspension of a suspect organism is added to each well, rehydrating the material as it is inoculated. After incubation, results are interpreted by noting the colour change in each well. The results can be recorded as a number by assigning positive and negative results in a binary fashion, as ones and zeroes. Sequential groups are then added together to produce a 'biogram' signature that reflects the activity of the organism in a wide range of substrates. The companies marketing these systems supply lists of numbers that correlate a specific biogram with ranked identity probabilities, determined from large databases of reference organisms. Several automated systems (e.g. Vitek) are available that handle all the steps from inoculation through to identification with a combination of mechanical, optical and computer technologies.

BACTERIAL AGENTS DETECTABLE IN CULTURE

Staphylococcus aureus

Laboratory confirmation involves demonstration of the organism in food or faeces, or the detection of staphylococcal enterotoxins by gel diffusion or radioimmunoassay (RIA) tests (Bryan, 1995).

Bacillus cereus and *Clostridium perfringens*

Both organisms cause food poisoning (*see* Chapter 18). Laboratory confirmation depends on the demonstration of high counts of bacteria in the faeces of affected individuals and in the ingested food (Bryan, 1995).

Clostridium difficile

This organism can be isolated from faeces using antibiotic-containing selective media, and identified by carbohydrate fermentation and gas–liquid chromatography of its metabolic products. Heat-shock treatment of the specimen to 75°C for 10 minutes enhances isolation of *C. difficile* by killing vegetative cells of non-spore-forming bacteria, promoting growth of spores and reducing the background contamination. Toxin detection methods include a cell-culture cytotoxicity technique on faecal extracts and the detection of an associated protein by a commercial latex particle agglutination on a faecal suspension (Isenberg, 1992).

Enteropathogenic, toxigenic, invasive, aggregative and haemorrhagic *E. coli*

E. coli is normally present in stool cultures in large numbers. Pathogenic strains are classified by their harbouring of plasmids or phages that encode for a variety of pathogenic mechanisms or virulence factors, including invasiveness, pathogenicity, secretion of enterotoxins and release of cytotoxins (Evans and Evans, 1983; Granum *et al.*, 1995).

Although certain sero groups have been associated with each of these classes of *E. coli*, the transmissible plasmid or phage-borne nature of their pathogenicity makes sero group detection unreliable. Such work is performed only in specialist reference laboratories that possess techniques including DNA probes and tissue culture assays for cytotoxins. There are no reliable and specific biochemical tests that allow the differentiation of pathogenic *E. coli* strains from normal non-pathogenic strains found in stools (Isenberg, 1992). The detection of these strains in the clinical laboratory therefore awaits the commercialization of new techniques in molecular biology.

Enteropathogenic and enterotoxigenic strains of *E. coli* commonly infect the small intestine, while enteroinvasive and enterohaemorrhagic *E. coli* infect both the distal small intestine and the colon. Strains classified as enteroaggregative usually involve only the colon (Guerrant, 1995) (*see* Chapter 18).

Salmonella

Many selective media have been produced that use the resistance of *Salmonella* to a range of compounds, including bile salts, selenium salts and dyes. The organisms are classically motile, non-lactose fermenters, oxidase and urease negative. Isolates of *Salmonella* are generally reported generically by laboratories as '*Salmonella* species'. A follow-up report is issued when the isolate is further identified by serological or other testing methods to one of 2000 or so known serotypes (Portnoy and Smith, 1992). This extra serotypic information may be useful in tracing a source of infection.

Where a fever is present in patients with *Salmonella*, the organism can frequently be isolated from blood cultures.

Shigella species

Molecular biology has revealed that the *Shigella* species and enteroinvasive strains of *E. coli* are closely related based on DNA sequencing (Karaolis *et al.*, 1994). *Shigella* species are isolated readily on the less selective enteric media such as XLD, and identified by carbohydrate reactions. Shigellae are non-motile, and are usually lactose non-fermenters, producing pale colonies on SS agar (Isenberg, 1992).

Yersinia enterocolitica

A specialized selective media, cefsulodin–irgasam–novobiocin (CIN) agar is available for the isolation of *Y. enterocolitica*. The organism is somewhat peculiar in that it grows better at lower temperatures (22–25°C) than other Enterobacteraceae (Isenberg, 1992). This characteristic is used to enhance isolation of pathogen by storing a saline emulsion of the stool at 4°C for 1–3 weeks and subculturing on to MacConkey agar at room temperature. Laboratories more commonly store a MacConkey agar plate at room temperature for 2–4 days and examine it for suspect colonies that have enlarged appreciably at the lower temperature on the bench. The organism is a motile lactose and oxidase-negative urease producer that does not deaminate phenylalanine. Test results change markedly between 22°C and 37°C, with motility, and various other reactions, being negative at the higher temperature. On CIN agar, the organism produces dark-red 'bullseye' colonies with a clear border. Both the small intestine and the colon can be involved in the infection.

While *Y. enterocolitica* is associated with blood-transfusion-related bacteraemia, it is primarily considered to be a food-borne pathogen of the gastrointestinal tract (Bottone, 1997).

Aeromonas hydrophila

This organism can be isolated from faeces using media that select for its usual resistance to ampicillin, but this characteristic is not invariable (Obi *et al.*, 1995). *Aeromonas* is motile, oxidase positive and variably ferments lactose (Isenberg, 1992; Janda *et al.*, 1995).

Vibrio cholerae and *Vibrio parahaemolyticus*

The reliable isolation of *Vibrio* species requires the use of specialized media such as thiosulphate–citrate–bile salts (TCBS) agar. The two species are oxidase positive, but differ in that *V. parahaemolyticus* is halophilic; that is, it has a requirement for sodium chloride. Both organisms are readily identified by carbohydrate fermentation: *V. cholerae* forms yellow colonies 2–3 mm in diameter, *V. parahaemolyticus* has blue or green colonies 3–5 mm in diameter, while non-vibrios are much smaller colonies (Isenberg, 1992).

Campylobacter

This microaerophilic, thermophilic organism requires an isolation medium that contains antibiotics as selective agents, and supplements of blood or charcoal to overcome the toxic effects of peroxides that occur in organic substrates exposed to air. Isolation media are incubated at 43°C in an atmosphere of 3–5 per cent oxygen in carbon dioxide or nitrogen for 48–72 hours. Isolates are identified by their curved, S-shaped or seagull-shaped rods, negative by Gram stain, a darting motility in wet preparation microscopy and a positive oxidase reaction (Isenberg, 1992). Colonies are typically effuse and tend to spread along the direction of the agar streak. Pus and blood is not uncommon in the stools of infected patients, and the organism may appear in blood cultures. These organisms predominantly infect the colon, but small intestinal infection can occur, producing a watery diarrhoea due to the secretion of a cholera-like toxin (*see* Chapter 18)

Plesiomonas shigelloides

This organism can be isolated from faeces using SS agar, where it manifests as oxidase-positive colonies. It does not grow well on *Vibrio* medium but a selective medium is inisotol brilliant-green bile-salts agar (Isenberg, 1992). Lactulose utilization, lysine decarboxylase, ornithine decarboxylase and arginine dihydrolase positivity are among the biochemical tests used to differentiate the organism from others with similar phenotypes (Janda *et al.*, 1995).

VIRAL AGENTS

Rotavirus

Enzyme-linked immunosorbent assay (ELISA) tests are the diagnostic tests routinely used. The virus can be cultured with difficulty.

Norwalk-like agents

Immune electron microscopy may be used to detect the infectious particle, but is usually regarded only as a research technique. Various RIA and ELISA methods under development may prove useful in the future.

REFERENCES

Ash, L.R., Orihel, T.C. 1994: *Atlas of human parasitology*, 3rd edn. Chicago: American Society of Clinical Pathologists Press.

Ash, L.R., Orihel, T.C. 1995: Intestinal helminths. In Murray, P.R. (ed.) *Manual of cinical microbiology*, 6th Ed. Washington: American Society of Microbiology, 1229–43.

Bottone, E.J. 1997: Yersinia enterocolitica: the charisma continues. *Clinical Microbiological Reviews* 10, 257–76.

Bryan, F.L. 1995: Procedures to use during outbreaks of food-borne disease. In Murray, P.R. (ed.) *Manual of clinical microbiology*, 6th ed. Washington: American Society of Microbiology, 209–26.

Evans, D.J., Jr., Evans, D.G. 1983: Classification of pathogenic Escherichia coli isolates according to serotype and the production of virulence factors, with special reference to colonization-factor antigens. *Reviews of Infectious Diseases* 5(Suppl. 4), S692–701.

Garcia, L.S., Shimizu, R.Y. 1993: Diagnostic parasitology: parasitic infections and the compromised host. *Laboratory Medicine* 24, 205–15.

Granum, P.E., Tomas, J.M., Alouf, J.E. 1995: A survey of bacterial toxins involved in food poisoning: a suggestion for bacterial food poisoning toxin nomenclature. *International Journal of Food Microbiology* 28, 129–44.

Guerrant, R.L. 1995: Principles and syndromes of enteric infection. In Mandel, G.L., Bennett, J.E., Dolin, R. (eds) *Principles and practice of infectious diseases*. 4th edn. New York: Churchill Livingstone, 940–60.

Isenberg, H.D. 1992: *Clinical microbiology procedures handbook*. Washington: American Society of Microbiology.

Janda, J.M., Abbott, S.L., Carnahan, A.M. 1995: Aeromonas and Plesiomonas. In Murray, P.R. (ed.) *Manual of clinical microbiology*, 6th edn. Washington: American Society of Microbiology, 477–82.

Karaolis, D.K., Lan, R., Reeves, P.R. 1994: Sequence variation in Shigella sonnei (Sonnei), a pathogenic clone of Escherichia coli, over four continents and 41 years. *Journal of Clinical Microbiology* 32, 796–802.

Nash, T.E. 1995: Visceral larvae migrans and other unusual helminth infections. In Mandel, G.L., Bennett, J.E., Dolin, R. (eds) *Principles and practice of infectious diseases*, 4th edn. New York: Churchill Livingstone, 2553–7.

Nishiyama, T., Araki, T., Mizuno, N., Wada, T., Ide, T., Yamaguchi, T. 1992: Detection of circulating antigens in human trichinellosis. *Transcripts of the Royal Society of Tropical Medicine and Hygiene* 86, 292–3.

Obi, C.L., Coker, A.O., Epoke, J., Ndip, R. 1995: Aeromonas and Plesiomonas species as bacterial agents of diarrhoea in urban and rural areas of Nigeria: antibiogram of isolates. *Central Africa Journal of Medicine* 41, 397–403.

Owen, R.L. 1989: Parasitic diseases. In Sleisenger, M., Fordtran, J.S. (eds) *Gastrointestinal disease: pathophysiology, diagnosis, management*, 4th edn. Philadelphia: W.B. Saunders Co., 1153–91.

Pearson, R.D., Guerrant, R.L. 1995: Enteric fever and other causes of abdominal symptoms with fever. In Mandel, G.L., Bennett, J.E., Dolin, R. (eds) *Principles and practice of infectious diseases*, 4th edn. New York: Churchill Livingstone, 998–1012.

Portnoy, D.A., Smith, G.A. 1992: Cell biology. Devious devices of Salmonella. *Nature* 357, 536–7.

13.5

Haematological tests

NICHOLAS WICKHAM

INTRODUCTION AND OVERVIEW

Blood is a curious juice. (Mephistopheles)

The small bowel is the pre-eminent organ of nutrient absorption and gastrointestinal secretion that provides an extremely intimate interface between ingested food and the blood. It is hardly surprising therefore that disturbances in the function of the small bowel may be detected by examination of the blood.

The blood count *per se* does not detect nutritional deficiencies or defects in absorption until a relatively late stage. The reason for this is that the healthy adult normally has adequate stores of iron, vitamin B_{12}, folate and other haematinic trace elements, and changes in cellular production take place only when these stores are considerably depleted. Exceptions to this rule occur either at the extremes of life (the neonate and the elderly) (Newland and Evans, 1997), or in debilitated patients who do not enjoy the luxury of such stores. In addition, increased demands in toddlers, adolescents (especially females) and women of child-bearing age may outstrip supplies, particularly of iron, so that subclinical iron deficiency is relatively common (Looker *et al.*, 1997). In one study in Sweden, in an otherwise healthy population, up to 40 per cent of adolescent girls and 15 per cent of boys had subclinical iron deficiency (Hallberg *et al.*, 1993).

HAEMOGLOBIN CONCENTRATION AND BLOOD COUNT

Haemoglobin concentration, reticulocyte count and red cell indices

HAEMOGLOBIN CONCENTRATION

The commonest cause of anaemia world-wide is iron deficiency (Scrimshaw, 1991), and in adult men and postmenopausal women the commonest cause is gastrointestinal blood loss (Fairbanks and Beutler, 1990). This is usually from the stomach, duodenum or the large bowel, and secondary to peptic ulceration or malignancy, respectively. The small bowel may be the site of blood loss in a variety of conditions as listed in Table 13.5.1.

RETICULOCYTE COUNT

This is one of the simplest and most valuable tests, which is all too often overlooked in the assessment of anaemia and of steady-state bone marrow function. Patients with bleeding, haemolysis, hypersplenism or other causes of peripheral red-cell destruction will have a raised reticulocyte count if marrow function is normal. A raised reticulocyte count with a normal haemoglobin indicates chronic low-grade loss or

Table 13.5.1 *Causes of small bowel blood loss*

Anatomical anomalies
Aberrant pancreas
Meckel's diverticulum
Volvulus
Intussusception
Polyps
Vascular anomalies
Angiodysplasia
Telangiectasia
Haemangioma
Vascular occlusions
Tumours
Carcinoma
Leiomyoma
Infections
Helminthiasis
Inflammation
Regional enteritis
Ulcers

After Fairbanks and Beutler (1990).

peripheral destruction that is fully compensated for by increased bone marrow activity. Patients with anaemia release reticulocytes earlier than normal from their bone marrow and a reasonably accurate adjustment can be made for this by dividing the reticulocyte percentage by two (Hillman and Finch, 1967). A normal or low reticulocyte count in the face of anaemia is direct evidence of bone marrow dysfunction.

RED CELL INDICES

Nowadays, the haemoglobin, red cell count and the classical indices of mean corpuscular volume (MCV), mean corpuscular haemoglobin (MCH) and mean corpuscular haemoglobin concentration (MCHC) are measured or derived electronically in automated analysers. This has permitted the calculation of other indices, such as the red-cell distribution width (RDW) and mean platelet volume (MPV), which provide further useful information in certain conditions, and an earlier indication of abnormal erythropoiesis, both congenital or acquired, than the haemoglobin concentration alone. In malabsorption, there may be complex deficiencies of all the haematinic vitamins and iron deficiency may mask the macrocytosis of associated folate or B_{12} deficiency (Lewis, 1976), although the presence of neutrophil hypersegmentation provides a clue (Das *et al.*, 1978).

Red-cell distribution width

This is a measure of the degree of variation in red-cell size or anisocytosis, which tends to increase in acquired haematinic deficiences. In a study of untreated pernicious anaemia, a raised RDW was found in two-thirds of cases examined, of whom approximately one-third had a normal MCV (Saxena *et al.*, 1988). Similarly, in iron deficiency, increasing anisocytosis with a progressive microcytosis is the earliest sign, but initially with a normal haemoglobin and a normal transferrin saturation. There follows a further decline in the MCH and MCV as the haemoglobin falls below 12 g/dL. Finally, when the haemoglobin becomes less than 9 g/dL, the MCHC will fall and the transferrin saturation will be less than 16 per cent (England *et al.*, 1976). The RDW reflects this early change in iron deficiency (Bessman and Feinstein, 1979), and thus helps in the diagnostic distinction between thalassaemia and iron deficiency.

Although the MCV will usually be low–normal in iron deficiency and low in thalassaemia, the RDW will tend to be high in iron deficiency but remain within the normal range in thalassaemia (Bessman *et al.*, 1983). Using discriminant functions, derived primarily from the MCH, MCV and RDW, increases the accuracy of making a correct distinction between iron deficiency and thalassaemia (Bessman *et al.*, 1989). According to an analysis of the usefulness of different indices in discriminant functions used in an epidemiological survey of microcytic anaemia, the combination of sensitivity and specificity was said to be best for the RDW and worst for the MCHC (Mahu *et al.*, 1990).

Mean platelet volume

The MPV varies independently of the platelet count in a variety of diseases. In coeliac disease, non-splenectomized patients have higher MPV values than normal subjects, although this does not depend on splenic function (O'Grady *et al.*, 1985). Patients with active inflammatory bowel disease have a lower MPV than normal subjects (Jaremo and Sandberg-Gertzen, 1996). The significance of these findings is uncertain, although in patients who have survived a myocardial infarction a raised MPV may be an independent risk factor for recurrence (Martin *et al.*, 1991).

White cell count

Inflammatory bowel disease is a potent stimulus as inflammation, bleeding and infection all provoke a leucocytosis, and, in combination, may produce a leukaemoid response in acute toxic episodes (Merrin and Lancaster Smith, 1989). In a recent Italian study of prognostic factors prior to surgery in 110 patients with Crohn's disease, a total preoperative white count greater than 9×10^9/L was associated with a significant ($P < 0.05$) increased risk of postsurgical recurrence (Caprilli *et al.*, 1996).

Platelet count

The platelet count, which varies normally between 150 and 400 $\times$ 10^9/L, also takes part in the acute phase response to bleeding and inflammation. It mirrors the erythrocyte sedimentation rate (ESR) and other markers of inflammatory bowel disease (Talstad *et al.*, 1973) and may be useful as a monitor of response to therapy (Harries *et al.*, 1983). Marked thrombocytosis (> 1000 $\times$ 10^9/L) has been reported in Whipple's disease (Chapter 22) (Nuzum *et al.*, 1981). A moderate rise occurs in chronic gastrointestinal blood loss and should alert the physician to investigate for iron deficiency and associated gastrointestinal lesions (Dinco and Aksoy, 1969). Conversely, thrombocytopenia and leucopenia are seen as a side-effect of immunosuppressive (and myelosuppressive) medication, but there are reports of immune thrombocytopenias occurring as part of an extraintestinal autoimmune dysregulation (Zlatanic *et al.*, 1997).

BLOOD FILM

Red cell morphology

Although patients with anaemia of chronic disease classically are described as having a mild normochromic normocytic anaemia, there are many who exhibit some degree of hypochromia and microcytosis (Cartwright, 1966). However, associated iron deficiency or bleeding should be suspected in those patients whose haemoglobin continues to fall or is below 9 g/dL. Features of patients with chronic bleeding may include polychromasia due to differential basophilic staining of younger red cells, and varying degrees of microcytosis and hypochromasia as iron deficiency results. In severe iron deficiency, the blood film may be extremely bizarre with fragments and poikilocytes, and may resemble a thalassaemia major. Bizarre fragmentation is a feature of microangiopathic films seen in patients with haemolytic–uraemic syndrome (associated especially in children with *E. coli* H:0157 enterotoxin and other toxic enteritides) (Kavi and Wise, 1989). Serological assays for verocytotoxins may identify exposure when stool cultures are negative (Chart and Rowe, 1990).

Hyposplenism associated with coeliac disease, or any other cause of asplenia, results in the appearance of target cells and Howell–Jolly bodies in the blood film. Red cell 'pits' or submembranous vacuoles can be seen in wet preparations of red cells using direct-interference microscopy and are the most sensitive indicator of hyposplenism (Reinhart and Chien, 1988). Basophilic stippling in the presence of a mild normochromic or hypochromic anaemia, and vague abdominal pain of a non-specific nature, should alert the clinician to the possiblity of lead poisoning (Albahary, 1972).

White cell differential

Inflammatory disorders in adults will usually be reflected by a rise in the relative and absolute numbers of neutrophils (an acute lymphocytosis is more often seen in young children). Although patients with a neutropenia may be suffering from severe folate or vitamin B_{12} deficiency, drug toxicity, hypoplasia, bone marrow infiltration, severe sepsis or an autoimmune disorder, it is important to remember that low white counts may be constitutional in patients of Afro-Caribbean and Middle Eastern extraction (Gilles, 1981). Parasitic infestations of the bowel may cause eosinophilia, although this is not associated with all parasites (Chapter 19), but mainly helminths and two enteric protozoans, *Isospora belli* and *Dientamoeba fragilis* (Rothenburg, 1998). Inflammatory bowel disease (Chapter 25) and eosinophilic gastroenteritis may or may not give rise to peripheral eosinophilia, although eosinophilic infiltrates will be found in the tissues.

ACUTE-PHASE RESPONSE

C-reactive protein

The International Committee on Standards in Haematology (ICSH) recommends the C-reactive protein (CRP) assay as being most suitable for the measurement of early changes in the acute-phase response as it is sensitive, has a wide range and responds rapidly within 24 hours to changes in inflammatory stimuli (ICSH, 1988). However, other more relevant and specific acute-phase proteins such as α1-antichymotrypsin may be particularly useful in monitoring inflammatory bowel disease (Thompson *et al.*, 1992).

Erythrocyte sedimentation rate

The ESR is non-specific but is particularly suited as a measure of chronic inflammation, depending as it does on a number of different acute-phase proteins and immunoglobulins. The normal range is < 10 mm in the first hour for men and < 12 mm for women. It increases slightly with age, but a value of > 19 mm for men or > 22 mm for women in patients over 50 is still worth investigating (Griffiths *et al.*, 1984). There are occasional patients, particularly among the elderly, who have a significantly elevated ESR (i.e. over 80 mm) and in whom investigation and follow-up over several years fails to reveal an underlying cause or disease (Zacharski, 1976). Children who are obese (weight/length index > 120) have an ESR that is twice the normal value for reasons that are not known (Kasapcopur *et al.*, 1991).

Plasma viscosity

Plasma viscosity is another non-specific measure of chronic inflammation that has several theoretical and practical advantages compared to the ESR, which are listed below.

1 It is independent of the number of red cells.
2 It is relatively free of sex and age bias.
3 It is a direct measure of acute-phase and other plasma proteins and immunoglobulins.
4 It can therefore detect hypoproteinaemias in patients with a normal ESR (Bradlow and Haggan, 1979).
5 It can be measured on plasma specimens stored for up to 6 days (ESR has to be measured within 2 hours of sample collection).
6 Finally, it gives a result in 15 minutes (ICSH, 1984).

However, in a concensus analysis of 31 different tests carried out in patients with rheumatoid arthritis, the ESR and plasma viscosity were found to be equally dependable, with the acute-phase serum protein orosomucoid judged the next most dependable acute-phase test (Bull *et al.*, 1986).

COAGULATION TESTS

Prothrombin time, vitamin K metabolism and malabsorption

The prothrombin time (PT) and its standardized ratio against a control plasma, the international normalized ratio (INR), is one of the most sensitive tests of liver function, depending as it does on the coagulation factors II, VII, IX and X, whose hepatic synthesis is dependent on vitamin K absorbed in the small intestine. Critically ill hospitalized patients are at risk of vitamin K deficiency and should be given prophylactic vitamin K (Alperin, 1987). Patients with malabsorption but normal liver function will respond to vitamin K given parenterally as the liver still produces the basic but inactive factors known as PIVKA (proteins formed in vitamin K's absence), whereas those patients with severe hepatic impairment will not only have acquired vitamin K deficiency, but will not be synthesizing enough factors for vitamin K to make any substantial difference (Blanchard *et al.*, 1981). A cautionary note for patients with small bowel dysfunction or malabsorption who are on warfarin and require parenteral feeding: solutions containing Intralipid (soybean oil emulsion) may interfere with the anticoagulant efficacy of warfarin (Lutomski *et al.*, 1987).

Activated partial thromboplastin time (APTT)

This clotting assay is sensitive to factors in the so-called intrinsic pathway, particularly factors VIII, IX, XI, XII as well as the common pathway factors, X, V and II. The APTT is particularly sensitive to heparin and is prolonged in haemophilia A or B and other intrinsic pathway factor deficiencies. Deficiencies in von Willebrand factor (vWF), the carrier molecule for factor VIII, may not be so severe in mild (Type 1) von Willebrand's disease (vWD) as to always prolong the APTT. In those patients with continued episodes of blood loss from the gut or elsewhere, it may be worth screening specifically for vWD and other congenital bleeding disorders. If only routine coagulation tests are employed, these diagnoses may be missed, as has been demonstrated recently in relation to menorrhagia (Kadir *et al.*, 1998). The ristocetin co-factor assay is said to be more sensitive than the vWF antigen assay in mild phenotypes with normal clotting screens (Rodeghiero *et al.*, 1990), which may nevertheless be revealed by bleeding from underlying vascular anomalies such as telangiectasia (Ahr *et al.*, 1977). High-dose gammaglobulin has been shown to be effective in resistant multifocal gastrointestinal haemorrhage due to vWD whether associated with inhibitors to vWF (Inbal *et al.*, 1997) or not (White and Chisholm, 1993). Acquired factor VIII (and, rarely, other) inhibitors occur in the elderly, either spontaneously or associated with occult malignancy, or in younger patients with connective tissue or autoimmune disorders. They are distinguished by a prolonged APTT that fails to correct significantly when repeated using a 50:50 mix of test plasma with normal plasma. They can cause severe bleeding and require urgent, expert haematological assessment and management (Morrison and Ludlam, 1995).

Markers of coagulation, fibrinolysis and thrombophilia in inflammatory bowel disease

Inflammatory bowel disease is invariably associated with evidence of a prothrombotic state with a rise in fibrinogen, factors V and VIII, and a fall in antithrombin III, all of which correlate with disease activity (Lake *et al.*, 1978). In 16 patients with Crohn's disease, elevated concentrations of fibrinopeptide A and prothrombin fragments (F1+2) were found in both active and inactive disease and D-dimer levels correlated closely with fibrinopeptide A (Hudson *et al.*, 1992). This suggested that both increased fibrin formation and reactive fibrinolysis continued even in apparent clinical remission. However, others have reported that raised fibrin degradation products did return towards normal with response to treatment in patients with both Crohn's disease and ulcerative colitis, suggesting that they may be another useful measure of disease activity (Kjeldsen *et al.*, 1998). In a larger study of 112 patients with inflammatory bowel disease (1/3 Crohn's and 2/3 ulcerative colitis), similar findings showed no differences between the two patient groups, but increased values of vWF and thrombomodulin, markers of endothelial cell damage and activation, were found during active disease (Souto *et al.*, 1995).

Thrombophilia, such as that associated with protein C resistance due to the Factor V Leiden mutation, has been reported as a cause of four cases of small bowel infarction (Herresbach *et al.*, 1997). Protein C is an important regulatory molecule in the clotting cascade, which inhibits activated factor V (and activated Factor VIII), and patients with factor V Leiden are resistant to this normal control mechanism (Middledorp and van der Meer, 1998). Protein C resistance, which is now known to underlie many cases of previously unexplained thrombosis, should always be considered as a cause of small bowel infarction as should other congenital causes of thrombophilia, such as protein C deficiency (Klar *et al.*, 1990), protein S deficiency (Crombleholme *et al.*, 1994) and antithrombin III deficiency (Guillou *et al.*, 1996).

HAEMATINICS

Tests of iron status

The serum iron, transferrin and transferrin saturation provide basic information about iron absorption and utilization. In patients on iron supplements, the serum iron will be high and can be used as a test of patient compliance, if small bowel function is normal. The serum ferritin is the best single guide to total body iron, but is an acute-phase response protein and therefore has to be interpreted in this light. A cut-off (lower limit of normal) of 50 μg/L has been suggested instead of 15 μg/L in patients with inflammatory bowel disease, in whom the diagnosis of iron deficiency is often associated with evidence of undernourishment (Harries *et al.*, 1984). However, in a recent retrospective survey of over 101 anaemic veterans in the USA who had both ferritin assays and bone marrow aspirates performed for any reason, an even higher cut-off point of 100 μg/L separated those with iron deficiency from those with other disorders (Kis and Carnes, 1998). Thus, iron deficiency should be suspected in any patient who has inflammatory bowel disease or other severe acute inflammation with a ferritin less than 100 μg/L. The variations in tests of iron status in various conditions are summarized in Table 13.5.2.

Folate and B_{12} absorption and deficiency

Serum folate varies in the short term with dietary intake, whereas red cell folate reflects a more long-term intake. However, in a large study involving 30 centres and over 1200 specimens, serum folate reflected accurately the true folate status of the patient (Phekoo *et al.*, 1997). The body does not have huge stores of folate, so this is the vitamin that is most likely to be deficient in patients who have had upper small bowel surgery or who have malnutrition, malabsorption, or a high consumption as in proliferative disorders of the skin, gut or bone marrow. However, in one study of surgical patients, folate absorption was adequate in all patients, whilst B_{12} absorption was low in those patients with Crohn's disease who had had an ileal resection of > 17 cm (Kennedy *et al.*, 1982). In patients with a well-functioning continent ileostomy, adequate B_{12} absorption occurs from the ileal reservoir (Jagenburg *et al.*, 1975). If malabsorption of B_{12} exists in a patient with ileostomy, stagnant loop syndrome should be considered (Schjonsby *et al.* 1977). In fact, bacterial contamination of the small intestine is an important cause of B_{12} malabsorption in the elderly and should be considered in those who present in an acute geriatric setting

Table 13.5.2 *Assessment of iron status in different disease states*

	Normal range	Iron deficiency	Chronic disease	Iron overload
Ferritin (μg/L)	10–150	< 10	> 150	> 250
Iron (μmol/L)	8–28	< 8	< 8	> 30
TIBC (μmol/L)	45–72	45–96	< 40	< 45
Transferrin (g/L)	2–3.9	> 4	< 2	< 2
Transferrin saturation (per cent)	15–48	< 15	< 25	> 60

TIBC, total iron binding capacity – used as an estimate of transferrin concentration; however, transferrin is now more commonly measured directly using an immunologic assay.

Note that anaemia of chronic disease is distinguished by a low serum iron with a raised or high–normal ferritin in association with a low transferrin and transferrin saturation.

Iron deficiency is associated with a low serum iron, a low ferritin with a raised transferrin but a low transferrin saturation, while iron overload has a raised ferritin, a high–normal iron, a low transferrin and an increased transferrin saturation.

even with non-gastrointestinal symptoms (McEvoy *et al.*, 1983).

Pernicious anaemia, the Schilling test, protein-bound B_{12} and malabsorption

Pernicious anaemia may be diagnosed with confidence in patients who have both a low serum B_{12} and antibodies to intrinsic factor (Lindenbaum, 1983). In other patients, the Schilling test is performed to establish whether there is true pernicious anaemia owing to lack of intrinsic factor production or whether there is malabsorption. It estimates B_{12} absorption by measuring the amount excreted in the urine after a test dose of radiolabelled oral B_{12} administered either bound to intrinsic factor or by itself. It is essential that the patient should have received adequate B_{12} parenterally for at least 2 weeks prior to performing the Schilling test. This is to ensure that any effects of B_{12} deficiency itself on the intestinal mucosa are reversed, otherwise a false impression of malabsorption may be gained. Interestingly, unlike B_{12} deficiency, severe folate deficiency does not have this adverse effect on vitamin B_{12} absorption as measured by the Schilling test (Cattan *et al.*, 1982). The other main cause of error is incomplete 24-hour urine collections. The Dicopak Schilling test utilizes the two isotopes ^{57}Co and ^{58}Co to estimate the absorption of both intrinsic factor-bound and unbound cyanocobalamin (B_{12}) simultaneously. This has the advantage of being quicker and making the results less dependent on a complete urine collection as the ratio of the two isotopes absorbed and excreted can be measured. However, there are some problems with this dual-tracer combined test which mean that, in doubtful cases, the classical two-stage test may be more accurate (Zuckier and Chervu, 1984). A flow chart outlining the procedure for conducting a standard two-stage Schilling test is given in Fig. 13.5.1.

In early pernicious anaemia, protein-bound B_{12} may be poorly absorbed while the Schilling test remains normal (Streeter *et al.*, 1976). In nearly 200 patient records analysed, 48 (25 per cent) with a low serum B_{12} had a normal Schilling test yet 25 of these patients had megaloblastic haemopoiesis. In ten patients from this group who were tested, protein-bound vitamin B_{12} absorption was abnormal in every case (Jones *et al.*, 1987). Although protein-bound vitamin B_{12} absorption is more common with increasing age after 55 years, and is associated with a high serum gastrin and hypochlorhydria, many patients maintain a normal serum cobalamin (Scarlett *et al.*, 1992). This lack of protein-bound B_{12} absorption may explain why many elderly patients, some with neuropsychiatric symptoms, have raised levels of intermediate metabolites that are dependent on B_{12}, folate and B_6, such as homocysteine and methylmalonic acid, which fall to normal after vitamin supplementation (Naurath *et al.*, 1995). The absorption block to B_{12} in pernicious anaemia can be overcome by taking relatively large doses of B_{12} by mouth and this is the preferred method of B_{12} supplementation in pernicious anaemia in Scandinavia (Lederle, 1991) (*see* Chapter 9).

Stage 1: Performed after finding a low serum vitamin B_{12} and giving vitamin B_{12} replacement for 2 weeks

The day prior to the test – fast from midnight moderate intake of fluids only permitted

↓

Attend clinic the next morning between 9 am and 10 am

↓

Empty bladder and note time

↓

Give 1 µg of oral cyanocobalamin (B_{12}) radiolabelled with ^{57}Co (at least 0.1 µCi activity)

↓

Give intramuscular 'flushing dose' of 1000 µg B_{12} to bind free transcobalamin receptors

↓

Patient may eat and drink normally half an hour after the injection

↓

Collect all urine passed over next 24 hours

↓

Assay for the per cent of radioactivity of initial dose excreted

A normal person will excrete 11–32 per cent of the total administered radioactive dose

Stage 2: Performed in a patient with a low excretion in Stage 1, after at least 5 days rest

Repeat the above procedure with the addition of 1000 units oral human intrinsic factor or equivalent hog intrinsic factor given with the test dose of radiolabelled ^{57}Co

In pernicious anaemia, excretion will return to within the normal range

Interpretation of results: percentage radioactivity excreted in 24 hours

	B_{12}	B_{12} + IF
Normal[a]	11–32	11–32
Pernicious anaemia[a]	0–6.8	3.1–30
Malabsorption	<11	<11
Blind-loop syndrome	Both values will be low (<11) but both will improve following antibiotics	
Suspect technical error such as incomplete urine collection	Normal	Low

[a]Data after Chanarin, I. 1979: The megaloblastic anaemias, 2nd edn. Oxford: Blackwell; as quoted in Chanarin (1989).

Figure 13.5.1 *Flow chart for the classical two-stage Schilling test.*

SPECIAL TESTS FOR GASTROINTESTINAL HAEMORRHAGE AND INFLAMMATORY BOWEL DISORDERS

Faecal occult blood tests and chromium-51 red cell labelling

Faecal occult blood tests are sensitive tests for detecting haemoglobin in faeces. They have been widely assessed mainly in the screening of patients for the early detection of colorectal cancer. However, over 80 per cent of positive tests on screening are false positives, although some of these false-positive results are subsequently found to be associated with other abnormalities such as adenomatous polyps (Towler *et al.*, 1998). Routine screening of the small bowel in general hospital patients with unexplained iron-deficiency anaemia is of questionable value in view of the low pick-up rate of positive findings (Bampton and Holloway, 1996). If small bowel disease is suspected and faecal occult blood tests are positive, but other upper gastrointestinal and large bowel investigations are negative, other methods of pinpointing the source of bleeding may be helpful, such as radioisotope red cell labelling (Oliver *et al.*, 1987). Labelling red cells with chromium-51 and assaying subsequent radioactivity in the stools quantifies gastrointestinal blood loss accurately. It is a more sensitive test for detecting occult gastrointestinal blood loss in unexplained iron deficiency when other methods fail (St John and Young, 1978). It is superior to other semiquantitative assays, such as the faecal haemporphyrin (HaemoQuant) assay in which some haem is reabsorbed (Young *et al.*, 1993).

Radionuclide labelling of red cells to detect angiodysplasia

Radioisotope labelling of autologous red cells with tracers such as technetium-99m, a gamma emitter with a short half-life but with sufficient energy to permit occult sites of active bleeding to be identified by scintigraphy. This method has identified bleeding from Meckel's diverticulum (Heyman *et al.*, 1979), from small bowel tumours (Oliver *et al.*, 1987), from small bowel anastomotic ulcers (Bosmans *et al.*, 1993), and small bowel haemorrhage even in the presence of barium (which would obscure conventional angiography) (Rehm *et al.*, 1996).

Radionuclide labelling of leucocytes for assessment of inflammatory bowel disease

Early imaging for inflammation and sepsis utilized gallium-67, but was cumbersome and required multiple imaging over several days. Indium-111-labelled neutrophils were subsequently introduced in 1976, providing same day results that correlated well with both clinical response to therapy (Saverymuttu *et al.*, 1983) and endoscopic findings (Froehlich and Field, 1988). More recently, white cell labelling with technetium-99m-hexamethyl propylene amine oxime (HMPAO), a lipophilic colloid, has become the method of choice, as it is a more convenient and accessible isotope and is more sensitive to the presence of active disease, especially of the small bowel (Arndt *et al.*, 1993). A negative scan excludes active disease (Allan *et al.*, 1993). Furthermore, using single photon emission computerized tomography (SPECT), the entire bowel may be visualized separate from the overlying structures, allowing measurement of segmental and whole-bowel white cell infiltration (Weldon *et al.*, 1996).

SPECIAL TESTS FOR RARE BLOOD DISORDERS THAT MAY PRESENT WITH GASTROINTESTINAL SYMPTOMS

Paroxysmal nocturnal haemoglobinuria

Paroxysmal nocturnal haemoglobinuria (PNH) is an acquired, somatic, bone marrow stem-cell mutation involving the phosphatidylinositol-glycan type A (PIG-A) gene, which is involved in the early processing of the glycosophosphatidylinositol (GPI) anchor for cell membranes (Miyata *et al.*, 1993). This anchor is important for the surface attachment of many different proteins including those associated with the neutralization of complement. Consequently, these patients have red cells that are prone to undergo complement-mediated intravascular haemolysis at the slightest provocation: minor infections, some drugs, surgery, blood transfusions or indeed anything that promotes complement activation. Patients are more prone to thrombosis. They often present with vague abdominal pain, episodes of apparent obstructive jaundice or hepatitis (due to haemolysis and occasionally veno-occlusive disease) and in some cases may undergo extensive gastrointestinal investigation for many months (and, on occasion, years) because this diagnosis has not been considered (Ware *et al.*, 1991). Intravascular haemolysis, from whatever cause, may be detected by the presence of urinary haemosiderin (Bunn and Jandl, 1969). The sucrose lysis test is a sensitive, but not entirely specific, screening test for PNH that makes use of the fact that low ionic strength iso-osmotic sugar solutions enhance the effect of complement on red cells (Hartmann and Jenkins, 1965).

The Ham–Dacie or acidified serum lysis test is the definitive test and depends on the fact that complement activity is enhanced at low pH. It is specific for PNH if it can be demonstrated that the patient's own serum is

(a)

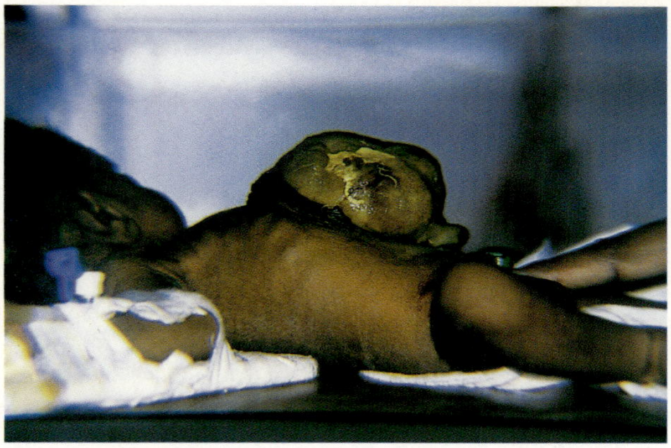

(b)

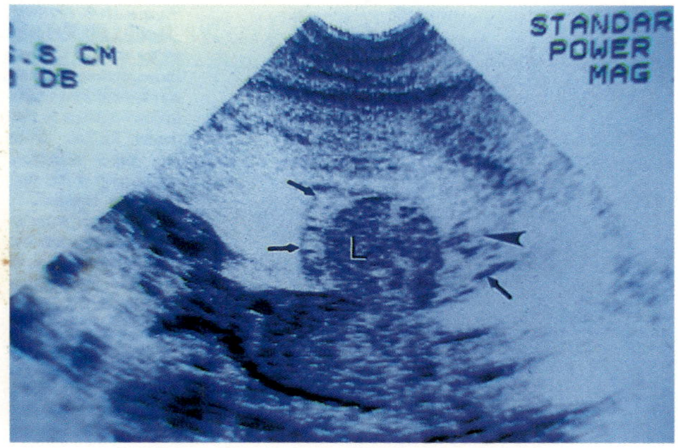

Plate 1.1 **(a)** *A photograph showing an example of exompholos major.* **(b)** *Ultrasound image. (Courtesy of Professor K. E. Mammen and Dr A. Pavai.)*

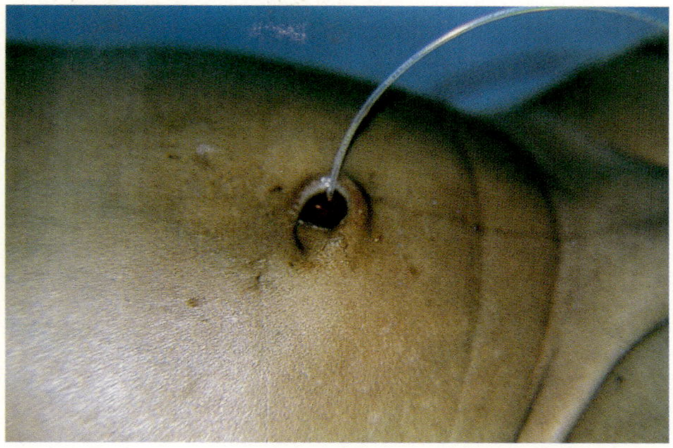

Plate 1.2 *Photograph of persistant vitellointestinal duct (with the catheter in) opening at the umbilicus. (Courtesy of Professor K. E. Mammen and Dr A. Pavai.)*

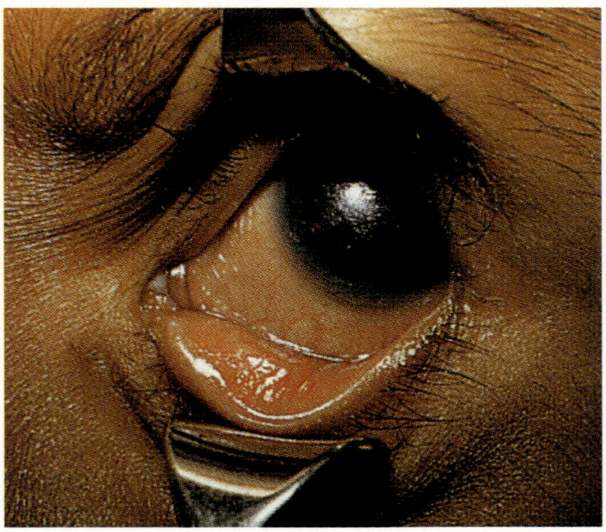

Plate 9.1 *Xerophthalmia. Excessive dryness of the conjunctiva and cornea gives the eye a dull, hazy appearance. (Photograph reproduced with permission of Professor W. Peters, reprinted from Peters, W., Gilles, H.M. 1995:* Colour atlas of tropical medicine and parasitology, *4th edn, with permission of the publisher, Mosby-Wolfe, London.)*

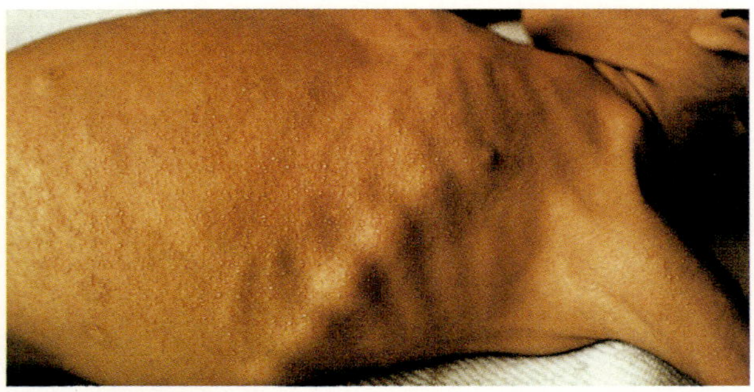

Plate 9.2 *Infantile rickets – 'rickety rosary'. The rounded swellings over the costochondrial junctions near the sternum give rise to the term 'rickety rosary'. (Photograph reproduced with permission of Professor W. Peters, reprinted from Peters, W., Gilles, H.M. 1995:* Colour atlas of tropical medicine and parasitology, *4th edn, with permission of the publisher, Mosby-Wolfe, London.)*

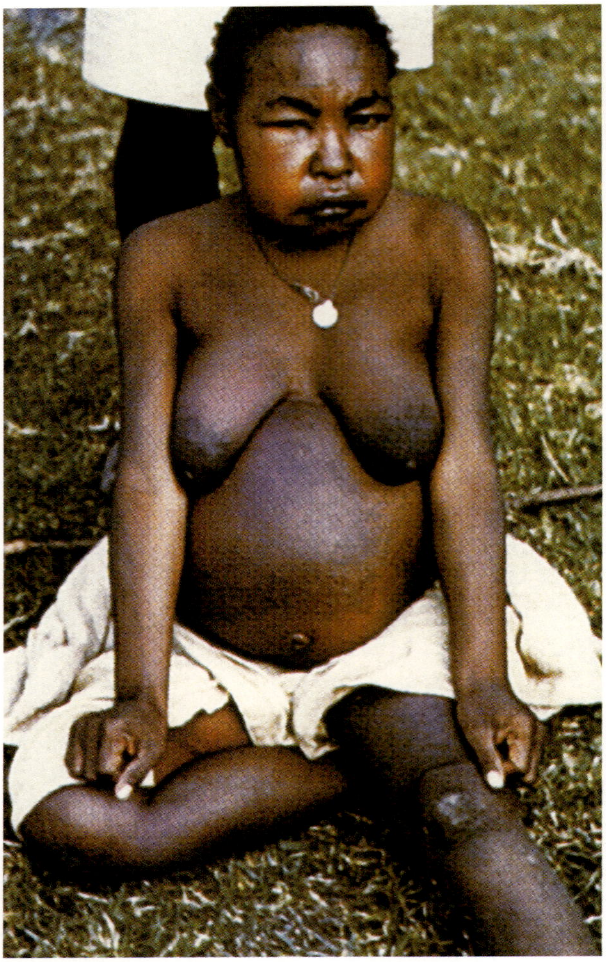

Plate 9.3 *Beriberi oedema. Generalized oedema in a patient with beriberi. (Photograph reproduced with permission of Professor A.J. Radford, reprinted from Peters, W., Gilles, H.M. 1995:* Colour atlas of tropical medicine and parasitology, *4th edn, with permission of the publisher, Mosby-Wolfe, London.)*

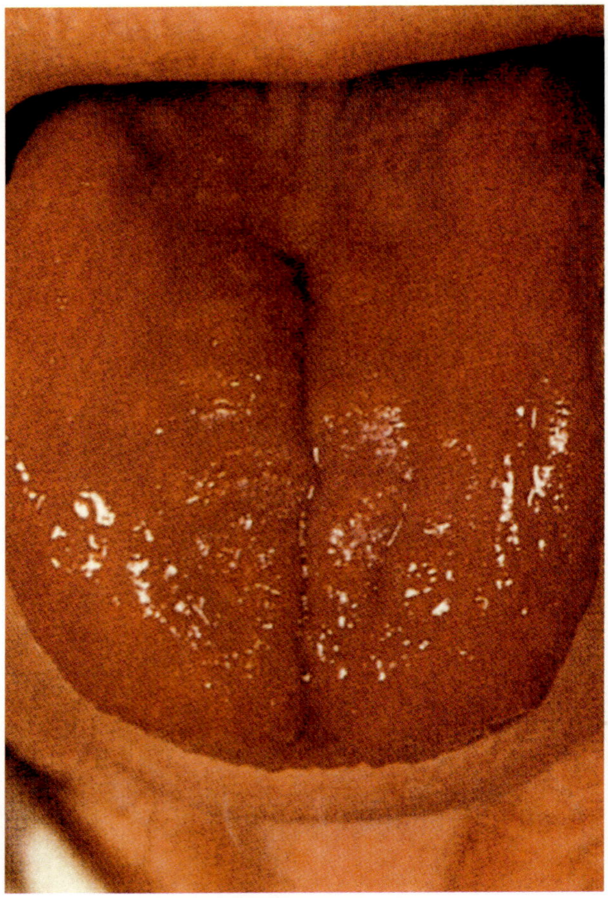

Plate 9.5 *Glossitis. Owing to inflammation, the tongue is sore, smooth and an abnormally deep red colour. (Photograph reproduced with permission of Professor C.D. Forbes and Dr W.F. Jackson, reprinted from Peters, W., Gilles, H.M. 1995:* Colour atlas of tropical medicine and parasitology, *4th edn, with permission of the publisher, Mosby-Wolfe, London.)*

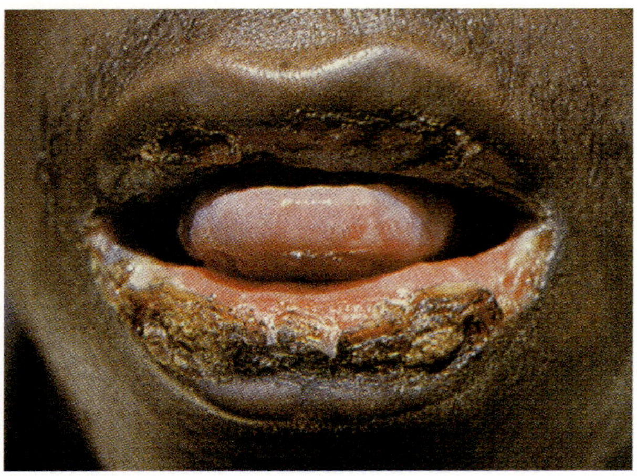

Plate 9.4 *Cheilosis, characterized by dry scaling and fissuring of lips. (Photograph reproduced with permission of Professor O.P. Arya, reprinted from Peters, W., Gilles, H.M. 1995:* Colour atlas of tropical medicine and parasitology, *4th edn, with permission of the publisher, Mosby-Wolfe, London.)*

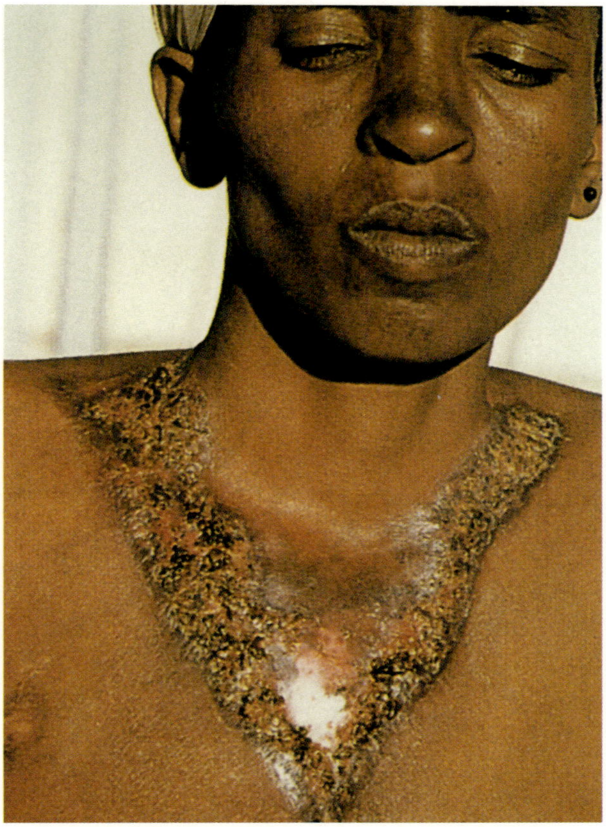

Plate 9.6 *'Casal's necklace' in a patient with severe pellagra. (Photograph reproduced with permission of Professor Dr K.F. Schaller, reprinted from Peters, W., Gilles, H.M. 1995:* Colour atlas of tropical medicine and parasitology, *4th edn, with permission of the publisher, Mosby-Wolfe, London.)*

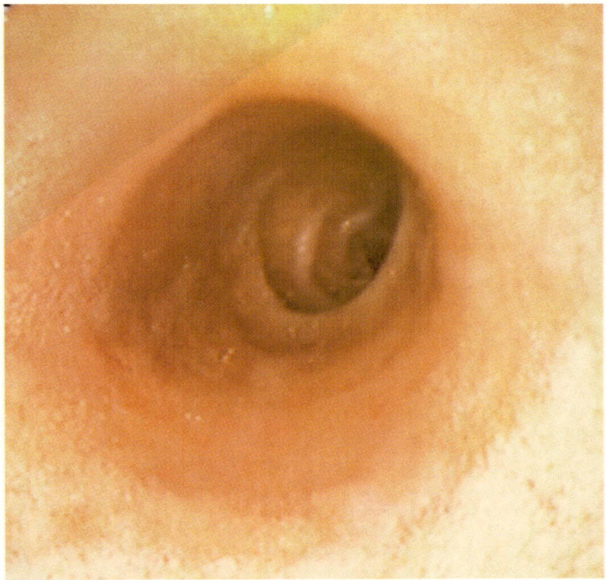

Plate 13.1.1 *A normal duodenal bulb showing a pale mucosa with tiny dots of reflected light.*

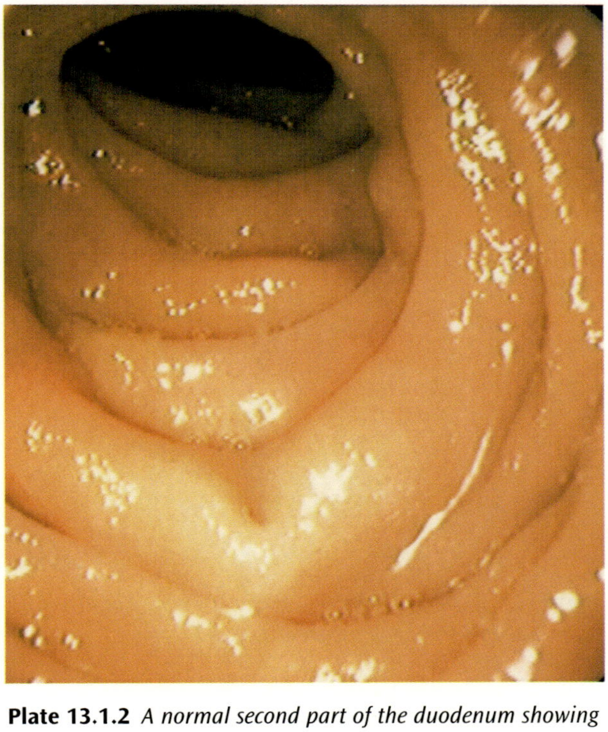

Plate 13.1.2 *A normal second part of the duodenum showing a yellow-orange mucosa and several circular folds (valvulae conniventes).*

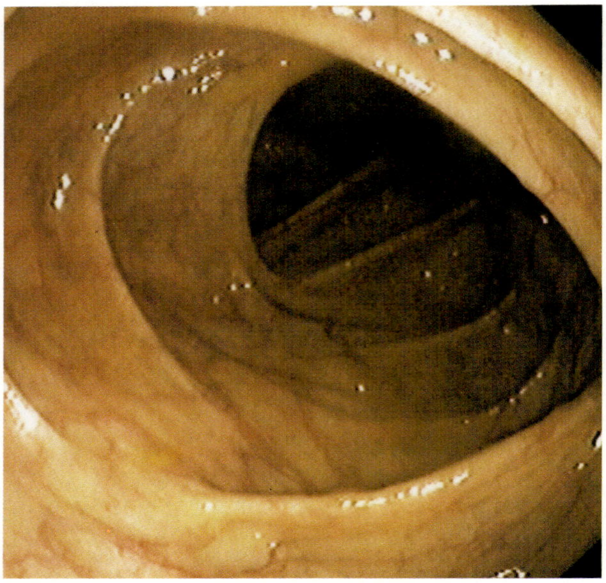

Plate 13.1.3 *A normal terminal ileum showing fewer circular folds than in the duodenum.*

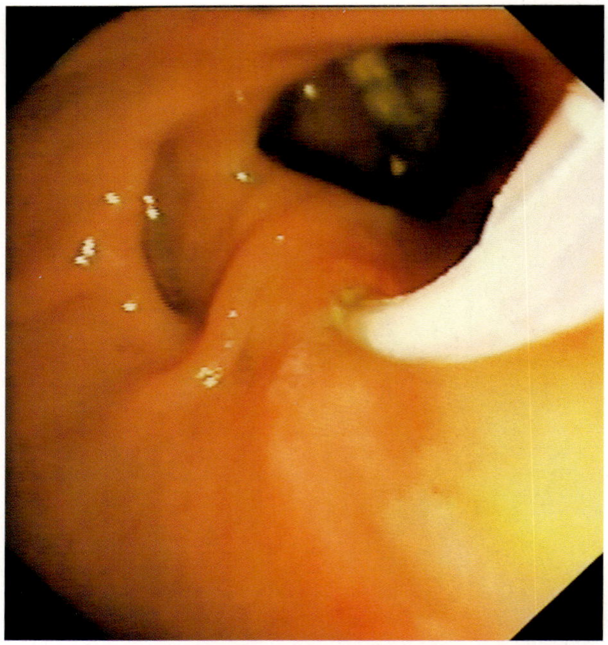

Plate 13.1.4 *Endoscopic view of a small (left) and larger diverticulum (right) where the bile duct enters the duodenum within a ridge of tissue that separates the diverticula.*

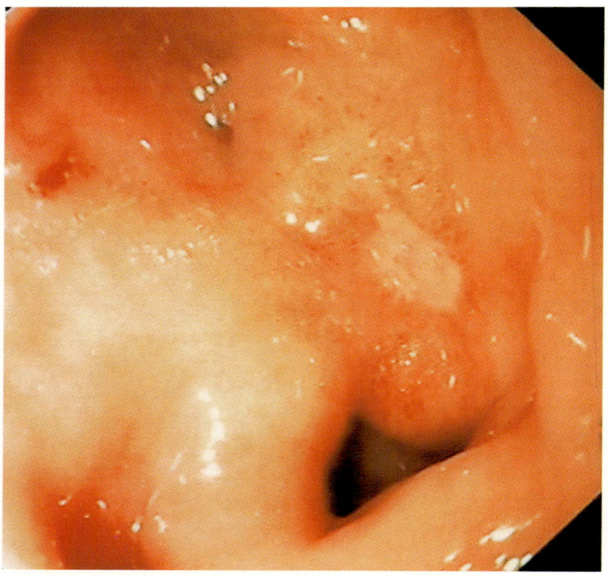

Plate 13.1.5 *A typical chronic duodenal ulcer associated with duodenal deformity and pseudodiverticula.*

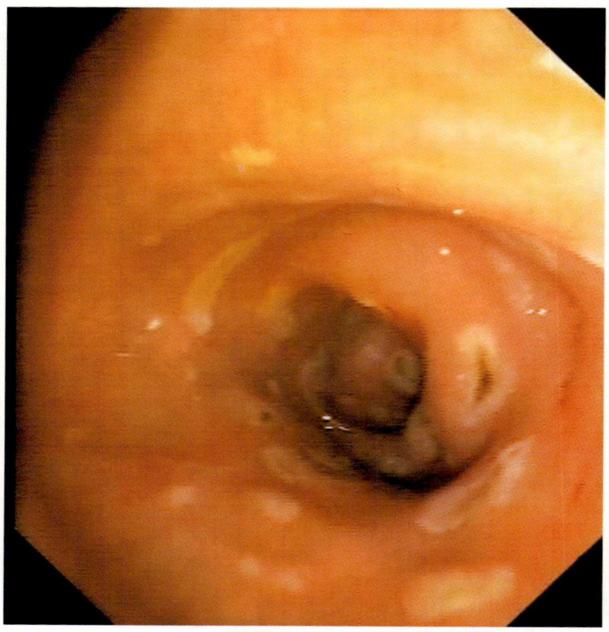

Plate 13.1.6 *Mulitple erosions in the duodenal cap without duodenal deformity.*

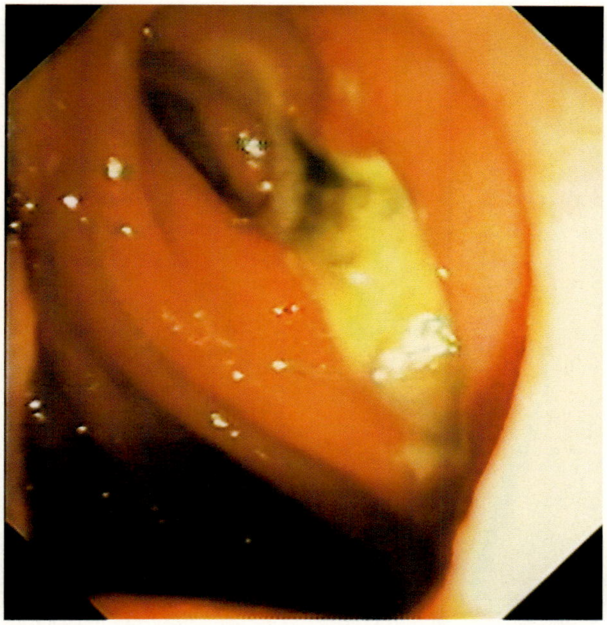

Plate 13.1.7 *Chronic ulcer in the afferent loop close to the stoma after a Billroth II gastrectomy.*

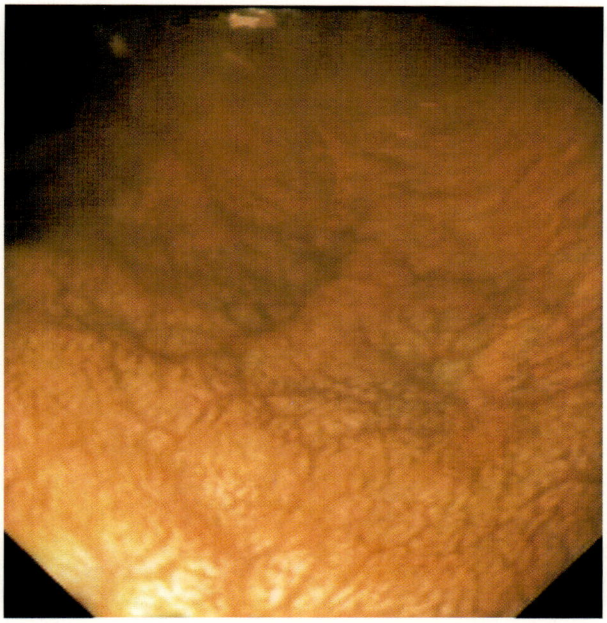

Plate 13.1.8 *Endoscopic appearance of coeliac disease highlighting a mosaic pattern and loss of valvulae conniventes.*

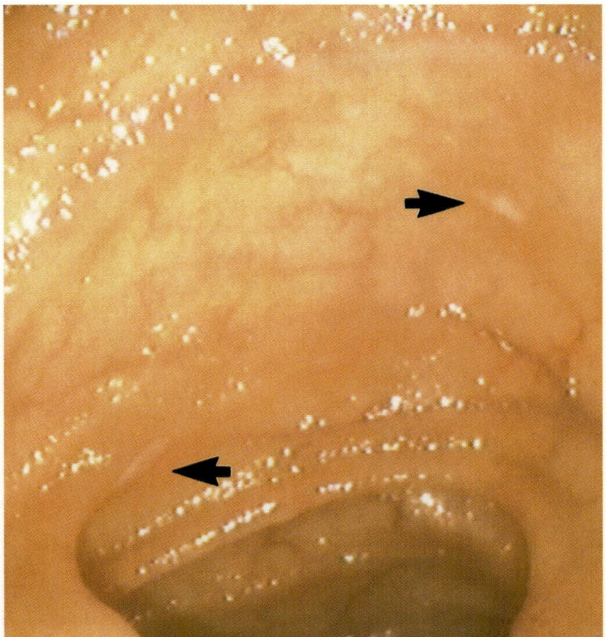

Plate 13.1.9 *Two small aphthous ulcers (arrows) in the terminal ileum of a patient previously treated with a small bowel resection of Crohn's disease.*

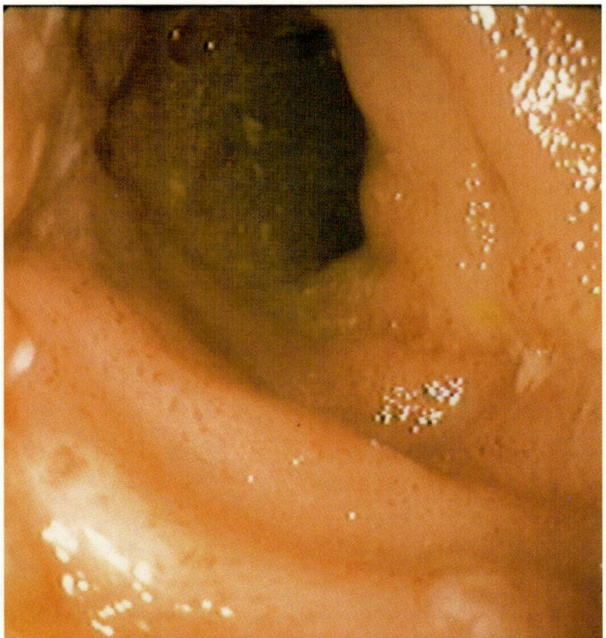

Plate 13.1.10 *Mild Crohn's disease of the terminal ileum showing inflammation, oedema and small areas of ulceration.*

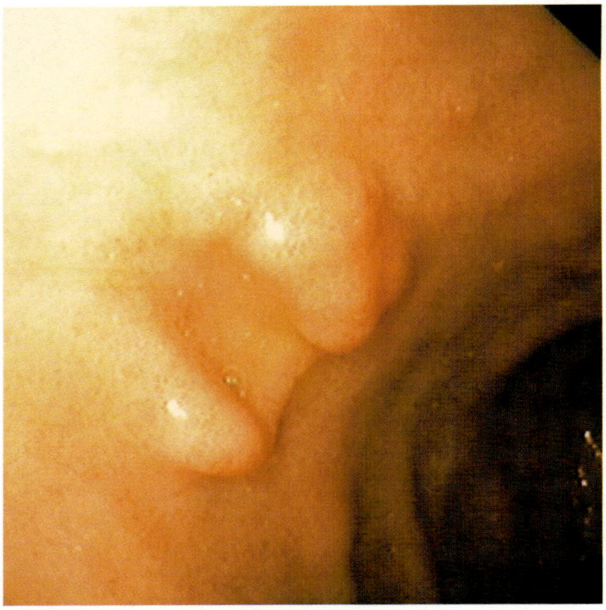

Plate 13.1.11 *Nodules in the duodenal bulb due to ectopic gastric mucosa.*

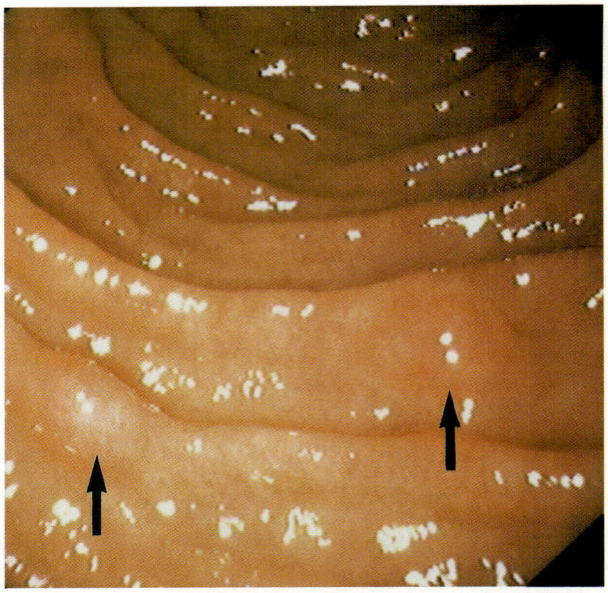

Plate 13.1.12 *Nodules (arrows) covered by normal mucosa in the second part of the duodenum which reflect hyperplasia of Brunner's glands.*

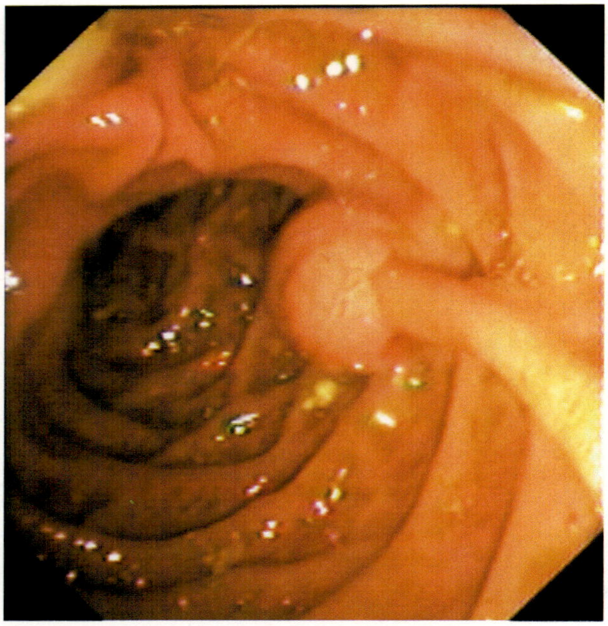

Plate 13.1.13 *An adenoma in the second part of the duodenum with a clearly-defined 'tuft' and a long stalk.*

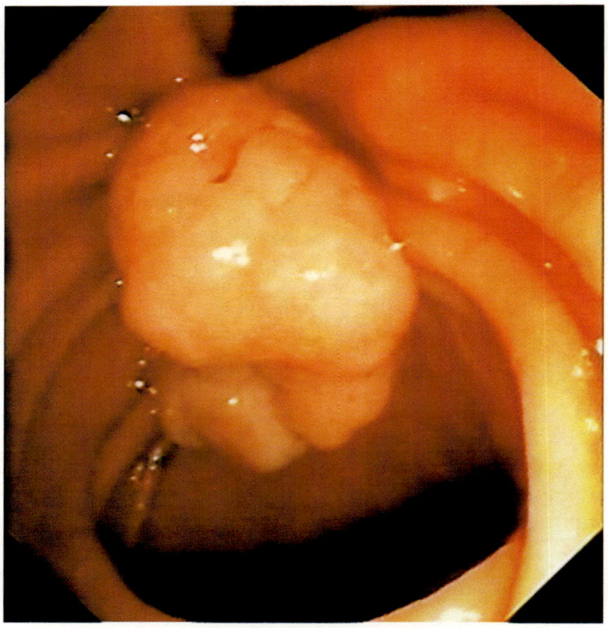

Plate 13.1.14 *Villous adenoma of moderate size in the second part of the duodenum.*

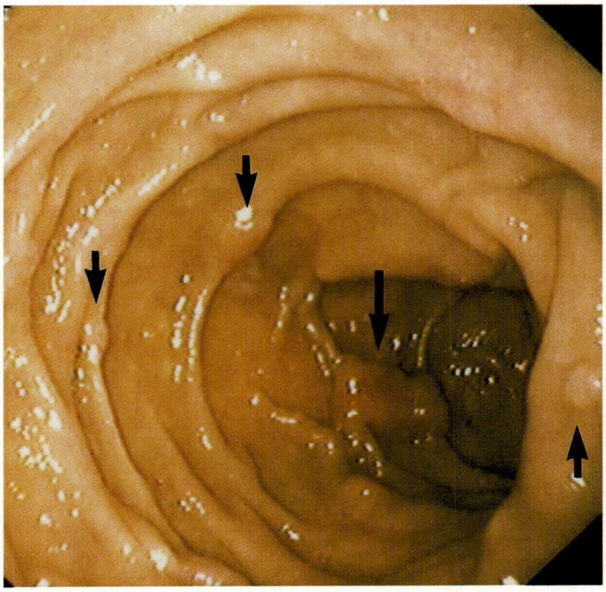

Plate 13.1.15 *Mulitple small adenomas (small arrows) and a larger adenoma (larger arrow) in the second part of the duodenum in a patient with familial adenomatous polyposis.*

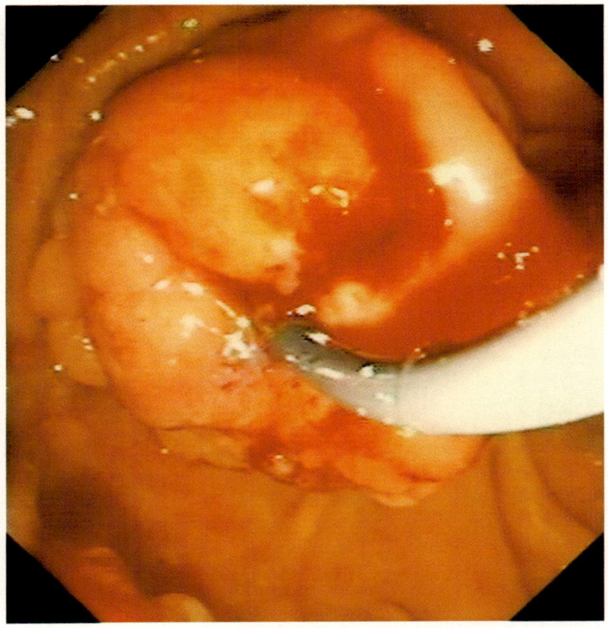

Plate 13.1.16 *A polypoid cancer of the papilla of Vater where the site of the orifice of the ampulla has been outlined with a catheter at the time of endoscopic retrograde cholangiopancreatography.*

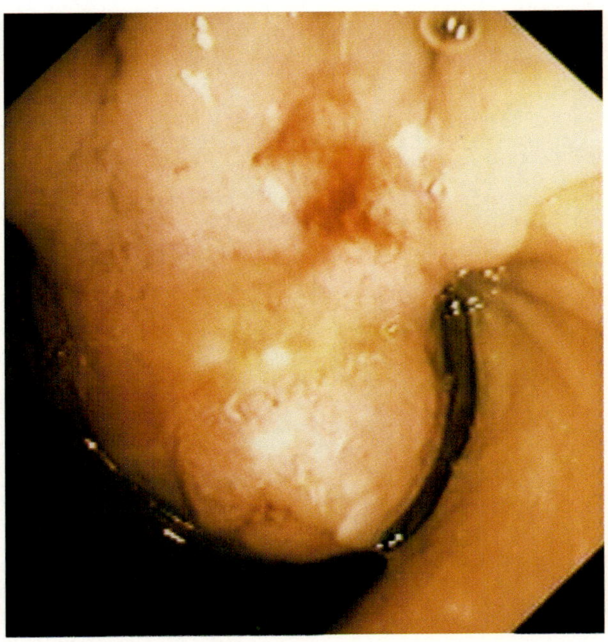

Plate 13.1.17 *A carcinoid tumour of the second part of the duodenum which is slightly irregular and covered by patchy red mucosa.*

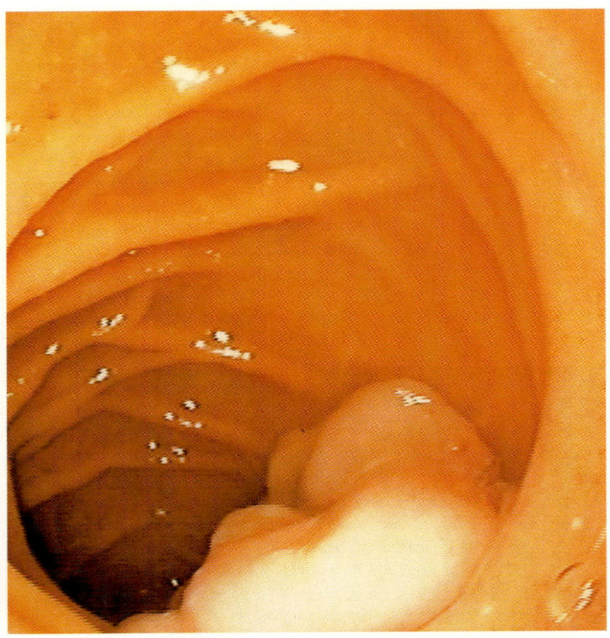

Plate 13.1.18 *Lymphomatous nodule in the second part of the duodenum in a patient with widespread B-cell lymphoma.*

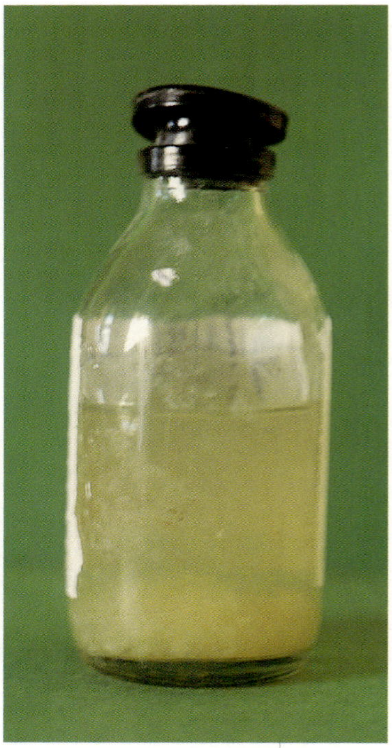

Plate 18.1 *'Rice water' stools in cholera. (Courtesy Professor B.V. Moses, Christian Medical College and Hospital, Vellore, India.)*

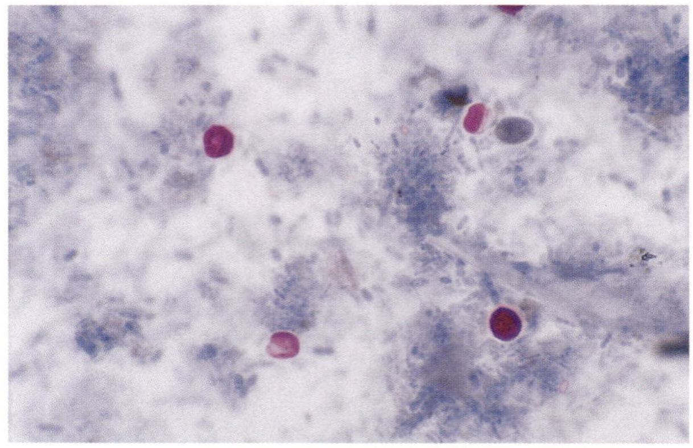

Plate 19.1 *Photomicrograph of faeces showing four red-staining oocysts of* Cryptosporidium *stained with a combination of modified Ziehl-Nielsen and iron-haematoxylin stains.*

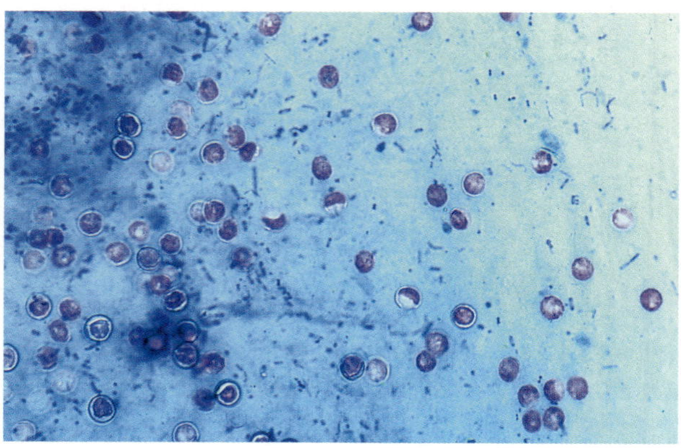

Plate 20.1 *Cryptosporidiosis. Modified acid fast stain of the stool with numerous cryptosporidial oocysts, measuring 4–6 μm in diameter. (Courtesy of Mr R. Lumb.)*

(a)

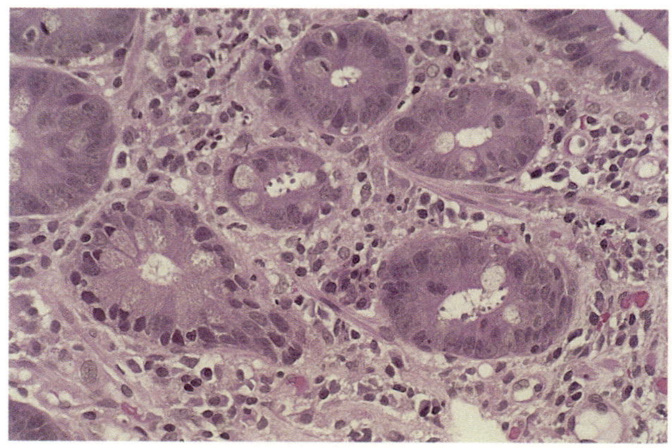

(b)

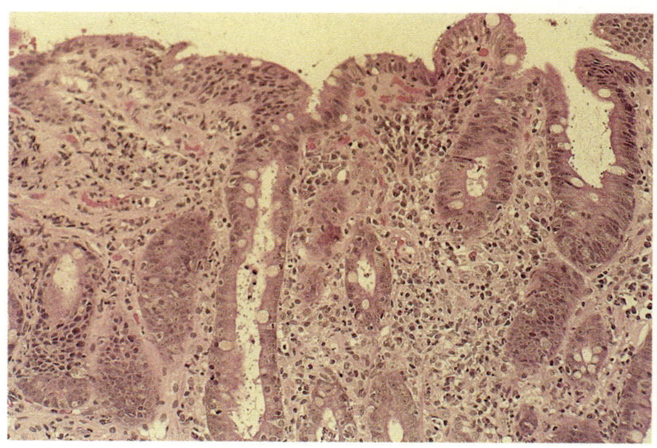

Plates 20.2 (a) and (b) *Cryptosporidial enteritis. Cryptosporidial organisms are evident on the luminal surface and in the crypts. The lamina propria contains an excess of inflammatory cells, especially plasma cells. There is focal attenuation of enterocytes. (Courtesy of Dr A. Ruszkiewicz.)*

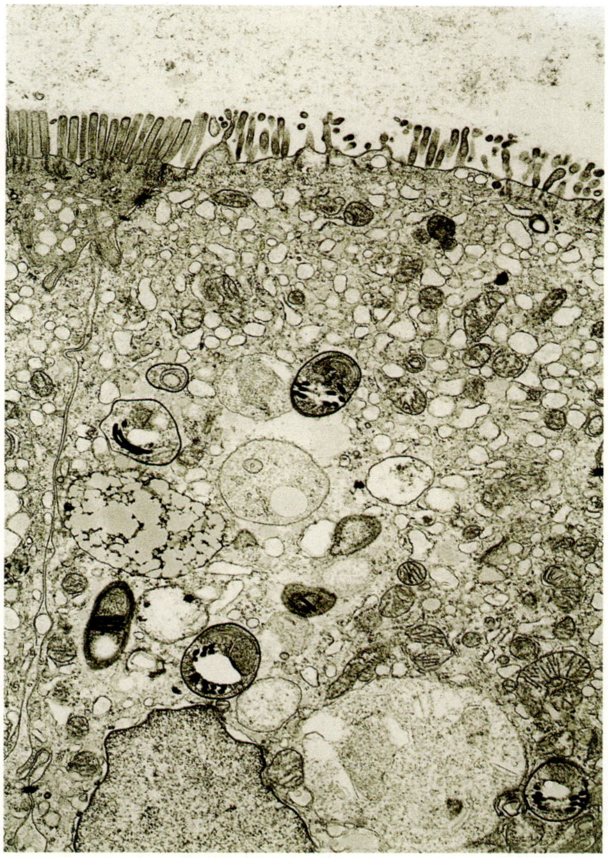

Plate 20.3 *Microsporidial enteritis. Electron micrograph of the developmental stages of* Enterocytozoon bieneusi *within the enterocyte. (Courtesy of Mr R. Lumb.)*

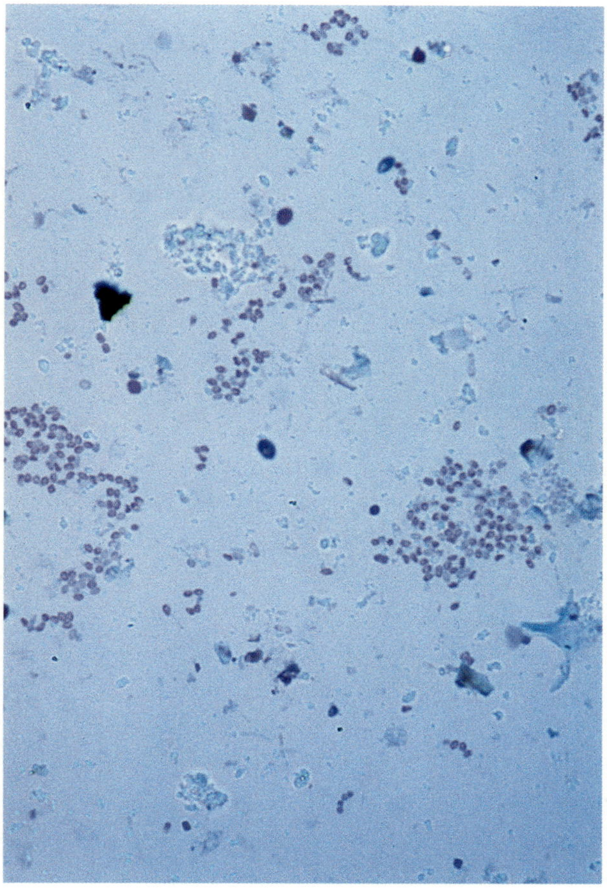

Plate 20.5 *Microsporidial spores in the stool stained by modified trichrome method. (Courtesy of Mr R. Lumb.)*

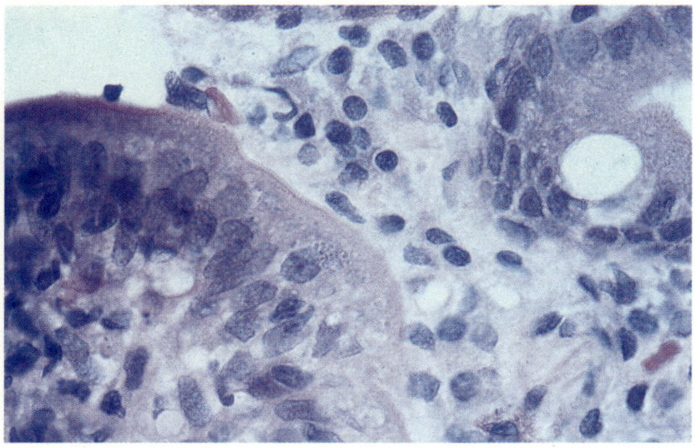

Plate 20.4 *Microsporidiosis. H&E section of duodenal mucosa showing the organisms as pale vacuoles in the apical part of the enterocyte.*

(a)

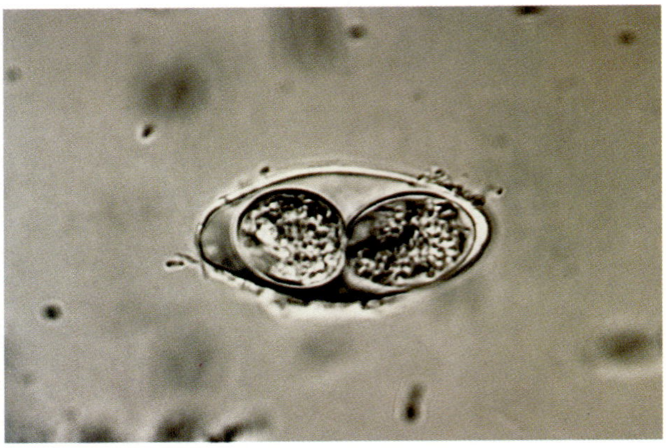

(b)

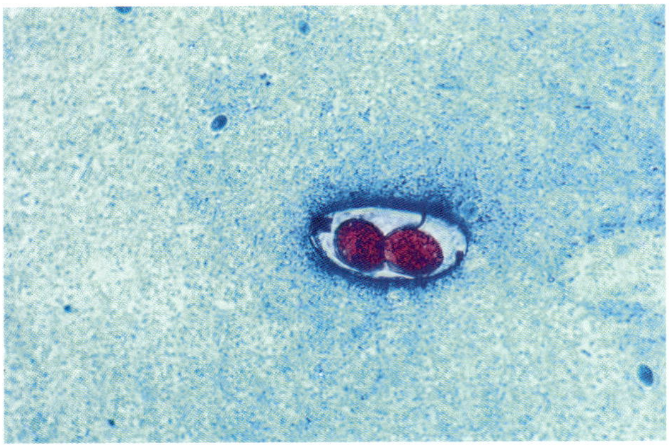

Plate 20.6 (a) and (b) Isospora belli. *Oocysts may be visible in faecal wet mounts as refractile oval structures. They are easily detected after modified Ziehl-Nielsen staining as ovoid structures, 30 μm in length, containing two sporocysts. (Courtesy of Mr R. Lumb.)*

(a)

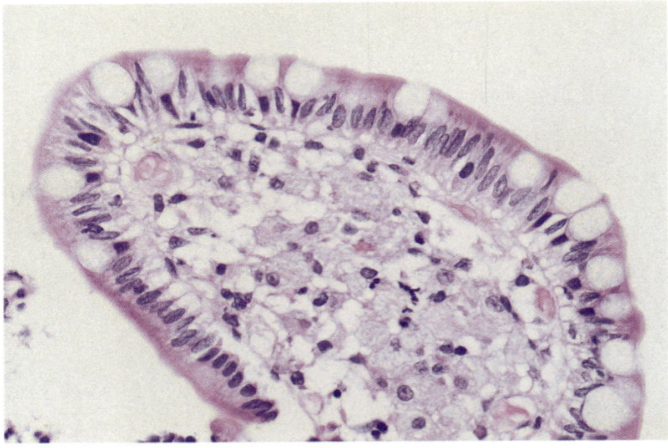

(b)

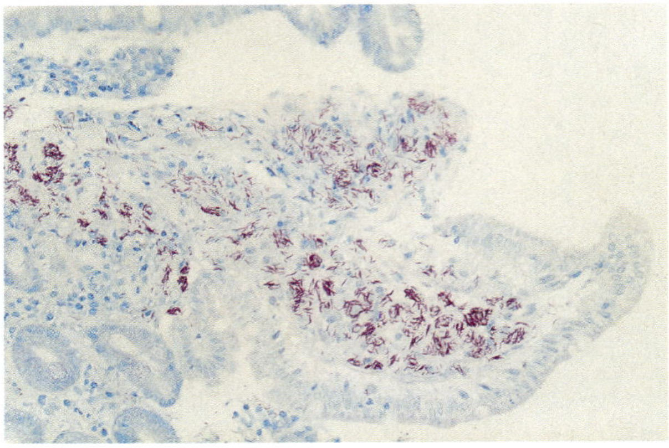

Plate 20.7 (a) and (b) Mycobacterium avium-intercellulare *complex enteritis. Intestinal villus filled with foamy macrophages which reveal acid-fast bacilli after Ziehl-Nielsen staining. (Courtesy of Dr A. Ruszkiewicz.)*

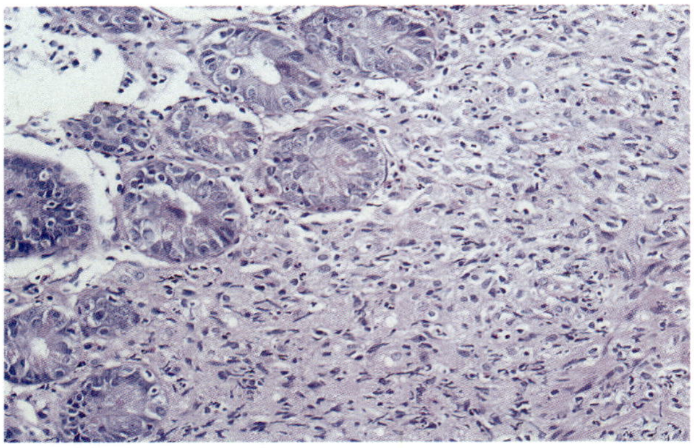

Plate 20.8 *Cytomegalovirus (CMV) enteritis. The lamina propria is hypercellular with many foamy macrophages. In addition, epithelial cells contain CMV inclusions. The villous architecture is lost. (Courtesy of Dr A. Ruszkiewicz.)*

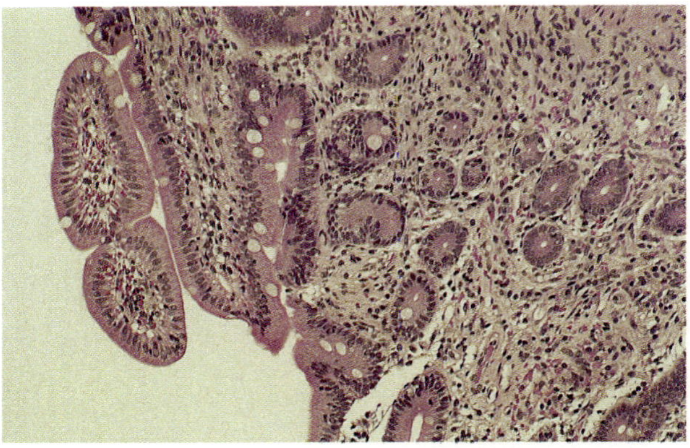

Plate 20.9 *Kaposi's sarcoma. The lamina propria is hypercellular with a spindle cell population, slit-like vascular space formation and extravasation of erythrocytes. (Courtesy of Dr A. Ruszkiewicz.)*

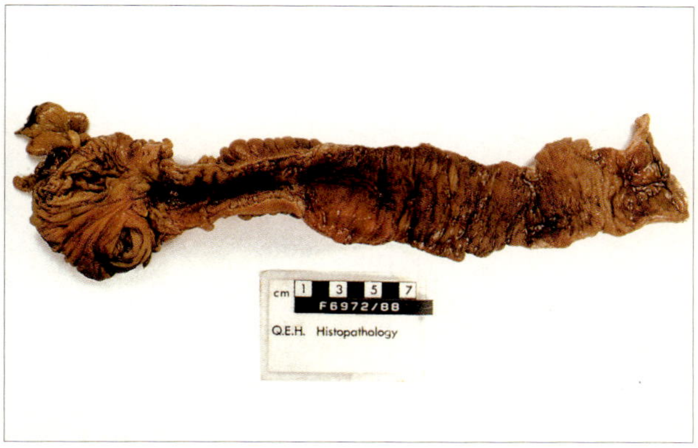

Plate 25.1 *An operative specimen of Crohn's ileitis showing the caecum on the left, a narrow segment of terminal ileum with a thick wall and an inflamed segment of terminal ileum with a 'cobblestone' appearance.*

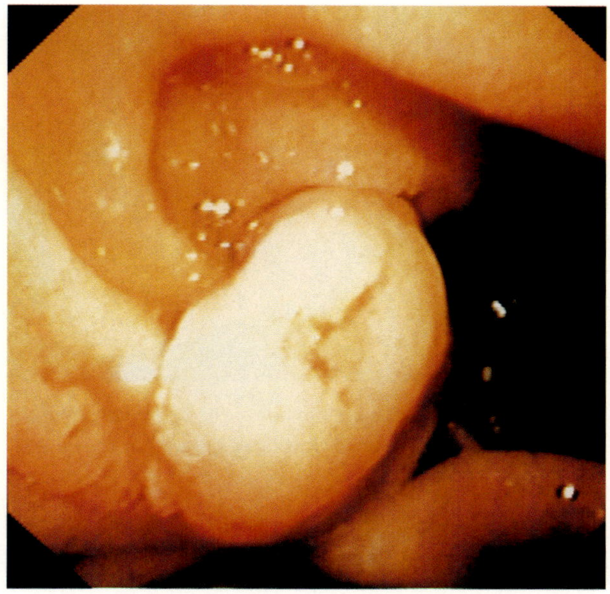

Plate 26.1 *Adenoma of the duodenum: endoscopic appearance. (Courtesy of Dr Reymond de Peyer, Geneva.)*

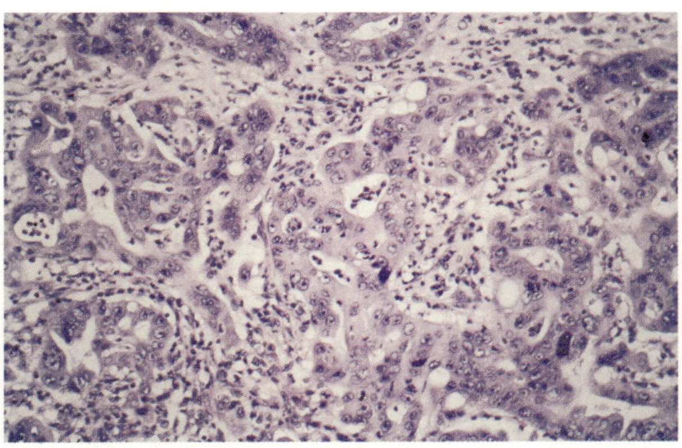

Plate 26.2 *Moderately differentiated adenocarcinoma of the duodenum (H&E)*

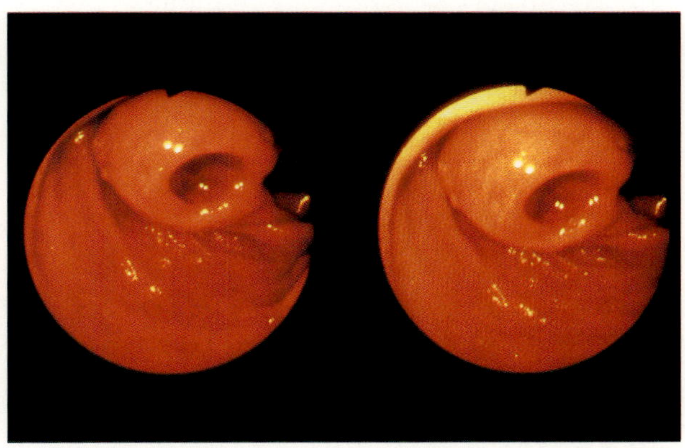

Plate 26.3 *Neuroendocrine tumour of the duodenum; endoscopic appearance. (Courtesy of Dr Reymond de Peyer, Geneva.)*

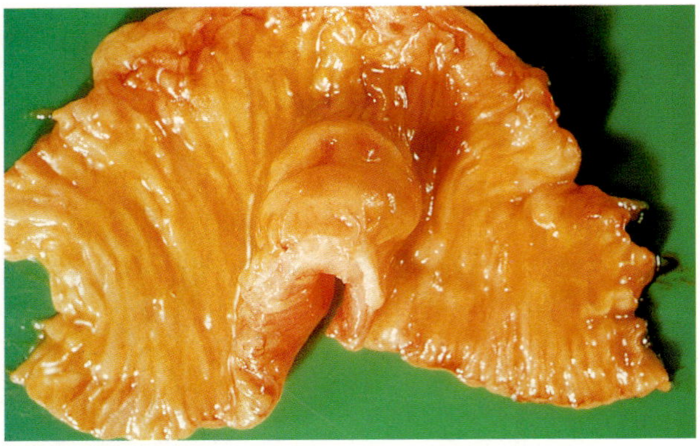

Plate 26.4 *Neuroendocrine tumour of the ileum bulging into the lumen; notice fibrotic thickening of the wall at the base of the tumour.*

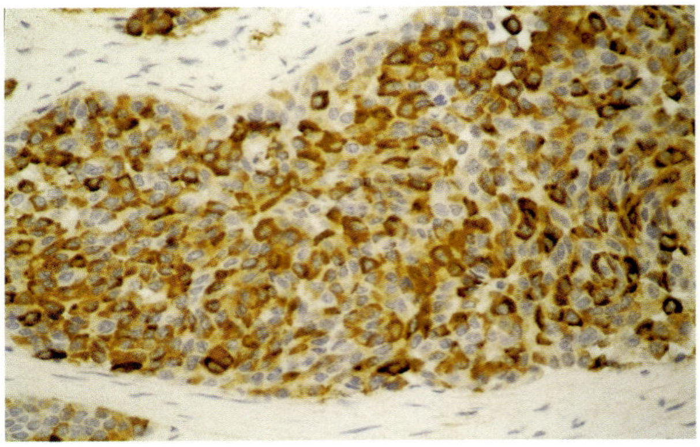

Plate 26.5 *Neuroendocrine tumour; immunohistochemical stain with chromogranin.*

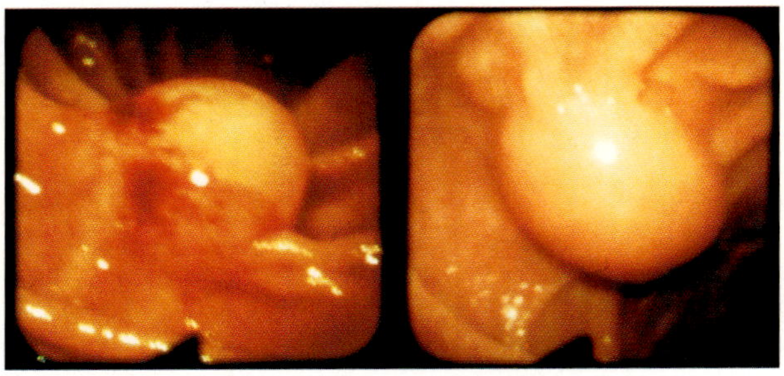

Plate 26.6 *Submucosal lipoma; endoscopic appearance. (Courtesy of Dr Reymond de Peyer, Geneva.)*

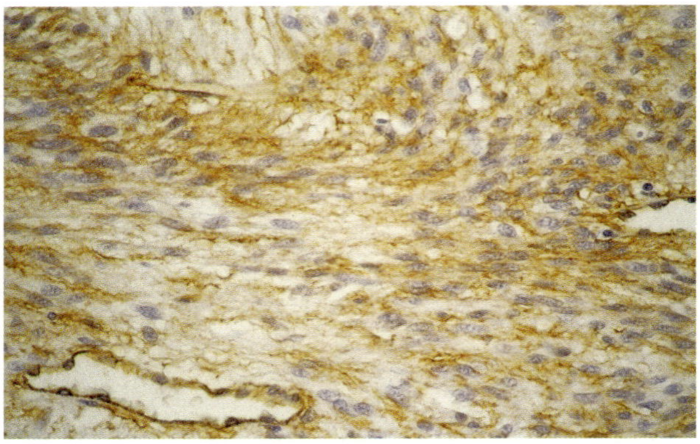

Plate 26.7 *Stromal tumour; immunohistochemical stain with CD 34 showing irregular staining of spindle cells.*

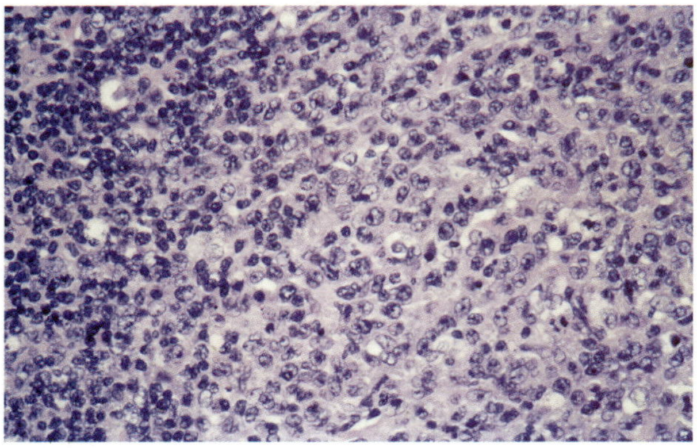

Plate 26.8 *Malignant lymphoma constituted partly of small cells on the left side and partly of large cells on the right (H&E).*

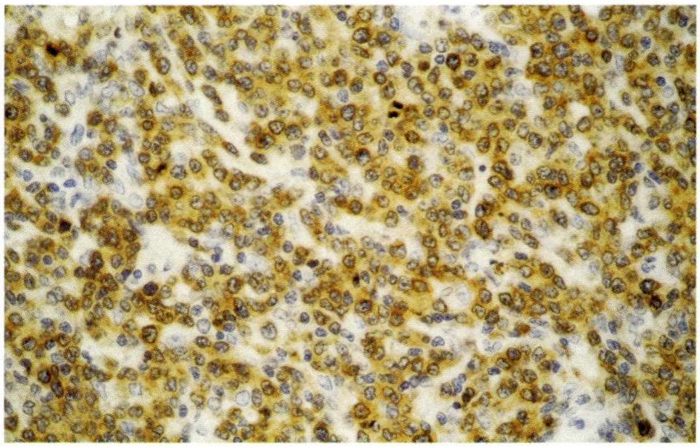

Plate 26.9 *Malignant lymphoma; immunohistochemical stain with CD79a showing a B-cell population.*

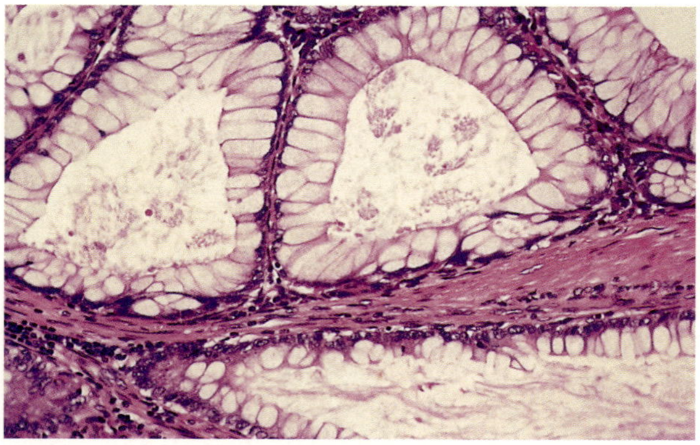

Plate 26.10 *Peutz–Jeghers polyp; histology showing smooth muscle bundles between glands (H&E).*

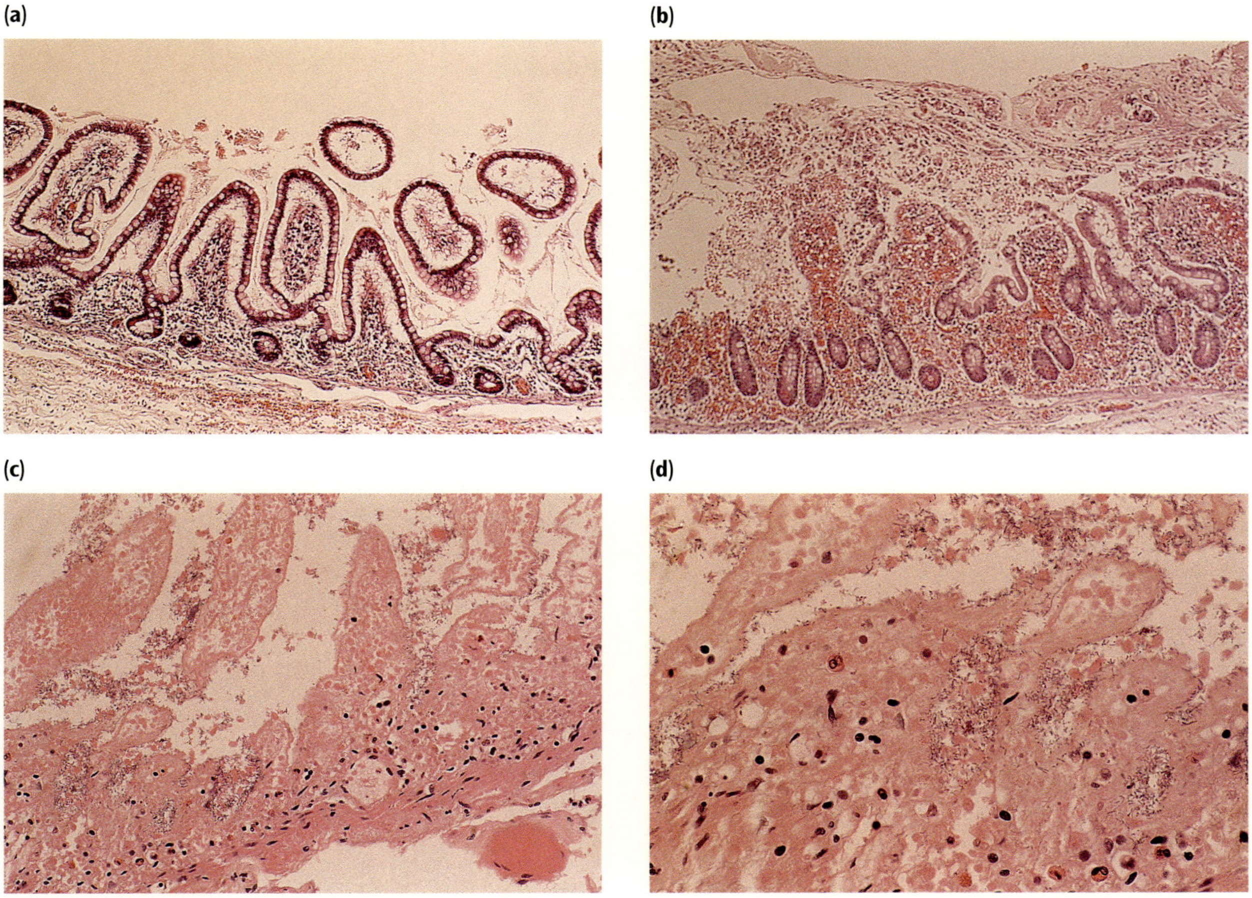

Plate 27.1 *Bowel ischaemia.* **(a)** *Normal villous architecture.* **(b)** *Early phase of ischaemia. There is severe congestion of the mucosa with early surface ulceration.* **(c)** *Later stage in which there is loss of the cellular details of the villi but the general architecture is still maintained. This is often referred to as 'mummification'.* **(d)** *A higher power to show the intestinal bacterial flora (deep purple bacilli) that are invading the lamina propria.*

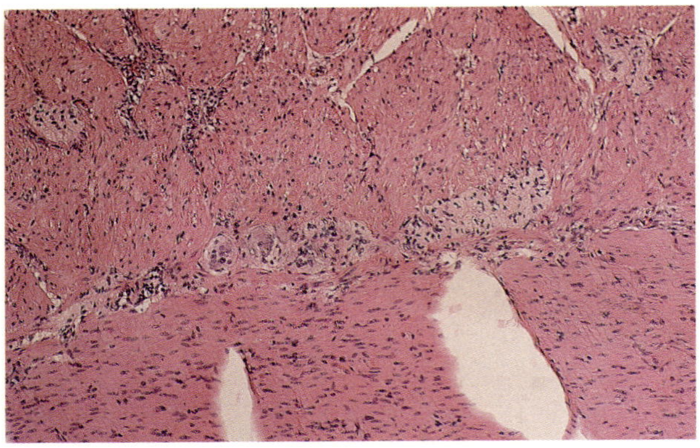

Plate 27.2 *Neuromuscular structure. The typical muscular structure of the intestine in which the ganglionated nerves lie between the inner circular and the outer longitudinal muscle.*

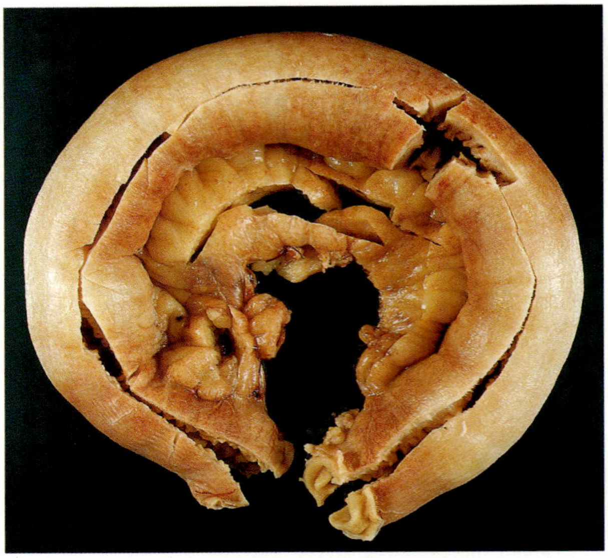

Plate 27.3 *Phlegmon. This is a portion of the jejunum from a patient who presented with intestinal obstruction and bleeding. The intestine is dilated, soft and covered by a thin layer of pus.*

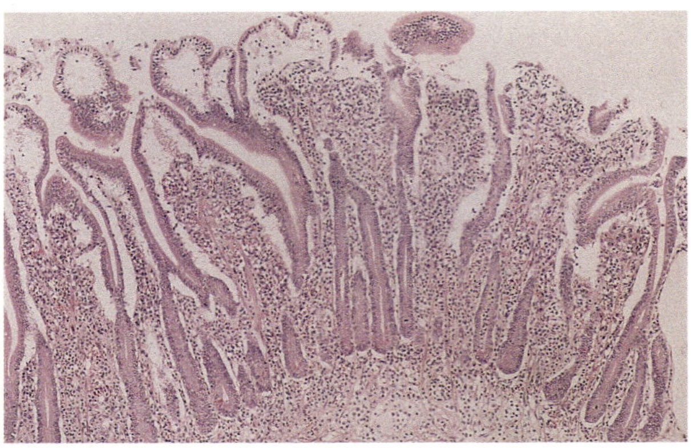

Plate 27.4 *Photomicrograph from the case described in Plate 27.3 showing dense active inflammation of the lamina propria without mucosal ulceration.*

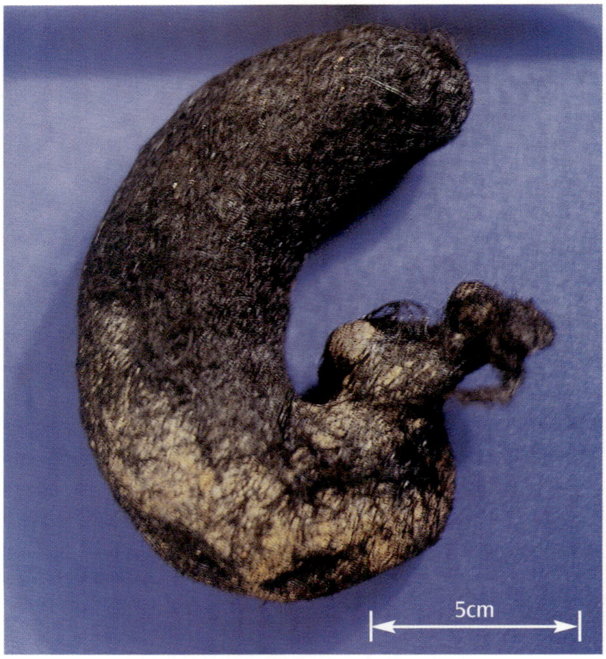

Plate 28.1 *Trichobezoar removed from a teenage girl.*

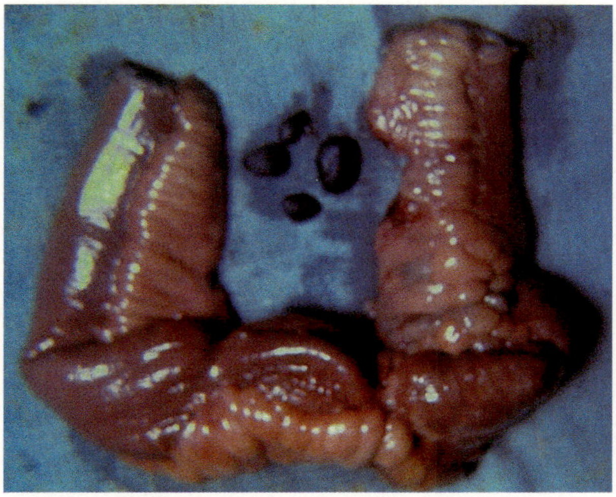

Plate 28.2 *Tuberculous stricture of intestine with enteroliths (nidus being pomegranate seeds).*

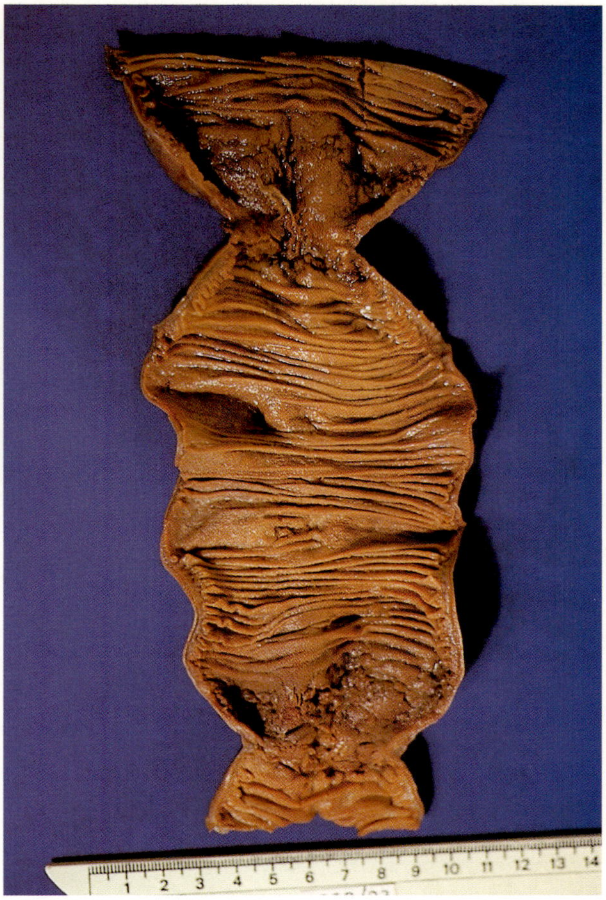

Plate 28.3 *Tuberculosis of ileum with stricture.*

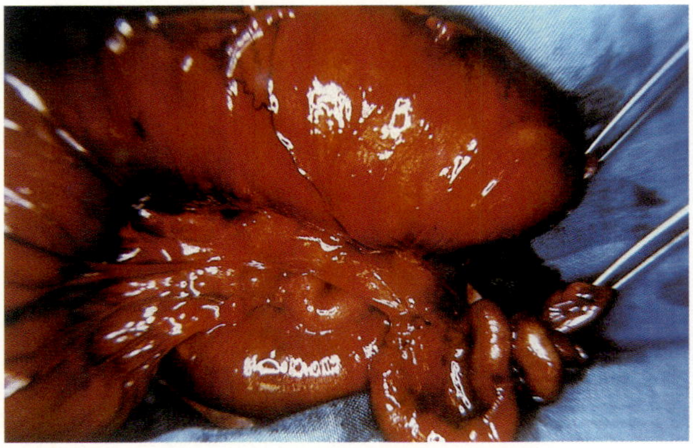

Plate 28.4 *Jejunal atresia showing proximal dilated and distal collapsed intestine.*

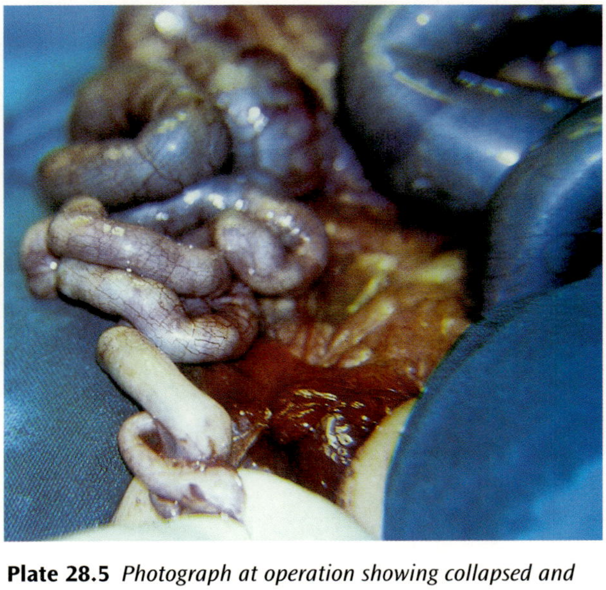

Plate 28.5 *Photograph at operation showing collapsed and dilated segment of ileum in meconium ileus.*

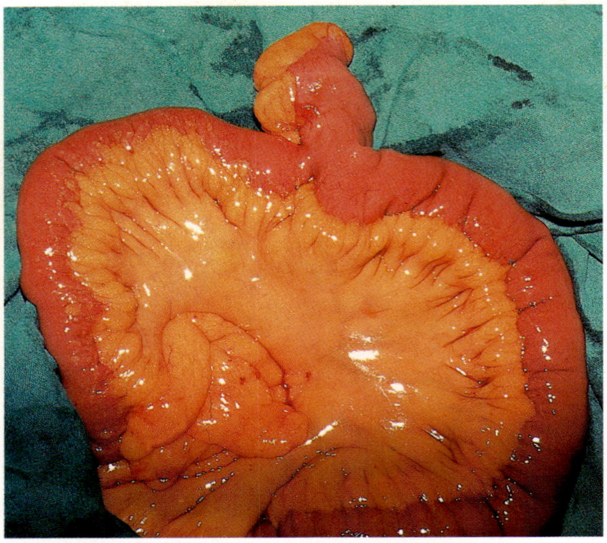

Plate 28.6 *Intraoperative appearance of Meckel's diverticulum.*

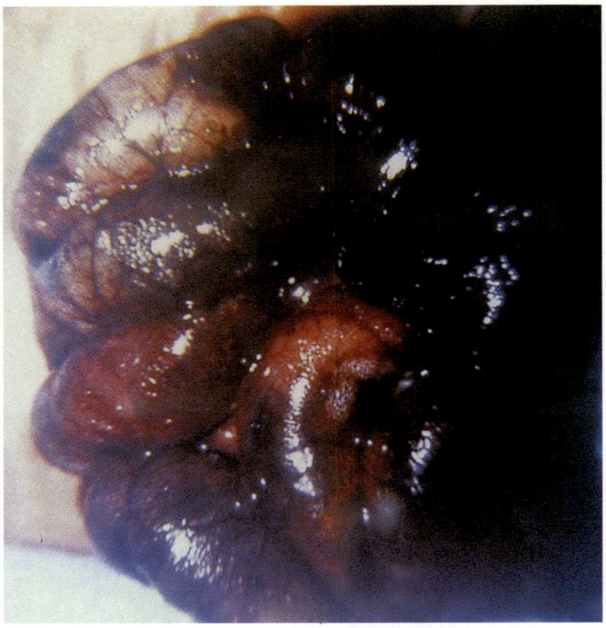

Plate 28.7 *Intestine affected by necrotizing enterocolitis.*

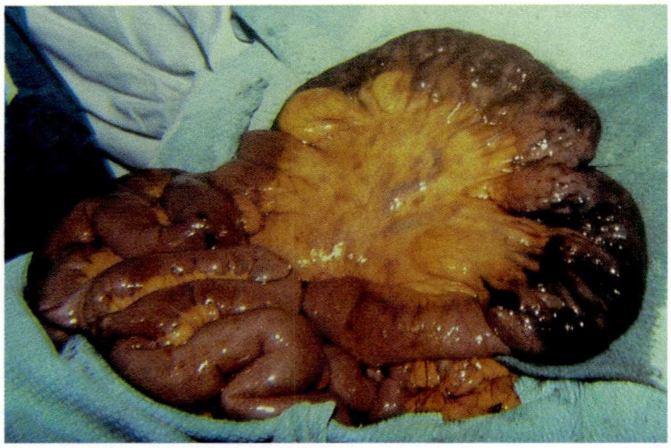

Plate 28.8 *Vascular malformation of jejunum (resected segment).*

capable of lysing his or her own red cells under acid conditions (Dacie, 1967).

Familial Mediterranean fever

This is an inherited recurrent polyserositis that is prevalent among (but not confined to) people in the Middle East: Arabs, Turks, Armenians and Sephardic Jews. It presents with symptoms of severe pleurisy or peritonitis and joint pain and swelling. In the past, it was a diagnosis of exclusion, although a deficiency of the inactivator of the chemotactic complement component C5a, C5a inhibitor, has been reported in peritoneal and synovial fluids (Matzner and Brzezinski, 1984). More recently, the FEMV gene on the short arm of chromosome 16, present in 85 per cent of patients, has been characterized and is the basis for making a diagnosis in the majority of suspected patients, although the precise mechanisms responsible for the acute inflammatory episodes are still unknown (Babior and Matzner, 1997).

Chronic granulomatous disease: NBT and DHR tests

This rare X-linked and autosomal recessive disorder of neutrophil superoxide generation increases susceptibility to, and causes, repeated bacterial and fungal infections, particularly of the lungs and skin (Smith and Curnutte, 1991). Infections leading to granuloma formation can occur anywhere, including the small and large bowel, and chronic enterocolitis can be particularly debilitating (Ament and Ochs, 1973). Blood film appearance of the white cells can be misleadingly normal, but the defect in superoxide generation can be detected, both in affected individuals and carriers, by measuring nitroblue tetrazolium reduction by activated neutrophils – the NBT test (Baehner and Nathan, 1968; Ochs and Igo, 1973). However, false positives may occur, and a recent alternative method using flow cytometry with dihydramine-123 as an indicator of neutrophil oxidase activity (DHR assay) is said to be more accurate (Vowells *et al.*, 1996).

Acute autosomal dominant porphyrias

Acute intermittent porphyria, hereditary coproporphyria and variegate porphyria all give rise to acute neurovisceral attacks that include severe abdominal pain over 90 per cent of the time. Once the diagnosis is considered during an acute attack, the urine should be screened for the presence of increased porphobilinogen, a positive finding confirmed with a specific, quantitative assay. A negative screening test does not exclude absolutely a diagnosis of porphyria and a definitive diagnosis is made by measuring faecal and plasma porphyrins (Elder *et al.*, 1997).

Bone marrow aspirate and trephine – iron stores, malignancy, other infiltration

The bone marrow aspirate stained with Perls potassium ferricyanide stain for iron will confirm the presence or absence of iron stores. Assessment of the aspirate will give further information as to whether there is effective erythropoiesis (Ellis, 1964). In severe malabsorption, starvation or anorexia, a striking lack of normal haemopoiesis is associated with large amounts of eosinophilic amorphous necrotic debris or hyaline ground substance (Smith and Spivak, 1985). Bone marrow trephines are best for assessing overall cellularity of the marrow as they provide information about the architecture of the marrow including the bony trabeculae. The appearance of the bone marrow in megaloblastic anaemia can be so deranged as to mimic acute leukaemia and it is important to be sure of the haematinic status of any elderly patient who presents with pancytopenia before making such a diagnosis (Dokal *et al.*, 1990). Infiltrations such as amyloid (Falk *et al.*, 1997) and metabolic storage disorders such as Gaucher's disease have characteristic marrow appearances, although pseudo-Gaucher-like cells are seen in a variety of proliferative disorders (Beutler, 1988).

SUMMARY AND CONCLUSIONS

Haematological investigations play an important role in the diagnosis and monitoring of disorders of the small bowel. Recent years have seen dramatic advances both in our understanding of disease pathology and, as has been briefly discussed in this section, the laboratory and associated clinical techniques available for the investigation of gut disorders. However, it must be remembered that the results of blood and other biochemical tests show a wide variation both biologically and analytically. It is important that all clinicians are aware of the degree of these variables, both in their community and their institution, with respect to each test, for the correct interpretation of laboratory results (Fraser and Fogarty, 1989).

REFERENCES

Ahr, D.J., Rickles, F.R., Hoyer, L.W., O'Leary, D.S., Conrad, M.E. 1977: von Willebrand's disease and hemorrhagic telangiectasia: association of two complex disorders of hemostasis resulting in life-threatening hemorrhage. *American Journal of Medicine* 62, 452–8.

Albahary, C. 1972: Lead and haemopoiesis. *American Journal of Medicine* 52, 367–78.

Allan, R.A., Sladen, G.E., Bassingham, S., Lazarus, C., Clarke, S.E., Fogelman, I. 1993: Comparison of simultaneous ^{99m}Tc-HMPAO and ^{111}In oxine labelled white cell scans in the assessment of inflammatory bowel disease. *European Journal of Nuclear Medicine* 20, 195–200.

Alperin, J.B. 1987: Coagulopathy caused by vitamin K deficiency in critically ill, hospitalized patients. *JAMA* 258, 1916–19.

Ament, M.E., Ochs, H.D. 1973: Gastrointestinal manifestations of chronic granulomatous disease. *New England Journal of Medicine* 288, 382–7.

Arndt, J.W., van der Sluys Veer, A., Blok, D., Griffoen, G., Verspaget, H.W., Lamers, C.B., Pauwels, E.K. 1993: Prospective comparative study of technetium-99m-WBCs and indium-111-granulocytes for the examination of patients with inflammatory bowel disease. *Journal of Nuclear Medicine* 34, 1052–7.

Babior, B.M., Matzner, Y. 1997: The familial Mediterranean fever gene – cloned at last. *New England Journal of Medicine*, 337, 1548–9.

Baehner, R.L., Nathan, D.G. 1968: Quantitative nitroblue tetrazolium test in chronic granulomatous disease. *New England Journal of Medicine* 278, 971–6.

Bampton, P.A., Holloway, R.H. 1996: A prospective study of the gastroenterological causes of iron deficiency anaemia in a general hospital. *Australia and New Zealand Journal of Medicine* 26, 793–9.

Bessman, J.D., Feinstein, D.I. 1979: Quantitative anisocytosis as a discriminant between iron deficiency and thalassaemia minor. *Blood* 53, 288.

Bessman, J.D., Gilmer, P.R., Gardner, F.H. 1983: Improved classification of anemias by MCV and RDW. *American Journal of Clinical Pathology* 80, 322–6.

Bessman, J.D., McClure, S., Bates, J. 1989: Distinction of microcytic disorders: comparison of expert, numerical-discriminant, and microcomputer analysis. *Blood Cells* 15, 533–40.

Beutler, E. 1988: Gaucher disease. *Blood Reviews* 2, 59–70.

Blanchard, R.A., Furie, B.C., Jorgensen, M.J. 1981: Acquired vitamin K-dependent carboxylation deficiency in liver disease. *New England Journal of Medicine* 305, 242.

Bosmans, L., Storms, P., Gruwez, J.A. 1993: Chronic anemia secondary to side-to-side distal small bowel anastomosis. *Acta Chirurgica Belgica* 93, 25–7.

Bradlow, B.A., Haggan, J.M. 1979: A comparison of the plasma viscosity and the erythrocyte sedimentation rate as screening tests. *South African Medical Journal* 55, 415–20.

Bull, B.S., Levy, W.C., Westengard, J.C. *et al.* 1986: Ranking of laboratory tests by consensus analysis. *Lancet* 2, 377–80.

Bunn, H.F., Jandl, J.H. 1969: The renal handling of hemoglobin. II. Catabolism. *Journal of Experimental Medicine* 129, 925–34.

Caprilli, R., Corrao, G., Taddei, G., Tonelli, F., Torchio, P., Viscido, A. 1996: Prognostic factors for postoperative recurrence of Crohn's disease. Gruppo Italiano per lo Studio del Colon e del Retto (GISC). *Diseases of the Colon and Rectum* 39, 335–41.

Cartwright, G.E. 1966: The anemia of chronic disorders. *Seminars in Hematology* 3, 351.

Cattan, D., Belaiche, J., Zittoun, J., Yvart, J. 1982: Effect of folate deficiency on vitamin B12 absorption. *Annals of Nutrition and Metabolism* 26, 367–73.

Chanarin, I. 1989: Megaloblastic anaemia. In Chanarin, I. (ed.) *Laboratory haematology*. Edinburgh: Churchill Livingstone, 115–52.

Chart, H., Rowe, B. 1990: Serological identification of infection by Vero cytotoxin producing *Escherichia coli* in patients with haemolytic uraemic syndrome. *Serodiagnosis and Immunotherapy in Infectious Disease* 4, 413–18.

Crombleholme, T.M., Harris, B.H., Rosenfield, C.G. 1994: Intestinal necrosis from congenital hypercoagulopathy. *Journal of Pediatric Surgery* 29, 235–6.

Dacie, J.V. 1967: *Paroxysmal nocturnal hemoglobinuria.*, London: Churchill.

Das, K.C., Herbert, V., Colman, N., Longo, D.L. 1978: Unmasking covert folate deficiency in iron-deficient subjects with neutrophil hypersegmentation: dU suppression tests on lymphocytes and bone marrow. *British Journal of Haematology* 39, 357–75.

Dinco, K., Aksoy, M. 1969: On the platelet leves in chronic iron deficiency anemia. *Acta Haematologica (Basel)* 41, 135–43.

Dokal, I.S., Cox, T.M., Galton, D.A.G. 1990: Vitamin B–12 and folate deficiency presenting as leukaemia. *British Medical Journal* 300, 1263–4.

Elder, G.H., Hift, R.J., Meissner, P.N. 1997: The acute porphyrias. *Lancet* 349, 1613–17.

Ellis, L.D. 1964: Marrow iron. An evaluation of depleted stores in a series of 1,332 needle biopsies. *Annals of Internal Medicine* 61, 44–9.

England, J.M., Ward, S.M., Down, M.C. 1976: Microcytosis, anisocytosis and the red cell indices in iron deficiency. *British Journal of Haematology* 34, 589–97.

Fairbanks, V.F., Beutler, E. 1990: Erythrocyte disorders: anemias related to disturbances of hemoglobin synthesis. In Williams, W.J., Beutler, E., Erslev, A.J., Lichtman, M.A. (eds) *Hematology*. New York: McGraw-Hill, 482–505.

Falk, R.H., Comenzo, R.L., Skinner, M. 1997: The systemic amyloidoses. *New England Journal of Medicine* 337, 898–909.

Fraser, C.G., Fogarty, Y. 1989: Interpreting laboratory results. *British Medical Journal* 298, 1659–60.

Froehlich, J.W., Field, S.A. 1988: The role of indium-111 white blood cells in inflammatory bowel disease. *Seminars in Nuclear Medicine* 18, 300–7.

Gilles, H.M. 1981: Normal haematological values in tropical areas. *Clinical Haematology* 10, 697–706.

Griffiths, R.A., Good, W.R., Watson, N.P., O'Donnell, H.F., Fell, P.J., Shakespeare, J.M. 1984: Normal erythrocyte sedimentation rate in the elderly. *British Medical Journal* 289, 724–5.

Guillou, Y.M., Bleichner, J.P., Gobron, F., Leroux, A., Le Calve, J.L., Malledant, Y. 1996: [Mesenteric vein infarction associated with congenital antithrombin III (ATIII) deficiency]. *Annales de Chirurgie* 50, 72–5.

Hallberg, L., Hulten, L., Lindstedt, G. *et al.* 1993: Prevalence of iron deficiency in Swedish adolescents. *Pediatric Research* 34, 680–7.

Harries, A.D., Fitzsimons, E., Fifield, R., Dew, M.J., Rhodes, J. 1983: Platelet count: a simple measure of activity in Crohn's disease. *British Medical Journal* 286, 1476.

Harries, A.D., Fitzsimons, E., Dew, M.J., Heatley, R.V., Rhodes, J. 1984: Association between iron deficiency anaemia and mid-arm circumference in Crohn's disease. *Human Nutrition and Clinical Nutrition* 38, 47–53.

Hartmann, R.C., Jenkins, D.E.J. 1965: The 'sugar-water' test for paroxysmal hemoglobinuria. *New England Journal of Medicine* 275, 155–7.

Herresbach, D., Pagenault, M., Gueret, P. *et al.* 1997: Leiden factor V mutation in four patients with small bowel infarctions. *Gastroenterology* 113, 322–5.

Heyman, S., Sacks, B., Khettry, J., Steer, M.L. 1979: Localization of bleeding small intestinal lesions using scanning techniques. *Surgery* 85, 372–6.

Hillman, R.S., Finch, C.A. 1967: Erythropoiesis normal and abnormal. *Seminars in Haematology* 4, 327–36.

Hudson, M., Hutton, R.A., Wakefield, A.J., Sawyerr, A.M., Pounder, R.E. 1992: Evidence for activation of coagulation in Crohn's disease. *Blood Coagulation and Fibrinolysis* 3, 773–8.

Inbal, A., Bank, I., Zivelin, A. *et al.* 1997: Acquired von Willebrand disease in a patient with angiodysplasia resulting from immune-mediated clearance of von Willebrand factor. *British Journal of Haematology* 96, 179–82.

International Committee on Standards in Haematology 1984: Recommendation for a selected method for the measurement of plasma viscosity. *Journal of Clinical Pathology* 37, 1147–52.

International Committee on Standards in Haematology 1988: Guidelines on selection of laboratory tests for monitoring the acute phase response. *Journal of Clinical Pathology* 41, 1203–12.

Jagenburg, R., Kock, N.G., Philipson, B. 1975: Vitamin B12 absorption in patients with continent ileostomy. *Scandinavian Journal of Gastroenterology* 10, 141–5.

Jaremo, P., Sandberg-Gertzen, H. 1996: Platelet density and size in inflammatory bowel disease [see comments]. *Thrombosis and Haemostasis* 75, 560–1.

Jones, B.P., Broomhead, A.F., Kwan, Y.L., Grace, C.S. 1987: Incidence and clinical significance of protein-bound vitamin B12 malabsorption. *European Journal of Haematology* 38, 131–6.

Kadir, R.A., Economides, D.L., Sabin, C.A., Owens, D., Lee, C.A. 1998: Frequency of inherited bleeding disorders in women with menorrhagia. *Lancet* 351, 485–9.

Kasapcopur, O., Ozdogan, H., Yazei, H. 1991: Obesity and erythrocyte sedimentation rate in children. *Journal of Pediatrics* 119, 773–5.

Kavi, J., Wise, R. 1989: Causes of the haemolytic uraemic syndrome. *British Medical Journal* 298, 65–6.

Kennedy, H.J., Callender, S.T., Truelove, S.C., Warner, G.T. 1982: Haematological aspects of life with an ileostomy. *British Journal of Haematology* 52, 445–54.

Kis, A.M., Carnes, M. 1998: Detecting iron deficiency in anemic patients with concomitant medical problems. *Journal of General Internal Medicine* 13, 455–61.

Kjeldsen, J., Lassen, J.F., Brandslund, I., Schaffalitzky de Muckadell, O.B. 1998: Markers of coagulation and fibrinolysis as measures of disease activity in inflammatory bowel disease. *Scandinavian Journal of Gastroenterology* 33, 637–43.

Klar, E., Buhr, H., Zimmermann, R. 1990: [Protein C deficiency with recurrent infarct of the small intestine]. *Chirurg* 61, 59–62.

Lake, A.M., Stauffer, J.Q., Stuart, M.J. 1978: Hemostatic alterations in inflammatory bowel disease: response to therapy. *American Journal of Digestive Diseases* 23, 897–902.

Lederle, F.A. 1991: Oral cobalamin for pernicious anemia. Medicine's best kept secret? *JAMA* 265, 94–5.

Lewis, R. 1976: Anemia – a common but never a normal concomitant of aging. *Geriatrics* 31, 53–60.

Lindenbaum, J. 1983: Status of laboratory testing in the diagnosis of megaloblastic anemia. *Blood* 61, 624–7.

Looker, A.C., Dallman, P.R., Carroll, M.D., Gunter, E.W., Johnson, C.L. 1997: Prevalence of iron deficiency in the United States. *JAMA* 277, 973–6.

Lutomski, D.M., Palascak, J.E., Bower, R.H. 1987: Warfarin resistance associated with intravenous lipid administration. *Journal of Parenteral and Enteral Nutrition* 11, 316–18.

Mahu, J.L., Leclercq, C., Suquet, J.P. 1990: Usefulness of red cell distribution width in association with biological parameters in an epidemiological survey of iron deficiency in children. *International Journal of Epidemiology* 19, 646–54.

Martin, J.F., Bath, P.M.W., Burr, M.L. 1991: Influence of platelet size on outcome after myocardial infarction. *Lancet* 338, 1409–11.

Matzner, Y., Brzezinski, A. 1984: C5a-inhibitor deficiency in peritoneal fluids from patients with familial Mediterranean fever. *New England Journal of Medicine* 311, 287–90.

McEvoy, A., Dutton, J., James, O.F.W. 1983: Bacterial contamination of the small intestine is an important cause of occult malabsorption in the elderly. *British Medical Journal* 287, 789–95.

Merrin, P., Lancaster Smith, M.J. 1989: Leukaemoid reaction and ulcerative colitis. *Gut* 30, 1154–5.

Middledorp, S., van der Meer, J. 1998: Factor V:Q506 mutation – resistance to activated protein C (APC): clinical implications with respect to family screening. *Seminars in Thrombosis and Hemostasis* 24, 363–6.

Miyata, T., Takeda, J., Iida, Y. *et al.* 1993: The cloning of PIG-A, a component in the early step of GPI-anchor synthesis. *Science* 259, 1318–20.

Morrison, A.E., Ludlam, C.A. 1995: Acquired haemophilia and its management. *British Journal of Haematology* 89, 231–6.

Naurath, H.J., Joosten, E., Riezler, R., Stabler, S.P., Allen, R.A., Lindenbaum, J. 1995: Effects of vitamin B12, folate, and vitamin B6 supplements in elderly people with normal serum vitamin concentrations. *Lancet* 346, 85–9.

Newland, A.C., Evans, T.G.J.R. 1997: Haematological disorders at the extremes of life. *British Medical Journal* 314, 1262–5.

Nuzum, C.T., Sandler, R.S., Paulk, H.T. 1981: Thrombocytosis in Whipple's disease. *Gastroenterology* 80, 1465–7.

Ochs, J.D., Igo, R.P. 1973: The NBT slide test: a simple screening method for detecting chronic granulomatous disease and female carriers. *Journal of Pediatrics* 83, 77–82.

O'Grady, J.G., Harding, B., Stevens, F.M., Egan, E.L., McCarthy, C.F. 1985: Influence of splenectomy and the functional hyposplenism of coeliac disease on platelet count and volume. *Scandinavian Journal of Haematology* 34, 425–8.

Oliver, G.C., Rubin, R.J., Park, Y.H., Ashton, J.K. 1987: Preoperative localization of intermittently bleeding small intestinal tumors using Tc–99m labeled red blood cell scanning. Report of two cases. *Diseases of the Colon and Rectum* 30, 715–20.

Phekoo, K., Williams, Y., Schey, S.A., Andrews, V.E., Dudley, J.M., Hoffbrand, A.V. 1997: Folate assays: serum or red cell? *Journal of the Royal College of Physicians of London* 31, 291–5.

Rehm, P.K., Atkins, F.B., Ziessman, H.A. 1996: Positive technetium-99m-red blood cell gastrointestinal bleeding scan after barium small-bowel study. *Journal of Nuclear Medicine* 37, 643–5.

Reinhart, W.H., Chien, S. 1988: Red cell vacuoles: their size and distribution under normal conditions and after splenectomy. *American Journal of Hematology* 27, 265–71.

Rodeghiero, F., Castaman, G., Tosetto, A. 1990: von Willebrand factor antigen is less sensitive than ristocetin cofactor for the diagnosis of type 1 von Willebrand disease – results based on an epidemiological investigation. *Thrombosis and Haemastasis* 64, 349–52.

Rothenburg, M.E. 1998: Eosinophilia. *New England Journal of Medicine* 338, 1592–600.

Saverymuttu, S.H., Lavender, P.J., Hodgson, H.J.F., Chadwick, V.S. 1983: Assessment of disease activity in inflammatory bowel disease: a new approach using 111 indium granulocyte scanning. *British Medical Journal* 287, 1751–3.

Saxena, S., Weiner, J.M., Carmel, R. 1988: Red blood cell distribution width in untreated pernicious anemia. *American Journal of Clinical Pathology* 89, 660–3.

Scarlett, J.D., Read, H., O'Dea, K. 1992: Protein-bound cobalamin absorption declines in the elderly. *American Journal of Hematology* 39, 79–83.

Schjonsby, H., Halvorsen, J.F., Hofstad, T., Hovdenak, N. 1977: Stagnant loop syndrome in patients with continent ileostomy (intra-abdominal ileal reservoir). *Gut* 18, 795–9.

Scrimshaw, N.S. 1991: Iron deficiency. *Scientific American* October, 24–30.

Smith, R.M., Curnutte, J.T. 1991: Molecular basis of chronic granulomatous disease. *Blood* 77, 673–86.

Smith, R.R.L., Spivak, J.L. 1985: Marrow cell necrosis in anorexia and involuntary starvation. *British Journal of Haematology* 60, 525–30.

Souto, J.C., Martinez, E., Roca, M., Mateo, J., Pujol, J., Gonzalez, D., Fontcuberta, J. 1995: Prothrombotic state and signs of endothelial lesion in plasma of patients with inflammatory bowel disease. *Digestive Diseases and Sciences* 40, 1883–9.

St John, D.J., Young, G.P. 1978: Evaluation of radiochromium blood loss studies in unexplained iron-deficiency anaemia. *Australian and New Zealand Journal of Medicine* 8, 121–6.

Streeter, A.M., Shum, H.Y., Duncombe, V.M., Hewson, J.W., Thorpe, M.E. 1976: Vitamin B12 malabsorption associated with a normal Schilling test result. *Medical Journal of Australia* 1, 54–5.

Talstad, I., Rootwelt, K., Gjone, E. 1973: Thrombocytosis in ulcerative colitis and Crohn's disease. *Scandinavian Journal of Gastroenterology* 8, 135–8.

Thompson, D., Milford-Ward, A., Whicher, J.T. 1992: The value of acute phase protein measurements in clinical practice. *Annals of Clinical Biochemistry* 29, 123–31.

Towler, B., Irwig, L., Glasziou, P., Kewenter, J., Weller, D., Silagy, C. 1998: A systematic review of the effect of screening for coloretal cancer using the faecal occult blood test, Hemoccult. *British Medical Journal* 317, 559–65.

Vowells, S.J., Fleisher, T.A., Malech, H.L. 1996: Testing for chronic granulomatous disease. *Lancet* 347, 1048–9.

Ware, R.E., Hall, S.E., Rosse, W.F. 1991: Paroxysmal nocturnal hemoglobinuria with onset in childhood and adolescence. *New England Journal of Medicine* 325, 991–6.

Weldon, M.J., Lowe, C., Joseph, A.E., Maxwell, J.D. 1996: Review article: quantitative leucocyte scanning in the assessment of inflammatory bowel disease activity and its response to therapy. *Alimentary Pharmacology and Therapeutics* 10, 123–32.

White, L.A., Chisholm, M. 1993: Gastro-intestinal bleeding in acquired von Willebrand's disease: efficacy of high-dose immuno-globulin where substitution treatments failed. *British Journal of Haematology* 84, 332–4.

Young, G.P., St John, D.J., Lynch, N.M., McHutchison, J.G., Barraclough, D. 1993: Measurement of occult upper gastrointestinal tract blood loss: a direct comparison of radiochromium and haem-porphyrin assay techniques. *Journal of Gastroenterology and Hepatology* 8, 328–33.

Zacharski, L. 1976: The erythrocyte sedimentation rate. *British Journal of Hospital Medicine* July, 53–62.

Zlatanic, J., Korelitz, B.I., Wisch, N. *et al.* 1997: Inflammatory bowel disease and immune thrombocytopenic purpura: is there a correlation? *American Journal of Gastroenterology* 92, 2285–8.

Zuckier, L.S., Chervu, L.R. 1984: Schilling evaluation of pernicious anemia: current status. *Journal of Nuclear Medicine* 25, 1032–9.

13.6

Radiology of the small intestine

ANIL B UTTURKAR

Imaging studies by their very nature are a visual description of pathological process. The conventional classification of pathological entities is adhered to and more common disorders are dealt with in greater detail. Less commonly occurring disorders are briefly discussed and salient features described so that they are not forgotten in differential diagnosis. A detailed account of many disorders is beyond the scope of this chapter.

With the advent of modern technology, there is proliferation of newer modalities like computed tomography (CT), ultrasound and nuclear medicine and, of late, magnetic resonance imaging (MRI). This section describes the scope, limitations and usefulness of these modalities to assist physicians in the selection process of various investigations. The importance of plain x-rays and appropriate barium studies is also stressed.

ANATOMY AND RADIOLOGICAL APPEARANCES

The small intestine is about 16 ft or 5 m in length. The proximal two-fifths constitutes jejunum, while the remaining three-fifths is ileum. It is attached to the posterior abdominal wall by its mesentery. The presence of mesentery allows it to be mobile.

The jejunum is about 3–3.5 cm in diameter and the ileum is about 2–2.5 cm. The circular jejunal mucosal folds are called valvulae conniventes and have an appearance resembling 'coiled spring' or 'stacked coin', while ileal folds are more or less featureless. Jejunal loops are predominantly in the left upper and central abdomen, and ileal loops occupy the lower abdomen and right iliac fossa (Fig. 13.6.1).

RADIOLOGICAL INVESTIGATIONS

Plain x-rays

The plain x-rays should be performed in suspected 'acute abdomen'. They are useful in the detection of free gas under the diaphragm from rupture of a hollow viscus, e.g. small intestine (Fig. 13.6.2). In cases of intestinal obstruction, they are the mainstay of radiological investigations. Small intestinal obstruction manifests as multiple gas-distended loops of small bowel with fluid levels in erect view and these are usually arranged in a 'stepladder pattern'. If an erect view of the abdomen is not possible, a decubitus view should be obtained (Fig. 13.6.3a,b). Plain x-ray of the chest in a sitting or erect position should be mandatory in the investigation of acute abdomen. Not only does it show free gas under the diaphragm, but it is also very useful as a baseline preoperative film. In the early stages, differentiation from paralytic ileus due to either inflammatory or vascular intra-abdominal pathology is

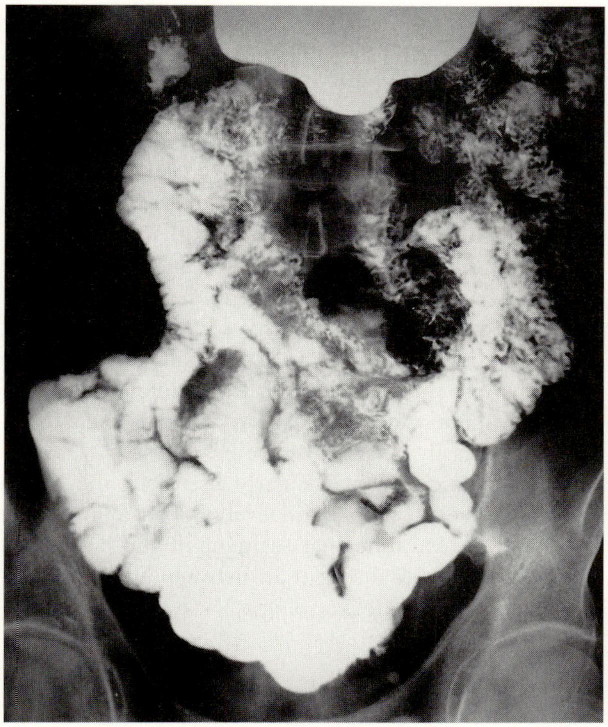

Figure 13.6.1 *Normal small bowel. Jejunal loops in the left upper and central abdomen, and ileal loops occupying the lower abdomen and right iliac fossa.*

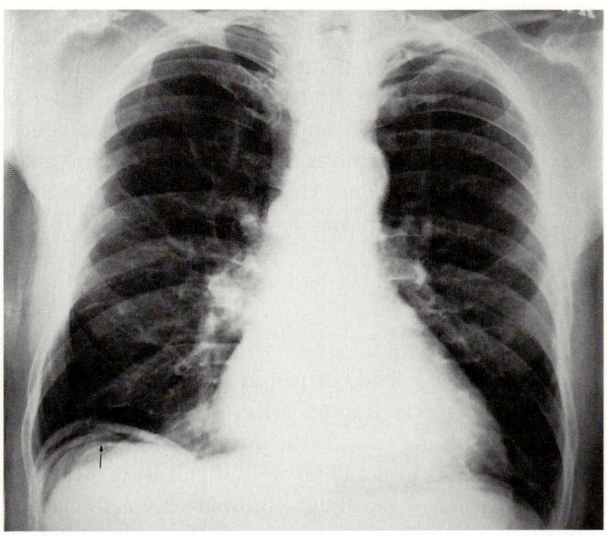

Figure 13.6.2 *Plain x-ray of the chest showing free gas under the diaphragm due to perforation of a hollow viscus.*

difficult and follow-up x-rays are necessary for further assessment.

The position of gas-filled bowel loops with fluid levels gives a clue to the underlying inflammatory pathology, e.g. pancreatitis, appendicitis. Mucosal oedema can point to inflammatory bowel disease or ischaemia (Fig. 13.6.4). An abdominal collection of 'gas

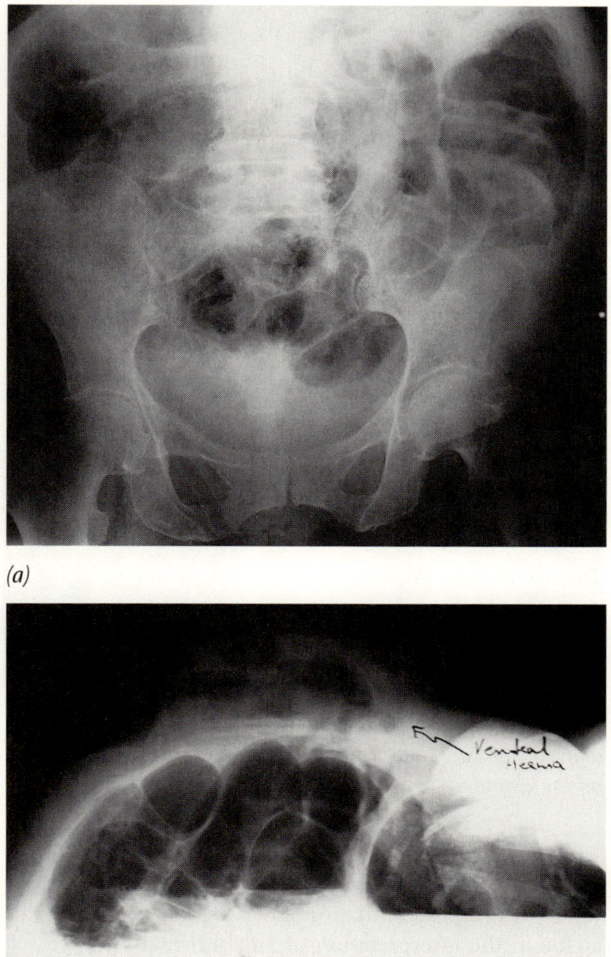

(a)

(b)

Figure 13.6.3 *(a) and (b) Supine and decubitus film shows multiple fluid levels due to small intestinal obstruction. The decubitus film shows obstructed ventral hernia.*

bubbles' that does not conform to the small bowel pattern often points to an intra-abdominal abscess. Soft tissue mass in the abdomen related to the bowel can point to obstructing intestinal pathology, e.g. a neoplasm or intussusception.

Barium studies

With the advent of endoscopic procedures the need for barium examination of the upper gastrointestinal tract and colon is becoming less frequent. However, the small bowel remains more or less 'unconquered' and barium studies are very useful.

SMALL BOWEL FOLLOW-THROUGH

Although this is the requested examination, it must be emphasized that the stomach and duodenum must also

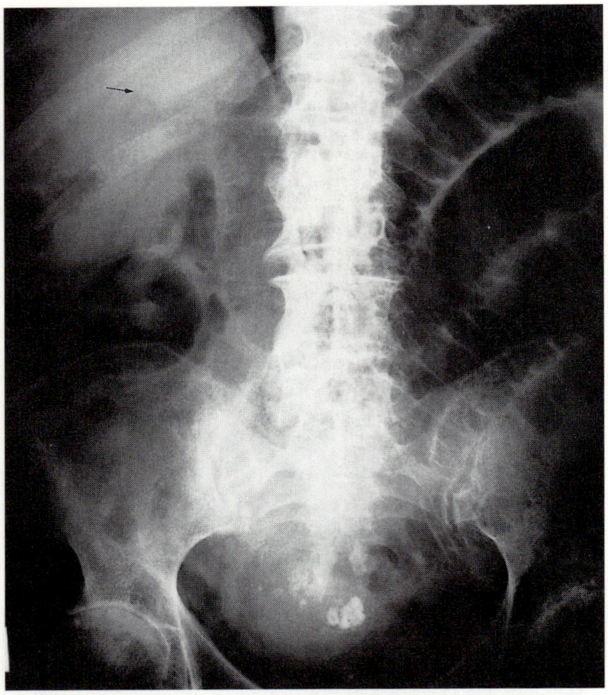

Figure 13.6.4 *Superior mesenteric ischaemia. Note dilatation and mucosal oedema of the jejunal loops and the gas-filled portal venous system (arrowed).*

be investigated as a matter of routine in any small bowel follow-through examination. Such examinations provide a clue in the interpretation of an abnormal finding.

The examination consists of rapid ingestion of about 500 mL of 30–40 per cent weight by volume barium sulphate suspension, which is micropulverized. The films are taken at 15–20-minute intervals to monitor the progress of the barium through the small bowel, and further cone compression spot films are taken as necessary to further evaluate segments of bowel. The length of the examination is dependent upon the transit time, which varies from 30 minutes to 4 hours. The passage of barium through the small bowel can be facilitated by oral or intravenous injection of Maxolon.

Double-contrast examination of the small intestine can be obtained by oral administration of effervescent tablets along with barium, which usually outlines upper to mid-jejunum. For demonstration of terminal ileum by double contrast, barium enema examination followed by air insufflation is sometimes employed. The success of this technique is, however, dependent upon incompetency of the ileo-caecal valve.

SMALL BOWEL ENEMA

This is a somewhat invasive technique that involves duodenal intubation with advancement of the tube as far as the duodenojejunal flexure, if possible. The success depends upon the patient's ability to tolerate intubation and sometimes mild sedation is required. The barium suspension used is much more dilute, about 20 per cent weight/volume, and injected through the duodenal tube via a syringe. Initially 400–500 mL are injected followed by water load or cold saline, which propulses the head of the barium column. This usually gives a good double-contrast view of the entire small bowel. Under fluoroscopic control, the head of the barium column is constantly watched and spot films are taken as necessary. In a conventional barium meal follow-through examination, there is often overlapping of bowel loops and sometimes a small lesion can be masked. With this technique, as the head of the barium column is continuously under surveillance, the pathology can be easily detected.

This technique is particularly useful in the delineation of the exact nature and level of obstruction in the small bowel. An abnormal segment of the bowel can also be evaluated to differentiate between inflammatory, vascular or neoplastic pathology.

Computed tomography

Serial axial slices are taken to demonstrate bowel and other intra-abdominal pathologies. It eliminates the problem of overlapping bowel loops and extrinsic bowel lesions are much better delineated. The site of pathology, especially obstruction, is easy to establish (Fig. 13.6.5a,b). In addition, assessment of the liver, spleen and abdominal lymph nodes gives a clue to the presence of neoplastic pathology (*see* Fig. 13.6.27). Internal and external fistulae (*see* Fig. 13.6.17) and abdominal collections help in establishing the diagnosis of Crohn's disease and allied inflammatory conditions. The involvement of mesentery is appreciated in inflammatory and neoplastic conditions.

Ultrasound

Owing to the presence of gas in the small bowel, this technique has very limited value in the assessment of small bowel, as gas refracts the ultrasound beam making visualization of the small bowel difficult. It is extremely useful in the assessment of radiologically 'silent abdomen', especially in children (Fig. 13.6.6) where there is fluid-filled bowel obstruction with very little gas present. Like CT it also gives a reasonably good assessment of liver, spleen and lymph nodes, and detects free fluid in the abdomen easily. The examination is cheap and easily available. It is non-invasive and does not involve radiation.

Srivastava *et al.* (1994) has reported features that differentiate between inflammatory and neoplastic strictures. Carcinomas appear as uneven thickening of bowel when seen in cross-section, while tuberculous strictures show circumferential symmetrical thickening.

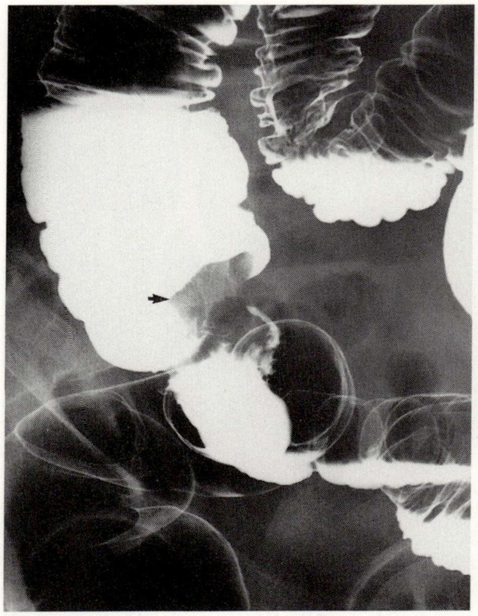

(a)

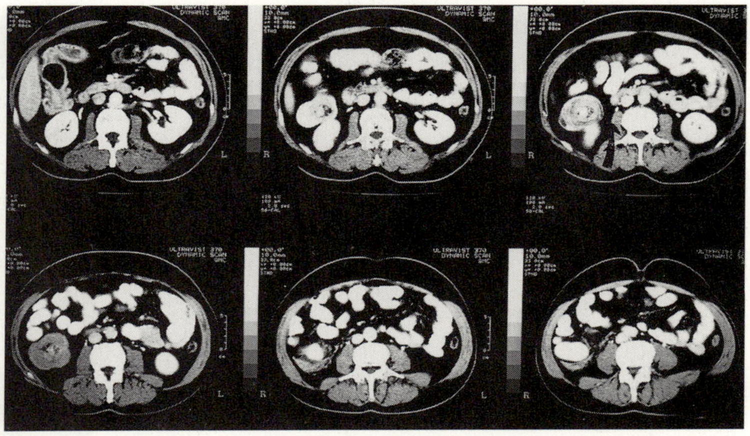

(b)

Figure 13.6.5 *(a) and (b) Barium meal follow-through. There is a mass effect (short arrow) in the caecum with shortening of the terminal ileum. CT scan shows a narrowed lumen of the caecum. The caecum is thick walled and shows concentric mucosal folds giving a clue to the diagnosis of ileo-colic intussusception (curved arrow).*

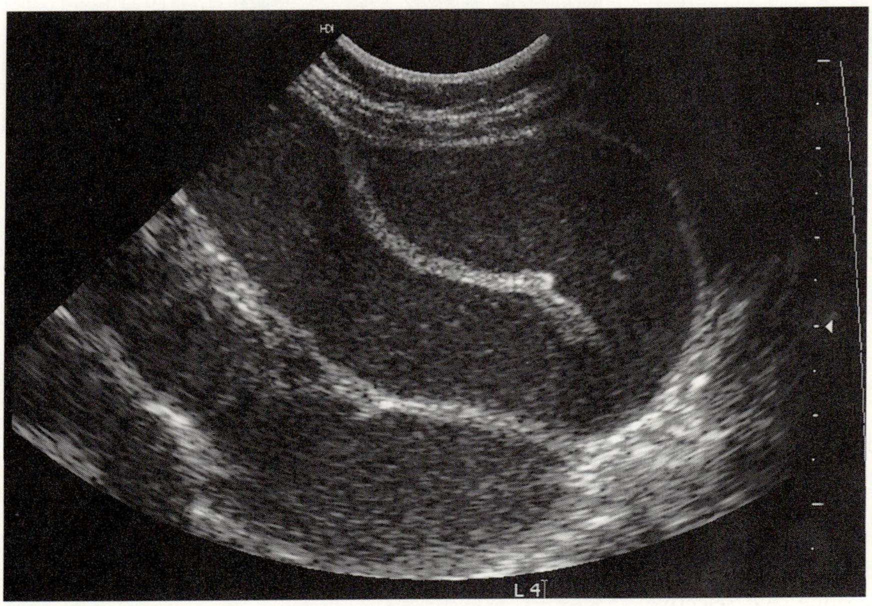

Figure 13.6.6 *Ultrasound examination of the small bowel. Fluid-filled dilated loops of small bowel due to obstruction.*

Bowel loops and mesentery tend to become matted in neoplastic and inflammatory processes, forming a palpable mass that can be appreciated by ultrasound as it disperses gas-filled loops of bowel away. These masses appear as echogenic bands containing superior mesenteric vessels surrounded by hypoechoic masses due to neoplasia, inflammation and lymph nodes (Fleisher *et al.*, 1989). They produce the 'sandwich sign' or the mesenteric 'cake sign' (*see* Fig. 13.6.47). Sonography may be useful in the assessment of afferent loop obstruction in which a dilated fluid-filled loop has 'U-shaped' configuration when scanned in the coronal plane (Hopens *et al.*, 1982). In a closed-loop obstruction, there is also a U-shaped appearance of fluid-filled dilated loop along with mural thickening owing to non-homogeneous echogenicity due to haemorrhage.

Radioisotope studies

The main use of this technique is in the detection of Meckel's diverticulum and determination of the bleeding site (Fig. 13.6.7; *see* also Chapter 14). Labelled leucocyte studies are useful in the detection of the site of inflammatory bowel disease.

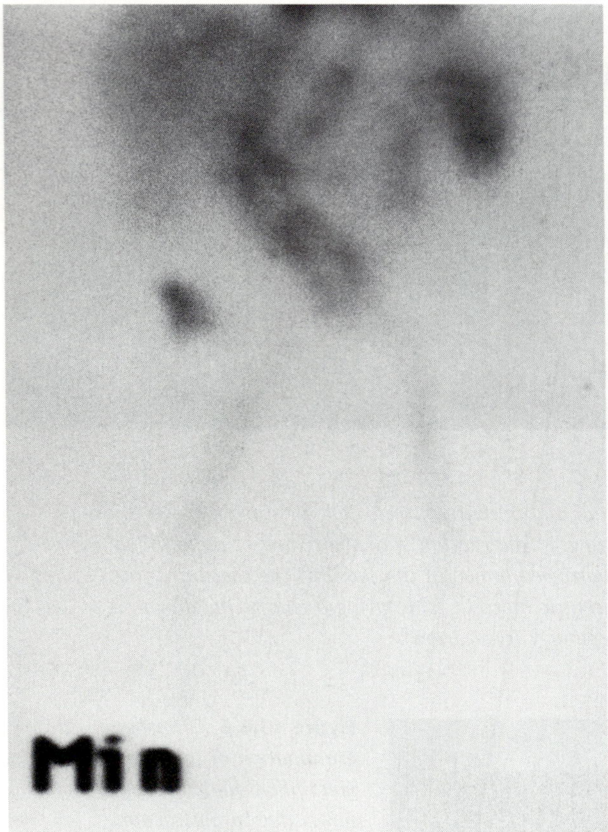

Figure 13.6.7 *Gastrointestinal bleed study for Meckel's diverticulum with technetium-99m-labelled red blood cells. The scan shows that the point of haemorrhage is in the right iliac fossa, which is consistent with Meckel's diverticulum.*

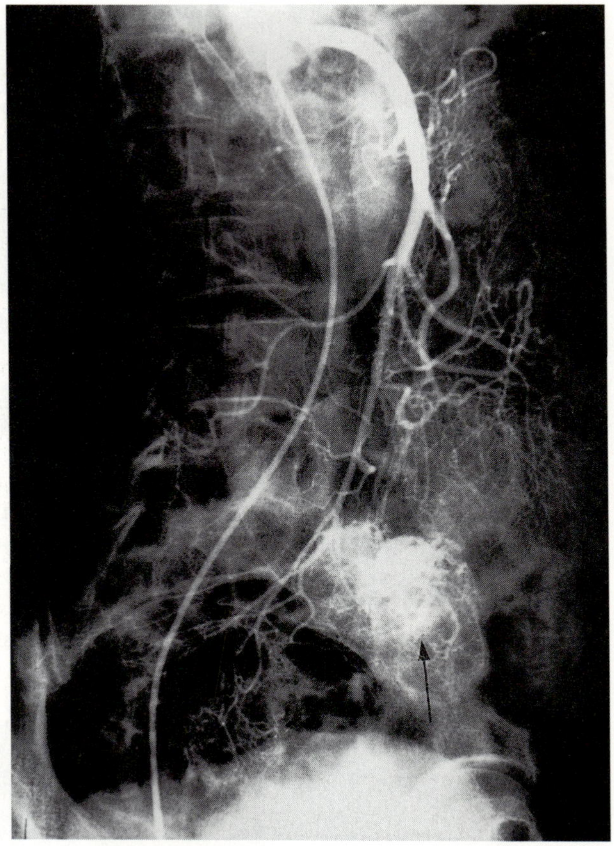

Figure 13.6.8 *Selective mesenteric angiography. Tumour blush of leiomyosarcoma of jejunum (arrowed).*

Angiography

Selective angiography of the superior mesenteric artery is useful in the detection of the bleeding site and in the assessment of the vascular supply of neoplastic lesions (Fig. 13.6.8). With the advancement in catheter technology as a logical extension of angiographic technique, radiological intervention can be done by selective catheterization of the third- and fourth-division vessels for tumour vessel embolization and containment of bleeding. However, this requires a highly skilled and experienced radiologist.

CONGENITAL ABNORMALITIES

Small bowel diverticulosis

These are often seen as incidental findings on barium meal follow-through examination. When present, they are more common in the jejunum than the ileum. When they are large, they can cause stasis and malabsorption. They are also a cause of infection due to stasis, lodgement of foreign bodies, etc. They are prone to rupture and bleeding. On plain x-ray they show fluid levels in erect view and should not be mistaken for small bowel obstruction (Fig. 13.6.9).

Meckel's diverticulum

This is not commonly detected by radiological investigation. It is situated 1–3 ft (0.3–1 m) from the ileocaecal valve. It occurs in 1:1000 population and clinically manifests as malaena as a result of ulceration in ectopic gastric mucosa in its wall. Sometimes it presents as an acute inflammatory process. Complications include perforation, intussusception, internal hernia, volvulus and adhesions. Small bowel studies are not generally useful in the demonstration of Meckel's diverticulum. Technetium–99m pertechnate studies are useful in the detection of ectopic gastric mucosa (Fig. 13.6.10). Labelled leucocyte studies enable detection of the acute inflammatory process. Angiography shows extravasation of contrast medium if there is active bleeding.

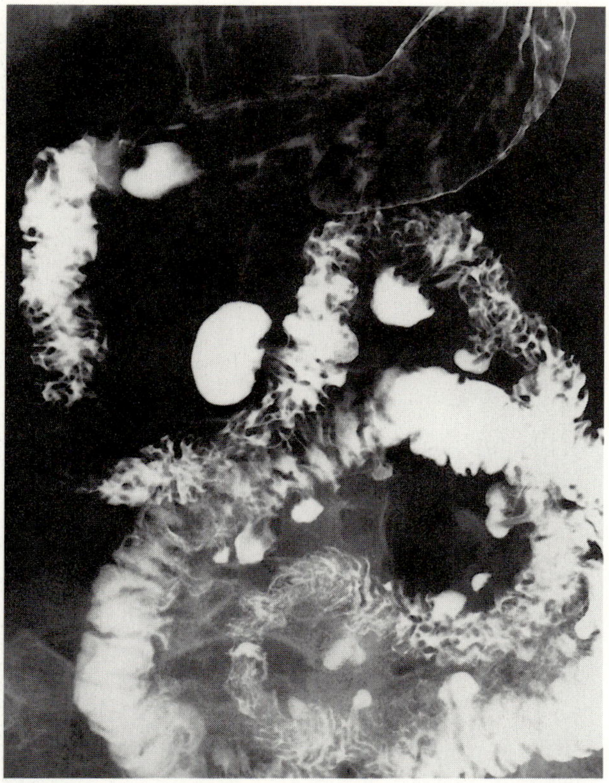

Figure 13.6.9 *Jejunal diverticulosis.*

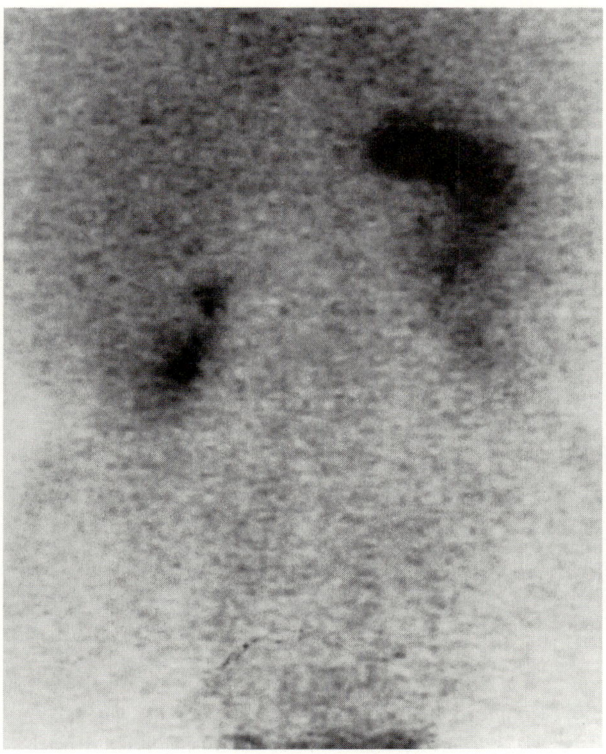

Figure 13.6.10 *Meckel's diverticulum scan with technetium-99m (Tc99m)-labelled pertechnate. There is focal accumulation of Tc99m in the right lower abdomen in the Meckel's diverticulum owing to ectopic gastric mucosa.*

MALROTATION

This can be complete or partial. In complete malrotation the colon lies on the left side of the abdomen and the small bowel loops are on the right side. Dextrocardia may be associated. In incomplete malrotation, the colon is displaced to the left side.

Internal herniation

This usually occurs in paraduodenal fossae or other peritoneal pockets. Immobility and fixity of intestinal loops usually points to this diagnosis. It is commonly seen adjacent to the second portion of the duodenum or the ligament of Treitz.

TRAUMATIC LESIONS

These are becoming common due to the use of safety belts in cars. The duodenum is commonly injured due to its relative fixity. An intramural haematoma can result due to the injury causing obstruction.

Laceration of the bowel or mesentery can result in a mucosal or extramural haematoma. Free gas under the diaphragm may point to bowel rupture and there may be signs of peritonitis. CT scan examination is very useful in the demonstration of subtle pathology, e.g. a small leakage of air due to rupture, mural haematomas and the detection of injury to other organs. Plain x-rays, however, should always be performed prior to CT scan to detect bony injury.

INFECTIONS AND INFLAMMATORY DISEASES

These usually present as acute inflammatory lesions. The most common inflammatory condition of small bowel is Crohn's disease. The infections affecting small bowel can be:

- bacterial – tuberculosis, yersiniosis, typhoid or paratyphoid;
- fungal – actinomycosis, South American blastomycosis;
- parasitic – giardiasis, ascariasis, tapeworms, strongyloidosis.

Crohn's disease

This is a chronic, usually progressive, granulomatous condition that most commonly occurs in Western populations (*see also* Chapter 25). The cause is unknown. Several separate areas of bowel may be affected. The bowel is thick walled and rigid, and the lumen is narrowed and the mucosa is ulcerated. Affected loops are matted, the mesentery is thickened and there are regional inflammatory lymph nodes. Fistulae to adjacent viscera are common as are sinuses to the abdominal wall. Abscess formation is frequent.

Abdomenal pain and diarrhoea are presenting symptoms. Low-grade fever, anaemia, anorexia and loss of weight follow if the condition is left untreated. Many present as an acute abdomen and subacute obstruction may result.

RADIOLOGICAL FINDINGS

Radiological appearances usually reflect an underlying pathological process. These include the following (Nolan and Gourtsoyiannis, 1980).

1 Thickening of mucosal folds due to oedema.
2 Rigidity of the walls due to muscular involvement and narrowing of the lumen.
3 Stenosis due to progressive thickening of bowel wall.
4 Prestenotic dilatation.
5 Ulceration – varieties of ulcers occur in Crohn's disease. These include deep 'rosethorn'-like ulcers or 'aphthoid' ulcers (Fig. 13.6.11), and fissured ulcers, or longitudinal and transverse ulcers, which have a pavement-like appearance or

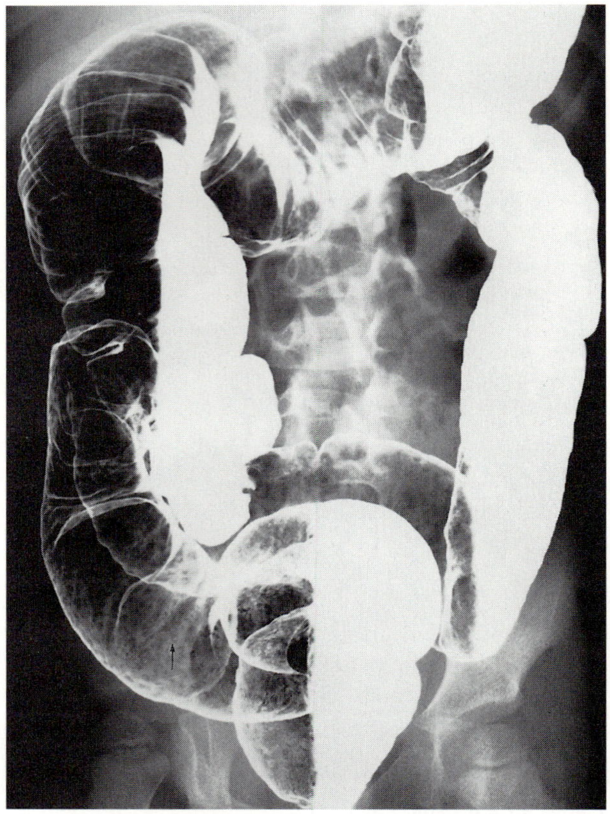

Figure 13.6.11 *Crohn's disease – aphthoid ulcers.*

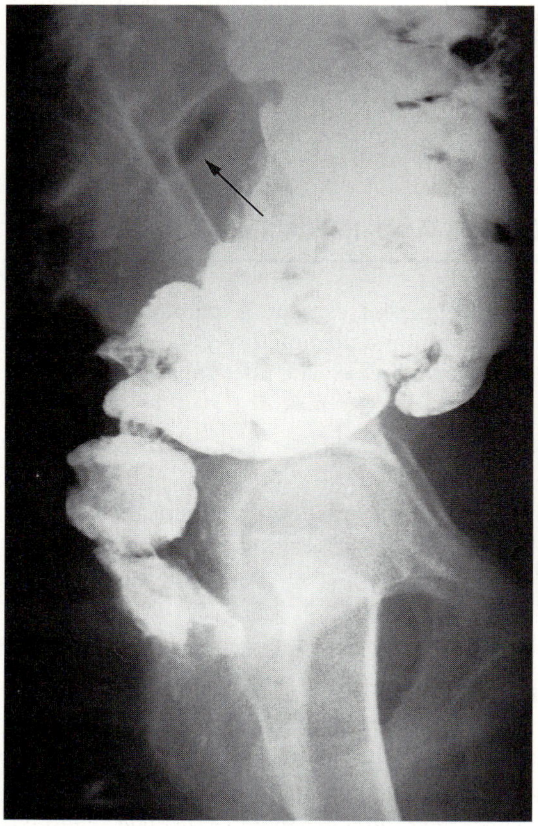

(a)

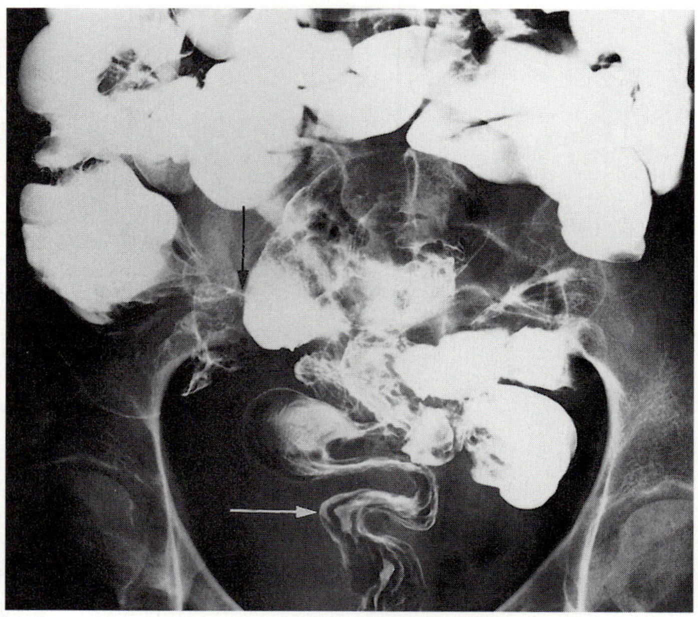

(b)

Figure 13.6.12 *Crohn's disease. (a) Lateral view shows a widened postrectal space due to an abscess with gas within it. (b) Sinus tract (black arrow) connecting the caecum with the rectum (white arrow). Note the absence of barium in the descending colon due to short circuiting.*

'cobblestoning' (*see* Fig. 13.6.15). They occur along the mesenteric border and therefore mesenteric involvement is common. 'Collar stud' ulcers are also seen commonly, although more often in colon (*see* Fig. 13.6.16).

6 Sinuses and fistulae – deep ulcers perforate the bowel, causing abscesses, and lead to sinus tract formation or fistulous communications (Fig. 13.6.12a,b).

7 Asymmetrical involvement – a typical feature of this disease process. One side of the bowel is affected, which results in contraction and therefore the involved side becomes shorter than the unaffected side and often 'pseudodiverticula' are seen.

8 Skip lesions – another characteristic feature of the disease process wherein long segments of unaffected bowel alternate with diseased bowel extending throughout the gastrointestinal tract (Fig. 13.6.13).

9 Inflammatory polyps – pseudopolyps seen as discrete, round, filling defects due to mucosal oedema and possibly lymphoid hyperplasia (Fig. 13.6.14).

10 The string sign of Kantor. This usually results from narrowing of the lumen due to the thick wall separating it from other loops and involves a long segment of terminal ileum resembling a 'long stretched string'. There is an element of spasm that contributes to this appearance and results in failure of the caecum to fill (Fig. 13.6.15).

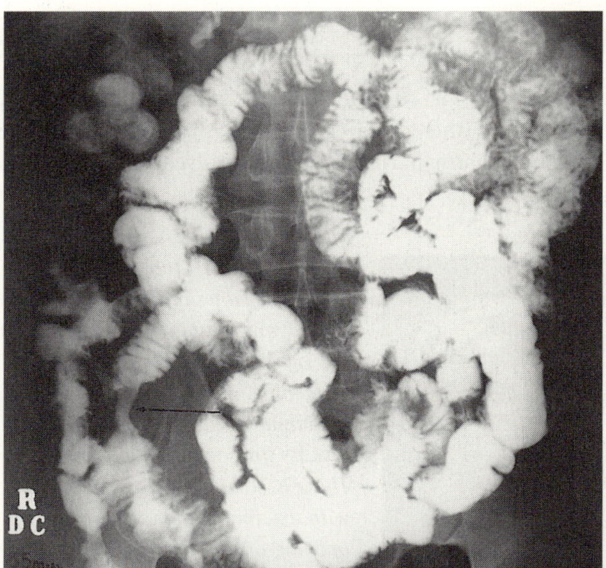

Figure 13.6.13 *Crohn's disease. Skip lesions – arrows showing strictures with normal intervening bowel loops. There is also evidence of extrinsic compression by enlarged lymph nodes.*

11 Mass and adhesions. These occur in the advanced stage of the disease as a result of thickening of bowel loops, mesenteric involvement, and local perforation with walled-off abscesses and

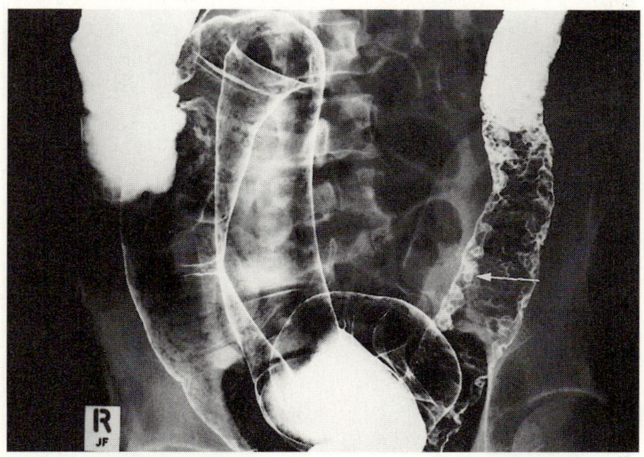

Figure 13.6.14 *Crohn's disease. Pseudopolyposis – multiple filling defects in the descending colon due to mucosal oedema and lymphoid hyperplasia (white arrow).*

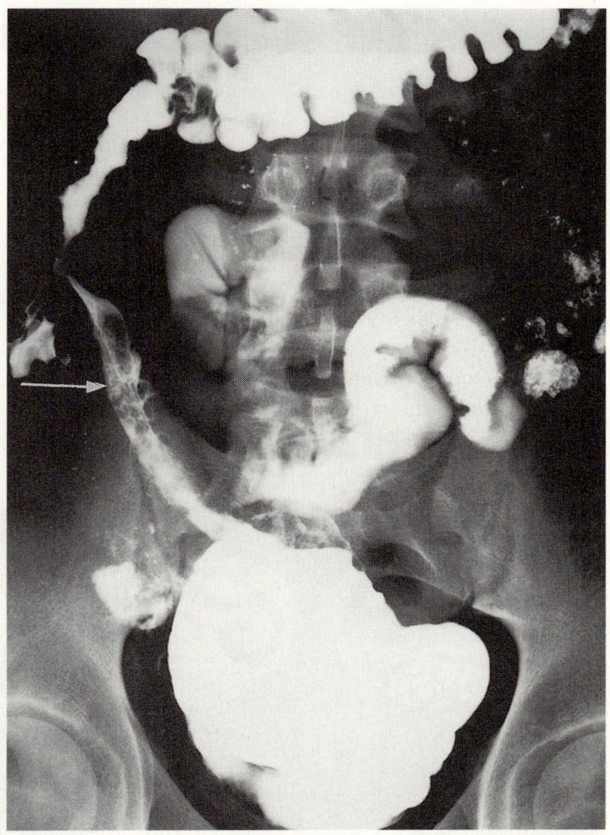

Figure 13.6.15 *Crohn's disease. String sign of Kantor – long segment of terminal ileum due to thickening of the bowel wall and narrowing of the lumen (white arrow). Also note cobblestoning due to criss-cross ulceration and failure of the caecum to fill.*

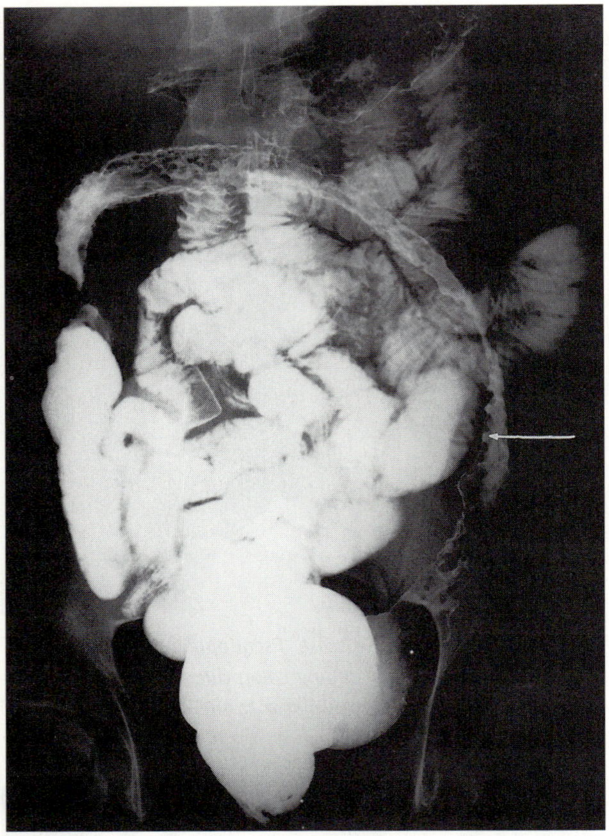

Figure 13.6.16 *Crohn's disease. Typical collar stud ulcers shown in the colon in this case (white arrow). The colon is fibrosed and shortened.*

superimposed fibrosis (Fig. 13.6.16) as chronicity supervenes (Fig. 13.6.17).

12 Signs of small intestinal obstruction due to luminal narrowing and adhesions.

13 Associated involvement of the colon and, less commonly, the stomach and duodenum.

Box 13.6.1 *Crohn's disease*

- Chronic granulomatous condition
- Acute abdomen or intestinal obstruction

Radiological signs
Thickened folds
Rigidity of wall
Stenotic segments
Prestenotic dilatation
Skip lesions (discontinuous involvement)
Asymmetric involvement
Inflammatory polyps
String sign of Kantor
Failure of caecum to fill

Ulceration
Longitudinal ulcers
Rosethorn ulcers
Aphthoid ulcers
Cobblestoning
Sinuses and fistulae
Abscess formation

Small intestinal obstruction

When confined to the terminal ileum and the caecum, the differential diagnosis includes tuberculosis, yersiniosis, amoebiasis, actinomycosis or even lymphosarcoma when stenosis is not a feature.

BACTERIAL INFECTIONS

Tuberculosis

Tuberculosis is common in the Indian subcontinent, and in Asia and Africa. The disease process involves the terminal ileum particularly. The presenting symptoms

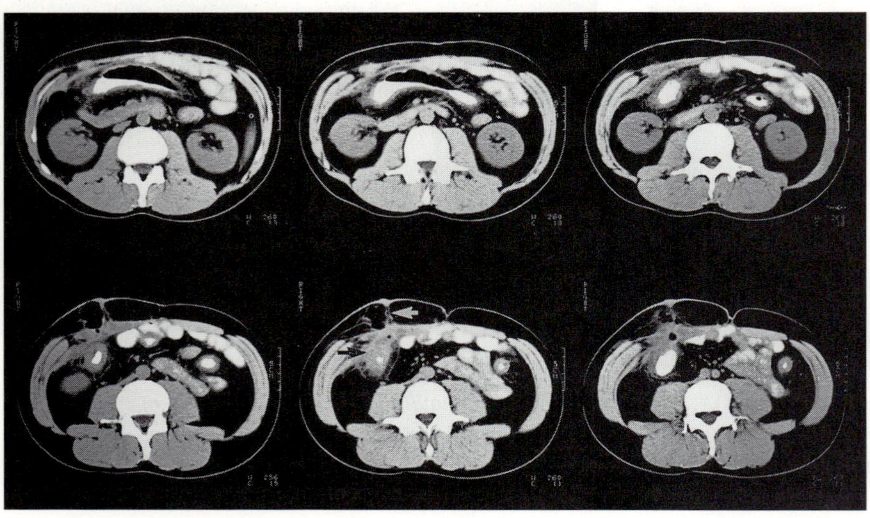

Figure 13.6.17 *Crohn's disease. Mass and adhesions. CT scan shows the advanced stage of the disease in the right iliac fossa with bowel wall thickening, adhesions with anterior abdominal wall muscles and abscess formation (black arrow). There is a sinus tract (white arrow) with external communication opening on the anterior abdominal wall.*

Box 13.6.2 *Tuberculosis*

Pain, diarrhoea, fever, weight loss
- Contracted, pulled-up caecum
- Narrowed, stretched terminal ileum
- Disturbed ileo-caecal angle
- Ileo-caecal valve patulous

are pain, diarrhoea, fever, anorexia, weight loss and, in the advanced stages, signs of intestinal obstruction. The infection is usually passed to humans through ingestion of infected cow's milk and pulmonary involvement is not necessarily always present (Vaidya and Sodhi, 1978).

The terminal ileum, caecum and ascending colon are affected in continuity, and the caecum may become extremely contracted and pulled up, and the ileo-caecal angle is disturbed. The terminal ileal segment involved is usually shorter (Fig. 13.6.18a,b). Asymmetric involvement, cobblestoning and longitudinal ulcers are absent.

Yersiniosis

This is caused by the Gram-negative bacilli *Yersinia enterocolitica*. It causes acute inflammation of the terminal ileum and is clinically indistinguishable from acute appendicitis with right iliac fossa pain, fever and diarrhoea. The mesentery is inflamed and the mesenteric lymph nodes are enlarged. The caecum and terminal ileum are oedematous, and there is hyperaemic swelling and local tenderness.

The mucosal folds are tortuous, increased in number and thickened with typically small, discrete, nodular filling defects of lymphoid hyperplasia. These changes are confined to the distal 20 cm of the terminal ileum. Radiologically, changes may be indistinguishable from other inflammatory pathologies.

Box 13.6.3 *Yersiniosis*

- Mimics acute appendicitis
- Distal 20 cm of terminal ileum involved
- Thickened mucosal folds
- Nodular filling defects of lymphoid hyperplasia and inflammatory oedema

Typhoid and paratyphoid infections

Radiological investigations are performed only if diagnosis of typhoid is not established. There are radiological signs of intestinal hurry and increased motility. On account of the diarrhoea, the x-ray examination shows an excess of gas in the bowel loops, and some mucosal oedema and fluid levels in the erect view. These radiological changes are not specific for this condition. Paralytic ileus may be present and signs of

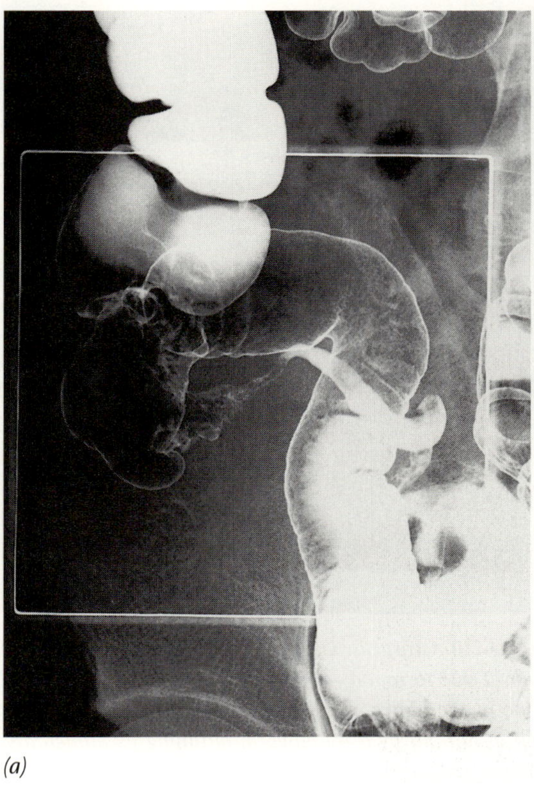

(a)

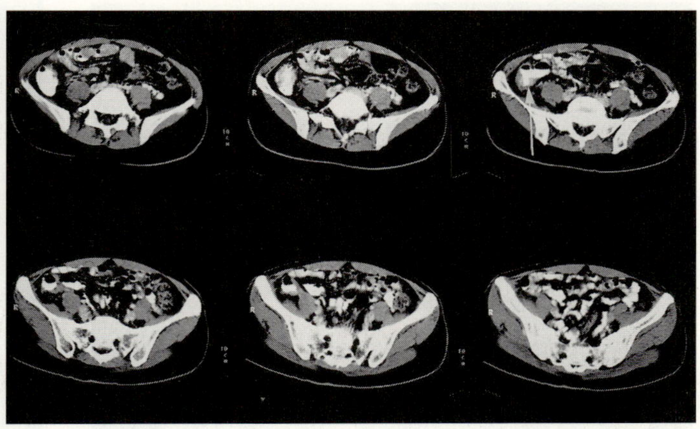

(b)

Figure 13.6.18 *Ileo-caecal tuberculosis. Hyperplastic tuberculosis (a) and (b) of the caecum showing a contracted narrow conical caecum and considerable thickening of its wall, which is better shown on CT scan (white arrow).*

peritonitis are seen. Perforation can occur. There can be ulceration of mucosa in bowel loops and, in such cases, haemorrhage may occur. In paratyphoid, changes are more diffuse and the large intestine is more commonly involved.

PARASITIC AND FUNGAL INFECTIONS (*see* Chapters 19 and 20)

Giardiasis

This is caused by a flagellate protozoan found in drinking water. Abdominal pain, diarrhoea, distension and soft offensive stools are common. Radiologically, there is thickening of the valvulae conniventes involving the duodenum and proximal jejunum, but appearances can be non-specific (Fig. 13.6.19). Malabsorption may supervene.

Ascariasis

This is caused by the parasite *Ascaris lumbricoides*, which is common in the tropics. Children may present with intestinal obstruction. A large collection of worms in the form of coiled shadows may be seen on plain x-rays. On barium studies, long, linear, tubular filling defects are seen in the small bowel loops. Sometimes a thin, linear, central, dense line is seen within these tubular filling defects if the barium is ingested by the worm, outlining its alimentary tract (Fig. 13.6.20). If these worms are present in large numbers, they can produce intestinal obstruction, especially in children.

Other parasitic infections involving the gastrointestinal tract are strongyloidosis, wherein the duodenum and proximal jejunum appear as a rigid pipestem with some irregularity. In anisakiasis there is concentric narrowing of the involved segment of ileum with proximal dilatation almost resembling Crohn's disease. This infection is common in The Netherlands and Japan, and is caused by eating pickled, infected, raw salt fish.

Actinomycosis

This rare infection is caused by the common saprophyte in the mouth, throat and gastrointestinal tract, *Actinomyces israelii*. Poor dental hygiene, diabetes, gastrointestinal perforations, steroid therapy, previous surgery and neoplasia predispose to this infection.

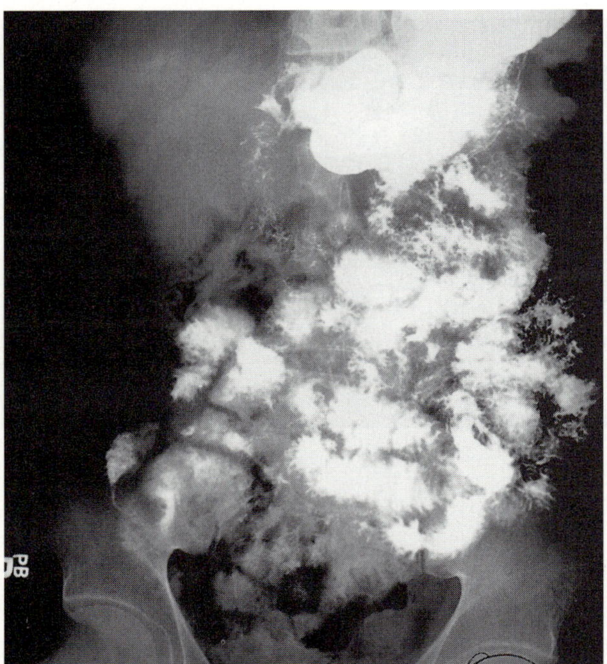

Figure 13.6.19 *Giardiasis. There is rather marked thickening and mucosal oedema involving the duodenum and jejunal loops. The duodenum shows some spasm.*

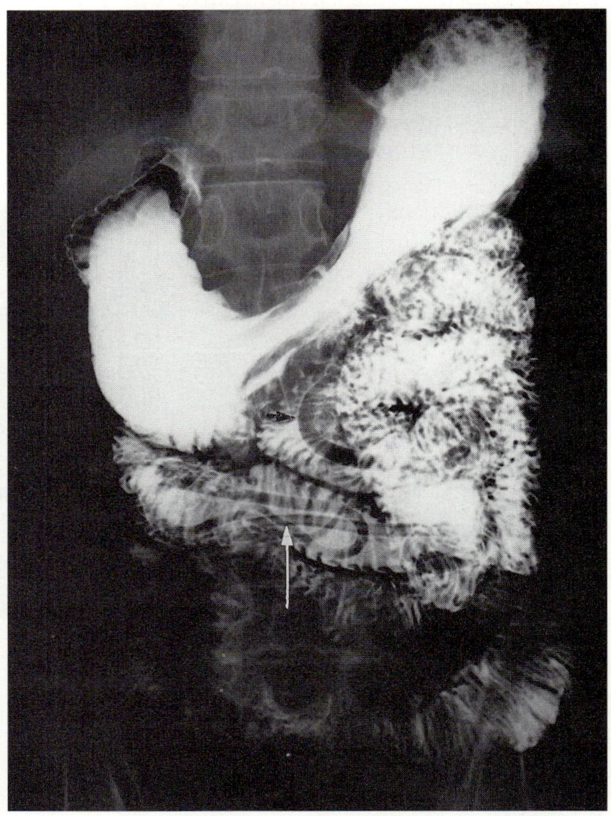

Figure 13.6.20 *Ascariasis. Linear tubular filling defects of the small bowel due to roundworms (black arrow). The thin dense line in the centre of these filling defects is due to the ingestion of barium by a roundworm outlining its alimentary canal (white arrow).*

It usually presents as a rapidly developing painful mass in the right iliac fossa. Appendicular involvement is common, as is a sinus tract discharging yellow pus. Radiologically, there is a mass in the right iliac fossa causing ileo-caecal compression. Enterocutaneous, enteroenteric and enterovesical fistulae are demonstrated (Reeder and Hamilton, 1969; Fower and Simpkins, 1983).

Box 13.6.4 *Actinomycosis*

- Painful mass in right iliac fossa
- Ileo-caecal compression
- Sinuses and fistulae with skin, urinary bladder and bowel loops

NEOPLASMS

Primary neoplasms of the small bowel are rare and constitute about 3–6 per cent of gastrointestinal tract tumours. They present with pain, malaise, iron-deficiency anaemia, obstruction and intussusception.

Benign neoplasm

Leiomyoma is the commonest benign neoplasm with a slight predilection for the jejunum. Leoimyomas can grow inward or outward or in both directions, and appear dumbell shaped. In such cases, the vascular supply is compromised, causing ulceration and bleeding, which is usually the presenting symptom along with pain. They are hypervascular and are seen on angiography in the capillary phase. They have malignant potential, which is related to their size and biological behaviour.

Adenomas and lipomas are uncommon, and are seen as polypoidal filling defects. They are of clinical significance because they form the apex of intussusception and present as recurrent abdominal pain. Haemangiomas are rare and present with bleeding; they can be shown on barium studies as distortion of small bowel segment but angiography is necessary for diagnosis. Hamartomatous polyps are multiple, and on barium studies are seen as multiple polypoidal filling defects. They occur in large numbers in Peutz–Jeghers syndrome and there is an associated mucocutaneous pigmentation.

Malignant neoplasm

Primary neoplasms are more common than secondary neoplasm. The primary neoplasms in their order of frequency are carcinoid, lymphoma, carcinoma and leiomyosarcoma.

CARCINOID TUMOUR

This is the commonest primary malignant neoplasm of the small intestine, commonly occurring in the distal ileum around ileo-caecal region and involving the appendix. Those occurring in the ileum are of low malignant potential but do have the potential to metastasize. The likelihood of metastasis is directly proportional to their size. Local, mesenteric, lymph node metastasis is common and disproportionate to the size of the primary tumour.

The tumours present with symptoms of intestinal obstruction, abdominal pain, diarrhoea, abdominal mass and sometimes intussusception. Hepatic metastasis is more likely if the patient presents with carcinoid syndrome associated with the production of serotonin. In such cases, the tumours have a higher malignant potential.

Radiologically, small bowel enema is the examination of choice in detecting primary ileal carcinoid. They can be single or multiple (Jeffree and Nolan, 1982) and are seen as smooth, rounded intramural or intraluminal filling defects 1–2 cm in size. They can ulcerate and cavitate giving rise to a 'bull's-eye' appearance on barium studies. Thickening of the bowel wall may occur due to muscle infiltration by the tumour. Narrowing of the lumen and stricture formation may be present. There may be separation of adjacent loops of bowel owing to thickening and mesenteric involvement by desmoplastic reaction.

CT scanning is useful in the demonstration of intestinal involvement, especially for the extrinsic component, and assessment of mesenteric lymph nodes and liver metastasis (Fig. 13.6.21a,b). The characteristic CT pattern is that of a mesenteric mass with curvilinear strands extending through the mesentery towards the surrounding bowel loops (Cockey *et al.*, 1985; Gould and Johnson, 1986).

Box 13.6.5 *Carcinoid tumour*

- Commonest small intestinal tumour
- Distal ileum and appendix
- Pain, mass, diarrhoea
- Intramural or intraluminal mass
- Cavitation, ulceration, 'bull's-eye' appearance
- Lymph node metastasis
- Hepatic metastasis when associated with carcinoid syndrome

LYMPHOMA

This is the second commonest tumour of the small intestine, accounting for 40 per cent of primary malig-

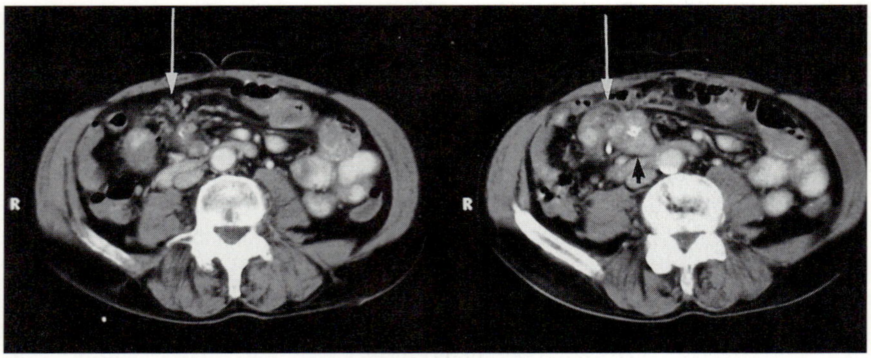

(a)

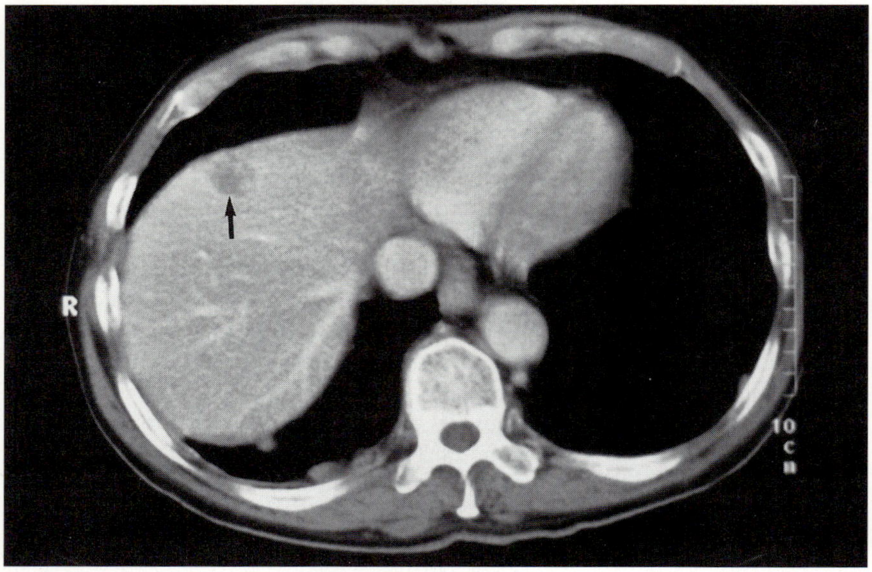

(b)

Figure 13.6.21 *Carcinoid tumour. (a) There are characteristic curvilinear strands in the mesentery extending to the small bowel loops (white arrow). They converge lower down and extend into a mesenteric mass as shown in the next slice (short black arrow). There is calcification in the mesenteric mass. (b) Hepatic metastasis (black arrow).*

nant neoplasms. Predisposing factors for secondary intestinal lymphomas are coeliac disease, immunoproliferative small intestinal disease, chronic lymphatic leukaemia and previous non-intestinal lymphoma. The tumours are more frequently seen in the ileum owing to predominance of lymphoid follicles in submucosa. Non-Hodgkin's lymphoma occurs in immunosuppressed patients, particularly as a complication of the acquired immunodeficiency syndrome (AIDS). Kaposi's sarcoma has also been reported involving small bowel.

Radiologically focal expansion of the small bowel by the disease process is supposed to be characteristic of this condition but is not commonly seen (Fig. 13.6.22). Mucosal destruction and luminal narrowing is also typically seen. Other less commonly seen features include thickened valvulae conniventes, ulceration, stricture formation, intraluminal filling defects and nodularity or polyposis. Proximal dilatation, owing to lymphomatous invasion and cavitation, and ileo-ileal fistula formation may occur (Fig. 13.6.23).

A CT scan is useful in assessing the extent of the spread of the mass, metastatic lymphadenopathy, and hepatic involvement.

Box 13.6.6 *Lymphomas*

- Local expansion of small bowel is characteristic
- Mucosal destruction and luminal narrowing is also typical
- Ulceration, cavitation and ileo-ileal fistula formation occurs
- CT is useful in the assessment of extraluminal involvement, lymph nodes and liver

PRIMARY CARCINOMA

Primary carcinomas constitute 15 per cent of small intestinal neoplasms, with jejunal involvement being far more common than that in the ileum. There is an increased incidence in cases of familial polyposis coli, coeliac disease and Crohn's disease. In the latter case, chronic intestinal obstruction, long duration of the illness and excluded loops of small bowel associated with bypass operation act as predisposing factors.

On barium examination, stricture formation with mucosal destruction and shouldering at margins are

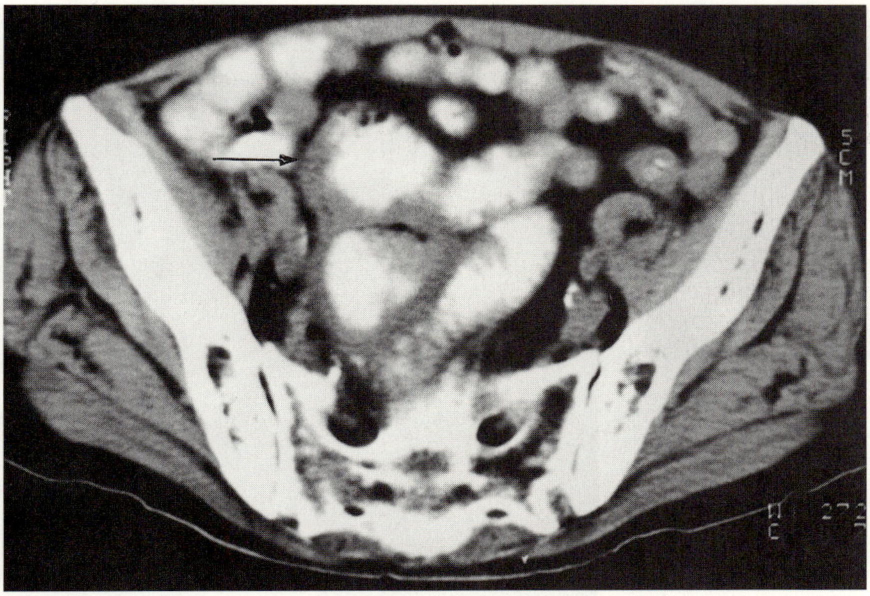

Figure 13.6.22 *Lymphoma. CT scan shows focal expansion of the small bowel, thickening of the wall and thick valvulae conniventes (black arrow).*

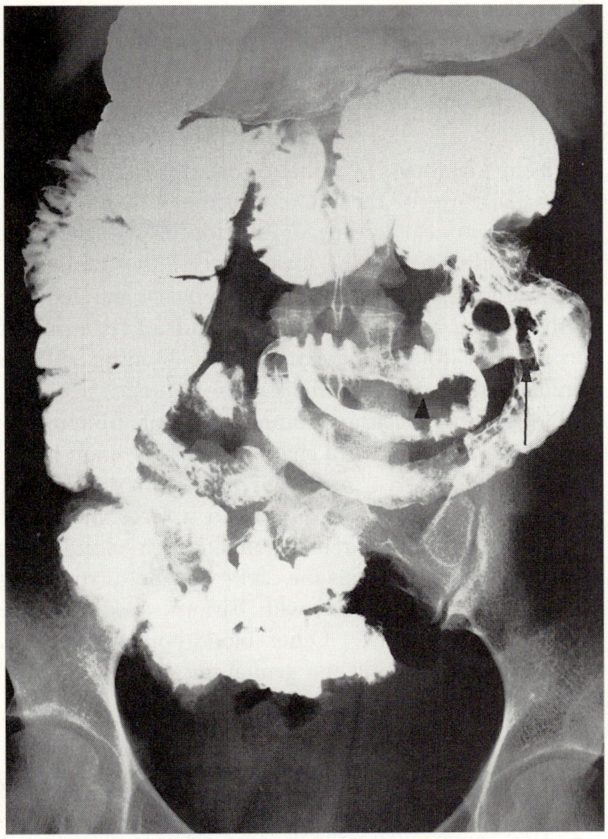

Figure 13.6.23 *Non-Hodgkin's lymphoma. Multiple loops of small bowel fixed in position. Separation of the loops has occurred by mesenteric thickening. There is ulceration of the bowel wall (arrowhead). Note the internal fistulation between adjacent loops (long arrow).*

common (Figs 13.6.24 and 13.6.25). Polypoid masses and ulceration are also commonly seen on good-quality, thin, collimated, contiguously obtained CT scans, and tend to be hypervascular on angiography. Polypoid masses can cause intussusception.

Box 13.6.7 *Primary carcinoma*
• More common in jejunum than ileum • Polypoidal or stenotic with shouldering • Can present with intussusception

LEIOMYOSARCOMA

This is one of the commonly occurring tumours in small intestine, the malignant tumour being more common than the benign tumour. It usually attains a large size and grows extraluminally. Cavitation is common and, on barium studies, a large cavity filled with barium is characteristic. CT scanning shows extraluminal spread quite well and shows enhancement of its lips. Acute bleeding is often the presenting symptom and can be massive.

Box 13.6.8 *Leiomyosarcoma*
• One of the sites of predilection • Large tumour with cavitation • CT shows extraluminal spread

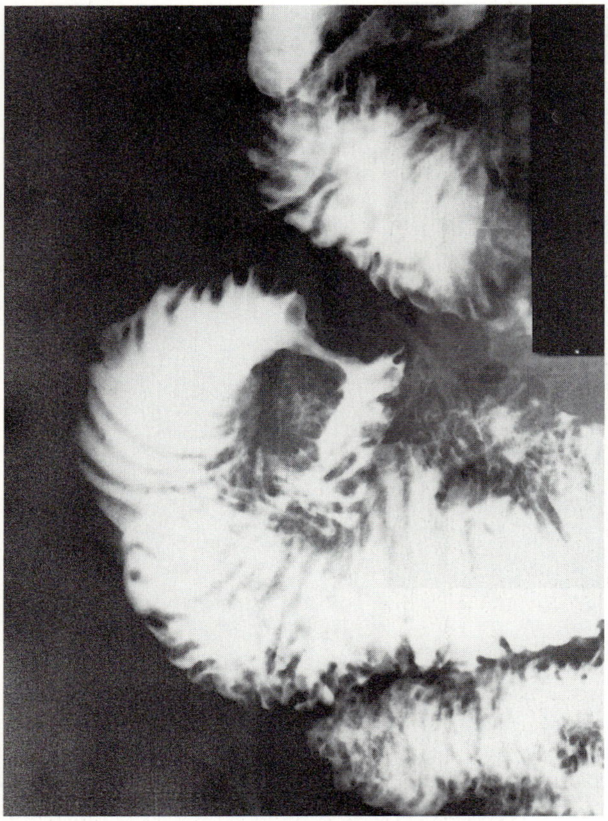

Figure 13.6.24 *Jejunal carcinoma. Stricture of the jejunum with pronounced shouldering. A classical 'applecore' lesion. Note the proximal dilatation due to obstruction.*

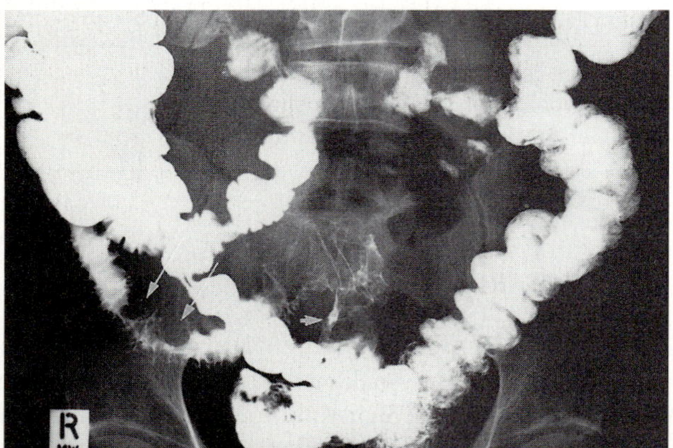

Figure 13.6.25 *Jejunal carcinoma. Stricture and 'applecore' lesion (short arrow). The extrinsic nodular impression on the small intestinal loop is due to lymph nodes (long arrows); there is also thickening and mucosal oedema of the small bowel loop involved.*

SECONDARY MALIGNANT NEOPLASMS

These are not very common but can occur. Various modes of invasion include direct extension from adjacent primary neoplasms of ovary, colon, prostate, uterus and kidneys. Lymphatic spread, when it occurs, is usually from the caecum and terminal ileum.

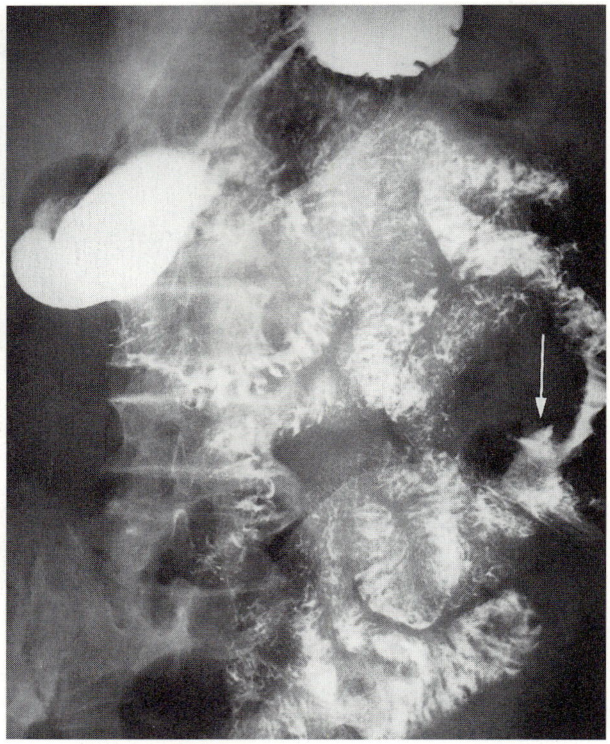

Figure 13.6.26 *Metastatic melanoma. Long narrow stricture without shouldering. There is a large surrounding soft tissue mass due to mesenteric involvement and lymphadenopathy, and ulceration within the mass (arrowed).*

Intraperitoneal seeding usually localizes to the right lower quadrant near the lower end of the mesentery. The ileal loops on barium studies appear separated due to thickening and angulated as a result of tethering of the mucosal folds. There may be 'palisading' due to parallel configuration of the narrowed loops.

Blood-borne metastasis commonly occurs from malignant melanoma and has a characteristic ulceration in the centre, giving rise to a 'target sign' on barium studies (Fig. 13.6.26). The 'target sign' refers to a large metastatic tumour usually from a melanoma, which ulcerates or cavitates. The barium fills the cavity but the surrounding tumour mass is not filled with barium, producing the 'target'-like appearance. Other blood-borne metastases come from breast, lung and genital tract.

Box 13.6.9 *Secondary malignant neoplasm*

- Most commonly from melanoma, showing ulceration and 'target sign'
- Direct invasion from adjacent neoplasms of ovary, colon, kidneys, prostate and uterus
- Lymphatic invasion from caecum
- Blood-borne metastasis from breast and lung

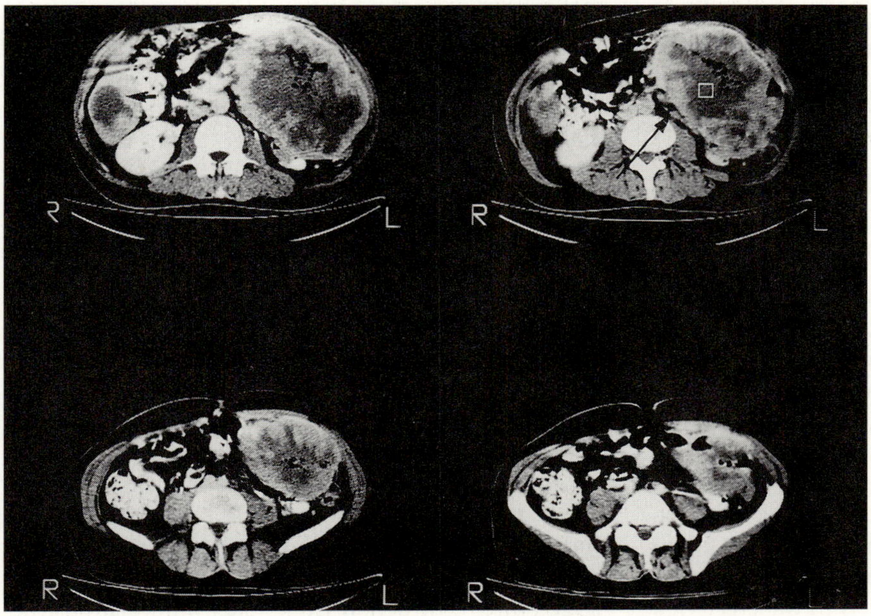

Figure 13.6.27 *Metastatic melanoma. Large metastatic deposit in the small bowel with extensive central necrosis (short long arrow). Note liver metastasis (long short arrow).*

A CT scan shows bowel wall thickening and encasement of bowel loops by a mesenteric mass (Fig. 13.6.27).

VASCULAR DISEASES

Ischaemia is the most common vascular disorder, which can be mesenteric occlusive disease or non-occlusive disease.

The causes of mesenteric occlusive disease include thrombosis and embolism, dissecting aneurysm, surgical trauma, strangulated hernia and intussusception. Venous occlusion could be a result of volvulus or blood dyscrasia.

Non-occlusive ischaemia results from cardiac failure, shock, drugs or severe bleeding. It is also associated with systemic diseases, such as polyarteritis nodosa, systemic lupus erthymatosis (Fig. 13.6.28), thromboangitis obliterans, radiation, etc. Clinically there is usually severe abdominal pain, fresh bleeding or malaena. Plain x-ray examination shows thick oedematous mucosal folds. Barium examination reveals separation of intestinal loops with oedema and marked thickening of valvulae conniventes. In severe cases, ulceration occurs. The changes are reversible, usually within 6 weeks, depending on the severity of the underlying process. Strictures may develop as a result of ischaemia.

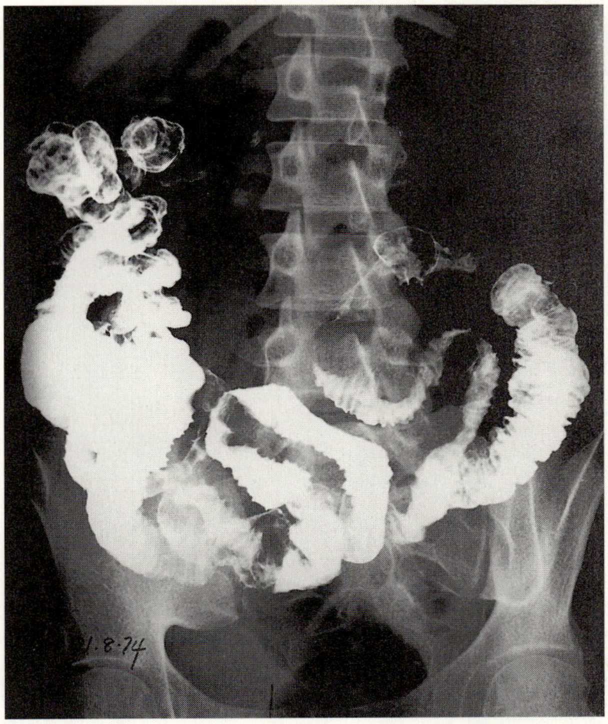

Figure 13.6.28 *Systemic lupus erythematosis. Barium meal follow-through examination showing thickening of valvulae conniventes and separation of intestinal loops. Note the fine ulceration. These changes reversed completely after 7 days of steroid therapy.*

Intramural haemorrhage

This is usually a result of anticoagulant therapy, abdominal trauma or bleeding diathesis. It may manifest as an intramural mass or diffuse segmental involvement. Pain and vomiting are presenting symptoms. Barium examination reveals thickened valvulae conniventes resembling 'stacked coins' (Khilnani *et al.*, 1964). There may be 'thumbprinting' due to submucosal bleeding. There may be single or multiple filling defects, scalloped contour of the bowel and, sometimes, narrowing of the lumen.

SMALL INTESTINAL OBSTRUCTION (*see* Chapter 28)

This is a very common problem in clinical practice and, if untreated, has a very high mortality (more than 50 per cent). Prompt diagnosis, fluid replacement and restoration of electrolyte imbalance is of paramount importance. Crampy abdominal pain, abdominal distension, nausea and vomiting are typical clinical features. Radiology plays an important role in the diagnosis of this condition. Most of the time, plain x-rays of the abdomen in the supine and erect positions are adequate in establishing a diagnosis. Gas-distended loops of small bowel with fluid levels in the erect view are characteristic (Fig. 13.6.29a,b). The fluid levels in the same distended loop are at different levels and are arranged in a stepladder pattern.

Small bowel loops are distended and occupy the central portion of the abdomen, and the colon, if filled with gas, is seen around the periphery of the abdomen. The number and size of the dilated loops of small bowel indicate the level of obstruction, either high (jejunal) or low (ileal). In complete mechanical small bowel obstruction, there is an absence of gas in the large bowel, which is a good differentiating feature from adynamic ileus. The presence of gas in the colon could be due to incomplete obstruction or as a result of putrefaction. If the amount of fluid is much larger than that of gas in the bowel loops, then a characteristic 'string of beads' appearance is produced (Fig. 13.6.30a,b). If a large amount of fluid is present in the bowel, then the water density of the bowel loops produces sausage-shaped shadows resembling pseudotumour – a feature of closed-loop obstruction. Clinically, there is no evidence of a 'palpable mass'. Ultrasound examination is useful in such an instance to show dilated loops.

Although in the majority of cases plain x-rays are adequate in establishing the level of obstruction, sometimes contrast studies are required for further assessment. Barium enema is helpful in differentiating large bowel obstruction from small intestinal obstruction. Oral barium meal examination, however, is the examination of choice in establishing the nature and level of obstruction. It is safe, as the barium does not dry up because there is a reasonable amount of fluid in dilated loops and does not make partial obstruction complete as is the case in large bowel obstruction. Water-soluble contrast examination is contraindicated

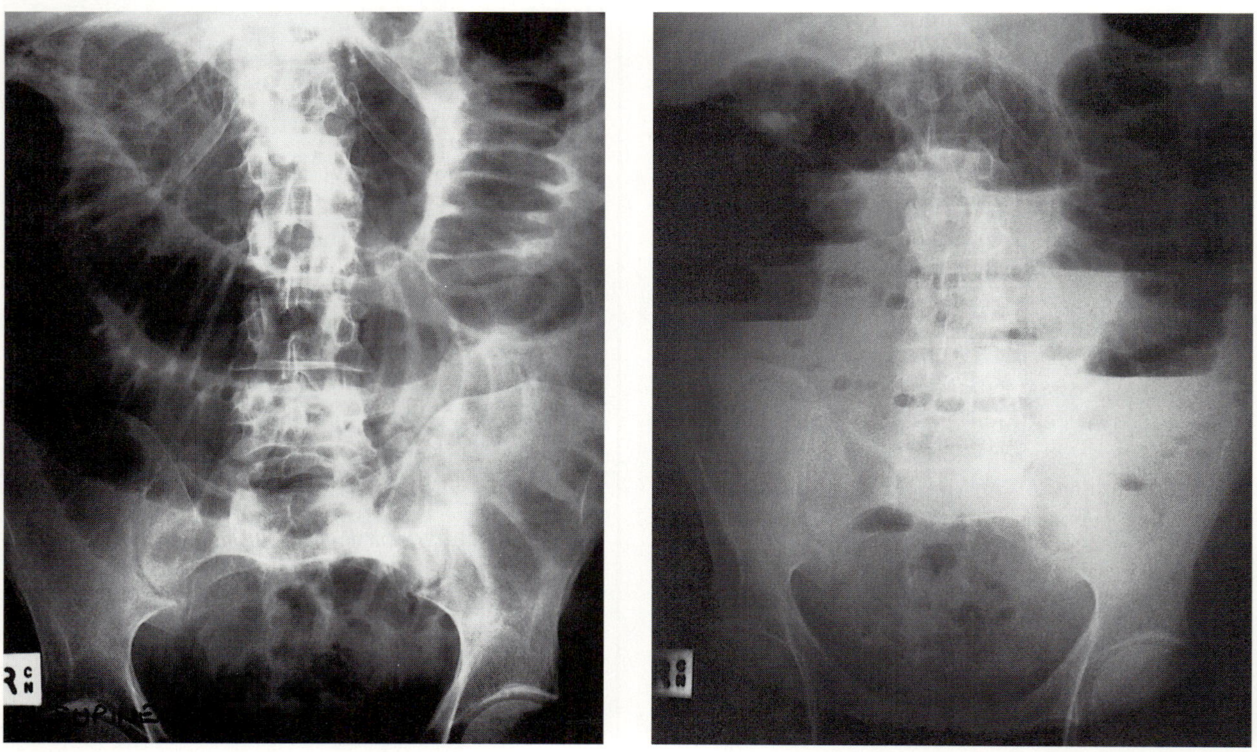

(a) *(b)*

Figure 13.6.29 *(a) and (b) Small intestinal obstruction. Supine and erect films show multiple gas-distended loops of small bowel with fluid levels in the erect view. Fluid levels are arranged in a 'stepladder' fashion.*

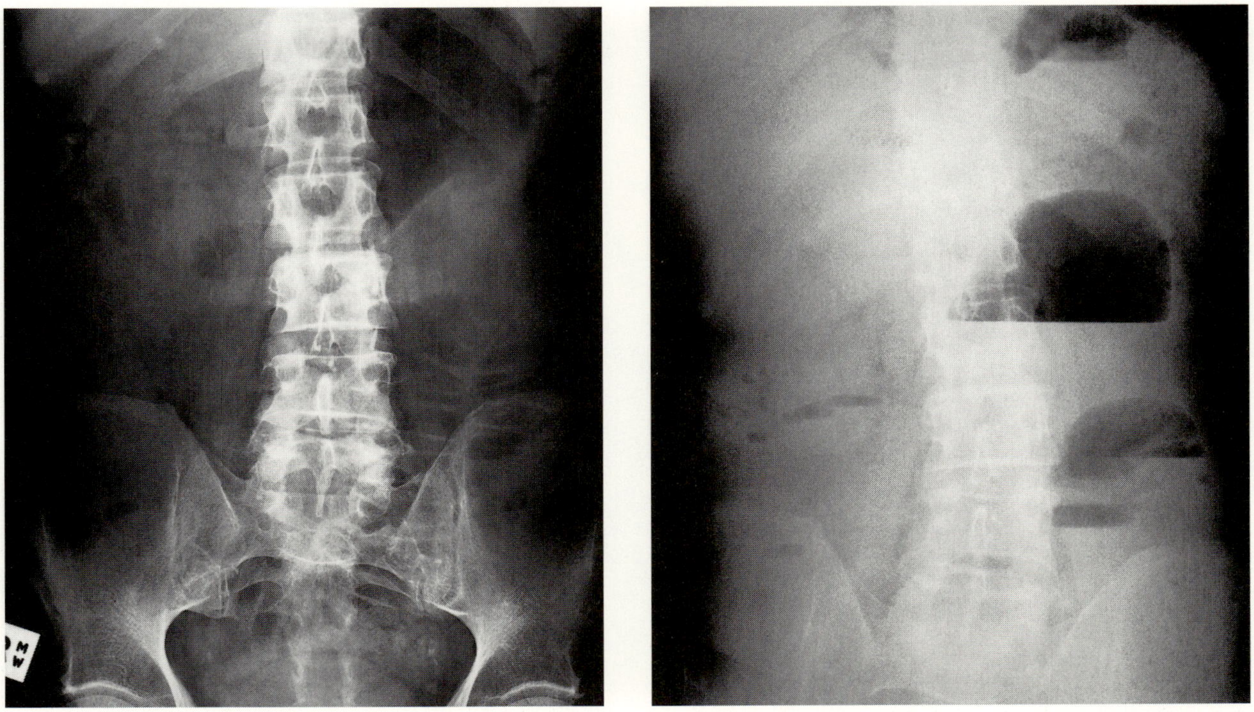

(a) (b)

Figure 13.6.30 *(a) and (b) Closed-loop small intestinal obstruction. Note the 'string of beads' appearance in the erect film due to 'fluid-filled' bowel loop obstruction. A large, featureless, gas-distended loop of bowel in the left upper abdomen suggests a closed-loop obstruction and resembles a 'coffee bean' in the supine film.*

as the hyperosmolarity of the contrast creates electrolyte imbalance and, owing to the dilution of contrast in the bowel loops that are already filled with fluid and dilated, the level and nature of the obstruction is difficult to establish. Oral barium meal examination should preferably be performed after excluding colonic obstruction by barium enema examination.

Box 13.6.10 *Small intestinal obstruction*

- Pain, abdominal distension, vomiting
- Gas-distended loops of small bowel with fluid levels arranged in a stepladder fashion
- 'String of beads' appearance in fluid-filled obstruction
- 'Coffee bean sign' in closed-loop obstruction

Strangulation

It is a special type of obstruction where there is interference with the blood supply, e.g. volvulus, incarcerated hernia, trapping of the small bowel by bands or small bowel entrapped by an abnormal loop in the mesentery. In these conditions, blockage of venous outflow occurs before mesenteric arterial ischaemia sets in, which results in necrosis of the bowel with sepsis and peritonitis. Perforation may also occur.

Radiologically obstructed closed loop is bent on itself and assumes a shape of a 'coffee bean'. Bowel loops are smooth and featureless and mucosal folds are flattened. Complications include exudate and free fluid in the peritoneal cavity, resulting in separation of the bowel loops and shifting of fluid density in the abdomen. Perforation can produce free gas and necrosis results in gas in the bowel wall or in the portal venous system.

Table 13.6.1 *Causes of small bowel obstruction*

Extrinsic to the bowel wall	Lesions in the lumen	Lesions of the bowel wall
Adhesions	Neoplasia	Strictures
Peritonitis	Gallstone	Neoplastic
Postsurgical	Foreign bodies	Inflammatory
Hernias	Bezoar	Chemical
Extrinsic masses	Intussusception	Anastomotic
Neoplasm	Meconium ileus	Radiation induced
Abscess		Vascular insufficiency
Volvulus		Congenital atresias
Congenital bands		

Fibrotic adhesions are the commonest cause of small intestinal obstruction (Table 13.6.1) and account for 75 per cent of all cases (Fig. 13.6.31a,b). The pelvis and the

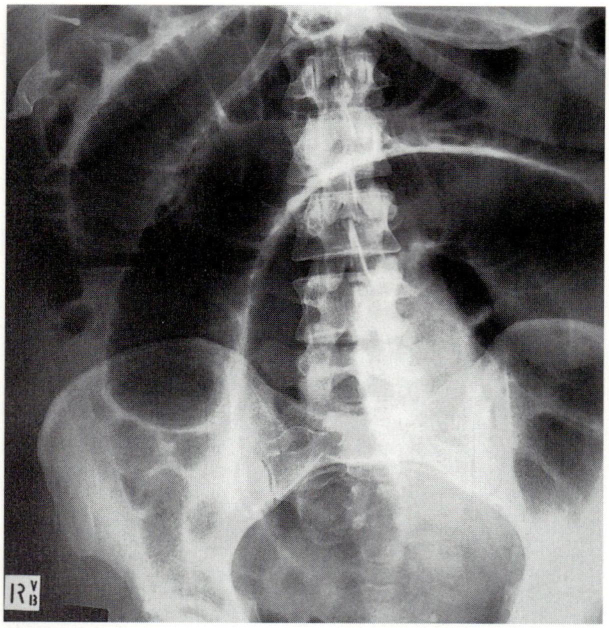

(a)

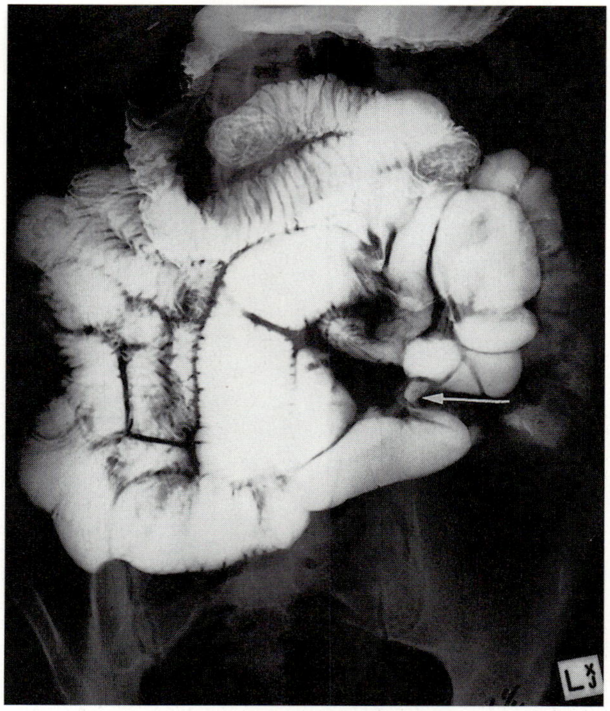

(b)

Figure 13.6.31 *(a) and (b) Small intestinal obstruction. Gross distension of jejunal loops due to obstruction, probably as a result of adhesion. Note the kink in the mid-jejunum on the barium meal follow-through examination (white arrow). There is proximal dilatation with a sudden change in calibre of the small bowel loops distally.*

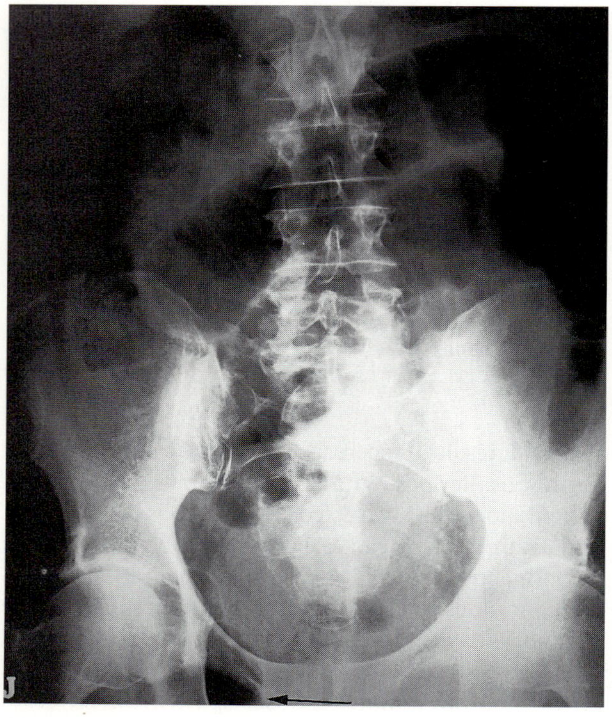

(a)

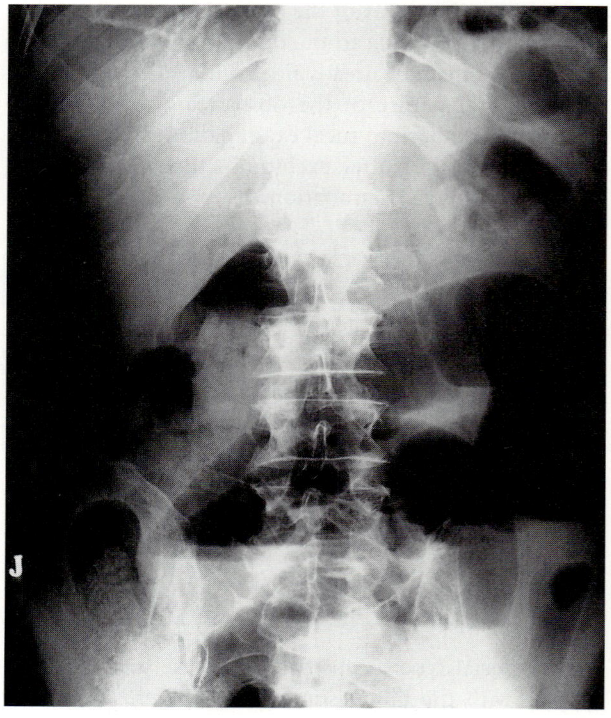

(b)

Figure 13.6.32 *(a) and (b) Small intestinal obstruction due to inguinal hernia. Note dilated loops with fluid levels extending towards the right inguinal region. An inguinal hernia is shown by the black arrow.*

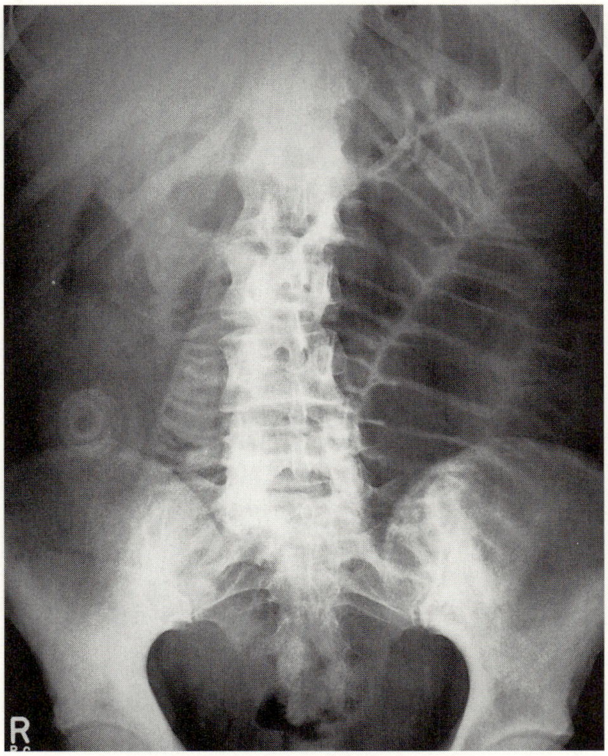

Figure 13.6.33 *Gallstone ileus. A large lamellated gallstone causing small bowel obstruction. The ileo-caecal junction is usually the commonest site of obstruction.*

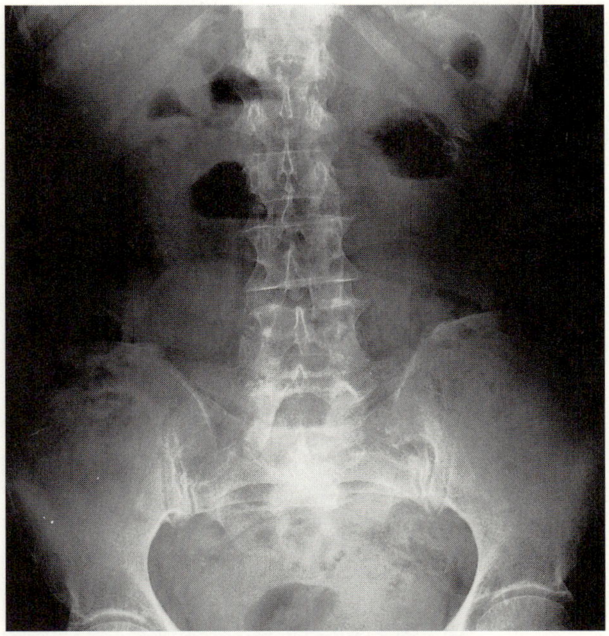

Figure 13.6.34 *Gallstone ileus. Gas-distended loops of small bowel in the left upper abdomen. Note the gas in the biliary tree due to a choledochoenteric fistula following the passage of the gallstone. The gallstone was impacted 15 cm distal to the duodeno-jejunal flexure.*

right lower quadrant are the most common sites for these adhesions, which most frequently affect the ileum.

External hernias, inguinal, umbilical, incisional or femoral, are the second most common cause of small intestinal obstruction (Fig. 13.6.32a,b). Internal hernias due to congenital abnormalities and surgical defects in the mesentery can also result in obstruction, with the commonest sites being paraduodenal and in the region of the foramen of Winslow.

Neoplastic and inflammatory lesions, involving bowel wall or mesentery, and volvulus are also not uncommonly encountered in clinical practice. Radiologically, the underlying causes of small intestinal obstruction in all these conditions cannot be separately identified except in volvulus, where twisting of the bowel can be seen.

Intraluminal causes of small bowel obstruction appear radiologically similar and a large smooth-walled filling defect is seen. In gallstone ileus, there may be gas in the biliary tree due to cholecystoenteric fistula. Sometimes a gallstone may be visible (Figs 13.6.33 and 13.6.34). Bezoars are irregular-shaped filling defects with a non-homogeneous appearance, and are common in mentally retarded and edentulous patients.

Intussusception has a characteristic coiled-spring appearance and is due to barium trapped between the intussusceptum and the surrounding bowel wall (Fig. 13.6.35). It is a result of invagination of a loop of proximal bowel into the distal portion due to peristaltic force. It can compromise vascular supply and produce ischaemic necrosis. Intussusception is very common in children, mostly in the region of the ileo-caecal valve. In adults there is usually a lead mass, such as a primary benign or malignant neoplasm, Meckel's diverticulum, chronic ulcers, foreign bodies, etc. In postoperative cases, intussusception at anastomic sites is not uncommon and is retrograde.

Meconium ileus is a cause of distal small bowel obstruction in infants due to thick, viscid, sticky meconium that cannot be propelled readily. It is frequently associated with cystic fibrosis of the pancreas (mucoviscidosis). On x-ray examination, there are dilated loops of small bowel with a bubbly, frothy appearance within.

In cases of obstruction by lesions in the bowel wall, the underlying pathology is usually visible on x-ray examination, e.g. neoplastic lesions, inflammatory strictures in Crohn's disease, tuberculosis, etc. Ischaemia may manifest as thumbprinting owing to submucosal bleeding or oedema. The radiation strictures are confined to the radiation field and show coarse, spiky, mucosal folds in the early stages (Fig. 13.6.36). In the late stage, there is straightening and rigidity of the mucosal folds or even complete loss of

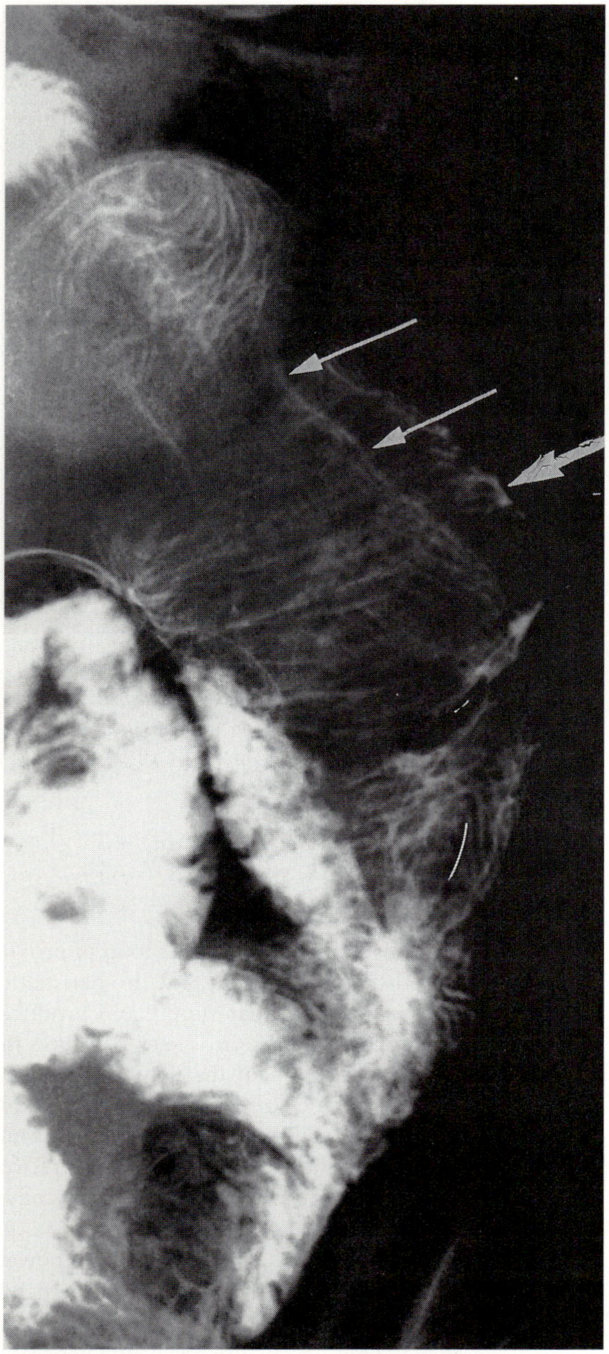

Figure 13.6.35 *Intussusception jejunum. The patient presented with small intestinal obstruction. A barium meal examination was performed to determine the cause of the obstruction. Note the intussuscipiens (bold arrow) and intussusceptum (thin arrows).*

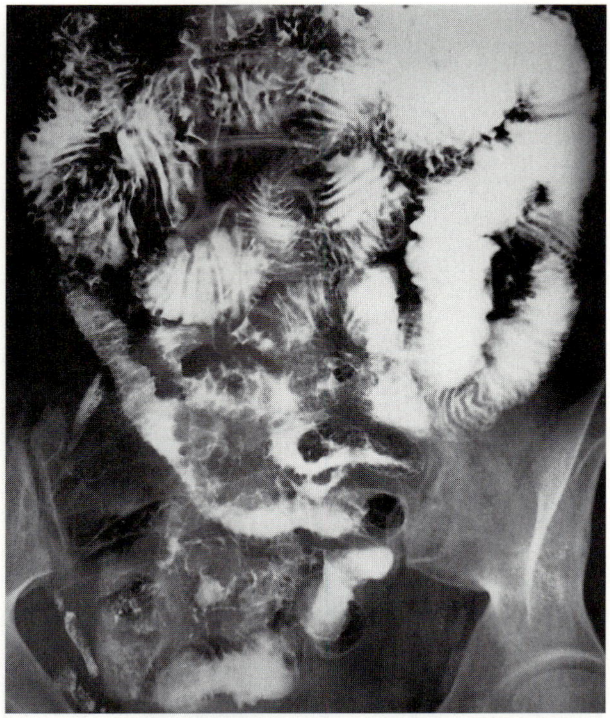

Figure 13.6.36 *Radiation enteritis. The patient presented with signs of small intestinal obstruction. A barium meal examination shows a sudden change in calibre of the small intestinal loops in the false and true pelvis. Note the narrowing due to radiation strictures. There is considerable mucosal oedema and thickening, and a spiky appearance of the mucosal folds due to vasculitis. The changes in the small bowel are confined to the radiation field in the lower abdomen.*

the mucosal fold pattern associated with fixity and loss of peristalsis.

While discussing small intestinal obstruction, it is appropriate that mention be made of the common disorder of adynamic or paralytic ileus. This is a disorder of motor activity in which gas and fluid in the bowel loops do not progress through unobstructed small and large bowel. This can be a result of a variety of neural, humoral or metabolic factors that inhibit intestinal mobility. Symptoms can be minimal compared to mechanical obstruction. On x-ray examination there is gaseous distension with fluid in dilated loops of small and large bowel. Bowel loops are uniformly dilated with no demonstrable cause of obstruction. The most common causes are peritonitis and the postoperative state. Other causes include medications, e.g. atropine, morphine, lomotil, L-dopa, barbiturates and other sympathomimetic agents. Electrolyte imbalances can also lead to adynamic ileus with hypokalaemia being the most common. Less frequently encountered causes include abdominal trauma, retroperitoneal haemorrhage, spinal or pelvic fractures, sepsis, shock, etc.

MALABSORPTION

The most important disorder that falls into this category is the malabsorption syndrome (*see* Chapter 16). It

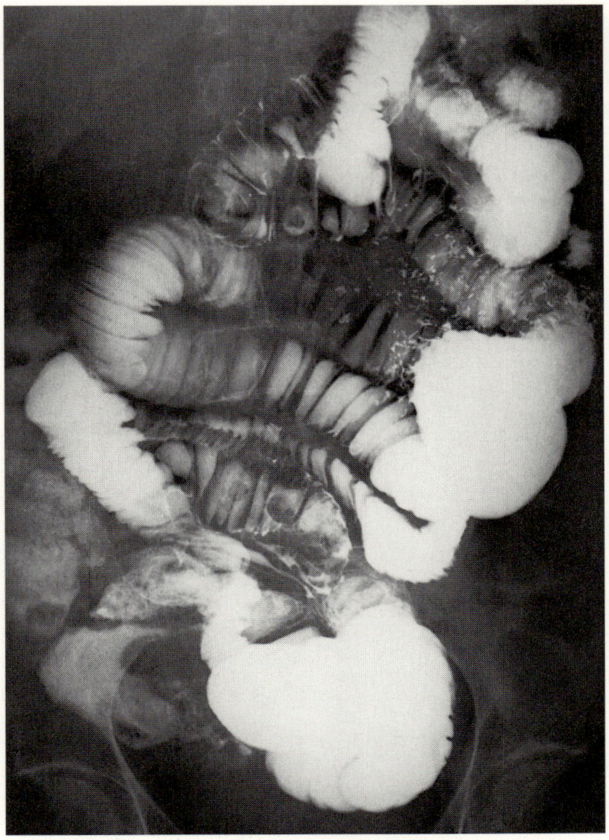

Figure 13.6.37 *Malabsorption. There is considerable dilatation of the small intestinal loops but no obstruction is shown. The terminal ileum is normal and barium has reached the ascending colon.*

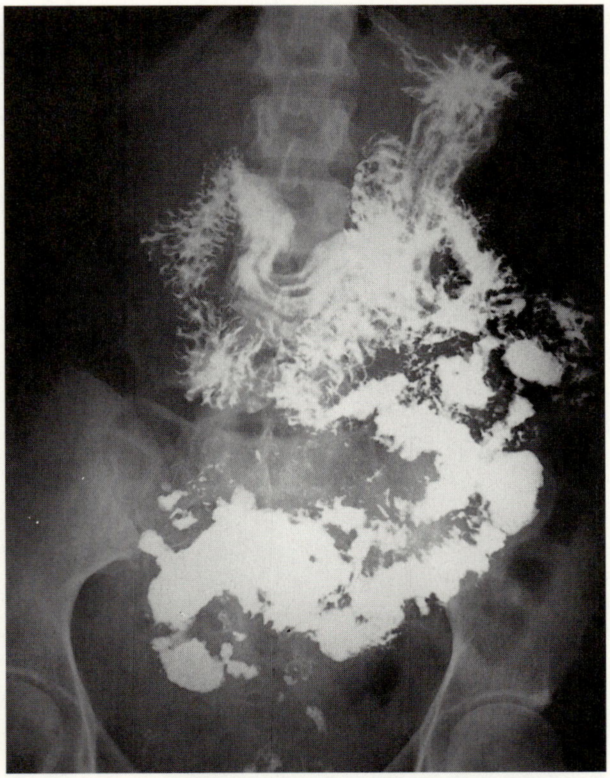

Figure 13.6.38 *Malabsorption. There is dilatation and coarsening of the mucosal folds of the jejunum. The barium shows clumping and flocculation, and there is segmentation of the barium column – all fairly typical features of malabsorption.*

refers to the patient's clinical status rather than being a definitive diagnosis. Before radiological investigation can be undertaken, it is important to assess the underlying clinical condition and to determine the patient's previous abdominal surgery, if any. Broadly speaking, radiologically the syndrome falls into two groups, i.e. those showing radiologic features of steatorrhoea and those with specific radiological features.

In lesions involving intestinal mucosa, radiological changes may suggest the diagnosis but intestinal biopsy is required for confirmation. Tropical sprue and gluten-induced enteropathy fall into this category. Radiologically there is dilatation (Fig. 13.6.37), segmentation and flocculation of the barium column, and there are areas of barium clumping due to the failure of coating (Fig. 13.6.38). The changes are not always proportional to the severity of the disease and the extent of villous atrophy. The changes can be reversible in gluten-induced enteropathy with an improvement in radiological appearances with gluten-free diets. On relapse, the small bowel calibre increases. Normal radiological appearances of the intestinal tract, however, do not exclude the diagnosis as, in early stages, the radiological changes are not manifest.

In Whipple's disease, similar changes are seen but in addition there are enlarged lymph nodes (better shown on CT scan) and bony changes resembling rheumatoid arthritis, and there is sclerosis of the sacro-iliac joints.

Whenever there are defects of digestion, as in obstructive jaundice or biliary cirrhosis, the radiological changes are not severe but their underlying cause, e.g. gallbladder or pancreatic cancer, may be demonstrable on CT scanning or ultrasound examination. Pancreatic calcification may point to chronic pancreatitis as the

Box 13.6.11 *Malabsorption*

Radiological features of steatorrhoea:

- Dilatation, segmentation, and flocculation and clumping of barium

Causes:

- Coeliac disease
- Tropical sprue
- Gluten-induced enteropathy
- Obstructive jaundice
- Chronic pancreatitis
- Pancreatectomy
- Postgastrectomy states

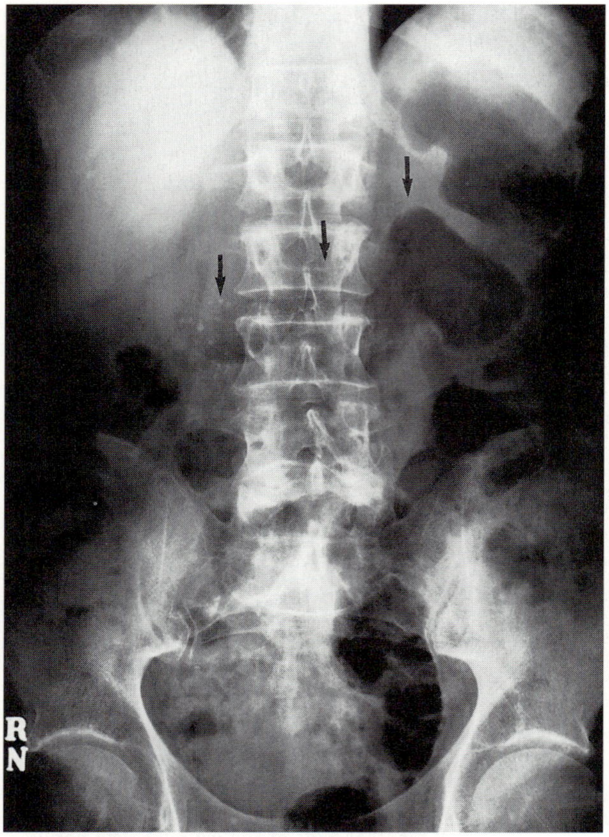

Figure 13.6.39 *Calcific pancreatitis. The foci of calcification are scattered throughout the pancreas (black arrows).*

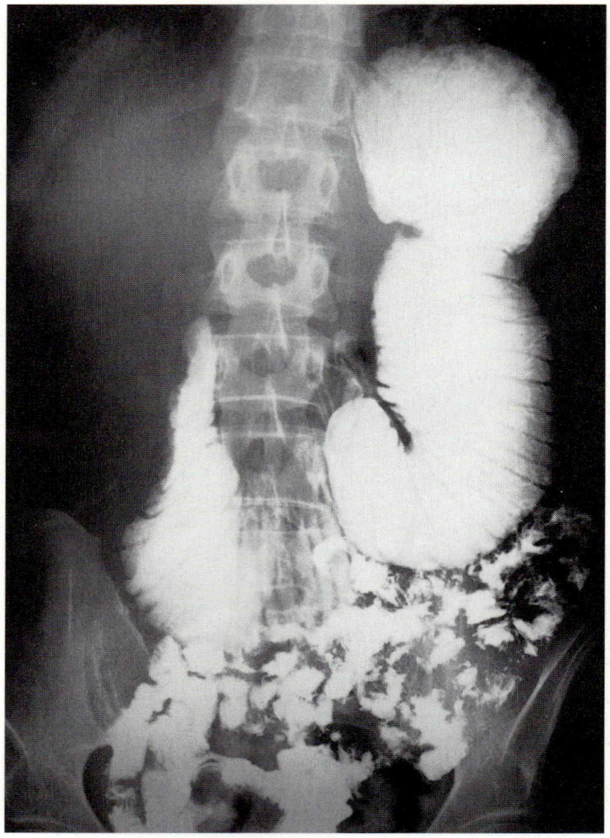

Figure 13.6.40 *Postgastrectomy blind loop causing malabsorption. Gross distension of the blind loop and stagnation of barium. Changes of malabsorption in the form of clumping segmentation and flocculation of barium are seen.*

underlying abnormality (Fig. 13.6.39). In defective digestion in postgastrectomy states, radiological changes are not usually seen but stagnation in an afferent loop may be demonstrable (Fig. 13.6.40).

In Crohn's disease, intestinal lymphoma or scleroderma can cause malabsorption, and there are usually multiple lesions causing stagnation with resultant malabsorption. The radiological changes with Crohn's disease are described elsewhere in this chapter (page 256). In intestinal lymphomas there is often localized dilatation of intestinal loops. Multiple ulcerated filling defects are present. In Hodgkin's disease there is villous atrophy. Rigid narrow areas may cause partial obstruction. A CT scan is useful in the assessment of any associated lymphadenopathy and enlargement of the liver and spleen.

When scleroderma is the underlying cause, the duodenum in particular is severely dilated, along with other small intestinal loops, but the folds are not thickened and there is no ulceration. Lack of peristalsis results in functional obstruction producing dilatation of loops.

Anatomical lesions such as the resection of bowel loops can cause malabsorption. The extent of bowel resection is directly proportional to the degree of malabsorption and malabsorption is more likely to occur in ileal resection than jejunal resection. These resections are more common in Crohn's disease, neoplastic lesions, adhesions, etc. With excision of the terminal ileum, malabsorption is more likely, owing to vitamin B_{12} deficiency.

Whenever there is stagnation of intestinal contents, as in jejunal diverticulosis (Fig. 13.6.41a,b), postoperative states resulting in blind loops, fistulous communications or small bowel strictures, etc., bacterial contamination supervenes and malabsorption results. Blind loops are common in side-to-side anastomosis following bowel resections. Strictures are usually a result of Crohn's disease, tuberculosis and adhesions. Fistulae

Box 13.6.12 *Malabsorption*

Conditions with specific x-ray features:

- Diseases of small intestine
- Crohn's disease
- Lymphomas
- Scleroderma
- Bowel resection
- Stagnant loops
- Jejunal diverticulosis
- Strictures, sinuses and fistulae
- Bacterial contamination

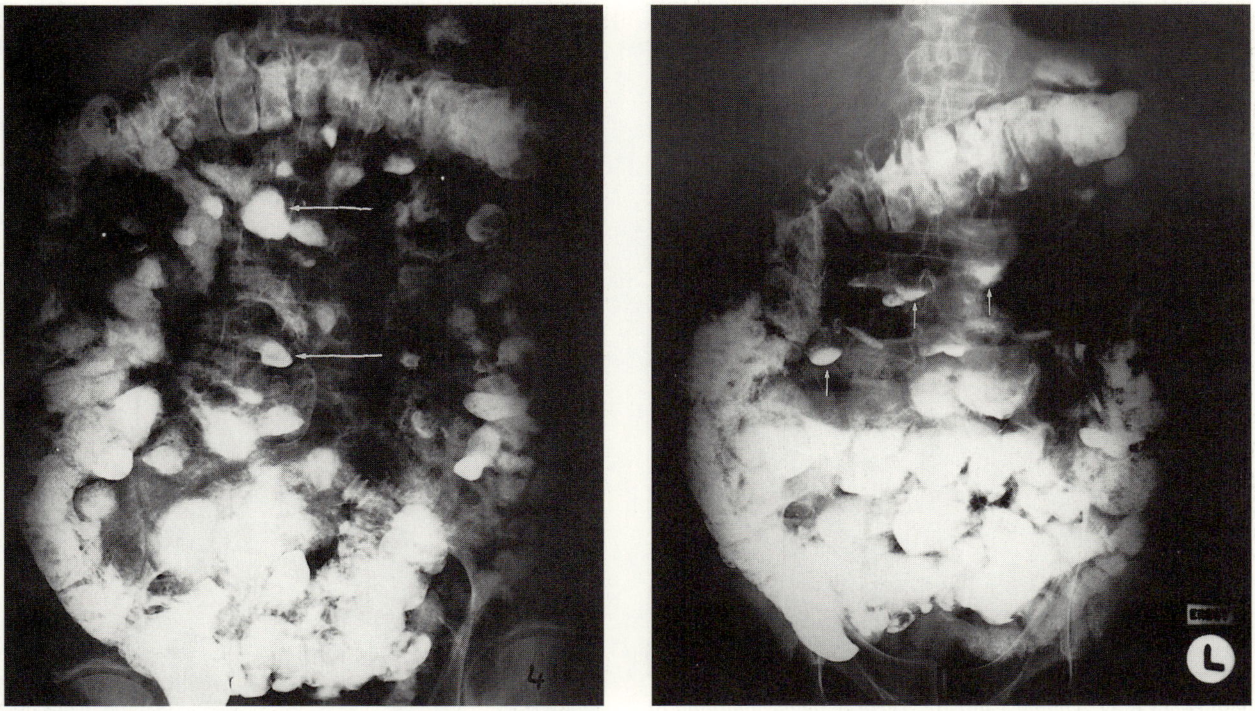

(a) *(b)*

Figure 13.6.41 *(a) and (b) Malabsorption due to jejunal diverticulosis. The erect film shows fluid levels within diverticula. The rest of the small bowel shows flocculation and clumping of barium suggesting malabsorption.*

are common in Crohn's disease, diverticular disease and neoplastic lesions. In these settings the diagnosis is usually obvious on a barium meal follow-through and barium enema examinations. Sometimes a combination of these factors can contribute to malabsorption.

Disaccharidase deficiency (*see* Chapter 24) is another cause of malabsorption, which is not commonly encountered in clinical practice. This condition results in an inability to break sucrose, maltose and lactose into monosaccharides and, subsequently, large unsplit molecules of sugar remain in the small bowel lumen increasing the osmotic load and leading to diarrhoea. Hyposucrasia is rare and hypomaltasia occurs as a part of multiple enzyme deficiency as in kwashiorkor syndrome.

Box 13.6.13 *Disaccharidase deficiency and idiopathic steatorrhoea*

Disaccharidase deficiency
Dilution of contrast in small bowel
Mucosal folds non-dilated or thickened
Rapid transit of contrast on barium meal follow-through examination with addition of test sugar

Idiopathic steatorrhoea
Dilution of contrast
Dilatation and thickening of mucosal folds
Segmentation and flocculation
Slow transit

Hypolactasia is the commonest form of disaccharidase deficiency and is commonest in Indians, Pakistanis and Greeks. These patients have diarrhoea, abdominal cramps, flatulence and distension. Biopsy of the jejunum is necessary to estimate enzyme activity. Radiological diagnosis is made by performing a barium meal follow-though examination with the addition of test sugar and observation of the small bowel. Twenty five grams of sugar is added to 4–6 oz of barium. If disaccharidase deficiency is present, there is a rather marked dilution of the contrast in the small bowel owing to osmotic overload, but mucosal folds are not thickened and there is no dilatation; however, the transit is rapid, which is obvious and diagnostic. In idiopathic steatorrhoea, although there is dilution of contrast, transit is slow, and the mucosal folds are thick and bowel loops are dilated.

IMMUNOLOGICAL DISORDERS

Acquired immunodeficiency syndrome (*see* Chapter 20)

Gastrointestinal tract involvement in AIDS is common, with small bowel involvement occurring in about 50 per cent of affected patients. Opportunistic infections such as *Mycobacterium avium-intracellulare* complex and *Cryptosporidium* are the most frequent. Kaposi's sarcoma and AIDS-related lymphomas are also seen.

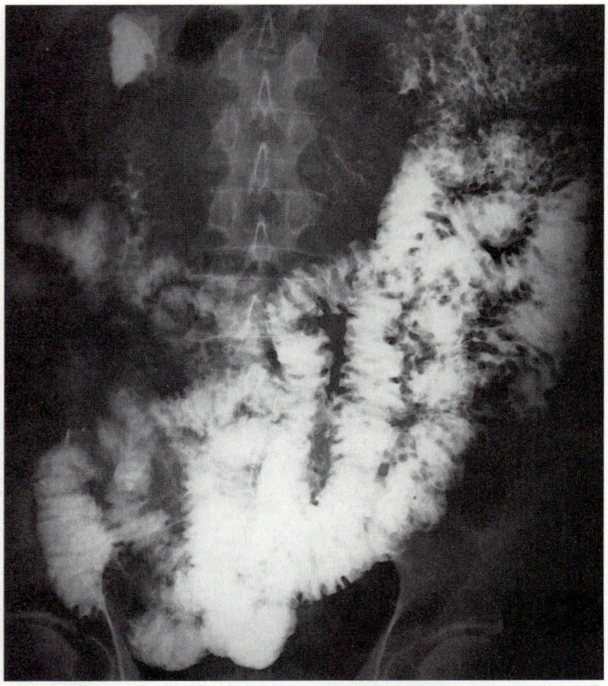

Figure 13.6.42 *Whipple's disease. There is slight dilatation of the bowel loops and thickening of valvulae conniventes.*

Clinical symptoms resemble Whipple's disease with profuse watery diarrhoea and malabsorption being common. Thickening and nodularity of the mucosal folds is a feature of Whipple's disease, and bulky retroperitoneal and mesenteric lymph nodes are present (Fig. 13.6.42). These are only shown on a CT scan. Sacro-iliac joint involvement may be present.

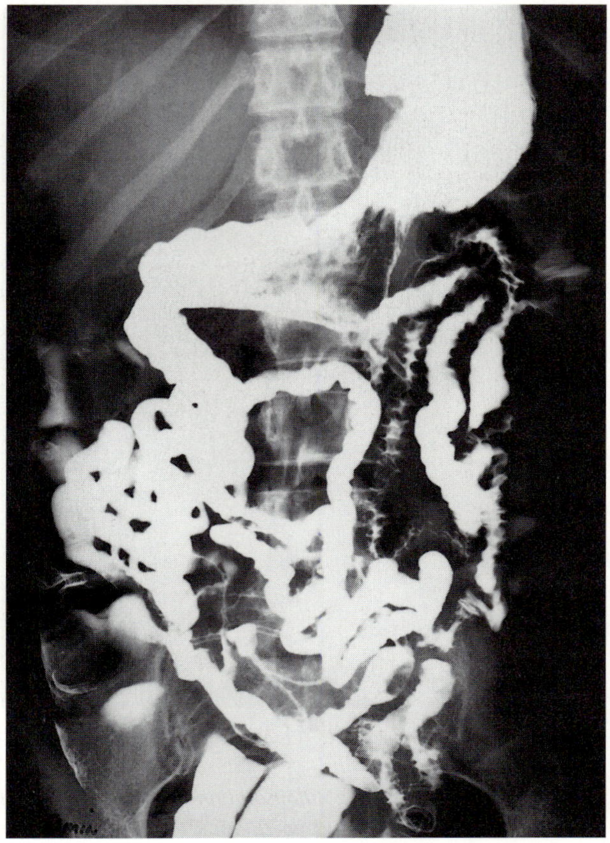

Figure 13.6.43 *Graft versus host disease. There is coarsening of the mucosal folds due to oedema and marked thickening of the intestinal wall causing a characteristic 'ribbon-like' appearance of the barium column. The bowel loops appear separated due to bowel wall thickening.*

Graft versus host disease (*see* Chapter 27)

The disease develops following allogenic bone marrow transplantation. The donor marrow evokes an immunological response against the host, particularly involving the gastrointestinal tract, skin, liver, lungs, etc.

In the acute stage, there is thickening of the mucosal folds and the intestinal wall, excessive intestinal fluid and rapid transit. Thickened intestinal wall may cause a ribbon-like appearance of the barium column in the intestinal tract (Fig. 13.6.43). Later on there is evidence of segmental distribution with eventual resolution but mural thickening may remain confined to the terminal ileum.

MISCELLANEOUS CONDITIONS AFFECTING THE SMALL BOWEL

Protein-losing enteropathy (*see* Chapter 14)

There are a variety of diseases in which protein loss occurs in excess with the result that the protein balance becomes negative. Most of these patients present with oedema but usually do not have intestinal symptoms. The common diseases involved are lymphatic obstruction, intestinal lymphangiectasis, venous causes, such as congestive cardiac failure (CCF), constrictive pericarditis, venous obstruction, and ulcerative conditions, such as in inflammatory and neoplastic lesions. Some other diseases such as tropical sprue, coeliac disease, gluten-induced enteropathy and eosinophilic enteropathy also have protein loss, but the exact mechanism is not known. Radiologically there is thickening of rugal folds owing to oedema of the intestinal wall. The other radiological features are those of the underlying diseases involved.

Eosinophilic gastroenteropathy (*see* Chapter 16)

This condition is characterized by eosinophilic infiltration of the small intestinal wall. Patients present with crampy pain, diarrhoea, abdominal distension and vomiting. Usually there is history of asthma and allergy.

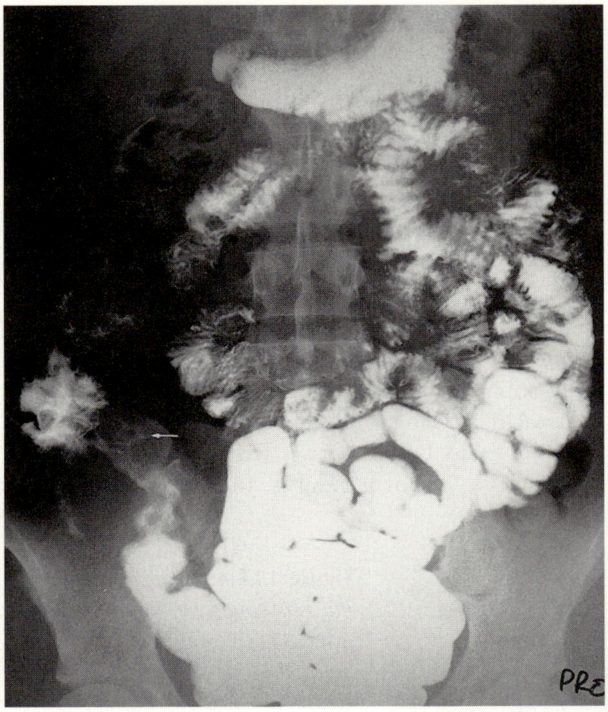

(a)

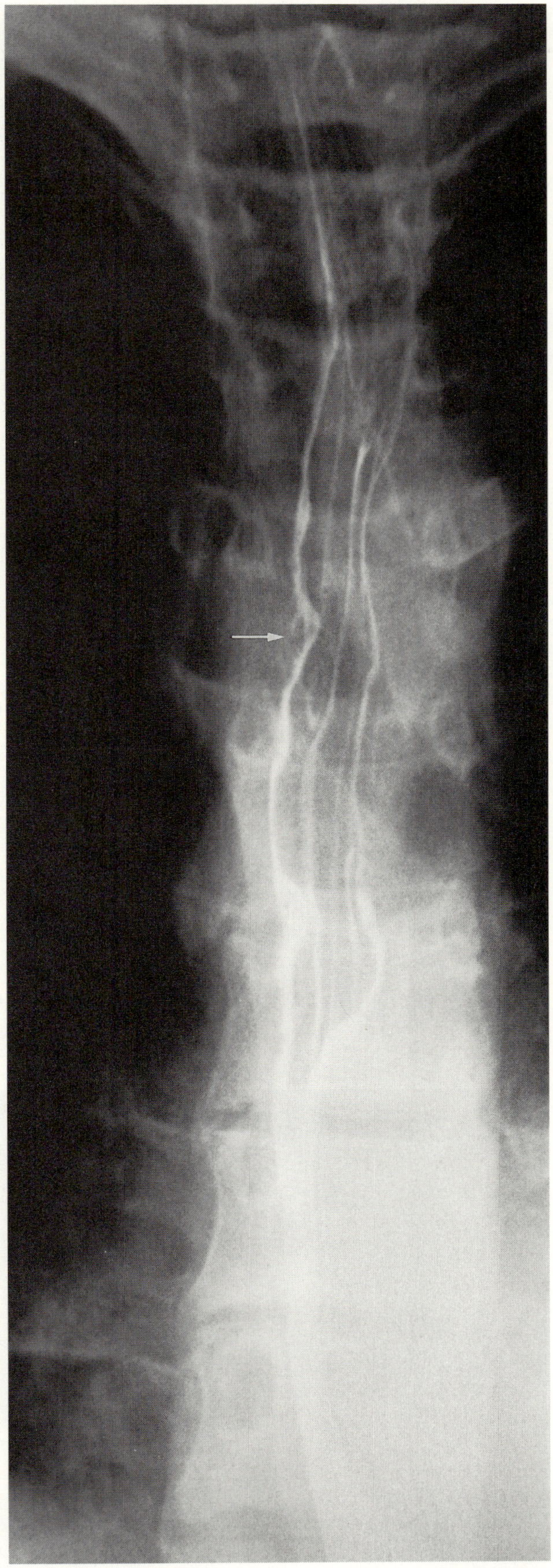

(b)

Figure 13.6.44 *(a) and (b) Behçet's syndrome. Characteristic involvement of ileo-caecal region. (a) The terminal ileum has gone into spasm due to ulceration (arrow). (b) A barium swallow shows oesophageal ulceration (arrow), which is typical and gives a clue to diagnosis. This 16-year-old Caucasian female presented with dysphagia and pain in the right iliac fossa; she had uveitis, arthritis, and central nervous system and pulmonary symptoms.*

Eosinophilia in peripheral blood is common. Patients respond to steroid therapy. Radiologically there is a thickening of the mucosal folds. Severe luminal narrowing may occur producing intestinal obstruction. Diagnosis is by jejunal biopsy.

Mastocytosis (*see* Chapter 16)

This condition is also known as urticaria pigmentosa owing to the characteristic rash. There is mast cell infiltration of skin and other tissues. Small intestinal involvement is common and manifests radiologically as thickening and nodularity of the mucosal folds with filling defects of about 2–5 mm. The bones appear sclerotic. The patient presents with pain, nausea and vomiting.

Amyloidosis (*see* Chapter 16)

There is infiltration of the gastrointestinal tract with amyloid. Amyloid is deposited in vessel walls and may produce vascular blockage. Mucosal and muscle layers of the intestine also are usually involved. Depending upon the extent of amyloid infiltration, the radiological changes vary from uniform thickening of folds to effacement. Intraluminal amyloid masses may also be seen in barium-filled intestine.

Behçet's disease (*see* Chapter 27)

In this condition there is a predilection for involvement of the ileo-caecal region. Barium examination shows evidence of ulceration and sometimes contraction of the lumen. Differential diagnosis involves tuberculosis and Crohn's disease. There is involvement of the oesophagus, which gives a clue to diagnosis (Fig. 13.6.44a,b).

Endometriosis

The terminal ileum is one of the ectopic sites of involvement by endometriosis. There is a localized stricture causing intestinal obstruction. Sometimes submucosal filling defects are seen encroaching on the lumen.

Radiation enteritis (*see* Chapter 16)

The changes in the small bowel are confined to those segments within the radiation field, and are oedema and congestion of the wall. Radiologically they manifest as luminal narrowing, and thick, rigid and straightened mucosal folds. Often there is fixity of the small bowel loops and a lack of peristalsis. In severe cases there is

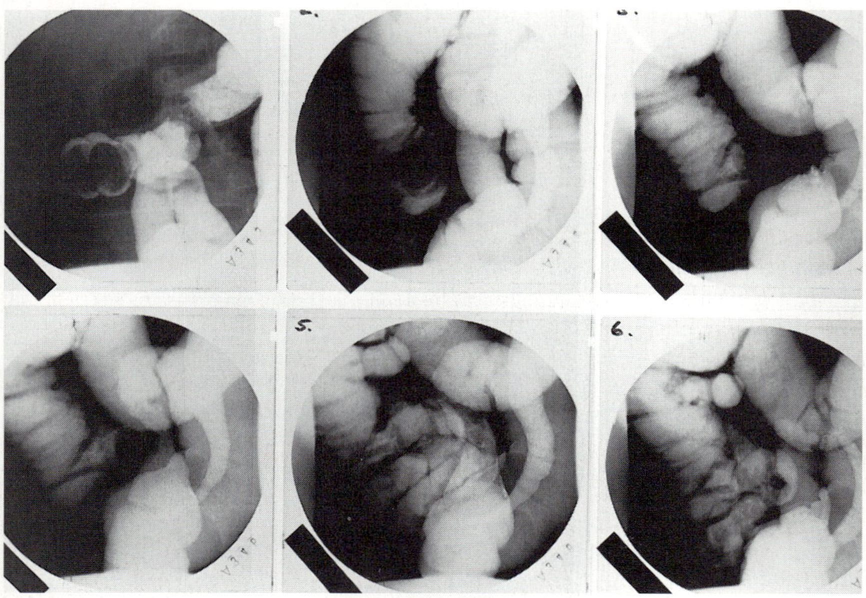

Figure 13.6.45 *Reduction of intussusception by a barium enema. A mass is seen to move backwards along the transverse colon up to the caecum. Reduction is complete when the mass disappears and barium flows into the terminal ileum. During reduction, the pressure should be low as the bowel is inflamed and is prone to perforation. If the intussusception has a long history, and if there are signs of intestinal obstruction or peritonitis, then therapeutic reduction is contraindicated.*

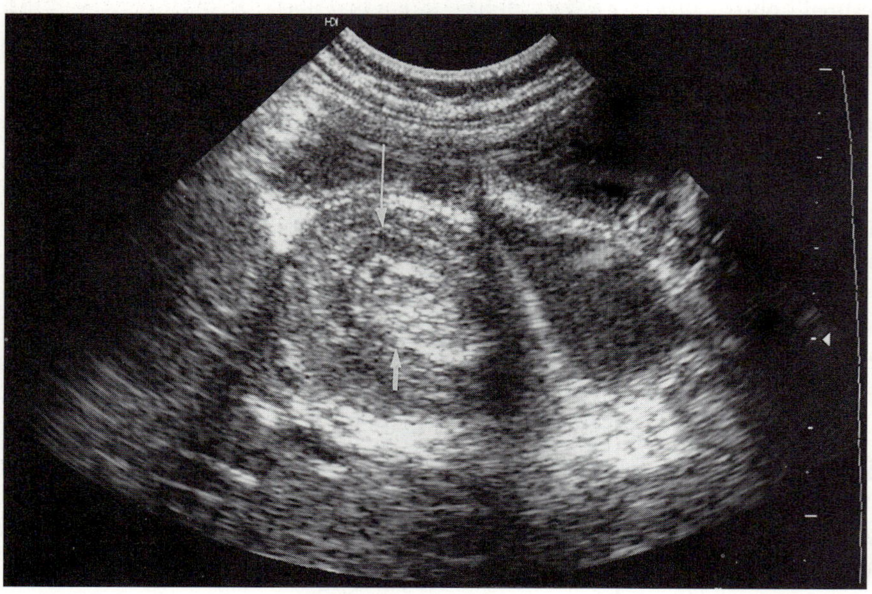

Figure 13.6.46 *Ultrasound examination of the small bowel showing intussusception. The intussuscipiens appears hypoechoic due to oedema. The intussusceptum appears echogenic due to many interfaces produced by the compacted mucosal folds.*

mucosal ulceration and gastrointestinal haemorrhage. Radiation strictures may develop in the later stages and there are adhesions with kinking of bowel loops, which may result in mechanical small bowel obstruction. Ischaemic fibrosis may occur in the later stages. The lower abdomen and pelvis are more commonly affected, predominantly in women treated for carcinoma of the cervix and urinary bladder (Fig. 13.6.36).

Paediatric conditions

This is not intended to be a detailed account of small bowel radiology in paediatrics and only some conditions will be outlined here.

Plain x-rays remain the mainstay of radiological investigation. Because of the danger of radiation in the paediatric population, ultrasound is more commonly used as an investigative tool and with great success. CT scans can certainly be performed but are reserved for problem-solving and for accurate assessment of the extent of the disease process, which is mainly neoplastic.

Small intestinal obstruction is shown well using ultrasound. Intussusception can be easily seen and its severity assessed and, depending upon its appearance on ultrasound, the suitability of therapeutic reduction with a barium enema can be determined (Fig. 13.6.45). Ultrasonically, it appears like a target (Fig. 13.6.46).

Lymphomas and inflammatory diseases such as Crohn's disease can also be diagnosed with ultrasound

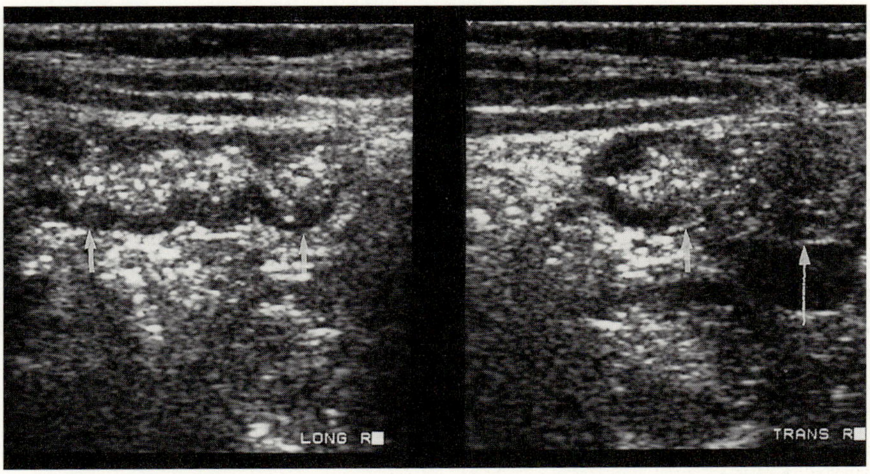

Figure 13.6.47 *Ultrasound examination of the small bowel in inflammatory and neoplastic lesions. A somewhat rounded, lobulated contour with a hypoechoic appearance in transverse scans suggests an inflammatory or neoplastic process, with matted mesentery and lymph nodes (long white arrow), producing a mesenteric 'sandwich' or 'cake'-like appearance. A linear thick-walled ileum is seen in longitudinal scans and as a target lesion in a transverse scan (short white arrows).*

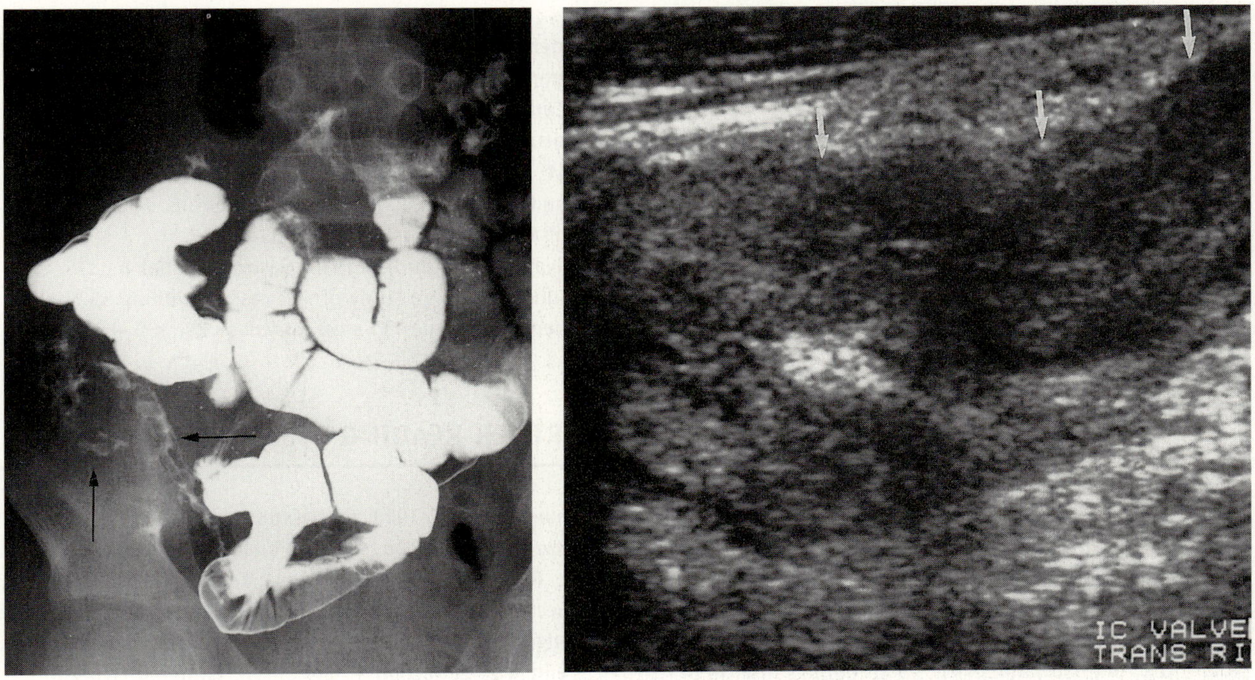

(a) *(b)*

Figure 13.6.48 *(a) and (b) Crohn's disease. Ultrasound examination showing a thick inflamed caecum and terminal ileum on x-ray (black arrows) and on ultrasound (white arrows).*

and their extent can be assessed. Thick hypoechoic segments are seen in longitudinal scans, while in transverse scans they appear as somewhat irregularly shaped, lobulated, roughly rounded masses of non-homogeneous but predominantly hypoechoic appearance. Their appearance is more irregular if there are surrounding lymph nodes and mesenteric involvement (Fig. 13.6.47).

Small intestinal obstruction due to congenital bands and atresias is common, and x-ray appearances are those of any other intestinal obstruction. Meconium ileus is a condition peculiar to the paediatric population, where inspissated meconium causes obstruction, although atresias can also coexist contributing to the obstruction.

Inflammatory diseases such as Crohn's disease are not uncommon in children (Fig. 13.6.48). Parasitic infestations occur with equal frequency in children and are more common in the tropics. Tuberculous enteritis is more common in endemic areas and can be due to primary bovine infection. Non-specific inflammation, such as acute jejunitis or ileitis, when it occurs, is more common in children than in adults.

Necrotizing enterocolitis occurs in infants and is a serious condition. There is often gas in the bowel wall extending into the portal venous system (Fig. 13.6.49).

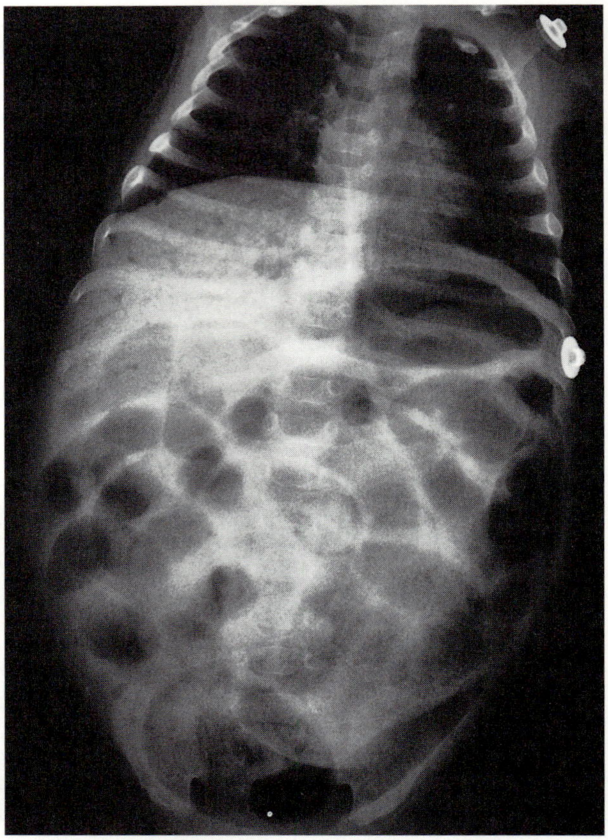

Figure 13.6.49 *Necrotizing enterocolitis. Dilated loops of the small and large bowel with gas in their wall. Gas is also present in the portal venous system.*

REFERENCES

Cockey, B.M., Fishman, E.K., Jones, B. 1985: Computed tomography of abdominal carcinoid tumour. *Journal of Computer Assisted Tomography* 9, 38–42.

Fleisher, A.C., Parulekar, S., Siebert, J.J. 1989: Sonography of the small bowel. In Herlinger, H., Maglinte, D. (eds) *Clinical radiology of the small intestine*. Philadelphia, W.B. Saunders, 153–9.

Fower, R.C., Simpkins, K.D. 1983: Abdominal actinomycosis: a report of three cases. *Clinical Radiology* 34, 301–7.

Gould, M., Johnson, R.J. 1986: Computed tomography of abdominal carcinoid tumour. *British Journal of Radiology* 59, 881–5.

Hopens, T., Coggs, G.C., Goldstein, H.M. *et al.* 1982: Sonographic diagnosis of afferent loop obstruction. *American Journal of Roentgenology* 138, 967–9.

Jeffree, M.A., Nolan, D.J. 1982: Multiple ileal carcinoid tumours. *British Journal of Radiology* 60, 402–3.

Khilnani, M.T., Marshak, R.H., Eliasoph, J., Wolf, B.S. 1964: Intramural intestinal haemorrhage. *American Journal of Roentgenology* 92, 1061–71.

Nolan, D.J., Gourtsoyiannis, N.C. 1980: Crohn's disease of small intestine – a review of radiological appearances in 100 consecutive patients examined by a barium infusion technique. *Clinical Radiology* 30, 596–603.

Reeder, M.M., Hamilton, L.C. 1969: Radiological diagnosis of tropical diseases of gastrointestinal tract. *Radiological Clinics of North America* 7, 57–81.

Srivastava, D.N., Shrestha, P., Vashisht, S., Gupta, R., Berry, M., Sharma, L.K. 1994: Comparative evaluation of US, CT and barium study in focal bowel lesions. *Indian Journal of Radiology and Imaging* 4, 31–6.

Vaidya, M.G., Sodhi, J.S. 1978: Gastrointestinal tract tuberculosis – a study of 102 cases including 55 hemicolectomies. *Clinical Radiology* 29, 189–95.

FURTHER READING

Eisenberg, R. (ed.) 1990: *Gastrointestinal radiology – a pattern approach*, 2nd edn, Part 5. Philadelphia: J.B. Lippincott.

Gore, R., Levine, M., Laufer, I. 1994: *Text book of G.I. radiology*, Section 7. Philadelphia: W.B. Saunders, 766–1027.

Grainger, R.G., Allison, D.J. 1992: *Diagnostic radiology,* 2nd edn, Vol. 2, Section 4. Edinburgh: Churchill Livingstone, 883–908.

Sutton, D. (ed.) 1980: *A text book of radiology and imaging*, 3rd edn. Edinburgh: Churchill Livingstone, 713–40.

14

Symptoms and signs of small intestinal disease

RANJIT N RATNAIKE

CLINICAL FEATURES

The major manifestations of small bowel disease are diarrhoea and its complications, abdominal pain and bleeding, and a variety of consequences of deranged digestive or absorptive processes.

SYMPTOMS

Nausea and vomiting

Nausea and vomiting are usually associated, although nausea may occur alone. Nausea is an unpleasant urge to vomit that is usually associated with salivation, sweating, pallor and tachycardia. Isolated vomiting occurs with pyloric obstruction or with elevated intracranial pressure. Drugs that are commonly associated with the side-effect of nausea include erythromycin, iron preparations, non-steroidal anti-inflammatory agents and chemotherapeutic agents.

Retching is an involuntary, ineffectual form of vomiting. Despite contractions of the stomach, the diaphragm and abdominal wall, the contents of the stomach are not expelled, as the lower oesophageal sphincter is not relaxed (Seigel and Longo, 1981).

Regurgitation of food due to oesophageal causes can occur without nausea or retching.

Vomiting

Although vomiting is primarily a gastric event, it may also occur with small intestinal dysfunction. Vomiting is a primitive defence mechanism that protects the gastrointestinal tract from noxious ingested substances or infections (*see* Chapter 5) . It involves the forceful expulsion of gastric or intestinal contents through the mouth (Koda-Kimble and Young, 1995). This powerful mechanism for 'clearing' and 'cleansing' occurs through vigorous retrograde propulsion. The act of vomiting is preceded by abnormal peristaltic activity of the small bowel and inhibition of gastric peristalsis. Table 14.1 lists the causes of vomiting related to the small intestine. Vomiting due to small intestinal pathology is often associated with abdominal pain (see below). It is unusual for ileal or colonic contents to be expelled during vomiting, although the large bowel may contract.

Table 14.1 *Small intestinal causes (intrinsic) of acute nausea and vomiting*

Viral gastroenteritis (*see* Chapter 17)
Bacterial infections (*see* Chapter 18)
Parasitic infections (*see* Chapter 19)
Mechanical obstruction (*see* Chapter 28)
Intestinal pseudo-obstruction (*see* Chapter 16)

VOMITING DUE TO INFECTIVE CAUSES

Gastroenteritis caused by rotavirus and Norwalk viral infections are associated with vomiting (*see* Chapter 17). Vomiting also occurs with food poisoning due to ingested toxins. Food poisoning is diagnosed when nausea, vomiting and diarrhoea occur after two or more persons have consumed the same food or beverage contaminated by a preformed toxin elaborated by a pathogen (*see* Chapter 18). The incubation period is short and the onset of symptoms is abrupt. The bacteria commonly implicated in food poisoning are *Staphylococcus aureus*, *Bacillus cereus*, *Clostridium perfringens* and *Vibrio parahaemolyticus*. Confusion often arises when vomiting is associated with symptoms and signs of a large bowel infection (tenesmus, diarrhoea with blood and mucus) as in *Shigella* infections. In shigellosis, the vomiting is due to the toxin secreted by the organism being absorbed during its passage through the small intestine. Parasitic infections of the small bowel can cause vomiting, as with *Sarcocystis* species, *Trichinella spiralis* and with heavy infection with *Fasciolopsis buski* (*see* Chapter 19).

VOMITING DUE TO NON-SMALL-INTESTINAL CAUSES

Table 14.2 shows the aetiology of vomiting unrelated to the small intestine. Vomiting may be due to pathology in the gastrointestinal tract that is separate from the small intestine, due to severe, acute pain, or arising from other abdominal organs, or organ systems. Therapeutic agents, chemical toxins and excessive alcohol ingestion are notable causes of vomiting. Vomiting is the most common side-effect of cancer chemotherapeutic agents, especially cisplatinum, dacarbazine and amsacrine. Other therapeutic agents associated with vomiting are opioids, theophylline, digoxin, anticholinergic drugs and antibiotics such as cotrimoxazole (Koda-Kimble and Young, 1995).

DISTINGUISHING FEATURES OF VOMITING AND VOMITUS

Vomiting after food occurs with:

- food poisoning;
- gastritis;
- gastric atony;
- pylorospasm;
- pyloric obstruction;
- small intestinal obstruction;
- psychogenic causes.

Other features of vomiting:

- early morning vomiting due to uraemia or pregnancy;
- 'coffee grounds' vomitus due to altered blood;
- putrid or faeculent vomitus owing to small bowel obstruction; with an infection or a gastrocolic fistula (*see* Chapter 28);
- undigested food apparent hours (usually 12 hours) after a meal owing to outlet obstruction (*see* Chapter 28);
- bile-stained vomitus due to small bowel obstruction (*see* Chapter 28);
- projectile vomiting in pyloric stenosis (*see* Chapter 28) and increased intracranial pressure.

Table 14.2 *Non-small-intestinal causes of vomiting*

Gastroenterological
Peptic ulcer disease
Gastric carcinoma
Gastric outlet obstruction (mechanical and functional)
Gastroparesis
Irritable bowel syndrome
Large bowel obstruction
Acute pancreatitis
Acute cholecystitis
Biliary colic
Acute appendicitis
Acute peritonitis
Visceral pain
Non-gastrointestinal
Visceral pain
Uterine cervix
Renal pelvis
Bladder
Testes
Myocardial infarction
Renal or biliary colic
Pancreatic carcinoma
Pancreatic pseudocyst
Drugs and toxic substances
Cancer chemotherapeutic agents
Cytotoxic agents
Anaesthetics
Analgesics
Anticholinergics
Antibiotics
Digoxin
Opioids
Theophylline
Alcohol excess
Toxic agents
Central nervous system
Raised intracranial pressure
Meningitis
Lower brainstem lesions
Migraine
Vestibular disorders
Acute labrynthitis
Menière's disease
Otitis interna
Motion sickness
Psychogenic causes
Anorexia nervosa
Bulimia nervosa
Metabolic causes
Uraemia
Diabetic ketoacidosis
Hypercalcaemia
Idiopathic cyclical vomiting
Adrenal insufficiency
Hyperparathyroidism
Miscellaneous
Acute radiation sickness
Pregnancy
Raised intracranial pressure

In pyloric stenosis, vomiting is characteristically projectile, of large volume and contains undigested food. In acute small bowel obstruction (*see* Chapter 28), vomiting is more severe if the obstruction is high and abdominal pain is an associated feature (*see* Chapter 28). A succussion splash may be present on abdominal auscultation.

VOMITING AND DIARRHOEA

Vomiting and diarrhoea occurring together are a common symptom complex of small intestinal disease. Table 14.3 shows the common infective causes of vomiting *and* diarrhoea. The sudden onset of vomiting and diarrhoea is characteristic of acute gastroenteritis (Walker-Smith, 1986).

Table 14.3 *Common infective causes of vomiting and diarrhoea*

Viral gastroenteritis
Bacterial infections
Staphylococcus aureus
Bacillus cereus
Clostridium perfringens
Vibrio parahaemolyticus
ETEC: enterotoxigenic *Escherichia coli*
EPEC: enteropathogenic *Escherichia coli*
Vibrio cholerae
Salmonella infections
Parasitic infections
Sarcocystis species
Fasciolopsis buski
Trichinella spiralis

COMPLICATIONS OF VOMITING

Biochemical abnormalities

The biochemical consequences of severe vomiting are due to loss of gastric acid, which causes hypokalaemia, hyponatraemia and hypochloraemic metabolic alkalosis. Volume depletion may cause increased albumin or raised urea concentrations.

Mechanical complications

Mallory–Weiss gastric prolapse syndrome A Mallory–Weiss tear (Fig. 14.1) is a consequence of severe retching or vomiting precipitated by excessive alcohol consumption, or the recent use of aspirin or other nonsteroidal anti-inflammatory agents. Gastric prolapse is a *forme fruste* that causes 'bruising' of mucosal folds of the cardia of the stomach owing to forceful prolapse into the oesophagus with vomiting without a mucosal tear. Initially, vomiting, retching or coughing is followed by haematemesis. In 10 per cent of patients, melaena is the only manifestation of bleeding.

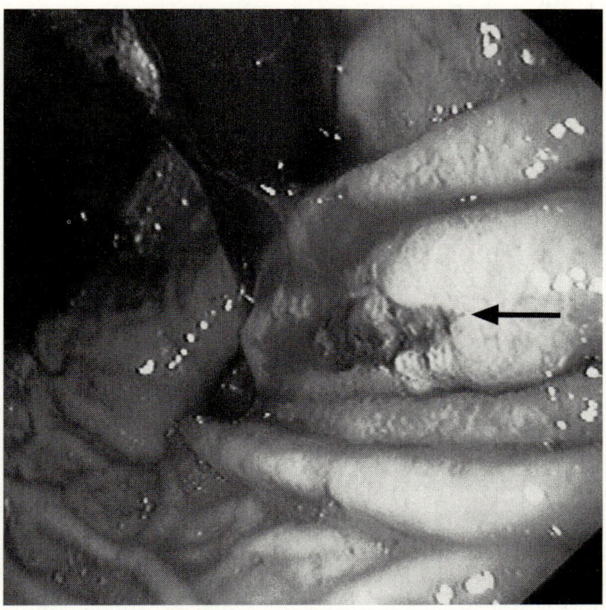

Figure 14.1 *Mallory–Weiss tear of the gastric cardia oozing with blood. The endoscope was retroflexed to obtain this observation. (Courtesy of Professor Ian Roberts-Thomson, Department of Gastroenterology, The Queen Elizabeth Hospital, Woodville, South Australia.)*

Mallory–Weiss tear accounts for 5–15 per cent of upper gastrointestinal tract bleeding. The lesion is a mucosal laceration of the gastric cardia or gastro-oesophageal junction along the longitudinal axis. In most instances, the tear is single, although three or, unusually, more may occur. Tears are most common just distal to the gastro-oesophageal junction on the lesser curve, although tears do occur on the greater curvature. Active intervention is rarely necessary. Blood loss is not great and bleeding resolves spontaneously in almost all patients (Katz and Salas, 1993). Patients at risk are, as in any acute bleed, those with abnormal coagulation and patients with portal hypertension. Octreotide infusion may be useful to lower splanchnic venous pressure and hence reduce bleeding. Persistent or severe bleeding may require endoscopic electrocoagulation (Bharucha *et al.*, 1997) or occasionally surgery.

Boerhaave's syndrome A less common complication of vomiting is Boerhaave's syndrome in which a *transmural* rupture of the oesophagus occurs. Spontaneous oesophageal rupture occurs as a result of a sudden rise in intraluminal pressure produced by actual or suppressed vomiting, with the stomach contents being ejected against a closed cricopharyngeus muscle. The diagnosis may be elusive: the symptoms mimic many common acute cardiac, thoracic or upper gastrointestinal tract conditions. The symptoms of Boerhaave's syndrome are vomiting followed by excruciating chest

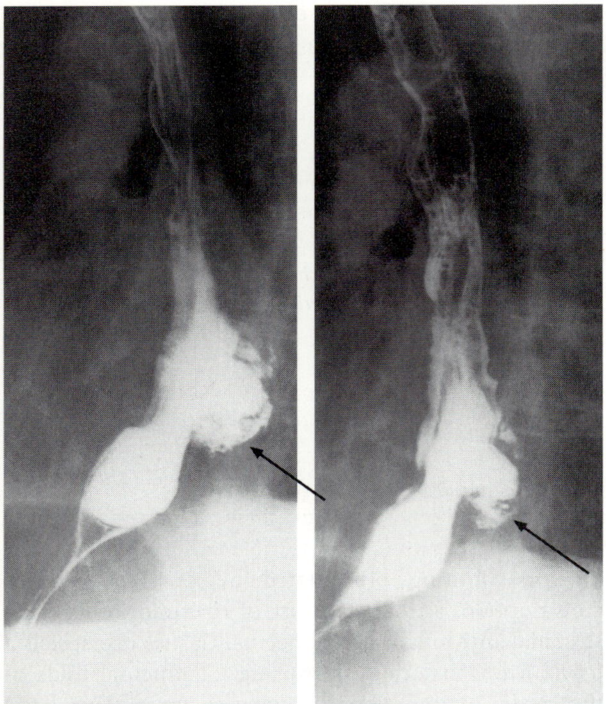

Figure 14.2 *Boerhaave's syndrome (barium swallow). The examination demonstrates extravasation of barium as a result of a full-thickness tear of the oesophagus. (Courtesy of Dr Anil B. Utturkar, Radiology Department, The Queen Elizabeth Hospital, Woodville, South Australia.)*

pain, dyspnoea, mediastinal or subcutaneous emphysema, and cardiovascular collapse (Janjua, 1997). Unusual clinical features include a change in voice, extreme swelling of the face and neck, pericarditis, pneumopericardium, pneumoperitoneum, proptosis and a ruptured diaphragm with hernia.

The diagnosis is based on the presence of a pleural effusion and pneumothorax, widening of the mediastinum and mediastinal emphysema (Fig. 14.2). A confirmatory investigation is a contrast study of the oesophagus or a computed tomography (CT) scan. The intervention of choice is surgery: open and wide mediastinal chest drainage, with or without oesophageal repair, resection or exclusion. Non-operative intervention consists of antibiotics, nasogastric suction, pleural drainage, H-2 receptor antagonists, a feeding enterostomy or total parental nutrition in selected patients (Janjua, 1997).

TREATMENT OF VOMITING

It is important that antiemetics should not be used unless the cause of vomiting is determined. Treatment of nausea and vomiting varies with the cause and severity. The commonly used antiemetic agents in chemotherapy-induced nausea and/or vomiting (and in other situations of severe and protracted vomiting where treatment with these drugs is considered appropriate) are metoclopramide, ondansetron, tropisetron and dexamethasone.

Diarrhoea

Diarrhoea is a common manifestation of small intestinal disease. 'Spurious diarrhoea' (also known as 'overflow diarrhoea') is a consequence of constipation, and should be considered when taking a history from an elderly patient with diarrhoea. Faecal incontinence should also be distinguished from true diarrhoea.

The causes of diarrhoea due to disease of the small intestine are discussed in detail in Chapters 15 and 16. The non-small-intestinal causes of diarrhoea include postvagotomy diarrhoea, colonic, pancreatic (*see* Chapter 16) or endocrine causes (*see* Chapter 16), and diarrhoea associated with drug therapy (*see* Chapter 15).

The diarrhoeal stools of small intestinal origin are not associated with the blood or mucus, nor the tenesmus, rectal pain or urgency, that characterize large bowel pathology. The nature of small intestinal diarrhoea varies with the cause and can be divided into secretory, osmotic, inflammatory and steatorrhoea. Often there are several mechanisms present. Large watery stools with little or no formed elements suggest secretory diarrhoea. Secretory diarrhoea continues after fasting (*see* Chapter 15). Secretory diarrhoea occurs with *V. cholerae* infection with severe voluminous diarrhoea. Watery diarrhoea is also a feature of cryptosporidial infection (*see* Chapter 19) and of the WDHA syndrome (watery diarrhoea, hypokalaemia and achlorhydria; 'pancreatic cholera') in patients with a vasoactive, inhibitory, peptide-secreting, islet cell tumour of the pancreas (Verner and Morrison, 1958). In viral infections, the diarrhoea is mild and self-limiting.

Maldigestion and malabsorption with emphasis on steatorrhoea are discussed in Chapter 16. The bowel actions due to steatorrhoea are greasy, large, frothy, foul smelling and difficult to flush. It improves on fasting. There is often a film of oil in the toilet pan even after flushing. Patients may complain of diarrhoea after a meal with a high fat content. The stools often float in malabsorptive diseases, not due to increased fat content, but due to increased buoyancy from carbon dioxide and hydrogen due to bacterial degradation of unabsorbed food. Undigested food in stools suggests intestinal hurry and is not usually a feature of a malabsorptive condition.

The maldigestion and the subsequent malabsorption of disaccharidases, most commonly lactose, is discussed in Chapter 24. Patients complain of abdominal discomfort, distension, the passage of flatus and diarrhoea after

Table 14.4 *The link between bacterial contamination and specific foods*

Food source	Bacterium	Reference
Fried rice	*Bacillus cereus*	Terranova and Blake (1978) (*see* Chapter 18)
Seafood	*Vibrio parahaemolyticus*	Barker (1974) (*see* Chapter 18)
Minced beef in fast foods	Enterohaemorrhagic *E. coli* O156:H7	Pavia *et al.* (1990) (*see* Chapter 18)
Poultry	*Campylobacter jejuni*	Skirrow (1991) (*see* Chapter 18)
Pork	*Trichinella spiralis*	Capo and Despommier (1996) (*see* Chapter 19)

consuming milk and milk-containing products. Yoghurt does not cause these symptoms because the lactase in the yoghurt is activated at body temperature (Kolars *et al.*, 1984). The threshold of symptoms may be set by a coincident irritable bowel syndrome.

ONSET AND DURATION

Acute diarrhoea is defined as being of less than 2 weeks duration (World Health Organization (WHO), 1993) and is usually self-limiting. Common causes of acute diarrhoea are dietary indiscretion, excessive alcohol intake and frequently a non-specific side-effect of medication. Viral or bacterial pathogens are also common causes (*see* Chapters 17 and 18). Low-grade fever, vomiting, myalgia, malaise, headache and a history of contact with a very young child with diarrhoea suggest a viral cause. The abrupt onset of vomiting and diarrhoea, especially if there is a clustering of cases, suggests food poisoning. Specific bacteria often contaminate a particular type of food, and this helps with the diagnosis (Table 14.4).

Chronic diarrhoea is defined as being over 3 weeks in duration in adults (Powell, 1991). A useful approach is to distinguish whether the diarrhoea is of small or large intestinal origin. Malabsorption is a predominant cause of small bowel diarrhoea (*see* Chapter 16). Colonic causes of chronic diarrhoea include the irritable bowel syndrome, a malignancy, bacterial infections such as *Mycobacterium tuberculosis* (*see* Chapter 18), or parasites, for example, *Entamoeba histolytica* (*see* Chapter 19). Large bowel diarrhoea may be associated with the passage of blood and mucus.

TEMPORAL PROFILE

The time at which diarrhoea occurs may suggest the aetiology. In patients with diabetes mellitus and autonomic neuropathy, diarrhoea occurs during the night. Early morning diarrhoea is a feature of the irritable bowel syndrome. Diarrhoea soon after a meal occurs with the irritable bowel syndrome, in some patients with amoebic colitis and with the dumping syndrome. Diarrhoea after a meal with a high fat content occurs in conditions of severe small bowel mucosal damage and pancreatic disease.

PAST MEDICAL HISTORY

The past medical history provides valuable information on drug-related and iatrogenic causes of diarrhoea. Diarrhoea may follow upper gastrointestinal surgery for peptic ulceration, cholecystectomy, resection of the intestines, especially the terminal ileum and colon, intestinal bypass procedures, pancreatic resection and radiation therapy (*see* Chapter 15). Chronic diarrhoea since childhood and failure to thrive suggest coeliac disease. Intolerance to milk and milk products suggests lactose intolerance (*see* Chapter 15).

CURRENT MEDICAL PROBLEMS

Awareness of the current medical condition for which the patient is receiving treatment is essential. Many systemic diseases involve the gastrointestinal tract and cause diarrhoea (*see* Chapter 27). Information on the patient's sexual preference is important. Patients with the acquired immunodeficiency syndrome (AIDS) (Chapter 20) and those on immunosuppressive agents are predisposed to pathogens that are not routinely requested, and the microbiology laboratory should be specifically asked to screen for these less common pathogens. Multiple infections can also occur in these patients.

DRUG HISTORY

Information on the patient's medication is an essential part of the clinical interview and should include a list of:

- proprietary drugs;
- non-proprietary drugs;
- over-the-counter medication;
- purchases from health food stores, not considered as drugs.

DRUG-RELATED CAUSES OF DIARRHOEA

Drugs often cause self-limiting diarrhoea as a side-effect. A common drug-induced cause of diarrhoea is antibiotic therapy, which induces a change to the bacterial flora in the colon.

Table 14.5 lists the drugs associated with diarrhoea. The antibiotics include almost all agents, especially broad-

Table 14.5 *Drugs associated with diarrhoea. (Adapted from Ratnaike, R.N., Jones, T.E. 1998: Mechanisms of drug-induced diarrhoea in the elderly.* Drugs and Aging *13, 245–53)*

Body system	Drugs
Cardiovascular	Methyldopa, digitalis, quinidine, propanolol, hydralazine, angiotensin-converting enzyme (ACE) inhibitors, procainamide, ethacrynic acid, amiloride, bretylium, guanethidine, triamterene
Gastrointestinal	Lactulose, antacids (Mg salts), cimetidine, proton pump inhibitors, H-2 receptor antagonists, cholestyramine, chenodeoxycholic acid, acarbose, bile salts, olsalazine, misoprostol, cathartics, laxatives
Musculoskeletal	Colchicine, non-steroidal anti-inflammatory agents, auranofin (an oral gold preparation), naproxen, indomethacin, phenylbutazone, mefenamic acid, diflunisal
Central nervous	Anticholinergic agents, levodopa, alprazolam, lithium, fluoxetine, tacrine, meprobamate
Endocrine	Oral hypoglycaemic agents, acarbose, clofibrate, thyroxine
Genitourinary	Propantheline
Miscellaneous	'Gastrografin', clofibrate, iron (usually causes constipation, but diarrhoea can occur)
	Antibiotics
	Clindamycin, amoxycillin, ampicillin, cephalosporins, neomycin
	Antimetabolites
	5-Fluorouracil, methotrexate
	Osmotic cathartics
	Mg-containing antacids, lactulose, sorbitol

spectrum drugs. The possibility of laxative abuse must not be disregarded in a patient with chronic diarrhoea of elusive aetiology. The mechanisms related to drug-induced diarrhoea are considered in detail in Chapter 15.

OTHER IATROGENIC CAUSES OF DIARRHOEA

Important iatrogenic causes to consider are surgery involving the gastrointestinal tract (*see* Chapters 16 and 29), and radiation enteritis (*see* Chapter 16).

PSYCHOSOCIAL HISTORY

The presence of psychosocial stressors should be explored. Events that are of importance are a recent bereavement, separation, divorce, relationship problems, financial difficulties, and features of depression and/or anxiety sought (Goh and Ratnaike, 1999).

FAMILY HISTORY

A family history of diarrhoea is associated with medullary carcinoma of the thyroid and coeliac disease (*see* Chapter 23).

TRAVEL ABROAD

Acute diarrhoea acquired during travel to the tropics or to areas of suboptimal hygiene is invariably infective in nature (*see* Chapters 18 and 19). Chronic diarrhoea after a visit to tropical and subtropical regions raises the possibility of parasitic causes (*see* Chapter 19), most importantly of *Giardia lamblia*. Postinfective irritable bowel syndrome can commonly persist after returning from overseas.

DIETARY HISTORY

Diarrhoea and abdominal discomfort with the ingestion of wheat products suggests coeliac disease (*see* Chapter 23), but may occur due to fermentation of fibre. Diarrhoea, abdominal discomfort, borborygmi and flatulence with milk products, except yoghurt, are usually diagnostic of lactose intolerance (*see* Chapter 15). Patients with malabsorption due to either small bowel or pancreatic pathology complain of diarrhoea after a meal with a high fat content (*see* Chapter 16).

COMPLICATIONS OF DIARRHOEA

Clinical signs of dehydration

The criteria for the clinical assessment of dehydration in paediatric populations are widely available. There is, however, little literature regarding elderly populations, even though dehydration is a common problem. A study on 55 subjects aged 60 or older found that the conventional signs and symptoms based on data from younger subjects are unreliable markers of dehydration (Gross *et al.*, 1992). The conventional signs include:

- reduction of skin turgor;
- increased thirst;
- decreased peripheral perfusion;
- postural hypotension;
- low jugular venous pressure;
- patient's sensations of thirst and dryness;
- tachycardia;
- elevated temperature.

None of these symptoms or signs ranked as strong correlates of dehydration in the elderly. The lack of correlation is due to normal age-related changes in these variables, and also the marked variation in physiological responses to dehydration between elderly and younger patients. For example, postural hypotension is a common sign in the elderly patient, independent of the state of hydration, due to a range of causes, including autonomic dysfunction and therapeutic agents.

Seven signs and symptoms strongly correlate with dehydration in the elderly, but do not exhibit a significant, independent, age-related change (Gross *et al.*, 1992). These are:

- dry tongue;
- longitudinal tongue furrows;
- dry mucous membranes of the nose and mouth;
- eyes that appear recessed in their sockets;
- upper body muscle weakness;
- speech difficulty;
- confusion.

Biochemical abnormalities

Most patients with severe diarrhoea will present with hypokalaemic hyperchloraemic metabolic acidosis. Potassium loss in the diarrhoeal fluid leads to hypokalaemia and, in situations of hypovolaemia, more potassium is lost in the urine due to secondary hyperaldosteronism.

Bicarbonate loss in diarrhoea decreases plasma bicarbonate concentration, lowering the blood pH (Henderson–Hasselbalch equation) and causing metabolic acidosis. In patients with a low bicarbonate concentration, acid–base status should be monitored by measuring blood pH and arterial blood gases. If acidosis is severe, bicarbonate therapy is indicated.

Diarrhoea causes the loss of water, although water loss is difficult to measure. Indirect tests to assess hypovolaemia are osmolality, plasma specific gravity, plasma proteins (albumin and globulins), urea and creatinine.

The measurement of plasma specific gravity has been re-evaluated, especially in older adults (Dauterman *et al.*, 1995). The test determines the plasma refractive index with a hand-held refractometer, and the specific gravity is determined using a standard conversion table. The test can be rapidly performed and is reported to be accurate. Since the refractive index of any fluid is a direct measure of the total mass of large molecules in solution, falsely elevated levels occur in hypergammaglobulinaemia and multiple myeloma.

Hypovolaemia increases the renal absorption of sodium and chloride, which tends to normalize the plasma sodium and increase the plasma chloride concentration. If dehydration is corrected with water only, which is non-isotonic, hyponatraemia can occur with normal plasma chloride concentration.

ISSUES OF MANAGEMENT

Oral rehydration therapy

Dehydration is responsible for an estimated 60–70 per cent of diarrhoeal deaths (WHO, 1985). Oral rehydration is used extensively to prevent or treat dehydration in patients, especially in developing countries where diarrhoea is an immense problem. Oral rehydration alone is an effective means of fluid and electrolyte replacement in nearly all cases of dehydration. After decades of use, controversy remains over the ideal composition of oral rehydration solutions. The most widely used solution is that recommended by the WHO, the composition of which is:

Sodium	90 mmol/L
Potassium	20 mmol/L
Glucose	111 mmol/L
Citrate	10 mmol/L
Chloride	80 mmol/L

The WHO formula (in g/L) is:

Sodium chloride	3.5
Trisodium citrate dihydrate	2.9
Potassium chloride	1.5
Glucose (anhydrous)	20.0

The measured weights of ingredients are added into a volume of 1 L of water (WHO, 1993). Sodium bicarbonate (baking soda) can be used *in place of* the trisodium citrate by adding 2.5 g/L. Boiled water is optimal but volume replacement must take priority, and drinking water is acceptable (Sack, 1991).

The rationale for the effectiveness of oral rehydration solutions is that, despite severe diarrhoea, the mechanisms of sodium and water absorption are not impaired. The presence of glucose in the solution enables the entry of sodium into the intestinal epithelial cell by co-transport. In many instances, hydration can be maintained by increasing the intake of fluids, such as water, mineral water, fruit juice and soft drinks. Large quantities of drinks with a high osmolality should not be used to treat dehydration. Examples of such drinks are Coca Cola (680 mosmol/kg), apple juice (870 mosmol/kg), orange juice (935 mosmol/kg) and grape juice (1170 mosmol/kg).

Intravenous therapy

Intravenous therapy is not always necessary, and is only indicated if oral intake is not possible or difficult to maintain. Intravenous therapy should be given to patients in shock, with hypovolaemia, and in those with persistent vomiting or problems of deglutition. Patients with less than 5 per cent (mild) and between 6 and 8 per cent (moderate) dehydration should be rehydrated orally. Those with 10 per cent or more dehydration should first be given intravenous fluids to correct the hypovolaemia, and then maintained on oral solutions.

Intravenous Ringer's lactate is considered the best commercially available fluid and can be used for patients in all age groups to treat dehydration due to acute diarrhoea of any cause (WHO, 1993). Normal saline is less appropriate because it does not correct the acidosis or replace the potassium. A dextrose solution has the disadvantage of not replacing electrolytes (Sack, 1991).

The amount of fluid to be given must replace previous and ongoing fluid losses and maintain optimal hydration. This requires measuring the volume of the stool as well as keeping an accurate fluid balance chart (Sack, 1991).

- Mild dehydration: oral therapy – 50 mL per kg of deficit (i.e. a loss of 1 kg body weight requires a replacement fluid volume of 50 mL).
- Moderate dehydration: oral therapy – 75 mL/kg.
- Severe dehydration: intravenous therapy – 100 mL/kg (over 2–4 hours).

Nutrition

The WHO guidelines promote feeding during diarrhoea to prevent undernutrition or the aggravation of existing undernutrition (WHO, 1989). Both malnutrition and undernutrition are common problems in children in the developing world and in the elderly even in developed countries. The nutritional status of the patient should be carefully assessed during episodes of both acute and chronic diarrhoea. Diarrhoea can lead to decreased food intake, impaired nutrient absorption and increased protein loss. In the elderly, in whom undernutrition or malnutrition is often an existing problem, fasting during an episode of diarrhoea can seriously worsen the state of nutrition. Protein loss during diarrhoea is a major problem, especially in the elderly, and may continue during convalescence. Malnutrition can easily result, more so when the diarrhoea occurs during another serious, debilitating illness or when the patient's nutritional status before the diarrhoea is inadequate. In children, a strong association between death from diarrhoea and hypoproteinaemia is reported (Islam and Khan, 1986).

Diarrhoea is not an indication for fasting and the notion that 'rest is best for the gut' is without foundation. Breast feeding of infants should continue. When small bowel mucosal damage has occurred, the duration of diarrhoeal episodes is reduced if nutrients and fluids and electrolytes are available for epithelial cell regeneration. Patients should be encouraged to eat food that can be tolerated. Foods to avoid are those with a high fat content, high roughage content, spicy food and raw food.

Antibiotics

The rationale for the cautious use of antibiotics in infectious diarrhoea is well founded. Many enteric pathogens such as viruses cause an acute episode of diarrhoea which is self-limiting and does not respond to antibiotics. The possibility of a parasitic cause of diarrhoea must always be considered (*see* Chapter 19). The decision to use an antibiotic should be based on the the possible aetiology, severity of diarrhoea, the current clinical circumstances of the patient, the potential side-effects and the presence of septicaemia. Treatment with antibiotics should be directed to the specific pathogen identified on stool culture.

Before the results of stool culture are available, if treatment is necessary, the choice of antibiotic should be based on the clinical picture and knowledge of the pathogens that commonly cause diarrhoea in the local setting. In these circumstances, trimethoprim-sulphamethoxazole or norfloxacin may be used. The clinical response to antibiotics may not parallel *in vitro* activity against the organism and resistant strains may emerge during treatment. Antibiotic treatment may itself cause antibiotic-associated diarrhoea, which is distinct from pseudomembraneous colitis. Suprainfection by *C. difficile* can present as a self-limiting illness with only mild diarrhoea or as a more severe syndrome of pseudomembraneous colitis (Bennett *et al.*, 1984).

Newer antibiotics such as norfloxacin and ciprofloxacin allay some of these concerns and have a broad spectrum of activity against the most common, important pathogens that cause dysentery. Antibiotics are indicated in dysentery, especially if systemic symptoms, such as fever, chills, headache and myalgia, are present.

Antimotility drugs

Loperamide and diphenoxylate delay the passage of the intestinal contents, allowing more time for fluid and electrolyte absorption. Loperamide is the preferred drug and is now available as an over-the-counter agent in 110 countries. The side-effects of loperamide are mild and temporary. The use of the drug is not recommended in inflammatory bowel disease, in infective diarrhoea with features of dysentery, and if fever or systemic toxic symptoms are present. Loperamide is a safe, effective drug in acute non-specific diarrhoea. The suggested dose is 8 mg in 24 hours.

Adsorbents

Kaolin increases the consistency of the stool by absorbing water. These compounds do not decrease the number of motions per day. A beneficial effect is the absorption of bacterial toxins, decreasing their luminal activity. In traveller's diarrhoea, bismuth subsalicylate (Pepto-Bismol) is a proven prophylactic agent and is useful in mild diarrhoea of less than four motions per day with neither blood nor mucus in the stools (Gorbach, 1990). Bismuth subsalicylate is a trivalent bismuth compound that forms salts that adversely affect bacterial metabolism. The salicylate is absorbed and therefore the concurrent ingestion of aspirin is not advised. The recommended duration of use is 3 weeks. The contraindications are similar to those for aspirin.

Antisecretory agents

Octreotide, a synthetic long-acting octapeptide analogue of somatostatin, is effective in the management of secretory diarrhoea (Harris *et al.*, 1995). Somatostatin stimulates the absorption of Na, Cl and water, and decreases Cl secretion by small intestinal epithelial cells. Net fluid absorption occurs. Octreotide has been particularly useful in treating severe refractory cases of the enteropathy caused by human immunodeficiency virus (HIV) infection (*see* Chapter 20) and in situations of elevated vasoactive intestinal polypeptide (VIP) secretion associated with watery diarrhoea, malabsorption and weight loss (*see* Chapter 6) (Manfredi *et al.*, 1996). It has also been used to reduce the duration of diarrhoea due to *Vibrio cholerae*, although the rate of stool output was unchanged (Abbas *et al.*, 1996).

Prevention of diarrhoea

Effective measures to prevent diarrhoea, especially in the developing world, are the availability and convenient access to adequate potable water, and sewage facilities. Community participation in programmes to increase personal, domestic and environmental hygiene has resulted in significant reductions in diarrhoea (Ratnaike and Chinner, 1994).

In infants and children, diarrhoea can be significantly reduced by specific *risk reduction behaviours* that should be promoted among mothers and carers. These are:

- breastfeeding;
- safe weaning practices;
- personal hygiene (especially the importance of handwashing after toileting, and before breast feeding or preparing food);
- domestic and environmental hygiene;
- the recognition and treatment of dehydration;
- continuation of feeding and hydration during episodes of diarrhoea.

In institutions such as nursing homes, rest homes or geriatric wards, inmates are at risk of acquiring diarrhoea from a point-source, food-borne outbreak or by person to person spread. Special attention to food preparation and storage is important (Telzak *et al.*, 1991). During cooking, care should be taken to prevent the cross-contamination of cooked and fresh food. Kitchen implements, utensils and surfaces used to prepare, for example, uncooked poultry, can harbour enteric pathogens that can contaminate fresh foods such as salads.

Patients most at risk are those who are immunocompromised, those whose personal hygiene is suboptimal due to a physical or mental infirmity, and patients who are highly dependent on staff. It is also recommended that patients at the greatest risk of acquiring diarrhoea, for example, those immunosuppressed, should avoid raw milk and uncooked animal products.

If an outbreak of diarrhoea occurs in an institution, measures must be set in place to prevent the spread of infection. This may be difficult in an institutional setting if there is overcrowding, patients with faecal incontinence, inadequate staff and if toilet facilities are shared. All patients and staff from the 'infected' ward or area should be restricted from contact with other patients. Control strategies include:

- an intensive educational programme on diarrhoeal infections;
- the thorough cleaning of toilets;
- the meticulous disposal of faeces and soiled linen;
- increased ward cleaning;
- increased handwashing with soap, especially after visiting the toilet, and before eating and handling medication;
- optimal food-handling practices.

Other precautions are to locate patients with diarrhoea near toilets, especially elderly patients with incontinence and/or dementia. Staff with diarrhoea should be advised not to attend work until the pathogen that caused the diarrhoea is no longer present in two consecutive stool samples.

Abdominal discomfort and pain

The 20 most common diagnoses found in a survey of 1000 patients with abdominal pain are listed in Table 14.6 (Brewer *et al.*, 1976).

Abdominal discomfort or pain is a common feature of small intestinal disease. The pain arising from different locations is referred to specific areas of the abdomen (Figs 14.3 and 14.4). Pain from the first and second part of the duodenum is referred to the epigastrium, and the periumbilical area is the site of referred pain from the third part of the duodenum, the jejunum and ileum. Owing to obstruction, spasm and distension of the proximal portion of the intestine, contractions occur to relieve the obstruction and have the characteristic of rhythmicity. Owing to increased dilatation of the intestine and loss of muscular tone, the colicky nature of the pain may become less prominent.

Upper small bowel pain lasts for 2–10 minutes and lower small bowel pain for 10–15 minutes. Gallbladder pain is prolonged and lasts for hours. Pain due to the involvement of the visceral or parietal peritoneum gives rise to a steady pain that is localized over the specific area that is inflamed. Guarding and rebound tenderness are also present. Abdominal pain is a feature of bacterial infections of the small intestine, especially *Clostridium perfringens* type C, which causes 'pig-bel' (*see* Chapter

Table 14.6 *Most commonly diagnosed causes of abdominal pain. (Reprinted from Brewer* et al., *1976)*

Diagnosis	Percentage of patients
Abdominal pain of unknown cause	41.3
Gastroenteritis	6.9
Pelvic inflammatory disease	6.7
Urinary tract infection	5.2
Ureteral stone	4.3
Appendicitis	4.3
Acute cholecystitis	2.5
Intestinal obstruction	2.5
Constipation	2.3
Duodenal ulcer	2.0
Dysmenorrhea	1.8
Simple pregnancy	1.8
Pyelonephritis	1.7
Gastritis	1.4
Chronic cholecystitis	1.2
Ovarian cyst	1.0
Incomplete abortion	1.0
Pancreatitis	0.9
Abdominal aneurysm	0.7
Epididymitis	0.7

Foregut structures:
- Stomach → **Epigastrium**
- Duodenum → **Epigastrium**
- Pancreas → **Epigastrium**

Midgut structures:
- Jejunum → **Periumbilical area**
- Ileum → **Periumbilical area**
- Right colon → **Periumbilical area**

Hindgut structures:
- Left colon → **Hypogastrium**

Figure 14.3 *Where pain is referred.*

Epigastric pain
Reflux oesophagitis
Hiatus hernia; paraoesophageal hernia
Oesophageal foreign body, obstruction, mass
Oesophageal perforation (Boerhaave's syndrome)
Gastritis
Gastric ulcer
Duodenal ulcer
Lesion of the transverse colon

Right upper quadrant
Duodenal ulcer
Retrocaecal, appendicitis
Lesion of the right colon (carcinoma, colitis)

Left Upper quadrant
Gastric perforation
Reflux oesophagitis
Hiatus hernia
Lesion of the left colon

Mid-abdominal pain
Ileus (small bowel)
Colonic
Non-specific enteritis, colitis
Ulcerative colitis
Crohn's disease
Mesenteric ischaemia
Infarction
Intussusception

Right lower quadrant
Acute appendicitis
Meckel's diverticulitis
Crohn's disease
Infectious colitis
Caecal carcinoma
Caecal volvulus
Duodenal, gastric perforation
Intra-abdominal haemorrhage
Inguinal hernia

Left lower quadrant
Sigmoid diverticulitis
Carcinoma, left colon
Sigmoid volvulus
Intra-abdominal haemorrhage
Inguinal hernia

Figure 14.4 *Common localizing patterns of abdominal pain in intestinal aetiology. (Adapted from Brazaitis, M.P., Dachman, A.H. 1993: Gastrointestinal emergencies.* Medical Clinics of North America *77, 939–61.)*

18), enteroinvasive *E. coli*, non-typhoidal salmonellae, *Campylobacter*, *Vibrio cholerae* and shigellae. Abdominal pain or discomfort occurs with parasitic infections of the small bowel such as *Giardia lamblia*, *Capillaria philippinensis* and *Fasciolopsis buski* (*see* Chapter 19)

Abdominal pain may occur 1–2 hours after meals in patients with Crohn's disease (*see* Chapter 25). Abdominal pain due to malabsorption of lactose results in cramping abdominal pain or discomfort, and diarrhoea (*see* Chapter 24).

Bleeding

Bleeding of small intestinal aetiology is uncommon. The prevalence of bleeding between the second part of the duodenum and the ileo-caecal valve occurs in 3–5 per cent of patients (Netterville *et al.*, 1968). This low figure may in part reflect the relative inaccessibility of the small intestine and the lack, until recently, of suitable diagnostic tests. Occult gastrointestinal bleeding is defined as acute or chronic blood loss from a source not identified by endoscopy or radiology (Mujica and Barkin, 1996). Haematemesis is rare and depends on the severity of the bleeding and whether or not the site of the bleeding is above the ligament of Treitz (Mujica and Barkin, 1996). The presence of bright blood in stools, or melaena, is dependent on the transit time of the blood bolus and the volume of blood.

Table 14.7 lists the main causes of bleeding in the small intestine. Most causes of bleeding that are detectable are due to angiodysplasia (Koga *et al.*, 1996; Akhrass *et al.*, 1997), which accounts for 70–80 per cent of bleeding (Lewis, 1994). Angiodysplasias are vascular ectasias, which

Table 14.7 *Causes of small intestinal bleeding*

Angiodysplasia
Neoplasia
Crohn's disease
Diverticulae
Meckle's diverticulum
Jejunal diverticulae
Ulceration
Zollinger–Ellison syndrome
Therapeutic agents
Non-steroidal anti-inflammatory drugs
Potassium chloride
6-Mercaptopurine
Infections
Radiation enteritis
Metastatic small bowel disease
Small bowel varices
Familial disorders
Polyposis
Telangiectasis
Osler–Weber–Rendu disease
Turner's syndrome
Other
Ehlers–Danlos syndrome
Pseudoxanthoma elasticum
Von Willebrand's disease
Henoch–Schönlein purpura
Peutz–Jeghers syndrome
Miscellaneous
Amyloidosis
Blue rubber bleb nevus syndrome
Aortoenteric fistula

include arterioles, capillaries and venules (Harford, 1988), and were previously termed arteriovenous malformations (AVMs). True AVMs are congenital lesions with thick-walled arteries and veins without intervening capillaries (Ottinger and Vickery, 1981). Other causes of bleeding are benign and malignant tumours (*see* Chapter 26), jejunal varices, small bowel diverticula and drug-related injury from non-steroidal anti-inflammatory agents. An infective cause of small bowel blood loss is due to *C. perfringens* type C, which causes 'pig-bel' associated with severe necrotizing enterocolitis (*see* Chapter 18). Enteroinvasive *E. coli* multiplies within the epithelial cells of the distal ileum and the colon, and leads to diarrhoea with blood and mucus, abdominal pain, tenesmus and systemic symptoms of fever and myalgia. Other pathogens that involve the terminal ileum that may cause blood loss are *Salmonella* and *Shigella* (Balthazar *et al.*, 1996), and *Mycobacterium tuberculosis.* In patients with AIDS, massive bleeding has resulted from cytomegalovirus enteritis (Soderlund *et al.*, 1994; Lai *et al.*, 1996). Other less common causes of bleeding are Crohn's disease (Anthony *et al.*, 1997) and radiation ileitis.

Radionuclide scans confirm occurrences of bleeding being of small bowel origin but are unreliable in accurately identifying the exact site. The use of technetium-99m-labelled red blood cells has significant advantages over previous technetium-99m-labelled sulphur colloid techniques in identifying blood loss. The labelled red blood cells have a much longer half-life in the body (24 hours), and imaging can be undertaken over several hours. Sequential scans increase the probability of determining the site of the bleeding. Bunker *et al.* (1982) in a study of 100 patients showed that technetium-99m-labelled red blood cells identified the bleeding site in 38 per cent but that labelled sulphur colloid was useful in only 5 per cent. In this study the labelled red blood cells had a sensitivity of 93 per cent, a specificity of 95 per cent, and an overall accuracy of 94 per cent.

The small bowel as the site of bleeding can be distinguished from the colon by the appearance over time of images of multiple loops (of small bowel) with labelled blood. However, localizing the point of bleeding *within* the small intestine may not be possible (Lewis, 1994). Other diagnostic procedures are angiography, endoscopy (*see* Chapter 13.1) and radiology (*see* Chapter 13.6).

Weight loss

Weight loss may be a prominent symptom in long-standing states of malabsorption, owing to a lack of calories from protein, carbohydrate and fat malabsorption. The major causes of weight loss related to the small intestine are:

- malignancy;
- malabsorption syndrome;
- inflammatory bowel disease;
- chronic infection.

Weight loss must be established on objective evidence, such as previous records, changes in the clothes size, or 'new' belt notches. A change in weight of 7–10 per cent or more of what the patient regards as the usual body weight is significant, and is of greater concern if the change occurred over weeks or months rather than in years.

Protein-losing enteropathy

The term protein-losing enteropathy denotes protein loss into the lumen of the gastrointestinal tract of sufficient severity to cause hypoproteinaemia. It is usually accompanied by lymphocytopenia and hypocholesterolaemia. Hypoproteinaemia of small intestinal origin should be considered if dietary protein intake is adequate, and hepatic and renal function are normal (*see* Chapter 16). In the elderly, a single episode of severe diarrhoea can lead to undernutrition and precipitate hypoproteinaemia. Besides malabsorptive conditions, protein loss

Table 14.8 *Symptoms and signs of malabsorption of nutrients*

System	Symptom or sign	Pathophysiology
Alimentary	Weight loss, wasting	Calorie loss due to malabsorption of fat, carbohydrate and protein
	Diarrhoea	Impaired absorption of sodium and water; effect of unabsorbed fatty acids and bile acids
	Oily, bulky stools	Malabsorption of fat
	Flatulence, borborygmi and abdominal distension	Maldigestion of lactose
	Frothy watery stools	Maldigestion of lactose
Haematopoietic	Anaemia	Impaired absorption of iron, folic acid, vitamin B12, pyridoxine
	Haemorrhagic phenomena (petechiae, ecchymoses, purpura and haematuria)	Vitamin K deficiency
	Glossitis, cheilosis, stomatitis	Deficiency of iron, vitamin B_{12}, folate and other vitamins
Nervous	Peripheral neuritis	Deficiency of vitamin B_{12}
	Bone pain, bone fractures	Protein depletion → impaired bone formation → osteoporosis Calcium malabsorption → demineralization of bone → osteomalacia
	Osteopenia, tetany and paraesthesia	Calcium malabsorption → hypocalcaemia Vitamin D malabsorption → osteomalacia (adults), rickets (children) Magnesium malabsorption → hypomagnesaemia
Skin	Oedema	Hypoproteinaemia due to decreased absorption of amino acids
	Petechiae, ecchymoses, purpura and haematuria	Malabsorption of vitamin K
	Dermatitis and hyperkeratosis	Malabsorption of vitamin A, niacin, zinc and fatty acids
Musculoskeletal	Weakness	Anaemia; electrolyte depletion (hypokalaemia)
Endocrine	Amenorrhoea	Protein depletion and 'caloric starvation' → secondary hypopituitarism
	Impotence, infertility amenorrhoea,	Generalized malnutrition
	hyperparathyroidism	Protracted calcium and vitamin D deficiency
	Nocturia	Delayed absorption of water

is associated with hookworm infection if the worm burden is significant and with very heavy infections of the fluke *Fasciolopsis buski* (*see* Chapter 19). In graft versus host disease, in addition to diarrhoea a severe protein-losing enteropathy can occur (Papadopoulou *et al.*, 1996). Luminal protein loss can be assessed by the faecal clearance of α_1-antitrypsin (*see* Chapter 13.3).

Vitamin and mineral deficiencies

Vitamin and mineral absorption is discussed in detail in Chapter 9. Vitamin and mineral deficiencies occur in conditions of small intestinal mucosal damage. Steatorrhoea, irrespective of the aetiology, impairs the absorption of the fat-soluble vitamins A, D, E and K (*see* Chapter 16). The occurrence and severity of the clinical, haematological and biochemical abnormalities due to the malabsorption of these nutrients depend on the nutrients malabsorbed, and the duration and severity of the problem. In small intestinal mucosal lesions, the site of the lesion determines the nutrient that is malabsorbed. Specific nutritional deficiencies are associated with lesions of the upper small intestine, such as anaemia due to iron or folate deficiency and deficiencies of the fat-soluble vitamins and minerals (*see* Chapter 9).

Lesions of the terminal ileum cause vitamin B_{12} malabsorption and impair reabsorption of bile salts. Bile salt malabsorption diminishes the bile salt pool required to maintain the enterohepatic circulation for adequate micellar concentration for the absorption of fats and fat-soluble vitamins. Other adverse influences on vitamin and mineral absorption are infection with a tapeworm, *Diphyllobothrium latum*, a cause of vitamin B_{12} deficiency, and heavy hookworm infection (*Ancylostoma duodenale* and *Necator americanus*), which can cause severe iron-deficiency anaemia.

The consequences of vitamin and mineral malabsorption are summarized in Table 14.8.

Flatulence

Flatus production occurs in the colon and is exaggerated with malabsorption of carbohydrates. The reported daily occurrence of flatulence in normal adult males is 14.6 times (Levitt *et al.*, 1976). Food that is normally digested and absorbed in the small intestine reaches the colon and is acted upon by colonic bacteria with the production of copious gas. The gases are hydrogen and carbon dioxide, and the dominant gas, mainly from air swallowing, is nitrogen. Excessive flatus occurs in patients with malabsorptive disorders and is a notable feature of carbohydrate malabsorption, especially in lactose intolerance (Welsh, 1970), where intraluminal fermentation by bacteria results in the production of hydrogen and carbon dioxide. Diffuse mucosal damage from many entities, notably severe bacterial infections (*see* Chapter 18), coeliac disease (*see* Chapter 23) and tropical sprue (*see* Chapter 21) reduce lactase concentration.

SIGNS OF SMALL INTESTINAL DISEASE

Systemic features

Fever may accompany acute viral or bacterial diarrhoea. Fever is a feature of *Shigella*, *Campylobacter* and *Salmonella* infections. In chronic diarrhoea, fever is associated with tuberculosis (*see* Chapter 18), Whipple's disease (*see* Chapter 22), some parasitic infections (*see* Chapter 19) and inflammatory bowel disease (*see* Chapter 25).

Lymphadenopathy

Lymphadenopathy should be sought for, especially in the left supraclavicular fossa for metastatic evidence of an abdominal malignancy, and may also reflect the presence of tuberculosis.

Skin

A variety of skin lesions may occur owing to vitamin and mineral malabsorption (Table 14.8). In inflammatory bowel disease, the skin lesions of mucosal ulceration, pyoderma gangrenosum, erythema nodosum, fistulas and anal tags specifically suggest Crohn's disease (Chapter 25). Hyperpigmentation occurs in Whipple's disease (*see* Chapter 22). Taut skin over the fingers that limits extension, telangiectasia and areas of depigmentation are suspicious of scleroderma, which can cause bacterial overgrowth of the small intestine (*see* Chapter 12). Dermatitis herpetiformis, associated with coeliac disease (*see* Chapter 23), causes intensely pruritic papulovesicular eruptions, which manifest as erythematous papules, vesicles or urticarial-like plaques. The lesions are symmetrically distributed in clusters on the extensor surfaces of the limbs, the back and the intergluteal folds (Fig. 14.5). Urticarial weals around the waist and on the buttocks and a transient urticarial rash that migrates are features of *Strongyloides stercoralis*. Urticaria pigmentosa (Fig. 14.6) occurs in systemic mastocytosis (*see* Chapter 16).

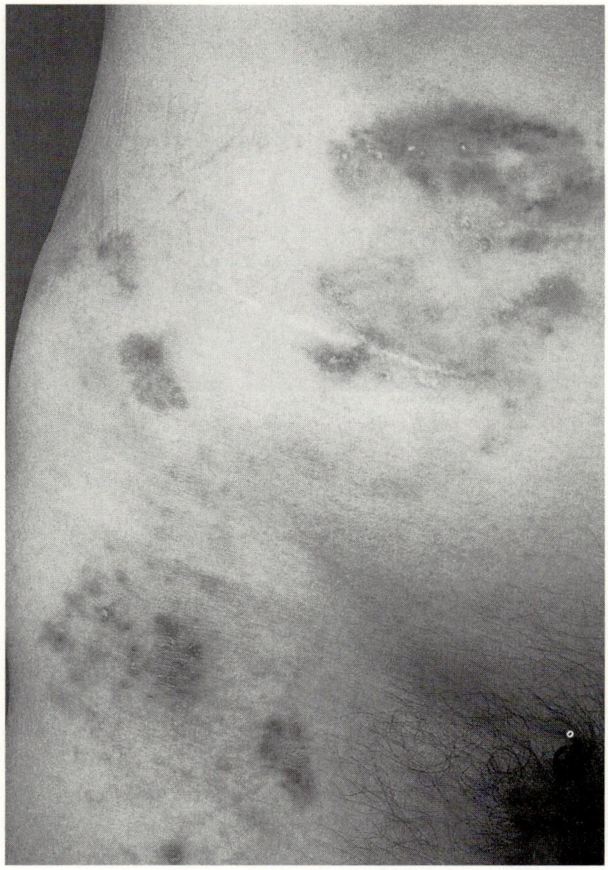

Figure 14.5 *Dermatitis herpetiformis.*

Abdominal examination

Abdominal distension may be the result of gas or ascites, due to severe hypoproteinaemia, or malignancy or tuberculosis. Abdominal distension in an acutely ill patient with inflammatory bowel disease requires the exclusion of a toxic megacolon. Abdominal distension that is limited to the upper abdomen suggests a high intestinal obstruction (*see* Chapter 28).

Abdominal rigidity due to involuntary muscle spasm of the abdominal wall denotes local peritonitis. Peritoneal seeding due to a malignancy may present as Sister Mary Joseph's node in the umbilicus. A 'doughy'

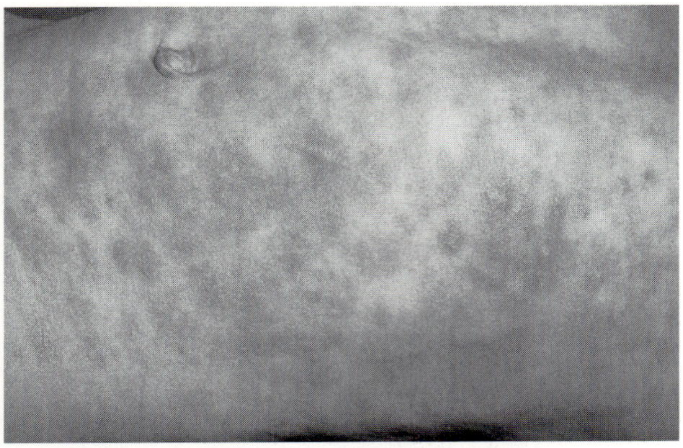

Figure 14.6 *Urticaria pigmentosa.*

feeling on palpation suggests oedematous intestines, which occur in patients with intestinal tuberculosis and typhoid fever. A mass may be palpable in Crohn's disease and in infection with the roundworm *Angiostrongylus costaricensis* (*see* Chapter 19). In a study of 85 patients with 89 small bowel tumours, only 18 per cent of primary malignant or metastatic tumours were palpable (Minardi *et al.*, 1998). The tumours included 11 adenocarcinomas, 10 carcinoids and 1 myxoliposarcoma. Benign tumours were not palpable and included adenomatous polyps, a lipoma, an arteriovenous malformation, a leiomyoma and a fundic polyp (Minardi *et al.*, 1998). In Whipple's disease, abdominal findings may include a mass due to lymph node involvement, splenomegaly or distended loops of intestine. Hepatosplenomegaly is a feature of systemic mastocytosis (*see* Chapter 16). Ascites due to hypoproteinaemia may occur (*see* Chapter 22). Abdominal auscultation may reveal borborygmi in patients with lactose intolerance after ingesting milk or milk products.

Rectal examination

Even if small intestinal disease is suspected, rectal examination is a rewarding exercise. Examination of the rectum should start with an inspection of the perianal area for signs of abscesses, fissures, fistulas and skin tags. The presence of mucus and/or blood in the rectum is suggestive of large bowel pathology. Digital examination of the rectum will reveal a palpable abnormality in approximately 90 per cent of cases with carcinoma of the rectum. It is also very useful to perform faecal occult blood tests using faeces on the examining glove. A proctoscope, not a sigmoidoscope, should be used to check for haemorrhoids. In patients with chronic diarrhoea, or diarrhoea associated with blood or mucus, examination with a sigmoidoscope is essential and should precede a barium enema.

Musculoskeletal system

Musculoskeletal changes include problems of the peripheral and axial joints. In Whipple's disease, peripheral rather than axial joint involvement occurs (*see* Chapter 22). Ankylosing spondylitis is seen in ulcerative colitis and in patients with the HLA-B27 haplotype; there is a male predominance. Single or multiple peripheral joints may be swollen and painful in patients with inflammatory bowel disease, especially Crohn's disease. Patients with the HLA-B27 haplotype infected with *Shigella* species, *Campylobacter jejuni* and *Yersinia enterocolitica* are predisposed to Reiter's syndrome (arthritis, urethritis and conjunctivitis). Bone pain, muscular weakness and tetany reflect malabsorption of vitamin D, calcium and magnesium. Muscle pain is a feature of the roundworm *Trichinella spiralis*.

REFERENCES

Abbas, Z., Moid, I., Khan, A.H., Jafri, S.M.W., Shah, S.H.A., Abid, S., Hamid, S. 1996: Efficacy of octreotide in diarrhoea due to *Vibrio cholerae*: a randomised, controlled trial. *Annals of Tropical Medicine and Parasitology* 90, 507–13.

Akhrass, R., Yaffe, M.B., Fischer, C., Ponsky, J., Shuck, J.M. 1997: Small bowel diverticulosis: perceptions and reality. *Journal of the American College of Surgeons* 184, 383–8.

Anthony, A., Dhillon, A.P., Pounder, R.E., Wakefield, A.J. 1997: Ulceration of the ileum in Crohn's disease: correlation with vascular anatomy. *Journal of Clinical Pathology* 50, 1013–17.

Balthazar, E.J., Charles, H.W., Megibow, A.J. 1996: Salmonella- and Shigella-induced ileitis: CT findings in four patients. *Journal of Computer Assisted Tomography* 20, 375–8.

Barker, W.H., Jr 1974: *Vibrio parahaemolyticus* outbreaks in the United States. *Lancet* 1, 551–4.

Bennett, G.C., Allen, E., Millard, P.H. 1984: *Clostridium difficile* diarrhoea: a highly infectious organism. *Age and Ageing* 13, 363–6.

Bharucha, A.E., Gostout, C.J., Balm, R.K. 1997: Clinical and endoscopic risk factors in the Mallory–Weiss syndrome. *American Journal of Gastroenterology* 92, 805–8.

Brewer, B.J., Golden, G.T., Hitch, D.C., Rudolf, L.E., Wangensteen, S.L. 1976: Abdominal pain. An analysis of 1,000 consecutive cases in a University Hospital emergency room. *American Journal of Surgery* 131, 219–23.

Bunker, S.R., Brown, J.M., McAuley, R.J., Lull, R.J., Jackson, J.H., Hattner, R.S., Huberty, J.P. 1982: Detection of gastrointestinal bleeding sites. Use of in vitro technetium Tc 99m-labeled RBCs. *Journal of the American Medical Association* 247, 789–92.

Capo, V., Despommier, D.D. 1996: Clinical aspects of infection with Trichinella spp. *Clinical Microbiology Reviews* 9, 47–54.

Dauterman, K.W., Bennett, R.G., Greenough, W.B., III, Redett, R.J., Gillespie, J.A., Applebaum, G., Schoenfeld, C.H. 1995: Plasma specific gravity for identifying hypovolaemia. *Journal of Diarrhoeal Disease and Research* 13, 33–8.

Goh, W.H., Ratnaike, R.N. 1999: Irritable bowel syndrome. In Ratnaike, R.N. (ed.) *Diarrhoea and constipation in geriatric practice*. Cambridge: Cambridge University Press, 162–70.

Gorbach, S.L. 1990: Bismuth therapy in gastrointestinal diseases. *Gastroenterology* 99, 863–75.

Gross, C.R., Lindquist, R.D., Woolley, A.C., Granieri, R., Allard, K., Webster, B. 1992: Clinical indicators of dehydration severity in elderly patients. *Journal of Emergency Medicine* 10, 267–74.

Harford, W. 1988: Gastrointestinal angiodysplasia: clinical features. *Endoscopy* 20, 144–8.

Harris, A.G., O'Dorisio, T.M., Woltering, E.A. *et al.* 1995: Consensus statement: octreotide dose titration in secretory diarrhea. Diarrhea Management Consensus Development Panel. *Digestive Diseases and Sciences* 40, 1464–73.

Islam, S.S., Khan, M.U. 1986: Risk factors for diarrhoeal deaths: a case-control study at a diarrhoeal disease hospital in Bangladesh. *International Journal of Epidemiology* 15, 116–21.

Janjua, K.J. 1997: Boerhaave's syndrome. *Postgraduate Medical Journal* 73, 265–70.

Katz, P.O., Salas, L. 1993: Less frequent causes of upper gastrointestinal bleeding. *Gastroenterology Clinics of North America* 88, 2056–8.

Koda-Kimble, M.A., Young, L.Y. 1995: Nausea and vomiting. In Young, L.Y., Koda-Kimble, M.A. (eds) *Applied therapeutics: the clinical use of drugs*, 6th edn. Vancouver, WA: Applied Therapeutics Inc., 1–11.

Koga, H., Iida, M., Nagai, E. *et al.* 1996: Jejunal angiodysplasia confirmed by intravascular injection technique in vitro. Report of a case and review of the literature. *Journal of Clinical Gastroenterology* 23, 139–44.

Kolars, J.C., Levitt, M.D., Aouji, M., Savaiano, D.A. 1984: Yoghurt – an autodigesting source of lactose. *New England Journal of Medicine* 310, 1–3.

Lai, I.R., Chen, K.M., Shun, C.T., Chen, M.Y. 1996: Cytomegalovirus enteritis causing massive bleeding in a patient with AIDS. *Hepatogastroenterology* 43, 987–91.

Levitt, M.D., Lasser, R.B., Schwartz, J.S., Bond, J.H. 1976: Studies of a flatulent patient. *New England Journal of Medicine* 295, 260.

Lewis, B.S. 1994: Small intestinal bleeding. *Gastroenterology Clinics of North America* 23, 67–91.

Manfredi, R., Mastroianni, A., Coronado, O., Chiodo, F. 1996: Effects of treatment with octreotide on vasoactive intestinal polypeptide (VIP) secretion and chronic AIDS-related diarrhoea. *AIDS* 10(Suppl. 2), S47, 116 (abstract).

Minardi, A.J., Zibari, G.B., Aultman, D.F., McMillan, R.W., McDonald, J.C. 1998: Small bowel tumours. *Journal of the American College of Surgeons* 186, 664–8.

Mujica, V.R., Barkin, J.S. 1996: Occult gastrointestinal bleeding: general overview and approach. *Gastrointestinal Endoscopy Clinics of North America* 6, 833–45.

Netterville, R., Hardy, J., Martin, R. 1968: Small bowel hemorrhage. *Annals of Surgery* 167, 949–57.

Ottinger, L., Vickery, A. 1981: A 30 year history of recurrent gastrointestinal bleeding. *New England Journal of Medicine* 305, 211–18.

Papadopoulou, A., Lloyd, D.R., Williams, M.D., Darbyshire, P.J., Booth, I.W. 1996: Gastrointestinal and nutritional sequelae of bone marrow transplantation. *Archives of Disease in Childhood* 75, 208–13.

Pavia, A.T., Nichols, C.R., Green, D.P. *et al.* 1990: Hemolytic–uremic syndrome during an outbreak of Escherichia coli O157:H7 infections in institutions for mentally retarded persons: clinical and epidemiologic observations. *Journal of Pediatrics* 116, 544–51.

Powell, D.W. 1991: Approach to the patient with diarrhea. In Yamada, T. (ed.) *Textbook of gastroenterology*. Philadelphia: J.B. Lippincott Co., 750.

Ratnaike, R.N., Chinner, T.L. 1994: The importance of health education in programs to control diarrhea: experiences in an Australian Aboriginal community. *Health Education* 25, 283–8.

Sack, D.A. 1991: Use of oral rehydration therapy in acute watery diarrhoea. A practical guide. *Drugs* 41, 566–73.

Seigel, L.J., Longo, D.L. 1981: The control of chemotherapy-induced emesis. *Annals of Internal Medicine* 95, 352–9.

Skirrow, M.B. 1991: Epidemiology of Campylobacter enteritis. *International Journal of Food Microbiology* 12, 9–16.

Soderlund, C., Bratt, G.A., Engstrom, L., Grutzmeier, S., Nilsson, R., Sjunnesson, M., Sandstrom, E. 1994: Surgical treatment of cytomegalovirus enterocolitis in severe human immunodeficiency virus infection. Report of eight cases. *Diseases of the Colon and Rectum* 37, 63–72.

Telzak, E.E., Greenberg, M.S.Z., Budnick, L.D., Singh, T., Blum, S. 1991: Diabetes mellitus – a newly described risk factor for infection from *Salmonella enteritidis*. *Journal of Infectious Diseases* 164, 538–41.

Terranova, W., Blake, P.A. 1978: *Bacillus cereus* food poisoning. *New England Journal of Medicine* 298, 143–4.

Verner, J.V., Morrison, A.B. 1958: Islet cell tumor and a syndrome of refractory watery diarrhea and hypokalemia. *American Journal of Medicine* 25, 374–80.

Walker-Smith, J.A. 1986: Acute gastroenteritis in childhood. In Manuel, P.D. Walker-Smith J.A., Tomkins, A. (eds) *Infections of the gastrointestinal tract*. Edinburgh: Churchill Livingstone, 87–97.

Welsh, J.D. 1970: Isolated lactase deficiency in humans: report on 100 patients. *Medicine (Baltimore)* 49, 257–77.

WHO 1985: *The management of diarrhoea and use of oral rehydration therapy. A joint WHO/UNICEF statement*, 2nd edn. Geneva: World Health Organization.
WHO 1989: *The treatment and prevention of acute diarrhoea. Practical guidelines*. Geneva: World Health Organization.
WHO 1993: *The management and prevention of diarrhoea*, 3rd edn. Programme for Control of Diarrhoeal Diseases. Geneva: World Health Organization.

15

Mechanisms of diarrhoea

RANJIT N RATNAIKE

TERMINOLOGY

In a healthy individual, the frequency of bowel actions varies from three motions a day to three per week. Diarrhoea is an increase in the frequency, fluidity or volume (weight) of bowel movements, relative to the usual habit for that individual (Phillips, 1972). The World Health Organization (WHO) defines diarrhoea as three or more unformed bowel actions in 24 hours (WHO, 1993). Acute diarrhoea is an episode of diarrhoea that lasts less than 2 weeks, while persistent diarrhoea is an episode that lasts for 2 weeks or longer (WHO, 1993). Chronic diarrhoea is defined as diarrhoea that lasts for at least 3–6 weeks (Powell, 1991).

Diarrhoea is also defined in terms of stool weight. Since the stool consists mostly of water, stool weight reflects water content. Dietary fibre increases stool weight by its water-holding property. In normal subjects on a Western diet, the stool weight is less than 200 g/day. However, significant differences in the diet, especially the high consumption of roughage in predominantly vegetable and plant-based diets common in parts of Asia and Africa, increases stool weight to greater than 200 g without diarrhoea.

FLUID ABSORPTION AND SECRETION

The basic mechanisms that cause diarrhoea are few, despite many aetiological factors. In the normal small and large intestine, active absorption and secretion of electrolytes and water results in net absorption (*see* Chapter 8). The small and large intestines absorb large quantities of fluid. About 10 L a day of fluid enters the small intestine, the sources of which are the diet and saliva, gastric juice, bile, and secretions of the small intestine and the pancreas (Matseshe and Phillips, 1978). The complex process of fluid absorption and secretion occurs throughout the gastrointestinal tract, influenced by a variety of factors that regulate the processes of absorption and secretion, and major fluxes of ions and fluid occur.

Depending on the type of food ingested, the luminal contents of the duodenum may be either hypertonic or hypotonic in relation to plasma. When fluid reaches the jejunum, the luminal contents are, under normal conditions, isotonic with plasma. In the small intestine, the jejunum (which has the largest surface area) absorbs most of the fluid. The ileum absorbs a lesser quantity of 3–5 L.

The principal function of the colon is the absorption of water and electrolytes. The contents from the ileum of up to 1500–2000 mL/day is reduced to less than 200 g of solid stool. Although the colon normally absorbs about 1–2 L, it has a reserve capacity to absorb up to 5 L.

It is important to note that water absorption occurs together with the absorption of solutes within the intestinal lumen. It is for this reason that osmotically active solutes in the lumen can impair water absorption or even lead to water secretion.

Diarrhoea may result from excessive secretion of water in the presence of *normal absorption*, or, in situations of normal secretion, decreased absorption may result in diarrhoea. Examples are diffuse mucosal disease of the small intestine or decreased surface area of the intestine due to surgical excision. Even when large volumes of fluid enter the colon, diarrhoea does not occur until the absorptive capacity of the colon is exceeded.

CLASSIFICATION OF DIARRHOEA

The causes of diarrhoea may be classified into several broad categories:

- secretory
- osmotic
- motility disorders
- multiple mechanisms.

How does a secretagogue and its receptor activate adenylate cyclase?

Preliminary information
The activation process involves two intermediaries:

1 the Gs protein;
2 guanosine triphosphate (GTP) or guanosine diphosphate (GDP).

The Gs protein is a peripheral membrane protein consisting of three subunits (α, β, γ subunits). The Gs protein can bind to either GTP or GDP. The Gs protein–GTP complex *activates* adenylate cyclase. The Gs protein–GDP complex *inhibits* adenylate cyclase.

The process of activation
When a secretagogue binds to its receptor the following events occur:

- The Gs protein binds to GTP by the α subunit as shown:

$$\alpha\beta\gamma + \text{GTP} \xrightarrow{\text{GTPase}} \alpha\text{GTP} + \beta\gamma$$

- αGTP now activates adenylate cyclase, which in turn forms cyclic adenosine monophosphate (cAMP) from adenosine triphosphate (ATP):

$$\text{ATP} \xrightarrow{\text{Adenylate cyclase}} \text{cAMP}$$

- Cyclic AMP ativates specific protein kinases that will bring about specific physiological responses.

How is adenylate cyclase deactivated?
The αGTP is slowly hydrolysed to αGDP and reforms the inactive protein GDP as shown:

$$\alpha\text{GTP} \xrightarrow[\searrow P_i]{} \alpha\text{GDP} \xrightarrow[\nearrow \beta_\gamma]{} \alpha\beta\gamma\text{GDP (inactive protein–GDP)}$$

Figure 15.1 *The process of activation and deactivation of adenylate cyclase. (Reproduced with permission from Ratnaike, R.N. 1999: Pathophysiology of diarrhoea. In Ratnaike, R.N. (ed.)* Diarrhoea and constipation in geriatric practice. *Cambridge: Cambridge University Press, 23–30.)*

SECRETORY DIARRHOEA

Normal homeostatic mechanisms ensure that intestinal absorption is greater than secretion (*see also* Chapter 8). Secretory diarrhoea primarily occurs in the small intestine and, less frequently, in the colon, when a secretagogue interacts with the mucosal epithelial cell to initiate a cascade of biochemical reactions as shown in Fig. 15.1. The secretagogue activates adenylate cyclase resulting in an increase in the concentration of cyclic AMP. This causes active secretion of Cl^- and HCO_3^-, a passive efflux of Na^+, K^+ and water, and inhibition of Na^+ and Cl^- entry to the cell (Field *et al.*, 1989). Less commonly a secretagogue elevates cyclic GMP, or secretory activity is mediated by an intracellular increase in calcium.

As shown in Fig. 15.1, secretory diarrhoea occurs as the culmination of a series of intracellular events. Cholera toxin, a powerful secretagogue, is the most extensively studied toxin on small intestinal epithelial cells and is an example of the mechanism by which secretory diarrhoea occurs (Grady and Keusch, 1971). Figure 15.2 shows the action of cholera toxin. The toxin binds to a receptor site on the cell surface. Adenylate cyclase is then activated. Adenylate cyclase reacts with ATP to generate cyclic AMP, which then activates a protein kinase that phosphorylates membrane proteins involved in active ion transport. The outcome is an increased secretion of Cl^- (predominantly) and HCO_3^- by the crypt cells, and decreased electroneutral Na and Cl and water absorption by more mature intestinal epithelial cells of the villi. In summary, a secretagogue acts to 'switch' the intestinal epithelial cells from a state of net absorption to net secretion. The mechanism

- The cholera toxin consists of an A subunit and five B subunits.
- The toxin enters intestinal mucosal cells and attaches to the Gs protein.
- Part of the A subunit of cholera toxin reacts and modifies the Gs protein by ribosylation. This involves the transfer of an ADP-ribose unit from NAD to a specific arginine on the α-Gs protein.
- This ribosylated complex is now unable to hydrolyse bound GTP to GDP and is locked in the active form.
- Adenylate cyclase is therefore persistently activated and cyclic AMP concentrations are consequently high.
- Specific protein kinases are activated, which will stimulate the active transport of ions leading to watery diarrhoea.

Figure 15.2 *The mechanism of action of cholera toxin. (Reproduced with permission from Ratnaike, R.N. 1999: Pathophysiology of diarrhoea. In Ratnaike, R.N. (ed.)* Diarrhoea and constipation in geriatric practice. *Cambridge: Cambridge University Press, 23–30.)*

Table 15.1 *Common secretagogues causing diarrhoea*

Bacterial enterotoxins
Vibrio cholerae
Escherichia coli
Staphylococcus aureus
Shigella species
Bacillus cereus
Clostridium perfringens
Therapeutic agents
Anthraquinone cathartics (e.g. senna, cascara)
Bisacodyl
Dioctyl sodium sulphosuccinate
Castor oil
Ricinoleic acid
Phenolphthalein
Misoprostol
Chenodeoxycholic acid
Endogenous agents
Long-chain fatty acids
Dihydroxy bile acids
Humoral agents
Vasoactive intestinal peptide (VIP)
Glucagon
Secretin
Calcitonin
Bradykinin
Prostaglandins
Serotonin

involves a series of *biochemical* intracellular events. The net fluid excretion results in diarrhoea. Since no cell damage occurs, blood in the faeces is not a feature in secretory diarrhoea.

Table 15.1 shows the common secretagogues that cause diarrhoea. Although in most instances secretory diarrhoea is due to bacterial toxins (*see* Chapter 18), other secretagogues include endogenous agents, therapeutic agents and humoral agents. An example of an endogenous secretagogue is chenodeoxycholic acid, a dihydroxy bile acid. These compounds may not be efficiently absorbed in terminal ileal disease (*see* Chapter 16). They reach the colon and act as secretagogues to cause increased secretion of water and electrolytes (Mekhjian *et al.*, 1971; Binder and Rawlins, 1973). Among the therapeutic agents, chenodeoxycholic acid, which is used for the dissolution of gallstones, causes diarrhoea as a side-effect in up to 49 per cent of patients (Iser *et al.*, 1975). Chenodeoxycholic acid stimulates cyclic AMP in the colonocytes causing net fluid secretion (Conley *et al.*, 1976). Long-chain fatty acids, which are malabsorbed in coeliac disease (*see* Chapter 23) and in other states of malabsorption due to small bowel mucosal damage, act as secretagogues in the colon.

The many humoral agents associated with secretory diarrhoea and their increasingly important role in the regulation of the gastrointestinal tract are discussed in detail in Chapter 7.

- The toxin forms a receptor–toxin complex before entering the cell (endocytosis)
- The toxin diffuses into the cytosol
- The toxin then catalyses the transfer of the ADP–ribosyl moiety to the peptide chain elongation factor 2 (EF-2)
- The ribosylated EF-2 is now inactivated and unable to synthesize protein
- Cell death eventually occurs

Figure 15.3 *The process of toxin-induced cell death. (Reproduced with permission from Ratnaike, R.N. 1999: Pathophysiology of diarrhoea. In Ratnaike, R.N. (ed.)* Diarrhoea and constipation in geriatric practice. *Cambridge: Cambridge University Press, 23–30.)*

A prominent cause of secretory diarrhoea is mucosal inflammation due to inflammatory bowel disease or due to invasive enteric pathogens that liberate cytotoxins, which cause cell death by a process detailed in Fig. 15.3. Inflammatory mediators with secretagogue properties released by damaged mast cells, macrophages, eosinophils and neutrophils are:

- prostaglandin E_2
- adenosine
- cytokines
- bradykinin
- histamine
- platelet-activating factor
- serotonin.

The presence or absence of secretory diarrhoea is established by measuring the osmotic gap. This is defined as the difference between the *measured* osmolality of stool and the *calculated* osmolality. Each of these measurements is determined by simple laboratory tests.

Measured osmolality

The osmolality of the stools is assumed to be equal to the *plasma* osmolality. This approximation is made because of the exchange of water and ions during the formation of stools, with the proviso that the stool is not retained in the colon where water absorption would occur (this of course does not happen during diarrhoea). The plasma osmolality is either measured directly or assumed to be approximately equal to the typical value of 290 mosmol/kg. This figure is often used rather than measuring the total plasma or stool osmolality.

Calculated osmolality

The calculated osmolality is determined by measuring the stool concentrations of sodium and potassium in milliosmoles per kilogram and multiplying their sum by two (owing to the presence of inorganic anions that also contribute to the osmotic value).

In normal subjects, the osmotic gap between plasma osmolality and stool osmolality is less than 50 mosmol/kg. In secretory diarrhoea, the two values, *measured* plasma and *calculated* stool osmolality, are essentially the same and no osmotic gap exists.

The characteristics of secretory diarrhoea are:

- voluminous watery stools, greater than 1 L a day;
- diarrhoea does *not* stop with fasting;
- stool osmolality parallels the plasma osmolality;
- intestinal mucosa may be normal;
- there is no pus or blood in the stools.

OSMOTIC DIARRHOEA

Osmotic diarrhoea is due to the presence of osmotically active compounds (hydrophilic solutes or dissolved substances that have the property of attracting water molecules) in the intestinal lumen. These substances are poorly absorbed (or not absorbed at all) and their high concentration increases the osmolality of the intestinal contents. This high luminal osmolality prevents the intestine from performing its normal physiological function of initiating or maintaining a water gradient. The osmotic effect causes fluid retention in the intestine and also fluid to be secreted into the lumen. Diarrhoea occurs when the absorptive capacity of the colon is exceeded. In contrast to secretory diarrhoea, where the process is biochemical due to the activation of enzymes within the enterocyte, in osmotic diarrhoea the mechanism is physiological.

The presence of osmotically active solutes within the intestinal lumen is due to the ingestion of osmotically active compounds (Table 15.2). Lactulose is an osmotic laxative used in decompensated liver disease to prevent hepatic encephalopathy. Sorbitol, another osmotic laxative, is also used in some liquid pharmaceutical preparations. Osmotic diarrhoea also occurs due to the presence of products of maldigestion and malabsorption owing to a variety of conditions (*see* Chapter 16).

Table 15.2 *Common osmotic agents causing diarrhoea*

Lactulose
Glycerol
Sorbitol
Mannitol
Magnesium-containing antacids
Magnesium sulphate (Epsom salts)
Sodium sulphate (Glauber's salt)
Sodium citrate
Monosaccharides and disaccharides

Conditions specifically associated with monosaccharide and/or disaccharide malabsorption, for example, congenital and acquired lactase deficiency, are discussed in detail in Chapter 24. Other specific causes of malabsorption are coeliac disease (Chapter 23), tropical sprue (Chapter 21), Whipple's disease (Chapter 22) and also a variety of viral (Chapter 17), bacterial (Chapter 18) and parasitic infections (Chapter 19) which include human immunodeficiency virus (HIV) and the acquired immunodeficiency syndrome (AIDS) (*see* Chapter 20).

Osmotic diarrhoea also occurs when large quantities of fruit and vegetables are ingested. Incomplete digestion may result in long-chain carbohydrate residues that can undergo bacterial degradation in the colon to short-chain compounds (for example, hydrophilic solutes), which cause an osmotic diarrhoea. Medications that are sweetened with sugars and poorly absorbed by the gastrointestinal tract (for example, sorbitol or fructose), and excessive consumption of candy, gum or foods containing similar sugars and sugar substitutes (for example, xylitol), also cause osmotic diarrhoea.

A self-inflicted cause of osmotic diarrhoea is the abuse of laxatives, some of which are osmotic agents. The excessive use of laxatives may or may not be surreptitious. Especially in the elderly, inadvertent ingestion of laxatives may occur due to problems of cognition. An examination of medications used by the patient with diarrhoea is useful (Ratnaike and Jones, 1998).

The key difference between secretory and osmotic diarrhoea is the osmotic gap. The small intestine can absorb Na^+ against a concentration gradient. The presence of large amounts of osmotically active compounds in the intestines induces retention of water, causing a drop in the *calculated* osmolality (determined only by the Na^+ and K^+ levels multiplied by two) to less than the *measured* osmolality. The consequence is that the osmotic gap is usually 50–100 mosmol/kg or even much higher. Since osmotic diarrhoea results from the presence of an osmotic load in the intestine the osmotic load is eliminated on fasting and the diarrhoea resolves.

The characteristics of osmotic diarrhoea are therefore:

- diarrhoea, which can be of large volume, that stops on fasting as the causative agent is removed;
- the osmotic gap in the stools is greater than 50 mosmol/kg.

The ideal collection period of faecal samples for measurement of the osmotic gap is 3 days, from a patient who is fasted and maintained on fluids, although, in practice, a 24-hour collection is widely used. A faecal volume of more than 500 mL should be collected for the test and stored (if necessary) in the refrigerator during the collection period to reduce the effects of bacterial metabolism, which can change the osmolality of the sample. The sample should be without urine contamination, as this increases the osmolality.

INTESTINAL MOTILITY DISORDERS

The role of altered intestinal motility as a *primary* mechanism of diarrhoea needs further study (*see* Chapter 11). Many diarrhoeal entities are associated with altered motility, but there is insufficient evidence that a causal relationship exists between intrinsic abnormalities in motility and diarrhoea. Motility affects intestinal absorption: decreased motility prolongs the time available for water and electrolyte absorption while increased motility decreases the time for intestinal absorption to occur and may lead to diarrhoea. Motility disorders may indirectly cause diarrhoea through intestinal stasis and bacterial overgrowth (*see also* Chapters 12 and 18). Bacteria deconjugate and metabolize bile salts, reducing the bile salt pool and decreasing micellar solubilization of fat (Donaldson, 1965). As previously mentioned, diarrhoea also occurs from dihydroxy bile salts that may reach the colon and act as secretagogues.

Diarrhoea may be associated with hypomotility due to systemic diseases or local conditions that affect the small intestine. Systemic conditions that cause hypomotility are:

- hypothyroidism
- diabetic autonomic neuropathy
- amyloidosis
- scleroderma
- myotonia dystrophica.

Local conditions include:

- intestinal pseudo-obstruction
- lymphoma (*see* Chapters 16 and 26)
- radiation enteritis.

Especially in the elderly, hypomotility due to hypothyroidism may cause bacterial overgrowth of the small intestine with the potential to cause diarrhoea. In hypothyroid elderly patients treated with thyroxine, the median orocaecal transit time increased from 75 to 135 minutes when thyroxine was withdrawn (Rahman *et al.*, 1991). Other prominent systemic causes of diarrhoea are diabetes mellitus and scleroderma (*see* also Chapters 16 and 27). In both conditions, diarrhoea can be attributed to bacterial overgrowth. In patients with diabetes mellitus, bacterial overgrowth may be responsible for a reduction in both intestinal contraction and transit time (Scarpello and Sladen, 1978). Another mechanism for diarrhoea in diabetes mellitus is a 'rapid' transit due to autonomic neuropathy. Scleroderma involves the small intestine where it causes fibrosis and subsequently stasis, which lead to bacterial overgrowth and malabsorption (*see also* Chapters 16 and 27).

Hypermotility also causes diarrhoea. In the small intestine, increased motility is associated with thyrotoxicosis, and thyroid replacement in hypothyroidism (Tobin *et al.*, 1989). Diarrhoea is the most severe side-effect of Tacrine, a cholinesterase inhibitor, used in Alzheimer's disease, owing to its cholinergic action (Antuono, 1995; Zemlan *et al.*, 1996). A new agent in treating colorectal cancer, irinotecan, causes severe diarrhoea, owing to a cholinergic-like syndrome caused by the inhibition of acetylcholinesterase (Bleiberg and Cvitkovic, 1996; Rivory, 1996).

Hypermotility may occur from enterotoxins liberated by bacterial pathogens and by bacterial mucosal invasion by *Shigella* species (La Brec *et al.*, 1964), *Salmonella* and strains of *E. coli* (Grady and Keusch, 1971).

MULTIPLE MECHANISMS

Diarrhoea of small intestinal origin is often multifactorial, especially in states of malabsorption. Secretory and osmotic diarrhoea may both operate, with one mechanism dominant, a contributory factor being altered motility. Inflammatory processes in the intestine liberate mediators that cause secretory diarrhoea and also alter intestinal motility. During the inflammatory process the secretion of fluid helps clear the mucosa of pathogens and other harmful products. Cell death results in blood and pus, which act as osmotic solutes to initiate an osmotic type of diarrhoea.

Diarrhoea in patients with diabetes mellitus is well documented and the mechanism is multifactorial. In diabetics with evidence of an autonomic neuropathy, derangement of the neural regulation of absorption and secretion may occur. Those susceptible to developing an autonomic neuropathy are patients on insulin treatment with poorly controlled blood glucose concentrations or with evidence of peripheral vascular disease. In patients with autonomic neuropathy, diarrhoea may occur since the autonomic nervous system is associated with the processes of intestinal absorption and secretion. The role of α_2-adrenergic receptors present on the enterocytes in the intestinal transport of ions is well established. Noradrenaline stimulates α_2-adrenergic receptors on the basolateral membrane of the enterocyte. This inhibits adenylate cyclase activity and decreases intracellular calcium concentration. The result is an increase in fluid and electrolyte absorption, and secretion is inhibited. In diabetics with severe autonomic neuropathy, diarrhoea is in part due to net fluid secretion. Treatment with α_2-adrenergic agonists such as clonidine and lidamidine is beneficial. These agents decrease cyclic AMP concentrations in the enterocyte and net water and electrolyte retention occurs. Unfortunately, central nervous and cardiovascular system side-effects, particularly in the elderly, limit their usefulness.

In coeliac disease (*see* Chapter 23), diarrhoea is due to both secretory and osmotic mechanisms. Mucosal damage, predominantly in the upper gastrointestinal tract, affects mucosal cells which secrete cholecystokinin (CCK), gastric inhibitory polypeptide (GIP) and secretin (*see* Chapter 7). Decreased concentration of these gut peptides impairs pancreatic function, since CCK and secretin are responsible for enzyme and bicarbonate secretion. Decreased CCK reduces gallbladder contraction and hence intraluminal bile salt concentrations. This consequently causes less micelle formation, decreasing fat absorption (*see* Chapter 16). Diarrhoea is therefore multifactorial.

SUMMARY OF MECHANISMS OF DRUG-INDUCED DIARRHOEA

The mechanisms by which drugs can cause diarrhoea have been reviewed by Ratnaike and Jones (1998). In addition to those mechanisms mentioned previously in this chapter, other mechanisms lead to drug-induced diarrhoea. Drugs can compromise both immune and non-immune responses of the gastrointestinal tract, predisposing to viral, bacterial and protozoal pathogens. Drug-induced hypomotility may result in bacterial overgrowth, deconjugation of bile salts and diarrhoea. Less commonly, diarrhoea may occur due to hypermotility because of a cholinergic-like syndrome. In the colon, the host-protective commensal bacteria provide a powerful defence against pathogens. Disruption of this commensal population by antibiotic therapy may result in *Clostridium difficile* suprainfection, which causes diarrhoea through toxin production. This is especially important in elderly patients on chemotherapy for malignancy and those with multiple diseases. The organism responds to vancomycin, metronidazole and bacitracin. Metronidazole is advocated as the drug of choice with vancomycin reserved for relapses.

Drugs also cause diarrhoea by interfering with normal physiological processes. Drugs impair fluid absorption by activating adenylate cyclase within the small intestinal enterocyte, increasing the concentration of cAMP. This causes active secretion of Cl^- and HCO_3^-, passive efflux of Na^+, K^+ and water, and inhibition of Na^+ and Cl^- into the enterocyte. Examples of these drugs (secretagogues) are bisacodyl, misoprostil and chenodeoxycholic acid.

Drugs may affect a second mechanism that regulates water and electrolyte transport, the Na^+–K^+ exchange pump. The energy for this pump is provided by the ATPase-mediated breakdown of ATP. ATPase may be inhibited by digoxin, auranofin, colchicine and olsalazine.

A number of drugs cause osmotic diarrhoea, including antacids containing magnesium trisilicate or hydroxide, lactulose and sorbitol. Another mechanism by which drugs cause diarrhoea is by mucosal damage of the small and large bowel. In the small intestine, mucosal damage causes diarrhoea and fat malabsorption, as may occur, for example, with neomycin and colchicine. In the colon, gold salts and penicillamine can cause colitis of varying severity.

Although the causes of diarrhoea are diverse, a drug-associated aetiology should always be considered, and actively sought and addressed to prevent the complications of dehydration, electrolyte imbalance and undernutrition.

There is now increasing interest and accumulating evidence regarding the enteric nervous system (*see* Chapters 1 and 7), and its dominant role and pervasive influence on the activities of the gastrointestinal tract. The autonomic nervous system regulates an array of mucosal and motor functions of the gut, and is composed of a dense plexus of afferent and efferent interneurones with cholinergic and non-cholinergic neurones. These regulate water and electrolyte transport crucial to maintaining homeostatic mechanisms. In inflammation, the inflammatory and immune mediators activate the secretomotor neurons of the enteric nervous system that result in a cascade of events affecting the processes of absorption and secretion. The large number and diverse nature of the neurotransmitters associated with the autonomic nervous system are discussed in Chapters 1 and 7.

The entire range of mechanisms that cause diarrhoea may yet be unknown. Further understanding of the role of both the enteric nervous system and the many specialized cells with exquisitely individual functions within the intestine will advance our knowledge of the pathophysiology of diarrhoea.

REFERENCES

Antuono, P.G. 1995: Effectiveness and safety of velnacrine for the treatment of Alzheimer's disease. A double-blind, placebo-controlled study. Mentane Study Group. *Archives of Internal Medicine* 155, 1766–72.

Binder, H.J., Rawlins, C.L. 1973: Effect of conjugated dihydroxy bile salts on electrolyte transport in rat colon. *Journal of Clinical Investigation* 52, 1460–6.

Bleiberg, H., Cvitkovic, E. 1996: Characterisation and clinical management of CPT-11 (irinotecan)-induced adverse events: the European perspective. *European Journal of Cancer* 32A, S18–23.

Conley, D.R., Coyne, M.J., Bonorris, G.G., Chung, A., Schoenfield, L.J. 1976: Bile acid stimulation of colonic adenylate cyclase and secretion in the rabbit. *American Journal of Digestive Diseases* 21, 453–8.

Donaldson, R.M., Jr 1965: Studies on the pathogenesis of steatorrhoea in the blind loop syndrome. *Journal of Clinical Investigation* 44, 1815–25.

Field, M., Rao, M.C., Chang, E.B. 1989: Intestinal electrolyte transport and diarrheal disease (1). *New England Journal of Medicine* 321, 800–6.

Grady, G.F., Keusch, G.T. 1971: Pathogenesis of bacterial diarrheas. I. *New England Journal of Medicine* 285, 831–41.

Iser, J.H., Dowling, R.H., Mok, H.Y., Bell, G.D. 1975: Chenodeoxycholic acid treatment of gallstones. A follow-up report and analysis of factors influencing response to therapy. *New England Journal of Medicine* 293, 378–83.

La Brec, E.H., Schneider, H., Magnani, T.J., Jr 1964: Epithelial cell penetration as an essential step in the pathogenesis of bacillary dysentery. *Journal of Bacteriology* 88, 1503.

Matseshe, J.W., Phillips, S.F. 1978: Chronic diarrhoea. A practical approach. *Medical Clinics of North America* 62, 141–54.

Mekhjian, H.S., Phillips, S.F., Hofmann, A.F. 1971: Colonic secretion of water and electrolytes induced by bile acids: perfusion studies in man. *Journal of Clinical Investigation* 50, 1569–77.

Phillips, S.F. 1972: Diarrhea: a current view of the pathophysiology. *Gastroenterology* 63, 495–518.

Powell, D.W. 1991: Approach to the patient with diarrhea. In Yamada, T. (ed.) *Textbook of gastroenterology.* Philadelphia: J.B. Lippincott Co., 750.

Rahman, Q., Haboubi, N.Y., Hudson, P.R., Lee, G.S., Shah, I.U. 1991: The effect of thyroxine on small intestinal motility in the elderly. *Clinical Endocrinology* 35, 443–6.

Ratnaike, R.N., Jones, T.E. 1998: Mechanisms of drug-induced diarrhoea in the elderly. *Drugs and Aging* 13, 245–53.

Rivory, L.P. 1996: Irinotecan (CPT-11): a brief overview. *Clinical and Experimental Pharmacology and Physiology* 23, 1000–4.

Scarpello, J.H., Sladen, G.E. 1978: Diabetes and the gut. *Gut* 19, 1153–62.

Tobin, M.V., Fisken, R.A., Diggory, R.T., Morris, A.I., Gilmore, I.T. 1989: Orocaecal transit time in health and in thyroid disease. *Gut* 30, 26–9.

WHO 1993: *The management and prevention of diarrhoea*, 3rd edn. Programme for Control of Diarrhoeal Diseases. Geneva: World Health Organization.

Zemlan, F.P., Keys, M., Richter, R.W., Strub, R.L. 1996: Double-blind placebo-controlled study of velnacrine in Alzheimer's disease. *Life Sciences* 58, 1823–32.

16

Maldigestion and malabsorption

RANJIT N RATNAIKE, ANGELA H BARBOUR

The major function of the small intestine is the digestion and absorption of food and nutrients. As commonly used, the term malabsorption includes disorders of both *maldigestion* and *malabsorption*, but the two processes are distinct. Maldigestion refers to problems relating to protein, carbohydrate and/or fat digestion and malabsorption refers to an impaired ability of these products of digestion to be absorbed by the small intestine. Malabsorption, in addition to the absent or suboptimal absorption of the breakdown products of proteins, fats and carbohydrates, also results in decreased absorption of vitamins and minerals, water and electrolytes.

The 'malabsorption syndrome' is characterized by excessive faecal excretion of fat (steatorrhoea), and variable malabsorption of fats, proteins, carbohydrates and other nutrients. In clinical practice, the terms malabsorption and the malabsorption syndrome focus primarily on fat malabsorption, or steatorrhoea, a word derived from the Greek words *stear* for fat and *rhoia* for flow, which is a common and often dominant feature. Malabsorption syndromes can result from a disorder of digestion, a functional decrease in the absorptive surface of the small intestine or from impaired transfer of absorbed nutrients from small intestinal enterocytes to the circulation. They may arise from intestinal disease or from extraintestinal disorders, such as pancreatic disease and obstruction of the common bile duct, which impairs the flow of bile into the intestine.

This chapter will focus on fat malabsorption. Carbohydrate and protein malabsorption are discussed in Chapters 10 and 24.

Digestion involves the breaking down or hydrolysis of nutrients to products that can easily be absorbed by the small intestinal mucosa. The process of digestion converts carbohydrates to monosaccharides and disaccharides, proteins to peptides and amino acids, and fats to fatty acids and monoglycerides. Salivary juice initiates these complex digestive activities that continue in the stomach and are completed in the upper small intestine. Gastric, pancreatic and biliary secretions are also necessary for digestion.

In the context of fat digestion, gastric juice is the least important of these secretions and pancreatic exocrine enzymes the most important. Pancreatic activity in relation to digestion is divided into three phases: the cephalic, gastric and intestinal phases. In the cephalic phase, the sight, smell or taste of food results in efferent vagal impulses that cause the secretion of pancreatic enzymes and bicarbonate. In the gastric phase, gastric distension due to food and amino acids and peptides in the lumen results predominantly in pancreatic enzyme secretion. The gastric phase contributes less than 10 per cent of pancreatic enzyme secretion. The intestinal phase of pancreatic secretion is the most important and occurs when gastric chyme (from the Greek word *chymos*, juice) enters the duodenum. Pancreatic lipase, in the presence of pancreatic co-lipase, hydrolyses triglycerides to monoglycerides, diglycerides and free fatty acids. At the same time, cholecystokinin (CCK), gastric inhibitory polypeptide and secretin are released from the upper small intestinal endocrine cells (*see* Chapter 7).

An adequate small intestinal surface area and an undamaged mucosa are necessary for optimal absorption of the products of digestion. After intraluminal digestion, further digestion and absorption of proteins and carbohydrates occurs at the brush border of the enterocyte. Nutrients enter the microvilli (*see* Chapter 2) and are then actively or passively transported across the mucosal cell. Following breakdown, efficient fat absorption occurs through micelle formation for which bile salts are essential (see below). A microvillus-membrane fatty acid-binding protein (FABP), which plays a role in the uptake of fatty acids, has been identified in animal and subsequently in human studies (Lieberman *et al.*, 1997).

The unstirred water layer of the small intestine has been considered a formidable barrier to fat absorption at the mucosal surface (Turnberg, 1978). The magnitude of the unstirred water layer, previously thought to be about 600 μm in depth, has recently been measured at 40 μm (Strocchi and Levitt, 1991). These authors suggest that, since the extent of the unstirred water layer is much less than previously estimated, its influence as a barrier to absorption may not be as significant as previously thought.

Fatty acids and monoglycerides enter the enterocytes via the microvilli and are re-esterified to triglycerides in the endoplasmic reticulum. These are then aggregated and coated with phospholipid, cholesterol ester and lipoprotein to form chylomicrons, which are transferred into the Golgi apparatus, and then into the lymphatic and subsequently the systemic circulations. Chylomicrons consist of triglyceride 90 per cent, phospholipid 7.5 per cent, cholesterol 1.6 per cent, and apolipoproteins 1.3 per cent by weight (Green *et al.*, 1979). Fats are predominantly absorbed in the proximal jejunum.

The absorption of water and electrolytes (Chapter 8), vitamins and minerals (Chapter 9) and further information on the digestion and absorption of fats, carbohydrates and proteins (Chapter 10) are discussed elsewhere in this text.

CLINICAL FEATURES OF MALABSORPTION

The clinical features of malabsorption are discussed in more detail in the chapter on the signs and symptoms of small bowel disease (*see* Chapter 14). Briefly, with steatorrhoea, the bowel actions are often bulky, greasy, difficult to flush and foul smelling, and a film of oil may be seen in the toilet pan. The stools may float, but this is due to air and not fat. Patients may complain of diarrhoea after a meal with a high fat content. However, the stools may appear normal despite increased faecal fat content.

Weight loss, and symptoms and signs due to deficiency of specific nutrients (e.g. iron, vitamin D or vitamin B_{12}), are often present, depending on the cause, severity and site of disease.

Undigested food in stools suggests intestinal hurry and not a malabsorptive condition. Diarrhoea with the passage of blood and mucus suggests large bowel pathology, and is not a feature of malabsorption. Carbohydrate malabsorption, as in lactose intolerance (*see* Chapter 24) is frequently associated with explosive diarrhoea, often precipitated by a meal containing lactose. Patients with lactose intolerance often complain of abdominal discomfort and distension, the passage of flatus, and diarrhoea after consuming milk and milk-containing products, although not yoghurt, as the lactase in the yoghurt is activated at body temperature (Kolars *et al.*, 1984).

CAUSES OF MALABSORPTION

Pancreatic disease

Steatorrhoea is a prominent feature of intrinsic pancreatic disease owing to the decreased secretion of enzymes or an obstruction to their flow. Table 16.1 summarizes the main pancreatic causes of steatorrhoea. Fat is ingested mainly as triglyceride and cholesterol. Pancreatic lipase hydrolyses triglyceride to two long-chain fatty acids, and the third (remaining) fatty acid combines with the glycerol to form β-monoglyceride (Kayden *et al.*, 1967) (Fig. 16.1). These products of hydrolysis need bile salts for micelle formation to enable solubilization and absorption within the aqueous environment of the small intestine.

Chronic pancreatitis is the most common pancreatic cause of adult steatorrhoea. Steatorrhoea occurs if destruction of the pancreas is extensive and a 90 per

Table 16.1 *Pancreatic causes of malabsorption*

Adults
Chronic pancreatitis
Pancreatic carcinoma
Pancreatic resection
Zollinger–Ellison syndrome (gastrinoma)
Somatostatinoma
Children
Cystic fibrosis
Shwachman–Diamond syndrome
Johanson–Blizzard syndrome

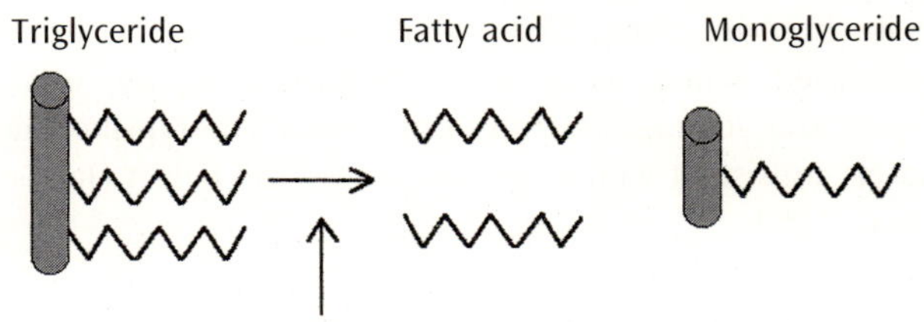

Figure 16.1 *The hydrolysis of triglyceride by pancreatic lipase. (Modified from Langman, M.J.S. 1982:* A concise textbook of gastroenterology, *2nd edn. Edinburgh: Churchill Livingstone, 57.)*

cent reduction of pancreatic lipase occurs (DiMagno *et al.*, 1973). Steatorrhoea is not inevitable but, when it does occur, the severity is such that about 50 per cent of patients report passing drops of oil per rectum. Carcinoma of the pancreas (resulting in tissue destruction and/or duct obstruction) and surgical resection are uncommon causes of steatorrhoea. Steatorrhoea may occur with the Zollinger–Ellison syndrome in patients with a gastrinoma. Excessive secretion of gastrin by the tumour causes gastric hypersecretion. This abnormal acid load exceeds the capacity of the pancreas to secrete adequate quantities of bicarbonate to effect a neutral pH in the duodenum and jejunum, which is necessary to both activate pancreatic enzymes and maintain their optimal function (King and Toskes, 1983). A very low intraluminal pH of the small intestine also impedes fat absorption by injury to the mucosa and by precipitating bile salts, impairing micelle formation. Thus a low intraluminal pH contributes to both maldigestion and malabsorption. Another non-beta islet cell tumour that can be associated with steatorrhoea is somatostatinoma. This neuroendocrine tumour causes diarrhoea and steatorrhoea by a variety of mechanisms, predominantly by inhibiting the pancreatic secretion of both enzymes and bicarbonate, and also by other mechanisms, which include deranged gallbladder motility affecting bile release and therefore fat absorption (Jensen and Norton, 1991). Both gastrinomas and somatostatinomas can occur in the duodenal wall, as well as in the pancreas. Steatorrhoea is much less common if the somatostatinoma is in the duodenum.

In children, cystic fibrosis is the commonest cause of pancreatic insufficiency, which results from chronic duct obstruction and atrophy. An inherited disorder, the Shwachman–Diamond syndrome is associated with absent trypsin and lipase owing to pancreatic hypoplasia (Shwachman *et al.*, 1964). The Johanson–Blizzard syndrome, an autosomal recessive disorder, is an extremely rare cause of pancreatic insufficiency and there are also numerous systemic abnormalities such as dwarfism, thyroid dysfunction, aplasia of the alae nasi, deafness and dental anomalies such as absence of permanent teeth (Johanson and Blizzard, 1971). Other abnormalities have also been described, including genitourinary and cardiac malformations (Gershoni-Baruch *et al.*, 1990). These patients are shown to have decreased acinar secretion of trypsin, co-lipase, total lipase and decreased serum immunoreactive trypsinogen levels consistent with a primary acinar cell defect (Jones *et al.*, 1994).

Bile salts

Fatty acids, β-monoglycerides and cholesterol are not water soluble. Bile salts, produced in the liver, are necessary for the absorption of the products of fat digestion and cholesterol by the formation of water-soluble micelles in the intestinal lumen (Hofmann and Small, 1967). The absorption of the fat-soluble vitamins A, D, E and K (*see* Chapter 9) also requires micelle formation for optimal absorption.

Cholic acid and chenodeoxycholic acid are the two primary bile acids. They constitute 80 per cent of the bile acids and are synthesized entirely within the liver from cholesterol. The primary bile acids are then conjugated with taurine or glycine in the liver to form primary bile salts. This functional grouping maximizes the bile salt activity within the intestinal lumen by increasing solubility at low pH, decreasing precipitation by ions and reducing loss from transfer across cell membranes. The bile salts are secreted into the biliary tract and stored in the gallbladder before release into the duodenum.

The bile salts initally remain in the lumen of the intestine, as they are not absorbed at the physiological pH of the upper small intestine, where micelle formation and fat absorption take place. Once in the terminal ileum, bile salts are reabsorbed via enterocytes by an active process against a concentration gradient and are then transported via the portal vein back to the liver, to be re-excreted in bile. A small proportion of bile salts are unabsorbed and reach the colon. Here, bacterial dehydroxylation results in the conversion of chenodeoxycholic acid to lithocholic acid, and cholic acid to deoxycholic acid. These secondary bile acids are reabsorbed and reconjugated to form bile salts, which comprise 20 per cent of the bile salt pool. While most are recirculated, a small amount (about 500 mg/day) of bile salts are lost in the faeces.

The bile salt pool is not large. The recirculation of bile, the enterohepatic circulation, takes place 6–8 times a day. On each occasion, 95 per cent of bile salts are reabsorbed. Up to 40 g are recycled every day to maintain efficient fat absorption. This recirculation of bile salts is important as the ability of the liver to synthesize bile salts is limited.

The SeHCAT test (using ^{75}Se-labelled homotaurocholate, an analogue of taurocholate) can be used to determine if there is a terminal ileal mucosal defect causing bile salt malabsorption (*see* Chapter 13.3).

MICELLE FORMATION

Bile salts aggregate to form spherical polymolecular micelles at or above a defined concentration (4 mmol/L), termed the critical micellar concentration, (Hofman and Borgström, 1963). These micelles, with the hydrophilic ends of their molecule outwards and the hydrophobic ends inwards, solubilize fatty acids and monoglycerides to form mixed micelles that are water soluble (Hofmann and Borgström, 1963) (Fig. 16.2). The micelles have a diameter of 40 Å and are able to pass between the microvilli (Senior, 1964). The lipids in

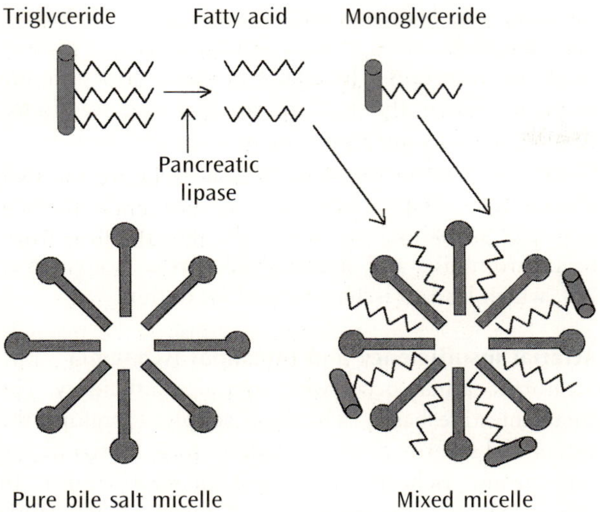

Figure 16.2 *The formation of mixed micelles. (Modified from Langman, M.J.S. 1982:* A concise textbook of gastroenterology, *2nd edn. Edinburgh: Churchill Livingstone, 57.)*

the mixed micelle are absorbed at the lumenal surface of the enterocyte.

Fat malabsorption due to a decreased critical micellar concentration can occur from reduced bile acid production, an obstruction to flow, excessive loss of bile salts or inactivation (within the intestinal lumen). The common causes are shown in Table 16.2. In situations of bacterial overgrowth of the small intestine, bile salts are dehydroxylated and deconjugated, and this results in decreased micellar concentrations and fat malabsorption (Tabaqchali *et al.*, 1968). The cholesterol-lowering drug cholestyramine, a basic anion-exchange resin, causes fat malabsorption by exchanging a chloride ion for bile acid to form a complex in the small intestine that is not digested nor absorbed, and hence depletes bile acids. Subsequently, the production of bile acids by the liver is increased. This results in a reduction in serum cholesterol, the substrate for bile acid production. The decrease in intraluminal bile salt concentration also causes malabsorption of the fat-soluble vitamins A, D, E and K (*see* Chapter 9).

Fat malabsorption due to bile salt depletion is modest compared to that due to pancreatic or small intestinal disease.

While most fats are not water soluble, about 30 per cent of medium-chain triglycerides (MCTs) (fatty acids with 6–10 carbon atoms) are somewhat water soluble and are thus absorbed directly, requiring neither pancreatic lipase for digestion nor bile salts for micellar solubilization (Clark and Holt, 1968). MCTs can even be absorbed by the small intestinal mucosa in the presence of mucosal damage. MCTs are not incorporated into chylomicrons in the enterocyte but are released directly into the portal vein unlike long-chain fatty acids, which are incorporated into chylomicrons and then transported by the lymphatic system. Owing to their ease of absorption and transport, MCTs are used in the treatment of conditions where digestion and absorption are impaired.

Table 16.2 *Conditions affecting intraluminal micellar concentration*

Decreased bile salt production
Hepatocellular disease
Decreased delivery of bile to the intestinal lumen
Biliary atresia
Biliary obstruction
Stone
Tumour
Stricture
Decreased enterohepatic circulation of bile salts
Ileal resection
Ileal disease
Ileal bypass (jejuno-ileostomy)
Depleted concentration of active intraluminal bile salts
Drugs
Cholestyramine
Calcium carbonate
Neomycin
Zollinger–Ellison syndrome
Intestinal bacterial overgrowth
Anatomical abnormalities
Duodenal and jejunal diverticula
Surgical anastomoses
Fistulae
Strictures
Bowel obstruction
Hypomotility
Intestinal pseudo-obstruction

Gastric conditions

A number of gastric conditions may contribute to fat malabsorption. The stomach serves three important functions in digestion. It is a reservoir for food from the oesophagus, it aids the process of digestion by secreting gastric juice and it emulsifies food. Importantly, the stomach also regulates the entry of food into the small intestine by gastric peristalsis. The mechanical activities of the stomach described above may be compromised by surgery and, depending on the nature and extent of the surgery, impair the process of digestion. Malabsorption has been described following procedures such as Billroth I (subtotal gastrectomy and duodenostomy) and Billroth II (gastrojejunostomy), and vagotomy and pyloroplasty. Steatorrhoea is most severe following a Billroth II anastomosis. Problems result from decreased gastric acid secretion and subsequent small bowel bacterial overgrowth (*see* Chapter 12).

Small bowel causes

The small intestinal epithelium, which covers the villi and the crypts, is only a single 20–30 μm barrier between the lumen and the host, is vulnerable to a variety of chemical and biological agents, and is easily accessible to the external environment. The small intestine has a vast absorptive surface (*see* Chapter 2). It is estimated that the villi increase the surface area by a factor of eight. Microvilli 1 μm in length and 0.1 μm wide project from the surface of the absorptive epithelial cells, further increasing the surface area considerably. Fat absorption occurs mainly in the proximal 100 cm of the jejunum (Booth *et al.*, 1961) at the brush border (microvilli) of the small intestinal enterocytes. Malabsorption is not an inevitable consequence of small intestinal disease. Both the reserve function and adaptability of the small intestine is considerable, as discussed in Chapter 29.

The causes of malabsorption related to the small intestine are extensive. It most commonly results from a reduction in the absorptive area of the intestine from mucosal disease or surgical resection. Less commonly, malabsorption results from impaired chylomicron formation within the enterocyte or in the transport of chylomicrons due to lymphatic obstruction. A variety of classifications of small bowel causes of malabsorption are possible as multiple mechanisms often overlap. In a single condition causing malabsorption, one pathophysiological mechanism may predominate but other processes may contribute significantly (*see* Chapter 15). The classification of malabsorption can be strictly physiological (related to the process of fat digestion, absorption and transport), anatomical (based on the site of the lesion), or aetiological. The classification in Table 16.3 incorporates a variety of approaches to provide a functional overview.

ANATOMICAL CAUSES

A decrease in surface area, not due to a mucosal lesion, can affect both digestion and absorption. These causes are listed in Table 16.3. Short bowel syndrome is dealt with in Chapter 29. In the congenital short bowel syndrome, there is malrotation of the bowel and the clinical features are similar to those of short bowel syndrome in general (*see* Chapter 29).

Small bowel resection

The consequences of malabsorption are most severe with ileal resection, rather than with jejunal or duodenal resection (Hardison and Rosenberg, 1967). Intestinal adaptation serves to minimize the effects of mild to moderate resection. The effects of major resection and the adaptation of the small intestine are discussed in the chapter on the short bowel syndrome (*see* Chapter 29). Common reasons for surgical resection are Crohn's disease (*see* Chapter 25) and vascular problems, for example, intestinal volvulus, intussusception, mesenteric thrombosis and strangulated hernia (*see* Chapter 28), which lead to ischaemia and infarction.

Arterial insufficiency and intestinal ischaemia

Steatorrhoea may occur with arterial insufficiency. The small intestine has a rich blood supply; therefore, the extent and severity of arterial disease must be significant for chronic ischaemia to result in steatorrhoea. In elderly persons, the possibility of intestinal ischaemia causing steatorrhoea is strengthened by evidence of peripheral vascular disease or other manifestations of atherosclerosis. A prominent symptom is abdominal pain after food. This may cause patients to minimize their food intake and severe weight loss may result.

MUCOSAL CAUSES

Coeliac disease and related entities

The most common cause of malabsorption of small intestinal mucosal origin in the West is coeliac disease (Chapter 23), although, globally, tropical sprue is more prevalent (*see* Chapter 21). Coeliac disease, tropical sprue and some of the other conditions listed below have the common feature of showing varying degrees of villous atrophy.

Collagenous sprue is a condition characterized by deposition of collagen beneath the epithelial basement membrane in the lamina propria, and villous atrophy. It is often seen in patients with a long history of coeliac disease and it is uncertain if this truly represents a separate entity. It has been reported in association with collagenous colitis (Eckstein *et al.*, 1988). In patients with chronic diarrhoea and progressive malabsorption, especially if resistant to gluten withdrawal, collagenous sprue is an essential consideration (Jarmay *et al.*, 1993).

It has been suggested that, in cases of coeliac disease refractory to treatment with gluten restriction, additional biopsies should be obtained from the proximal jejunum and possibly also from the terminal ileum to rule out collagenous sprue. If the diagnosis of collagenous sprue can be established, therapy with steroids should be attempted (Guller *et al.*, 1986). Sulphasalazine therapy may be of benefit. The prognosis is worse compared to uncomplicated coeliac disease. The development of ulcerative jejuno-ileitis in patients with coeliac disease may also result in their becoming refractory to gluten restriction.

Dermatitis herpetiformis is another condition associated with coeliac disease. The dominant feature is the

Table 16.3 *Small bowel causes of malabsorption*

Anatomical causes
- Short bowel syndrome
  - Small bowel resection
  - Congenital
- Arterial insufficiency and intestinal ischaemia

Mucosal causes
- Coeliac disease and related entities
- Tropical sprue
- Eosinophilic gastroenteritis
- Regional enteritis (Crohn's disease)
- Whipple's disease
- Therapeutic agents
  - Neomycin
  - Colchicine
  - Methotrexate
- Microvillus inclusion disease
- Abetalipoproteinaemia
- Acrodermatitis enteropathica
- Macroglobuliaemia
- Radiation injury
- Infections
  - Acute
    - Bacterial
    - Viral
    - Fungal
    - Parasitic
  - Chronic
    - Tuberculosis
    - Tropical sprue
    - Whipple's disease
  - HIV/AIDS enteropathy
- Miscellaneous
  - Malnutrition
  - Zollinger–Ellison syndrome

Submucosal causes
- Infiltrative conditions
  - Amyloidosis
  - Systemic mastocytosis
  - Lymphoma
- Fibrosis
  - Radiation enteritis
  - Systemic sclerosis
- Lymphatic obstruction
  - Intestinal lymphangiectasia
    - Primary
    - Secondary
- Vascular
  - Atherosclerosis
  - Vasculitides
  - Radiation injury

Motility disorders
- Endocrine and metabolic causes
  - Diabetes mellitus
  - Hyperthyroidism
  - Hypothyroidism
  - Hypoadrenalism (Addison's disease)
  - Hypoparathyroidism
- Infiltrative conditions (see above)
- Intestinal pseudo-obstruction (*see also* Table 16.4)
- Therapeutic agents
  - Anticholinergics
- Fibrosis
  - Radiation enteritis
  - Systemic sclerosis

Genetic causes
- Abetalipoproteinaemia
- Microvillus inclusion disease
- Acrodermatitis enteropathica

Miscellaneous causes
- Hypogammaglobulinaemia
- Alcohol

intensely pruritic lesions that are symmetrically distributed on the extensor surfaces of the limbs, over the scalp, buttocks and back. Excoriation is common. Not all patients experience diarrhoea and malabsorption; indeed, only a small proportion do so. The diagnosis is established by the clinical features and an abnormal small intestinal mucosa, both of which improve on gluten withdrawal from the diet (van der Meer, 1990). A skin biopsy shows deposits of immunoglobulin A (IgA) on direct immunofluorescence (Olbricht *et al.*, 1986). As in coeliac disease, antiendomysial, antireticulin and antigliadin antibodies are present in the serum. Resolution of the skin lesions occurs with dapsone therapy but the drug has no influence on the intestinal lesions. Once resolution of the skin lesions and small intestinal pathology has occurred, the reintroduction of gluten to the diet, as with coeliac disease, precipitates a recurrence of the condition (Leonard *et al.*, 1983).

Eosinophilic gastroenteritis

This is an uncommon but important entity. Numerous eosinophils infiltrate the stomach and sometimes the small intestine. In the stomach the gastric antrum and the pylorus are predominantly involved. The eosinophil infiltration occurs predominantly in the submucosa; however, mucosal and muscle layer involvement may be prominent. There is associated oedema, fibrosis and often vascular dilatation, resulting in distortion of the villous architecture. Ulceration is uncommon. Involvement of the oesophagus (Dobbins *et al.*, 1977; Talley *et al.*, 1990), pancreas (Vazquez-Rodriguez *et al.*, 1973), appendix (Jona *et al.*, 1976), urinary bladder (Gregg and Utz, 1974) and colon have also been described.

The majority of patients are between 30 and 40 years of age, but the disease may present in infancy or older ages. The cause is obscure but evidence suggests an allergic aetiology as many patients have a history of atopy. There are elevated IgE concentrations, data from skin tests is supportive and there is a dramatic response to corticosteroids. Food allergy is sometimes implicated as symptoms worsen on challenge to specific foods (Katz *et al.*, 1984). However, generally, elimination diets have been of no significant value (Leinbach and Rubin, 1970). There is no evidence of intrinsic immunological abnormalities (Thomas *et al.*, 1975; Katz *et al.*, 1984).

Clinical features depend on the main site of involvement. Vomiting due to narrowing of the antrum and pylorus may occur. The small bowel may become obstructed. Abdominal pain is a common feature. Depending on the extent of small intestinal involvement, diarrhoea, malabsorption and weight loss may occur. Protein loss may be significant, and rectal bleeding may result if the colon is involved. Serosal involvement leads to ascites and peritonitis (Klein *et al.*, 1970). Peripheral eosinophilia is also a feature.

The diagnosis is established by gastric and/or jejunal biopsy. There is eosinophilic infiltration and villous atrophy of varying severity. Since the small intestinal involvement can be patchy, multiple biopsies may be necessary to establish the diagnosis. Numerous eosinophils in small bowel biopsies may also be seen in a range of other conditions, including some lymphomas, Crohn's disease, parasitic infections (*see* Chapter 19), vasculitides, and conditions in which an elevated peripheral blood eosinophil count occurs. The symptoms resolve after treatment with prednisolone (Lee *et al.*, 1993).

Regional enteritis (Crohn's disease)

Crohn's disease (*see* Chapter 25) most commonly affects the terminal ileum but can involve any part of the gastrointestinal tract. Small intestinal biopsy can show a range of changes including inflammation, ulceration, villous distortion, granulomata, pyloric metaplasia and hyperplasia of the muscularis mucosae. About one-third of patients have steatorrhoea, the extent and severity of malabsorption correlating with the site and extent of lesions. The mechanism of malabsorption may be multifactorial and relates to mucosal damage, bacterial overgrowth owing to a fistula or stricture, or from secondary amyloidosis (uncommon). Contributory factors to malabsorption are rapid intestinal transit and suboptimal functioning of the bowel proximal to an obstructing lesion (*see* Chapters 2 and 25).

Whipple's disease

Whipple's disease is discussed in detail in Chapter 22. In their recent review, Durand *et al.* (1997) reported that this rare, multisystem illness (previously thought to occur usually in middle-aged White males) had an extended age range at diagnosis of 20–80 years. The mean age of the patients was 50 years for males and 55 years for females. In Whipple's disease the dominant symptoms relate to the gastrointestinal tract, and malabsorption and weight loss are prominent features. Small intestinal villous abnormalities are variable (*see* Chapters 2 and 22).

Recently, the Gram-positive, periodic acid–Schiff (PAS)-positive bacillus associated with the disease has been identified using the polymerase chain reaction (PCR) and the causative organism has been named *Tropheryma whippelii* (Relman *et al.*, 1992; Relman and Persing, 1997). The diagnosis has been based on small bowel biopsy with evidence of PAS-positive macrophages infiltrating the lamina propria and the presence of bacilliform organisms best demonstrated by electron microscopy. The PCR has been shown to be the diagnostic tool of choice. The test is highly sensitive and specific, and is now invaluable not only in diagnosis but also to monitor the response to treatment. The role of PCR is especially important as relapse occurs in about a third of patients treated with antibiotics.

Therapeutic agents

The list of therapeutic agents associated with malabsorption is increasing. Drugs can cause this problem in a number of ways, including by direct damage to the small intestinal mucosa. In most instances the effect is dose dependent and temporary, with complete reversal on discontinuing treatment. Some drugs, such as neomycin, colchicine and methotrexate (which cause mucosal damage) and cholestyramine (which depletes bile salts) invariably cause fat malabsorption. These drugs may also induce malabsorption of other nutrients. Fat malabsorption is also reported to occur with phenformin (Stowers and Bewsher, 1969) and with phenindione (Juel-Jensen, 1959).

Folate malabsorption (*see* Chapter 9) can occur with phenformin (Stowers and Bewsher, 1969), phenobarbitone, phenytoin (Reynolds *et al.*, 1965) and the contraceptive pill (Necheles and Snyder, 1970). Vitamin B_{12} malabsorption (*see* Chapter 9) may occur with methotrexate (Trier, 1962; Faloon, 1970) and colchicine (Race *et al.*, 1970). Para-aminosalicylic acid can cause both folate and vitamin B_{12} malabsorption (Heinivaara and Palva, 1965).

Malabsorption secondary to patchy partial villous atrophy or even subtotal villous atrophy may result from neomycin (Jacobson *et al.*, 1960; Faloon *et al.*, 1966) and large doses of colchicine used in the treatment of gout (Race *et al.*, 1970). Antineoplastic drugs such as methotrexate can cause malabsorption by damaging immature epithelial cells in the crypts, with reduced formation of mature absorptive cells. Drugs may also cause diarrhoea and less commonly malabsorption by altering intestinal motility (*see* Chapter 15).

Microvillous inclusion disease, abetalipoproteinaemia and acrodermatitis enteropathica

These are considered later, in the section on genetic causes.

Infectious causes

A variety of acute and chronic infections (*see* Chapters 17–19) can damage small intestinal villi leading to malabsorption. The severity ranges from mild, patchy, partial villous atrophy to severe villous atrophy. The common infectious aetiological agents are discussed individually in Chapters 17–19. Although most episodes of acute infective diarrhoea resolve with no ill-effects, a small proportion of patients may develop a malabsorptive syndrome. Young children may develop transient intolerance to cow's milk, gluten or lactose as a sequel to the infection.

In patients with malaria, biopsies of the small intestine may show congestion and oedema of the lamina propria, and even parasitized erythrocytes in capillaries (Olsson and Johnston, 1969; Cook, 1975). This raises the possibility that alterations of the small intestinal microcirculation by the parasite may interfere with absorption (Olsson and Johnston, 1969; Cook, 1975).

Chronic infections associated with malabsorption include tuberculosis (*see* Chapter 18), tropical sprue (Chapter 21) and Whipple's disease (Chapter 22). Overgrowth of commensal bacteria can arise following stasis of small intestinal contents due to duodenal or jejunal diverticula, surgical anastomoses, fistulae, strictures and small bowel obstruction (*see* Chapter 12). The resulting malabsorption is multifactorial in origin and relates to excessive bacterial load competing for essential nutrients, deconjugation of bile salts, bacterial inactivation of lipase and mucosal damage.

HIV enteropathy is discussed in Chapters 2 and 20.

Macroglobulinaemia

There is a well-documented association between Waldenstrom's macroglobulinaemia and gastrointestinal manifestations. Malabsorption occurs due to extensive mucosal and submucosal lymphangiectasia caused by surrounding immunoglobulin deposition (Tait *et al.*, 1993). Small intestinal dilatation may occur (Brandt *et al.*, 1981). The severity of the malabsorption can lead to severe steatorrhoea, marked protein-losing enteropathy, hypoalbuminaemia, weight loss and excessive endogenous faecal calcium clearance (Krawitt and Beeken, 1978).

Miscellaneous

Malnutrition. Changes in villous architecture occur in patients with marasmus, although this feature is not invariable. Villous atrophy similar to that in coeliac disease has been reported in kwashiorkor (Brunser *et al.*, 1966). In both marasmus and kwashiorkor, increased intraepithelial lymphocytes are a feature (Barbezat *et al.*, 1967).

Zollinger–Ellison syndrome. The mechanism of malabsorption associated with Zollinger–Ellison syndrome is discussed earlier in this chapter. A consistent abnormality of patchy villous atrophy has been shown in patients with the Zollinger–Ellison syndrome (Fang *et al.*, 1979). Zollinger–Ellison syndrome can occur as an isolated phenomenon or as part of the multiple endocrine neoplasia type I (MEN-I) syndrome, an autosomal dominant disorder characterized by endocrine tumours of the pituitary, pancreas and parathyroids, as well as other manifestations, including lipomata and less common tumours of other organs, such as the adrenals and thyroid. MEN-I is due to a mutation of the recently isolated MENIN gene located on chromosome 11 (11q13) (Chandrasekharappa *et al.*, 1997).

SUBMUCOSAL CAUSES

Infiltrative conditions

Amyloidosis. Both primary and secondary amyloidosis can involve the small intestine to cause malabsorption owing to submucosal vascular involvement. Histological evidence of amyloidosis on small intestinal biopsy is a late feature. The diagnosis of amyloidosis is best made on rectal biopsy (*see* Chapter 27).

Systemic mastocytosis. This is an uncommon disorder. An abnormal accumulation of mast cells associated with increased histamine production occurs in the skin, liver, spleen and bone marrow. In about 50 per cent of cases, the gastrointestinal tract is involved (Fishman and Flemming, 1979).

The small intestinal mucosa shows variable villous atrophy, with mast cell infiltration. Gastrointestinal symptoms include vomiting, abdominal pain and diarrhoea, which may be intermittent or chronic, and may be associated with steatorrhoea. Increased gastric acid secretion can lead to peptic ulceration and, for the reasons described previously, also contribute to steatorrhoea. Attacks of flushing, tachycardia, pruritus and headache may occur.

Suspected proliferation of mast cells in bone is confirmed by a radionuclide bone scan. An H-2 receptor antagonist and disodium cromoglycate control the diarrhoea (Frieri *et al.*, 1985).

Lymphoma. The small intestine is second only to the stomach as the major site of gastrointestinal lymphoma (*see* Chapter 26). Non-Hodgkin's lymphomas may occur primarily in the small intestine or they may occur here as part of systemic disease. Primary Hodgkin's disease in the small bowel is rare. In the elderly patient with malabsorption, lymphoma is an essential diagnostic consideration. Weight loss, steatorrhoea and severe nutrient malabsorption are common features when the small intestine is involved. Other clinical features include finger clubbing, fever, abdominal pain or discomfort, and a palpable abdominal mass. A high small bowel obstruction may lead to abdominal distension and vomiting.

T-cell lymphomas may arise in association with long-standing coeliac disease (enteropathy associated T-cell lymphoma; EATL) (*see* Chapter 23). This tends to involve the jejunum. Ulcerative jejuno-ileitis occurring in a patient with coeliac disease is thought by some to be a manifestation of EATL.

Other non-Hodgkin's lymphomas that occur in the small bowel include mucosa-associated lymphoid tissue (MALT) lymphomas, mantle cell lymphoma and Burkitt's lymphoma.

Fibrosis

Radiation enteritis. This may cause significant steatorrhoea. Supravoltage radiation, which is now available, delivers high doses of radiation with minimal or absent skin damage, and has increased side-effects, such as radiation enteritis (Berken, 1985). The small intestine is particularly vulnerable to radiation damage, although the colon and rectum are affected more frequently as they are in close proximity to organs, such as the cervix, which not uncommonly receive radiotherapy to treat malignancy. The initial vulnerability of the small intestine to ionizing radiation is partly due to the rapid turnover of epithelial cells (Berthrong and Fajardo, 1981). Diarrhoea may occur soon after therapy as a result of epithelial damage. Recovery is often spontaneous (Anonymous, 1983).

Long-term effects include ulceration and fibrosis, altered mucosal blood flow and villous atrophy. Lactase deficiency and bacterial overgrowth contribute to the pathogenesis of malabsorption. Damage to the less mobile duodenum and terminal ileum and areas fixed by adhesions may be severe.

Systemic sclerosis. Malabsorption is not uncommon in systemic sclerosis. Fibrosis of the muscularis propria and submucosa results in disordered motility. The decreased motility leads to stasis and bacterial overgrowth, and subsequent malabsorption (Chapters 12 and 15). Villous atrophy may also contribute.

Lymphatic obstruction

Intestinal lymphangiectasia. This may be primary, or secondary to obstruction of the lymphatics (Waldmann, 1966; Dobbins, 1991). In adults, intestinal lymphangiectasia is due to mechanical factors as diverse as intestinal malignancy, retroperitoneal fibrosis, sarcoidosis and constrictive pericarditis (Waldmann, 1966; Perera *et al.*, 1975; Popovic *et al.*, 1980; Harris *et al.*, 1983; Dobbins, 1991). Obstruction or hypoplasia of small intestinal lymph vessels cause an increase in intestinal lymph pressure and dilatation of mucosal, submucosal and subserosal lymph vessels results. The dilatation of the lymph vessels may be so severe that villous architecture becomes distorted. Both rupture and/or seepage of lymph can cause considerable loss of protein and fat into the lumen of the small intestine. The consequent hypoproteinaemia and steatorrhoea are significant. Decreased absorption of fats contributes to steatorrhoea. The hypoproteinaemia may be of sufficient severity to cause peripheral oedema.

Vascular

Intestinal ischaemia may occur from a variety of causes, including atheroma, vasculitis and radiation injury. Vasculitides that can affect the small intestine (*see also* Chapter 27) include Behçet's disease, Henoch–Schönlein purpura, giant cell arteritis, polyarteritis nodosa and Köhlmeier–Degos disease (malignant atrophic papulosis). Köhlmeier–Degos disease involves the skin and sometimes other organs, including the gastrointestinal tract.

MOTILITY DISORDERS

Endocrine and metabolic disorders

A number of endocrine and metabolic conditions are associated with steatorrhoea. Thyroid function disorders and diabetes mellitus are the best documented. The gastrointestinal tract interacts actively with the thyroid hormones. It is a reservoir for the thyroid hormones, especially for T3, and participates in the regulation of T4 and T3. Hypomotility associated with diabetes mellitus and hypothyroidism can cause steatorrhoea via bacterial overgrowth (*see* Chapters 12 and 15). Diarrhoea is a well-recognized feature of hyperthyroidism (Kristensson *et al.*, 1971) and increased gastrointestinal transit is a suggested mechanism (Wiley *et al.*, 1978).

Other endocrine disorders reported to be associated with malabsorption, although the evidence available is not substantial, are hypoadrenalism (Neil and Weinstock, 1991; Weber and Ryan, 1993) and hypoparathyroidism (Beardwood, 1935).

Infiltrative conditions

Amyloidosis, systemic mastocytosis and lymphoma are discussed above.

Intestinal pseudo-obstruction

Intestinal pseudo-obstruction is a condition in which clinical features of chronic bowel obstruction are present in the absence of a demonstrable mechanical cause. Primary intestinal pseudo-obstruction is due to degenerative changes in the myenteric plexus of the intestine and results in a dysfunction of intestinal motility. Table 16.4 shows the many causes of secondary intestinal pseudo-obstruction due to systemic disease (Greenberger *et al.*, 1968; Legge *et al.*, 1970), local disease such as coeliac disease (Naish *et al.*, 1960) and drug therapy.

Vomiting, abdominal pain and, in a subset of patients, dysphagia, are significant problems. Owing to the motor disorder of the intestine, bacterial overgrowth and its consequences, diarrhoea, steatorrhoea and vitamin B_{12} deficiency, are possible complications. Barium studies demonstrate distension of segments of the small intestine or colon.

Therapeutic agents

Drugs with anticholinergic effects including propantheline (prescribed for the treatment of urinary incontinence), benztropine (prescribed for Parkinson's disease) and tricyclic antidepressants have the potential to cause diarrhoea, although more often the predominant side-effect is constipation. The mechanism of diarrhoea and malabsorption is due to decreased intestinal motility leading to bacterial overgrowth. These drugs should be considered as possible contributory factors if the aetiology of diarrhoea is obscure.

GENETIC CAUSES

Abetalipoproteinaemia, microvillus inclusion disease and acrodermatitis enteropathica are three inherited conditions associated with fat malabsorption.

Abetalipoproteinaemia

Abetalipoproteinaemia is a rare autosomal recessive disorder first described by Isselbacher *et al.* in 1964. In affected patients the fatty acids and monoglycerides absorbed from the small intestine are re-esterified as normal to triglycerides in enterocytes. However, the subsequent step of chylomicron formation does not occur within these cells. This is due to the absence of apolipoprotein B-48 (apo B-48), which is not synthesized in this condition (Rader and Brewer, 1993). Accumulated triglycerides are seen on electron microscopy as numerous intracytoplasmic lipid droplets, especially in enterocytes at the tips of villi (*see* Figs 2.32 and 2.33 in Chapter 2). Triglycerides also accumulate in hepatocytes. Patients have very low plasma apo B concentrations, and lack the fat-soluble vitamins A, D, E and K.

Since chylomicrons are not available to transport essential nutrients to tissues, these patients fail to thrive and diarrhoea and mild steatorrhoea occur. Owing to vitamin E deficiency, lipid membrane abnormalities result in acanthocytosis, although the most serious consequences are the significant neurological abnormalities of progressive spinocerebellar ataxia, atypical retinitis pigmentosa (Fig. 16.3) and a polyneuropathy. In abetalipoproteinaemia, high doses of vitamin E may prevent neurological complications and also arrest or even improve the neurological symptoms, which are best monitored by sensory evoked potentials (Muller *et al.*, 1983; Fagan and Taylor, 1987).

Table 16.4 *Systemic and local causes of secondary intestinal pseudo-obstruction*

Systemic diseases
Systemic sclerosis
Amyloidosis
Diabetes mellitus
Hypothyroidism
Polymyositis
Parkinson's disease
Local causes
Coeliac disease
Therapeutic agents
Tricyclic antidepressants
Phenothiazines

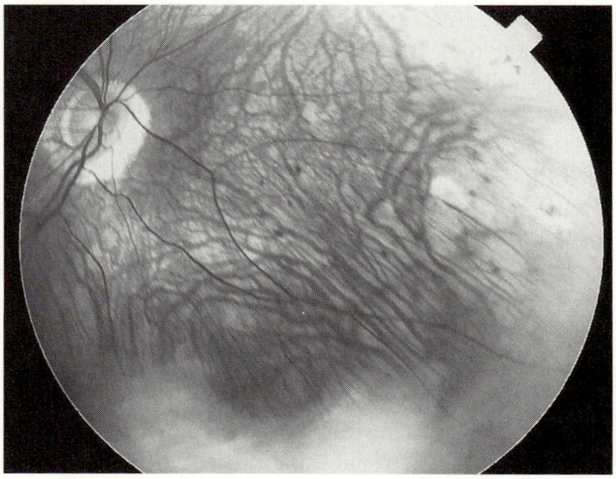

Figure 16.3 *Atypical retinitis pigmentosa due to abetalipoproteinaemia. Pigmentary retinopathy associated with abetalipoproteinaemia is characterized by peripheral 'bone spickule' pigmentation and loss of choroidal retinal pigmentation. The loss of choroidal pigmentation results in the extensive choroidal vasculature becoming visible. (Courtesy of Dr Michael Goggin and Mr Anton Drew, Department of Ophthalmology, The Queen Elizabeth Hospital, Woodville, South Australia.)*

Microvillus inclusion disease

This autosomal recessive condition is characterized by abnormal microvillus architecture and apical intracytoplasmic inclusions (Cutz *et al.*, 1989; Bell *et al.*, 1991). Severe diarrhoea, steatorrhoea and death occur at a young age.

Acrodermatitis enteropathica

Acrodermatitis enteropathica is inherited as an autosomal recessive trait and manifestations are thought to relate to zinc deficiency (Chapter 9). The salient features are cutaneous lesions and malabsorption. All these features respond to zinc therapy (Chapter 9).

MISCELLANEOUS CAUSES

Hypogammaglobulinaemia

Hypogammaglobulinaemia is a rare cause of steatorrhoea. The steatorrhoea is probably multifactorial in origin, but infection, particularly by *Giardia*, plays a significant role. In a 35-year-old woman with primary hypogammaglobulinaemia, intestinal villous atrophy, osteomalacia and protein-losing enteropathy, there was no response to antibiotics, vitamin therapy or a gluten-free diet. The intravenous administration of a native immunoglobulin preparation resulted in continuous elevation of IgG serum levels, and a rapid resolution of the clinical symptoms and small bowel histology (Layer *et al.*, 1985).

Alcohol

Alcohol is often mentioned as a cause of small intestinal malabsorption. Ultrastructral changes in the architecture of the microvilli have the potential to lead to 'brush border' maldigestion and malabsorption. Whether alcohol alone leads to small intestinal damage sufficient to cause diarrhoea and steatorrhoea in human subjects needs more evidence to be conclusive. Chronic alcoholics may develop diarrhoea from rapid mouth to caecal transit, and steatorrhoea as a result of pancreatic insufficiency and decreased bile acid production, which impedes micelle formation and therefore fat absorption.

INVESTIGATION OF FAT MALABSORPTION (*see also* Chapter 13.3)

The purpose of investigating patients with suspected malabsorption is to confirm the diagnosis, to determine the site of the problem, and the aetiology, and to establish the consequences of malabsorption, such as nutritional deficiencies and their severity.

Tests to determine the presence and site of fat malabsorption

These are the faecal fat estimation and the D-xylose absorption test (*see* Chapter 13.3).

Intestinal permeability tests

The permeability of the small bowel mucosa in disease states is assessed by the tests discussed in Chapter 13.3.

Radiological investigations

The major radiological abnormalities associated with malabsorption are discussed in Chapter 13.6. A preliminary radiological examination that may be rewarding in patients with steatorrhoea is a plain x-ray of the abdomen to detect pancreatic calcification in patients with pancreatitis. Barium studies can provide non-specific evidence of malabsorption from the detection of small bowel abnormalities, such as diverticula, fistulae and surgical alterations.

Tests to determine the aetiology of small intestinal causes of fat malabsorption

SMALL BOWEL BIOPSY

The small bowel biopsy is performed to help in diagnosis, for assessing severity and to determine the extent of disease and response to treatment.

An abnormal small bowel biopsy localizes the lesion and can help to eliminate a pancreatic or, less commonly, biliary cause of steatorrhoea. The small bowel biopsy (*see* Chapter 13.2) is now most conveniently done at endoscopy (*see* Chapter 13.1). This has eliminated the time-consuming and uncomfortable process of positioning the biopsy capsule of the suction biopsy tubes used in the past. The specimens at endoscopy, although smaller than from a biopsy capsule, are adequate to make a diagnosis. An additional advantage of endoscopy is that it provides a view of the upper gastrointestinal tract, and intestinal juice can be conveniently obtained for bacteriological culture and examination for parasitic pathogens. Further infomation on biopsy features can be found in Chapter 13.2.

Tests for enteric pathogens

The tests to determine the presence of enteric pathogens are discussed in chapters 13.3 and 13.4. Steatorrhoea may result from a variety of viral, bacterial and parasitic infections (*see* Chapters 17–20). In regard to bacterial overgrowth of the small bowel (*see* Chapter 12), the most valid examination is purported to be intubation of the upper small intestine with bacteriological culture of the aspirated fluid (King and Toskes, 1983). Standard breath tests are now widely used based on the metabolic processing of a radioactively labelled compound by bacteria (*see* Chapter 13.3).

Tests to determine nutritional deficiencies and their severity

Proximal mucosal damage affects the absorption of minerals and the non-fat-soluble vitamins except vitamin B_{12}, which is absorbed by the terminal ileum. Steatorrhoea primarily affects absorption of the fat-soluble vitamins A, D, E and K. The tests to determine the presence of nutritional deficiencies and their severity are discussed in Chapters 9 and 13.5.

HAEMATOLOGICAL TESTS

Haematological methods for detecting and monitoring nutritional deficiencies include tests for haemoglobin, folate, iron, vitamin K and the Schilling test for vitamin B_{12} (*see* Chapter 13.5). The differential blood count may be helpful. Eosinophilia may be seen with primary inflammatory bowel disease, non-Hodgkin's lymphoma involving the gut, eosinophilic gastroenteritis and some parasitic infections (*see* Chapter 19). It is important to note that giardiasis does not cause eosinophilia.

BIOCHEMICAL TESTS

Biochemical tests include those for the concentration of minerals, such as calcium and zinc, which are useful markers of malabsorption (Chapter 9). D-xylose absorption is discussed in Chapter 13.3. A low albumin level may reflect long-standing protein malabsorption or, less commonly, a protein-losing enteropathy (*see* Chapter 14). Faecal clearance of endogenous α1-antitrypsin is a useful marker of protein loss (*see* Chapter 13.3).

Miscellaneous tests

Immunological tests that are useful are detailed in Chapter 23:

- serum immunoglobulin levels
- endomysial antibodies
- antigliadin antibodies
- antireticulin antibodies.

REFERENCES

Anonymous 1983: Radiation induced proctosigmoiditis. *Lancet* 1, 1082–3.

Barbezat, G.O., Bowie, M.D., Kaschula, R.O.C., Hansen, J.D.L. 1967: Studies on the small intestinal mucosa of children with protein-calorie malnutrition. *South African Medical Journal* 41, 1031–6.

Beardwood, J.T. 1935: The abdominal symptomatology of diabetic acidosis. *JAMA* 105, 1168.

Bell, S.W., Kerner, J.A., Jr., Sibley, R.K. 1991: Microvillus inclusion disease. The importance of electron microscopy for diagnosis. *American Journal of Surgical Pathology* 15, 1157–64.

Berken, C.A. 1985: Nd:YAG laser therapy for gastrointestinal bleeding due to radiation colitis. *American Journal of Gastroenterology* 80, 730–1.

Berthrong, M., Fajardo, L.F. 1981: Radiation injury in surgical pathology. Part II. Alimentary tract. *American Journal of Surgical Pathology* 5, 153–78.

Booth, C.C., Alldis, D., Read, A.E. 1961: Studies on the site of fat absorption. 2. Fat balances after resection of varying amounts of the small intestine in man. *Gut* 2, 168.

Brandt, L.J., Davidoff, A., Bernstein, L.H., Biempica, L., Rindfleisch, B., Goldstein, M.L. 1981: Small-intestine involvement in Waldenstrom's macroglobulinemia. Case report and review of the literature. *Digestive Diseases and Sciences* 26, 174–80.

Brunser, O., Reid, A., Monckeberg, F., Maccioni, A., Contreres, I. 1966: Jejunal biopsies in infant malnutrition: with special reference to mitotic index. *Pediatrics* 38, 605–11.

Chandrasekharappa, S.C., Guru, S.C., Manickam, P. *et al.* 1997: Positional cloning of the gene for multiple endocrine neoplasia type 1. *Science* 276, 404–7.

Clark, S.B., Holt, P.R. 1968: Rate-limiting steps in steady-state intestinal absorption of trioctanoin-1-14C. Effect of biliary and pancreatic flow diversion. *Journal of Clinical Investigation* 47, 612–23.

Cook, G.C. 1975: Relation between malaria, serum globulin concentration and the D-xylose absorption test. *Transactions of the Royal Society of Tropical Medicine and Hygiene* 69, 143.

Cutz, E., Rhoades, J.M., Drumm, B., Sherman, P.N., Durie, P.R. 1989: Microvillus inclusion disease: an inherited defect of brush-border assembly and differentiation. *New England Journal of Medicine* 320, 646–51.

DiMagno, E.P., Go, V.L.W., Summerskill, W.H.J. 1973: Relations between pancreatic enzyme outputs and malabsorption in severe pancreatic insufficiency. *New England Journal of Medicine* 288, 813–15.

Dobbins, J.W., Sheahan, D.G., Behar, J. 1977: Eosinophilic gastroenteritis with esophageal involvement. *Gastroenterology* 72, 1312–16.

Dobbins, W.O., III. 1991: Small bowel biopsy in malabsorptive states. In Norris, H.T. (ed.) *Pathology of the colon, small intestine, and anus.* New York: Churchill Livingstone, 137–88.

Durand, D.V., Lecomte, C., Cathebras, P., Rousset, H., Godeau, P. 1997 : Whipple disease. Clinical review of 52 cases. The SNFMI Research Group on Whipple Disease. Société Nationale Française de Médecine Interne. *Medicine (Baltimore)* 76, 170–84.

Eckstein, R.P., Dowsett, J.F., Riley, J.W. 1988: Collagenous enterocolitis: a case of collagenous colitis with involvement of the small intestine. *American Journal of Gastroenterology* 83, 767–71.

Fagan, E.R., Taylor, M.J. 1987: Longitudinal multimodal evoked potential studies in abetalipoproteinaemia. *Canadian Journal of Neurological Science* 14, 617–21.

Faloon, W.W. 1970: Drug production of intestinal malabsorption. *New York State Journal of Medicine* 70, 2189–92.

Faloon, W.W., Paes, I.C., Woolfolk, D., Nankin, H., Wallace, K., Haro, E.N. 1966: Effect of neomycin and kanamycin upon intestinal absorption. *Annals of the New York Academy of Science* 132, 879–87.

Fang, M., Ginsburg, A.L., Glassman, L. *et al.*, 1979: Zollinger–Ellison syndrome with diarrhea as the predominant clinical feature. *Gastroenterology* 76, 378–87.

Fishman, R.S., Flemming, C.R., Li, C. 1979: Systemic mastocytosis with review of gastrointestinal manifestations. *Mayo Clinic Proceedings* 54, 51–4.

Frieri, M., Alling, D.W., Metcalfe, D.D. 1985: Comparison of the therapeutic efficacy of cromolyn sodium with that of combined chlorpheniramine and cimetidine in systemic mastocytosis. Results of a double-blind clinical trial. *American Journal of Medicine* 78, 9–14.

Gershoni-Baruch, R., Lerner, A., Braun, J., Katzir, Y., Iancu, T.C., Benderly, A. 1990: Johanson–Blizzard syndrome: clinical spectrum and further delineation of the syndrome. *American Journal of Medicine and Genetics* 35, 546.

Green, P.H.R., Glickman, R.M., Saudek, C.D., Blum, C.B., Tall, A.R. 1979: Human intestinal lipoproteins. Studies in chyluric subjects. *Journal of Clinical Investigation* 64, 233–42.

Greenberger, N.J., Dobbins, W.O., III, Ruppert, R.D., Jesseph, J.E. 1968: Intestinal atony in progressive systemic sclerosis (scleroderma). *American Journal of Medicine* 45, 301.

Gregg, J.A., Utz, D.C. 1974: Eosinophil cystitis associated with eosinophilic gastroenteritis. *Mayo Clinic Proceedings* 49, 185–7.

Guller, R., Anabitarte, M., Mayer, M. 1986: Kollagensprue und ulzerierende Jejunoileitis bei einem Patienten mit gluteninduzierter Enteropathie. [Collagenous sprue and ulcerative jejuno-ileitis in a patient with gluten-induced enteropathy.] *Schweiz Medicine Wochenschrift* 116, 1343–9.

Hardison, W.G., Rosenberg, I.H. 1967: Bile-salt deficiency in the steatorrhoea following resection of the ileum and proximal colon. *New England Journal of Medicine* 277, 337–42.

Harris, M., Burton, I.E., Scarffe, J.H. 1983: Macroglobulinaemia and intestinal lymphangiectasia: a rare occasion. *Journal of Clinical Pathology* 36, 30–6.

Heinivaara, O., Palva, I.P. 1965: Malabsorption and deficiency of vitamin B_{12} caused by treatment with para-aminosalicylic acid. *Acta Medica Scandinavica* 177, 337.

Hofmann, A.F., Borgström, B. 1963: Physiochemical state of intestinal contents during their digestion and absorption. *Federation Proceedings: Federation of American Societies for Experimental Biology* 21, 43.

Hofmann, A.F., Small, D.M. 1967: Detergent properties of bile salts: correlation with physiological function. *Annual Review of Medicine* 18, 333–76.

Isaacson, P., Wright, D.H. 1978. Malignant histiocytosis of the intestine. Its relationship to malabsorption and ulcerative jejunitis. *Human Pathology* 9, 661–77.

Isselbacher, K.J., Scheig, R., Plotkin, G.R. *et al.* 1964: Congenital β-lipoprotein deficiency: an hereditary disorder involving a defect in the absorption and transport of lipids. *Medicine* 43, 347.

Jacobson, E.D., Chodos, R.B., Faloon, W.W. 1960: An experimental malabsorption syndrome induced by neomycin. *American Journal of Medicine* 28, 524.

Jarmay, K., Varkonyi, T., Hajnal-Papp, R. 1993: Die kollagene Sprue – eine seltene Form der Zoliakie im Erwachsenenalter. [Collagenous sprue – a rare form of celiac disease in adulthood.] *Zeitschrift für Gastroenterologie* 31, 144–6.

Jensen, R.T., Norton, J.A. 1991: Endocrine neoplasms of the pancreas. In Yamada, T. (ed.) *Textbook of gastroenterology,* Vol. 2. Philadelphia: J.B. Lippincott Co., 1912–37.

Johanson, A., Blizzard, R. 1971: A syndrome of congenital aplasia of the alae nasi, deafness, hypothyroidism, dwarfism, absent permanent teeth, and malabsorption. *Journal of Pediatrics* 79, 982.

Jona, J.Z., Belin, R.P., Burke, J.A. 1976: Eosinophilic infiltration of the gastrointestinal tract in children. *American Journal of Diseases of Children* 130, 1136–9.

Jones, N.L., Hofley, P.M., Durie, P.R. 1994: Pathophysiology of the pancreatic defect in Johanson–Blizzard syndrome: a disorder of acinar development. *Journal of Pediatrics* 125, 406.

Juel-Jensen, B.E. 1959: Sensitivity to phenindione. Report of a case of severe diarrhoea. *British Medical Journal* 2, 173.

Katz, A.J., Twarog, F.J., Zeiger, R.S., Falchuk, Z.M. 1984: Milk-sensitive and eosinophilic gastroenteropathy: similar clinical features with contrasting mechanisms and clinical course. *Journal of Allergy and Clinical Immunology* 74, 72–8.

Kayden, H.J. Senior, J.R., Mattson, F.H. 1967: The monoglyceride pathway of fat absorption in man. *Journal of Clinical Investigation* 46, 1695–703.

King, C.E., Toskes, P.P. 1983: Nutrient absorption in the Zollinger–Ellison syndrome. *Archives of Internal Medicine* 143, 349.

Klein, N.C., Hargrove, R.L., Sleisenger, M.H., Jeffries, G.H. 1970: Eosinophilic gastroenteritis. *Medicine* 49, 299–319.

Kolars, J.C., Levitt, M.D., Aouji, M., Savaiano, D.A. 1984: Yoghurt – an autodigesting source of lactose. *New England Journal of Medicine* 310, 1–3.

Krawitt, E.L., Beeken, W.L. 1978: Case report: intestinal clearance of calcium and protein in Waldenstrom's macroglobulinemia. *American Journal of Medical Sciences* 276, 349–52.

Kristensson, K., Nordborg, C., Olsson, Y., Sourander, P. 1971: Changes in the vagus nerve in diabetes mellitus. *Acta Pathologica et Microbiologica Scandinavica: Section A, Pathology* 79, 684–5.

Layer, P., Balzer, K., Goebell, H.Z. 1985: Schweres Malabsorptionssyndrom und exsudative Enteropathie bei Hypogammaglobulinamie: Vollige Ruckbildung unter intravenoser Immunglobulin-Substitution. [Severe malabsorption syndrome and exudative enteropathy in hypogammaglobulinemia: complete involution with intravenous immunoglobulin substitution.] *Zeitschrift für Gastroenterology* 23, 412–17.

Lee, C.M., Changchien, C.S., Chen, P.C. *et al.* 1993: Eosinophilic gastroenteritis: 10 years experience. *American Journal of Gastroenterology* 88, 70–4.

Legge, D.A., Wollaeger, E.E., Carlson, H.C. 1970: Intestinal pseudo-obstruction in systemic amyloidosis. *Gut* 11, 764.

Leinbach, G.E., Rubin, C.E. 1970: Eosinophilic gastroenteritis: a simple reaction to food allergens? *Gastroenterology* 59, 874–89.

Leonard, J.N., Haffenden, G., Tucker, W. *et al.* 1983: Gluten challenge in dermatitis herpetiformis. *New England Journal of Medicine* 308, 816–19.

Lieberman, J.M., Sacchettini, J., Marks, C., Marks, W.H. 1997: Human intestinal fatty acid binding protein: report of an assay with studies in normal volunteers and intestinal ischemia. *Surgery* 121, 335.

Muller, D.P., Lloyd, J.K., Wollf, O.H. 1983: Vitamin E and neurological function. *Lancet* 1, 225–8.

Naish, J.M., Capper, W.M., Brown, N.J. 1960: Intestinal pseudo-obstruction with steatorrhoea. *Gut* 1, 62.

Necheles, T.F., Snyder, L.M. 1970: Malabsorption of folate polyglutamates associated with oral contraceptive therapy. *New England Journal of Medicine* 282, 858.

Neil, G.A., Weinstock, J.V. 1991: Gastrointestinal manifestations of systemic diseases. In Yamada, T. (ed.) *Textbook of gastroenterology*, Vol. II. Philadelphia: J.B. Lippincott Co., 2135–57.

Olbricht, S.M., Flotte, T.J., Collins, A.B., Chapman, C.M., Harrist, T.J. 1986: Dermatitis herpetiformis. Cutaneous deposition of polyclonal IgA_1. *Archives of Dermatology* 122, 418.

Olsson, R.A., Johnston, E.H. 1969: Histopathologic changes and small-bowel absorption in falciparum malaria. *American Journal of Tropical Medicine and Hygiene* 18, 355.

Perera, D.R., Weinstein, W.M., Rubin, C.E. 1975: Small intestinal biopsy. *Human Pathology* 6, 157–217.

Popovic, O.S., Brkic, S., Bojic, P., Kenic, V., Jojic, N., Djuric, V., Djordevic, N. 1980: Sarcoidosis and protein-losing enteropathy. *Gastroenterology* 78, 119.

Race, T.F., Paes, I.C., Faloon, W.W. 1970: Intestinal malabsorption induced by oral colchicine. Comparison with neomycin and cathartic agents. *American Journal of Medical Sciences* 259, 32–41.

Rader, D.J., Brewer, H.B. 1993: Abetalipoproteinemia. New insights into lipoprotein assembly and vitamin E metabolism from a rare genetic disease [clinical conference]. *JAMA* 270, 865–9.

Relman, D.A., Persing, D.H. 1997: Diagnosis and monitoring of Whipple disease by polymerase chain reaction. *Annual Internal Medicine* 126, 520–7.

Relman, D.A., Schmidt, T.M., MacDermott, R.P., Falkow, S. 1992: Identification of the uncultured bacillus of Whipple's disease. *New England Journal of Medicine* 327, 293–301.

Reynolds, E.H., Hallpike, J.F., Phillips, B.M., Matthews, D.M. 1965: Reversible absorptive defects in anticonvulsant megaloblastic anaemia. *Journal of Pathology* 18, 593.

Senior, J.R. 1964: Intestinal absorption of fats. *Journal of Lipid Research* 5, 495.

Shwachman, H., Diamond, L.K., Oski, F.A., Khaw, K.T. 1964: The syndrome of pancreatic insufficiency and bone marrow dysfunction. *Journal of Pediatrics* 65, 645.

Stowers, J.M., Bewsher, P.D. 1969: Studies on the mechanism of weight reduction by phenformin. *Postgraduate Medical Journal* 45, 12.

Strocchi, A., Levitt, M.D. 1991: A reappraisal of the magnitude and implications of the intestinal unstirred layer. *Gastroenterology* 101, 843–7.

Tabaqchali, S., Hatgioannou, J., Booth, C.C. 1968: Bile salt deconjugation and steatorrhoea in patients with stagnant loop syndrome. *Lancet* 2, 12–16.

Tait, R.C., Oogarah, P.K., Houghton, J.B., Farrand, S.E., Haeney, M.R. 1993: Waldenstrom's macroglobulinaemia secreting a paraprotein with lupus anticoagulant activity: possible association with gastrointestinal tract disease and malabsorption. *Journal of Clinical Pathology* 46, 678–80.

Talley, N.J., Shorter, R.G., Phillips, S.F., Zinsmeister, A.R. 1990: Eosinophilic gastroenteritis: a clinicopathological study of patients with disease of the mucosa, muscle layer, and subserosal tissues. *Gut* 31, 54–8.

Thomas, E., Lev, R., McCahan, J.F., Pitchumoni, C.S. 1975: Eosinophilic gastroenteritis with malabsorption, extensive villous atrophy, recurrent hemorrhage and chronic pulmonary fibrosis. *American Journal of Medical Sciences* 269, 259–65.

Trier, J.S. 1962: Morphologic alterations induced by methotrexate in the mucosa of the human proximal intestine. *Gastroenterology* 42, 295.

Turnberg, L.A. 1978: Intestinal transport of salt and water. *Clinical Science and Molecular Medicine* 54, 337–48.

van der Meer, J.B. 1990: Gluten-free diet and elemental diet in dermatitis herpetiformis. *International Journal of Dermatology* 29, 679.

Vazquez-Rodriguez, J.J., Saez, E.S., Vega, J.S., Serrano, M.C.L. 1973: Pancreatitis and eosinophilic gastroenteritis. *International Surgery* 58, 415–19.

Waldmann, T.A. 1966: Protein-losing enteropathy. *Gastroenterology* 50, 422–43.

Weber, J.R., Ryan, J.C. 1993: Effects on the gut of systemic disease and other extraintestinal conditions. In Feldman, M., Scharschmidt, B.F. Sleisenger, M.H. (eds) *Sleisenger and Fordtran's gastrointestinal and liver disease*, Vol. I. Philadelphia: W.B. Saunders Co., 411–38.

Wiley, Z.D., Lavigne, M.E., Liu, K.M., MacGregor, I.L. 1978: The effect of hyperthyroidism on gastric emptying rates and pancreatic exocrine and biliary secretion in man. *American Journal of Digestive Diseases* 23, 1003–8.

17

Viral infections

GEOFFREY DAVIDSON

INTRODUCTION

Viral diarrhoea is an important disease globally, especially in developing countries, with the young, the elderly and the immunocompromised being the most vulnerable. Viruses are the commonest cause of infectious diarrhoea in infants and young children in both the developed and the developing world. In developing countries, they are responsible for up to 25 per cent of deaths among children less than 5 years old, with rotavirus alone being responsible for nearly 800 000 deaths per year (Bern and Glass, 1994). In developed countries, diarrhoeal disease is a major cause of morbidity (Jin *et al.*, 1996), and hospitalization (Jin *et al.*,1996; Carlin *et al.*, 1998), but few deaths (Glass *et al.*, 1991).

In discussing viral diarrhoea in this chapter, other terminology has been encompassed that may be in more common use, such as infectious diarrhoea, gastroenteritis or viral gastroenteritis. The illness is defined as one of acute onset of fever, diarrhoea and/or vomiting of less than 10 days duration. An important proviso is the absence of another obvious cause for the symptomatology, implying correctly that the diagnosis is often one of exclusion.

Serum antibody studies have shown that by the time a child reaches the age of 5, he or she will have been infected by many viral pathogens causing infectious diarrhoea (Table 17.1). Adults are also susceptible to many of these viral pathogens, particularly when they have their own children, travel, or reach old age where the pathogens may be fatal (Hrdy, 1987).

Table 17.1 *Viruses causing infectious diarrhoea*

Rotavirus
Enteric adenoviruses
Caliciviridae
Human calicivirus
Norwalk and Norwalk-like viruses
Astroviridae
Coronaviridae

Viruses as a cause of diarrhoea were suspected from the late 1930s. However, it was the advent of the electron microscope in the 1960s that led to the first discovery of a viral aetiology for diarrhoea by Kapikian and others (1972), who described the Norwalk agent, and Bishop *et al.* (1973a,b), who discovered rotavirus. Prior to these discoveries, a causative agent for infectious diarrhoea had been found in less than 20 per cent of cases.

AETIOLOGY AND EPIDEMIOLOGY

Rotavirus

Rotavirus, initially discovered in Melbourne, Australia, 25 years ago (Bishop *et al.*, 1973a,b) by electron microscopic examination of duodenal mucosal biopsies from infected children, is the major cause of acute sporadic gastroenteritis in young children and also causes diarrhoeal illness in adults (Hrdy, 1987) and travellers (Black, 1990).

Rotaviruses are double-stranded RNA viruses with a genome of 11 segments made up of six viral proteins (VP) and five non-structural proteins (NSP). There are at least seven antigenically distinct rotavirus groups (Groups A–G), which are morphologically identical. More than 90 per cent of human disease is caused by group A rotaviruses, mainly serotypes (G types 1–4). Viruses in groups B and C have also caused outbreaks of diarrhoea in both adults (Fang *et al.*, 1987) and children (Grice *et al.*, 1994).

In temperate climates, rotavirus is a winter disease but can be present for up to 8 months of the year (LeBaron *et al.*, 1990). In tropical areas, seasonal variation is less evident. Rotavirus is transmitted by the faecal–oral route possibly enhanced by aerosol formation (Ansari *et al.*, 1988). The number of particles required to cause disease is unknown but may be as low as 10 particles per millilitre (Ward *et al.*, 1989).

Bishop (1994) highlighted the age-related epidemiology of rotavirus infection. Neonatal infections are often acquired in hospital, occurring within days of birth and affecting up to 60 per cent of all infants with over 90 per cent being asymptomatic. Infants and older children acquire rotavirus infection in the community, peaking at between 6 and 18 months of age. Most primary rotavirus infections are symptomatic, resulting in a high rate of hospitalization (Fearson, 1996; Carlin *et al.*, 1998). Group A serotype G1 is the most common cause and usually only one serotype circulates during any season.

Nosocomial rotavirus infections are a major problem in paediatric hospitals (Ringenberg *et al.*, 1989), neonatal nurseries (Cameron *et al.*, 1978), day care centres (Ferson *et al.*, 1997), hospitals and homes for the elderly (Hrdy, 1987), and significantly within families (Grimwood *et al.*, 1983). Rotavirus has a very high attack rate compared to other pathogens, with high secondary attack rates in families (Guerrant and Bobak, 1991). Hospital-acquired infections can result in up to one in every five children admitted with another illness acquiring rotavirus infection (Ringenberg *et al.*, 1989). This may be related to poor handwashing techniques (Ansari *et al.*, 1988), prolonged excretion of rotavirus after infection (Richardson *et al.*, 1998), asymptomatic rotavirus excretion (Champsaur *et al.*, 1984) and the massive excretion of rotavirus in stools together with possible aerosol formation (Ansari *et al.*, 1988).

Enteric adenoviruses (EAds)

These are the second most commonly identified viral cause of infectious diarrhoea in children. They are morphologically identical to adenoviruses, causing respiratory and other illness, but have been categorized into a separate group (F), comprising two distinct serotypes 40 and 41.

EAds cause gastroenteritis with no respiratory symptoms. The incidence of adenovirus infection in adults is not known but, according to hospital studies, the frequency of infection varies from 6 to 17 per cent of all cases of paediatric diarrhoea (Kotloff *et al.*, 1989). Unlike rotavirus infection, there does not appear to be a seasonal variation with adenovirus infection.

The route of transmission is most likely faecal–oral with a long incubation period of 8–10 days. Virus excretion can last up to 14 days and nosocomial infections are not uncommon, particularly in hospitals and day care centres (Lew *et al.*, 1991). The infection rate in adults is not known but it is likely to be a problem, particularly in the parents of young children.

Caliciviridae

These are a family of non-cultivatable viruses that have a characteristic electron microscopic surface appearance composed of 32 cups (calices); they have been shown to be non-enveloped, single-stranded RNA viruses. With the development of recent techniques and gene sequencing, the Norwalk and Norwalk-like viruses have been shown to be caliciviruses (Jiang *et al.*, 1993).

HUMAN CALICIVIRUS

These animal pathogens were first noted to be a cause of diarrhoea in infants by Madeley and Cosgrove (1976). There are at least five human calcivirus (HuCV) serotypes affecting all age groups and often occurring in epidemics. Cross-infection within hospitals, day care centres and homes for the elderly results in both symptomatic and asymptomatic infection (Grohmann *et al.*, 1991).

NORWALK VIRUS (NV) AND NORWALK-LIKE VIRUS (NLV)

The NV was the first major human gastroenteritis virus discovered by using the technique of immune electron microscopy in 1972 (Kapikian *et al.*, 1972). The spherical 27 nm virus-like particle was isolated from an epidemic of diarrhoea in students in an elementary school in Norwalk, Ohio, USA. It became the prototype of a group of morphologically similar but antigenically distinct aetiologic agents of epidemic diarrhoea. NV and NLV viruses are the major aetiologic agents for epidemics of non-bacterial gastroenteritis in adults and older children, which occur world-wide at any time of the year and in various settings, e.g. families, recreation camps, cruise ships, schools, nursing homes and after ingestion of contaminated food or water (Blacklow and Greenberg, 1991). Both viruses are transmitted by the faecal–oral route, although rapid secondary spread suggests that the airborne route is also likely.

Astroviridae

Astroviruses are cultivable, small, round, non-enveloped, single-stranded RNA viruses, 28–30 nm first seen by electron microscopy in stool samples of children with diarrhoea by Appleton and Higgins (1975). They were named by Madeley and Cosgrove (1975) for their star-shaped appearance and there are at least five distinct human serotypes. They are also a common cause of cross-infection in hospitals, day care centres (Lew *et al.*, 1991) and geriatric centres (Lewis *et al.*, 1989) with a very high attack rate and prolonged virus excretion (Mitchell *et al.*, 1995). Astrovirus is also the most common cause of diarrhoea in immunocompromised adults with human immunodeficiency virus (HIV) infection (Grohmann *et al.*, 1993).

Coronaviridae

HUMAN CORONAVIRUSES

These are enveloped viruses, with a round or pleomorphic shape, which cause severe diarrhoea in various animal species, but their role as a cause of diarrhoea in humans remains to be determined because of the difficulties of isolation and propagation in cell culture (Caul, 1994).

TOROVIRIDAE

This group, previously classified under Coronaviridae, have now been recognized as a separate entity. Toroviruses are recognized pathogens in cattle (Breda virus) and horses (Berne virus), and have recently been seen by electron microscopy in the faeces of children and adults with diarrhoea (Woode, 1994). They are distinguished from coronaviruses by their marked pleomorphism. These torovirus-like particles (TVLPs) were found more commonly in patients with diarrhoea than those without and were a particular problem in immunocompromised patients who shed the virus for prolonged periods (Koopmans *et al.*, 1993; Jamieson *et al.*, 1998).

PATHOGENESIS

Rotavirus

Following ingestion, rotavirus invades only mature epithelial cells initially in the duodenum, multiplies, causes cell rupture and then moves progressively down the intestine, resulting in mild to severe structural abnormalities (Davidson and Barnes, 1979). Earlier studies have indicated that the diarrhoea in rotavirus enteritis is not related to direct viral damage but produces a delay in the normal differentiation of villus enterocytes. This results in a decreased capacity for water, electrolyte and glucose absorption, and disaccharidase deficiency leading to carbohydrate malabsorption and subsequent osmotic diarrhoea (Davidson *et al.*, 1977; Shepherd *et al.*, 1979; Telch *et al.*, 1981). The extent of mucosal damage as well as factors that control epithelial cell differentiation and renewal, such as adequate nutrition, may determine the severity of the clinical illness.

More recent evidence suggests that rotavirus diarrhoea can occur in the absence of epithelial damage (Glass *et al.*, 1996). A non-structural glycoprotein of rotavirus (NSP 4) produces an enterotoxin-like effect that mediates calcium-dependent chloride secretion, although its importance in the clinical syndrome remains to be elucidated (Ward *et al.*, 1997).

Enteric adenoviruses

The mechanism whereby EAds cause diarrhoea remains unknown, although the presence of massive viral shedding during acute infection suggests that active multiplication in the gut is most likely within the mucosa. In a fatal case of adenovirus gastroenteritis, Whitelaw *et al.* (1977) did note the presence of adenovirus particles in the nucleus of intestinal epithelial cells. Uhnoo *et al.* (1984) have shown persistent lactose intolerance following enteric adenovirus infection, suggesting it may have a role in the aetiology of chronic diarrhoea and malnutrition.

Caliciviruses

There is no information available on the histopathology of HuCV, but in animals it causes mucosal atrophy in the duodenum and small intestine. Reversible structural damage to the intestinal mucosa has been shown in human volunteers infected with NV or NVL. The damage appears within 48 hours of infection and has completely resolved by 10–14 days.

Malabsorption of fat and depression of mucosal disaccharidase levels have also been shown during the acute illness. There is no information on the pathogenesis of the diarrhoea or the functional changes induced by these viruses (Dolin *et al.*, 1987).

CLINICAL FEATURES

Rotavirus

Symptomatic rotavirus infection has an incubation period of 1–3 days and produces an illness of fever and vomiting, which usually precedes the onset of diarrhoea and lasts 1–3 days. The diarrhoea can last for up to 7 days. Community-based studies suggest that symptoms are milder than in hospital-based studies (Hjelt, 1988). The duration and severity of symptoms are more significant in children during the first 18 months of life. Rotavirus infection causes more severe vomiting and dehydration than in non-rotavirus diarrhoeal illnesses or bacterial causes in both developed and developing countries (Yolken and Curlin, 1980). The clinical severity of the illness varies from asymptomatic infection (Champsaur *et al.*, 1984) to a severe fatal illness (Bern and Glass, 1994) and does not appear to be influenced by the rotavirus serotype (Barnes *et al.*, 1992).

Rotavirus infection may lead to a more prolonged illness due to secondary carbohydrate malabsorption (Davidson *et al.*, 1984). Rotavirus has also been described in association with necrotizing enterocolitis, intussusception, sudden infant death syndrome, aseptic meningitis and exanthem subitum (Blacklow and Greenberg, 1991). The recent findings of prolonged rotavirus excretion following infection suggest that it may also be an important cause of persistent diarrhoea (Richardson *et al.*, 1998).

Enteric adenoviruses

The clinical manifestations of enteric adenovirus infection are similar to those noted for rotavirus infection, although the disease is characteristically milder, with 1 or 2 days of vomiting and fever, followed by watery diarrhoea, which is significantly longer in duration than for rotavirus infection (Uhnoo *et al.*, 1986). Virus shedding can occur for several weeks. The illness lasts for 8–12 days.

Human caliciviruses

Most of these viruses have a similar clinical pattern with an incubation period of 1–3 days and a similar duration of symptoms, which are generally mild, with watery diarrhoea, abdominal cramps and vomiting. Compared to rotavirus infection the illnesses are relatively mild with a high rate of subclinical infection and prolonged viral shedding well after symptoms have settled.

Astroviridae

Astrovirus is predominantly a winter disease and generally produces a mild clinical illness with watery diarrhoea lasting 1–2 days. It has recently been shown to be a more common agent of gastroenteritis than previously thought (Oishi *et al.*, 1994). There is also some evidence emerging to suggest it may be a more common cause of severe diarrhoea and hospitalization than previously suspected (Palombo and Bishop, 1996).

IMMUNITY

Rotavirus

A recent study from Mexico suggested that natural rotavirus infection conferred protection against subsequent infections and that the protection was greatest against severe infection and increased with repeated exposures (Velazquez *et al.*, 1996). This suggests that widespread immunization with an effective immunogen could prevent severe disease and, in fact, there is now evidence to support this being the case (Kapikian *et al.*, 1996). Despite this progress and the identification of the viral proteins that can neutralize rotavirus and provide host protection, the factors that determine susceptibility and illness in humans are not known. There is also a poor correlation between serotype-specific human immunity and protection, and the role of cellular immunity remains unclear.

Breast feeding seems to provide protection against rotavirus in totally breast-fed infants, although rotavirus infections are also common in societies where exclusive breast feeding is practised.

Enteric adenovirus

Most of the information on immunity relates to sero surveys, although a recent report has been published suggesting that enteric adenovirus infection, unlike rotavirus infection, does not protect against subsequent symptomatic infection (Unicomb *et al.*, 1996). In some population groups, 50 per cent of children have antibodies to enteric adenoviruses by the age of 4 (Shinozaki *et al.*, 1987).

Caliciviridae

Earlier volunteer studies have shown that, although antibody may play a part in short-term immunity over 1–2 months, long-term immunity appears to be independent of antibody, as both serum and intestinal antibody fail to correlate with resistance to infection (Kapikian, 1994). A recent Finnish study showed the presence of antibodies to NV in infants and young children, suggesting that NV infections are more common in this age group than had previously been suspected and that antibody to NV may be protective against reinfection (Lew *et al.*, 1994). There is no information about the immunity to human calicivirus infection. The recent development of more sensitive polymerase chain reaction (PCR) techniques for diagnosis should help our understanding of the immune response.

Astroviridae

There is no information on immunity to this infection, although most children have antibodies to one of the five astrovirus serotypes by the age of 5 (Kurtz and Lee, 1978).

VIRAL DIARRHOEA IN THE IMMUNOCOMPROMISED PATIENT

Severely immunocompromised patients, both adults and children, are susceptible to severe and protracted infections with known gut pathogens, or with infections with viruses that do not normally cause gastroenteritis as their primary manifestation, but which may cause diarrhoea as part of their symptom complex.

Both rotavirus and adenovirus have been shown to be chronically excreted in immunocompromised patients, most commonly following bone marrow transplant, where there is a very high morbidity and mortality (Saulsbury *et al.*, 1980; Yolken *et al.*, 1982). Cytomegalovirus (CMV) infection of the gastrointestinal tract also occurs in the severely immunocompromised, either associated with organ transplantation or as a complication of infection. CMV infection involves both the small bowel, where it causes villus atrophy, malabsorption and chronic diarrhoea, or the large intestine, causing a colitis with bloody diarrhoea (Escudero-Fabre *et al.*, 1992).

Many opportunistic infections can cause diarrhoea in patients with HIV infection, but it also appears that HIV itself can cause an enteropathy with watery diarrhoea, malabsorption and weight loss (Friedman, 1994). It is still possible, however, that this condition may also be related to an as yet undiagnosed opportunistic infection.

DIAGNOSIS

Table 17.2 shows the current techniques used for the diagnosis of the common human viral pathogens. The recent introduction of reverse transcriptase–polymerase chain reaction (RT-PCR) technology to the detection of these diarrhoeal viruses will increase our knowledge, and help to clarify their epidemiology and also their overall importance as human pathogens. At the present time routine testing using an enzyme immunosorbent assay (EIA) is used for rotavirus enteric adenoviruses and recently astroviruses. It is expected that RT-PCR techniques should soon become available to study the NV and NVL, which will help provide more information on these common causes of epidemics of diarrhoeal disease.

TREATMENT AND PREVENTION

Most causes of viral diarrhoea are self-limited and the mainstay of treatment is the management of dehydration, which is best achieved with oral rehydration solutions (Sack, 1991). These have been life saving, and are simple to use and effective for all but the most severe diarrhoeal dehydration with shock. Recent modifications to these solutions using different substrates (e.g. rice) have improved efficacy, as reduction in diarrhoea was a problem with earlier solutions (Pizarro *et al.*, 1991). If there are no clinical signs of dehydration, then increasing the fluid intake using hypotonic solutions, such as diluted fruit juice or cordial are satisfactory. In breast-fed infants, breast feeding should be continued and extra fluid given.

Following rehydration, if children are hungry, they should be fed, as starvation leads to prolongation of the diarrhoea. There is also no need to use diluted formula or milk. Full-strength milk should be restarted as soon as the child is hungry and this will be well tolerated in the majority of cases. Lactase deficiency, which can occur following rotavirus gastroenteritis, is relatively uncommon but, if the diarrhoea does not settle, this should be looked for (Davidson *et al.*, 1984).

Table 17.2 *Viral agents and their mode of diagnosis*

	Electron microscopy	Immune electron microscopy	EIA	RT-PCR	Culture
Rotavirus	+	—	+	+	+
Enteric adenoviruses	+	—	+	—	+
Human caliciviruses	+	—	+	—	—
Norwalk virus and Norwalk like-virus	—	+	+	+	—
Astroviruses	+	—	+	+	+
Coronavirus-like particles (TVLP)	+	—	+	+	—

EIA, enzyme immunosorbent assay; RT-PCR, reverse transcriptase–polymerase chain reaction; +, diagnostic tests available; —, no diagnostic test developed or available.

Recently, there have been attempts to use oral immunoglobulin and hyperimmune bovine colostrum as treatments for acute rotavirus gastroenteritis in children. They have been shown to reduce the duration and severity of the diarrhoea (Ylitalo *et al.*, 1998).

Prevention is obviously the major aim in the management of diarrhoea and has led to the search for active vaccines. The first licensed rotavirus vaccine became available in North America in August 1998. This tetravalent rhesus rotavirus reassortant vaccine has been shown to provide more than 80 per cent efficacy against severe rotavirus infection but only 50 per cent efficacy against mild to moderate infection (Kapikian *et al.*, 1996). Unfortunately, the vaccine was withdrawn in late 1999 because of a suspected causal increased link between intussusception and rotavirus vaccine use (Barnes, 1999).

Passive protection against diarrhoeal disease using hyperimmune bovine colostrum or bovine immunoglobulin concentrate has also been shown to be successful in trials both for the prevention of rotavirus cross-infection in hospitals and also community acquisition of rotavirus (Davidson, 1996). This simple approach may have wider application to other enteric pathogens, particularly as there are no totally effective active vaccines available for any enteric pathogen.

The use of passive protection has also been of value in managing immunocompromised patients with viral gastroenteritis (Losonsky *et al.*, 1985). This is important as this group of patients may not be suitable for active vaccines.

CONCLUSION

Since their discovery 35 years ago, viral infections of the gastrointestinal tract have been shown to be the major cause of diarrhoeal disease in infants and young children, and a very important cause of diarrhoea in adults, particularly in the elderly. The development of newer more specific and sensitive techniques for diagnosis should provide new information on the relative importance of these pathogens, their pathogenesis, epidemiology, transmission and immunity, which will hopefully lead to more effective treatment and prevention of these medically important infections.

REFERENCES

Ansari, S.A., Sattar, S.A., Springthorpe, V.S., Wells, G.A., Tostowary, K.W. 1988: Rotavirus survival on human hands and transfer of infectious virus to animate and nonporous inanimate surfaces. *Journal of Clinical Microbiology* 20, 1464–9.

Appleton, H., Higgins, P.G. 1975: Viruses and gastroenteritis in infants. *Lancet* 2, 1297.

Barnes, G.L. 1999: Intussesception and rotavirus vaccine. *Journal of Pediatric Gastroenterology and Nutrition* 29, 375.

Barnes, G.L., Unicomb, L., Bishop, R.F. 1992: Severity of rotavirus infection in relation to serotype, monotype and electropherotype. *Journal of Pediatrics and Child Health* 28, 54–8.

Bern, C., Glass, R.I. 1994: Impact of diarrheal diseases worldwide. In Kapikian, A.Z., (ed) *Viral infections of the gastrointestinal tract*, 2nd edn. New York: Marcel Dekker, 1–26.

Bishop, R.F. 1994: Natural history of human rotavirus infections. In Kapikian, A.Z., (ed) *Viral infections of the gastrointestinal tract*, 2nd edn. New York: Marcel Dekker, 131–67.

Bishop, R.F., Davidson, G.P., Holmes, I.H., Ruck, B.J. 1973a: Evidence for viral gastroenteritis. *New England Journal of Medicine* 289, 1096–7.

Bishop, R.F., Davidson, G.P., Holmes, I.H., Ruck, B.J. 1973b: Virus particles in epithelial cells of duodenal mucosa from children with acute non-bacterial gastroenteritis. *Lancet* 1, 149–51.

Black, R.E. 1990: Epidemiology of travellers diarrhoea and relative importance of various pathogens. *Journal of Infectious Diseases* 12, 573–4.

Blacklow, N.R., Greenberg, H.B. 1991: Viral gastroenteritis. *New England Journal of Medicine* 325, 252–64.

Cameron, D.J.S., Bishop, R.F., Veenstra, A.A., Barnes, G.L. 1978: Non-cultivable viruses and neonatal diarrhoea: fifteen month survey in a newborn special care nursery. *Journal of Clinical Microbiology* 8, 93–8.

Carlin, J.B., Chondros, P., Masendycz, P., Bugg, H., Bishop, R.F., Barnes, G.L. 1998: Rotavirus infection and rates of hospitalization for acute gastroenteritis in young children in Australia, 1993–1996. *Medical Journal of Australia*, 169, 252–6.

Caul, E.O. 1994: Human coronavirus. In Kapikian, A.Z. (ed.) *Viral infections of the gastrointestinal tract*, 2nd edn. New York: Marcel Dekker, 603–25.

Champsaur, H., Questiaux, E., Prevot, J. *et al.* 1984: Rotavirus carriage, asymptomatic infection and disease in the first two years of life. 1. Virus shedding. *Journal of Infectious Diseases* 140, 667–74.

Davidson, G.P. 1996: Passive protection against diarrhoeal disease. *Journal of Pediatric Gastroenterology and Nutrition* 23, 207–12.

Davidson, G.P., Barnes, G.L. 1979: Structural and functional abnormalities of the small intestine in infants and young children with rotavirus enteritis. *Acta Paediatrica Scandinavica* 68, 181–6.

Davidson, G.P., Gall, D.G., Butler, D.G., Petric, M., Hamilton, J.R. 1977: Human rotavirus enteritis induced in conventional piglets. Intestinal structure and transport. *Journal of Clinical Investigation* 60, 1402–9.

Davidson, G.P., Goodwin, D., Robb, T.A. 1984: Incidence and duration of lactose malabsorption in children hospitalized with acute enteritis: a study in a well nourished urban population. *Journal of Pediatrics* 105, 587–90.

Dolin, R., Treanor, J.J., Madore, P.H. 1987: Novel agents of viral enteritis in humans. *Journal of Infectious Diseases* 15, 365–76.

Escudero-Fabre, A., Cummings, O., Kirklin, J.K., Bourge, R.C., Aldrete, J.S. 1992: Cytomegalovirus colitis presenting as hematochezia and requiring resection. *Archives of Surgery* 127, 102–4.

Fang, Z., Ye, Q., Ho, M. *et al.* 1987: Investigations of an outbreak of adult diarrhoea virus in China. *Journal of Infectious Diseases* 160, 948–53.

Ferson, M.J. 1996: Hospitalizations for rotavirus gastroenteritis among children under five years of age in New South Wales. *Medical Journal of Australia* 18, 71–8.

Ferson, M.J., Strangfellow, S., McPhie, K., McIvor, C.J., Simos, A. 1997: Longitudinal study of rotavirus infection in child care centres. *Journal of Pediatric and Child Health* 33, 157–60.

Friedman, S.L., 1994: Diarrhea. In Cohen, P.T., Sande, M.A., Volderding, P.A. (eds) *The AIDS knowledge base*. Boston: Little Brown and Co., 5.19.1–19.

Glass, R.I., Lew, J.F., Gangerosa, R.E., Le Baron, C.W., Ho, M.S. 1991: Estimates of morbidity and mortality rates of diarrheal diseases in American children. *Journal of Pediatrics* 118, 27–33.

Glass, R.I., Gentsch, J.R., Ivanoff, B. 1996: New lessons for rotavirus vaccines. *Science* 272, 46–8.

Grice, A.S., Lambden, P.R., Caul, O.E., Clarke, I.N. 1994: Sequence conservation of the major outer capsid glycoprotein of human group C rotaviruses. *Journal of Medicine and Virology* 44, 166–71.

Grimwood, K., Abbot, G.D., Fergusson, D.M., Jennings, L.C., Allan, J.M. 1983: Spread of rotavirus within families: a community based study. *British Medical Journal* 287, 575–7.

Grohmann, G., Glass, R.I., Gold, R. *et al.* 1991: An outbreak of human calicivirus gastroenteritis in a day care centre in Sydney, Australia. *Journal of Clinical Microbiology* 159, 71–8.

Grohmann, G., Glass, R.I., Pereira, H.G. *et al.* 1993: Enteric viruses and diarrhea in HIV infected patients. *New England Journal of Medicine* 329, 14–20.

Guerrant, R.L., Bobak, D.A. 1991: Bacterial and protozoal gastroenteritis. *New England Journal of Medicine* 325, 327–40.

Hjelt, K., 1988: Acute rotavirus gastroenteritis in children. Clinical, epidemiological and immunological aspects. *Danish Medical Bulletin* 35, 222–36.

Hrdy, D.B. 1987: Epidemiology of rotavirus infection in adults. *Reviews of Infectious Diseases* 9, 461–9.

Jamieson, F.B., Wang, E.E.L., Bain, C., Good, J., Duckmanton, L., Petric, M. 1998: Human Torovirus: a new nosocomial gastrointestinal pathogen. *Journal of Infectious Diseases* 178, 1263–9.

Jiang, X., Wang, M., Estes, M.K. 1993: Sequences and genomic organization of Norwalk virus. *Virology* 195, 51–61.

Jin, S., Kilgore, P.E., Holman, P.C., Clarke, M.J., Gangarosa, E.J., Glass, R.I. 1996: Trends in hospitalizations for diarrhea in United States children from 1979 through 1992: estimates of the morbidity associated with rotavirus. *Pediatric Infectious Diseases Journal* 15, 397–404.

Kapikian, A.Z. 1994. Norwalk and Norwalk-like viruses. In Kapikian, A.Z. (ed.) *Viral infections of the gastrointestinal tract*, 2nd edn. New York: Marcel Dekker, 471–518.

Kapikian, A.Z., Wyatt, R.G., Dolin, R., Thornbill, T.S., Kalica, A.R., Chanock, R.M. 1972: Visualization by immune electron microscopy of a 27 nm particle associated with acute infectious non-bacterial gastroenteritis. *Journal of Virology* 10, 1075–81.

Kapikian, A.Z., Hoshino, Y., Chanock, R.M., Perez-Schael, I. 1996. Efficacy of a quadrivalent rhesus rotavirus-based human rotavirus vaccine aimed at preventing severe rotavirus diarrhea in infants and young children. *Journal of Infectious Diseases* 174(Suppl), 565–72.

Koopmans, M., Petric, M., Glass, R.I., Munroe, S.S. 1993: Enzyme linked immunosorbent assay of Torovirus-like particles in faecal specimens from humans with diarrhoea. *Journal of Clinical Microbiology* 31, 2738–44.

Kotloff, K.L., Losonsky, G.A., Morris, J.G., Jr. *et al.* 1989: Enteric adenovirus infection and childhood diarrhea: an epidemiologic study in three clinical settings. *Pediatrics* 84, 219–25.

Kurtz, J.B., Lee, T.W., 1978: Astrovirus gastroenteritis. Age distribution of antibody. *Medical Microbiology and Immunology* 166, 227–30.

LeBaron, C.W., Lew, J., Glass, R.I., Weber, J.M., Ruiz Palacios, G.M. 1990: The Rotavirus Study Group. Annual rotavirus epidemic patterns in NA. *JAMA* 264, 983–8.

Lew, J.F., Moe, C.L., Monroe, S.S. *et al.* 1991: Astrovirus and adenovirus associated with diarrhea in children in day care settings. *Journal of Infectious Diseases* 164, 673–8.

Lew, J.F., Valdesuso, J., Vesikari, T. *et al.* 1994: Detection of Norwalk virus or Norwalk-like virus infections in Finnish infants and young children. *Journal of Infectious Diseases* 169, 364–7.

Lewis, D.C., Lightfoot, N.F., Cubit, W.D., Wilson, S.A. 1989: Outbreaks of astrovirus type 1 and rotavirus gastroenteritis in a geriatric inpatient population. *Journal of Hospital Infection* 14, 9–14.

Losonsky, G., Johnson, J.P., Winkelstein, J.A., Yolken, R.H., 1985. Oral administration of human serum immunoglobulin in immunodeficient patients with viral gastroenteritis. A pharmacokinetic and functional analysis. *Journal of Clinical Investigation* 76, 2362–7.

Madeley, C.R., Cosgrove, B.P. 1975: 28 nm particles in faeces in infantile gastroenteritis. *Lancet* 2, 451–2.

Madeley, C.R., Cosgrove, B.P. 1976: Caliciviruses in man. *Lancet* 1, 199–200.

Mitchell, D.K., Monroe, S.S., Jiang, X. *et al.* 1995: Virologic features of an astrovirus diarrhea outbreak in a day care center revealed by reverse transcriptase–polymerase chain reaction. *Journal of Infectious Diseases* 172, 1437–44.

Oishi, I., Yamazaki, K., Kimoto, T. *et al.* 1994: A large outbreak of acute gastroenteritis associated with astrovirus among students and teachers in Osaka. *Journal of Infectious Diseases* 170, 439–43.

Palombo, E.A., Bishop, R.F. 1996: Annual incidence serotype distribution and genetic diversity of human astrovirus isolates from hospitalized children in Melbourne, Australia. *Journal of Clinical Microbiology* 34, 1750–3.

Pizzaro, D., Prosada, G., Sandi, L., Moran, J.R. 1991: Rice based oral rehydration solutions for the management of infantile diarrhea. *New England Journal of Medicine* 324, 517–21.

Richardson, S., Grimwood, K., Gorrell, R., Palombo, E., Barnes, G.L., Bishop, R.F. 1998: Extended excretion of rotavirus after severe diarrhoea in young children. *Lancet* 351, 1844–8.

Ringenberg, M., Davidson, G.P., Spence, J., Morris, S. 1989: Prospective study of nosocomial rotavirus infection in a paediatric hospital. *Australian Paediatric Journal* 139, 935–9.

Sack, D.A., 1991: Use of oral rehydration therapy in acute watery diarrhea. Practical guide. *Drugs* 41, 566–73.

Saulsbury, F.T., Winkelstein, J.A., Yolken, R.H. 1980: Chronic rotavirus infection in immunodeficiency. *Journal of Pediatrics* 97, 61–5.

Shepherd, R.W., Gall, D.G., Butler, D.G., Hamilton, J.R. 1979: Determinants of diarrhoea in viral enteritis: the role of ion transport and epithelial changes in the ileum in transmissible gastroenteritis in piglets. *Gastroenterology* 76, 20–4.

Shinozaki, T., Araki, K., Ushijima, H., Fujii, R. 1987: Antibody response to enteric adenovirus types 40 and 41 in sera from people in various age groups. *Journal of Clinical Microbiology* 25, 1679–82.

Telch, J., Shepherd, R.W., Butler, D.G. 1981: Jejunal glucose transport in acute invasive viral enteritis. *Clinical Science* 61, 29–34.

Uhnoo, I., Wadell, G., Svensson, L., Johansson, M.E. 1984: Importance of enteric adenoviruses 40 and 41 in acute gastroenteritis in infants and young children. *Journal of Clinical Microbiology* 20, 365–72.

Uhnoo, I., Olding-Stenkvist, E., Kreuger, A. 1986: Clinical features of acute gastroenteritis associated with rotavirus, enteric adenoviruses and bacteria. *Archives of the Diseases of Childhood* 61, 732–8.

Unicomb, L., Jarecki-Khan, K., Hall, A., Podder, G., 1996: Previous enteric adenovirus infection does not protect against subsequent symptomatic infection: longitudinal follow up of eight infants. *Microbiology and Immunology* 40, 161–8.

Velazquez, F.R., Matson, D.O., Calva, J.J. *et al.* 1996: Rotavirus infection in infants as protection against subsequent infections. *New England Journal of Medicine* 335, 1022–8.

Ward, R.L., Bernstein, D.I., Shukla, R. *et al.* 1989: Effects of antibody on adults challenged with a human rotavirus. *Journal of Infectious Diseases* 159, 79–88.

Ward, R.L., Mason, B.B., Bernstein, D.I. *et al.* 1997: Attenuation of a human rotavirus vaccine candidate did not correlate with mutations in the NSP4 protein gene. *Journal of Virology* 71, 6267–70.

Whitelaw, A., Davies, H., Parry, J. 1977: Electron microscopy of fatal adenovirus gastroenteritis. *Lancet* 1, 361.

Woode, G.N. 1994: The Toroviruses: bovine (Breda virus) and equine (Berne virus) and the Torovirus-like agents of humans and animals. In Kapikian, A.Z. (ed.) *Viral infections of the gastrointestinal tract*, 2nd edn. New York: Marcel Dekker, 581–602.

Ylitalo, S., Uhari, M., Rasi, S., Pudas, J., Leppaluoto, J. 1998: Rotaviral antibodies in the treatment of acute rotavirus gastroenteritis. *Acta Paediatrica* 87, 264–7.

Yolken, R.H., Curlin, G.T. 1980: A two-year study of bacterial, viral and parasitic agents associated with diarrhea in rural Bangladesh. *Journal of Infectious Diseases* 142, 660–4.

Yolken, R.H., Bishop, C.A., Townsend, T.R. *et al.* 1982: Infectious gastroenteritis in bone marrow transplant recipients. *New England Journal of Medicine* 306, 1009–12.

18

Bacterial infections

RANJIT N RATNAIKE, KELLY PAPANAOUM

Bacterial infections are a major cause of acute and, less often, of chronic diarrhoea. The mechanisms that protect the host against invasive pathogens have been discussed in Chapters 4 and 5. Diarrhoea due to the ingestion of a pathogen is not invariable. The occurrence of diarrhoea reflects the size of the inoculum, the virulence of the organism and the resistance of the host (Grady and Keusch, 1971). Many bacteria that cause diarrhoea have common features in regard to their mechanism of action, site of action and extraintestinal manifestations. For example, patients with the HLA-B27 haplotype infected with *Shigella* species, *Campylobacter jejuni* and *Yersinia enterocolitica* are predisposed to Reiter's syndrome (arthritis, urethritis and conjunctivitis). Fever is a particular feature of *Shigella*, *Campylobacter* and *Salmonella* infections. The haemolytic uraemic syndrome is associated with Gram-negative enteric infections, usually due to enterohaemorrhagic *Escherichia coli* (Siegler, 1995), particularly *E. coli* O157:H7 (Griffin *et al.*, 1988; Wall *et al.*, 1996), but is occasionally caused by *Campylobacter* (Delans *et al.*, 1984), *Salmonella* and *Shigella* (Mariani-Kurkdjian and Bingen, 1995).

MECHANISMS OF DIARRHOEA

The several mechanisms in the pathogenesis of diarrhoeal disease are discussed in Chapter 15. In general, bacteria cause diarrhoea by the elaboration of a toxin, which may act as a secretagogue (secretory agent) or as a cytotoxin, or by mucosal invasion, or a combination of these factors. The same pathogen may cause diarrhoea through more than one mechanism.

Enterotoxins

Bacterial enterotoxins are polypeptides released from bacteria, and intestinal mucosal cells are their site of action. Bacterial enterotoxins include:

1. toxins that cause diarrhoea by increased secretion of fluids and electrolytes, for example, secretagogues such as cholera toxin;
2. cytotoxins that cause diarrhoea by damaging mucosal tissue through cell death, for example, the colonic mucosal damage caused by the verocytotoxins of enterohaemorrhagic *E. coli* (Hart *et al.*, 1993);
3. toxins produced after the bacteria invade the cells of the intestinal mucosa, for example, the Shiga toxin released by invasive *Shigella dysenteriae* type 1 (Gemmell, 1984; Keusch *et al.*, 1985).

Some toxins are preformed in food (previously cooked meat, poultry or gravy, which is not refrigerated adequately), and then act on the intestine, usually within a characteristically short time after ingestion of the contaminated food. Most enterotoxins are secreted by bacteria during the process of infection. For example, the toxin produced by *Vibrio cholerae* in the small intestine is a powerful secretagogue that causes severe watery diarrhoea by activating adenylate cyclase in the enterocyte.

Toxins produced *in situ*

- *Vibrio cholerae*
- *Vibrio parahaemolyticus*
- Enterotoxigenic *E. coli* (ETEC)

- Enteropathogenic *E. coli* (EPEC)
- *Shigella* species
- *Salmonella* species
- *Yersinia enterocolitica*
- *Clostridium perfringens* (this also produces a preformed toxin)
- *Bacillus cereus* (enterotoxins)
- *Plesiomonas* species
- *Aeromonas* species.

Secretagogue production

These toxins may be preformed in food prior to ingestion or can also be elaborated by the organism once established in the gastrointestinal tract. In the latter instance, exemplified by *Vibrio cholerae*, the bacteria produces a powerful toxin and merely attaches itself superficially to the mucosa for this purpose. Mucosal penetration and damage is not a feature. Diarrhoea occurs due to the significant derangement in fluid and electrolyte absorption and secretion in the small intestine (Sharp, 1973). In secretory diarrhoea, the diarrhoea is mediated through an increase in the concentration of intracellular cyclic AMP or less commonly cyclic GMP (Gemmell, 1984; Ganguly and Kaur, 1996). The diarrhoea is secretory in nature (*see* Chapter 15) and is characterized by bowel actions that are voluminous and watery. Nausea and vomiting with cramping periumbilical abdominal pain may be present.

Cytotoxin production

The bacteria listed below produce cytotoxins. Unlike toxins, which act as secretagogues, these cytotoxins do *not* cause diarrhoea by intracellular enzyme activation (which induces net electrolyte and water secretion), but as a result of cell injury and cell death.

- *Shigella* species
  - *Shigella dysenteriae 1*
  - *Shigella sonnei* (some strains)
  - *Shigella flexneri* (some strains)
- *Clostridium difficile*
- Enterohaemorrhagic *Escherichia coli* (EHEC)
- *Campylobacter jejuni*.

Mucosal invasion

Bacterial invasion of epithelial cells is the third major mechanism by which bacteria cause diarrhoea and it occurs mainly in the colon. However, the small intestine is frequently involved (Hart *et al.*, 1993). Although these bacteria ultimately cause cell death by the elaboration of a cytotoxin, invasion is the primary event. These bacteria (which invade the mucosa) overcome the need to proliferate in the lumen of the gut by attaching themselves to the intestinal epithelium and they then penetrate into the cells and multiply within them. This mucosal invasion and replication of bacteria inside the epithelial cells causes tissue death and in some instances submucosal invasion and further tissue damage.

Once within the cell, intracellular division occurs rapidly and the bacteria spread actively and with ease to adjacent cells (Ogawa *et al.*, 1968). The cytotoxin produced causes cell injury and death. When the dead cells are shed, microulcers or microabscesses are formed in the mucosa, and an extensive inflammatory reaction occurs in the lamina propria. Invasion of the colonic epithelium is the predominant mechanism by which *Shigella* and enteroinvasive *E. coli* cause dysentery (LaBrec *et al.*, 1964).

Dysentery is a term that refers to diarrhoea with blood and mucus, and implies severe *colonic* infection characterized by small, frequent bowel actions with pus, mucus and often blood; tenesmus, urgency, cramping and infraumbilical abdominal pain are associated features. The loss of brush-border enzymes and reduced absorptive surface as tissue damage occurs decreases fluid absorption, resulting in diarrhoea. The diarrhoeal stool consists of an inflammatory exudate, sloughed cells and cell debris, copious mucus from goblet cells, pus and blood.

The bacteria listed below predominantly affect the colon to produce dysentery:

- enteroinvasive *Escherichia coli* (EIEC)
- *Shigella* species
- *Campylobacter jejuni*
- *Yersinia enterocolitica*
- enterohaemorrhagic *Escherichia coli* (EHEC)
- enteroaggregative *Escherichia coli* (EAggEC).

ACUTE DIARRHOEA

Vibrio cholerae

Vibrio cholerae is a comma-shaped, Gram-negative, motile bacillus. Two biotypes are recognized, the *classical* biotype and the *El Tor* biotype. The two main serotypes based on the O antigen are Ogawa and Inaba. The infection is spread by contaminated food and drink. Person to person spread is unlikely, as the inoculum for infection is large, unlike in *Shigella* species. Carrier states exist and the gallbladder is the site of infection. The *El Tor* biotype causes a milder or asymptomatic infection with spontaneous resolution.

The toxin of *V. cholerae* is the same in all strains. It is a powerful secretagogue, which causes severe watery diarrhoea by activating adenylate cyclase in the enterocyte (Finkelstein, 1973; *see* Chapter 15). Cholera toxin has a molecular weight of 84 000 Da and consists of one A subunit of molecular weight 29 000 Da and five smaller B subunits, which surround the A subunit (Gill, 1976). Mucosal penetration does not occur and no significant mucosal lesions are evident on light microscopy.

Seafood is an important source of infection. Cholera is most common in south Asia (Bangladesh, India, Pakistan and Sri Lanka). An outbreak of cholera in Peru in 1991 spread to seven other South American countries (Glass *et al.*, 1991). In the USA, cholera has occurred in Texas and Louisiana (Morris and Black, 1985). The presence of the organism around the Bay of Bengal in India and the Gulf coast of the USA reflects its preference to live in environments with a high concentration of salt.

Cholera is a rare cause of traveller's diarrhoea and an unlikely cause of diarrhoea in the developed world, although sporadic cases occur. In the clinical setting of voluminous, diarrhoeal stools, which resemble 'rice water' owing to the slightly turbid opalescent appearance (Plate 18.1), the probability of cholera should be considered, especially in a patient from an endemic area. The incubation period is about 48 hours and the onset of the illness is associated with vomiting, which lasts for about 1 day. The massive outpouring of watery stools, on occasion exceeding 5 L a day, are maximal during the first 48 hours. Death from dehydration and electrolyte loss may occur even within the first 24 hours of the illness. Hypoglycaemia has been described in children (Bennish *et al.*, 1990).

The characteristic morphology and motility of *V. cholerae* may be seen in a fresh stool specimen on dark ground microscopy, but this is not specific. Diagnosis is confirmed by culture.

Antibiotic therapy with tetracycline rapidly resolves the illness (Greenough *et al.*, 1964). Owing to the development of resistance to tetracycline, other antibiotics have been used. A single 300 mg dose of doxycycline was found to be as effective as the standard multiple-dose tetracycline treatment (Alam *et al.*, 1990). A 5-day treatment with erythromycin (50 mg/kg per day in four equally divided doses) or with co-trimoxazole (a combination of sulphamethoxazole and trimethoprim, given as 50 mg/kg and 10 mg/kg, respectively, per day in two equally divided doses) are both effective, and of particular value, specifically in younger children in whom tetracycline is contraindicated or when there is resistance (Grados *et al.*, 1996; Kabir *et al.*, 1996). Fluoroquinolones are also useful, particularly with increasing resistance to tetracycline and sulphamethoxazole– trimethoprim.

A hallmark of the illness is severe watery diarrhoea, progressing rapidly to dehydration. Substantial rapid fluid and electrolyte replacement are an essential part of management.

The use of oral rehydration solutions (ORS) is the treatment of choice for mild to moderate dehydration (WHO, 1984; Greenough and Khin-Maung, 1991). It is important to note that, despite the continuing diarrhoea, ORS is absorbed and helps enterocyte regeneration. Fluids, however, need not be confined to ORS. Water and other suitable drinks may be used, although not drinks with a high osmolality, for example, Coca Cola (680 mosmol/kg), apple juice (870 mosmol/kg), orange juice (935 mosmol/kg) and grape juice (1170 mosmol/kg). ORS formulae and guidelines for rehydration are given in Chapter 14.

VACCINES

The original parenteral cholera vaccines were not satisfactory for public use, but new oral vaccines are now under trial or in commercial production in several countries. One vaccine consists of killed whole *V. cholerae* O1 in combination with purified recombinant B-subunit of cholera toxin (WC/rBS). Two doses of this vaccine a week apart confer 85–90 per cent protection for 6 months, and 50 per cent after 3 years. This vaccine is licensed in Sweden, Norway, Peru, Argentina, Guatemala, Salvador, Honduras and Nicaragua (WHO, 1998).

A variant of the above toxin vaccine without the B subunit is produced in Vietnam and showed an efficacy of 66 per cent at 8 months, but is only licensed in Vietnam (WHO, 1998).

A third oral vaccine consists of an attenuated, live, genetically manipulated *V. cholerae* O1 strain CVD 103-HgR. Trials have been performed in Indonesia for 4 years. Preliminary results have been disappointing, although, in adult volunteers in the USA, a single oral dose conferred 95 per cent protection after 1 week against *V. cholerae classical* biotype and 65 per cent against *El Tor* biotypes. This vaccine is licensed in Switzerland, Canada, Finland, Argentina, Peru and The Philippines (WHO, 1998).

Vibrio cholerae non-01

This group of strains are identical morphologically and biochemically to *V. cholerae* but do not react with the O-group 1 antisera, which the *V. cholerae* organisms agglutinate. The organisms, previously called non-cholera vibrios, are also found in salty surface waters, and shellfish are a major source of infection. They cause watery diarrhoea, which tends to be milder than the disease caused by O1 strains, and also extraintestinal infections such as soft tissue wound infections.

A new pathogenic serotype, *V. cholerae* O139, was identified in India in 1992 and is spreading around the world (Dalsgaard and Larsen, 1995). It is a non-O1 strain, but behaves differently from other non-O1 strains by its ability to cause epidemic cholera-like disease. It has the same register of virulence factors as the O1 strain, and is genetically closely related to the *El Tor* biotype of *V.*

cholerae O1. A 1-g oral dose of ciprofloxacin is effective against *V. cholera* O1 or O139 (Khan *et al.*, 1996).

Vibrio parahaemolyticus

V. parahaemolyticus causes food poisoning from contaminated seafood. Shellfish or fish eaten raw or inadequately cooked are common sources of contamination. Outbreaks are common in Japan, due to the custom of eating raw seafood, but have also occurred in coastal states of the USA (Barker, 1974). Sporadic cases occur more frequently. The organism, which is found worldwide in marine waters, elaborates an enterotoxin which acts on the small intestine. The majority of patients suffer from watery diarrhoea with abdominal cramps, nausea and vomiting, headache, fever and chills, which resolve within 3 days. Less commonly, a dysenteric form of illness may occur reflecting colonic involvement, owing to the liberation of a cytotoxin or mucosal invasion. The diagnosis is established on stool culture. The treatment is symptomatic.

Escherichia coli

There is an ever-changing taxonomic status as increasing numbers of strains of *E. coli* that cause diarrhoea are being described. Serologically, *E. coli* strains are classified by their surface antigenic components:

- the O (somatic or body) antigen of the lipopolysaccharide molecule;
- the H (hauch) antigen (hauch = German for flagella);
- the K (kapsule) antigen of the bacterial capsule.

A more disease-related classification is based on pathogenic mechanisms that cause disease: a categorization of patterns of attachment to host cells; the effects of attachment; the toxins produced; and the invasiveness of the bacteria. This is because most bacterial toxins and adherence factors are virulence factors that are genetically coded by infectious plasmids, bacteriophages and sometimes host chromosomes, properties that can be transferred between individual strains of bacteria.

Disease-producing virotypes of *E. coli* that cause diarrhoea are:

- enterotoxigenic *E. coli* (ETEC);
- enteropathogenic *E. coli* (EPEC);
- enteroinvasive *E. coli* (EIEC);
- enterohaemorrhagic *E. coli* O157:H7 (EHEC);
- enteroaggregative *E. coli* (EAggEC).

Enterotoxigenic *E. coli* and enteropathogenic *E. coli* infect the small intestine to cause watery, non-inflammatory diarrhoea. Infections of the colon and sometimes the distal ileum occur with enteroinvasive *E. coli* and enterohaemorrhagic *E. coli* O157:H7 (EHEC), while enteroaggregative *E. coli* (EAggEC) infections cause inflammatory diarrhoea by damaging the colonic epithelium.

Enterotoxigenic *E. coli*

Infection occurs by ingestion of contaminated food or water. ETEC are the commonest cause of traveller's diarrhoea and are associated primarily with diarrhoea in young children in the developing world. The major symptom is profuse watery diarrhoea due to a heat-labile cholera-like toxin. Damage to the intestinal mucosa does not occur, as mucosal invasion is not a feature. The disease is usually self-limiting, although treatment with antibiotics, such as sulphamethoxazole–trimethoprim or a quinolone, such as norfloxacin, significantly shortens the duration of illness.

Enteropathogenic *E. coli*

Diarrhoea occurs due to cell damage by the organism first adhering to the microvilli of the epithelial cell using a plasmid-encoded adherence factor and then liberating a cytotoxin. This causes the effacement of the brush border in the jejunum and ileum, decreased disaccharidase enzymes and loss of large areas of absorptive surface, resulting in a characteristically watery diarrhoea.

Enteroaggregative *E. coli*

The category 'enteroaggregative' was suggested to replace a previously confusing description–'enteroadhesive'. EAggEC are a prime cause of persistent diarrhoea in children, particularly in the developing world (Levine, 1987). EAggEC damage the epithelial cell through adherence. They are a less common cause of traveller's diarrhoea. The mechanism of damage to the colonic epithelium is not yet determined, but the bacteria do produce toxins (Hart *et al.*, 1993). Although adherence is specifically to colonic epithelium in adults, in children these strains adhere to jejunal mucosa, with only limited adhesion to ileum and colon (Hicks *et al.*, 1996). This may be due to a change in the distribution of mucosal sites of adhesion as the gut matures, and could explain the predominance of diarrhoea caused by EAggEC in children. The increased ability to adhere to human intestinal epithelium is an important factor in the virulence of pathogenic *E. coli* (Paton *et al.*, 1998).

Enteroinvasive *E. coli*

This invasive pathogen multiplies within the epithelial cells of the distal ileum and the colon, resulting in necrosis and stripping of large areas of epithelium. EIEC closely resemble *Shigella* and contain a plasmid that codes for several membrane proteins that are required for invasiveness (Levine, 1987). The major site of infection is the colon. Although an infrequent cause of diarrhoea, EIEC are implicated in food-borne infectious diarrhoea and traveller's diarrhoea. The clinical picture is of inflammatory diarrhoea with blood and mucus, abdominal pain, tenesmus and systemic symptoms of fever and myalgia, indistinguishable clinically from *Salmonella* or *Campylobacter* or *Shigella*. Treatment is with sulphamethoxazole–trimethoprim or norfloxacin.

Enterohaemorrhagic *E. coli* 0157:H7

The major site of infection is the terminal ileum and the colon. The natural reservoir is the gastrointestinal tract of animals, and infection is from contaminated animal products. Inadequately cooked ground beef in fast foods, such as hamburgers, meat pies and tacos, is the commonest source of infection (Doyle, 1991). Serious infections and several outbreaks have occurred in the USA from undercooked minced beef foods (Pavia *et al.*, 1990). The bacterium can also be spread from person to person (Wall *et al.*, 1996). The most vulnerable are the elderly and the very young. An outbreak in a nursing home in Canada highlighted the high mortality associated with this entity (Carter *et al.*, 1987).

E. coli O157:H7 is the recently identified predominant serotype of enterohaemorrhagic *E. coli* and is responsible for severe haemorrhagic colitis due to two toxins, Verotoxin I and Verotoxin II. These are almost identical in structure to shigatoxin, and are therefore often referred to as Shiga-like toxins. The organism attaches and effaces the mucosa of the terminal ileum and colonic mucosa (Cohen and Giannella, 1992), damaging the vascular endothelial cells, and also other body organs, especially the renal glomeruli and blood vessels of the nervous system.

The disease spectrum caused by *E. coli* O157:H7 is thus very wide (Griffin *et al.*, 1988). The initial symptoms are those of watery diarrhoea and abdominal pain. Subsequently, owing to colonic involvement, bloody diarrhoea and abdominal cramps may follow. Fever is not a part of the illness. The organism may also cause an asymptomatic infection or a mild non-bloody diarrhoea. The haemolytic uraemic syndrome and thrombotic thrombocytopenic purpura are major life-threatening complications (Obrig *et al.*, 1988; Louise and Obrig, 1992). At present, there is no evidence that antibiotic therapy shortens the course of illness or prevents development of complications.

Recent Australian cases of haemolytic uraemic syndrome were caused by strains of *E. coli* that are associated with Shiga-like toxins. Although the contaminated sausages, which were the source of the infection, contained multiple, Shiga-like, toxin-producing strains of *E. coli*, only strains with a high adherence to human intestinal epithelium, all of *E. coli* O111:H7 serotype, were found in the stools of affected patients (Paton *et al.*, 1997). This demonstrates well the link between adherence and virulence (Paton *et al.*, 1998). Adherence was inhibited almost completely by antibodies to lipopolysaccharide, which suggests a future basis for an early treatment for infection by interfering with the colonization process using suitable antibodies to block adherence (Paton *et al.*, 1998).

Shigella

The *Shigella* organism is highly contagious and an inoculum may be as small as 200 organisms (DuPont *et al.*, 1972). Thus person to person spread of the infection is more common with shigellosis than other bacterial causes of diarrhoea. Infection also occurs from contaminated food and water. Shigella dysentery occurred in 3000 women at a music festival in Michigan in 1988 due to contaminated tofu salad. The risk of *Shigella* infection continues to be a problem in areas that do not have optimal sewage and potable water facilities and in environments where it is difficult to impose adequate standards of personal hygiene, as in institutions for the mentally retarded (DuPont *et al.*, 1970).

The four serogroups are *S. sonnei*, common in the developing world, *S. dysenteriae 1*, *S. flexneri* and *S. boydii*. The most virulent of the organisms, *S. dysenteriae 1*, is also associated with a protein-losing enteropathy. All strains of *Shigella* cause dysentery, and dysentery due to *Shigella* is termed shigellosis and is the preferred term to 'bacillary dysentery'.

Diarrhoea occurs when the organisms attach themselves initially to the small intestinal mucosa, where they multiply and liberate an enterotoxin. Vomiting may occur during this phase. The onset of the illness is abrupt and the dominant symptoms are watery, non-bloody diarrhoea and fever. The infection may be confined to the small intestine and, if so, the symptoms resolve in less than a week.

The mechanism of action of the enterotoxin (which causes fluid and electrolyte loss) is not due to activation of adenylate cyclase, as in secretory diarrhoea, but by inhibition of protein biosythesis via inactivation of ribosomes (Gemmell, 1984; Keusch *et al.*, 1985). This appears to inhibit the maintenance of cell integrity, leading to cell death and destructive lesions of the epithelium.

At a later stage in the colon, the organism penetrates the mucosa and liberates a cytotoxin that causes cell death. Mucosal inflammation, ulceration and crypt abscesses, and dysentery characterized by bloody diarrhoea, mucus, tenesmus, urgency and rectal pain occur. Bloody diarrhoea is not invariable and in one series occurred in less than half the patients (Rosenstein, 1964). The motions are small and frequent. Proctoscopy and sigmoidoscopy are unnecessary and are extremely painful, but demonstrate an oedematous, erythematous mucosa with mucus and possibly small ulcers.

In a study in Israel on shigellosis over a 10-year period, 32 of 116 patients were over 70 years old and the most frequent extragastrointestinal symptom was confusion. The protein-losing enteropathy that occurs with *S. dysenteriae 1* has implications in undernourished or malnourished patients. Shiga toxin can also cause the haemolytic uraemic syndrome (Koster *et al.*, 1984), as its action is similar to the verotoxin produced by EHEC. A variety of extraintestinal complications are reported, and include fever and a runny nose and cough. Neurological symptoms can be prominent in children, often preceding the diarrhoeal symptoms. During the acute phase, a rash may appear. Arthritis, usually asymmetrical and involving the large joints can appear 2–3 weeks after the onset. Patients with the HLA-B27 haplotype are predisposed to develop Reiter's syndrome (Calin and Fries, 1976). Autoantibodies to HLA-B27 antigens will cross-react with *Shigella* proteins and cause the circulation of antigen–antibody complexes (Koster *et al.*, 1978). Bacteraemia is not a feature of shigellosis.

The chronic carrier state with *Shigella* is rare. When it does occur, the organisms persist in the colon rather than the gallbladder as with cholera and salmonellosis.

The treatment is with sulphamethoxazole–trimethoprim or a quinolone (e.g. norfloxacin). Antimotility drugs are not recommended as with patients with dysentery. The prevention of spread of the organism is important and personal hygiene, especially adequate handwashing, should be rigorously promoted.

Salmonella infections

Salmonella species are motile, non-spore-forming bacilli and invasive pathogens, which infect humans, animals and insects. Recent taxonomy of the genus *Salmonella* recognizes two primary species: *S. enterica* and *S. bongori*; the vast majority of serotypes fall into the *S. enterica* species, which has over 2000 serotypes. Formally, a serotype would therefore be *S. enterica* serovar Typhi, but for convenience this is called *Salmonella typhi*.

Salmonellosis refers to the entire disease spectrum due to infection with *Salmonella*. Non-typhoidal salmonellosis is an illness due to any serotype belonging to the genus of *Salmonella* except *S. typhi*. The organisms are frequent in polluted water and sewage.

In common with other Gram-negative bacteria, *Salmonella* species possess an endotoxin that is released on the death of the bacteria. In the gastrointestinal tract the common site of infection is the ileum and less commonly the colon. *Salmonella* invade the intestinal mucosa through the M-cells of the Peyer's patches and lymphoid aggregates. In severe cases, systemic infection can occur via the lymphatic system (Gaines *et al.*, 1968).

The risk factors to acquiring salmonella infections are as follows.

- A decrease in gastric acidity associated with ageing (*see* Chapter 5).
- The ingestion of the organism with agents that reduce gastric acidity, such as milk and milk products, or therapeutic agents, such as antacids, H-2 antagonists or proton pump inhibitors.
- Concurrent treatment with antibiotics. Patients on antibiotics to which *Salmonella* are resistant are more susceptible to infection due to suppression of the protective normal bacterial flora of the colon.
- Malignancy.
- States of decreased immunity.
- Sickle cell anaemia.

There are four major disease entities that may overlap. These are described below. Each is due predominantly to a particular serotype of *Salmonella*.

SALMONELLA GASTROENTERITIS

Gastroenteritis is an acute infection of the gastrointestinal tract characterized by the clinical syndrome of diarrhoea and/or vomiting. The small intestine is the principal organ affected, although the stomach and the colon may be involved (Barnes and Townley, 1973). In *Salmonella* gastroenteritis, the most frequent causative organisms include *S. typhimurium*, *S. enteritidis* and *S. newport*.

In most instances, human *Salmonella* gastroenteritis is due to contaminated food. Poultry constitute the largest reservoir of *Salmonella* (Hobbs, 1961). *S. enteritidis* infects the ovaries of hens, although they appear to be healthy and contamination of the egg occurs before the shell is formed. *S. enteritidis* is present in albumin and predominantly in the yolk where they multiply (Humphrey *et al.*, 1991). Food preparations with raw eggs are therefore especially dangerous (Mishu *et al.*, 1991). Eggs (unpasteurized) that are not refrigerated, not thoroughly cooked, and not promptly eaten carry the risk of infection. Chickens are readily infected and transmission to humans has occurred from baby chickens sold as pets at Easter (Anderson *et al.*, 1955). Pet turtles have also been incriminated as *Salmonella* carriers. Person to person spread, although rare, may occur. Contamination of young children occurs by faeco–oral spread (Kaufmann *et al.*, 1967). Although isolated cases occur, *Salmonella* gastroenteritis is often epidemic, with a history of a single source outbreak.

The incubation period is about 24 hours, with a range of 6–48 hours. The illness lasts from 1 to 5 days. The onset is sudden, with nausea, vomiting and diarrhoea and severe colicky abdominal pain. Other symptoms include fever with chills and headache. The infection may spread to the colon, presenting as dysentery.

Salmonella gastroenteritis is a self-limited disease. Despite the organism penetrating the enterocytes and lodging in the lamina propria, the defence mechanisms of the small intestine (*see* Chapters 4 and 5) contain the spread of infection. Pyrexia that persists should raise the possibility of a complication outside the gastrointestinal tract. In children, pneumonitis and rarely meningitis may occur (Berkowitz, 1984). The well-established complication of *Salmonella* osteomyelitis in patients with sickle cell disease may be due to due to a deficiency in the alternative pathway of complement activation (Hook *et al.*, 1957; Hand and King, 1977). Recent intestinal tract surgery predisposes to acquiring salmonella (Sanders *et al.*, 1963).

The diagnosis is established by identifying the organism on stool culture or occasionally in the vomitus. Blood culture is unrewarding.

Since the illness is usually a self-limiting entity, antibiotic therapy does not alter the course of the disease (Aserkoff and Bennett, 1969). Treatment with antibiotics may result in patients becoming carriers and the emergence of antibiotic-resistant organisms. Indeed, early studies demonstrated that *Salmonella* may persist within cells despite adequate concentrations of antibiotics to which the organisms were sensitive (Smadel, 1963).

Antibiotic therapy is warranted in patients at risk of complications, such as the very young, the elderly and immunocompromised patients, in whom bacteraemia is a serious complication. Antibiotics, such as ciprofloxacin, amoxycillin or sulphamethoxazole–trimethoprim, for susceptible organisms are also recommended in these patients.

ENTERIC FEVER

Enteric fever is an older term, which includes typhoid fever due to infection with *S. typhi* and paratyphoid fever due to *S. paratyphi A*, and also much less commonly *S. schottmuelleri* (formerly *S. paratyphoid* B) or *S. hirschfeldii* (formerly *S. paratyphi* C).

Typhoid fever is due to *Salmonella typhi* and is an acute, severe, systemic illness characterized by fever and bacteraemia, abdominal pain and tenderness, hepatosplenomegaly and rose spots (salmon-coloured, erythematous maculopapular lesions), a characteristic rash that occurs during the first or second week of infection. The incubation period depends on the size of the infective inoculum and is usually from 10 to 20 days (Cvjetanovic *et al.*, 1971). Typhoid fever is more notable as a severe systemic illness rather than one with significant gastrointestinal manifestations.

Salmonella (uniquely) penetrate the epithelial cells of the small intestine, particularly the distal ileum, without destruction to reach and damage the lamina propria (Takeuchi, 1967). Bacteria are taken up by the Peyer's patches, spread to the mesenteric glands and from this site reach the general circulation (Gaines *et al.*, 1968). The organism proliferates within mononuclear phagocytic cells in the liver, spleen and lymph nodes, and again enters the blood stream to give rise to a second, more intense wave of bacteraemia. The patient is febrile, the pulse rate is slow in comparison to the fever (relative bradycardia) during the first week of the illness and increases in a characteristic stepwise pattern (Fig. 18.1). Right lower quadrant pain or more diffuse abdominal pain may occur.

Initially, constipation is followed by diarrhoea, described as 'pea soup' in consistency in about half the patients. The diarrhoeal component of the illness has been underestimated and recent reports from many countries emphasize the extent of the problem. The severity of diarrhoea in individual patients is reported to range from 3 to 30 stools per day.

During the second or third week in untreated cases, perforation of the ileum may occur (Bohrer, 1966). Enterocolitis is a feature of variable severity. Toxic megacolon is a potential complication (Gonzalez *et al.*, 1985). Other complications are severe haemorrhage and

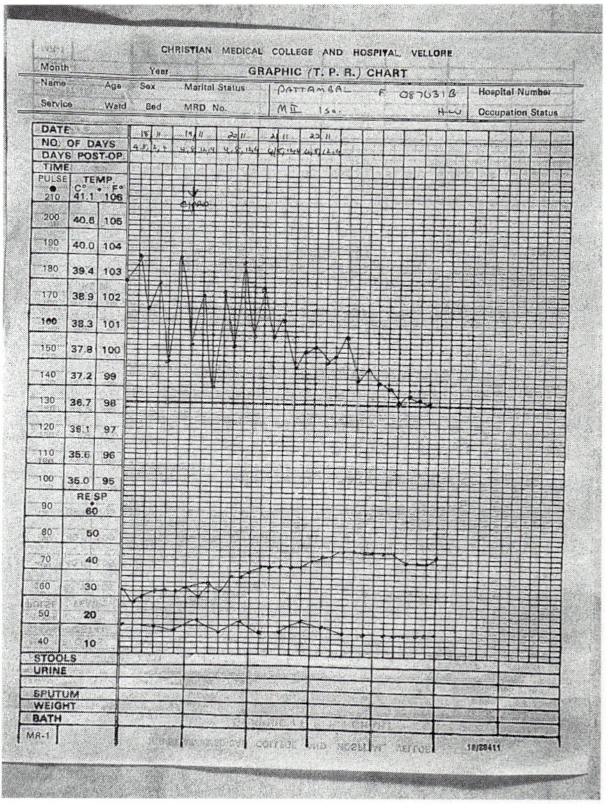

Figure 18.1 *Temperature chart in typhoid fever, which shows a characteristic 'stepwise' pattern and demonstrates (middle line) relative bradycardia. (Courtesy of Professor B.V. Moses, Christian Medical College and Hospital, Vellore, India.)*

bowel perforation. The abdomen feels 'doughy' and loops of small intestine may be easily palpable. Other features are rebound tenderness due to peritonitis, splenomegaly during the second week, and, in a minority, hepatomegaly.

The diagnosis of typhoid fever is made by isolation of *S. typhi* in blood cultures, which are positive in over 90 per cent of cases. The sigmoidoscopic appearances in severe cases are hyperaemia, contact bleeding, granularity, friability and ulceration of the colonic mucosa, indistinguishable from ulcerative colitis (Dertinger *et al.*, 1991).

In typhoid fever, treatment with ciprofloxacin, chloramphenicol, ampicillin or sulphamethoxazole–trimethoprim is effective in sensitive organisms. Early treatment with systemic antimicrobials, such as ampicillin 50–100 mg/kg per day in divided doses for 10–14 days, or co-trimoxazole, effectively reduces the morbidity and mortality. Ciprofloxacin is now the treatment of choice, particularly in areas of multidrug resistance, although quinolone resistance is also being reported. Ceftriaxone, 2–3 g daily for 5–10 days, is an alternative.

In a study from Ghana, Mock *et al.* (1992) reported that, if the ileum is perforated, mortality is reduced by a factor of three by double-layer closure of the perforation and treatment with chloramphenicol, metronidazole and gentamicin.

Vaccines

Both live attenuated, killed and subunit vaccines are available against *S. typhi*. The efficacy is about 70 per cent and vaccination is recommended before travel to areas where the disease is endemic. Vaccination does not guarantee immunity from typhoid illness if the inoculum of the organism is large and the patient is from a high-risk group.

EXTRAINTESTINAL INFECTIONS

In the past, most extraintestinal *Salmonella* infections were caused by *S. choleraesuis* and *S. dublin*; however, *S. typhimurium* was the predominant serotype in a recent study (Cohen *et al.*, 1987). Local areas of infection tend to occur in areas of ischaemia and necrosis, possibly due to poor microcirculation, which permits the growth of the organism (Hook *et al.*, 1957).

Extraintestinal complications may also result from the rare occurrence of bacteraemia as a complication of non-typhoidal food-borne illness. Local infections are usually in the form of abscesses and occur in a variety of organs and sites (Cohen *et al.*, 1987):

- cardiac prostheses;
- vascular grafts;
- damaged cardiovascular endothelial surfaces;
- infrarenal atherosclerotic aortic aneurysms;
- mural thrombi;
- necrotic tumours;
- haematomas;
- skeletal prostheses;
- axial and peripheral joints;
- long bones – joints commonly involved in suppurative arthritis are the knee, shoulder, hip and sacroiliac joints; aseptic polyarthritis also occurs;
- central nervous system – encephalitis with a severe confusional state (Ramachandran *et al.*, 1975), a neuropsychiatric syndrome, and lesions in the basal ganglia and pyramidal tract signs have been reported (Osuntoken *et al.*, 1972).

Extraintestinal complications, especially in the elderly, may require extensive investigations to establish the extent of infection before treatment. The therapy may involve surgical intervention together with intravenous ampicillin or ciprofloxacin.

ASYMPTOMATIC *SALMONELLA* CARRIER STATE

About 3 per cent of adults infected with *S. typhi* continue to harbour the organism for a year or more, and become chronic asymptomatic carriers. The source of infection is the gallbladder or intestine. The carrier state is more common among the elderly, especially females, and those with biliary tract abnormalities or cholelithiasis. Urinary tract carriage of the organism occurs with an obstructive uropathy. In patients with schistosomiasis, *Salmonella* can penetrate and multiply within the parasite (Rocha *et al.*, 1971).

Some carriers spontaneously remit the carrier state. In contrast to the carriers of *Shigella* (an unusual occurrence), carriers of *Salmonella* may infect themselves with the strain they carry. Chronic asymptomatic carriers should be monitored for 1 year and, if excretion of the organism persists, be treated with ciprofloxacin or amoxycillin for 4–6 weeks. If this therapy fails, a cholecystectomy under antibiotic cover, and ampicillin or amoxycillin for 2 weeks, resolves the problem in 90 per cent or more cases (Tynes and Utz, 1962).

Yersinia enterocolitica

Yersinia enterocolitica is a common diarrhoeal pathogen that infects the colon but small intestinal involvement also occurs. In an Australian study on adult diarrhoea in the community, *Y. enterocolitica* was the third commonest bacterial pathogen identified after *C. jejuni* and non-typhoidal *Salmonella* (Feeney *et al.*, 1987).

Infected food, particularly pork, is the commonest source of infection, although the organism may be present in natural water sources. Unlike other pathogens, the organism can grow at 4°C, the temperature of a refrigerator. As with *Campylobacter jejuni*, *Y. enterocolitica* has been isolated from domestic pets and farm animals. Epidemics have been reported after the ingestion of contaminated chocolate milk (Black *et al.*, 1978), contaminated pasteurized milk, and dairy produce, meat, shellfish and tofu (a soya bean preparation).

At the onset of the illness, a profuse watery diarrhoea may occur due to the action of the enterotoxin on the small intestine. Terminal ileal involvement mimics Crohn's disease. In some patients with dysentery, right lower quadrant pain may mimic appendicitis. In the elderly, septicaemia is an uncommon but serious complication, and may also occur after blood transfusion (Bottone, 1997). Extraintestinal multisystem infection can occur in patients with predisposing factors, such as immunosuppression, iron overload or treatment with desferrioxamine, and recurrences are reported in a proportion of patients. Metastatic foci following extraintestinal infection are common and often involve the liver and spleen (Bottone, 1997). A rash and arthralgia occur in individuals with the HLA-B27 haplotype. A 10-year study from Norway (Saebo and Lassen, 1992) highlights the chronicity of colitis, and a higher prevalence of ulcerative colitis.

Infection with *Y. enterocolitica* is self-limiting in healthy persons. In the elderly person at risk or if complications of extraintestinal infection occur, the drugs of choice are either gentamicin or ciprofloxacin. Chloramphenicol, sulphamethoxazole–trimethoprim and doxycycline are alternatives.

Campylobacter jejuni

This organism predominantly infects the colon, but the small intestine is infected at the onset. The incidence of infections due to this pathogen is increasing. Fifty to 70 per cent of infections with *C. jejuni* are associated with undercooked and cross-contaminated poultry (Skirrow, 1991). Important non-poultry sources of infection are raw milk and milk products, raw meat and meat products, and unchlorinated water (Skirrow, 1991). Other sources of infection are pets such as dogs and cats with diarrhoea that transmit *Campylobacter* (Moreno *et al.*, 1993). A study from Washington State found 63 per cent of 218 cases of *Campylobacter* were attributable to exposure to domestic animals (Altekruse *et al.*, 1994). In a study from Norway, the risk factors for *Campylobacter* were eating sausages at a barbecue (OR = 7.64; $P = 0.005$), daily contact with a dog (OR = 4.26; $P = 0.024$) and eating poultry 'brought into the house raw' (frozen or refrigerated, OR = 2.42; $P = 0.042$).

Campylobacter jejuni produces a heat-labile enterotoxin that is blocked by cholera antitoxin (Ruiz-Palacios *et al.*, 1983). In the majority of healthy persons, diarrhoea is invariably self-limiting and settles within 7 days. The disease spectrum ranges from mild watery diarrhoea and cramping abdominal pain due to small intestinal involvement, to fulminating colitis associated with fatalities. The colonic lesions are similar to Crohn's colitis and ulcerative colitis. Toxic megacolon is a potential complication (Vyas *et al.*, 1993; Larvol *et al.*, 1994). In patients with the HLA-B27 haplotype, reactive arthritis or Reiter's syndrome may occur (Peterson, 1994). Other extraintestinal manifestations include carditis (Ponka *et al.*, 1984), pneumonia (Ponka and Kosunen, 1982), infections of the urinary tract (Smith and Blaser, 1985) and the Guillain–Barré syndrome (Ropper, 1988; Mishu and Blaser, 1993).

Treatment is warranted if the diarrhoea is prolonged, if blood is present in the stools and in patients with pyrexia, severe concomitant illnesses, and those who are debilitated. The drug of choice at present is erythromycin. Ciprofloxacin is an alternative, but resistance is widespread.

A study from Norway by Kapperud (1994) suggests that the preventive measures with the greatest impact against infection with *Campylobacter* are a potable water supply, good hygienic practices when in contact with dogs and cats, a high standard of kitchen hygiene while dealing with poultry, and adequate preparation of meat (sausages) during barbecues.

Aeromonas species

Aeromonas-associated diarrhoea most often occurs in children under 5 years old (Agger *et al.*, 1985; Ashdown and Koehler, 1993), and clinical features include fever, nausea, vomiting, abdominal cramps and watery diarrhoea, sometimes containing blood (Agger *et al.*, 1985; Challapalli *et al.*, 1988). Diarrhoea can last for up to 10 days. *Aeromonas* species are increasingly being detected in cases of diarrhoea as the sole organism isolated, and are also often present with other enteropathogens in diarrhoeal stools. Between 1978–79 and 1986–87, the isolation rate of *Aeromonas* species from diarrhoeal patients increased from 0.2 per cent to 5.0 per cent in one study from India (Jesudason and Koshi, 1990), while in another increases occurred from 0.2 per cent in 1986 to 6.0 per cent in 1990 (Verenkar *et al.*, 1995). *Aeromonas* was also the fourth most common isolate in Japanese travellers with diarrhoea returning from developing countries, with *A. veronii* biovar *sobria* most frequently isolated, followed by *A. hydrophila* and *A. caviae* (Yamada *et al.*, 1997).

The organism is water borne and can be transmitted by food. It has a world-wide distribution, with cases reported from the USA, Mexico, Finland, Morocco, Nigeria, India, Thailand and tropical Australia. Enterotoxin is produced by most *Aeromonas* strains, and more than half of the diarrhoeal isolates secrete a cytotoxin that is a haemolysin (Agger *et al.*, 1985; Ljungh and Waldstrom, 1985).

The infection responds well to gentamicin, sulphamethoxazole–trimethoprim, fluoroquinolones and chloramphenicol, but is resistant to ampicillin (Obi *et al.*, 1995).

Plesiomonas shigelloides

Clinical features of *Plesiomonas*-associated diarrhoea include fever, vomiting, abdominal pain and watery diarrhoea, sometimes containing blood (Obi *et al.*, 1995). *P. shigelloides* is a water-borne organism with a world-wide distribution (Obi *et al.*, 1995), but cases occur at higher frequency in diarrhoeal stools of travellers from the tropics (Kain and Kelly, 1989). It was the third most common isolate in Japanese travellers with diarrhoea returning from developing countries (Yamada *et al.*, 1997). Non-travellers with episodes of diarrhoea-associated infection have a history of recently consuming seafood and/or drinking untreated water (Kain and Kelly, 1989). Although often present with other enteropathogens, the organism is often the sole isolate from diarrhoeal stools. It is not reported to be enteroinvasive but some isolates can show cytotoxic activity (Olsvik *et al.*, 1990).

Antimicrobial therapy significantly reduces the duration of the illness (Kain and Kelly, 1989). *P. shigelloides* is usually susceptible to quinolones, cephalosporins and sulphamethoxazole–trimethoprim, according to a recent Thai study; however, no significant decrease in the duration of fever and diarrhoea after treatment was found (Visitsunthorn and Komolpis, 1995). Resistance is often found to ampicillin, gentamicin, erythromycin, kanamycin and streptomycin (Olsvik *et al.*, 1990).

Food-borne illness and food poisoning

The term 'food-borne illness', through frequent usage, includes the term 'food poisoning'. True food-borne illness requires the presence of the pathogen for the symptoms to occur. A food-borne illness outbreak is considered to have occurred if the following criteria are met:

- two or more people experience the same symptoms, usually referrable to the gastrointestinal tract, after the consumption of the same dietary item;
- the dietary item is implicated as the common source by epidemiological investigation.

Food poisoning implies the presence of a toxin in food, which may be preformed by a pathogen, or due to contamination with toxic chemicals. It is usually characterized by gastrointestinal symptoms, although neurological symptoms occur in some instances. Food poisoning is diagnosed when nausea, vomiting and diarrhoea occur after 2–3 persons have consumed the same food or beverage contaminated by a preformed toxin elaborated by a pathogen. The incubation period is short and the onset of symptoms is abrupt. The bacteria commonly implicated in food poisoning are those which produce a preformed toxin in food:

- *Staphylococcus aureus*;
- *Bacillus cereus* (one of the spore coat proteins is an emetic toxin);
- *Clostridium perfringens* (this also produces another toxin *in situ*);
- *Clostridium botulinum*.

Staphylococcus aureus

Illness due to *Staphylococcus aureus* is mediated by one or more toxins (Marrack and Kappler, 1990). Several enterotoxins have been identified, many with the ability to cause fever, hypotension and shock, and with implications in multiorgan failure. Some of these exert their action through stimulation of T-lymphocyte populations, and are called bacterial superantigens. They have a high affinity for histocompatibility antigens on monocytes, macrophages and mast cells, activating the immune system activation and releasing cytokines, which are pathogenic at high concentrations, causing fever and osmotic imbalances (Schlievert, 1993). Some *S. aureus* toxins have a direct effect upon biological membranes, causing disruption, and increasing permeability to cations (Rogolsky, 1979).

The immediate occurrence of nausea and vomiting is due to a neurotoxic effect of enterotoxin B, which is a heat-stable toxin, produced by about half of the strains of *S. aureus*. The source is invariably contaminated food that has been inadequately cooked or refrigerated. A food handler with a pustule or paronychia, is often the source of contamination. Foods most commonly incriminated have a high content of protein, sugar and salt (custards, salads with mayonnaise, cottage cheese and canned meat).

Profuse nausea, vomiting and diarrhoea 1–6 hours after a meal suggests ingestion of this preformed toxin elaborated by *S. aureus*. Vomiting is severe and is the major symptom, associated with diarrhoea, which is watery and profuse. Neurological symptoms such as numbness, tingling and vertigo may occur infrequently. The symptoms resolve within 24–48 hours. Since the illness is due to the toxin which is already elaborated in the food, antibiotics are irrelevant in the management. Treatment should be directed to prevent dehydration.

Bacillus cereus

Bacillus cereus is a Gram-positive, spore-forming organism that produces two symptom complexes: a severe emetic illness (or vomiting syndrome) and a diarrhoeal syndrome. These two entities are due to separate toxins (Melling *et al.*, 1976). The vomiting syndrome is due to a heat-stable emetic toxin (Granum and Lund, 1997), is of rapid onset, usually with a 2-hour incubation period, lasts for about 8–10 hours and is usually self-limiting. It is often associated with eating inadequately reheated fried rice (Terranova and Blake, 1978). The temperature reached during 'flash frying' to reheat cold rice is insufficient to destroy the heat-stable toxin. *B. cereus* is present in soil and contaminates uncooked rice. The process of cooking rice does not destroy the spores of the organism and, when cooked rice is left to cool at room temperature, the spores germinate and produce toxin as more spores are formed. It is therefore important that cooked rice is refrigerated as soon as possible.

In the second symptom complex, diarrhoea dominates the clinical picture with, in a small number of patients, abdominal cramps and vomiting. The diarrhoea is secretory in nature as the organism produces a secretagogue, which, like cholera toxin, activates adenylate cyclase in the small intestine enterocytes (Turnbull, 1976; Beecher *et al.*, 1995). The incubation time after ingestion of the contaminated food is between 6 and 14 hours (with an average of 9 hours), and the symptoms last for between 20 and 36 hours. The food sources implicated include cream, sauces, puddings and even spices (Gilbert and Parry, 1977). Since the illness is self-limiting, drug therapy is not warranted.

Clostridium perfringens

C. perfringens is widely distributed and contaminates particularly meat, poultry and gravies, and is responsible for numerous outbreaks of food poisoning. The infection occurs after ingestion of inadequately reheated cooked meat. Most human infections arise from *C. perfringens* type A. Although many toxins are formed, the gastrointestinal symptoms are due to an enterotoxin that is an integral part of the spore structure produced by the organism during sporulation (Frieben and Duncan, 1973). The toxin may be preformed in food or elaborated in the small intestine (McDonel, 1980). The toxin causes a secretory type of diarrhoea (Duncan and Strong, 1971) but, unlike cholera toxin, acts predominantly on the ileum, causing protein loss and mucosal damage (McDonel and Duncan, 1977).

The vehicle of infection is usually a meat or poultry dish that was cooked, allowed to cool at room temperature (enabling the organism to multiply in the anaerobic conditions present and form more spores), and served a day or two later. The incubation period is 6–24 hours and the duration of illness about 1 day. Prominent symptoms are cramping abdominal pain and diarrhoea. Vomiting is infrequent. Constitutional symptoms are absent.

Antibiotic-associated diarrhoea, although rare, can occur with *C. perfringens* (Samuel *et al.*, 1991; Borriello *et al.*, 1984) and an outbreak has been reported in a geriatric unit (Williams *et al.*, 1985). An enterocolitis similar to that due to *C. difficile* is reported, although pseudomembrane formation is not a feature (Bartlett, 1994). The treatment is with metronidazole.

C. perfringens type C is the cause of necrotizing enterocolitis called 'pig-bel' in Papua New Guinea. This condition arises from eating undercooked pork and sweet potato at the same meal (Murrell *et al.*, 1966). The toxin is heat labile, so infections rely upon incomplete cooking of meat, which is common during roasting of whole pigs at village feasts (Sakurai and Duncan, 1978). The toxin would usually be degraded by the proteolytic enzymes present in normal people. Those susceptible are deficient in digestive proteases because of a traditional low-protein diet, which is worsened by the presence of a protease inhibitor in sweet potato. Inadequately roasted pork can harbour *C. perfringens*, which causes severe toxaemia and haemorrhagic necrosis of bowel due to the action of the beta toxin released by *C. perfringens* type C. Necrotizing enterocolitis may go undiagnosed when it occurs in unexpected circumstances and cases have been reported in developed countries (Watson *et al.*, 1991).

The lesion is in the jejunum and is characterized by a patchy gangrenous enteritis. The symptoms are anorexia, vomiting, severe abdominal pain and bloody diarrhoea, associated with a high mortality. A major preventive measure has been the development of the Wellcome Pig-bel toxoid vaccine (Lawrence *et al.*, 1979). Hospital admissions for pig-bel in Papua New Guinea highland hospitals have dropped to less than 20 per cent of the preimmunization figures (Lawrence *et al.*, 1990).

Clostridium botulinum

Food-borne botulism due to *C. botulinum* is often associated with home-canning kits used to preserve vegetables and fruit, and sometimes meat and fish. If the food is contaminated with spores of *C. botulinum*, or the temperature used to prepare the food is inadequate, spores can germinate. The organism proliferates, particularly in conditions of low acidity, and produces toxin, which is a strong neurotoxin. Food must be heated to 100°C for at least 10 minutes to destroy the toxin, and 120°C to inactivate the spores.

Although *C. botulinum* infection involves a preformed toxin, in infants it is known to cause botulism by producing toxin *in vivo* in the infant gut. Honey is the single most frequently involved source of infecting bacteria in these infant cases (Arnon *et al.*, 1979). This infant variant of food-borne botulism is currently the most frequently reported form (Cherington, 1998).

The incubation period is usually about 18–36 hours, with a range from a few hours to several days, depending upon the amount of preformed toxin ingested. The illness is characterized by a symmetrical descending weakness or paralysis, which can lead to respiratory failure and death. Paralysis can present asymmetrically and may be preceded or followed by nausea, vomiting and abdominal pain. Fever is *not* a feature. Other symptoms include functional impairment of the cranial nerves, starting with blurring of vision and double vision, dizziness, slurring of speech, difficulty in swallowing and a dry mouth and throat. Paralysis may impair the gag reflex and deep tendon reflexes may be normal or decreased. Constipation due to gastric paralysis and/or intestinal pseudo-obstruction is common, along with urinary retention.

The diagnosis is established by identifying the organism in samples of vomitus, gastric contents or stools, or by detecting the toxin in stool or blood samples. Patients should be hospitalized and mechanically ventilated if respiratory capacity falls below 30 per cent of that expected. Equine antitoxin should be given as soon as specimens are taken for analysis, and therapy should commence without laboratory confirmation of the diagnosis, owing to the time required to confirm the infection and the urgency of the condition. If only a few hours have elapsed since ingestion of the contaminated meal, gastric lavage can be performed. Cathartics and enemas can be used if paralytic ileus is not a feature.

Traveller's diarrhoea

Euphemisms for traveller's diarrhoea abound: 'Aztec two-step', 'Delhi belly', 'Ho Chi Minh's', 'Hong Kong Dog', 'Montezuma's revenge', 'Rangoon runs', 'Seeping slickness', 'Tourist trots' and 'Turkey trots'. Diarrhoea due to *Giardia lamblia* infection acquired in Russia is called 'the Trotskys' (Gorbach, 1998).

The risk of acquiring traveller's diarrhoea depends on the destination of travel. Geographical areas are designated according to the potential risk they pose to visitors (Kendrick, 1972; Lowenstein *et al.*, 1973; Ryder *et al.*, 1977):

- high risk – Africa, Latin America, Asia;
- moderate risk – Southern Europe, Middle East, some Caribbean islands, China;
- low risk – Northern Europe, North America, Australia and New Zealand, Japan, some Caribbean Islands.

On the information available, the chance of a traveller from a developed country acquiring diarrhoea during travel to a high-risk area is 20–50 per cent, although the standard of hygiene may differ markedly in a particular geographical region or a single country. Food is the major vehicle through which infection occurs (Tjoa *et al.*, 1977; Ericsson *et al.*, 1980).

A recent study from Pakistan showed that flies and water were reservoirs of pathogenic *Campylobacter*, enterotoxigenic *E. coli*, *Shigella* and *Salmonella* (Khalil *et al.*, 1994). Verocytotoxin-secreting *E. coli* (VTEC) can be spread from person to person, or via food and water, and cattle are a natural reservoir (Wall *et al.*, 1996).

The aetiology of diarrhoea is known in only 80 per cent of patients despite intense study. The evidence points to bacteria, protozoa and helminths as the major cause of traveller's diarrhoea.

The common causative bacteria are:

- enterotoxigenic *E. coli* (ETEC)
- enteroadherent *E. coli* (EAEC)
- enteroinvasive *E. coli* (EIEC)
- *Salmonella* species
- *Shigella* species
- *Campylobacter jejuni*
- *Vibrio parahaemolyticus*
- *Plesiomonas shigelloides*
- *Aeromonas hydrophila.*

The parasites that cause traveller's diarrhoea are *Giardia lamblia*, *Entamoeba histolytica*, *Cryptosporidium* and *Strongyloides stercoralis*. Rotavirus is the most frequent viral agent.

Enterotoxigenic *E. coli* is one of the most common aetiological agents. The symptoms of diarrhoea vary with the pathogen. Diarrhoea of a secretory nature with watery motions with no evidence of blood in the stools occurs with ETEC, EAEC, *Cryptosporidium* and Rotavirus. Dysentery is a feature of infectious *Shigella* spp., especially *S. dysenteriae* type 1 and EIEC. *Aeromonas hydrophila* and the protozoan parasite *Cryptosporidium* are identified increasingly as aetiological agents in traveller's diarrhoea. As more sophisticated laboratory techniques for the identification of enteric pathogens are developed, 'newer' pathogens can be identified.

The causative organism varies with the geographical area. *Giardia* and *Cryptosporidium* are frequent causes of diarrhoea in tourists who visit St Petersburg (Leningrad), Russia. *Salmonella* spp. are commonly acquired during travel in the Indian subcontinent and South Asia. In Thailand and Bangladesh, *Campylobacter jejuni* is a more common cause of traveller's diarrhoea than in Mexico, where *E. coli* (ETEC) is frequently isolated.

A recent very large study from Japan of over 29 000 travellers returning to Osaka and Kansai Airport Quarantine Station with diarrhoea reported that, in 9766 cases (33 per cent), enteropathogenic bacteria were isolated from stool samples (Ueda *et al.*, 1997). Of these, 33.1 per cent were *Plesiomonas shigelloides*, 22.9 per cent were *Salmonella* species, 20.1 per cent were *Vibrio parahaemolyticus*, ETEC accounted for 16.6 per cent and 12.7 per cent were *Shigella* species, mostly *S. sonnei* and *S. flexneri*. The largest number of travellers were infected in India (53.4 per cent).

Travellers to areas of inadequate hygiene and sanitation should take sensible steps to prevent infection, summed up by the advice: 'if you can't peel it, shell it, boil it or cook it, don't eat it'. Depending on where one travels, these criteria may not be easy to fulfil. In most developing countries, 'safe', 'Western food' is not easy to obtain and, if available, is expensive.

Dietary items to avoid especially are dairy products, raw seafood, unpeeled raw fruit, and fruit and vegetable salads. Foods that may have been cooked and left unrefrigerated should not be eaten. Food from street vendors is associated with a high degree of enteric infections. Western visitors to developing countries often forget that refrigeration is expensive, power supplies capricious and the quantity of water available to practise optimal hygiene is limited. There is no guarantee that tap water is safe water. The most meticulous travellers who drink only bottled water may unwittingly 'slip up': add ice to bottled water or bottled soft drinks; eat a salad; have a milk-based local confectionary, ice cream or fruit salad for dessert. It is safe to drink bottled carbonated beverages, hot tea, coffee, water boiled or treated with chlorine or iodine, and alcohol, such as local beer. The traveller should not be lulled into being less wary of enteric infection by the grand appearance of a hotel building and its liveried staff, or if the establishment belongs to a chain they are familiar with and for which they have a high regard.

The cause of diarrhoea is not always an infection. Non-infective causes include:

- overindulgence of free airline food and alcohol;
- fear of flying and thoughts of the return flight;
- overindulgence of local fruit;
- the stress of living abroad, delays, frustrations, not being in control and problems with travel companions;
- spicy food, e.g. hot curries;
- prophylaxis.

The question of prophylaxis is important, especially in elderly patients. Advice on how to minimize the risk of diarrhoea, and what steps should be taken if diarrhoea occurs and the dangers of dehydration and the prevention of dehydration are important issues. While abroad, the importance of seeking early medical attention, particularly if dysentery or if more than four bowel actions a day or vomiting occur, must be emphasized. Oral rehydration salts packets can be carried and reconstituted when required.

Extensive studies have demonstrated the efficacy of bismuth subsalicylate as a prophylactic agent against traveller's diarrhoea. In regard to antibiotics based on cost-effectiveness studies, their prophylactic use is justified. In addition to benefits to health, travel would not be disrupted and additional expense is not incurred nor time wasted. These advantages have to be weighed against the possibility of adverse drug reactions and the emergence of resistant organisms. Suitable antimicrobials for prophylaxis are sulphamethoxazole–trimethoprim, norfloxacin and ciprofloxacin. Doxycycline is no longer recommended, owing to resistant ETEC, *Salmonella* species and *Shigella* species.

The sale of drugs that are ineffective and expensive is widespread in the developing world. Compounds prescribed for diarrhoea, such as iodochlorhydroxyquin (Enterorioform, Elioquinol) and other halogenated hydroxyquinolone derivatives, have dubious therapeutic value but are established causes of myelo-optic neuropathy.

The traveller should be warned against the purchase of over-the-counter medication for diarrhoea and to be extremely cautious of therapy prescribed locally. If diarrhoea occurs, the patient should be advised to increase fluid intake. In addition to carbonated soft drinks, commercially available oral rehydration solutions should be used.

Antimotility drugs, such as loperamide or diphenoxylate, provide effective relief of symptoms. Contraindications are fever, and blood and mucus in the stools, or if the diarrhoea continues for longer than 48 hours. These drugs should not be prescribed to patients with dysentery associated with high fever and evidence of toxaemia due to shigellosis or salmonellosis (DuPont and Hornick, 1973).

Antibiotics are indicated in patients with dysentery or if the diarrhoea persists for longer than 48 hours. The antibiotics which may be used are sulphamethoxazole–trimethoprim, norfloxacin and ciprofloxacin.

In patients who develop chronic diarrhoea after travel abroad, the possibility of a parasitic infection, especially *Giardia lamblia* (since the incubation period is 14–21 days) and *Entamoeba histolytica*, should be vigorously pursued.

CHRONIC DIARRHOEA

Mycobacterium tuberculosis

Although intestinal tuberculosis is still prevalent in many less industrialized countries, it is becoming less frequent due to the availability and increased accessibility of effective chemotherapy to treat pulmonary tuberculosis. Intestinal tuberculosis is invariably the result of swallowed tubercle bacilli infecting the small intestine, the site of predilection in the gastrointestinal tract. Owing to the predominance of lymphatic tissue in the terminal ileum and the ileo-caecal valve, these two sites are most often involved. The caecum is also commonly involved. The lesions are an annular or oval ulcer. In time, small intestinal narrowing, stricture formation, fistulas and bacterial overgrowth may occur. The histologically characteristic finding is a granuloma.

Mycobacterium tuberculosis should be considered as a cause of chronic diarrhoea associated with significant weight loss, fever and night sweats. An important feature is abdominal pain or discomfort, often, although not necessarily, localized to the right lower quadrant. On abdominal palpation there may be a 'doughy' feeling due to oedematous intestines. The complications include bacterial overgrowth and consequent malabsorption as a result of scarring, fibrosis and stricture formation. Disseminated tuberculosis may develop in the untreated patient.

DIAGNOSIS

The diagnosis is based on the suspicion of tuberculosis on radiology confirmed by the presence of acid-fast bacilli in intestinal biopies. The treatment consists of antituberculous therapy as for pulmonary tuberculosis. Combination therapy should include isoniazid, rifampicin, ethambutol and pyrazinamide until drug sensitivities are known. Therapy should be given for a minimum of 6 months.

Other causes

The other infectious causes of chronic diarrhoea are tropical sprue (*see* Chapter 21), Whipple's disease (*see* Chapter 22) and parasitic infections (*see* Chapter 19).

REFERENCES

Agger, W.A., McCormick, J.D., Gurwith, M.J. 1985: Clinical and microbiological features of Aeromonas hydrophila-associated diarrhea. *Journal of Clinical Microbiology* 21, 909–13.

Alam, A.N., Alam, N.H., Ahmed, T., Sack, D.A. 1990: Randomised double blind trial of a single dose of doxycycline for treating cholera in adults. *British Medical Journal* 300, 1619–21.

Altekruse, S.F., Hunt, J.M., Tollefson, L.K., Madden, J.M. 1994: Food and animal sources of human Campylobacter jejuni infection. *Journal of the American Veterinary Medical Association* 204, 57–61.

Anderson, A.S., Bauer, H., Nelson, C.B. 1955: Salmonellosis due to *Salmonella typhimurium* with Easter chicks as likely source. *JAMA* 158, 1153.

Arnon, S.S., Midura, T.F., Damus, K., Thompson, B., Wood, R.M., Chin, J. 1979: Honey and other environmental risk factors for infant botulism. *Journal of Pediatrics* 94, 331–6.

Aserkoff, B., Bennett, J.V. 1969: Effect of antibiotic therapy in acute salmonellosis on the fecal excretion of salmonellae. *New England Journal of Medicine* 281, 636.

Ashdown, L.R., Koehler, J.M. 1993: The spectrum of Aeromonas-associated diarrhea in tropical Queensland, Australia. *Southeast Asian Journal of Tropical Medicine and Public Health* 24, 347–53.

Barker, W.H., Jr 1974: *Vibrio parahaemolyticus* outbreaks in the United States. *Lancet* 1, 551–4.

Barnes, G.L., Townley, R.R.W. 1973: Duodenal mucosal damage in 31 infants with gastroenteritis. *Archives of Disease in Childhood* 48, 343–9.

Bartlett, J.G. 1994: *Clostridium difficile*: history of its role as an enteric pathogen and the current state of knowledge about the organism. *Clinical Infectious Diseases* 18(Suppl 4), S265–72.

Beecher, D.J., Schoeni, J.L., Wong, A.C. 1995: Enterotoxic activity of hemolysin BL from Bacillus cereus. *Infection and Immunity* 63, 4423–8.

Bennish, M.L., Azad, A.K., Rahman, O., Phillips, R.E. 1990: Hypoglycemia during diarrhea in childhood. Prevalence, pathophysiology, and outcome. *New England Journal of Medicine* 322, 1357–63.

Berkowitz, F.E. 1984: Bacteremia in hospitalized black South African children. A one-year study emphasizing nosocomial bacteremia and bacteremia in severely malnourished children. *American Journal of the Diseases of Childhood* 138, 551–6.

Black, R.E., Jackson, R.J., Tsai, T. *et al.* 1978: Epidemic *Yersinia enterocolitica* infection due to contaminated chocolate milk. *New England Journal of Medicine* 298, 76–9.

Bohrer, S.P. 1966: Typhoid perforation of the ileum. *British Journal of Radiology* 39, 37–41.

Borriello, S.P., Larson, H.E., Welch, A.R., Barclay, F., Stringer, M.F., Bartholomew, B.A. 1984: Enterotoxigenic *Clostridium perfringens*: a possible cause of antibiotic associated diarrhoea. *Lancet* 8372, 305–7.

Bottone, E.J. 1997: *Yersinia enterocolitica*: the charisma continues. *Clinical Microbiological Reviews* 10, 257–76.

Calin, A., Fries, J.F. 1976: An 'experimental' epidemic of Reiter's syndrome revisited. Follow-up evidence on genetic and environmental factors. *Annals of Internal Medicine* 84, 564–6.

Carter, A.O., Borczyk, A.A., Carlson, J.A. *et al.* 1987: A severe outbreak of *Escherichia coli* 0157:H7-associated hemorrhagic colitis in a nursing home. *New England Journal of Medicine* 317, 1496–500.

Challapalli, M., Tess, B.R., Cunningham, D.G., Chopra, A.K., Houston, C.W. 1988: Aeromonas-associated diarrhea in children. *Pediatrics and Infectious Diseases Journal* 7, 693–8.

Cherington, M. 1998: Clinical spectrum of botulism. *Muscle and Nerve* 21, 701–10.

Cohen, J.I., Bartlett, J.A., Corey, G.R. 1987: Extra-intestinal manifestations of Salmonella infections. *Medicine* 66, 349–88.

Cohen, M.B., Giannella, R.A. 1992: Haemorrhagic colitis associated with *Escherichia coli* 0157:H7. *Advances in Internal Medicine* 37, 173–95.

Cvjetanovic, B., Grab, B., Uemura, K. 1971: Epidemiological model of typhoid fever and its use in the planning and evaluation programmes. *Bulletin of the World Health Organization* 44, 667.

Dalsgaard, D.A., Larsen, J.L. 1995: Is Vibrio cholerae serotype 0139 a potential cause of a new pandemic? (in Danish) *Ugeskr Laeger* 157, 280–3.

Delans, R.J., Biuso, J.D., Saba, S.R., Ramirez, G. 1984: Hemolytic uremic syndrome after Campylobacter-induced diarrhea in an adult. *Archives of Internal Medicine* 144, 1074–6.

Dertinger, S., Scheubel, R., Kekos, G. 1991: Guaiac-positive stools and ulceration of the colon associated with salmonellosis. *Endoscopy* 23, 306–7.

Doyle, M.P. 1991: *Escherichia coli* 0157:H7 and its significance in foods. *International Journal of Food Microbiology* 12, 289–302.

Duncan, C.L., Strong, D. 1971: *Clostridium perfringens* Type A food poisoning. I. Response of the rabbit ileum as an indication of enteropathogenicity of strains of *Clostridium perfringens* in monkeys. *Infectious Immunology* 3, 167.

DuPont, H.L., Hornick, R.B. 1973: Adverse effect of lomotil therapy in shigellosis. *JAMA* 226, 1525–8.

DuPont, H.L., Gangarosa, E.J., Reller, L.B. *et al.* 1970: Shigellosis in custodial institutions. *American Journal of Epidemiology* 92, 172–9.

DuPont, H.L., Hornick, R.B., Snyder, M.J., Libonati, J.P., Formal, S.B., Gangarosa, E.J. 1972: Immunity in shigellosis. II. Protection induced by oral live vaccine or primary infection. *Journal of Infectious Diseases* 125, 12–16.

Ericsson, C.D., Pickering, L.K., Sullivan, P., DuPont, H.L. 1980: The role of location of food consumption in the prevention of travelers' diarrhea in Mexico. *Gastroenterology* 79, 812–16.

Feeney, G.F.X., Kerlin, P., Sampson, J.A. 1987: Clinical aspects of infection with *Yersinia enterocolitica* in adults. *Australian and New Zealand Journal of Medicine* 17, 216–19.

Finkelstein, R.A. 1973: Cholera. *Critical Reviews in Microbiology* 2, 553.

Frieben, W.R., Duncan, C.L. 1973: Homology between enterotoxin protein and spore structural protein in *Clostridium perfringens* type A. *European Journal of Biochemistry* 39, 393–401.

Gaines, S., Sprinz, H., Tully, J.G., Tigertt, W.D. 1968: Studies on infection and immunity in experimental typhoid fever: VII The distribution of Salmonella typhi in chimpanzee tissue following oral challenge, and the relationship between the numbers of bacilli and morphologic lesions. *Journal of Infectious Diseases* 118, 293–306.

Ganguly, N.K., Kaur, T. 1996: Mechanism of action of cholera toxin and other toxins. *Indian Journal of Medical Research* 104, 28–37.

Gemmell, C.G. 1984: Comparative study of the nature and biological activities of bacterial endotoxins. *Journal of Medical Microbiology* 17, 217–35.

Gilbert, R.J., Parry, J.M. 1977: Serotypes of *Bacillus cereus* from outbreaks of food poisoning and from routine foods. *Journal of Hygiene* 78, 69–74.

Gill, D.M. 1976: The arrangement of subunits in cholera toxin. *Biochemistry* 15, 1242–8.

Glass, R.I., Claeson, M., Blake, P.A., Waldman, R.J., Pierce, N.F. 1991: Cholera in Africa: lessons on transmission and control for Latin America. *Lancet* 338(8770), 791–5.

Gonzalez, A., Vargas, V., Guarner, L., Accarino, A., Guardia, J. 1985: Toxic megacolon in typhoid fever. *Archives of Internal Medicine* 145, 2120.

Gorbach, S.L. 1998: Infectious diarrhoea and bacterial food poisoning. In Sleisenger, M., Fordtran, J.S. (eds) *Gastrointestinal disease: pathophysiology, diagnosis, management*, 6th edn. Philadelphia: W.B. Saunders Co., 1594–632.

Grados, P., Bravo, N., Battilana, C. 1996: Comparative effectiveness of co-trimoxazole and tetracycline in the treatment of cholera. *Bulletin of the Pan American Health Organization* 30, 36–42.

Grady, G.F., Keusch, G.T. 1971: Pathogenesis of bacterial diarrheas. I. *New England Journal of Medicine* 285, 831–41.

Granum, P.E., Lund, T. 1997: Bacillus cereus and its food poisoning toxins. *FEMS Microbiological Letters* 157, 223–8.

Greenough, W.B., 3rd, Khin-Maung, U. 1991: Oral rehydration therapy. In Field, M. (ed.) *Diarrheal diseases.* New York: Elsevier, 485–99.

Greenough, W.B., Gordon, R.S., Rosenberg, I.S. *et al.* 1964: Tetracycline in the treatment of cholera. *Lancet* 1, 355.

Griffin, P.M., Ostroff, S.M., Tauxe, R.V., Greene, K.D., Wells, J.G., Lewis, J.H., Blake, P.A. 1988: Illness associated with *Escherichia coli* 0157:H7 infections. A broad clinical spectrum. *Annals of Internal Medicine* 109, 705–12.

Hand, W.L., King, N.L. 1977: Serum opsonization of salmonella in sickle cell anemia. *American Journal of Medicine* 64, 388–95.

Hart, C.A., Batt, R.M., Saunders, J.R. 1993: Diarrhoea caused by *Escherichia coli. Annals of Tropical Paediatrics* 13, 121–31.

Hicks, S., Candy, D.C., Phillips, A.D. 1996: Adhesion of enteroaggregative *Escherichia coli* to formalin-fixed intestinal and ureteric epithelia from children. *Journal of Medicine and Microbiology* 44, 362–71.

Hobbs, B.C. 1961: Public health significance of salmonella carriers in livestock and birds. *Journal of Applied Bacteriology* 24, 340.

Hook, E.W., Campbell, C.G., Weens, H.S. *et al.* 1957: Salmonella osteomyelitis in patients with sickle cell anaemia. *New England Journal of Medicine* 257, 403.

Humphrey, T.J., Whitehead, A., Gawler, A.H., Henley, A., Rowe, B. 1991: Numbers of Salmonella enteritidis in the contents of naturally contaminated hens' eggs. *Epidemiology and Infection* 106, 489–96.

Jesudason, M.V., Koshi, G. 1990: Aeromonas species in human septicaemia and diarrhoea. *Indian Journal of Medical Research* 91, 174–6.

Kabir, I., Khan, W.A., Haider, R., Mitra, A.K., Alam, A.N. 1996: Erythromycin and trimethoprim-sulphamethoxazole in the treatment of cholera in children. *Journal of Diarrhoeal Diseases Research* 14, 243–7.

Kain, K.C., Kelly, M.T. 1989: Clinical features, epidemiology, and treatment of *Plesiomonas shigelloides* diarrhea. *Journal of Clinical Microbiology* 27, 998–1001.

Kapperud, G. 1994: Campylobacter infection. Epidemiology,

risk factors and preventive measures (in Norwegian). *Tidsskrift for den Norske Laegeforening* 114, 795–9.

Kaufmann, A.F., Feeley, J.C., DeWitt, W.E. 1967: Salmonella excretion by turtles. *Public Health Reports* 82, 840–2.

Kendrick, M.A. 1972: Study of illness among Americans returning from international travel, July 11–August 24, 1971. *Journal of Infectious Diseases* 126, 684–5.

Keusch, G.T., Donohue-Rolfe, A., Jacewicz, M. 1985: Shigella toxin and the pathogenesis of shigellosis. *Ciba Foundation Symposia* 112, 193–214.

Khalil, K., Lindblom, G.B., Mazhar, K., Kaijser, B. 1994: Flies and water as reservoirs for bacterial enteropathogens in urban and rural areas in and around Lahore, Pakistan. *Epidemiology and Infection* 113, 435–44.

Khan, W.A., Bennish, M.L., Seas, C. *et al.* 1996: Randomised controlled comparison of single-dose ciprofloxacin and doxycycline for cholera caused by Vibrio cholera 01 or 0139. *Lancet* 348, 296–300.

Koster, F., Levin, J., Walker, L. *et al.* 1978: Hemolytic-uremic syndrome after shigellosis. Relation to endotoxemia and circulation immune complexes. *New England Journal of Medicine* 298, 927–33.

Koster, F.T., Boonpucknavig, V., Sujaho, S., Gilman, R.H., Rahaman, M.M. 1984: Renal histopathology in the hemolytic-uremic syndrome following shigellosis. *Clinical Nephrology* 21, 126–33.

LaBrec, E.H., Schneider, H., Magnani, T.J., Jr 1964: Epithelial cell penetration as an essential step in the pathogenesis of bacillary dysentery. *Journal of Bacteriology* 88, 1503.

Larvol, L., Zeitoun, E., Barge, J., Valverde, A., Delaroque, I., Soule, J.C. 1994: Toxic megacolon with colonic perforation complicating Campylobacter jejuni ileo-colitis (in French). *Gastroenterologie Clinique et Biologique* 18, 281–4.

Lawrence, G., Shann, F., Freestone, D.S., Walker, P.D. 1979: Prevention of necrotising enteritis in Papua New Guinea by active immunisation. *Lancet* 1(8110), 227–30.

Lawrence, G.W., Lehmann, D., Anian, G., Coakley, C.A., Saleu, G., Barker, M.J., Davis, M.W. 1990: Impact of active immunisation against enteritis necroticans in Papua New Guinea. *Lancet* 336(8724), 1165–7.

Levine, M.M. 1987: Escherichia coli that cause diarrhea: enterotoxigenic, enteropathogenic, enteroinvasive, enterohemorrhagic, and enteroadherent. *Journal of Infectious Diseases* 155, 377–89.

Ljungh, A., Waldstrom, T. 1985: Aeromonas and Plesiomonas as possible causes of diarrhoea. *Infection* 13, 169–73.

Louise, C.B., Obrig, T.G. 1992: Shiga toxin-associated hemolytic uremic syndrome: combined cytotoxic effects of shiga toxin and lipopolysaccharide (endotoxin) on human vascular endothelial cells in vitro. *Infection and Immunity* 60, 1536–43.

Lowenstein, M.S., Ballows, A., Gangarosa, E.J. 1973: Turista at an international congress in Mexico. *Lancet* 1, 529–31.

Mariani-Kurkdjian, P., Bingen, E. 1995: Hemolytic–uremic syndrome after verotoxin-producing Escherichia coli infection (in French). *Presse Medicale* 24, 99–101.

Marrack, P., Kappler, J. 1990: The staphylococcal enterotoxins and their relatives. *Science* 248, 705–11.

McDonel, J.L. 1980: Mechanism of action of *Clostridium perfringens* enterotoxin. *Food Technology* 34, 91.

McDonel, J.L., Duncan, C.L. 1977: Regional localization of activity of *Clostridium perfringens* Type A enterotoxin in the rabbit ileum, jejunum, and duodenum. *Journal of Infectious Diseases* 136, 661–6.

Melling, J., Capel, B.J., Turnbull, P.C., Gilbert, R.J. 1976: Identification of a novel enterotoxigenic activity associated with Bacillus cereus. *Journal of Clinical Pathology* 29, 938–40.

Mishu, B., Blaser, M.J. 1993: The role of *Campylobacter jejuni* infection in the initiation of Guillain–Barre syndrome. *Clinics in Infectious Diseases* 17, 104–8.

Mishu, B, Griffin, P.M., Tauxe, R.V. 1991: Salmonella enteritidis gastroenteritis transmitted by intact chicken eggs. *Annals of Internal Medicine* 115, 190–4.

Mock, C.N., Amaral, J., Visser, L.E. 1992: Improvement in survival from typhoid ileal perforation. Results of 221 operative cases. *Annals of Surgery* 215, 244–9.

Moreno, G.S., Griffiths, P.L., Connerton, I.F., Park, R.W. 1993: Occurrence of campylobacters in small domestic and laboratory animals. *Journal of Applied Bacteriology* 75, 49–54.

Morris, J.G., Black, R.E. 1985: Cholera and other vibrioses in the United States. *New England Journal of Medicine* 312, 343–50.

Murrell, T.G.C., Roth, L., Egerton, J. *et al.* 1966: Pig-bel: enteritis necroticans. A study in diagnosis and management. *Lancet* 1, 217.

Obi, C.L., Coker, A.O., Epoke, J., Ndip, R. 1995: Aeromonas and Plesiomonas species as bacterial agents of diarrhoea in urban and rural areas of Nigeria: antibiogram of isolates. *Central Africa Journal of Medicine* 41, 397–403.

Obrig, T.G., Del-Vecchio, P.J., Brown, J.E., Moran, T.P., Rowland, B.M., Judge, T.K., Rothman, S.W. 1988: Direct cytotoxic action of Shiga toxin on human vascular endothelial cells. *Infection and Immunity* 56, 2373–8.

Ogawa, H., Nakamura, A., Nakaya, R. 1968: Cinemicroscopic study of tissue cell cultures infected with *Shigella flexneri*. *Japanese Journal of Medical Science and Biology* 21, 259–73.

Olsvik, O., Wachsmuth, K., Kay, B., Birkness, K.A., Yi, A., Sack, B. 1990: Laboratory observations on *Plesiomonas shigelloides* strains isolated from children with diarrhea in Peru. *Journal of Clinical Microbiology* 28, 886–9.

Osuntoken, B.O., Bademosi, O., Ogunremi, K. *et al.* 1972: Neuropsychiatric manifestations of typhoid fever in 959 patients. *Archives of Neurology* 27, 7–13.

Paton, A.W., Voss, E., Manning, P.A., Paton, J.C. 1997: Shiga toxin-producing *Escherichia coli* isolates from cases of human disease show enhanced adherence to intestinal epithelial (Henle 407) cells. *Infection and Immunity* 65, 3799–805.

Paton, A.W., Voss, E., Manning, P.A., Paton, J.C. 1998: Antibodies to lipopolysaccharide block adherence of

Shiga toxin-producing *Escherichia coli* to human intestinal epithelial (Henle 407) cells. *Microbial Pathogenesis* 24, 57–63.

Pavia, A.T., Nichols, C.R., Green, D.P. *et al.* 1990: Hemolytic–uremic syndrome during an outbreak of Escherichia coli O157:H7 infections in institutions for mentally retarded persons: clinical and epidemiologic observations. *Journal of Pediatrics* 116, 544–51.

Peterson, M.C. 1994: Clinical aspects of *Campylobacter jejuni* infections in adults. *Western Journal of Medicine* 161, 148–52.

Ponka, A., Kosunen, T.U. 1982: Pneumonia associated with enteritis due to *Campylobacter fetus* ssp *jejuni*. *Annals of Clinical Research* 14, 137–9.

Ponka, A., Pitkanen, T., Sarna, S. *et al.* 1984: Infection due to *Campylobacter jejuni*: a report of 524 outpatients. *Infection* 12, 175–8.

Ramachandran, S., Wickremasinghe, H.R., Perera, M.V. 1975: Acute disseminated encephalomyelitis in typhoid fever. *British Medical Journal* 1, 494–5.

Rocha, H., Kirl, J.W., Hearey, C.D. 1971: Prolonged Salmonella bacteremia in patients with *Schistosoma mansoni* infection. *Archives of Internal Medicine* 128, 254–7.

Rogolsky, M. 1979: Nonenteric toxins of *Staphylococcus aureus*. *Microbiological Reviews* 43, 320–60.

Ropper, A.H. 1988: Campylobacter diarrhea and Guillain–Barré syndrome. *ARCL Neurology* 45, 655.

Rosenstein, B.J. 1964: Shigella and salmonella enteritis in infants and children. *Bulletin of the Johns Hopkins Hospital* 115, 407.

Ruiz-Palacios, G.M., Torres, J., Torres, N.I., Escamilla, E., Ruiz-Palacios, B.R., Tamayo, J. 1983: Cholera-like enterotoxin produced by Campylobacter jejuni. Characterisation and clinical significance. *Lancet* 2(8344), 250–3.

Ryder, R.W., Wells, J.G., Gangarosa, E.J. 1977: From the Center for Disease Control: A study of travelers' diarrhea in foreign visitors to the United States. *Journal of Infectious Diseases* 136, 605–7.

Saebo, A., Lassen, J. 1992: Acute and chronic gastrointestinal manifestations associated with *Yersinia enterocolitica* infection. A Norwegian follow-up study on 458 hospitalized patients. *Annals of Surgery* 215, 250–5.

Sakurai, J., Duncan, C.L. 1978: Some properties of beta-toxin produced by Clostridium perfringens type C. *Infection and Immunity* 21, 678–80.

Samuel, S.C., Hancock, P., Leigh, D.A. 1991: An investigation into *Clostridium perfringens* enterotoxin-associated diarrhoea. *Journal of Hospital Infections* 18, 219–30.

Sanders, E., Sweeny, F.J., Friedman, E.A. *et al.* 1963: An outbreak of hospital associated infections due to *Salmonella derby*. *JAMA* 186, 984.

Schlievert, P.M. 1993: Role of Superantigens in human disease. *Journal of Infectious Diseases* 167, 997–1002.

Sharp, G.W.G. 1973: Action of cholera toxin on fluid and electrolyte movement in the small intestine. *Annual Review of Medicine* 24, 19–23.

Siegler, R.L 1995: The hemolytic uremic syndrome. *Pediatric Clinics of North America* 42, 1505–29.

Skirrow, M.B. 1991: Epidemiology of Campylobacter enteritis. *International Journal of Food Microbiology* 12, 9–16.

Smadel, J.E. 1963: Intracellular infection and the carrier state. *Science* 140, 153.

Smith, G.S., Blaser, M.J. 1985: Fatalities associated with Campylobacter jejuni infections. *JAMA* 253, 2873–5.

Takeuchi, A. 1967: Electron microscope studies of experimental Salmonella infection. I. Penetration into the intestinal epithelium by Salmonella typhimurium. *American Journal of Pathology* 50, 109–36.

Terranova, W., Blake, P.A. 1978: *Bacillus cereus* food poisoning. *New England Journal of Medicine* 298, 143–4.

Tjoa, W., DuPont, H.L., Sullivan, P. *et al.* 1977: Location of food consumption and travelers' diarrhea. *American Journal of Epidemiology* 106, 61–6.

Turnbull, P.C.B. 1976: Studies on the production of enterotoxins by *Bacillus cereus*. *Journal of Clinical Pathology* 29, 941–8.

Tynes, B.S., Utz, J.P. 1962: Factors influencing the cure of salmonella carriers. *Annals of Internal Medicine* 57, 871.

Ueda, Y., Suzuki, N., Miyagi, K. *et al.* 1997: Studies on bacillary dysentery cases of overseas travellers – during 1979 to 1995 (in Japanese) *Nippon Saikingaku Zasshi* 52, 735–46.

Verenkar, M., Naik, V., Rodrigues, S., Singh, I. 1995: Aeromonas species and *Plesiomonas shigelloides* in diarrhoea in Goa. *Indian Journal of Pathology and Microbiology* 38, 169–71.

Visitsunthorn, N., Komolpis, P. 1995: Antimicrobial therapy in *Plesiomonas shigelloides*-associated diarrhea in Thai children. *Southeast Asian Journal of Tropical Medicine and Public Health* 26, 86–90.

Vyas, S.K., Law, N.N., Hill, S. *et al.* 1993: Toxic megacolon with late perforation in Campylobacter colitis – a cautionary tale. *Postgraduate Medical Journal* 69, 322–4.

Wall, P.G., McDonnell, R.J., Adak, G.K., Cheasty, T., Smith, H.R., Rowe, B. 1996: General outbreaks of vero cytotoxin producing Escherichia coli O157 in England and Wales from 1992 to 1994. *Communicable Disease Report CDR Review* 6, R26–33.

Watson, D.A.R., Andrew, J.H., Banting, S. *et al.* 1991: Pig-bel but no pig: enteritis necroticans acquired in Australia. *Medical Journal of Australia* 155: 47–50.

WHO 1984: *A manual for the treatment of acute diarrhea*. Geneva: World Health Organization.

WHO 1998: *Cholera vaccines update*. Global Task Force on Cholera Control. Division of Emerging and other Communicable Diseases Surveillance and Control. Geneva: World Health Organization.

Williams, R., Piper, M., Borriello, P. *et al.* 1985: Diarrhoea due to enterotoxigenic *Clostridium perfringens*: clinical features and management of a cluster of ten cases. *Age and Ageing* 14, 296–302.

Yamada, S., Matsushita, S., Dejsirilert, S., Kudoh, Y. 1997: Incidence and clinical symptoms of Aeromonas-associated traveller's diarrhoea in Tokyo. *Epidemiology and Infection* 119, 121–6.

19

Parasitic infections

DAVID I GROVE

The human gastrointestinal tract plays host to a large number of protozoal and helminthic parasites. Protozoa are unicellular eukaryotic organisms (in contrast to the prokaryotic bacteria), while worms are multicellular animals with various differentiated cells. All of the protozoa and some of the worms simply gain entry to the gut following ingestion of infective forms. Some worms penetrate the intact skin and pass to the bowel via the blood stream and the lungs. Many parasites infect only the small bowel, while others infect both the small intestine as well as other parts of the gastrointestinal tract (Fig. 19.1). Yet others, such as the protozoan, *Entamoeba histolytica*, or the worm, *Enterobius vermicularis*, merely pass through the small bowel on their way to their destination in the large intestine; these organisms are not considered further.

Details of the morphological appearances of these parasites are beyond the scope of this book. Descriptions of cysts and ova in faeces can be found in standard texts of parasitology. Superb illustrations of the parasites in the tissues of the gastrointestinal tract may be seen in two recent books (Orihel and Ash, 1995; Connor *et al.*, 1997).

PROTOZOAL INFECTIONS

Protozoal parasites of the four major groups including flagellates, amoebae, ciliates and spore-formers infect the gastrointestinal tract, but only flagellates and spore-formers inhabit the small bowel (Table 19.1). The sole flagellate infecting humans is *Giardia lamblia* whereas infections are known with five spore-formers: *Cryptosporidium*, *Isospora*, *Cyclospora*, Microsporidia and *Sarcocystis*. Whereas *Giardia* lines the surface of the small bowel and trophozoites generally encyst in the lower bowel, the other organisms are coccidian parasites that invade small bowel enterocytes, reproduce and are excreted in the stools as spores. Although the non-microsporidial parasites may cause symptomatic infection in normal individuals, such infections are usually self-limiting. On the other hand, apart from *Sarcocystis* with which it has not yet been described, all the coccidian parasites may produce severe, prolonged infections in immunocompromised patients, particularly those suffering from acquired immunodeficiency syndrome (AIDS). Conversely, many infections with each of these parasites in immunocompetent individuals are asymptomatic. The key manifestation of these infections is diarrhoea without blood or mucus. How these organisms cause diarrhoea is poorly understood. Infections

Table 19.1 *Protozoal pathogens of the gastrointestinal tract*

Flagellates
Giardia lamblia[a]

Amoebae
Entamoeba histolytica

Ciliates
Balantidium coli

Spore-formers
Cryptosporidium parvum[b]
Cyclospora cayetanensis[a]
Enterocytozoon bieneusi[a]
Encephalitozoon intestinalis[a]
Isospora belli[a]
Sarcocystis species[a]

[a]Only or primarily involves the small bowel and is discussed in this chapter.
[b]Involves both the small bowel and other parts of the gastrointestinal tract, and is discussed in this chapter.

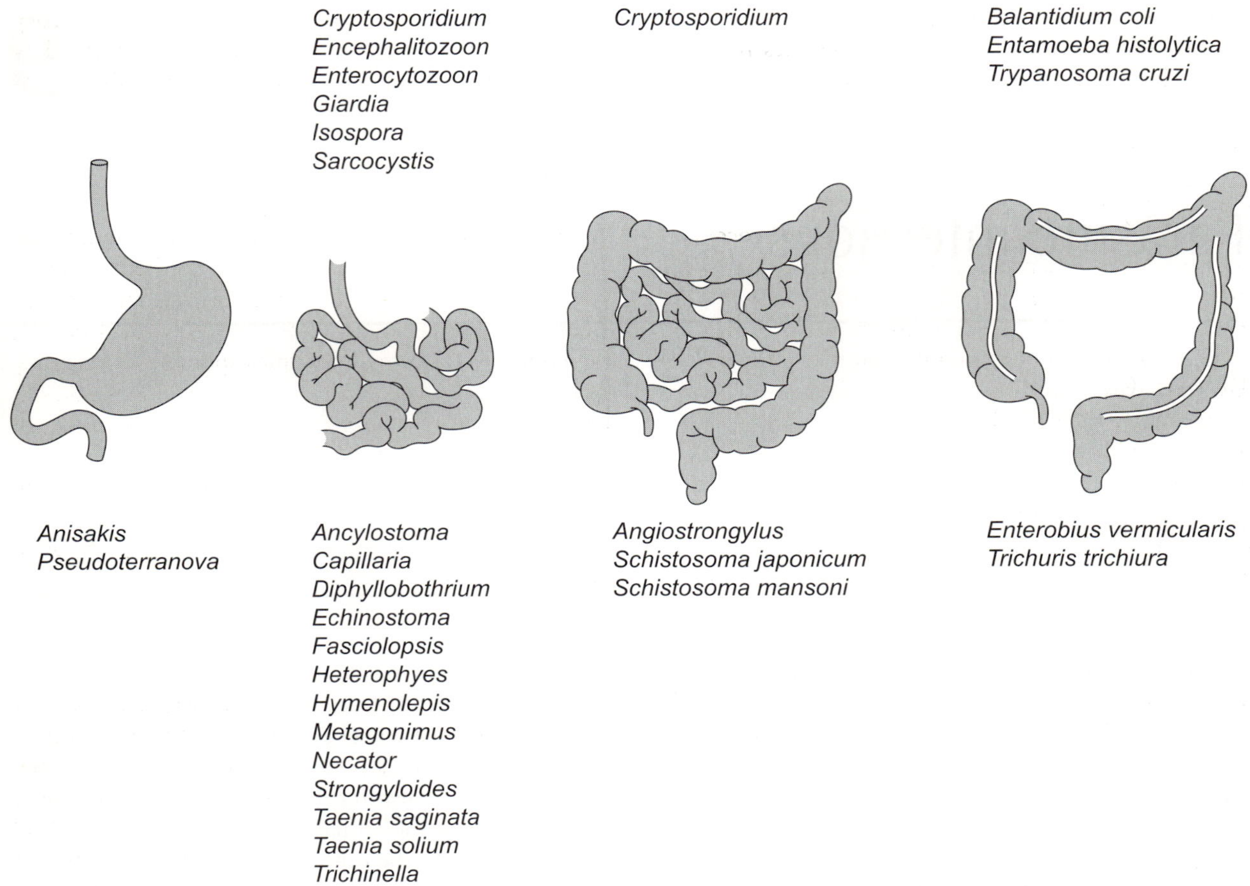

Figure 19.1 *Parasites infecting primarily (from left), stomach and small bowel, small bowel alone, small bowel and large bowel, and large bowel alone. Protozoa are listed above and worms are indicated below.*

may be associated with impaired absorption of fats, xylose and vitamin B_{12}. In some patients, the small bowel morphology is relatively normal despite heavy infections, whereas in others there may be shortening or flattening of the villi, hyperplasia of the crypts and leucocytic infiltration of the mucosa.

Giardia lamblia

EPIDEMIOLOGY

Giardia lamblia is a cosmopolitan parasite with estimates of prevalence of infection in temperate areas of the world ranging from 2 to 5 per cent compared with 20–30 per cent in the tropics (Ortega and Adam, 1997). In developed countries such as Australia, infection is most common in preschool children and in adults aged 20–39 years – the age group that would be expected to contain most parents of toddlers. These figures suggest that, in developed countries, transmission is mostly occurring in two situations: between children in day-care centres and among family members of these children at home. In developing countries in the tropics, where sanitation is much poorer and water supplies are inadequate, there is increased transmission among all levels of the population.

There has been considerable controversy about whether humans and various species of animals are infected with the same or different species of *Giardia*, and whether there is transmission between these various hosts. In all probability, humans can be infected from humans or other animals, including cats, dogs, sheep, cattle, goats, rats and beavers. Which source of infection is most important may depend upon the environment in which the person lives. Infection may be acquired via contaminated water, food, fomites or direct person to person transfer, particularly in child-care centres. Cysts may survive for several months in water and are relatively resistant to chlorination.

LIFE CYCLE

Infection may result from ingestion of 10 or fewer cysts (Adam, 1991). In the upper small bowel, cysts hatch motile trophozoites, which multiply asexually, particularly in the crypts. Some parasites pass down the intestinal tract and develop a protective cyst wall. They are then eliminated in the faeces, sometimes reaching tens of thousands of cysts per gram of stool.

PATHOLOGY

Many trophozoites attach to the epithelial surface via a powerful sucking disc; in contrast to the coccidian parasites to be described, there is generally no tissue invasion. The histological appearances of the small bowel are variable. In some patients, there are no obvious abnormalities despite large numbers of parasites, while in others there is variable villous blunting and lymphocytic infiltration. Precisely how *Giardia* causes diarrhoea is uncertain (Farthing, 1996), but possible mechanisms include damage to the mucosa (particularly disruption of the microvilli), mucosal inflammation, inhibition of enzyme (disaccharidase) activity and bacterial overgrowth within the bowel lumen (which may in turn interfere with the action of bile salts). Humoral immunity may be important in control of infection because giardiasis is more severe in patients with hypogammaglobulinaemia and possibly those with isolated immunoglobulin A (IgA) deficiency.

CLINICAL FEATURES

The spectrum of presentation in giardiasis is extremely wide. Acute illness is most marked in those who are infected for the first time. After an incubation period of 1–3 weeks, there is often a sudden onset of explosive, watery diarrhoea, abdominal distension and discomfort, anorexia, nausea and flatulence. Rarely, in extremely heavy infections, a malabsorption syndrome develops with the frequent passage of pale, bulky, foul-smelling stools. In most patients, symptoms resolve spontaneously over a few weeks or subside into chronic low-grade infection with mild diarrhoea, debility and weight loss, which may last for weeks or months. On the other hand, patients living in endemic areas with a high prevalence of infection are constantly reinfected. They tend to come to terms with the organism and have low parasite burdens that do not excite much in the way of symptoms.

DIAGNOSIS

The usual way of making the diagnosis is by finding the distinctive organisms in the stools. In formed faeces they appear as cysts 8×10 μm in size, whereas trophozoites may be seen in diarrhoeic stools. Unfortunately, excretion of *Giardia* is sometimes sporadic – cysts may be there one day but not the next. In various studies, it has been estimated that 70–88 per cent of patients may be diagnosed with a single specimen, whereas 80–95 per cent are diagnosed if three stools are assessed. Some patients undergo upper gastrointestinal endoscopy, and trophozoites may be found in duodenal aspirate or in duodenal biopsies.

TREATMENT

Drugs available for the treatment of giardiasis vary in different countries. First-line treatment is usually with a nitroimidazole agent, such metronidazole or tinidazole, either as a large single dose or a prolonged course of smaller doses (Table 19.2). Over 90 per cent of patients will respond to one of these regimens. There is usually cross-resistance between the nitroimidazoles but, if a patient fails to respond to single-dose therapy with tinidazole, it is reasonable to try a longer course with metronidazole. Citrus-flavoured benzoyl metronidazole 5 mg/kg three times daily for several days is a palatable preparation for children. Second-line agents are more problematic; there are no clear-cut clinical trials for comparison and some suggestions rely upon *in vitro* susceptibility evidence rather than clinical evidence. Table 19.2 lists drugs in the order in which I would use them; however, they may not be available in all countries. It may be necessary to try one after

Table 19.2 *Drugs used in the treatment of giardiasis*

Drug	Dose
First-line regimens	
Tinidazole	2 g as a single dose
Metronidazole	2 g as a single dose
Metronidazole	200 mg three times daily for 7 days
Second-line regimens	
Quinacrine (mepacrine)	250 mg three times daily for 5 days
Albendazole	200 mg twice daily for 5 days
Mebendazole	100 mg twice daily for 5 days
Doxycycline	100 mg daily for 7 days
Furazolidone	100 mg four times daily for 7 days
Paromomycin	10 mg/kg three times daily for 7 days
Mefloquine	500 mg as a single dose
Rifampicin (rifampin)	150 mg twice daily for 3 days

another until success is achieved. Doxycycline and other tetracyclines should not be used in children and all the drugs listed are best avoided in pregnancy.

Cryptosporidium parvum

EPIDEMIOLOGY

Cryptosporidiosis is a zoonotic infection that has been recognized in humans since 1976. Prevalence surveys have found < 1–10 per cent of the population to be infected. Infections are common in domesticated livestock, particularly cattle. The organism may cause sporadic self-limiting infections in immunocompetent humans, especially children living in rural areas and in elderly patients (Neill *et al.*, 1996). Sometimes epidemics occur. For example, a recent outbreak due to contamination of the water supply was estimated to afflict over 400 000 people living in Milwaukee in the United States (Mackenzie *et al.*, 1994). In that outbreak, the risk of secondary infection within a household was less than 5 per cent (Mackenzie *et al.*, 1995). In immunocompromised patients, prolonged unremitting infections are sometimes seen.

LIFE CYCLE

Infection is usually acquired by ingestion of oocysts in food or water. Studies in volunteers have shown that 88 per cent of those who ingested 300 or more cysts became infected (Dupont *et al.*, 1995). Sporozoites are released in the lumen of the gut and then penetrate the apical tip of enterocytes in the small bowel. They remain in the microvillous brush border, separated from the intestinal lumen by a tent-like membrane of host origin. Within the enterocyte, the sporozoite matures into a trophozoite, which multiplies asexually to produce merozoites, some of which develop into sexual forms, which unite to produce cysts that are excreted in the faeces.

PATHOLOGY

The mechanisms by which *C. parvum* cause diarrhoea are poorly understood. There is excessive secretion of fluid (up to 6 L/day) into the proximal small intestine. Heavy infections produce marked partial villous atrophy and cellular infiltration of the lamina propria. Immunocompetent individuals develop protective immunity but the roles of antibody and cell-mediated immunity are unclear. Prolonged infections have been seen in patients with hypogammaglobulinaemia and those with AIDS. Moreover, in the latter group of patients especially, infection is not restricted to the small bowel and parasites may be found in the epithelial cells of the stomach, biliary and pancreatic ducts, colon and occasionally in the respiratory tract.

CLINICAL FEATURES

Watery diarrhoea is the key feature of cryptosporidial infection. In immunocompetent individuals, symptoms usually resolve within several weeks. In patients with AIDS, however, diarrhoea may be prolonged and profuse leading to severe dehydration and electrolyte disturbances.

DIAGNOSIS

Cysts may be found in faeces stained with special stains, such as the Ziehl–Nielsen technique (Goodgame, 1996). In the latter, they appear as red cysts 4–6 μm in diameter (Plate 19.1). Alternatively, parasites may be seen within enterocytes in biopsies; they appear as 4 μm blue dots on the apical membrane. In a series of 30 patients with AIDS and cryptosporidiosis, parasites were seen in duodenum (53 per cent), terminal ileum (91 per cent) and colon (60 per cent) (Greenberg *et al.*, 1996).

TREATMENT

Therapy with this infection is difficult. Spiramycin, clarithromycin and paromomycin have been suggested as specific therapeutic agents, but response rates are poor. Paromomycin is given in a dose of 500 mg four times daily for several weeks followed by maintenance therapy of 500 mg twice daily in patients with AIDS and cryptosporidiosis (Hoepelman, 1996). More success has been claimed recently for nitazoxanide, a drug which is not generally available (Doumbo *et al.*, 1997). Bovine colostrum holds some promise (Greenberg and Cello, 1996). Patients with severe dehydration may require intravenous fluids. Octreotide is of little value.

Cyclospora cayetanensis

EPIDEMIOLOGY

This organism was first recognized in humans in 1979 and was for a time termed 'cyanobacteria-like bodies' or blue–green algae (Soave, 1996); it was given its current name in 1994 (Ortega *et al.*, 1998). Infection is most common in developing countries. The sources of infection are unclear but include contaminated water and food. One outbreak in the USA was due to the consumption of contaminated raspberries imported from Guatemala (Herwaldt and Ackers, 1997). Currently, it is thought that this parasite only infects humans.

LIFE CYCLE

The life cycle is similar to that of cryptosporidia, with oocysts being ingested, sporozoites penetrating the small bowel mucosa, where asexual and sexual multiplication occur, followed by the passage of oocysts in the faeces.

PATHOLOGY

Jejunal biopsy discloses partial villous atrophy and lymphocytic infiltration in some patients. Investigation may reveal impaired absorption of xylose and vitamin B_{12}, and increased faecal fat excretion.

CLINICAL FEATURES

After an incubation period of several days, immunocompetent individuals often develop an abrupt onset of watery diarrhoea, fatigue and anorexia, which may be associated with myalgias and weight loss. The illness often lasts 4–8 weeks and may be prolonged even further in patients with AIDS.

DIAGNOSIS

Like cryptosporidia, *Cyclospora* stains pinkish red with carbol–fuchsin in modified Ziehl–Nielsen and haematoxylin–eosin stains, but the organisms are larger, measuring 8–9 μm in size. Parasites are difficult to find within the enterocytes in small bowel biopsies and are best seen with electron microscopy (Goodgame, 1996).

TREATMENT

In immunocompetent patients, the disease is usually self-limiting but responds to therapy with one double-strength tablet (160/800 mg) of trimethoprim–sulphamethoxazole twice daily for 10 days (Hoge *et al.*, 1995). Prolonged therapy at a lower dosage may be necessary in patients with AIDS.

Enterocytozoon and *Encephalitozoon* species

EPIDEMIOLOGY

Microsporidia, so-called because they belong to the phylum Microsporidia, have long been known as ubiquitous parasites of invertebrates, fish and various mammals (Weber *et al.*, 1994). Human infections were not recognized until the AIDS era (Croft *et al.*, 1997; Kotler and Orenstein, 1998). Species of Microsporidia that are known to infect the human bowel are *Enterocytozoon bieneusi* and *Encephalitozoon (Septata) intestinalis.* So far they have only been isolated from humans but they still may represent zoonotic infections.

LIFE CYCLE

The parasites are small, obligate intracellular protozoa without mitochondria. The spore contains a coiled polar tube. When a spore is ingested, the tube first everts then injects the sporoplasm into an enterocyte. Within the epithelial cell, multiplication occurs, culminating in the release of spores, which are passed in the stools.

PATHOLOGY

Microsporidia usually infect the villi of the small bowel and are often associated with partial villous atrophy, crypt hyperplasia and increased numbers of intraepithelial lymphocytes. *E. bieneusi* has a strong preference for the distal duodenum and proximal jejunum. *E. intestinalis* is similar but has more spillover into the colon. In patients with AIDS, parasites may also be seen in the biliary tract and liver, kidney and respiratory tract.

CLINICAL FEATURES

Microsporidiosis is rarely seen except in patients with AIDS in whom it may produce a very troublesome diarrhoea.

DIAGNOSIS

Occasionally, spores may be found in faeces stained with trichrome or Giemsa, but they are very small and difficult to see, being about the size of a bacterium (about 1 μm) (Goodgame, 1996). More commonly, they are observed as 2 μm inclusions, often containing clear clefts, in the apical cytoplasm of small bowel enterocytes. In disseminated infections, they may be found in other organs. It is likely that, in the near future, polymerase chain reaction-based tests will speed and simplify diagnosis.

TREATMENT

Specific therapy is generally unsatisfactory, although claims have been made for albendazole (an anthelmintic) (Soule *et al.*, 1997), itraconazole (an antifungal) and thalidomide (Sharpstone *et al.*, 1997). Dehydration requires symptomatic therapy.

Isospora belli

EPIDEMIOLOGY

This organism has been known since the First World War (hence its name) but has come into prominence with the recognition of infections in patients with AIDS. The parasite is more prevalent in tropical countries. Infection is relatively uncommon and appears to be restricted to humans.

LIFE CYCLE

Infection is acquired by ingestion of oocysts (Lindsay *et al.*, 1997). Sporozoites are released in the small intestinal lumen, and invade the enterocytes of the distal duodenum and proximal jejunum. As with *Cryptosporidium*, asexual and sexual multiplication occur, culminating in the production of oocysts, which are passed in the stools.

PATHOLOGY

Infection in the small bowel may be associated with reduction in the length of villi and elongation of the crypts. Infection is generally restricted to the small bowel, but, rarely, dissemination occurs in patients with AIDS, with organisms being found in colon, mesenteric lymph nodes, liver, spleen and the biliary system (Orenstein, 1997).

CLINICAL FEATURES

After an incubation period of 1–2 weeks, diarrhoea with up to 10 bowel actions per day develops. In immunocompetent patients, the illness usually settles in a couple of weeks. In patients with AIDS, however, there is often prolonged infection, which may also be associated with abdominal pain, steatorrhoea and low-grade fever.

DIAGNOSIS

The diagnosis is usually made by seeing the characteristic ova, 24 × 15 μm in size, in the stools. Sometimes parasites may be seen in jejunal biopsies as 20 μm blue inclusions in the enterocyte cytoplasm (Goodgame, 1996).

TREATMENT

This infection often responds to therapy with one double-strength tablet (160/800 mg) of trimethoprim–sulphamethoxazole twice daily for 10 days. Maintenance therapy is often needed in patients with AIDS.

Sarcocystis species

Human intestinal sarcocystosis (= sarcosporidiosis) rarely follows ingestion of undercooked infected beef (*S. bovihominis*) or pork (*S. suihominis*). Parasites invade the mucosal cells, transform into gametes, then fertilize with oocyst formation and minimal host reaction. Infection is generally characterized by transient fever, vomiting and diarrhoea, which require no treatment. It is possible that infection may rarely cause severe necrotizing enteritis (Bunyaratvej *et al.*, 1982).

HELMINTH INFECTIONS

Worms of the three major groups, nematodes (roundworms), trematodes (flukes) and cestodes (tapeworms) infect the gastrointestinal tract, with some of them affecting primarily the small bowel (Table 19.3). However, many of these worms migrate through other parts of the body at some stage during their life cycle. Thus, hookworm larvae penetrate the skin and pass via the blood stream and the lungs to the small bowel where they develop into adult worms. Conversely, cysts of *Trichinella spiralis* are ingested and mature in the small intestine into adult worms, which in turn produce newborn larvae that seed the muscles via the blood stream. Then there are some worms, such as the schistosomes, which produce lesions in both the small and large intestines.

In contrast to protozoa and all other infectious agents, most worms are not able to multiply in the human host. Whereas one *Giardia* cyst can release several trophozoites, which multiply many times to produce enormous numbers of parasites, one hookworm larva or one *Ascaris* egg can only become one adult worm. This has several implications. Firstly, many worm infections have a limited life span. Secondly, once a person has left an endemic area, the worm numbers cannot increase. Finally, when treating patients with worm infections, it is often necessary only to reduce the worm burden rather than eradicate infection, since severity of disease is generally proportional to the worm burden.

Table 19.3 *Major helminthic parasites of the gastrointestinal tract*

Roundworms
Ancylostoma duodenale[a]
Angiostrongylus costaricensis[b]
Anisakis species[b]
Ascaris lumbricoides[a]
Capillaria philippinensis[a]
Enterobius vermicularis
Necator americanus[a]
Strongyloides stercoralis[a]
Trichinella spiralis[a]
Trichuris trichiura
Flukes
Echinostoma species[a]
Fasciolopsis buski[a]
Heterophyes heterophyes[a]
Metagonimus yokogawai[a]
Schistosoma japonicum[b]
Schistosoma mansoni[b]
Tapeworms
Diphyllobothrium latum[a]
Hymenolepis diminuta[a]
Hymenolepis nana[a]
Taenia saginata[a]
Taenia solium[a]

[a]Only or primarily involves the small bowel, and is discussed in this chapter.
[b]Involves both the small bowel and other parts of the gastrointestinal tract, and is discussed in this chapter.

Hookworm infection

EPIDEMIOLOGY

Ancylostoma duodenale and *Necator americanus* are spread widely throughout the tropics and subtropics with hundreds of millions being infected. Humans are the reservoir of infection. Infection is most prevalent in areas where sanitation is poor and people walk barefoot.

LIFE CYCLE

Infection occurs when infective larvae on the ground penetrate the intact skin and pass via the blood stream to the lungs, where they break into the alveolar spaces, ascend the airways, are swallowed and move to the small bowel where they mature. Adult worms, about 1 cm long, attach to the mucosa and may live for several years. Egg excretion begins 3–6 weeks after skin penetration. Ova deposited in the faeces hatch larvae, which moult twice over 1–2 weeks to become infective larvae.

PATHOLOGY

A mild inflammatory infiltrate together with haemorrhage develops in the mucosa around the sites of worm attachment. Hookworms suck blood; the average daily blood loss for *A. duodenale* is about 0.2 mL per worm compared to 0.03 mL for *N. americanus*. Whether or not hookworm infection results in disease depends on the one hand upon the worm burden, which determines the amount of blood loss, and on the other, the patient's nutritional status, which modifies the ability to replace lost blood.

CLINICAL FEATURES

The majority of people with chronic light infections are asymptomatic. Those with heavy worm burdens, particularly if they are malnourished, develop iron-deficiency anaemia and hypoalbuminaemia with their attendant symptoms and signs. Acute infections are sometimes associated with a pruritic rash, where larvae penetrate the skin, or pulmonary infiltrates with eosinophilia reflecting migration of larvae through the lungs.

DIAGNOSIS

Eggs $40 \times 60\ \mu m$ in size can be detected in faecal smears. The intensity of infection should be quantified as disease is more likely if there are more than 2000 eggs per gram of faeces.

TREATMENT

Hookworm disease can be treated with one of the agents indicated in Table 19.4. Light infections in asymptomatic individuals do not really need to be treated, particularly if they live in an endemic area and are likely to be reinfected. Patients with anaemia may need iron and protein supplements, or, rarely, blood transfusion.

There are two other species of hookworm that sometimes produce intestinal infections. *A. ceylanicum* is a parasite of dogs that is able to produce patent infections in humans similar to those caused by *A. duodenale. A. caninum* is the common dog hookworm. It has recently been shown in northern Australia that infection with this parasite can cause eosinophilic enteritis (Prociv and Croese, 1996). Larvae infect humans in the usual way and some develop into adult worms in the small and large bowel, but they are infertile and eggs are not passed in the stools. Clinically, patients present with abdominal pain and diarrhoea. Severe infections may cause intestinal obstruction that requires a laparotomy. Diagnosis is difficult but worms are sometimes seen on endoscopy. If recognized, the infection usually responds to mebendazole or albendazole.

Table 19.4 *Drugs used in the treatment of roundworm (nematode) infections*

	Albendazole	Ivermectin	Levamisole	Mebendazole	Pyrantel	Thiabendazole
Ascariasis	2–5 years: 200 mg once $>$ 5 years: 400 mg once	0.2 mg/kg once	5 mg/kg once	100 mg twice daily for 1 day	10 mg/kg once	
Hookworm infection	400 mg daily for 2 days	0.2 mg/kg once	5 mg/kg once	100 mg twice daily for 3 days	10 mg/kg once	
Strongyloidiasis	400 mg daily for 3 or 21 days	0.2 mg/kg once		100 mg daily for 21 days		25 mg/kg twice daily for 3 days
Trichinosis[a]	200 mg daily for 7 days					25 mg/kg daily for 7 days
Trichostrongyliasis	400 mg once[b]	0.2 mg/kg once[b]	2.5 mg/kg once			

[a]Intestinal phase only.
[b]Effective in animals but not approved for use in humans.

Angiostrongylus costaricensis

This parasite, also called *Parastrongylus costaricensis*, is restricted to parts of Central and South America. Infection is acquired by ingestion of slugs, usually contaminating vegetables. Rats are the usual definitive hosts and slugs are intermediate hosts. Worms reside in the mesenteric blood vessels in the ileo-caecal region. They may produce fever, abdominal pain and an abdominal mass, an illness which may be mistaken for Crohn's disease (Liacouras *et al.*, 1993). Eggs, often surrounded by a granulomatous inflammatory reaction and a necrotizing arteritis, are found in the ileum and adjacent large bowel, but neither eggs nor larvae are usually seen in human faeces. There is no proven satisfactory treatment. It may be reasonable to try repeated doses of mebendazole (Terada *et al.*, 1993) or albendazole.

Anisakis and *Pseudoterranova* species

These worms occur world-wide. They are acquired by ingestion of infected, raw saltwater fish. They may be found in the lumen or the mucosa of the stomach and the small bowel. They may cause abdominal pain. Occasionally patients have urticaria or an anaphylactic reaction. Sometimes they are seen on gastroduodenoscopy. These worms are immature, hence eggs are not produced. There is no satisfactory treatment for anisakiasis other than endoscopic or surgical removal when required (Bouree *et al.*, 1995).

Ascaris lumbricoides

EPIDEMIOLOGY

The common roundworm is widespread in the tropics and subtropics with over one billion people being infected. Humans are the only reservoir infection. Infection is most common in areas where sanitation is poor, particularly in regions where human faeces are used as a fertilizer. Infection is acquired by ingestion of contaminated food. The eggs are highly resistant and may survive in the soil for months. Development of the embryo within the egg to the larval stage occurs during moist conditions, so transmission occurs mostly during the rainy seasons.

LIFE CYCLE

When eggs are ingested, larvae hatch in the small bowel, but then penetrate the intestinal mucosa and pass via the blood stream to the lungs. Here they break into the alveolar spaces, ascend the airways, are swallowed and return to the small bowel where they mature. The adult worms, 15–35 cm long, dwell within the gut lumen, particularly in the jejunum, and live for 1–2 years. After about 2 months, egg production begins. Under warm, moist shady conditions, eggs excreted in the faeces become infective after 2–3 weeks.

PATHOLOGY

There is usually little reaction to migrating larvae but sometimes granulomatous inflammation develops around larvae in the lungs. Adult worms in the small bowel rarely produce any pathological changes.

CLINICAL FEATURES

Most persons with small worm loads are either asymptomatic or have vague, ill-defined abdominal discomfort. When many worms are present, they may gather into a bolus, which can cause intestinal obstruction, especially in young children. Whether or not ascarids are associated with subnutrition is controversial. Occasionally worms wander into aberrant sites, such as the bile duct (where they may cause obstructive jaundice) or the pancreatic ducts (where they may precipitate pancreatitis). Pulmonary infiltrates with eosinophilia may sometimes be seen, usually in areas where transmission is seasonal.

DIAGNOSIS

Female worms produce an enormous number of eggs, 45×65 μm in size, so infection is easily diagnosed with a simple smear of faeces. Occasionally, adult worms are passed spontaneously.

TREATMENT

Any person with intestinal ascariasis should be treated with one of the drugs listed in Table 19.4. In children thought to have early intestinal obstruction due to ascariasis, a trial of conservative management with nasogastric suction, and fluid and electrolyte replacement, is warranted before laparotomy. If available, piperazine should be given as it paralyses the worms and may aid their passage under the action of peristalsis; it can be given as a syrup through a nasogastric tube. Alternatively, the administration of 15–30 mL Gastrografin (diatrizoate meglumine 66 per cent and diatrizoate sodium 10 per cent) through a nasogastric tube has been advocated for partial bowel obstruction. Gastrografin is hyperosmolar and accumulation of fluid around the worm mass may lead to their separation (Khuroo, 1996).

Capillaria philippinensis

This worm is generally restricted to the Philippines and Thailand. Infection is acquired by ingestion of infected, raw, freshwater fish. Worms are partly embedded in the mucosa of the small bowel and may produce abdominal pain, diarrhoea and malabsorption. *C. philippinensis* is unusual in that, like *S. stercoralis*, it is able to replicate within infected humans. The diagnosis is made by finding eggs in the stools. Untreated severe infections may be fatal. Infection generally responds to treatment with 100–200 mg mebendazole or albendazole daily for 10–20 days (Lee *et al.*, 1993; Grencis and Cooper, 1996).

Strongyloides stercoralis

EPIDEMIOLOGY

Strongyloidiasis is common in tropical and some temperate areas with tens or hundreds of millions of people being infected. Humans are the prime reservoir of infection. Conditions favouring the transmission of this parasite are similar to those applying in hookworm infection.

LIFE CYCLE

Like hookworms, *S. stercoralis* larvae penetrate the intact skin and pass to the gastrointestinal tract via the blood stream and the lungs, or possibly directly through the connective tissues. In the small bowel, larvae burrow into a tunnel in the enterocytes, mature and produce eggs by parthenogenesis. The eggs hatch in the lumen of the small bowel and are passed in the stools as first-stage larvae, beginning 3 weeks or so after the acquisition of infection. In the soil, these larvae either moult twice to become infective larvae or develop into free-living adult worms, which in turn produce eggs that ultimately develop into infective larvae. Unlike most worms, however, *S. stercoralis* can replicate within the human host. Some first-stage larvae in the bowel lumen appear to moult twice to become infective larvae, which then either penetrate the intestinal mucosa or the perianal skin, and undergo the usual migration. This process is called autoinfection and allows infection to persist for many years.

PATHOLOGY

Occasionally there is a mild inflammatory reaction around worms in the intestinal mucosa and, in mild infections, there is no partial villous atrophy. In immunocompetent individuals, the worm and host come to relative terms with each other and the infection is contained with the prime clinical manifestations limited to the skin and gut. If a person becomes immunosuppressed for one reason or another, then massive multiplication of worms occurs with dissemination throughout the body, often with concomitant septicaemia, which may terminate in death.

CLINICAL FEATURES

Many patients with strongyloidiasis are asymptomatic. Some patients complain of stationary urticarial weals located particularly around the waist and on the buttocks that recur at irregular intervals. Others have a transient pathognomonic urticarial rash called larva currens that migrates in a serpiginous fashion at the rate of several centimetres per hour. Gastrointestinal features include mild diarrhoea, abdominal pain and pruritus ani. In severe infections there may be malabsorption or a protein-losing enteropathy. Disseminated strongyloidiasis in immunosuppressed patients is characterized by intestinal obstruction, Gram-negative septicaemia, pneumonia and meningitis. Over 50 per cent of patients with such massive, overwhelming infections die.

DIAGNOSIS

Strongyloidiasis is generally diagnosed by finding first-stage larvae, 20×400 μm in size, either in the stools or in duodenal aspirates or biopsies. It is often difficult to find larvae in faeces as parasite loads are usually low; consequently, multiple specimens may need to be examined. In disseminated infections, larvae may be found in other body fluids or in biopsied tissues.

TREATMENT

The aim of treatment is to eradicate infection to prevent recurrence of disease due to autoinfection. Unfortunately, this parasite is relatively resistant to treatment. Ivermectin or benzimidazole agents, such as thiabendazole or albendazole, may be tried (Table 19.4). If a short course fails to eradicate infection in an immunosuppressed patient, then it is worth trying a 4-week course of therapy with mebendazole or albendazole. If such a patient is still infected, then a single dose of thiabendazole or albendazole should be given each month (Grove, 1996).

Trichinella spiralis

EPIDEMIOLOGY

T. spiralis is found throughout the world apart from Australia and New Zealand. There are a number of related species that are found in Africa, and temperate and Arctic zones. Humans are incidental hosts. Parasites are widespread in pigs, rats, horses, bears, hyenas and panthers as well as birds in the case of *T. pseudospiralis*. Epidemics occur when families or small communities consume trichinous meat from a common source.

LIFE CYCLE

Infection is acquired by ingestion of cysts in undercooked meat. Larvae hatch in the stomach and pass into the small intestine, where they invade the columnar epithelium at the bases of the villi and develop over 2 weeks into adult worms about 2–3 mm in length; they are obligate intracellular parasites occupying the cytoplasm of a row of enterocytes. The fertilized female adult worms produce newborn larvae, which seed the muscles via the blood stream; here they develop over several weeks into cysts which remain viable for several years (Capo and Despommier, 1996). The adult worms in the bowel are expelled in the faeces after a few weeks.

PATHOLOGY

When worms are in the bowel, the small intestine shows a mild partial villous atrophy, and an inflammatory infiltrate of polymorphs, eosinophils and mononuclear cells in the mucosa and submucosa. Skeletal muscle fibres host coiled worms, each surrounded by a cyst wall and an inflammatory infiltrate.

CLINICAL FEATURES

Most infections are subclinical with symptoms only developing if there is ingestion of a heavy inoculum of cysts. Gastrointestinal symptoms are prominent in the first week or two of the infection, with patients complaining of diarrhoea, abdominal pain and vomiting. Invasion of muscles is associated with fever, myositis and periorbital oedema. These systemic symptoms peak after 2–3 weeks, then slowly subside.

DIAGNOSIS

It is usually impossible to diagnose trichinosis during the intestinal phase of infection. Definitive diagnosis later in the illness is by finding worms on muscle biopsy.

TREATMENT

There is no satisfactory treatment for established trichinosis when the muscles are already seeded with worms, although thiabendazole or albendazole, which are active against intestinal but not muscle worms, is often given. In the rare instance where a patient is known to have ingested trichinous meat within the past week or so, thiabendazole or albendazole should be administered daily for 1 week (Table 19.4).

Trichostrongylus species

A number of species of *Trichostrongylus* are found throughout the world where they infect humans, sheep, goats and cattle. Infection is usually acquired by ingestion of infective larvae. The worms live embedded in the mucosa of the small bowel and eggs are passed in the faeces. In the soil, larvae hatch and moult twice to become infective forms. Infections are usually asymptomatic but may be associated with abdominal pain. The diagnosis is made by finding eggs in the stools. Infection may be treated with one of the drugs listed in Table 19.4.

Echinostoma species

A number of species of *Echinostoma* are found in tropical countries, particularly Southeast Asia, and infect various birds and mammals. Humans are infected by eating undercooked second intermediate hosts (snails and fish); adult worms develop in the small bowel. Eggs passed in the stools hatch larvae (miracidia), which infect certain species of snails. Infected snails release a new form of larva (cercaria), which infects other large snails and fish, and develops into a metacercaria. Light infections are usually asymptomatic but heavy infections may cause abdominal pain, nausea and diarrhoea. The diagnosis is established by finding eggs in the stools. Praziquantel is the drug of choice (Table 19.5) (Liu and Harinasuta, 1996).

Fasciolopsis buski

This parasite is found in Southeast Asia, China and the eastern part of the Indian subcontinent. It infects both humans and pigs. Infection is acquired by ingestion of plants, usually watercress, water chestnuts or water bamboo shoots, contaminated with cysts containing

Table 19.5 *Drugs used in the treatment of fluke (trematode) infections*

	Praziquantel	Oxamniquine
Echinostomiasis	15 mg/kg once	
Fasciolopsiasis	15 mg/kg once	
Heterophyiasis	15 mg/kg once or twice	
Metagonimiasis	15 mg/kg once	
Schistosomiasis japonica	30 mg/kg repeated 6 hours later	
Schistosomiasis mansoni		
Africa:	30 mg/kg repeated 6 hours later	15 mg/kg twice daily for 2 days
South America	30 mg/kg repeated 6 hours later	15 mg/kg once

metacercariae. These hatch in the duodenum and mature over 3 months. When eggs are passed in the stools, they hatch miracidia, which infect snails. Subsequently, cercariae escape from the snail and encyst on water plants. Adult worms, which live for about 1 year, attach to the small bowel mucosa, especially in the duodenum, where they may cause inflammation and ulceration. Light infections are usually asymptomatic, but heavy infections, often with more than 500 worms, may cause abdominal pain, nausea, vomiting and diarrhoea. Extreme cases may have a protein-losing enteropathy. The diagnosis is made by finding characteristic eggs in the stools. Praziquantel is the drug of choice (Table 19.5) (Liu and Harinasuta, 1996).

Heterophyes heterophyes

This fluke is found in eastern Asia and the Middle East. It infects humans, dogs, cats and foxes. Human infection is acquired by ingestion of undercooked infected fish. Worms mature in the small bowel and attach to the mucosa, sometimes causing ulceration. Eggs passed in the stools hatch larvae, which infect freshwater snails. These release cercariae, which infect various freshwater fish in which they develop into infective metacercariae. Symptoms may include anorexia, nausea and abdominal pain. The diagnosis is made by finding eggs in the stools. The infection usually responds to treatment with praziquantel (Table 19.5) (Liu and Harinasuta, 1996).

Metagonimus yokogawai

This worm is found in eastern Asia. Its life cycle, clinical manifestations, diagnosis and treatment are similar to those of *H. heterophyes.*

Schistosoma japonicum

EPIDEMIOLOGY

This fluke is found in parts of China, Indonesia (Sulawesi) and the Philippines. A related parasite, *S. mekongi*, occurs in Laos and Cambodia. *S. japonicum* infects humans, cows, pigs, water buffalo, rats and various other animals. Infection is only prevalent in areas where susceptible snail intermediate hosts of the genus *Oncomelania* are also found.

LIFE CYCLE

Infection is usually acquired when walking in wet paddy fields. Infective larvae (cercariae) penetrate the intact skin and pass via the blood stream to the superior and inferior mesenteric venous systems, where they mature over 6 weeks or so and live for 5–10 years. Fertilized female adult worms produce eggs, many of which are deposited in the mucosa of the gastrointestinal tract including the small bowel, although this is relatively lightly infected. Others embolize to the liver. Some of the eggs in the bowel mucosa breach the epithelium and are passed in the faeces. When eggs are passed in the stools, miracidia hatch and invade susceptible snails. These in turn release cercariae that are able to infect human and other definitive hosts directly.

PATHOLOGY

Macroscopic changes seen in the bowel include mucosal hyperplasia, pseudopolyposis, ulceration and thickening of the intestinal wall. In severe, long-standing disease, bands of fibrosis may be seen in the portal tracts of the liver. Microscopically, the characteristic lesion is a granulomatous inflammatory lesion surrounding each egg. Occasionally, such granulomas are found in the brain or spinal cord.

CLINICAL FEATURES

Acute infection may cause Katayama fever. This usually begins 4–6 weeks after exposure and is characterized by fever, headache, myalgias and an urticarial rash. Chronic infections are commonly asymptomatic. Patients with heavy infections may have non-specific abdominal discomfort and diarrhoea. Large numbers of eggs in the liver cause presinusoidal portal hypertension with splenomegaly and ascites.

DIAGNOSIS

The diagnosis is usually made by finding eggs in faeces or in a biopsy of bowel (usually rectum) or liver. Ultrasound or computed tomography (CT) scanning may be useful in defining macroscopic liver disease.

TREATMENT

Praziquantel is the only drug with significant activity against *S. japonicum* (Table 19.5) (Davis, 1996). The aim should be to reduce egg output by at least 90 per cent of pretreatment levels. Patients with severe portal hypertension may benefit from propranolol prophylaxis, sclerotherapy of bleeding varices or decompressive surgery (Elliott, 1996).

Schistosoma mansoni

EPIDEMIOLOGY

This fluke is found in many countries in Africa, in Madagascar, parts of the Arabian peninsula and in

Brazil, Surinam, Venezuela and a number of Caribbean islands (Elliott, 1996). Humans are the prime reservoir of infection, although a number of animal species can be infected. The snail intermediate hosts belong to the genus *Biomphalaria*. Infection is common where sanitation is poor and people come in contact with infected water as in rivers, streams and dams.

LIFE CYCLE AND PATHOLOGY

These are similar to that described for *S. japonicum*.

CLINICAL FEATURES

Patients with light infections are generally asymptomatic. Heavy infections may be associated with abdominal discomfort. The most important complication is periportal hepatic fibrosis with portal hypertension manifesting as hepatosplenomegaly and ascites. Embolization of eggs to the lungs may lead to cor pulmonale. A mild glomerulonephritis may follow deposition of schistosomal antigens in the kidneys. A myelopathy with paraparesis may result from egg deposition in the spinal cord.

DIAGNOSIS

This is achieved by demonstration of the characteristic eggs in faeces or in a biopsy.

TREATMENT

Praziquantel is the drug of choice but oxamniquine is also effective (Table 19.5) (Davis, 1996).

Diphyllobothrium latum

EPIDEMIOLOGY

The fish tapeworm has been reported from parts of Europe, Asia and the Americas, but most transmission occurs in Russia (Baily, 1996a). Humans are the prime reservoir of infection of *D. latum*. There are a number of other species of *Diphyllobothrium* that infect various birds, bears and marine mammals that occasionally infect humans. Infection occurs when people eat raw or undercooked infected freshwater fish, particularly pike, perch and burbot (Schantz, 1996).

LIFE CYCLE

Humans are infected by ingesting undercooked, infected fish. The larva attaches to the mucosa of the small bowel, develops into an adult worm, which may grow up to 10 m in length, and after 3–5 weeks begins to produce eggs. Adult worms may live for 10 years or more. Eggs passed in the faeces into fresh water each hatch a larva (coracidium), which infects a microscopic crustacean (*Cyclops* or *Diaptomus*) in which it develops into a procercoid larva. Infected crustaceans are in turn ingested by freshwater fishes in which the procercoid larva migrates to the muscles and becomes a plerocercoid larva; this process is repeated when small infected fish are eaten by larger fish.

PATHOLOGY

The worm is not invasive and there is little pathological damage other than where the head of the worm attaches to the small bowel mucosa.

CLINICAL FEATURES

Most patients are asymptomatic, although the worm may cause abdominal discomfort. The worm is composed of individual sections called proglottids, which may be passed in the stools and are seen by the patient as semimotile, yellow bodies 10 × 20 mm in size. In the past, some patients have developed pernicious anaemia as a consequence of the worms competing for vitamin B_{12}.

DIAGNOSIS

The diagnosis is made by finding the characteristic eggs, 60 × 40 μm in size, in the stools.

TREATMENT

Infection may be treated with praziquantel or niclosamide (Table 19.6). Diphyllobothriasis may be prevented by ensuring that fish is cooked adequately.

Hymenolepis species

Infection with the dwarf tapeworm, *Hymenolepis nana*, is most common in the tropics; infection is generally acquired by ingestion of eggs. They invade the small bowel mucosa and encyst within a villus, developing into adult worms 3–4 cm long after a month, then eggs are excreted in the stools. However, this worm is unique among cestodes in that autoinfection often occurs in the bowel or a person may be reinfected by their own eggs. Infection may cause anorexia or abdominal discomfort. The diagnosis is made by finding the characteristic eggs, 30–50 μm in size, in the stools. Praziquantel and niclosamide are generally effective (Table 19.6).

Hymenolepis diminuta, the rat tapeworm, is primarily an infection of rodents with fleas as intermediate hosts. Infection is usually acquired by ingestion of infected fleas. Adult worms grow to 9 cm in length and produce eggs 80 μm in size. The clinical manifestations,

Table 19.6 *Drugs used in the treatment of tapeworm (cestode) infections*

	Praziquantel	Niclosamide
Diphyllobothriasis	10 mg/kg once	2 g[a] once
Hymenolepiasis	40 mg/kg once	2 g[a] daily for 7 days
Taeniasis saginata	10 mg/kg once	2 g[a] once
Taeniasis solium (intestinal phase only)	10 mg/kg once	2 g[a] once

[a]< 2 years, 0.5 g; 2–6 years, 1 g; > 6 years, 2 g.

diagnosis and treatment are similar to those described for *H. nana*.

Taenia saginata

EPIDEMIOLOGY

The beef tapeworm is found in most parts of the world. Man is the only definitive host and cattle are the intermediate hosts. Infection occurs where sanitation is poor and undercooked beef is eaten (Schantz, 1996).

LIFE CYCLE

Humans are infected by ingesting undercooked beef containing small cystic worms up to 1 cm in size called cysticerci. The head of the cysticercus everts its head and attaches to the mucosa of the small bowel, develops into an hermaphroditic adult worm, which may grow 5–10 m in length, and after 2–4 months begins to produce eggs. Adult worms may live for 10 years or more. Eggs passed in the faeces are ingested by grazing cattle; a larva hatches and passes to the tissues, especially the muscles, where it develops into a cysticercus.

PATHOLOGY

The worm is not invasive and there is little pathological damage other than where the head of the worm attaches to the small bowel mucosa.

CLINICAL FEATURES

Most patients are asymptomatic, but others may complain of vague abdominal pain, nausea and distension. Sometimes, individual proglottids or groups of proglottids called segments are observed in the stools.

DIAGNOSIS

A diagnosis of taeniasis can be made by finding the distinctive eggs 30–40 μm in size in the stools but it is not possible to differentiate those of *T. saginata* from those of *T. solium*. The definitive diagnosis of taeniasis saginata relies on finding typical morphology on examination of proglottids 5 × 12–20 mm in size.

TREATMENT

Infection may be treated with praziquantel, the drug of choice, or niclosamide (Table 19.6). Infection is prevented by ensuring that all beef is properly cooked.

Taenia solium

EPIDEMIOLOGY

The pork tapeworm is found world-wide apart from Australia and adjacent regions of Oceania. Man is the only definitive host and pigs are the intermediate hosts. Infection occurs where sanitation is poor and undercooked pork is eaten (Schantz, 1996).

LIFE CYCLE

In many respects, this is similar to that of *T. saginata* except that pigs rather than cattle are intermediate hosts. However, whereas *T. saginata* is found only in the tapeworm form in humans, *T. solium* may occur as both tapeworms in the bowel and as cysticerci in the tissues. The latter occurs when eggs are ingested, usually in vegetables or ground fruits that have been contaminated with human faeces. A larva hatches in the small bowel and passes through the mucosa to the blood stream and seeds the tissues, particularly the muscles, brain and eye.

PATHOLOGY

Intestinal tapeworms produce similar effects to *T. saginata*. Cysticerci in the tissues that are neither actively growing or degenerating elicit little host response.

CLINICAL FEATURES

Patients with *T. solium* intestinal tapeworms have similar symptoms to those who harbour *T. saginata*. Cysticerci are often asymptomatic. Those in the subcutaneous tissues are of only cosmetic importance. However, cysts in the brain may cause epilepsy or the features of a space-occupying lesion. Cysticerci in the eye may cause visual disturbance.

DIAGNOSIS

T. solium intestinal tapeworm infection is diagnosed by finding eggs in the stools but they cannot be differentiated from those of *T. saginata*. Species identification relies on examination of proglottids. Imaging techniques including plain radiographs (which show calcified lesions), and CT and magnetic resonance imaging scanning demonstrate lesions; serology may lend specificity to the diagnosis.

TREATMENT

T. solium intestinal tapeworms are treated in the same manner as *T. saginata* (Table 19.6). It is no longer recommended that a purgative be given as well as an anthelmintic (Baily, 1996a). Symptomatic treatment of neurocysticercosis may require administration of antiepileptic drugs. Patients with calcified lesions are unlikely to benefit from anthelmintic treatment. Those with growing cysticerci may benefit from treatment with 50 mg/kg praziquantel daily for 15 days, but this may be associated with exacerbation of inflammation and cerebral oedema, which may be controlled by concomitant administration of corticosteroids. Alternatively, 15 mg/kg albendazole daily for 2–4 weeks may be tried (Baily, 1996b). Intestinal taeniasis solium can be prevented by avoiding eating undercooked pork. Prevention of cysticercosis is more problematic unless consumption of salads and unwashed ground fruits is proscribed.

REFERENCES

Adam, R.D. 1991: The biology of Giardia spp. *Microbiological Reviews* 55, 706–32.

Baily, G.G. 1996a: Intestinal cestodes. In Cook, G.C. (ed.) *Manson's tropical diseases*, 20th edn. London: W.B. Saunders, 1477–85.

Baily, G.G. 1996b: Cysticercosis. In Cook, G.C. (ed.) *Manson's tropical diseases*, 20th edn. London: W.B. Saunders, 1508–16.

Bouree, P., Paugam, A., Petithory, J.C. 1995: Anisakidosis: report of 25 cases and review of the literature. *Comparative Immunology, Microbiology and Infectious Diseases* 18, 75–84.

Bunyaratvej, S., Bunyawongwiroj, P., Nitiyanant, P. 1982: Human intestinal sarcosporidiosis – report of 6 cases. *American Journal of Tropical Medicine and Hygiene* 31, 36–41.

Capo, V., Despommier, D.D. 1996: Clinical aspects of infection with Trichinella spp. *Clinical Microbiology Reviews* 9, 47–54.

Connor, D.H., Chandler, F.W., Schwartz, D.A., Manz, H.J., Lack, E.E. (eds) 1997: *Pathology of infectious diseases*. Stamford: Appleton and Lange.

Croft, S.L., Williams, J., McGowan, I. 1997: Intestinal microsporidiosis. *Seminars in Gastrointestinal Diseases* 8, 45–55.

Davis, A. 1996: Schistosomiasis. In Cook, G.C. (ed.) *Manson's tropical diseases*, 20th edn. London: W.B. Saunders, 1413–56.

Doumbo, O., Rossignol, J.F., Pichard, E. *et al.* 1997: Nitazoxanide in the treatment of cryptosporidial diarrhea and other intestinal parasitic infections associated with AIDS in tropical Africa. *American Journal of Tropical Medicine and Hygiene* 56, 637–9.

Dupont, H.L., Chappell, C.L., Sterling, C.R., Okhuysen, P.C., Rose, J.B., Jakubowski, W. 1995: The infectivity of Cryptosporidium parvum in healthy volunteers. *New England Journal of Medicine* 332, 855–9.

Elliott, D.E. 1996: Schistosomiasis: pathophysiology, diagnosis and treatment. *Gastroenterology Clinics of North America* 25, 599–625.

Farthing, M.J.G. 1996: Giardiasis. *Gastroenterology Clinics of North America* 25, 493–515.

Goodgame, R.W. 1996: Understanding intestinal spore-forming protozoa: Cryptosporidia, Microsporidia, Isospora and Cyclospora. *Annals of Internal Medicine* 124, 429–41.

Greenberg, P.D., Cello, J.P. 1996: Treatment of severe diarrhea caused by Cryptosporidium parvum with oral bovine immunoglobulin concentrate in patients with AIDS. *Journal of Acquired Immune Deficiency Syndromes and Human Retrovirology* 13, 348–54.

Greenberg, P.D. Koch, J., Cello, J.P. 1996: Diagnosis of Cryptosporidium parvum in patients with severe diarrhea and AIDS. *Digestive Diseases and Sciences* 41, 2286–90.

Grencis, R.K., Cooper, E.S. 1996: Enterobius, Trichuris, Capillaria, and hookworm including Ancylostoma caninum. *Gastroenterology Clinics of North America* 25, 579–97.

Grove, D.I. 1996: Human strongyloidiasis. *Advances in Parasitology* 38, 251–309.

Herwaldt, B.L., Ackers, M.L. 1997: An outbreak in 1996 of cyclosporiasis associated with imported raspberries: The Cyclospora Working Group. *New England Journal of Medicine* 336, 1548–65.

Hoepelman, A.I. 1996: Current therapeutic approaches to cryptosporidiosis in immunocompromised patients. *Journal of Antimicrobial Chemotherapy* 37, 871–80.

Hoge, C.W., Schlim, D.R., Ghimire, M. *et al.* 1995: Placebo-controlled trial of co-trimoxazole for Cyclospora infections among travellers and foreign residents in Nepal. *Lancet* 345, 691–3.

Khuroo, M.S. 1996: Ascariasis. *Gastroenterology Clinics of North America* 25, 553–77.

Lee, S.H., Hong, S.T., Chai, J.Y. *et al.* 1993: A case of intestinal capillariasis in the Republic of Korea. *American Journal of Tropical Medicine and Hygiene* 48, 542–6.

Kotler, D.P., Orenstein, J.M. 1998: Clinical syndromes associated with microsporidiosis. *Advances in Parasitology* 40, 321–49.

Liacouras, C.A., Bell, L.M., Aljabi, M.C., Piccoli, D.A. 1993: Angiostrongylus costaricensis enterocolitis mimics Crohn's disease. *Journal of Pediatric Gastroenterology and Nutrition* 16, 203–7.

Lindsay, J.S., Dubey, J.P., Blagburn, B.L. 1997: Biology of Isospora spp. from humans, non-human primates, and domestic animals. *Clinical Microbiology Reviews* 10, 19–34.

Liu, L.X., Harinasuta, K.T. 1996: Liver and intestinal flukes. *Gastroenterology Clinics of North America* 25, 627–36.

Mackenzie, W.R., Hoxie, N.J., Proctor, M.E. *et al.* 1994: A massive outbreak in Milwaukee of Cryptosporidium infection transmitted through the public water supply. *New England Journal of Medicine* 331, 161–7.

Mackenzie, W.R., Schell, W.L., Blair, K.A. *et al.* 1995: Massive outbreak of waterborne Cryptosporidium infection in Milwaukee, Wisconsin: recurrence of illness and risk of secondary transmission. *Clinical Infectious Diseases* 21, 57–62.

Neill, M.A., Rice, S.K., Ahmad, N.V., Flanagan, T.P. 1996: Cryptosporidiosis: an unrecognized caused of diarrhea in elderly patients. *Clinical Infectious Diseases* 22, 168–70.

Orenstein, J.M. 1997: Isosporiasis. In Connor, D.H., Chandler, F.W., Schwartz, D.A., Manz, H.J., Lack, E.E. (eds) *Pathology of infectious diseases*. Stamford: Appleton and Lange, 1185–90.

Orihel, T.C., Ash, L.R. 1995: *Parasites in human tissues*. Chicago: ASCP Press.

Ortega, Y.R., Adam, R.D. 1997: Giardia: an update. *Clinical Infectious Diseases* 25, 545–50.

Ortega, Y.R., Sterling, C.R., Gilman, R.H. 1998: Cyclospora caretanensis. *Advances in Parasitology* 40, 399–418.

Prociv, P., Croese, J. 1996: Human enteric infection with Ancylostoma caninum: hookworms reappraised in the light of a 'new' zoonosis. *Acta Tropica* 62, 23–44.

Schantz, P.M. 1996: Tapeworms (cestodiasis). *Gastroenterology Clinics of North America* 25, 637–53.

Sharpstone, D., Rowbottom, A., Francis, N., Tovey, G., Ellis, D., Barrett, M., Gazzard, B. 1997: Thalidomide: a novel therapy for microsporidiosis. *Gastroenterology* 112, 1823–9.

Soave, R. 1996: Cyclospora: an overview. *Clinical Infectious Diseases* 23, 429–35.

Soule, J.B., Jalverson, A.L., Becker, R.B., Pistole, M.C., Orenstein, J.M. 1997: A patient with AIDS and untreated Encephalitozoon (Septata) intestinalis microsporidiosis leading to small bowel perforation. Response to albendazole. *Archives of Pathology and Laboratory Medicine* 121, 880–7.

Terada, M., Kiro, H., Akyol, C., Sano, M. 1993: Effects of mebendazole on Angiostrongylus costaricensis in mice, with special reference to timing of treatment. *Parasitology Research* 79, 441–3.

Weber, R., Bryan, R.T., Schwartz, D.A., Owen, R.L. 1994: Human microsporidial infections. *Clinical Microbiology Reviews* 7, 426–61.

20

HIV/AIDS and the small bowel

KELLY PAPANAOUM, DAVID R SHAW, F DYLAN L BARTHOLOMEUSZ

INTRODUCTION

The pandemic of human immunodeficiency virus (HIV) infection continues to create a major impact on global morbidity and mortality. The World Health Organization estimated that, by 1998, over 30 million individuals were infected with HIV and that 11.7 million had died of the acquired immunodeficiency syndrome (AIDS) (UNAIDS, 1998). Nearly 90 per cent of people with HIV infection live in sub-Saharan Africa and Asia, and have little or no access to antiretroviral therapy.

Gastrointestinal disease is an extremely important manifestation of HIV infection, which is symptomatic in the majority of patients. Small intestinal involvement by HIV or enteric opportunistic pathogens often leads to diarrhoea, malnutrition and the severe wasting syndrome characteristic of the late-stage HIV infection or AIDS. Furthermore, the absorption of potent antiretroviral drugs may be compromised in the presence of small bowel disease. AIDS-associated malignancies also frequently develop in the intestinal tract. This chapter reviews the natural history of HIV infections and immunodeficiency, the various opportunistic pathogens and secondary malignancies that affect the small intestine during HIV infection, and their management, malabsorption and wasting, and an approach to the efficient diagnosis and management of small intestinal disease.

NATURAL HISTORY OF HIV INFECTION

Infection by the retrovirus HIV results in an inexorable progressive decline in immune function over many years. The hallmark of progression is the decline in peripheral CD4 lymphocytes. The course of HIV infection may be divided into four stages: primary infection or seroconversion; early immunodeficiency (CD4 counts greater than 500/μL of plasma); intermediate immunodeficiency (CD4 counts 200–500/μL); and advanced immunodeficiency (CD4 counts less than 200/μL), which defines the development of AIDS.

Following initial infection, viral particles are taken up by regional lymph nodes where stimulation of both cellular and humoral responses begins. Within days there is active viral replication, high levels of viraemia, infection of CD4-positive cells and a lymphopenia with reduction in circulating CD4-positive T cells. As well as T cells, a variety of cell types expressing CD4 are infected, including macrophages in the gut and elsewhere. This may be accompanied by a seroconverting illness mimicking infectious mononucleosis. As this acute phase resolves, the level of viraemia dramatically falls. The major mechanism of this drop is by CD8-positive cytotoxic T cells, which cause the lysis of HIV-infected cells and release cytokines that inhibit viral replication in CD4-positive cells.

During the ensuing early phase of HIV infection, patients may be asymptomatic for years. However, there remains a large turnover of virus and CD4-positive cells, mostly occurring within lymphoid tissue. The level of plasma viraemia remains fairly constant within an individual and, when quantified by nucleic acid amplification, can predict the rate of progression towards AIDS (Mellors *et al.*, 1996).

During the middle phase of infection (CD4 count 200–500/μL), subtle features of immunodeficiency, such as herpes zoster and oral candidiasis, can appear. The fall

Table 20.1 *Small intestinal pathogens associated with HIV*

Protozoa
Cryptosporidium parvum
Isospora belli
Microsporidia
Enterocytozoon bieneusi
Encephalitozoon intestinalis
Cyclospora cayatanensis
Giardia lamblia
Leishmania spp.

Helminth
Strongyloides stercoralis

Bacteria
Mycobacterium avium complex
Mycobacterium tuberculosis
Salmonella spp.
Enteroadherent *Escherichia coli*
Campylobacter spp.
Shigella spp.
Bacterial overgrowth

Viruses
HIV
Cytomegalovirus
Adenovirus
Rotavirus
Astrovirus
Coronavirus
Picobirnaviruses
Small round viruses

in CD4-positive T cells accelerates towards the end of this phase as the immune system begins to fail. With advanced immunodeficiency (CD4 < 200/μL), the immune system becomes overwhelmed by the rapidly replicating virus. At this point, particularly when CD4 cell counts fall below 100/μL, major opportunistic infections and HIV-related malignancies develop, which eventually lead to death.

Gastrointestinal cellular immunity is also impaired with the observation of the depletion of CD4 lymphocytes in the lamina propria of the intestinal epithelium and an inverted CD4:CD8 ratio. This decline is often earlier and more severe than that seen in the peripheral blood. CD4+ memory cells (CD45 RO+) are lost earlier than CD4+ naïve cells (CD45 RA+) as in the peripheral circulation. The role of declining humoral immunity is less well defined. A decrease in immunoglobulin A (IgA) plasma cells and mucosal IgA deficiency has been demonstrated by some investigators but not others (Janoff *et al.*, 1994; Benhamou *et al.*, 1995). Response to oral vaccination has shown suboptimal antibody responses, especially if CD4 counts are below 200/μL (Eriksson *et al.*, 1993). Cytokine dysregulation in the small intestinal mucosa has also been shown with increased levels of the pro-inflammatory cytokines interferon-γ (IFN-γ) and interleukin-1β (IL-1β) (McGowan *et al.*, 1994).

Treatment with highly active antiretroviral therapy, when available, has benefited survival and reduced the frequency of secondary infections. The three classes of antiretroviral drugs currently licensed are the nucleoside and non-nucleoside reverse transcriptase inhibitors and the protease inhibitors.

OPPORTUNISTIC INFECTIONS OF THE SMALL INTESTINE

Opportunistic gastrointestinal infections are extremely frequent during HIV infection, particularly during its advanced stages. The range of pathogens that may occur is listed in Table 20.1. Table 20.2 summarizes the treatment of choice for the more common infections encountered.

Table 20.2 *Specific treatment of common infections in HIV (see text for details)*

Infection	Treatment
Protozoal	
Cryptosporidiosis	Paromomycin 500 mg orally 8 hourly for 14 days
Microsporidiosis	Albendazole 400 mg orally twice daily for 14 days
Cyclospora	Trimethoprim–sulphamethoxazole 160/800 mg orally twice daily for 10 days
Isosporiasis	Trimethoprim–sulphamethoxazole 160/800 mg orally four times daily for 10 days, then twice daily for 21 days
Giardiasis	Metronidazole 400 mg orally 8 hourly for 5–7 days
Bacterial	
Mycobacterium avium complex	Clarithromycin 500 mg orally twice daily plus rifabutin 300 mg orally daily plus ethambutol 400 mg orally twice daily – given lifelong
Salmonella/Shigella	Ciprofloxacin 500 mg orally twice daily for 14 days
Campylobacter spp.	Erythromycin 500 mg orally four times daily for 7–14 days
Viral	
Cytomegalovirus	Ganciclovir 5 mg/kg intravenously twice daily for 14–21 days; if intolerant and/or resistant, foscarnet 90 mg/kg intravenously twice daily for 14–21 days

Parasitic infections

CRYPTOSPORIDIOSIS

Cryptosporidial enteric infection is caused by the coccidian protozoal parasite *Cryptosporidium parvum*. It is a common cause of chronic diarrhoea in patients with HIV infection, affecting 10–20 per cent of patients with AIDS in Britain and the USA, and 30–50 per cent in Africa and Asia (Petersen, 1992; Blanshard *et al.*, 1996; Lanjewar *et al.*, 1996). Infection in immunocompetent hosts has also been increasingly recognized, partly due to greater awareness of the organism as a significant cause of diarrhoea. Several large outbreaks have been reported in recent years as a result of contamination of swimming pools and public water supplies (Hayes *et al.*, 1989; Hazen, 1993).

Infection occurs by the ingestion of oocysts from contaminated water, by person to person contact or, less frequently, from infected animals. Transmission of the organism is facilitated by the hardy nature of the oocysts, which can survive in the environment for several months and resist sterilization by routine chlorination and ozone purification processes (Wittner *et al.*, 1993). Furthermore, infection may result after exposure to as few as 10 organisms. After ingestion the oocysts excyst in the small intestine. The newly hatched sporozoites invade the enterocytes and undergo further division, sexual multiplication and then eventual release of oocysts into the intestinal lumen. Oocysts then reinvade the intestinal mucosa to repeat this cycle. Thus, both asexual and sexual phases of the life cycle occur within one host (Ungar, 1995).

The jejunum and ileum are the prime targets of infection; the colon, duodenum and stomach may also be affected. Following an incubation period of 2–14 days, a diarrhoeal illness characterized by voluminous watery stools, cramping epigastric pain, anorexia, nausea and vomiting develops. In immunocompetent hosts the diarrhoea usually lasts between 4 and 20 days. However, patients with advanced HIV infection may have chronic persistent diarrhoea passing up to 17 L daily. Ensuing dehydration, generalized wasting, malabsorption and lactose intolerance are common (Soave and Johnson, 1988). Flanigan *et al.* (1992) defined a relationship between the degree of HIV-related immunosuppression and chronicity of cryptosporidiosis with nearly 90 per cent of patients with CD4 counts below 180 cells/μL developing chronic unremitting diarrhoea. Patients with counts over 180 cells/μL had self-limited disease. Biliary involvement occurs in up to 10 per cent of patients with cryptosporidiosis (Soave and Johnson, 1988).

Microscopic examination of faecal specimens is usually negative for leucocytes and red blood cells. The most widely used method for detection of cryptosporidial oocysts in stool samples is the modified acid-fast stain, performed after concentration of the specimen. The small 4–6 μm oocysts appear red against the green counterstain, distinguishing them from faecal yeasts and debris (Plate 20.1). This provides a sensitivity of detection of approximately 75 per cent when multiple stool specimens are submitted (Greenberg *et al.*, 1996). Other techniques for detection of cryptosporidial oocysts include fluorescent stains, monoclonal and polyclonal immunofluorescence assays, and enzyme immunoassays. These have a similar or better sensitivity to the modified acid-fast stain, although they are more expensive and cumbersome to perform (MacPherson and McQueen, 1993). An *in situ* polymerase chain reaction (PCR) assay has been developed, which has a superior sensitivity (Talal *et al.*, 1997).

Endoscopic intestinal biopsy was shown to detect the organisms in the terminal ileum in 91 per cent of cases compared to 53 per cent from duodenal biopsies, 60 per cent of colonic biopsies and 11 per cent of gastric biopsies (Greenberg *et al.*, 1996). The organisms may be seen on haematoxylin and eosin stains as rounded basophilic excrescences protruding from the luminal border of the enterocytes (Wittner *et al.*, 1993). Their location is intracytoplasmic but extracellular (Plate 20.2a). Small intestinal biopsies may show normal villous architecture, with a normal or only mildly inflamed lamina propria (Genta *et al.*, 1993) (Plate 20.2b). The presence of organisms in the crypts, villous atrophy and crypt hyperplasia are associated with particularly severe clinical infection (Clayton *et al.*, 1994).

Treatment of cryptosporidiosis remains problematic with few agents that are only partially successful in controlling the diarrhoea. Paromomycin, a poorly absorbed aminoglycoside given orally 500 mg three times daily for 14 days results in clinical improvement but eradication is not achieved even with high dosages (Clezy *et al.*, 1991; White *et al.*, 1994; Verdon *et al.*, 1995). Azithromycin has shown activity in sporadic cases, although a recent study found it to be ineffective at a dosage of 500 mg daily (Blanshard *et al.*, 1997). Octreotide, a somatostatin analogue, has been used for control of the secretory diarrhoea with varying success (Romeu *et al.*, 1991). Improvement in immune function with anti-HIV therapy is important in attempting to control cryptosporidial infection. Interestingly, HIV-infected patients receiving clarithromycin or rifabutin for chemoprophylaxis of mycobacterial infection were observed to develop cryptosporidiosis less frequently than patients not receiving these drugs (Holmberg *et al.*, 1998). Letrazuril, a benzene-acetonitrile derivative, has been shown to reduce the diarrhoea in 40 per cent of patients treated, although organisms persisted in duodenal biopsies (Blanshard *et al.*, 1997). Hyperimmune bovine colostrum and bovine dialysable leucocyte extract given orally have been used in small series, with improvement, but the availability of these agents is limited (McMeeking *et al.*, 1989; Ritchie and Becker, 1994).

MICROSPORIDIOSIS

Microsporidia are eukaryotic intracellular spore-forming parasites lacking mitochondria that are found in a number of invertebrate and vertebrate hosts. Human infection had been rarely reported prior to the HIV epidemic. Five genera have been identified in humans: *Nosema* spp., *Pleistophora* spp., *Enterocytozoon* sp., *Septata* spp. and *Encephalitozoon* spp. (Weber *et al.*, 1994). Microsporidial infection was first reported in a patient with HIV infection in 1985 and within several years the importance of this organism as a cause of AIDS-associated diarrhoea was recognized. Two species are commonly identified in small intestinal infection associated with HIV: *Enterocytozoon bieneusi* and *Encephalitozoon* (formerly *Septata*) *intestinalis* (Desportes-Livage, 1996).

Microsporidia have been found to be the cause for between 7 and 50 per cent of unexplained chronic diarrhoea for which no other pathogen is identified after extensive evaluation (Molina *et al.*, 1993). Recent studies have confirmed a strong correlation between the presence of microsporidia in stool or intestinal biopsies and symptomatic diarrhoea (Wuhib *et al.*, 1994; Sobottka *et al.*, 1998). This had been questioned by an earlier report that found no association with diarrhoea (Rabeneck *et al.*, 1993).

The source of microsporidial infection and routes of transmission are unclear. Zoonotic or arthropod-borne infection have been postulated but have not been confirmed. Spores have been found in surface water, although not of species known to infect humans. Transmission probably occurs via the oral–faecal route, following the ingestion of spores. However, transmission via aerosols, sexually and the transplacental route have also been suggested. Infection in immunocompetent hosts is probably common, asymptomatic and self-limited, based on the high prevalence of microsporidial antibodies in serological surveys of normal individuals (Weber *et al.*, 1994).

Both *E. bieneusi* and *E. intestinalis* principally cause infection in the small intestinal epithelium, although biliary tract involvement with cholangitis and cholecystitis may occur. *E. bieneusi* is the more common of the two species, accounting for 60–90 per cent of cases (Dore *et al.*, 1995; Lambl *et al.*, 1996; Sobottka *et al.*, 1998). The predominant gastrointestinal symptoms are of chronic watery diarrhoea occurring up to 20 times per day, which may be associated with abdominal pain, nausea, vomiting and bloating. Weight loss is common and malabsorption of fat, D-xylose, vitamin B_{12} and zinc have been demonstrated (Lambl *et al.*, 1996). Self-limited diarrhoea may occur in individuals with higher CD4 counts. *Encephalitozoon* spp. also infects macrophages and may cause systemic infection with resultant keratoconjunctivitis, bronchiolitis, sinusitis, nephritis and hepatitis (Weber *et al.*, 1994).

Electron microscopy of tissue biopsies is the gold standard for confirmation of microsporidiosis. It allows the visualization of the organism's developmental stages and tiny spores, which range from 1 to 2.5 μm, thereby enabling species identification (Plate 20.3). Scant organisms may be overlooked in routine histological sections by inexperienced observers. Microsporidia are visualized in haematoxylin and eosin stained sections of duodenal or ileal mucosal biopsies as pale vacuoles of 4–5 μm in diameter in the peripheral cytoplasm of enterocytes, mainly in the villi (Plate 20.4). Other changes include a reduction in the villus:crypt ratio with villus blunting, mild crypt hyperplasia and macrophage infiltration of the lamina propria (Field *et al.*, 1993). Schmidt *et al.* (1997) found a 40 per cent reduction in mean villus surface area in duodenal biopsies, implying increased apical enterocyte desquamation. Warthin–Starry staining and tissue Gram stains of mucosal biopsies demonstrate greater numbers of organisms, which are seen as aggregates or clusters in the enterocytes. *E. intestinalis* may also be seen within lamina propria macrophages (Field *et al.*, 1993). Microsporidial infection is associated with significantly reduced activities of the brush-border enzymes lactase, alkaline phosphatase and α-glucosidase by histochemical staining of duodenal biopsies, suggesting malabsorption plays a significant role in the mechanism of diarrhoea (Schmidt *et al.*, 1997).

Diagnosis of microsporidiosis by stool microscopy is hampered by the very small size of the spores. Detection has been greatly enhanced by the use of the modified trichrome stain or the chemofluorescent agent Uvitex 2B (Plate 20.5). These stains may also be used to detect spores from duodenal aspirates. Evaluation of these methods has shown similar sensitivity and specificity to detection from tissue biopsies. However, strict adherence to diagnostic criteria is important to avoid false-positive results (DeGirolami *et al.*, 1995).

More recently, PCR has been shown to be a sensitive method for identifying microsporidia from stool specimens. Following DNA extraction from stool specimens, amplification of the ribosomal RNA genes of *E. bieneusi* and *E. intestinalis*, using two primer pairs, allowed both the diagnosis and speciation of microsporidial enteritis (Liguory *et al.*, 1997). Species identification is useful to predict the response to therapy.

Trials for a number of agents in the treatment of microsporidiosis have been carried out with limited success. Albendazole, a benzimidazole derivative, 400 mg twice daily for 2–4 weeks has shown excellent efficacy for the treatment of infection due to *E. intestinalis*, eradicating the organism in most cases (Dore *et al.*, 1995). However, the response of *E. bieneusi*, which is more common, is less dramatic. Responses to atovaquone, azithromycin and paromomycin have been noted in uncontrolled studies, but patients frequently relapse (Weber *et al.*, 1994; Anwar-Bruni *et al.*, 1996). Recently, fumagillin, a compound derived from the mould *Aspergillus fumigatus*, demonstrated potent antimicrosporidial activity in patients with HIV infection (Molina *et al.*, 1997), although thrombocytopenia was a frequent dose-limiting side-effect. Thalidomide, a suppressor of tumour necrosis factor-α (TNF-α), has also had anecdotal success against microsporidia, on the basis of the finding of elevated TNF-α levels in the stools in microsporidiosis (Sharpstone *et al.*, 1995). Immune reconstitution with the use of potent antiretroviral therapy against HIV has resulted in lasting remission of microsporidial infection, particularly when a protease inhibitor drug is included (Goguel *et al.*, 1997).

ISOSPORIASIS

Isospora belli is an intracellular coccidian protozoon, closely related to *Cryptosporidium* spp. Like cryptosporidiosis, infection is self-limited in normal hosts, but causes chronic life-threatening diarrhoea in patients with AIDS. Isosporiasis is uncommon in Britain and in the USA, affecting less than 1 per cent of individuals with HIV infection (Soave and Johnson, 1988; Blanshard *et al.*, 1996). However, its recognition is vital as it readily responds to treatment. *Isospora* spp. are endemic in tropical and subtropical climates, especially in areas with poor sanitation. A study from Haiti revealed the parasite in 15 per cent of patients with AIDS (Dehovitz *et al.*, 1986).

Diarrhoea develops around 1 week following the ingestion of mature oocysts of *I. belli* in contaminated water or food. Sporozoites released from the oocyst invade the enterocytes of the proximal small bowel, undergoing both asexual and sexual multiplication (Wittner *et al.*, 1993). The oocysts excreted in the stool mature in the environment for 2–3 days before becoming infectious. The resulting profuse, non-bloody diarrhoea is associated with symptoms of anorexia, abdominal cramping and foul-smelling gas. Malabsorption of fat, vitamin B_{12} and lactose are reported, and peripheral eosinophilia is common (Lew *et al.*, 1997).

The diagnosis of isosporiasis is usually based on the identification of the oocysts in stool specimens. The oocysts are occasionally seen in unstained wet mounts as elongated oval structures that take up iodine poorly. The modified acid-fast stain is most widely used, allowing detection of the large, bright-red, elliptical oocysts, approximately 12 × 30 μm each containing two sporocysts (Plates 20.6a,b). These are easily distinguished from the smaller rounder cryptosporidial oocysts measuring around 5 μm. Concentration of the stool by the laboratory is recommended as oocysts may be few in number and shed only intermittently. There are no serological or molecular tests that have been developed for the detection of *Isospora* spp. Endoscopic biopsies are diagnostic with organisms visible within cytoplasmic vacuoles. The small intestinal changes in severe infection include flattening of the villi with inflammatory cells, including eosinophils infiltrating the lamina propria (Wittner *et al.*, 1993; Lew *et al.*, 1997).

Therapy of isosporiasis with trimethoprim 160 mg/sulphamethoxazole 800 mg four times daily for 10 days, then twice daily for 3 weeks is effective; however, relapse occurs in 50 per cent of patients (Soave and Johnson, 1988). Shorter courses of 7–10 days seem to have similar efficacy (Peterson and Wofsy, 1994). Relapsing infection responds to retreatment and patients should receive subsequent long-term prophylaxis with one double-strength tablet three times a week. Patients who are allergic to sulphonamides may be treated with high-dose pyrimethamine 75 mg daily plus folinic acid 15 mg daily, followed by pyrimethamine 25 mg daily plus folinic acid 5–10 mg daily (Wittner *et al.*, 1993). Alternatively, the combination of albendazole 400 mg three times daily for 20 days plus ornidazole 2 g daily given on days 1, 10 and 20 has been reported to be effective (Dionisio *et al.*, 1996).

CYCLOSPORA

The genus *Cyclospora* spp. was established in the late 19th century but, until recently, species affecting humans had not been described. The first report of this novel intestinal organism in humans was in 1986 by Soave *et al.* Early reports classified the agent as a cyanobacterium-like body (blue-green alga). Recently, it was speciated as a coccidian protozoan, *Cyclospora cayetanensis*, on the demonstration of oocysts containing two sporocysts each with two sporozoites (Ortega *et al.*, 1993). Human infection was initially identified in Haiti, Nepal and Peru, and is now known to occur widely in most continents. Groups commonly affected are children in countries having a high prevalence of the disease, travellers and HIV-infected persons. Transmission is presumed to occur via the oral–faecal route, usually following the ingestion of contaminated water. Direct faecal to oral transmission is unlikely as the oocysts excreted in faeces are unsporulated and not initially infective.

Infection with *C. cayatanensis* produces persistent watery diarrhoea, which is difficult to distinguish on clinical grounds from cryptosporidiosis or isosporiasis. Weight loss, fatigue, anorexia and nausea are frequent. Patients with lower CD4 counts tend to have more prolonged diarrhoea and weight loss. This was reflected in a Mexican study of *C. cayatanensis* infections including patients with AIDS, most with CD4 cells below 50/μL, who had diarrhoea for a mean of 120 days and weight loss of 7 kg (Sifuentes-Osornio *et al.*, 1995). Cholecystitis was also reported in association with the enteritis. The organism may cause diarrhoea in immunocompetent individuals lasting for up to 12 weeks, although asymptomatic carriage is also described (Pollok *et al.*, 1992).

Diagnosis is best confirmed by a stool examination using a modified Ziehl–Nielsen smear. The variable acid-fast oocysts appear as spherical bodies 8–10 mm in diameter, intermediate in size between the smaller oocysts of *Cryptosporidium* spp. and the larger ones of *Isospora* spp. (Ortega *et al.*, 1993). The organisms may also autofluoresce blue when examined by ultraviolet epifluorescence microscopy. Small intestinal biopsy reveals an inflammatory reaction with surface epithelial disarray, partial villous atrophy and crypt hyperplasia. Organisms are visible within intestinal epithelial cells only by electron microscopy. D-Xylose absorption is impaired, suggesting that malabsorption plays a significant role in the causation of diarrhoea (Connor *et al.*, 1993).

The illness responds promptly to treatment with co-trimoxazole (trimethoprim 160 mg/sulphamethoxazole 800 mg) orally four times daily for 10 days (Pape *et al.*, 1994). Long-term prophylaxis with one tablet three times a week may be required as there is a high rate of recurrent infection.

OTHER PARASITES

Infection with *Giardia lamblia* has been found to occur at a similar frequency in HIV-infected patients compared to HIV-negative homosexual men and thus is not considered to be predictive of HIV infection (Smith *et al.*, 1992). A recent Italian study found that giardiasis during HIV infection occurred in all HIV risk groups and was associated with severe immunodeficiency with a mean CD4 count of 27/μL (Angarano *et al.*, 1997). Response to imidazole therapy, with metronidazole 200–400 mg orally 8 hourly for 5–7 days is in general similar to that in immunocompetent hosts.

Visceral leishmaniasis is an important opportunistic infection for HIV-infected individuals living in Mediterranean areas endemic for *Leishmania* spp. It follows reactivation of latent infection by the intracellular protozoan *Leishmania donovani*, acquired through the bites of infected female sandflies. The parasite infects macrophages of the spleen, bone marrow, lymph nodes, liver and bowel, resulting in fever, pancytopenia, splenomegaly, diarrhoea, malabsorption and weight loss. Visceral leishmaniasis has been reported to occur in up to 5 per cent of HIV-infected individuals residing in endemic areas (Gradoni *et al.*, 1996) and was the cause of gastrointestinal symptoms in 3 per cent of individuals presenting for endoscopy at a Spanish clinic (Laguna *et al.*, 1994). Small bowel involvement is well described and may lead to malabsorption and diarrhoea (Muigai *et al.*, 1983; Albrecht *et al.*, 1996). Diagnosis may be obtained by duodenal biopsy with the visualization of leishmania amastigotes in the intestinal mucosa. Serology is of limited value, owing to frequent false-negative results. Treatment with pentavalent antimonials (e.g. sodium stibogluconate) has been the mainstay of treatment of leishmaniasis for decades, but has a failure rate approaching 50 per cent in patients with HIV infection. Alternatives are pentamidine and amphotericin B. Short-course therapy with liposomal formulations of amphotericin show promising efficacy with little toxicity (Davidson *et al.*, 1994). Relapsing infection occurs in up to 80 per cent of individuals without ongoing prophylactic medication (Albrecht *et al.*, 1996).

Infestation with the intestinal helminth *Strongyloides stercoralis* is common in many tropical and subtropical regions of the world. An African study found the organism present in the stools of 3 per cent of patients with AIDS (Colebunders *et al.*, 1988). The hyperinfection syndrome described in immunocompromised patients has only rarely been reported in patients with HIV infection (Harcourt-Webster *et al.*, 1991). This illness is characterized by autoinfection with dissemination of large numbers of larvae to the lungs and other organs. Death from Gram-negative septicaemia is common and due to the larvae carrying coliform bacteria as they migrate from the intestine. Diagnosis of intestinal strongyloidiasis infection in patients from endemic areas is important to enable therapy and prevent hyperinfection. Larvae may be identified in the stool by wet mount and, occasionally, in respiratory specimens and urine.

Entamoeba histolytica is commonly detected in stools of certain populations of homosexual men. However, invasive disease is rare in HIV infection, presumably due to the predominance of non-pathogenic strains observed in this group of patients. The identification of *E. histolytica* and other amoebae is not associated with the existence of diarrhoea or other symptoms. Similarly, *Blastocystis hominis* has not been convincingly shown to cause diarrhoea in AIDS (Smith *et al.*, 1992).

Bacterial infections

MYCOBACTERIUM AVIUM-INTRACELLULARE COMPLEX

Mycobacterium avium-intracellulare complex (MAC) infection is extremely frequent in advanced HIV infection, occurring in approximately 25 per cent of patients living with AIDS and up to 50 per cent of patients in autopsy series. The risk of developing MAC infection rises with progressive immune dysfunction and is most significant when the CD4 count is less than 50 cells/μL (Chin, 1994).

The organism is commonly encountered in the environment, largely in soil and water; however, infection in immunocompetent hosts is rare. In patients with

AIDS, the usual portal of entry is the gastrointestinal tract, with ingestion of the organism resulting in initial intestinal and mesenteric lymph node infection. Inhalation of mycobacteria is a less common mode of entry. Subsequent systemic infection of the liver, spleen, bone marrow and blood results in the classic syndrome of MAC infection. The organism is phagocytosed by macrophages but intracellular lysis is defective, allowing unchecked replication. Malabsorption and diarrhoea result from diffuse involvement of the intestinal villi and obstruction of lymphatic drainage. Small bowel involvement is most frequent followed by colonic then oesophageal disease (Smith *et al.*, 1992).

Characteristically, patients complain of chronic diarrhoea, which is of mild to moderate severity and is associated with symptoms of fever, night sweats, fatigue, weight loss and abdominal pain. Affected individuals usually are wasted, with lymphadenopathy, hepatosplenomegaly and anaemia. Less common gastrointestinal manifestations include gastrointestinal bleeding, bowel obstruction and, in children, appendicitis and intussusception.

At endoscopy the duodenal mucosa may be erythematous, oedematous and granular with fine white to yellow nodules measuring 1–4 mm surrounded by a rim of erythema. Alternatively, the mucosa may appear normal (Gray and Rabenek, 1989; Cappell and Philogene, 1995). Mucosal biopsies show the lamina propria is packed with foamy macrophages that are periodic acid–Schiff positive, reminiscent of Whipple's disease. Ziehl–Nielsen staining reveals acid-fast bacilli within these macrophages (Plates 20.7a,b). Mycobacterial cultures of intestinal biopsies are important to increase the sensitivity of detection and for confirming a species diagnosis but may take several weeks to grow. Blood cultures taken in specific media, e.g. Bactec 13A (Becton Dickinson), are usually positive within 2 weeks and are the least invasive method of diagnosis of systemic infection with a sensitivity of up to 98 per cent if two cultures are taken (Lew *et al.*, 1997). Faecal smears and cultures may also be positive for acid-fast bacilli but are of little diagnostic value as they do not confirm invasive disease. Endoscopy may still be necessary to exclude concomitant enteric pathogens.

MAC is resistant to many standard antituberculous drugs and early therapies often failed to induce lasting remission. In recent years, combination therapies containing macrolide antibiotics have been more effective in suppressing MAC infection as well as prolonging survival of patients. These regimens combine clarithromycin 500 mg twice daily or azithromycin 300–600 mg daily, with rifabutin 450 mg daily and ethambutol 15 mg/kg daily. Other agents that may be included are clofazimine, ciprofloxacin, ofloxacin or amikacin. Treatment is continued for life as relapse is inevitable if therapy is stopped (Chin, 1994).

Primary chemoprophylaxis of MAC infection is now advocated to avoid the toxicity associated with long-term multiple drug therapy, and has been shown to prolong survival. The agents of choice are clarithromycin 500 mg twice daily or azithromycin 1.2 g once weekly, which should be commenced when the CD4 count drops to below 100 cells per microlitre (Havlir *et al.*, 1996; Pierce *et al.*, 1996).

MYCOBACTERIUM TUBERCULOSIS

The resurgence of tuberculosis (TB) noted in the last 15 years has been attributable in part to the AIDS epidemic. In patients with HIV infection, the clinical presentation of tuberculosis is often atypical with frequent extrapulmonary involvement (Schecter, 1994). Although infrequently encountered in developed nations, the incidence of gastrointestinal tuberculosis has been rising in some urban areas such as New York City (Horvath and Whelan, 1998). The impact of TB is more dramatic in developing countries, as exemplified in a report from Thailand, which found that 18 per cent of HIV-infected patients presenting with chronic diarrhoea had tuberculous enteritis or colitis (Manatsathit *et al.*, 1996). Gastrointestinal *Mycobacterium tuberculosis* infection most commonly involves the ileocaecum, followed by the jejunum and colon. Common presenting symptoms are colicky mid-abdominal or right lower quadrant pain, weight loss, fever and altered bowel habit. Complications of intestinal obstruction and perforation, which is rare in non-AIDS patients, may develop (Friedenberg *et al.*, 1993). Chest x-rays may reveal coexisting pulmonary TB.

Colonoscopy with ileal intubation is the most valuable method of diagnosing intestinal tuberculosis. Infection is usually granulomatous and segmental, unlike MAC, which is diffuse. Lesions are usually ulcerative, but hypertrophic masses and fibrotic strictures may occur. The ileo-caecal valve is often deformed and incompetent. Multiple biopsies should be taken with fresh and fixed specimens all submitted for smear, culture and histology, respectively. Each method individually has a low sensitivity and a combination of diagnostic methods is thus required. PCR methods that amplify a repetitive DNA sequence of the IS 6110 region of the genome have been applied to intestinal biopsy specimens with success (Anand *et al.*, 1994). However, a study from Korea in non-HIV-infected patients showed an overall sensitivity of approximately 40 per cent, although a rapid diagnosis was obtained (Kim *et al.*, 1998).

Therapy should be started empirically when intestinal TB is suspected, using the four drug combination of isoniazid, rifampicin, pyrazinamide, and ethambutol or streptomycin. A symptomatic response is observed within 1–2 weeks, thus bowel obstruction should be managed conservatively if the patient is stable. Surgery may be necessary to establish a diagnosis, or to manage the complications of intestinal perforation, or bowel obstruction that is unresponsive to antituberculous drug therapy.

ENTERIC BACTERIA

Bacterial gastroenteritis is generally more common, severe, prolonged and prone to recurrence when it occurs in HIV infection. As in normal hosts, it is characterized by fever, abdominal pain and diarrhoea, which may be bloody. *Salmonella* gastroenteritis during HIV infection is frequently complicated by bacteraemia, the latter occurring up to 100 times more commonly than in the general population. Gastrointestinal symptoms are absent in about 50 per cent of cases of bacteraemia (Sperber and Schleupner, 1987). Persistence of the organism in the intestine is common due to the impairment of T-cell function and macrophage killing, leading to long-term carriage and relapsing infection. Treatment of gastroenteritis is with ampicillin, co-trimoxazole, ciprofloxacin or ceftriaxone.

Campylobacter jejuni enteritis may also be prolonged, severe and recurrent, especially when CD4 counts are depressed. *Campylobacter* bacteraemia was found to occur in 8 per cent of HIV-seropositive patients with *Campylobacter* enteritis, compared with < 2 per cent of seronegative patients with enteritis (Tee and Mijch, 1998). Ciprofloxacin and multidrug-resistant strains are frequent, especially in relapsing infections. Erythromycin is recommended as first-line therapy, as antibiotic resistance develops less commonly than with quinolone therapy.

The role of enteropathogenic *E. coli* in HIV-related diarrhoea is still being defined. Enteroadherent or enteroaggregative *E. coli* have been found in HIV-positive subjects in African and US studies, and were associated with diarrhoea in patients with low CD4 counts (Mathewson *et al.*, 1995; Orenstein and Kotler, 1995; Wanke *et al.*, 1998a). Enteroadherent *E. coli*, most with a diffuse pattern of adherence, were seen in 24 per cent of HIV patients with diarrhoea (Mathewson *et al.*, 1998). The right colon is most commonly involved, with small intestinal involvement confined to the ileum. A recent trial demonstrated symptomatic improvement following treatment with ciprofloxacin (Wanke *et al.*, 1998b).

Helicobacter pylori has a lower prevalence in HIV-seropositive individuals compared with seronegative subjects. This difference is largely accounted for by the lower frequency in patients with CD4 counts below 200 cells/μL. A similar disparity in the frequency of peptic ulceration has been noted (Cacciarelli *et al.*, 1996). The potential explanations for the reduced colonization with *H. pylori* include the increased frequency of achlorhydria, inadequate mucosal immune response and prior antibiotic usage.

Bacterial overgrowth in the small intestine has been reported and is attributed to hypochlorhydria (Lake-Bakaar *et al.*, 1988). Reduced upper gastrointestinal motility has also been described in HIV infection and may contribute to this (Papanaoum *et al.*, 1992). If suspected, a broad-spectrum antibiotic, such as tetracycline 500 mg four times daily or ciprofloxacin 500 mg twice daily for 7–14 days, may be administered.

Fungal infections

Histoplasmosis occurs as a generalized systemic infection in patients with AIDS who are severely immunosuppressed individuals with CD4 counts usually below 150/μl, following either recent exposure to the fungus or reactivation of latent infection (McKinsey *et al.*, 1997). Infection is most frequent in individuals residing in areas endemic for *Histoplasma capsulatum*, such as central USA and parts of South America, occurring in 5 per cent of AIDS patients from endemic regions (Hajjeh, 1995).

Gastrointestinal involvement occurs as part of a progressive disseminated infection in 70 per cent of AIDS patients with histoplasmosis but is only symptomatic in 10 per cent (Smith *et al.*, 1992). It may present as a mass lesion (particularly in the colon), with ulceration (often in the oropharynx) or as serosal disease. Obstruction, perforation and intussuception of the small bowel are described, mostly involving the ileum (Sarosi and Johnson, 1992). Diagnosis is by microscopy, showing yeast-like organisms within gut macrophages, and is confirmed by fungal cultures of blood, bone marrow and infected tissues. Amphotericin B or itraconazole are indicated for initial treatment followed by long-term suppressive therapy.

Colonization of the intestine with *Candida albicans* or other yeasts is extremely common. Although it frequently causes oral and oesophageal disease in HIV infection, there is no convincing evidence that it contributes to diarrhoea or is anything more than a commensal organism of the bowel (Smith *et al.*, 1992; Hazen, 1993).

Viral infections

CYTOMEGALOVIRUS

Cytomegalovirus (CMV) infection in patients with AIDS is a disseminated disease, which may involve the eyes, central nervous system and gastrointestinal tract. Disease is due to reactivation of latent CMV infection during advanced immunodeficiency, usually emerging when the CD4 count is below 100 cells/μL. Gastrointestinal CMV disease is reported in up to one-third of patients with AIDS (Dieterich and Rahmin, 1991). The entire intestinal tract from mouth to anus may be involved as well as the biliary tract, liver and pancreas. The most common sites affected are the colon, oesophagus and distal small bowel. Small intestinal CMV rarely occurs without the involvement of other gastrointestinal sites. Infection of the vascular endothelium of the intestine leads to a vasculitis, which results in focal thrombosis, mucosal ischaemia and ulceration. Clinically, patients with CMV enteritis experience fevers, abdominal pain and watery diarrhoea. Diffuse involvement of the duodenum and jejunum leads to malabsorption and wasting. As the disease progresses, there may be complications of gastrointestinal bleeding, intestinal perforation and, less frequently, toxic megacolon and bowel obstruction. CMV-induced perforation is the commonest reason for emergency surgery in patients with AIDS.

At colonoscopy or endoscopy, there is usually patchy or diffuse inflammation with a friable erythematous mucosa and ulceration, which is discrete or confluent in severe cases. Intestinal biopsies are required to confirm the diagnosis of CMV infection. The mucosa may appear normal in up to 25 per cent of cases; therefore, multiple biopsies from normal mucosa should be taken (Dieterich *et al.*, 1993). Haematoxylin and eosin staining depicts the characteristic changes of CMV infection with the intranuclear 'owl's eye' inclusion surrounded by a clear halo in an enlarged cell (Plate 20.8). Smudge cells may be present. Immunostaining and DNA *in situ* hybridization increase the sensitivity of histologic diagnosis (Francis *et al.*, 1989). PCR has also been used to detect CMV in intestinal biopsy tissue with high sensitivity (Cotte *et al.*, 1993; Goodgame *et al.*, 1993). Viral culture of intestinal biopsies may be falsely positive due to contamination by blood. Detection of the virus in the blood by culture or PCR is common in AIDS, but is not specific for visceral disease. Measurement of a high CMV load in the plasma by quantitative PCR appears to be more predictive of clinical disease (Kuhn *et al.*, 1995). Viral culture of the stool for CMV infection is inappropriate, owing to its poor sensitivity. Serological diagnosis is generally useless in this setting, as virtually all patients with HIV infection are CMV IgG-positive, indicating previous exposure to the virus. CMV IgM rises are unpredictable and of little value.

The diagnosis of CMV disease in patients with AIDS portends a poor long-term survival. Without therapy, the median time to death was reported to be 2 months (Holland *et al.*, 1990). However, this has been significantly improved with treatment of both the CMV and underlying HIV infection. Initial therapy is with ganciclovir, an acyclic nucleoside structurally related to acyclovir. The induction dosage is 5 mg/kg intravenously twice daily for 14–21 days. Approximately 80 per cent of patients respond to initial treatment (Dieterich *et al.*, 1993). In patients with a partial or delayed response, 4 weeks of therapy may be required. The main toxicity of ganciclovir is neutropenia and thrombocytopenia, occurring in up to 40 per cent of patients. If this is dose limiting, the co-administration of granulocyte colony-stimulating factor (G-CSF) may be required. Foscarnet, a pyrophosphate analogue inhibiting viral DNA polymerase, is also active against CMV, and may be used if patients are intolerant or resistant to ganciclovir. Its efficacy and effect on survival is similar to ganciclovir (Blanshard *et al.*, 1995). The dosage is 60 mg/kg three times daily or 90 mg/kg twice daily intravenously with adverse events including nephrotoxicity, electrolyte imbalance and seizures. Maintenance therapy with either agent may be considered in patients with frequent relapsing disease, although its benefit in preventing relapse is not as established as for CMV retinitis. Resistance to both agents has been reported, usually associated with prolonged treatment. Concurrent therapy may be considered in this setting. Cidofavir, a nucleotide analogue, may be required for salvage treatment of CMV disease. It is active against ganciclovir- and foscarnet-resistant strains of CMV *in vitro*, although it has significant dose-limiting nephrotoxicity (Lalezari *et al.*, 1995).

OTHER GASTROINTESTINAL VIRUSES

Adenovirus infection has been found in up to 9 per cent of patients with diarrhoea, usually affecting the colon. Most studies have found that there is a correlation with diarrhoea with prolonged infection when the CD4 count is less than 200/μL (Grohmann *et al.*, 1993; Schmidt *et al.*, 1996). Diagnosis is made by intestinal biopsy or stool examination by electron microscopy, enzyme immunoassay or viral culture. Response to therapy is generally poor, although case reports showing a response to ribavirin have been described (Kapelushnik *et al.*, 1995; Maslo *et al.*, 1997). Schmidt *et al.* (1996) found that patients with adenoviruses had a higher rate of co-infection with other enteropathogens and postulated that adenovirus may facilitate infection by other intestinal pathogens.

Rotavirus is a common enteric pathogen in HIV-infected children, where it may cause severe and protracted diarrhoea. In adults, its significance is less clear, with rates of 0–18 per cent reported in AIDS patients with diarrhoea (Cunningham *et al.*, 1988; Grohmann *et al.*, 1993). Anecdotal improvement in chronic infection has been reported with orally administered human serum immunoglobulin (Guarino *et al.*, 1996).

Other viruses that have been detected in patients with HIV infection include astroviruses, coronaviruses, picobirnaviruses and caliciviruses (Grohmann *et al.*, 1993). Intensive investigation for viruses in AIDS patients with diarrhoea in a German study revealed a rate of detection of 17 per cent, but the rate of pathogen-negative diarrhoea decreased by only 5 per cent as most contained other enteropathogens (Schmidt *et al.*, 1996).

HIV ENTEROPATHY

Infection of the gut directly by HIV has been proposed as the cause for symptoms of diarrhoea, malabsorption, wasting and alteration of bowel function. Although HIV-infected persons with gut symptomatology are most likely to have other pathogens co-infecting the gastrointestinal tract, approximately 30 per cent of those with diarrhoea have no opportunistic infection detectable (Kotler *et al.*, 1984). Diarrhoea may occur very early in the course of HIV infection, well before severe immune deficiency has occurred, and it is not uncommonly a manifestation of the illness associated with the initial infection during the phase of seroconversion. Therefore, there is strong evidence that HIV infection of the gut itself plays a role in diarrhoea and wasting; the clinical diagnosis attached to these cases is HIV enteropathy.

A number of histopathologic and functional abnormalities have been described in the small intestine during HIV infection. The relationship between symptom severity, histologic changes and functional defects, such as D-xylose absorption, has not been clearly established (Carlson *et al.*, 1994; Rabeneck *et al.*, 1996). Villous atrophy with and without crypt hyperplasia has been the most frequent finding on biopsy of the small bowel, but both case-controlled and observational studies have failed to find an association with asymptomatic or symptomatic HIV-infected persons (Greenson *et al.*, 1991; Rabeneck *et al.*, 1996). Other histologic abnormalities described include abnormal lipid accumulation (Benhamou *et al.*, 1994), crypt epithelial cell apoptosis (Kotler *et al.*, 1986), lamina propria inflammation (Kotler *et al.*, 1993) and enterocyte cytoplasmic vacuolation (Patterson *et al.*, 1993). Characterization of active ion transport mechanisms and epithelial barrier function utilizing a miniaturized Ussing device has recently demonstrated impaired epithelial barrier function, which could contribute to the diarrhoea by a leak flux mechanism, without evidence of active ion secretion or sodium/glucose malabsorption (Stockmann *et al.*, 1998).

The cells in the gut tissues identified to be primarily infected by HIV have been CD4 lymphocytes or macrophages within the lamina propria, but there are also reports that HIV itself can be isolated from enterocytes or colonic cells *in vitro* and *in vivo* (Bigornia *et al.*, 1992; Fleming *et al.*, 1992). Infection can be initiated in foetal small bowel explants; the cells sustaining HIV replication are of lymphocytic or monocytic lineage. The mechanism for gut injury may be a direct cytopathic effect within the intestinal mucosa (Dobbins and Weinstein, 1985) or mediated by cytokines. T-cell activation and cytokine release (TNF, IL-1) have been associated with structural changes, and modulation of ion and water flux through colonic mucosa (Chang *et al.*, 1990; Kotler *et al.*, 1993). Dysregulation of cytokine gene expression occurs in the intestinal mucosa; increased expression of pro-inflammatory cytokine mRNA (IL-10, INF-γ) and reduced expression of IL-10 and IL-2 has been demonstrated (McGowan *et al.*, 1994). Epithelial cell and lamina propria mononuclear cell apoptosis occurs presumably secondarily to autocrine dysregulation (Lu *et al.*, 1996).

The significance of HIV replication within gut tissue may far outweigh the direct gut-related disease it produces, as it has been found that, while HIV proviral load is similar in gut tissues and peripheral blood, high levels of HIV p-24 antigen exist within the gut, suggesting that the intestinal mucosa is a major reservoir for HIV production, and a site of accelerated infection and destruction of CD4+ lymphocytes. This reservoir will therefore need to be targeted in drug therapy aiming at viral eradication or long-term suppression (Fackler *et al.*, 1998).

The effect of highly active antiretroviral therapy on gut symptoms and function associated with HIV enteropathy has been reported recently. Improvement of chronic diarrhoea, abdominal bloating and cramps has been noted in cases without identifiable pathogens, as well as in those with microsporidial and cryptosporidial infection, presumably secondarily to a degree of immune reconstitution (Foudraine *et al.*, 1998). Antiretroviral therapy reduces HIV RNA levels in both the blood and gut mucosa to a similar extent, with increases in CD4 lymphocyte counts in both compartments. Treatment is associated with a reduction in mononuclear cell apoptosis (Kotler *et al.*, 1998).

HIV-ASSOCIATED MALIGNANCY

The two most frequent HIV-associated malignancies are Kaposi's sarcoma and non-Hodgkin's lymphoma. Both of these neoplasms constitute AIDS-defining illnesses, usually occurring when infection is advanced. Gastrointestinal involvement by both diseases is common and is frequently the site of presentation.

Kaposi's sarcoma

Kaposi's sarcoma (KS) was one of the earliest reported manifestations of AIDS identified at the beginning of the epidemic. It is a multicentric angioproliferative tumour and an AIDS-defining condition. The cause was long suspected to be due to a sexually transmitted agent because of the observation that KS was mainly a disease of homosexual men, occurring rarely in other risk groups. Recently, the newly recognized human herpes virus 8 (HHV-8) has been found to have a key role in the causation of KS, both in HIV infection and the rarer indolent tumour described in HIV-negative elderly European men (Chang *et al.*, 1994). The incidence of KS in AIDS has declined since the early 1980s, possibly reflecting a change in high-risk sexual behaviour in homosexual men. KS most commonly involves the skin, where it causes violaceous nodules and plaques. The visceral organs most often involved are the gastrointestinal tract, the lungs and pleura.

KS of the gastrointestinal tract was found in up to 70 per cent of patients with KS in autopsy series (Guarda *et al.*, 1984; Welch *et al.*, 1984). Lesions may be widely disseminated through the entire gut but usually cause few symptoms. Oral KS is a frequent finding but is not predictive of disease in the rest of the gastrointestinal tract. Likewise, cutaneous lesions may be absent. Kaposi's sarcoma lesions in the gut are usually small and submucosal, rarely causing clinical symptoms (Friedman *et al.*, 1985). Occasionally the tumours may ulcerate and bleed, but serious gastrointestinal haemorrhage is uncommon. Perforation and obstruction are extremely rare.

At endoscopy, the lesions of KS in the lumen are maculopapular, polypoid or nodular in appearance. Endoscopic biopsy has only a 23 per cent positive yield owing to the tumour's submucosal location (Friedman *et al.*, 1985). Barium contrast x-rays are not useful for diagnosis because of their low specificity and sensitivity. Histologically, KS lesions contain a proliferation of spindle-shaped cells, which form slit-like vascular spaces lined by atypical endothelial cells. Extravasated red blood cells and haemosiderin are often seen in these vascular spaces (Plate 20.9). Eosinophilic cytoplasmic inclusions are seen in 60 per cent of biopsies and help establish the diagnosis.

Patients with few lesions that are asymptomatic are best observed without specific therapy. Individuals with symptomatic disease may be treated with radiotherapy for localized symptomatic lesions or, if disseminated, with cytotoxic drugs. The drugs most commonly used are vincristine, bleomycin and doxorubicin, usually in combination. Liposomal doxorubicin is associated with less toxicity and results in higher intralesional concentrations. Paclitaxel has also shown reasonable efficacy (Lin, 1998). Interferon-α has antitumour activity, but is less effective than chemotherapy and is frequently limited by side-effects. Immune reconstitution with highly active antiretroviral therapy directed towards HIV has recently been shown to cause regression of KS lesions and should be the first therapy tried. Since the discovery of HHV-8 as a causal factor in KS, there has been interest in the use of specific antiviral therapy. In retrospective studies, patients receiving ganciclovir or foscarnet were less likely to develop KS (Mocroft *et al.*, 1996). However, prospective data are so far lacking. Hormonal therapy with β-human chorionic gonadotrophin (β-HCG) is also being studied following the discovery of its antitumour effect in KS (Gill *et al.*, 1996). This may account for the rarity of this tumour in women.

Non-Hodgkin's lymphoma

Non-Hodgkin's lymphoma (NHL) occurs in approximately 10 per cent of people with HIV infection. The two main types are systemic lymphoma and primary central nervous system (CNS) lymphoma, the latter usually featuring in advanced AIDS when CD4 counts are less than 50/μL. In contrast, approximately one-third of patients with systemic NHL have a CD4 count greater than 200 cells/μL. The vast majority of these are B cell in lineage and of high grade. Between 30 and 60 per cent of systemic lymphomas (and all CNS lymphomas) contain Epstein–Barr virus sequences. Coexpression of viral DNA with the oncogene c-*myc*, detected in most HIV-related NHLs, plays a key role in lymphomagenesis.

Extranodal disease is very common in HIV-related NHL. The gastrointestinal tract, liver and biliary tract are frequent sites of presentation, occurring in up to 30 per cent of all cases (Ziegler *et al.*, 1984). Gastrointestinal lymphoma usually presents with enteric bleeding, abdominal pain, bowel obstruction, ascites or an altered bowel habit. Endoscopically, they appear nodular and may be ulcerated. Tissue should be submitted frozen for immunostaining. Most gastrointestinal lymphomas are immunoblastic large non-cleaved cell lymphomas or, less often, Burkitt's. Factors that result in a better prognosis are a polyclonal rather than monoclonal phenotype, peripheral blood CD4 count of 200 cells/μL or greater, and no prior AIDS diagnosis, absence of extranodal and bone marrow involvement and intermediate-grade large cell lymphoma.

Treatment of systemic lymphoma with cytotoxic drugs is difficult in people already immunosuppressed by their HIV infection. Drug interactions with antiretroviral medication may also be problematic. Although average survival is rarely more than 6–12 months, chemotherapy is usually required for palliation of symptoms. CHOP (cyclophosphamide, doxorubicin, vincristine, prednisolone) results in remission rates of up to 70 per cent. Myelosuppression is minimized by using lower dosages of cytotoxics, administering G-CSF and avoiding concomitant zidovudine therapy. Palliative therapy is advised in patients who are severely immunocompromised with a poor performance status.

WEIGHT LOSS AND MALABSORPTION ASSOCIATED WITH HIV

Weight loss and malnutrition are major complications associated with advancing HIV infection and AIDS, causing both morbidity and mortality. Body cell mass depletion and weight loss have been shown to be associated with an increased risk of mortality, which may be independent of the CD4 lymphocyte count (Chlebowski *et al.*, 1989; Kotler *et al.*, 1989; Guenter *et al.*, 1993; Palenicek *et al.*, 1995; Babameto and Kotler, 1997). The aetiology of malnutrition in AIDS patients is often multifactorial, and may be due to reduced food intake, intestinal malabsorption and other metabolic alterations. Oropharangeal and oesophageal pathology, malignancy, fatigue, cytokine or drug-induced anorexia and neurological complications, such as dementia, can all contribute to reduced oral intake. Gastroparesis may be a further factor limiting food intake (Papanaoum *et al.*, 1992; Konturek *et al.*, 1997).

The small intestine is an important and common target of infection in patients with AIDS. Infections, which in immunocompetent individuals are self-limiting, can cause severe diarrhoeal diseases and result in significant malabsorption and weight loss in immunocompromised AIDS patients. Opportunistic infections account for most cases of chronic diarrhoea and malnutrition. While approximately 60 per cent of HIV-infected patients in developed countries have diarrhoea lasting longer than 1 week, this approaches 100 per cent in underdeveloped countries (Babameto and Kotler, 1997). Searching for the pathogen is useful as yields of from 83 to 100 per cent in patients with severe immune depletion have been described (Kotler and Orenstein, 1994). Early studies in non-HIV-infected male homosexuals revealed a high carriage rate of standard enteropathogens (Quinn *et al.*, 1983), but, in advanced HIV infection, stool enteropathogens are likely to be of more clinical significance (Griffin, 1990). Thirty per cent may have three or more enteric pathogens (Kotler and Orenstein, 1994).

The mechanisms of diarrhoea and malabsorption are diverse. The villous atrophy seen in HIV enteropathy has been shown to correlate with fat malabsorption and the ^{14}C-labelled triolein breath test (Miller *et al.*, 1988). Lactose intolerance is common and can be detected by the lactose breath test (Kapembwa *et al.*, 1989). Carbohydrate malabsorption has been shown in children and adults with HIV wasting syndrome using the D-xylose absorption test (Guarino *et al.*, 1991; Ehrenpreis *et al.*, 1992a). Abnormal D-xylose absorption is associated with more profound impairment of body composition, lipids and protein (Ott *et al.*, 1993). In addition to proximal bowel abnormalities, there is emerging evidence that distal small bowel function may also be reduced, resulting in bile acid malabsorption, measured by ^{75}Se-homocholic acid taurine (HCAT) absorption, and vitamin B_{12} malabsorption in chronic diarrhoea (Ehrenpreis *et al.*, 1994; Sciarretta *et al.*, 1994). Up to 39 per cent of HIV-infected patients with chronic diarrhoea were noted to have vitamin B_{12} deficiency in the study by Ehrenpreis. This is important as the sequelae of vitamin B_{12} deficiency, particularly in the neurological system, may be reversible. Increased intestinal permeability, measured using tests of sugar absorption with glucose/rhamnose/lactulose, has been noted in patients with AIDS and malabsorption (Keating *et al.*, 1995). Lymphatic obstruction has also been described and may be another cause of protein loss and malabsorption (Ehrenpreis *et al.*, 1992b). Autonomic neuropathy may also contribute to gastric and intestinal dysmotility, chronic diarrhoea and malabsorption. In addition to causing malnutrition, diarrhoea and malabsorption may result in variable absorption of antiretroviral drugs, such as zidovudine, although data to date have not confirmed a significant reduction in drug efficacy (Kapembwa *et al.*, 1996; Macnab *et al.*, 1996). Metabolic alterations found during HIV infection include fasting hypertriglyceridaemia, low serum cholesterol and reduced endogenous anabolic steroids, such as testosterone and dehydroepiandrosterone (DHEA), which may contribute to protein depletion (Coodley *et al.*, 1994; Zangerle *et al.*, 1994). Micronutrient deficiencies in vitamin B_6 and vitamin B_{12} have been demonstrated (Harriman *et al.*, 1989; Herzlich *et al.*, 1992). There is interest in the role of cytokines in the cause of cachexia of infection, particularly tumour necrosis factor-α and interleukin-1, which may be released from cells involved in the immune system, particularly during infection (Lahdevirta *et al.*, 1988).

As malnutrition, malabsorption and wasting are major complications of HIV infection associated with a worsening prognosis, it is important to provide early nutritional intervention and aim to educate patients on the importance of maintaining nutrition. There are multiple causes that can result in reduced oral intake, malabsorption and altered metabolic states. Infections and diarrhoea are major factors and the therapeutic goals are to identify all treatable disorders that may be contributing to weight loss. Oral and enteral supplementation via nasoenteric tube or percutaneous gastrostomy (PEG) may be necessary in patients with intractable diarrhoea and weight loss. PEG feeding may be needed, especially in patients requiring long-term feeding. A small number of studies have shown improvement in body mass and albumin after enteral nutrition (Kotler *et al.*, 1991; Cappel and Godil, 1993). The use of medium-chain triglycerides and short peptides in patients with major small bowel dysfunction may also reduce malabsorption and diarrhoea (Wanke *et al.*, 1996). Parenteral nutrition is probably best considered in patients with severe small bowel dysfunction and malabsorption. With improved medical control of HIV infection, there is interest in longer term parenteral nutrition. Although it has been shown to increase weight, particularly over periods of 6–8 weeks in AIDS patients, the effect on survival is unclear (Melchior *et al.*, 1996; Babameto and Kotler, 1997). It seems that the rate of wound infections relating to PEG and central line insertion is only slightly increased in AIDS patients (Raviglione *et al.*, 1989). The role of anabolic agents, such as testosterone and growth hormone, and cytokine modulators, such as thalidomide, is not established (Babameto and Kotler, 1997).

DIAGNOSTIC EVALUATION OF DIARRHOEA

Initial evaluation of diarrhoea in HIV-infected patients requires a detailed history and examination. A travel history is important to identify not only recent travel to areas endemic for pathogens, such as *Cyclospora* sp. and *Isospora* sp., but also prior residence in areas endemic for tuberculosis, leishmaniasis or strongyloidiasis, which may reactivate years after initial exposure. A dietary history, including intake of raw or unpasteurized foods and lactose, should be taken. Some antiretroviral drugs, including didanosine and protease inhibitors, such as ritonavir, frequently cause diarrhoea and may need to be withdrawn if it is prolonged. The nature of the diarrhoeal symptoms is important to assist in localization of the disease process. Infrequent, large-volume, watery stools associated with bloating are indicative of small intestinal disease, whereas frequent small-volume stools containing blood and mucus, tenesmus and cramping lower abdominal pain are suggestive of colitis. Frequently, the clinical situation is difficult to distinguish clearly as some pathogens may involve both sites, or, alternatively, multiple pathogens may be present concurrently.

The investigations performed should be guided by the severity of the diarrhoea and the degree of immunosuppression. Patients with CD4 counts below 200/μL should be extensively evaluated for the opportunistic pathogens previously outlined. Patients with more intact immunity should initially have bacterial enteropathogens excluded prior to repeated examinations for stool parasites. A diagnostic algorithm for the evaluation of diarrhoea is outlined in Fig. 20.1. Faecal specimens should be submitted for microscopy for leucocytes and parasites, and cultured for bacterial pathogens. The *Clostridium difficile* toxin assay should be requested. Viral studies should be performed using enzyme immunoassay or electron microscopy when available. Modified acid-fast staining of the stool is the method most commonly used to detect *Cryptosporidium* sp., *Isospora* sp. and *Cyclospora* sp. infections. Modified trichrome staining to identify the spores of microsporidia should also be performed in severely immunosuppressed patients. Some laboratories may perform enzyme immunoassays, immunofluorescence or PCR for detection of some of these organisms. If the patient is febrile, blood cultures should be obtained in standard liquid media, as bacteraemia frequently complicates bacterial gastroenteritis. In patients with CD4 cell counts below 100/μL, blood should also be inoculated into mycobacterial media, such as BACTEC 13 A (Becton Dickinson™).

Endoscopic examination should follow if stool specimens fail to provide a diagnosis. Upper endoscopy with multiple small bowel biopsies should be performed first if the history is consistent with an enteritis.

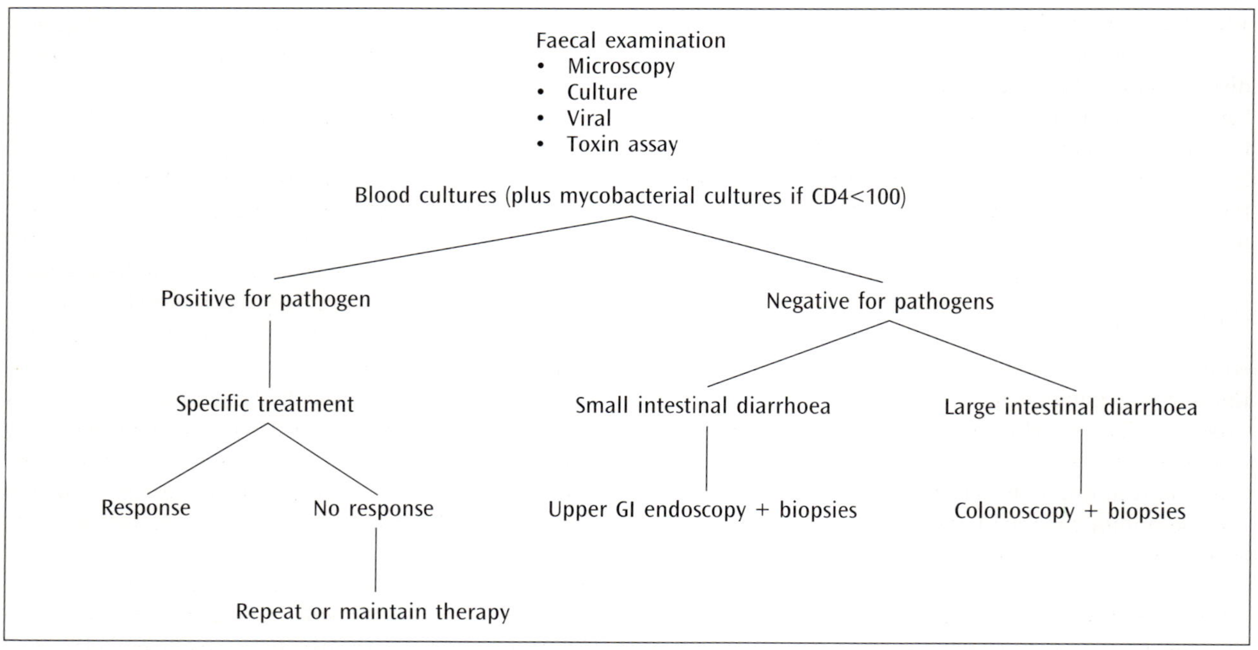

Figure 20.1 *Evaluation of HIV-related diarrhoea. GI, gastrointestinal.*

Colonoscopy or flexible sigmoidoscopy should be performed if a diagnosis is not obtained, or could be done at the same visit as the endoscopy if the clinical distinction between enteritis and colitis is blurred. Intestinal biopsies should be sent for histopathology with haematoxylin–eosin, Grocott methenamine-silver and Ziehl–Nielsen staining. In addition, mycobacterial cultures and viral studies, including CMV, should be performed on unfixed tissue. Between 15 and 40 per cent of patients with diarrhoea do not have an identifiable pathogen despite extensive evaluation. Many of these individuals have an enteropathy due to HIV *per se* and will respond to the commencement of highly active antiretroviral medication. If patients have end-stage disease that is resistant to antiretrovirals or are infected with untreatable opportunistic pathogens, symptomatic therapy is the only available option. Antimotility agents, such as loperamide, diphenoxylate hydrochloride or codeine phosphate, should be used initially; if these are ineffective, morphine or its derivatives may be added. In the event of severe unremitting secretory diarrhoea, octreotide should be considered, beginning with 50 mg subcutaneously 8 hourly, titrating the dose every 48 hours to a maximum of 500 mg every 8 hours.

CONCLUSION

A great deal of knowledge has been acquired regarding the nature and treatment of HIV-related intestinal complications. In many cases, this has led to improvements in the care of immunosuppressed patients without HIV. However, there remain gaps in the understanding of the biology of HIV, including its exact role in the gut, and the role of the intestine as a reservoir of HIV infection. Advances in anti-HIV therapy with immune reconstitution have led to a reduction in the frequency of many complications of HIV, although for the majority of the worlds' HIV sufferers this is beyond their grasp. Future developments in antiretroviral therapy should include targeting the intestine specifically.

REFERENCES

Albrecht, H., Sobottka, I., Emminger, C. *et al.* 1996: Visceral leishmaniasis emerging as an important opportunistic infection in HIV infected persons living in areas nonendemic for *Leishmania donovani*. *Archives of Pathology and Laboratory Medicine* 120, 189–98.

Anand, B.S., Schneider, F.R., El-Zaatari, F.A., Shawar, R.M., Clarridge, J.E., Graham, D.Y. 1994: Diagnosis of intestinal tuberculosis by polymerase chain reaction on endoscopic biopsy specimens. *American Journal of Gastroenterology* 89, 2248–9.

Angarano, G., Maggi, P., DiBari, M.A. *et al.* 1997: Giardiasis in HIV: a possible role in patients with severe immunodeficiency. *European Journal of Epidemiology* 13, 485–7.

Anwar-Bruni, D.M., Hogan, S.E., Schwartz, D.A., Wilcox, C.M., Bryan, R.T., Lennox, J.L. 1996: Atovaquone is effective treatment for the symptoms of gastrointestinal microsporidiosis in HIV-1 infected patients. *AIDS* 10, 619–23.

Babameto, G., Kotler, D.P. 1997: Malnutrition in HIV infection. *Gastroenterology Clinics of North America* 26, 393–415.

Benhamou, Y., Hilmarsdottir, I., Desportes-Livage, I. *et al.* 1994: Association of lipid accumulation in small intestinal mucosa with decreased serum triglyceride and cholesterol levels in AIDS. *Digestive Diseases and Sciences* 39, 2163–9.

Benhamou, Y., Kapel, N., Hoang, C. *et al.* 1995: Inefficacy of intestinal secretory immune response to *Cryptosporidium* in acquired immunodeficiency syndrome. *Gastroenterology* 108, 627–35.

Bigornia, E., Simon, D., Weiss, L.M. *et al.* 1992: Detection of HIV-1 protein and nucleic acid in enterochromaffin cells of HIV-1 seropositive patients. *American Jounal of Gastroenterology* 87, 1624–9.

Blanshard, C., Benhamou, Y., Dohin, E., Lernestedt, J.O., Gazzard, B.G., Katlama, C. 1995: Treatment of AIDS associated gastrointestinal CMV infection with foscarnet and ganciclovir: a randomised comparison. *Journal of Infectious Diseases* 172, 622–8.

Blanshard, C., Francis, N., Gazzard, B.G. 1996: Investigation of chronic diarrhoea in acquired immunodeficiency syndrome. A prospective study of 155 patients. *Gut* 39, 824–32.

Blanshard, C., Shanson, D.C., Gazzard, V.G. 1997: Pilot studies of azithromycin, letrazuril and paromomycin in the treatment of cryptosporidiosis. *International Journal of STDs and AIDS* 8, 124–9.

Cacciarelli, A.G., Marano, B.J., Gualtieri, N.M., Zuretti, A.R., Torres, R.A., Starpoli, A.A., Robilotti, J.G. 1996: Lower *Helicobacter pylori* infection and peptic ulcer disease in patients with AIDS and suppressed CD4 counts. *American Journal of Gastroenterology* 91, 1783–4.

Cappell, M.S., Godil, A. 1993: A multicentre case controlled study of percutaneous endoscopic gastrostomy in HIV seropositive patients. *American Journal of Gastroenterology* 88, 2059.

Cappell, M.S., Philogene, C. 1995: The endoscopic appearance of severe intestinal Mycobacterium avium complex infection and a coarsely granular mucosa due to massive infiltration and expansion of intestinal villi without mucosal exudation. *Journal of Clinical Gastroenterology* 21, 323–6.

Carlson, S., Yokoo, H., Craig, R. 1994: Small intestinal HIV associated enteropathy: evidence for panintestinal enterocyte dysfunction. *Journal of Laboratory and Clinical Medicine* 124, 652–9.

Chang, E.B., Musch, M.W., Mayer, L. 1990: Interleukins 1 and 3 stimulate anion secretion in chicken intestine. *Gastroenterology* 98, 1518–23.

Chang, Y., Cesarman, E., Pessin, M.S., Lee, F., Culpepper, J., Knowles, D.M., Moore, P.S. 1994: Identification of herpesvirus-like DNA sequences in AIDS-associated Kaposi's sarcoma. *Science* 266, 1865–9.

Chin, D.P. 1994: Mycobacterium avium complex. In Cohen, P.T., Sande, M.A., Volberding, P.A. (eds) *The AIDS knowledge base*, 2nd edn. Little, Brown and Co., 6.4-1–14.

Chlebowski, R.T., Grosvenor, M.B., Bernhard, N.H. 1989: Nutritional status, gastrointestinal dysfunction and survival in patients with AIDS. *American Journal of Gastroenterology* 84, 1288–93.

Clayton, F., Heller, T., Kotler, D.P. 1994: Variation in the enteric distribution of cryptosporidia in acquired immunodeficiency syndrome. *American Journal of Clinical Pathology* 102, 420–5.

Clezy, K., Gold, J., Blaze, J., Jones, P. 1991: Paromomycin for the treatment of cryptococcal diarrhoea in AIDS patients. *AIDS* 5, 1146–7.

Colebunders, R., Lusakumuni, K., Nelson, A.M. *et al.* 1988: Persistent diarrhoea in Zairian AIDS patients: an endoscopic and histological study. *Gut* 29, 1687–91.

Connor, B.A., Shlim, D.R., Scholes, J.V., Rayburn, J.L., Reidy, J., Rajah, R. 1993: Pathologic changes in the small bowel in 9 patients with diarrhea associated with a coccidia-like body. *Annals of Internal Medicine* 119, 377–82.

Coodley, G.O., Loveless, M.O., Nelson, H.D., Coodley, M.K. 1994: Endocrine function in the HIV wasting syndrome. *Journal of Acquired Immune Deficiency Syndrome* 7, 46–51.

Cotte, L., Drouet, E., Bissuel, F., Denoyel, G.A., Trepo, C. 1993: Diagnostic value of amplification of human cytomegalovirus DNA from gastrointestinal biopsies in HIV infected patients. *Journal of Clinical Microbiology* 31, 2066–9.

Cunningham, A.L., Grohman, G.S., Harkness, J., Law, C., Marriott, D., Tindall, B., Cooper, D.A. 1988: Gastrointestinal viral infections in homosexual men who were symptomatic and seropositive for HIV. *Journal of Infectious Diseases* 158, 386–91.

Davidson, R.N., DiMartino, L., Gradoni, L. *et al.* 1994: Liposomal amphotericin in Mediterranean visceral leishmaniasis: a multi-centre trial. *Quarterly Journal of Medicine* 87, 75–81.

DeGirolami, P.C., Ezratty, C.R., Desai, G., McCullough, A., Asmuth, D., Wanke, C., Federman, M. 1995: Diagnosis of intestinal microsporidiosis by examination of stool and duodenal aspirate with Weber's modified trichrome and Uvitex B stain. *Journal of Clinical Microbiology* 33, 805–10.

Dehovitz, J.A., Pape, J.W., Boncy, M., Johnson, W.D. 1986: Clinical manifestations and therapy of Isospora belli infections in patients with the acquired immunodeficiency syndrome. *New England Journal of Medicine* 315, 87–90.

Desportes-Livage, I. 1996: Human microsporidioses and AIDS: recent advances. *Parasite* 3, 107–13.

Dieterich, D.T., Rahmin, M. 1991: Cytomegalovirus colitis in AIDS: presentation in 44 patients and a review of the literature. *Journal of the Acquired Immune Deficiency Syndrome* 4(Suppl), S29–35.

Dieterich, D.T., Kotler, D.P., Busch, D.F., Crumpacker, C., DuMond, C., Dearmand, B., Buhles, W. 1993: Ganciclovir treatment of cytomegalovirus colitis in AIDS: a randomized double blind placebo controlled multicentre study. *Journal of Infectious Diseases* 167, 278–82.

Dionisio, D., Sterrantino, G., Meli, M., Leoncini, F., Orsi, A., Nicholetti, P. 1996: Treatment of isosporiasis with combined albendazole and ornidazole in patients with AIDS. *AIDS* 10, 1301–2.

Dobbins, W.O., Weinstein, W.M. 1985: Electron microscopy of the intestine and rectum in acquired immunodeficiency syndrome. *Gastroenterology* 88, 738–42.

Dore, G.J., Marriott, D.J., Hing, M.C., Harkness, J.S., Field, A.S. 1995: Disseminated microsporidiosis due to *S. intestinalis* in nine patients with the human immunodeficiency virus: response to therapy with albendazole. *Clinical Infectious Diseases* 21, 70–6.

Ehrenpreis, E.D., Ganger, D.R., Kochvar, G.T., Patterson, B.K., Craig, R.M. 1992a: D-xylose malabsorption : characteristic findings in patients with the AIDS wasting syndrome and chronic diarrhoea. *Journal of the Acquired Immune Deficiency Syndrome* 10, 1047–50.

Ehrenpreis, E.D., Patterson, B.K., Brainer, J.A. *et al.* 1992b: Histopathological findings of duodenal biopsy specimens in HIV infected patients with and without diarrhoea and malabsorption. *American Journal of Clinical Pathology*, 97, 21–8.

Ehrenpreis, E.D., Carlson, S.J., Boorstein, H.L., Craig, R.M. 1994: Malabsorption and deficiency of vitamin B12 in HIV infected patients with chronic diarrhoea. *Digestive Diseases and Sciences* 39, 2159–62.

Eriksson, K., Kilander, A., Hagberg, L., Norkrans, G., Holmgren, J., Czerkinsky, C. 1993: Intestinal antibody responses to oral vaccination in HIV infected individuals. *AIDS* 7, 1087–91.

Fackler, O., Schafer, M., Schmidt, W. *et al.* 1998: HIV-1 p24 but not proviral load is increased in the intestinal mucosa compared with the peripheral blood in HIV-infected patients. *AIDS* 12, 139–46.

Field, A.S., Hing, M.C., Milliken, S.T., Marriott, D.J. 1993: Microsporidia in the small intestine of HIV infected patients. *Medical Journal of Australia* 158, 390–4.

Flanigan, T., Whalen, C., Turner, J., Soave, R., Toerner, J., Havli, D., Kotler, D. 1992: Cryptosporidium infection and CD4 counts. *Annals of Internal Medicine* 116, 840–2.

Fleming, S.C., Kapembwa, M.S., McDonald, T.T., Griffin. G.E. 1992: Direct in vitro infection of human intestine with HIV. *AIDS* 6, 1099–104.

Foudraine, N., Weverling, G., van Gool, T. *et al.* 1998: Improvement in chronic diarrhoea in patients with advanced HIV-1 infection during potent anti-retroviral therapy. *AIDS* 12, 35–41.

Francis, N.D., Boylston, A.W., Roberts, A.H., Parkin, J.M., Pinching, A.J. 1989: Cytomegalovirus infection in gastrointestinal tracts of patients infected with HIV-1 or AIDS. *Journal of Clinical Pathology* 42, 1055–64.

Friedenberg, K.A., Draguesku, J.O., Kiyabu, M., Valenzuela, J.E. 1993: Intestinal perforation due to *M. tuberculosis* in HIV infected individuals: report of two cases. *American Journal of Gastroenterology* 88, 604–7.

Friedman, S., Wright, T., Altman, D. 1985: Gastrointestinal manifestations of Kaposi's sarcoma in acquired immunodeficiency syndrome: endoscopic and autopsy findings. *Gastroenterology* 89, 102–8.

Genta, R.M., Chappell, C.L., White, A.C., Kimball, K.T., Goodgame, R.W. 1993: Duodenal morphology and intensity of infection in AIDS related intestinal cryptosporidiosis. *Gastroenterology* 105, 1769–75.

Gill, P.S., Lunardi-Iskander, Y., Louie, S. *et al.* 1996: The effects of preparations of human chorionic gonadotrophin on AIDS related Kaposi's sarcoma. *New England Journal of Medicine* 335, 1261–9.

Goguel, J., Katlama, C., Sarfati, C., Maslo, C., Leport, C., Molina, J.M. 1997: Remission of AIDS-associated intestinal microsporidiosis with highly active antiretroviral therapy. *AIDS* 11, 1658–9.

Goodgame, R.W., Genta, R.M., Estrada, R., Demmler, G., Buffone, G. 1993: Frequency of positive tests for cytomegalovirus in AIDS patients: endoscopic lesions compared with normal mucosa. *American Journal of Gastroenterology* 88, 338–43.

Gradoni, L., Scalone, A., Gramiccia, M., Troiani, M. 1996: Epidemiological surveillance of leishmaniasis in HIV-1 infected individuals in Italy. *AIDS* 10, 785–91.

Gray, J.R., Rabeneck, L. 1989: Atypical mycobacterial infection of the gastrointestinal tract in AIDS patients. *American Journal of Gastroenterology* 88, 604–7.

Greenberg, P.D., Koch, J., Cello, J.P. 1996: Diagnosis of Cryptosporidium parvum in patients with severe diarrhoea and AIDS. *Digestive Diseases and Sciences* 41, 2286–90.

Greenson, J., Belitsas, P., Yardley, J., Bartlett, J. 1991: AIDS enteropathy: occult enteric infection and duodenal mucosal alterations in chronic diarrhoea. *Annals of Internal Medicine* 114, 366–72.

Griffin, G.E. 1990: Malabsorption, malnutrition and HIV disease. *Bailliere's Clinical Gastroenterology* 4(2), 361–73.

Grohmann, G.S., Glass, R.I., Pereira, H.G., Monroe, S.S., Hightower, A.W., Weber, R., Bryan, R.T. 1993: Enteric viruses and diarrhea in HIV infected patients. *New England Journal of Medicine* 329, 14–20.

Guarda, L.A., Luna, M.A., Smith, J.L., Mansell, P.W., Gyorkey, F., Roca, A.N. 1984: Acquired immune deficiency syndrome: autopsy findings. *American Journal of Clinical Pathology* 81, 549–57.

Guarino, A., Tarallo, L., Guandalini, S., Troncone, R., Albano, F., Rubino, A. 1991: Impaired intestinal function in symptomatic HIV infection. *Journal of Paediatric Gastroenterology and Nutrition* 12, 453–8.

Guarino, A., Russo, S., Castaldo, A,, Spagnuolo, M.I., Tarallo, L., Rubino, A. 1996: Passive immunotherapy for rotavirus induced diarrhoea in children with HIV infection. *AIDS* 10, 1176–7.

Guenter, P., Muurahainen, N., Simons, G., Kosok, A., Cohan, G.R., Redenstein, R., Turner, J.L. 1993: Relationships among nutritional status, disease progression and survival in HIV infection. *Journal of Acquired Immune Deficiency Syndrome* 6, 1130.

Hajjeh, R.A. 1995: Disseminated histoplasmosis in persons infected with HIV. *Clinical Infectious Diseases* 21(Suppl 1), S108–10.

Harcourt-Webster, J.N., Scaravilli, F., Darwish, A.H. 1991: *Strongyloides stercoralis* hyperinfection in an HIV-positive patient. *Journal of Clinical Pathology* 44, 346–8.

Harriman, G.R., Smith, P.D., Horne, M.K. *et al.* 1989: Vitamin B12 malabsorption in patients with the acquired immunodeficiency syndrome. *Archives of Internal Medicine* 149, 2039–41.

Havlir, D.V., Dube, M.P., Sattler, F.R. *et al.* 1996: Prophylaxis against disseminated *Mycobacterium avium* complex infection with weekly azithromycin, daily rifabutin or both. *New England Journal of Medicine* 335, 392–8.

Hayes, E.B., Matte, T.D., O'Brien, T.R. *et al.* 1989: Large community outbreak of cryptosporidiosis due to contamination of a filtered public water supply. *New England Journal of Medicine* 320, 1372–6.

Hazen, K.C. 1993: Controversial fungal and protozoan gastrointestinal infections. *Current Opinion in Infectious Diseases* 6, 77–82.

Herzlich, B.C., Schiano, T.D., Moussa, Z., Zimbalist, E., Panagopoulos, G., Ast, A., Nawabi, I. 1992: Decreased intrinsic factor secretion in AIDS: relation to parietal cell acid secretory capacity and vitamin B12 malabsorption. *American Journal of Gastroenterology* 87, 1781–8.

Holland, G.N., Sison, R.F., Jatulis, D.E., Haslop, M.G., Sakamoto, M.J., Wheeler, N.C. 1990: Survival of patients with acquired immunodeficiency syndrome after development of CMV retinopathy. *Ophthalmology* 97, 204–11.

Holmberg, S.D., Moorman, A.C., VonBargen, J.C., Palella, F.J., Loveless, M.O., Ward, D.J., Navin, T.R. 1998: Possible effectiveness of clarithromycin and rifabutin for cryptosporidiosis for chemo prophylaxis in HIV disease. *JAMA* 279, 384–6.

Horvath, K.D., Whelan. R.L. 1998: Intestinal tuberculosis: return of an old disease. *American Journal of Gastroenterology* 93, 692–6.

Janoff, E.N., Jackson, S., Wahl, S.M., Thomas, K., Peterman, J.H., Smith. P.D. 1994: Intestinal immunoglobulins during human immunodeficiency virus type 1 infection. *Journal of Infectious Diseases* 170, 299–307.

Kapelushnik, J., Or, R., Delukina, M., Nagler, A., Livni, N., Engelhard, D. 1995: Intravenous ribavirin therapy for adenovirus gastroenteritis after bone marrow transplantation. *Journal of Pediatric Gastroenterology and Nutrition* 21, 110–12.

Kapembwa, M.S., Batman, P.A., Fleming, S.C., Griffin, G.E. 1989: HIV enteropathy. *Lancet* 2, 1521–2.

Kapembwa, M.S., Fleming, S.C., Orr, M., Wells, C., Bland, M., Back D., Griffin, G.E. 1996: Impaired absorption of zidovudine in patients with AIDS related small intestinal disease. *AIDS* 10, 1509–14.

Keating, J., Bjarnason, I., Somasundaram, S. *et al.* 1995: Intestinal absorptive capacity, intestinal permeability and jejunal histology in HIV and their relation to diarrhoea. *Gut* 37, 623–9.

Kim, K.M., Lee, A., Choi, K.Y., Lee, K.Y., Kwak, J.J. 1998: Intestinal tuberculosis: clinicopathologic analysis and diagnosis by endoscopic biopsy. *American Journal of Gastroenterology* 93, 606–9.

Konturek, J.W., Fischer, H., Van Der Voort, I.R., Domschke, W. 1997: Disturbed gastric motor activity in patients with human immunodeficiency virus infection. *Scandinavian Journal of Gastroenterology* 32, 221–5.

Kotler, D.P., Orenstein, J.M. 1994: Prevalence of intestinal microsporidiosis in HIV infected individuals referred for gastroenterological evaluation. *American Journal of Gastroenterology* 89, 1998.

Kotler, D.P., Gaetz, H.P., Lange, M., Klein, E., Holt, D.R. 1984: Enteropathy associated with the acquired immunodeficiency syndrome. *Annals of Internal Medicine* 101, 421–8.

Kotler, D., Weaver, S., Terzakis, J. 1986: Ultrastructural features of epithelial cells degeneration in rectal crypts of patients with AIDS. *American Journal of Surgical Pathology* 10, 531–8.

Kotler, D.P., Tierney, A.R., Wang, J., Pierson, R.N. 1989: The magnitude of body cell mass depletion and the timing of death from wasting in AIDS. *American Journal of Clinical Nutrition* 50, 444–7.

Kotler, D.P., Tierney, A.R., Ferraro, R., Cuff, P., Wang, J., Pierson, R.N., Heymsfield, S.B. 1991: Enteral feeding and repletion of body cell mass in malnourished patients with acquired immunodeficiency syndrome. *American Journal of Clinical Nutrition* 53, 149–54.

Kotler, D., Reka, S., Clayton, F. 1993: Intestinal mucosal inflammation associated with HIV infection. *Digestive Diseases and Sciences* 38, 1119–27.

Kotler, D., Terumasa, S., Snow, G. *et al.* 1998: Effect of combination antiretroviral therapy upon rectal mucosal HIV RNA burden and mononuclear cell apoptosis. *AIDS* 12, 597–604.

Kuhn, J.C., Wendland, T., Eggers, H.J. *et al.* 1995: Quantitation of human cytomegalovirus genomes in the brain of AIDS patients. *Journal of Medical Virology* 47, 70.

Laguna, F., Garcia-Samaniego, J., Moreno, V., Gonzalez-Lahoz, J.M. 1994: Prevalence of gastrointestinal leishmaniasis in Spanish HIV positive patients with digestive symptoms. *American Journal of Gastroenterology* 89, 1606.

Lahdevirta, J., Maury, C.P.J., Teppo, A.M., Repo, H. 1988: Elevated levels of circulating cachectin/tumour necrosis factor in patients with acquired immunodeficiency syndrome. *American Journal of Medicine* 85, 289–91.

Lake-Bakaar, G., Quadros, E., Beidas, S. *et al.* 1988: Gastric secretory failure in patients with the acquired immunodeficiency syndrome (AIDS). *Annals of Internal Medicine* 109, 502–4.

Lalezari, J.P., Drew, W.L., Glutzer, E. *et al.* 1995: Cidofovir: results of a phase I/II study of a novel antiviral nucleotide analogue. *Journal of Infectious Diseases* 171, 788–96.

Lambl, B.B., Federman, M., Pleskow, D., Wanke, C. 1996: Malabsorption and wasting in AIDS patients with microsporidia and pathogen negative diarrhoea. *AIDS* 10, 739–44.

Lanjewar, D.A., Rodrigues, C., Saple, D.G., Hira, S.K., DuPont, H.L. 1996: Cryptosporidium, Isospora and Strongyloides in AIDS. *National Medical Journal of India* 9, 17–19.

Lew, E.A., Poles, M.A., Dieterich, D.T. 1997: Diarrheal diseases associated with HIV infection. *Gastroenterology Clinics of North America* 26, 259–90.

Liguory, O., David, F., Sarfati, C. *et al.* 1997: Diagnosis of infections caused by *Enterocytozoon bieneusi* and *Encephalitozoon intestinalis* using polymerase chain reaction in stool specimens. *AIDS* 11, 723–6.

Lin, J.-C. 1998: Kaposi's sarcoma and HHV-8: implications for therapy. *Infections in Medicine* 15, 337–43.

Lu, S., Chen, W., Kotler, D. 1996: Variation in mucosal apoptosis along the length of the intestine in HIV (+) subjects (abstract). *Gastroenterology* 2, 70A.

Macnab, K.A., Gill, M.J., Sutherland, L.R., Murphy, A., Brant, R. 1996: Zidovudine absorption and small intestinal function in HIV sero-positive patients. *Journal of Antimicrobial Chemotherapy* 37, 825–9.

MacPherson, D.W., McQueen, R. 1993: Cryptosporidiosis: multiattribute evaluation of six diagnostic methods. *Journal of Clinical Microbiology* 31, 198–202.

Manatsathit, S., Tansupasawasdikul, S., Wanachiwanawin, D. *et al.* 1996: Causes of chronic diarrhoea in patients with AIDS in Thailand: a prospective clinical and microbioligical study. *Journal of Gastroenterology* 31, 533–7.

Maslo, C., Girard P.M., Urban, T., Guessant, S., Rozenbaum, W. 1997: Ribavirin therapy for adenovirus pneumonia in an AIDS patient. *American Journal of Respiratory and Critical Care Medicine* 156, 1263–4.

Mathewson, J.J., Jiang, Z.D., Zumla, A. *et al.* 1995: HEp-2 cell adherent *Escherichia coli* in patients with human immunodeficiency virus associated diarrhoea. *Journal of Infectious Diseases* 171, 1636–9.

Mathewson, J.J., Salameh, B.M., Dupont, H.L. *et al.* 1998: HEp-2 cell adherent *Escherichia coli* and intestinal secretory immune response to human immunodeficiency virus (HIV) in outpatients with HIV associated diarrhoea. *Clinical Diagnostic Laboratory Immunology* 5, 87–90.

McGowan, I., Radford-Smith, G., Jewell, D.P. 1994: Cytokine gene expression in HIV-infected intestinal mucosa. *AIDS* 8, 1569–75.

McKinsey, D.S., Spiegel, R.A., Hutwagner, L. *et al.* 1997: Prospective study of histoplasmosis in patients infected with HIV: incidence, risk factors, and pathophysiology. *Clinical Infectious Diseases* 24, 1195–203.

McMeeking, A., Borkowsky, W., Klesius, P.H., Bonk, S., Holzman, R.S., Lawrence, H.S. 1989: A controlled trial of bovine dialyzable leucocyte extract for cryptosporidiosis in patients with AIDS. *Journal of Infectious Diseases* 161, 108–12.

Melchior, J.C., Chastang, C., Gelas, P. *et al.* 1996: Efficacy of two month total parenteral nutrition in AIDS patients: controlled, randomised prospective trial. *AIDS* 10, 379–84.

Mellors, J.W., Rinaldo, C.R., Gupta, P., White, R.M., Todd, J.A., Kingsley, L.A. 1996: Prognosis in HIV-1 infection predicted by the quantity of virus in plasma. *Science* 272(5265), 1167–70.

Miller, A.R., Griffen, G.E., Batman, P., Farquar, C., Forster, S.M., Pinching, A.J., Harris, J.R. 1988: Jejunal mucosal architecture and fat malabsorption in male homosexuals infected with human immuno-deficiency virus. *Quarterly Journal of Medicine* 69, 1009–119.

Mocroft, A., Youle, M., Gazzard, B., Morcinek, J., Halai, R., Phillips, A.N. 1996: Anti-herpesvirus treatment and risk of Kaposi's sarcoma in HIV infection. *AIDS* 10, 1101–5.

Molina, J.M., Sarfati, C., Beauvaisa, B. *et al.* 1993: Intestinal microsporidiosis in human immunodeficiency virus infected patients with chronic unexplained diarrhoea: prevalence and clinical and biologic features. *Journal of Infectious Diseases* 167, 217–21.

Molina, J.M., Goguel, J., Sarfati, C. *et al.* 1997: Potential efficacy of fumagillin in intestinal microsporidiosis due to *Enterocytozoon bieneusi* in patients with HIV infection; results of a drug screening study. *AIDS* 11, 1603–10.

Muigai, R., Gatei, D.G., Shaunak, S., Wozniak, A., Bryceson, A.D.M. 1983: Jejunal function and pathology in visceral leishmaniasis. *Lancet* ii, 476–9.

Orenstein, J.M., Kotler, D.P. 1995: Diarrhoegeneic bacterial enteritis in acquired immune deficiency syndrome: a light and electron microscopy study of 52 cases. *Human Pathology* 26, 481–92.

Ott, M., Wegner, A., Caspary, W.F., Lembcke, B. 1993: Intestinal absorption and malnutrition in patients with the acquired immunodeficiency syndrome (AIDS). *Zeitschrift für Gastroenterologie* 11, 661–5.

Ortega, Y.R., Sterling, C.R., Gilman, R.H., Cama, V.A., Diaz, F. 1993: Cyclospora species, a new protozoan pathogen of humans. *New England Journal of Medicine* 328, 1308–12.

Palenicek, J.G., Graham, N.M., He, Y.D., Hoover, D.A., Oishi, J.S., Kingsley, L., Saah, A.J. 1995: Weight loss prior to clinical AIDS as a predictor of survival. *Journal of Acquired Immune Deficiency Syndrome* 10, 366.

Papanaoum, K., Collins, P.J., Manning, J., Bartholomeusz, F.D.L., Horowitz, M., Shaw, D.R. 1992: Delayed gastric emptying in patients with HIV infection. *Australian and New Zealand Journal of Medicine* 22, 762.

Pape, J.W., Verdier, R.I., Boncy, M., Boncy, J., Johnson, W.D. 1994: Cyclospora infection in adults infected with HIV: clinical manifestations, treatment and prophylaxis. *Annals of Internal Medicine* 121, 654–7.

Patterson, B., Ehrenpreis, E., Yokoo, H. 1993: Focal enterocyte vacuolization: a new microscopic finding in acquired immune deficiency wasting syndrome. *American Journal of Clinical Pathology* 99, 24–7.

Petersen, C. 1992: Cryptosporidiosis in patients infected with the human immunodeficiency virus. *Clinical Infectious Diseases* 15, 903–9.

Petersen, C., Wofsy, C.B. 1994: Isosporiasis. In Cohen, P.T., Sande, M.A., Volberding, P.A. (eds) *The AIDS knowledge base*, 2nd edn. Little Brown and Co., 6.20.1–5.

Pierce, M., Crampton, S., Henry, D. *et al.* 1996: A randomized trial of clarithromycin as prophylaxis against disseminated *Mycobacterium avium* complex infection in patients with advanced acquired immunodeficiency syndrome. *New England Journal of Medicine* 335, 384–91.

Pollok, R.C., Bendall, R.P., Moody, A., Chiodini, P.L., Churchill, D.R. 1992: Traveller's diarrhoea associated with cyanobacterium-like bodies. *Lancet* 340, 556–7.

Quinn, T.C., Stamm, W.E., Goodell, S.E. *et al.* 1983: The polymicrobial origin of intestinal infections in homosexual men. *New England Journal of Medicine* 309, 576–82.

Rabeneck, L., Gyorkey, F., Genta, R.M., Gyorkey, P., Foote, L.W., Risser, J.M.H. 1993: The role of microsporidia in the pathogenesis of HIV related chronic diarrhoea. *Annals of Internal Medicine* 119, 895–9.

Rabeneck, L., Genta, R., Risser, J., Bailey, M., Clarridge, J., Gyorkey, F. 1996: Uncertain clinical significance of duodenal mucosal abnormalities in HIV infected individuals. *Journal of Clinical Gastroenterology* 23, 11–14.

Raviglione, M.C., Battan, R., Pablos-Mendez, A., Aceves-Casillas, P., Mullen, M.P., Taranta, A. 1989: Infections associated with Hickman's catheters in patients with acquired immunodeficiency syndrome. *American Journal of Medicine* 86, 780–6.

Ritchie, D.J., Becker, E.S. 1994: Update on the management of intestinal cryptosporidiosis in AIDS. *Annals of Pharmacotherapy* 28, 767–78.

Romeu, J., Miro, J.M., Sirea, G. *et al.* 1991: Efficacy of octreotide in the management of chronic diarrhoea in AIDS. *AIDS* 5, 1495–9.

Sarosi, G.A., Johnson, P.C. 1992: Disseminated histoplasmosis in patients infected with HIV. *Clinical Infectious Diseases* 14 (Suppl 1), S60–7.

Schecter, G.F. 1994: Mycobacterium tuberculosis infection.

In Cohen, P.T., Sande, M.A., Volberding, P.A. (eds) *The AIDS knowledge base*, 2nd edn. Little Brown and Co., 6.5.1–6.

Schmidt, W., Schneider, T., Heise, W. *et al.* 1996: Stool viruses, coinfections and diarrhoea in HIV infected patients. *Journal of Acquired Immune Deficiency Syndromes and Human Retrovirology* 13, 33–8.

Schmidt, W., Schneider, T., Heise, W. *et al.* 1997: Mucosal abnormalities in microsporidiosis. *AIDS* 11, 1589–94.

Sciarretta, G., Bonazzi, L., Monti, M. *et al.* 1994: Bile acid malabsorption in AIDS associated chronic diarrhoea: prospective one year study. *American Journal of Gastroenterology* 89, 379–81.

Sharpstone, D., Rowbottom, A., Nelson, M. *et al.* 1995: The treatment of microsporidial diarrhoea with thalidomide. *AIDS* 9, 658.

Sifuentes-Osornio, J., Porras-Cortes, G., Bendall, R.P., Morales-Villareal, F., Reyes-Teran, G., Ruiz-Palacios, G.M. 1995: *Cyclospora cayatenensis* infection in patients with and without AIDS: biliary disease as another clinical manifestation. *Clinical Infectious Diseases* 21, 1092–7.

Smith, P.D., Quinn, T.C., Strober, W,, Janoff, E.N., Masur, H. 1992: Gastrointestinal infections in AIDS. *Annals of Internal Medicine* 116, 63–77.

Soave, R., Johnson, W.D. 1988: *Cryptosporidium* and *Isospora belli* infections. *Journal of Infectious Diseases* 157, 225–9.

Soave, R., Dubey, J.P., Ramos, L.J., Tummings, M. 1986: A new intestinal pathogen? *Clinical Research* 34, 533.

Sobottka, I., Schwartz, D.A., Schottelius, J. *et al.* 1998: Prevalence and clinical significance of intestinal microsporidiosis in human immunodeficiency virus infected patients with and without diarrhoea in Germany: a prospective coprodiagnostic study. *Clinical Infectious Diseases* 26, 475–80.

Sperber, S.J., Schleupner, C.J. 1987: Salmonellosis during infection with human immunodeficiency virus. *Reviews of Infectious Diseases* 9, 925–32.

Stockmann, M., Fromm, M., Schmitz, H., Schmidt, W., Reichen, E., Schulzhe, J. 1998: Duodenal biopsies of HIV-infected patients with diarrhoea exhibit epithelial barrier defects but no active secretion. *AIDS* 12, 43–51.

Talal, A.H., Weiss, L.M., Vanderhorst, C. 1997: Molecular diagnosis of gastrointestinal infections associated with HIV infection. *Gastroenterology Clinics of North America* 26, 417–44.

Tee, W., Mijch, A. 1998: *Camylobacter jejeuni* bacteraemia in human immuno-deficiency virus infected and non HIV infected patients: comparison of clinical features and review. *Clinical Infectious Diseases* 26, 91–6.

UNAIDS 1998: *Report on the global HIV/AIDS epidemic.* Geneva: UNAIDS, World Health Organization, June 1998.

Ungar, B.L.P. 1995: Cryptosporidium. In Mandell, G.L., Bennett, J.E., Dolin, R. (eds) *Principles and practice of infectious diseases,* 4th edn, New York: Churchill Livingstone, 2500–10.

Verdon, R., Polianski, J., Gaudebout, C., Marche, C., Garry, L., Carbon, C., Pocidalo, J.J. 1995: Evaluation of high dose regimen of paromomycin against cryptosporidiosis in the dexamethasone treated rat model. *Antimicrobial Agents and Chemotherapy* 39, 2155–7.

Wanke, C.A., Pleskow, D., Degirolami, P.C., Lamb, B.B., Merkel, K., Akrabawi, S. 1996: A medium chain triglyceride based diet in patients with HIV and chronic diarrhoea reduces diarrhoea and malabsorption: a prospective controlled trial. *Nutrition* 12, 766–71.

Wanke, C.A., Mayer, H., Weber, R., Zbinden, R., Watson, D.A., Acheson, D. 1998a: Enteroaggregative *Escherichia coli* as a potential cause of diarrhoeal disease in adults infected with human immunodeficiency virus. *Journal of Infectious Diseases* 178, 185–90.

Wanke, C.A., Gerrior, J., Blais, V., Mayer, H., Acheson, D. 1998b: Successful treatment of diarrhoeal disease associated with enteroaggregative *Escherichia coli* in adults infected with human immunodeficiency virus. *Journal of Infectious Diseases* 178, 1369–72.

Weber, R., Bryan, R.T., Schwartz, D.A., Owen, R.L. 1994: Human microsporidial infections. *Clinical Microbiology Reviews* 7, 426–61.

Welch, K., Finkbeiner, W., Alpers, C.E., Blumenfeld, W., Davis, R.L., Smuckler, E.A., Beckstead, J.H. 1984: Autopsy findings in the acquired immune deficiency syndrome. *JAMA* 252, 1152–9.

White, A.C., Chappell, C.L., Hayat, C., Kimball, K.T., Flanigan, T.P., Goodgame, R.W. 1994: Paromomycin for cryptosporidiosis in AIDS: a prospective double-blind trial. *Journal of Infectious Diseases* 170, 419–24.

Wittner, M., Tanowitz, H.B., Weiss, L.M. 1993: Parasitic infections in AIDS patients. *Infectious Disease Clinics of North America* 7, 569–86.

Wuhib, T., Silva, T.M.J., Newman, R.D. *et al.* 1994: Cryptosporidial and microsporidial infections in human immunodeficiency virus infected patients in north-eastern Brazil. *Journal of Infectious Diseases* 170, 494–7.

Zangerle, R., Sarcletti, M., Gallati, H., Reibnegger, G., Wachter, H., Fuchs, D. 1994: Decreased plasma concentration of HDL cholesterol in HIV infected individuals is associated with immune activation. *Journal of Acquired Immune Deficiency Syndrome* 7, 1149–56.

Ziegler, J.L., Beckstead, J.A., Volberding, P.A. *et al.* 1984: Non-Hodgkin's lymphoma in 90 homosexual men: relation to generalized lymphadenopathy and the acquired immunodeficiency syndrome. *New England Journal of Medicine* 311, 565–70.

21

Tropical sprue

VI MATHAN, MINNIE M MATHAN

INTRODUCTION

Failure of the primary function of the small intestine, the absorption of nutrients, leads to malabsorption syndromes. Malabsorption can result from abnormalities affecting any of the stages of digestion and absorption of nutrients. The underlying causes may be defects in intestinal luminal digestion, failure of the external secretions essential for digestion (liver, pancreas), alteration in the mucosal phase of absorption and obstruction to the transport of nutrients from the intestine to the rest of the body. There are many conditions, dealt with elsewhere (*see* Chapter 16), where the aetiology and pathogenesis of malabsorption is well understood and is secondary to the primary pathology. Examples of such diseases are coeliac disease (*see* Chapter 23), abetalipoproteinaemia (*see* Chapter 16), and Whipple's disease (*see* Chapter 22), which can be diagnosed by detailed investigations. Patients with malabsorption in whom no underlying causative disease is found have a primary or idiopathic malabsorption syndrome. Residents of or visitors to certain tropical regions who develop a primary malabsorption syndrome are diagnosed as having tropical sprue (Klipstein and Baker, 1970).

DEFINITION

Since the aetiology of this syndrome is not yet understood, there is still some confusion as to the correct definition. This is further complicated by the differences between patients with tropical sprue in different geographical regions, and between expatriates or travellers from temperate climates who visit sprue endemic regions and the syndrome developing in indigenous populations. It has been suggested (Cook, 1984) that a postinfective bacterial overgrowth syndrome is responsible for the clinical presentation of tropical sprue. Other workers (Tompkins and Booth, 1985; Klipstein and Baker, 1970) have felt that if, in an individual patient suspected to have tropical sprue, significant luminal bacterial overgrowth can be demonstrated and its therapy results in a return to normal intestinal function, then the patient is a case of secondary malabsorption due to bacterial overgrowth, and not a patient with tropical sprue.

The most appropriate working definition is 'a primary malabsorption syndrome affecting residents of or visitors to certain tropical regions' (Klipstein and Baker, 1970; The Wellcome Trust, 1971). While this is a good working definition, it raises the question of the role of tropical enteropathy. The finger-like villi in the jejunal mucosa are replaced by broader leaf-shaped or ridge-like villi, with some reduction in villus height, an increase of crypt height and an increase in the mononuclear cell infiltrate in the epithelium and lamina propria in the indigenous populations of many tropical developing countries (Baker and Mathan, 1972; Baker, 1973; Wood *et al.*, 1991). These morphological changes are associated with mild degrees of malabsorption of fat and carbohydrate, as shown by decreased calorie and xylose absorption. The individuals in whom tropical enteropathy has been demonstrated are apparently healthy and asymptomatic. The available evidence suggests that tropical enteropathy is an adaptation of the gut to the contaminated tropical environment and frequent enteric infections with increased enterocyte turnover (Mathan *et al.*, 1982). In contrast to this, tropical sprue is a clear clinical entity with persistent diarrhoea, characteristic enterocyte damage and the nutritional sequelae of continuing malabsorption (Mathan, 1988).

HISTORY

An ancient Indian treatise of medicine, the *Charaka-Samhita*, describes patients in whom the 'digestive fire is weakened and food is expelled from the body without contributing to growth'. This was called 'Grahani vyadhi' or disease of the organ of assimilation. The clinical description of these patients, written around 600 BC, is remarkably similar to that of patients with tropical sprue seen currently in India. William Hillary described the disease in European expatriates in Barbados in 1759 and suggested that the disease attained epidemic proportions 3 years after he reached there. With colonization of South and Southeast Asia by the European maritime powers, the syndrome in the expatriate was well recognized by British and Dutch physicians. The term 'sprue' is derived from the Dutch term 'Indische sprouw' describing the glossitis and aphthous ulcers that develop consequent to nutritional deficiency. Sprue was also described in the French in Indochina and Europeans in China, and in American expatriates in the Philippines and Puerto Rico. However, no cases were reported from tropical Africa. The colonial physicians did not usually report cases in the indigenous population, probably because they were not seeing the indigenous patients! It was, therefore, generally accepted that tropical sprue does not affect indigenous populations, in spite of the early description in *Charaka-Samhita*. In fact, the district health officer of a district in the Madras Presidency of India, reporting an epidemic of a peculiar diarrhoea, wrote in 1926 'these patients resemble the cases of tropical sprue I have seen as a student in the Madras General Hospital. However, since tropical sprue does not affect Indians, I am at a loss as to a diagnosis'!

The work of Baker and colleagues in southern India, and Klipstein in Puerto Rico and Haiti in the 1960s and 1970s clearly established that tropical sprue is a significant problem in indigenous populations. Much of the early work on sprue was from the haematological perspective, since severe megaloblastic anaemia, due to malabsorption of vitamin B_{12} and folic acid, had a high prevalence in these patients. In southern India and Puerto Rico, malabsorption was an inevitable finding in almost all non-pregnant adults with megaloblastic anaemia. Epidemic tropical sprue was a major medical problem affecting Indian and European troops in the Assam and Burma theatre during the Second World War. Major epidemics of tropical sprue in the indigenous population were described in southern India from 1960 (Mathan and Baker, 1968, 1970, 1971).

EPIDEMIOLOGY

Tropical sprue occurs in two epidemiologically distinct forms, endemic cases in indigenous and expatriate populations, and epidemic tropical sprue in indigenous populations (Baker, 1982).

Endemic tropical sprue is reportedly geographically restricted to South and Southeast Asia and the Caribbean Islands other than Jamaica. There are only a limited number of reports from Central and South America and from Africa (Falaye, 1970; Thomas and Clain, 1976). This geographic restriction to certain tropical areas suggests that the causal factor or factors may be related to some environmental factors. The fact that most of the literature is limited to expatriate personnel in these regions and that, in India, tropical sprue has only been documented from two large and well-developed medical centres, with excellent laboratory facilities for detecting malabsorption, could suggest that, especially in marginally nourished indigenous populations, many cases are missed due to poor diagnostic facilities. In fact, it could be instructive to study in detail the innumerable patients who are labelled 'intestinal tuberculosis' because of wasting and diarrhoea! (Baker and Mathan, 1968).

Although Hillary reported that sprue in Barbados approached epidemic proportions in the 1750s, well-documented epidemics have been reported only from the Indian subcontinent. During the Second World War in the Assam–Burma theatre of war, epidemics of tropical sprue affected both British and indigenous troops. Italian prisoners of war were also affected in a camp in the Yol-Kangra valley. Detailed studies of epidemics affecting the indigenous populations have been reported from southern India since 1960. The first reported epidemic in 1960–1961 affected an area roughly 150 km north–south and 60 km east–west in the North and South Arcot districts of Tamil Nadu. It was estimated to have affected at least 100 000 individuals with a mortality of 40 per cent (Baker and Mathan, 1970). Further epidemics usually confined to one or two villages have been reported, the last such in 1978. In all these epidemics the attack rate in adults was significantly higher than in children, and adults were affected earlier during the course of the epidemic. The epidemics evolved over a period of several months to years. Although initially the patients presented with acute diarrhoea with vomiting in about 30 per cent and fever in 25 per cent, unlike other diarrhoeal illnesses, which are self-limited, the symptoms persisted with 50 per cent or more having diarrhoea for longer than a month. Much of the epidemiologic data suggests an infectious aetiology, but no recognized viral, bacterial or parasitic agent has been convincingly identified. There was an association between the prevalence of fringed, pleomorphic, virus-like particles in the stool of patients and the presence of malabsorption. All attempts to establish that these particles are similar to coronaviridae to date have failed (Mathan *et al.*, 1975b).

CLINICAL PRESENTATION

The individual patient with tropical sprue is usually an adult with a history of loose or watery stools for several weeks or months, and with symptoms and signs of nutritional deficiency. There is usually anorexia, a feeling of abdominal distension and loud abnormal borborygmi. The signs of nutritional deficiency include pallor due to anaemia, angular stomatitis, glossitis, oedema, and skin and hair changes of severe hypoproteinaemia. In a large group of patients it can be shown that the prevalence of nutritional deficiency measured by clinical or laboratory parameters is higher with longer duration of symptoms. In the epidemic situation, the prevalence of nutritional deficiency in patients during the first month of illness was not different from that in the unaffected people in the same village. However, in patients affected in the epidemics, persistent malabsorption begins during the first few days of illness (Baker and Mathan, 1971).

The diarrhoea can be severe enough to produce life-threatening dehydration and, in the epidemics, the early deaths were mainly due to fluid and electrolyte imbalance. These could be prevented by the maintenance of hydration. As the disease progresses, the sequelae of severe malnutrition and consequential acute infections, especially of the respiratory tract, contribute to mortality.

The natural history of the illness shows periods of remission, and relapses and spontaneous recovery, which make an evaluation of specific therapy difficult. Although patients have been followed up for up to 25 years in southern India, there was no evidence of development of intestinal neoplasms.

Tropical sprue can also affect children. In the epidemics reported from southern India, the attack rate was significantly lower in children. Detailed clinical and laboratory evaluation showed that the illness in children, including the intestinal mucosal changes, was similar to that in adults (Mathan *et al.*, 1969).

INVESTIGATIONS

The absorption of a variety of nutrients can be tested to establish intestinal malabsorption. While a fat balance study with faecal fat estimation would confirm steatorrhoea, in most situations a Sudan 3 stain of a faecal smear for fat droplets and fatty-acid crystals can be an effective screening test. Where facilities are available, ^{13}C breath triolein tests can be used. A good measure of carbohydrate absorption is a calorie balance study. Measuring the 5- or 8-hour urinary excretion of D-xylose, a pentose, is considered a measure of carbohydrate malabsorption. It is relevant to remember that, in indigenous populations with tropical enteropathy, up to 40 per cent of adults may have mild D-xylose malabsorption and 10 per cent mild steatorrhoea. Another useful test of absorption is that of vitamin B_{12}. A total of 60–90 per cent of patients with tropical sprue have vitamin B_{12} malabsorption. Rarely, this may be due only to defective intrinsic factor secretion by a damaged gastric mucosa, but in the vast majority of patients it is the result of the intestinal lesion affecting the ileal enterocytes.

Jejunal mucosal biopsy is an important part of the evaluation of a patient (Baker *et al.*, 1962; Swanson and Thomassen, 1963; Mathan *et al.*, 1975a). The biopsies have to be evaluated against the changes of tropical enteropathy for the particular population. At the light microscopic level, the characteristic features are non-specific shortening of the villi and hypertrophy of the crypts with increased infiltration of the lamina propria and the epithelium by mononuclear cells. These changes, while not diagnostic, can be graded as mild, moderate and severe. The severity of the malabsorption correlates well with the severity of the mucosal lesion, but not with the duration of illness or nutritional status of the patient. At the ultrastructural level it is possible to detect individual damaged and degenerated enterocytes especially in the crypts (Figs 21.1 and 21.2).

Radiological examination of the small and large bowel is an important part of the full clinical evaluation, particularly to exclude anatomical abnormalities, such as strictures, fistulae, etc., which could be associated with malabsorption (Maclean *et al.*, 1982).

PATHOGENESIS

Autopsy examination of the intestines suggested that the primary lesion in tropical sprue was in the intestinal mucosa (Manson-Bahr, 1924). The availability of peroral mucosal biopsy instruments has enabled detailed studies of the jejunal mucosa. Ultrastructural studies have confirmed the presence of damage to enterocytes in the crypt and villus compartments (Mathan *et al.*, 1975a). This is likely to be the primary

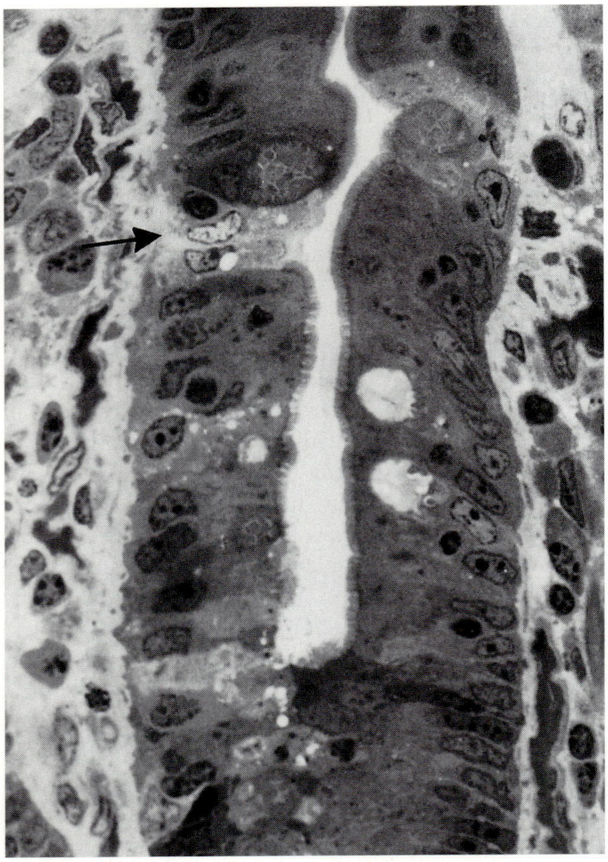

Figure 21.1 *Crypt region of jejunal mucosa in a biopsy from a patient with tropical sprue. Note focal degeneration of enterocytes (arrow between apparently normal cells). Resin-embedded section stained with toluidene blue (× 1100).*

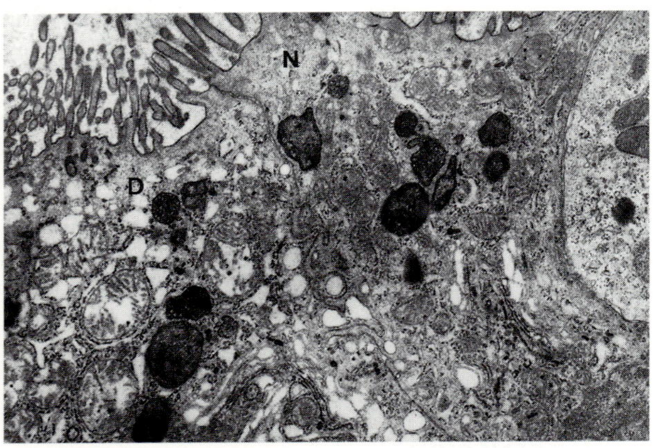

Figure 21.2 *Electron micrograph of jejunal biopsy from same patient showing damaged enterocyte (D) adjacent to a relatively normal enterocyte (N). Both cells show increase in lysosomal bodies (× 14 000).*

lesion and can be detected even during the first week of illness in patients affected in epidemics (Marsh *et al.*, 1983). Pulse labelling of *in vitro* organ cultures of jejunal mucosa with tritiated thymidine has shown accelerated cell turnover in the crypt, the regenerative compartment, and increased loss of enterocytes from the functional compartment, the villus. This is responsible for the villus shortening and increase in crypt height (Mathan *et al.*, 1986). The enterocyte damage leads to decreased membrane digestion and absorption of disaccharides and peptides. There is a hold-up of fat transport in enterocytes, although resynthesis into triglycerides of absorbed fatty acids and monoglycerides appears intact (Mathan *et al.*, 1975a).

The ileal lesion (Wheby *et al.*, 1971), which causes vitamin B_{12} malabsorption, also interrupts the enterohepatic circulation of bile salts contributing to steatorrhoea. This is increased by deconjugation of bile salts in the event of bacterial colonization of the small bowel.

It was originally thought that the lesion in tropical sprue affected only the small intestine. Atrophic gastritis with low gastric acid output has a higher prevalence in patients with tropical sprue compared to age-matched controls (Vaish *et al.*, 1965). Significant malabsorption of water and sodium from the colon has been demonstrated, suggesting that colonic functional abnormalities contribute to the volume of diarrhoea in this disease. Detailed studies have shown that, in addition to a colonocyte lesion similar to the enterocyte damage, unabsorbed unsaturated fatty acids in the colonic content can inhibit the enzyme Na^+K^+-ATPase in colonocyte basolateral membranes. This enzyme is the biochemical equivalent of the sodium pump, and plays a key role in water and electrolyte absorption (Ramakrishna and Mathan, 1982; Ramakrishan *et al.*, 1994).

REGIONAL DIFFERENCES

The syndrome of tropical sprue has been clearly documented in indigenous populations of southern India, European expatriates to South and Southeast Asia, and indigenous and expatriate populations in Puerto Rico and Haiti. While all patients have malabsorption, vitamin B_{12} malabsorption is found only in about 70 per cent of patients in southern India, while it is present in almost all expatriate and Caribbean patients. In Haiti and Puerto Rico, a seasonal incidence of tropical sprue is ascribed to small intestinal colonization by toxin-producing coliforms, secondary to the consumption of rancid pork fat (Klipstein *et al.*, 1978). In southern India, however, the extent and the severity of small bowel colonization by toxin-producing coliforms is no higher than in appropriate controls. These apparent differences between patients with tropical sprue in different regions can be fully understood once an aetiological agent is identified. The crypt enterocyte lesion described in southern Indian patients has not been described elsewhere, as ultrastructural studies were not performed.

DIAGNOSIS AND DIFFERENTIAL DIAGNOSIS

The diagnosis of tropical sprue is essentially dependent on the exclusion of conditions that can give rise to secondary malabsorption syndromes. The investigation in the individual patient should establish the pattern of malabsorption (fat, D-xylose, calories, vitamin B_{12}), investigate for underlying causes (barium meal follow-through and small bowel enema, jejunal mucosal biopsy, quantification of bacterial flora, specific tests for immunoglobulin deficiency, etc.) and establish the extent of nutritional deficiencies.

Prior to the onset of the human immunodeficiency virus (HIV) epidemic, the majority of patients with chronic diarrhoea and malabsorption in endemic areas in the tropics were ultimately diagnosed as tropical sprue. HIV can by itself cause an enteropathy with malabsorption and, in addition, persistent opportunistic infections of the small bowel also give rise to a wasting chronic diarrhoea leading to 'slim disease' as in many parts of Africa. This would, therefore, be an important differential diagnosis in most regions (Mathan *et al.*, 1990; Farthing *et al.*, 1996).

The most common diagnosis arrived at in patients with malabsorption, particularly in South Asia, is intestinal tuberculosis. However, malabsorption occurs in tuberculosis only under two circumstances: intestinal strictures with bacterial overgrowth and a stagnant bowel syndrome, or due to significant lymphatic obstruction associated with tabes mesenterica. A careful radiological examination is essential to differentiate.

TREATMENT

The three cardinal principles of treatment of these patients is to provide symptomatic therapy for diarrhoea, correct nutritional deficiencies and attempt specific therapy for the malabsorption. Loperamide tablets can be given to control diarrhoea. The feeling of abdominal distension can be helped by judicious use of dimethyl polysiloxane. These symptomatic measures give the patients considerable relief. Increasing the intake of nutrients is the first step in the correction of deficiencies. Therapeutic supplementation with iron, folic acid and vitamin B_{12} is often necessary for the correction of the widely prevalent anaemia. Other nutrient supplementation can be given as indicated (Guerra *et al.*, 1965; Klipstein *et al.*, 1966).

The role of specific therapy to cure the malabsorption has to await the elucidation of the aetiologies of tropical sprue. However, empirical evidence in patients in the Caribbean and in European expatriates indicates that, in patients where duration is less than 2 months, folic acid leads to alleviation of symptoms, while in those with longer duration, the addition of 3–6 months of tetracycline, orally, leads to clearing of the malabsorption. The exact mode by which these therapies are effective is not known. In southern Indian patients, the results of specific therapy were not so clear-cut. While folic acid, vitamin B_{12} and tetracycline were apparently helpful in some patients, in others there was spontaneous remission. A few patients were resistant to all therapy.

The maintenance of fluid and electrolyte balance is of critical importance, especially when there is significant watery diarrhoea. In epidemics, this saves many lives.

CONCLUSIONS

Tropical sprue was a major problem in expatriates to several tropical regions. The availability of a good water supply and environmental sanitation has apparently reduced the occurrence of tropical sprue. In Puerto Rico and southern India, there is also an apparent decrease in the prevalence of tropical sprue in the indigenous population. Klipstein (communication at a meeting) noted in Puerto Rico that, with improvement in nutrition and hygiene, the number of cases were decreasing and attributed this to patients possibly self-medicating with folic acid and antibiotics early in the course of their diarrhoeal illness. In southern India also there is a reduction in serious cases of tropical sprue and this correlates with an improvement in the nutritional status of the rural population. Clearly, when the nutrient intake is more than adequate, a proportional malabsorption can be accepted by the individual. Why after five epidemics between 1960 and 1978 there have been no further epidemics of tropical sprue in southern India is an enigma.

REFERENCES

Baker, S.J. 1973: Geographical variation in the morphology of the small intestinal mucosa in apparently healthy individuals. *Pathology and Microbiology* 39, 222–37.

Baker, S.J. 1982: Idiopathic small intestinal disease in the tropics. In Chandra, R.K. (ed.) *Critical reviews in tropical medicine*. New York: Plenum, 147–245.

Baker, S.J., Mathan V.I. 1968: The syndrome of tropical sprue in South India. *American Journal of Clinical Nutrition* 21, 984–93.

Baker, S.J., Mathan, V.I. 1970: An epidemic of tropical sprue in Southern India. II. Epidemiology. *Annals of Tropical Medicine and Parasitology* 64, 453–67.

Baker, S.J., Mathan, V.I. 1971: Tropical sprue in Southern India. In The Wellcome Trust (ed.) *Tropical sprue and megaloblastic anaemia*. London: Churchill Livingstone, 189–260.

Baker, S.J., Mathan, V.I. 1972: Tropical enteropathy and tropical sprue. *American Journal of Clinical Nutrition* 25, 1047–55.

Baker, S.J., Ignatium, M., Mathan, V.I., Vaish, S.K., Chacko, C.E. 1962: Intestinal biopsy in tropical sprue. In Wolstenholme, G.E.W., Cameron, M.P. (eds) *Intestinal biopsy*. London: Churchill, 84–101.

Cook, G.C. 1984: Aetiology and pathogenesis of post infective tropical malabsorption (tropical sprue). *Lancet* 1, 721–3.

Falaye, J.M. 1970: Tropical sprue in Nigeria. *Journal of Tropical Medicine and Hygiene* 73, 119–25.

Farthing, M.J.G., Kelly, M.P., Veitch, A.M. 1996: Recently recognised microbial enteropathies in HIV infection. *Journal of Antimicrobials and Chemotherapy* 37, 61–6.

Guerra, R., Wheby, M.S., Bayless, T.M. 1965: Long term antibiotic therapy in tropical sprue. *Annals of Internal Medicine* 63, 619–33.

Klipstein, F.A., Baker, S.J. 1970: Regarding the definition of tropical sprue. *Gastroenterology* 58, 717–21.

Klipstein, F.A., Schenk, E.A., Samloff, I.M. 1966: Folate repletion associated with oral tetracycline therapy in tropical sprue. *Gastroenterology* 51, 317–29.

Klipstein, F.A., Engert, A.F., Short, H.B. 1978: Enterotoxigenicity of colonising coliform bacteria in tropical sprue and blind loop syndrome. *Lancet* 2, 342–4.

Maclean, A.M., Farthing, M.J.G., Kurien, G., Mathan, V.I. 1982: The relationship between hypoalbuminaemia and the radiological appearances of the jejunum in tropical sprue. *British Journal of Radiology* 55, 725–8.

Manson-Bahr, P.H. 1924: The morbid anatomy and pathology of sprue and their bearing upon aetiology. *Lancet* 1, 1148–51.

Marsh, M.N., Mathan, M., Mathan, V.I. 1983: Studies on intestinal lymphoid tissue VII. The secondary nature of lymphoid cell 'activation' in the jejunal tissues of tropical sprue. *American Journal of Pathology* 112, 302–12.

Mathan, M., Mathan, V.I., Baker S.J. 1975a: An electronmicroscopic study of jejunal mucosal morphology in control subjects and patients with tropical sprue in southern India. *Gastroenterology* 68, 17–32.

Mathan, M., Mathan, V.I., Swaminathan, S.P., Yesudoss, S., Baker, S.J. 1975b: Pleomorphic virus like particles in human faeces. *Lancet* 1, 1068.

Mathan, M., Ponniah, J., Mathan, V.I. 1986: Epithelial cell renewal and turnover and its relationship to the morphological abnormalities in the jejunal mucosa in tropical sprue. *Digestive Diseases and Sciences* 31, 586–93.

Mathan, M., Griffin, G.E., Miller, A., Batman, P., Forster, S., Pinching, A.S., Harris, W. 1990: Ultrastructure of the jejunal mucosa in human immunodeficiency virus infection. *Journal of Pathology* 161, 119–27.

Mathan V.I. 1988: Tropical sprue in southern India. *Transactions of the Royal Society of Tropical Medicine and Hygiene* 82, 10–14.

Mathan, V.I., Baker, S.J. 1968: Epidemic tropical sprue and other epidemics of diarrhoea in south Indian villages. A comparative study. *American Journal of Clinical Nutrition* 21, 1077–87.

Mathan, V.I., Baker S.J. 1970: An epidemic of tropical sprue in southern India 1. Clinical features. *Annals of Tropical Medicine and Parasitology* 64, 439–51.

Mathan, V.I., Baker, S.J. 1971: The epidemiology of tropical sprue. In The Wellcome Trust (ed.) *Tropical sprue and megaloblastic anaemia*. London: Churchill Livingstone, 159–88.

Mathan, V.I., Joseph, S., Baker, S.J. 1969: Tropical sprue in children. A syndrome of idiopathic malabsorption. *Gastroenterology* 56, 556–78.

Mathan, V.I., Ponniah, J., Mathan, M. 1982: Tropical enteropathy: an adaptation of the small intestine to accelerated cell loss in 'contaminated' environments. In Robinson, J.W.L., Dowling, R.H., Riecken, E.O. (eds) *Mechanisms of intestinal adaptation*. Lancaster: MTP Press, 609–10.

Ramakrishna, B.S., Mathan, V.I. 1982: Water and electrolyte absorption by the colon in tropical sprue. *Gut* 23, 843–6.

Ramakrishna, B.S., Mathan, M., Mathan, V.I. 1994: Alteration of colonic absorption by long-chain unsaturated fatty acid. *Scandinavian Journal of Gastroenterology* 29, 54–8.

Swanson, V.L., Thomassen, R.W. 1963: Pathology of the jejunal mucosa in tropical sprue. *American Journal of Pathology* 46, 511–51.

Thomas, G., Clain, D.J. 1976: Endemic tropical sprue in Rhodesia. *Gut* 12, 877–87.

Tompkins, A., Booth, C.C. 1985: Tropical sprue. In Booth, C.C., Neale, G. (eds) *Disorders of the small intestine*. Oxford: Blackwell, 311–32.

Vaish, S.K., Sampathkumar, J., Jacob, R., Baker, S.J. 1965: The stomach in tropical sprue. *Gut* 6, 458–65.

Wellcome Trust, The 1971: *Tropical sprue and megaloblastic anaemias*. London: Churchill Livingstone.

Wheby, M.S., Swanson, V.L., Bayless, T.M. 1971: Comparison of jejunal and ileal biopsies in tropical sprue. *American Journal of Clinical Nutrition* 24, 117–23.

Wood, G.M., Gearty, J.C., Cooper, B.T. 1991: Small bowel morphology in British, Indian and Afro-Caribbean subjects: evidence of tropical enteropathy. *Gut* 32, 256–61.

22

Whipple's disease

RANJIT N RATNAIKE

The first report of what is now termed Whipple's disease is attributed to Allchin and Hebb, who described a case in 1895 (Morgan, 1961). In 1907, George Hoyt Whipple, the first American to receive the Nobel Prize in physiology, reported the case of a 36-year-old medical missionary with intestinal lipodystrophy. The patient presented with transient polyarthritis, fever, tiredness and weight loss, and subsequently developed 3–4 loose bowel actions a day. Whipple's view was that the pathophysiology of the disease was due to altered fat metabolism. This view was revised when patients responded to antibiotic therapy (Paulley, 1952) and 'bacillary bodies' were described (Chears and Ashworth, 1961; Yardley and Hendrix, 1961).

In 1991, Wilson's group reported the results of nucleotide sequencing and amplification using the polymerase chain reaction (PCR) of bacterial 16S ribosomal RNA from the small intestinal biopsy of a patient with Whipple's disease. These 'bacillary bodies' have now been termed *Tropheryma whippelii*, a name derived from the Greek words *trophe* (nourishment) and *eryma* (barrier) and George Whipple's surname (Relman *et al.*, 1992).

Although the number of cases of Whipple's disease is small, there is now sufficient evidence that the disease is multisystem in nature. The predominant manifestations of Whipple's disease are usually due to small intestinal involvement that leads to malabsorption and its consequences (Dobbins, 1985). However, in some patients with Whipple's disease, small intestine involvement is patchy and not a major feature (Moorthy *et al.*, 1977; Mansbach *et al.*, 1978; Wilcox *et al.*, 1987). Intestinal involvement may even be absent (Lynch *et al.*, 1997). Infrequently, the presenting and most severe features of Whipple's disease are non-gastrointestinal. Musculoskeletal symptoms of polyarthralgia may predate other manifestations of Whipple's disease by months or even years, and cause diagnostic problems. Indeed, a commonly described triad of symptoms is steatorrhoea, wasting and polyarthralgia.

DEFINITION

Whipple's disease is a chronic multisystem disease, due to infection by *Tropheryma whippelii* (Relman *et al.*, 1992), and intestinal malabsorption is a common feature.

EPIDEMIOLOGY

Whipple's disease is extremely rare and is estimated to have occurred in 1500–2000 patients (Dobbins, 1985). The disease is most frequent in Caucasians and predominantly in males (Gaist and Ladefoged, 1994; Durand *et al.*, 1997). The age range at diagnosis in 52 patients was 20–82 years (mean 55 years); in male patients the mean age was 50 years and in females 58 years (Durand *et al.*, 1997). The predominance of male patients continues to hold true, with 73 per cent of patients in the series by Durand *et al.* (1997). Whipple's disease has been reported in siblings (Gross *et al.*, 1959; Dobbins, 1987; Durand *et al.*, 1997).

AETIOLOGY

Whipple's disease is due to Gram-positive bacteria found as periodic acid–Schiff (PAS)-positive, diastase-resistant inclusions in macrophages from involved tissues (Relman *et al.*, 1992). DNA sequencing on samples of the organism taken from infected tissues demonstrate a lack of similarity to any known genus, and therefore, on the basis of phylogenetic relationships and its distinct morphology, the bacillus was assigned to a new genus and species termed *Tropheryma whippelii* (Relman *et al.*, 1992).

PATHOLOGY

There is diffuse small bowel involvement that predominantly involves the jejunum. Macroscopically the small intestine may be dilated, thickened and rigid, and the peritoneal surface covered with a fibrinous exudate (Isenberg *et al.*, 1971). The mesenteric and para-aortic lymph nodes are enlarged (Chears *et al.*, 1959).

Histologically there is distension of the normal villous architecture by an infiltrate of foamy macrophages, which replaces the lamina propria and often extends into the muscularis mucosa or submucosa (Fig. 22.1). The macrophages have a coarsely granular cytoplasm, which is intensely PAS-positive, staining a brilliant magenta colour (Fig. 22.2). By electron microscopy the cytoplasmic granules are seen as clumps of *Tropheryma whippelii* and their degradation products. These bacilliform bodies measure approximately 2 μm in length and 0.2 μm in diameter. They may also be seen in the epithelial cells, polymorphonuclear leucocytes and plasma cells.

An additional feature seen in small bowel biopsies is the presence of rounded empty spaces scattered through the lamina propria. They contain neutral fat and were described by Whipple (1907) in his original report as intestinal lipodystrophy. Despite the infective nature of the disease, there is usually no marked inflammatory response. In a small number of patients, non-caseating granulomas may be identified in the intestine, mesenteric and peripheral lymph nodes, the liver, lungs, brain and meninges. The histological differential diagnosis includes histoplasmosis and the *Mycobacterium avium-intercellulare* complex.

Reflecting the multisystem nature of the disease, the pathognomonic PAS-positive macrophages may also be seen in the peripheral and mesenteric lymph nodes, liver, spleen, heart valves, brain and lungs (Clancy *et al.*, 1975; Johnson and Diamond, 1980), and occasionally in the synovium (Hawkins *et al.*, 1976).

CLINICAL FEATURES

Owing to the involvement of various organ systems, Whipple's disease has numerous clinical features. The most common manifestations are related to the small intestine. The musculoskeletal, cardiovascular and the central nervous systems (CNS) are also frequently involved. Systemic manifestations include a low-grade fever in about 54 per cent of patients, and this may be the only manifestation of the illness for many years (Pirola *et al.*, 1967).

Gastrointestinal tract

The major symptoms are due to the involvement of the small intestine and the consequent malabsorption.

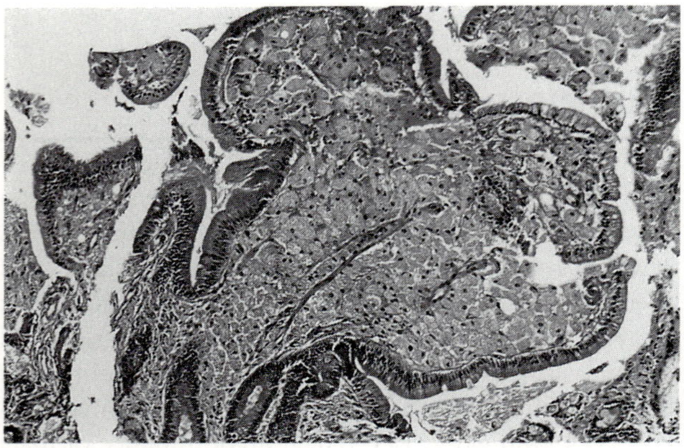

Figure 22.1 *Expansion of lamina propria by foamy macrophages. (Courtesy of Dr John E. Cooper, Department of Histopathology, The Queen Elizabeth Hospital, Woodville, South Australia.)*

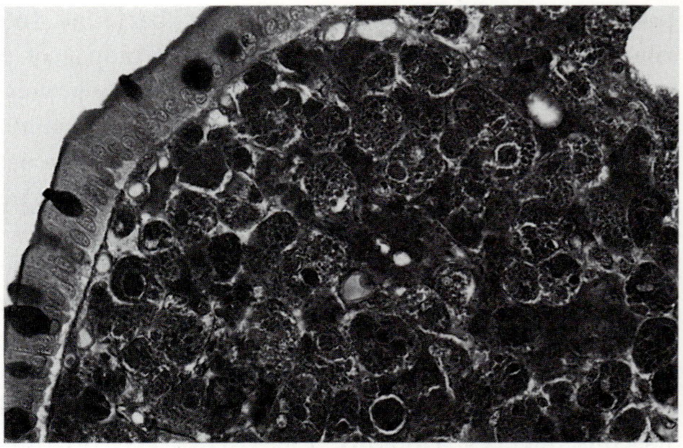

Figure 22.2 *Macrophages are intensely PAS-positive and the cytoplasm has a coarse granular quality. (Courtesy of Dr John E. Cooper, Department of Histopathology, The Queen Elizabeth Hospital, Woodville, South Australia.)*

Diarrhoea due to steatorrhoea is the commonest symptom in almost all patients and may be nocturnal (Gross *et al.*, 1959; Durand *et al.*, 1997). The stools, typical of malabsorption, are bulky, greasy and malodorous, and difficult to flush away. Besides diarrhoea, weight loss is invariably present. Anorexia and flatulence are other features.

As a result of malabsorption, the manifestations of a variety of nutrient deficiencies may occur. Vitamin deficiencies (*see* Chapter 9) can cause anaemia, bleeding and clotting disorders. Both occult and, rarely, gross gastrointestinal bleeding may occur, and cause or worsen iron-deficiency anaemia (James *et al.*, 1984; Dobbins 1987; Feldman and Price, 1989). Mineral malabsorption could cause osteopenia (*see* Chapter 9). Oedema and ascites may occur due to protein malabsorption.

Abdominal pain is non-specific and may occur in the epigastric area, especially after meals, mimicking peptic ulcer or gallbladder disease. Abdominal findings may also include a mass due to lymph node involvement, splenomegaly or distended loops of intestine. Peritonitis may be a feature.

Endoscopic findings in Whipple's disease have been described (Mayberry *et al.*, 1986). The endoscopic appearances in 12 patients with Whipple's disease at the time of diagnosis were: oesophagitis (1/12); erosive gastritis (4/12); atrophic gastritis (2/12); severe erosive bulbitis (3/10); and pathognomonic postbulbar duodenal lesions (9/12) (Geboes *et al.*, 1992). In 20 per cent of the patients the endoscopic lesions resolved after antibiotics. PAS- positive macrophages can persist in endoscopic biopsies for years (Geboes *et al.*, 1992).

Musculoskeletal system

Arthralgia and or arthritis occurs in about 80–90 per cent of patients (Durand *et al.*, 1997). These symptoms may be the only manifestations of ill-health for many years and precede other symptoms and signs. In Whipple's disease, the polyarthritis is mild, migratory and episodic, lasting for a few days to a few weeks, followed by long periods of remission. The joints most frequently affected are the limb and girdle joints (Durand *et al.*, 1997). In 35 of 52 patients in the series by Durand *et al.* (1997), peripheral joint involvement occurred in all patients and axial involvement in five. These five patients were all males and complained of back pain, with 'stiffness' in three, although none showed radiological evidence of spinal involvement. Ankylosing spondylitis is rare (Canoso *et al.*, 1978). In patients with axial arthritis, HLA-B27 is present in 8 per cent to 33 per cent. In Whipple's disease neither chronicity nor permanent joint damage or deformity is a feature (LeVine and Dobbins, 1973; Durand *et al.*, 1997). A myopathy has been described in a small number of patients (Swash *et al.*, 1977; Cruz-Martinez *et al.*, 1987).

Cardiovascular system

A common finding is low blood pressure. Significant cardiovascular lesions are endocarditis, myocarditis and pericarditis (Smith *et al.*, 1965; Vlietstra *et al.*, 1978; Durand *et al.*, 1997). Endocarditis involving the mitral valve is a common complication (Smith *et al.*, 1965; Durand *et al.*, 1997) and the lesion resembles that in rheumatic valvular disease. The characteristic PAS-positive macrophages and bacteria are present (Kraunz, 1969; McAllister and Fenoglio, 1975). Whipple's disease may cause mitral stenosis. In a series of 19 patients, 11 (58 per cent) presented with clinical signs of cardiac involvement and, at autopsy, 15 (79 per cent) had evidence of adhesive pericarditis, myocardial fibrosis and valvular deformity (McAllister and Fenoglio, 1975).

Central nervous system

A variety of psychiatric and neurological manifestations are described (Sieracki *et al.*, 1960; Durand *et al.*, 1997). Common abnormalities are dementia, seizures, cerebellar ataxia, visual disturbances, supranuclear ophthalmoplegia, myoclonia and myelopathy in 25–50 per cent of patients (Dobbins, 1987; Durand *et al.*, 1997). Other neurological features include confusional states, pyramidal signs, coma and brainstem syndromes (Knox *et al.*, 1976; Romanul *et al.*, 1977; Durand *et al.*, 1997), intellectual deterioration and hypothalamic manifestations (Hausser-Hauw *et al.*, 1988; Lynch *et al.*, 1997). Polyuria and polydipsia due to involvement of the hypothalamic–pituitary axis are reported (Dobbins, 1987).

Owing to possible peripheral labyrinthine or cranial nerve involvement, hearing loss and vestibulo-ocular reflex impairment occur (Verhagen *et al.*, 1996). A unique finding is oculomasticatory myorhythmia (Silbert *et al.*, 1976; Schwartz *et al.*, 1986; Grotta *et al.*, 1987), where a synchronicity occurs between contractions of the masticatory muscles and convergence of the eyes. Another form of myorhythmia has also been described: oculo-facial-skeletal myorhythmia, a slow smooth convergent–divergent pendular nystagmus associated with synchronous contractions of other body parts (Hausser-Hauw *et al.*, 1988; Adler and Galetta, 1990; Simpson *et al.*, 1995). These synchronous myorhythmic signs occur in 20 per cent of patients with CNS disease and are always associated with a supranuclear vertical gaze palsy (Louis *et al.*, 1996). Both signs are rare but pathognomonic of Whipple's disease (Schwartz *et al.*, 1986; Mendel *et al.*, 1999) and of equal diagnostic value to a positive biopsy or positive PCR assay for the bacterial RNA (Lynch *et al.*, 1997).

Although uncommon, Whipple's disease can cause chronic and recurrent meningitis (Feldman *et al.*, 1980). Involvement of the peripheral nervous system is also described. Polyneuritis is reported in one patient and mononeuritis involving the external popliteal sciatic nerve in another (Durand *et al.*, 1997). In patients with CNS involvment, cerebrospinal fluid PCR for *T. whippelii* is positive and abnormal findings on magnetic resonance imaging (MRI) are described.

Ocular manifestations of Whipple's disease result from CNS involvement, specific intraocular pathology, or both. Uveitis and ophthalmoplegia are common findings in patients with Whipple's disease.

Skin

In about 50 per cent of patients, a generalized hyperpigmentation occurs most frequently in exposed areas, but not in the buccal mucosa as in Addison's disease. Subcutaneous nodules that resemble rheumatoid nodules are described and on biopsy may show the diagnostic features of Whipple's disease (Durand *et al.*, 1997). Other skin manifestations are purpuric lesions not due to thrombocytopenia.

Haemopoietic system

Lymphadenopathy may occur in the mesenteric, retroperitoneal, mediastinal and lymph nodes (Samuels *et al.*, 1990; Durand *et al.*, 1997). Haematological abnormalities include anaemia, a common finding due mainly to iron deficiency (less often due to folate deficiency), and disorders of bleeding and clotting.

Respiratory system

Respiratory tract symptoms and signs include a chronic cough and pleural pain associated with pleural effusions, hilar lymphadenopathy or pulmonary infiltrates (Pirola *et al.*, 1967; Durand *et al.*, 1997).

Immune system

Abnormalities of immune function in patients with Whipple's disease may predispose to infection with *T. whippelii* (Bjerknes *et al.*, 1988; Ectors *et al.*, 1994; Marth *et al.*, 1994; Bai *et al.*, 1996). An *in vitro* defect in the intracellular killing function of monocytes and macrophages persists in patients even in remission (Bjerknes *et al.*, 1988; Marth *et al.*, 1994; Bai *et al.*, 1996). A primary defect in monocyte production of interleukin-12 reduces interferon-γ production by T lymphocytes (Marth *et al.*, 1997). Other immunological abnormalities include suppressed delayed-type hypersensitivity responses *in vivo*, decreased *in vitro* T-cell responses and altered lymphocyte subpopulations (Marth and Strober, 1996). However, some immune abnormalities may be epiphenomena of disease. MHC class II antigens are constitutively expressed on small intestinal enterocytes. In 20 patients with Whipple's disease, MHC class II antigen expression was reduced or absent, but restored after treatment (Ectors *et al.*, 1994). This reduction in MHC class II antigen expression is attributed to a deficiency in the inflammatory or immune response and not due to damage of intestinal epithelial cells. Dobbins has noted that 'the Whipple bacillus has an unusual ability to enter cells and the mucosa while failing to provoke injury or an intense immune reaction' (Dobbins, 1987). IgA-bearing plasma cells in the intraepithelial lymphocyte subpopulation of the small intestine are also destroyed in Whipple's disease, but return to normal after treatment (Eck *et al.*, 1997).

INVESTIGATIONS AND DIAGNOSIS

The erythrocyte sedimentation rate (ESR) is invariably elevated at the time of diagnosis. Owing to malabsorption, vitamin and mineral deficiencies occur. Since the gastrointestinal tract lesion in Whipple's disease is primarily in the upper small intestine, iron and folate concentrations may be decreased, although vitamin B_{12} concentrations are rarely abnormal as the terminal ileum is infrequently affected. Anaemia in the majority of cases is due to iron-deficiency anaemia. Severe hypoproteinaemia is common. Biochemical tests of malabsorption (*see* Chapter 13.3), such as the D-xylose absorption test and 3-day faecal fat excretion, are abnormal. These tests may now be unnecessary to perform owing to the ease of making a definitive histological diagnosis with an endoscopic small intestinal biopsy.

Barium studies of the small intestine show thickening of mucosal folds and other typical features of malabsorption (Chapter 13.6). Computed tomography (CT) scan and/or MRI demonstrate localized lesions and also serve to monitor response to resolution on treatment. On x-ray, features of rheumatoid arthritis may be seen in the hands and of ankylosing spondylitis in the sacroiliac joint (Rice *et al.*, 1967). Synovial biopsy and synovial fluid examination show mild non-specific inflammatory changes. Rheumatoid factor and antinuclear antibodies are absent.

The diagnosis of Whipple's disease is usually established histologically on small bowel biopsy.

A recent important diagnostic test is the polymerase chain reaction of the 16S ribosomal RNA of

Tropheryma whippelii. In 1997 this test was reported to be positive in 29 of 30 patients with histological evidence of Whipple's disease (Ramzan *et al.*, 1997).

MANAGEMENT

Untreated, Whipple's disease is lethal. Antibiotic therapy offers a dramatic improvement in Whipple's disease and was described as early as 1952, pointing to an infective aetiology (Paulley, 1952). The dramatic changes in the small bowel mucosa after antibiotic treatment are well documented (Maizel *et al.*, 1970; Denholm *et al.*, 1981). The resolution of gastrointestinal symptoms occurs and, for those due to arthritis, it is rapid, often within days. Complete histological recovery occurs in about 2 years, although radiological abnormalities may take 6–9 years to resolve (Davis *et al.*, 1963). Clinical relapses are common and are associated with the reappearance of the organism (Morningstar, 1975). In a series of 88 patients with Whipple's disease, 31 experienced relapses (Fleming *et al.*, 1988).

Treatment with tetracycline or penicillin as the sole agent has resulted in a high relapse rate. The treatment of choice is long-term trimethoprim–sulphamethoxazole because it crosses the blood–brain barrier. Since this drug is associated with folate malabsorption (a problem which could also occur in Whipple's disease from small bowel involvement), folate supplementation is advisable.

The treatment of Whipple's disease involving the CNS requires a more vigorous approach. A recommendation for treatment is as follows (Schnider *et al.*, 1997): initial treatment with intravenous ceftriaxone (instead of penicillin), 2 g twice daily, plus streptomycin, 1 g once daily for 2 weeks, or alternatively intravenous trimethoprim–sulphamethoxazole, 960 mg twice daily for 1–2 weeks. Follow-up treatment for 1 year should consist of oral trimethoprim–sulphamethoxazole (TMP-SMX), 960 mg once daily, or oral cefixime, 400 mg twice daily.

Singer (1998) recommends a treatment regime beginning with an initial daily parenteral administration of streptomycin 1 g and benzylpenicillin (penicillin G) 1.2 million units over a period of 14 days, followed by oral TMP-SMX 960 mg twice daily for 1 year, or at least 2 years if there is a 'supplementary impairment' of the immune system, with follow-up of the patient for a minimum of 10 years. Alternative treatments are (Singer, 1998):

1 TMP-SMX 960 mg three times daily for 14 days, then twice a day at the same dosage for another year.
2 Parenteral treatment for 14 days with ampicillin 2 g three times daily and ceftriaxone 2 g daily, followed by TMP-SMX 960 mg twice daily for 1 year.
3 Parenteral administration of ceftriaxone 2 g twice daily and streptomycin 1 g per day for 2 weeks, followed by a daily dose of TMP-SMX 960 mg or cefixime 400 mg orally for 1 year.

The response to therapy has been monitored by the improvement of clinical signs and symptoms, and the absence of *Tropheryma whippelii* on histological examination. The study from the Mayo Clinic (Ramzan *et al.*, 1997) reports the usefulness of PCR to monitor the response to therapy. This approach is particularly valuable as the relapse rate is high in Whipple's disease. Patients with CNS involvement, in particular, need careful monitoring. Treatment should begin and end with a PCR analysis of cerebrospinal fluid, in order to definitively diagnose infection of the CNS with Whipple's disease and to document the disappearance of the bacillus (Singer, 1998).

REFERENCES

Adler, C.H., Galetta, S.L. 1990: Oculo-facial-skeletal myorhythmia in Whipple disease: treatment with ceftriaxone. *Annals of Internal Medicine* 112, 467–9.

Bai, J.C., Sen, L., Diez, R. *et al.* 1996: Impaired monocyte function in patients successfully treated for Whipple's disease. *Acta Gastroenterologica Latinoamericana* 26, 85–9.

Bjerknes, R., Odegaard, S., Bjerkvig, R., Borkje, B., Laerum, O.D. 1988: Whipple's disease. Demonstration of a persisting monocyte and macrophage dysfunction. *Scandinavian Journal of Gastroenterology* 23, 611–19.

Canoso, J.J., Saini, M., Hermos, J.A. 1978: Whipple's disease and ankylosing spondylitis simultaneous occurrence in HLA-B27 positive male. *Journal of Rheumatology* 5, 79–84.

Chears, W.C., Jr, Ashworth, C.T., 1961: Electron microscopic study of the intestinal mucosa in Whipple's disease. Demonstration of encapsulated bacilliform bodies in the lesion. *Gastroenterology*, 41, 129.

Chears, W.C., Jr, Smith, A.G., Ruffin, J.M. 1959: Diagnosis of Whipple's disease by peripheral lymph node biopsy: report of a case. *American Journal of Medicine* 27, 351–3.

Clancy, R.L., Tomkins, W.A., Muckle, T.J., Richardson, H., Rawls, W.E. 1975: Isolation and characterization of an aetiological agent in Whipple's disease. *British Medical Journal* 33, 568–70.

Cruz-Martinez, A., Gonzalez, P., Garza, E., Bescansa, E., Anciones, B. 1987: Electrophysiologic follow-up in Whipple's disease. *Muscle-Nerve* 10, 616–20.

Davis, T.D., Jr, McBee, J.W., Borland, J.L. *et al.* 1963: The effect of antibiotics and steriod therapy on Whipple's disease. *Gastroenterology* 44, 112.

Denholm, R.B., Mills, P.R., More I.A. 1981: Electron microscopy in the long-term follow-up of Whipple's disease. Effect of antibiotics. *American Journal of Surgical Pathology* 5, 507–16.

Dobbins, W.O., 3rd 1985: Whipple's disease: an historical perspective. *Quarterly Journal of Medicine* 56, 523–31.

Dobbins, W.O., 3rd 1987: *Whipple's disease.* Springfield, IL: Charles C. Thomas.

Durand, D.V., Lecomte, C., Cathebras, P., Rousset, H., Godeau, P. 1997: Whipple disease. Clinical review of 52 cases. The SNFMI Research Group on Whipple Disease. *Medicine* 76, 170–84.

Eck, M., Kreipe, H., Harmsen, D., Muller-Hermelink, H.K. 1997: Invasion and destruction of mucosal plasma cells by Tropheryma whippelii. *Human Pathology* 28, 1424–8.

Ectors, N.L., Geboes, K.J., de Vos, R.M. *et al.* 1994: Whipple's disease: a histological, immunocytochemical, and electron microscopic study of the small intestinal epithelium. *Journal of Pathology* 172, 73–9.

Feldman, M., Price, G. 1989: Intestinal bleeding in patients with Whipple's disease. *Gastroenterology* 96, 1207–9.

Feldman, M., Hendler, R.S., Morrison, E.B. 1980: Acute meningoencephalitis after withdrawal of antibiotics in Whipple's disease. *Annals of Internal Medicine* 93, 709–11.

Fleming, J.L., Wiesner, R.H., Shorter, R.G. 1988: Whipple's disease: clinical, biochemical, and histopathological features and assessment of treatment in 29 patients. *Mayo Clinic Proceedings* 63, 539–51.

Gaist, D., Ladefoged, K. 1994: Whipple's disease [review]. *Scandinavian Journal of Gastroenterology* 29, 97–101.

Geboes, K., Ectors, N., Heidbuchel, H., Rutgeerts, P., Desmet, V., Vantrappen, G. 1992: Whipple's disease: the value of upper gastrointestinal endoscopy for the diagnosis and follow-up. *Acta Gastroenterologica Belgica* 55, 209–19.

Gross, J.B., Wollaeger, E.E., Sauer, W.G., Huizenga K.A., Dahlin, D.C., Power, M.H. 1959: Whipple's disease. Report of four cases including two in brothers, with observations on pathologic physiology, diagnosis and treatment. *Gastroenterology* 36, 65.

Grotta, J.C., Pettigrew, L.C., Schmidt, W.A., Friedman, G., Snatic, S. 1987: Oculomasticatory myorhythmia [letter]. *Annals of Neurology* 22, 395–6.

Hausser-Hauw, C., Roullet, E., Robert, R., Marteau, R., 1988: Oculo-facio-skeletal myorhythmia as a cerebral complication of systemic Whipple's disease. *Movement Disorders* 3, 179–84.

Hawkins, C.F., Farr, M., Morris, C.J., Hoare, A.M., Williamson, N. 1976: Detection by electron microscope of rod-shaped organisms in synovial membrane from a patient with the arthritis of Whipple's disease. *Annals of the Rheumatic Diseases* 35, 502–9.

Isenberg J.I., Gilbert S.B., Pitcher J.L. 1971: Ascites with peritoneal involvement in Whipple's disease. Report of a case. *Gastroenterology* 60, 305–10.

James, T.N., Bulkley, B.H., Kent, S.P. 1984: Vascular lesions of the gastrointestinal system in Whipple's disease. *American Journal of the Medical Sciences*, 288, 125–9.

Johnson, L., Diamond, I. 1980: Cerebral Whipple's disease. Diagnosis by brain biopsy. *American Journal of Clinical Pathology*, 74, 486–90.

Knox, D.L., Bayless, T.M., Pittman, F.E. 1976: Neurologic disease in patients with treated Whipple's disease. *Medicine,* 55, 467–76.

Kraunz, R.F. 1969: Whipple's disease with cardiac and renal abnormalities. *Archives of Internal Medicine* 123, 701–6.

LeVine, M.E., Dobbins, W.O. 1973: Joint changes in Whipple's disease. *Seminars in Arthritis and Rheumatism* 3, 79–93.

Louis, E.D., Lynch, T., Kaufman, P., Fahn, S., Odel, J. 1996: Diagnostic guidelines in central nervous system Whipple's disease. *Annals of Neurology* 40, 561–8.

Lynch, T., Odel, J., Fredericks, D.N. *et al.* 1997: Tropheryma whippelii in central nervous system Whipple's disease. *Annals of Neurology*. 42, 120–4.

Maizel, H., Ruffin, J.M., Dobbins, W.O., 3rd 1970: Whipple's disease: a review of 19 patients from one hospital and a review of the literature since 1950. *Medicine* 49, 175–205.

Mansbach, C.M., 2nd, Shelburne, J.D., Stevens, R.D., Dobbins, W.O., 3rd 1978: Lymph-node bacilliform bodies resembling those of Whipple's disease in a patient without intestinal involvement. *Annals of Internal Medicine* 89, 64–6.

Marth, T., Strober, W. 1996: Whipple's disease. *Seminars in Gastroenterological Disease* 7, 41–8.

Marth, T., Roux, M., von Herbay, A., Meuer, S.C., Feurle, G.E. 1994: Persistent reduction of complement receptor 3 α-chain expressing mononuclear blood cells and transient inhibitory serum factor in Whipple's disease. *Clinical Immunology and Immunopathology* 72, 217–26.

Marth, T., Nuerath, M., Cuccerini, B. *et al.* 1997: Defects of monocyte interleukin-12 production and humoral immunity in Whipple's disease. *Gastroenterology* 113, 442–8.

Mayberry, J., Furness, P., Austin, M., Toghill, P. 1986: Endoscopic appearances in Whipple's disease. *Journal of the Royal Society of Medicine* 79, 483–5.

McAllister, H.A., Jr, Fenoglio, J.J., Jr 1975: Cardiac involvements in Whipple's disease. *Circulation* 52, 152–6.

Mendel, E., Khoo, L.T., Go, J.L., Hinton, D., Zee, C.S., Apuzzo, M.L. 1999: Intracerebral Whipple's disease diagnosed by stereotactic biopsy: a case report and review of the literature. *Neurosurgery* 44, 203–9.

Moorthy, S., Nolley, G., Hermos, J.A. 1977: Whipple's disease with minimal intestinal involvement. *Gut* 18, 152–5.

Morgan, A.D. 1961: The first recorded case of Whipple's disease. *Gut* 2, 370–2.

Morningstar, W.A. 1975: Whipple's disease. An example of the value of the electron microscope in diagnosis, follow-up, and correlation of a pathologic process. *Human Pathology* 6, 443–54.

Paulley, J.W. 1952: A case of Whipple's disease (intestinal lipodystrophy). *Gastroenterology* 22, 128.

Pirola, R.C., Mishkel, M.A., Macdonald, G.J., Liddelow, A.G. 1967: Whipple's disease. *Medical Journal of Australia* 2, 985–8.

Ramzan, N.N., Loftus, E., Jr, Burgart, L.J. *et al.* 1997: Diagnosis and monitoring of Whipple's disease by polymerase chain reaction. *Annals of Internal Medicine* 126, 520–7.

Relman, D.A., Schmidt, T.M., MacDermott, R.P., Falcow, S. 1992: Identification of the uncultured bacillus of Whipple's disease. *New England Journal of Medicine* 327, 293–301.

Rice, R.P., Roufail, W.M., Reeves, R.J. 1967: The roentgen diagnosis of Whipple's disease (intestinal lipodystrophy), with emphasis on improvement following antibiotic therapy. *Radiology* 88, 295–301.

Romanul, F.C.A., Radvany, J., Rosales, R.K. 1977: Whipple's disease confined to the brain: a case studied clinically and pathologically. *Journal of Neurology, Neurosurgery and Psychiatry* 40, 901–9.

Samuels, T., Hamilton, P., Shaw, P. 1990: Whipple disease of the mediastinum. *American Journal of Roentgenology* 154, 1187–8.

Schnider, P.J., Rersinger, E.C., Berger, T., Krejs, G.J., Auff, E. 1997: Treatment guidelines in central nervous system Whipple's disease [letter]. *Annals of Neurology* 41, 560–1.

Schwartz, M.A., Selhorst, J.B., Ochs, A.L. *et al.* 1986: Oculomasticatory myorhythmia: a unique movement disorder occurring in Whipple's disease. *Annals of Neurology* 20, 677–83.

Sieracki, J.C., Fine, G., Hain, J.C., Jr, Babin, J. 1960: Central nervous system involvment in Whipple's disease. *Journal of Neuropathology and Clinical Neurology* 19, 70.

Silbert, S.W., Parker, E., Horenstein, S. 1976: Whipple's disease of the central nervous system. *Acta Neuropathologica* 36, 31–8.

Simpson, D.A., Wishnow, R., Gargulinski, R.B., Pawlak, A.M. 1995: Oculofacial-skeletal myorhythmia in central nervous system Whipple's disease: additional case and review of the literature. *Movement Disorders* 10, 195–200.

Singer, R. 1998: Diagnosis and treatment of Whipple's disease [review]. *Drugs* 55, 699–704.

Smith, W.T., French, J.M., Gattsman, M. *et al.* 1965: Cerebral complications of Whipple's disease. *Brain* 88, 137.

Swash, M., Schwartz, M.S., Vandenburg. M.J., Pollock, D.J. 1977: Myopathy in Whipple's disease. *Gut* 18, 800–4.

Verhagen, W.I.M., Huygen, P.L.M., Dalman, J.E., Schuurmans, M.M.J. 1996: Whipple's disease and the central nervous system. A case report and review of the literature. *Clinical Neurology and Neurosurgery* 98, 299–304.

Vlietstra, R.E., Lie, J.T., Kuhl, W.E., Danielson, G.K., Roberts, M.K. 1978: Whipple's disease involving the pericardium: pathological confirmation during life. *Australian and New Zealand Journal of Medicine* 8, 649–51.

Whipple, G.H. 1907: A hitherto undescribed disease characterised anatomically by deposits of fats and fatty acids in the intestinal mesenteric lymphatic tissues. *Johns Hopkins Hospital Bulletin* 17, 382–91.

Wilcox, G.M., Tronic, B.S., Schecter, D.J., Arron, M.J., Righi, D.F., Weiner, N.J. 1987: Periodic acid–Schiff-negative granulomatous lymphadenopathy in patients with Whipple's disease. Localization of the Whipple bacillus to noncaseating granulomas by electron microscopy. *American Journal of Medicine* 83, 165–70.

Wilson, K.H., Blitchington, R., Frothingham, R., Wilson, J.A. 1991: Phylogeny of the Whipple's-disease-associated bacterium. *Lancet* 328, 474–5.

Yardley, J.H., Hendrix, T.R. 1961: Combined electron and light microscopy in Whipple's disease – demonstration of 'bacillary bodies' in the intestine. *Bulletin of the Johns Hopkins Hospital* 109, 80–98.

23

Coeliac disease

PAUL J CICLITIRA

INTRODUCTION

Coeliac disease is defined as a condition in which there is an abnormal small intestinal mucosa, which improves morphologically when treated with a gluten-free diet and relapses when gluten is reintroduced (Booth, 1974). The condition was first described by Samuel Gee (Gee, 1888), but it was not until more than 60 years later that Dicke and co-workers observed the toxicity of wheat to individuals with this condition (Dicke *et al.*, 1953; van de Kamer *et al.*, 1953).

Coeliac disease is essentially a disorder of Europeans, and also affects those countries to which they have emigrated, including North America and Australasia. The prevalence in England is reported to be 1:1200, although more recent screening data suggests that the true figure may lie closer to 1:300, as reported around Galway Bay in Southern Ireland (Mylotte *et al.*, 1973). In mainland Europe, the prevalence is thought to vary between 1:300 and 1:1000. Coeliac disease occurs in non-Caucasians, although the prevalence is probably much lower.

It has been suggested that the female–male ratio is 2:1 but in other series the sexes are more equally affected (Cooke and Holmes, 1983). Concordance in identical or apparently identical twins is well documented, but discordance has been reported in infancy with biopsy findings, although for monozygous twins the evidence is not good.

The outlook for individuals with coeliac disease prior to the introduction of a gluten-free diet was poor, with published mortality rates being approximately 20 per cent. Following the introduction of a gluten-free diet, the mortality fell to 0.4 per cent (Sheldon, 1959). Statistics suggest that this mortality may be twice that of a matched control population (Holmes *et al.*, 1976).

PATHOLOGY

Coeliac disease affects the mucosa of the small intestine, particularly the proximal region, with damage gradually decreasing in severity towards the distal small intestine, although in severe cases the lesion extends to the ileum (Rubin *et al.*, 1962). Abnormalities of the rectal mucosa may be observed in some severe cases (Kiln *et al.*, 1980). The presence of complicating lymphocytic colitis and gastritis has been reported.

The characteristic histological appearance of the jejunal mucosa in normal individuals is shown in Fig. 23.1; this compares with the appearance of a jejunal mucosa from a patient with untreated coeliac disease in Fig. 23.2. The classic flat mucosa exhibits no villi, a loss of the normal villous architecture, and a reduction in the normal villus height:crypt depth ratio of between 5:1 and 3:1 (Shiner and Doniach, 1960). There is a flattening of the mucosa, which can vary from mild

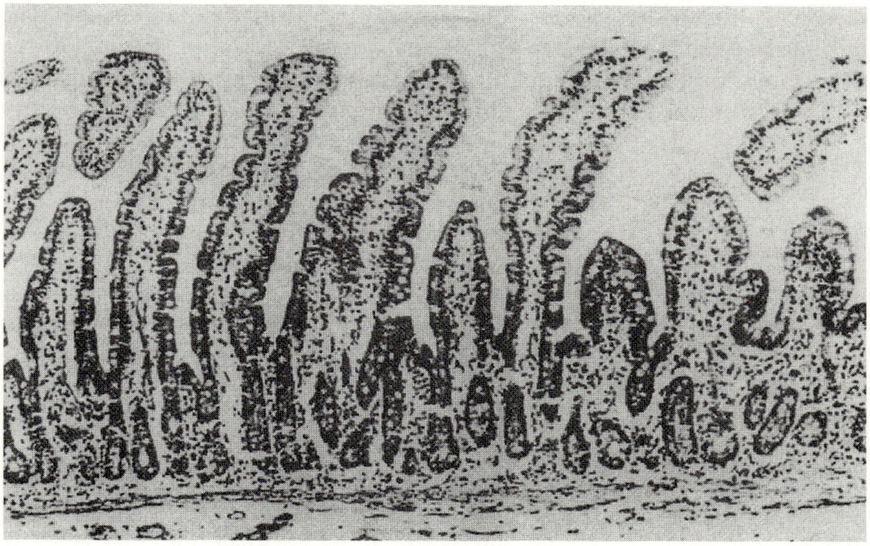

Figure 23.1 *Histological appearance of the jejunal mucosa from a normal subject.*

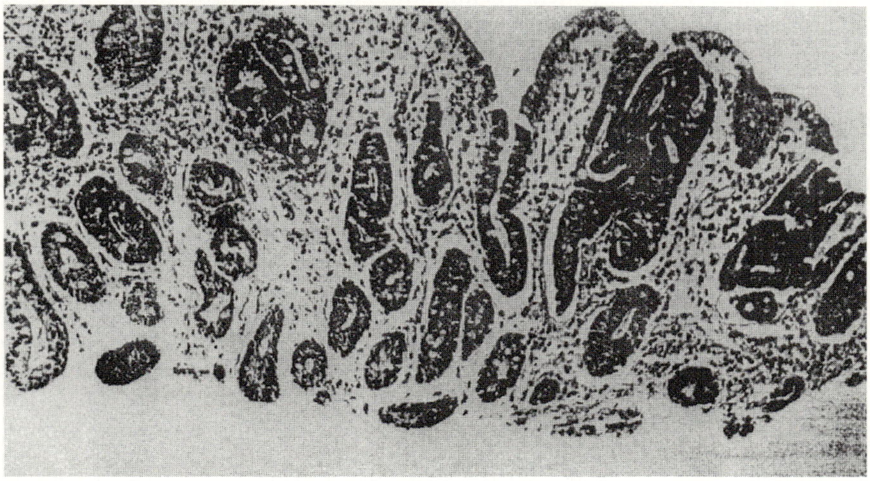

Figure 23.2 *Histological appearances of the jejunal mucosa from a patient with untreated coeliac disease. Note the absence of villi, expanded mononuclear cell population and increased intraepithelial lymphocytes.*

through partial villous atrophy to a total absence of villi. The total thickness of the mucosa may be increased because of crypt hyperplasia and infiltration of the lamina propria by plasma cells and lymphocytes. The surface epithelial cells become pseudostratified compared to their normal tall columnar shape. Enterocyte surface cell height is reduced. Crypt mitotic activity is normally confined to the lower third of the crypt, but in coeliac disease this activity may be increased and continue to the crypt surface, although the histological appearance of the crypt appears normal.

The time taken for cells to migrate from the crypt to the surface is reduced from the normal time of 3–5 days to between 1 and 2 days. The number of intraepithelial lymphocytes in relation to the number of surface cell enterocytes is increased in patients with active disease. Crypt abscesses have been described and small ulcers may be encountered. These ulcers may become problematical, developing into the small intestinal T-cell lymphoma that complicates approximately 10 per cent of cases.

Goblet cells are evident throughout the crypts along the surface of the epithelium. Paneth cells in coeliac disease may more readily discharge their contents into the crypt lumen, making recognition difficult, and resulting in an apparent reduction in their numbers. There have been reports of both increased and decreased numbers of endocrine-secreting cells in the small intestine of patients with untreated coeliac disease. The basement membrane may be thickened, this change often being patchy and having the staining characteristics of collagen rather than reticulin.

Chronic inflammatory cells infiltrate the jejunal mucosa in untreated coeliac disease. Increased numbers of plasma cells are found in the lamina propria (Lancaster-Smith *et al.*, 1974) and lymphocytes in the surface epithelium. The majority of intraepithelial lymphocytes express the common lymphocyte antigen CD3, 70 per cent express the supressor-cytotoxic phenotypic CD8, 5 per cent express the helper-inducer CD4 phenotype, and 20 per cent of the cells, while they are $CD3^+$, are $CD4^-$ and $CD8^-$ (Jenkins *et al.*, 1986;

Freedman *et al.*, 1987; Spencer *et al.*, 1989a). There are also increases in the number of intraepithelial lymphocytes expressing the more primitive γ-δ T-cell receptor in both treated and untreated coeliac disease, compared to controls (Spencer *et al.*, 1989b).

Electron microscopy

Electron microscopy reveals the surface of villi from normal subjects to be traversed by a series of furrows. In contrast, in untreated coeliac disease, shallow depressions on the surface of the mucosa can be seen into which 2–4 crypts open. Higher magnification shows that the microvilli are thicker than normal and appear as rounded projections. Transmission electron microscopic studies of normal enterocytes reveal the brush border is composed of tall regular microvilli covered by a glycocalyx. Below this is found the terminal web, where the cells appear tightly bound together by an apparent fusion of the lateral cell membranes. The epithelium in untreated coeliac disease reveals stratified cells (Marsh *et al.*, 1970), with the microvilli showing varying degrees of abnormality from shortening to gross disorganization and disappearance. Abnormalities within the enterocytes include an increase in the number of lysosome-like bodies, swelling of the mitochondria, increased vacuolation and evidence of cellular degeneration.

Dermatitis herpetiformis

Skin disorders are common, including psoriasis, eczema and pustular dermatitis (Cooke and Holmes, 1984). Atopic eczema in coeliac patients may respond to a gluten-free diet. There are a number of rare skin disorders that have been reported in association with the condition including cutaneous amyloid, cutaneous vasculitis, nodular prurigo, acquired icthyosis, epidermal necrolysis, pityriasis rubra pilaris and mycosis fungoides. The most important skin disorder associated with coeliac disease, however, is dermatitis herpetiformis. This is because the enteropathy is common to both conditions and the possible mucosal mechanism linking gluten to the development of skin lesions.

Dermatitis herpetiformis is characterized by an itchy patchy vesicular eruption, usually located symmetrically on the elbows, knees, buttocks, sacrum, face, neck, trunk and, occasionally, within the mouth (Duhring, 1884).

The majority of patients with dermatitis herpetiformis have abnormal small intestinal mucosae, which reaches nearly 100 per cent if several biopsies are taken, suggesting that the lesion is patchy (Scott and Losowsky, 1976). Some patients have apparently normal jejunal mucosa biopsies but have increased lymphocyte counts in the epithelium. The numbers fall towards normal following treatment with a gluten-free diet. The degree of mucosal change appears to depend on the amount of gluten ingested, as well as individual sensitivity. The exact relationship of gluten-sensitive enteropathy found in patients with dermatitis herpetiformis to that found in coeliac disease remains unclear. The pathogenesis of the condition remains poorly understood, although it has been suggested that antibodies form in the gut as a result of stimulation by gluten, which then circulate to the skin where they fix and create the conditions for the skin lesion to develop.

The treatment of dermatitis herpetiformis is dapsone at a dose of 50–100 mg/day. Patients should also be advised to take a gluten-free diet as this results in a significant improvement, but not until after 6–12 months, permitting the discontinuation of dapsone on a long-term basis. Months or years are usually required for the full benefit to be obtained, resulting in many patients being unwilling to cooperate with continuing the diet.

CHARACTERIZATION OF TOXIC CEREAL PEPTIDES

Classification of cereal proteins

Wheat grains have three major constituents, which are separated by milling: the outer husk or bran, the germ, and the endosperm or white flour, which constitutes 72 per cent of the whole grain by weight (Fig. 23.3). The storage proteins of cereals fall into two major groups, the ethanol-soluble fraction, termed prolamins, and the

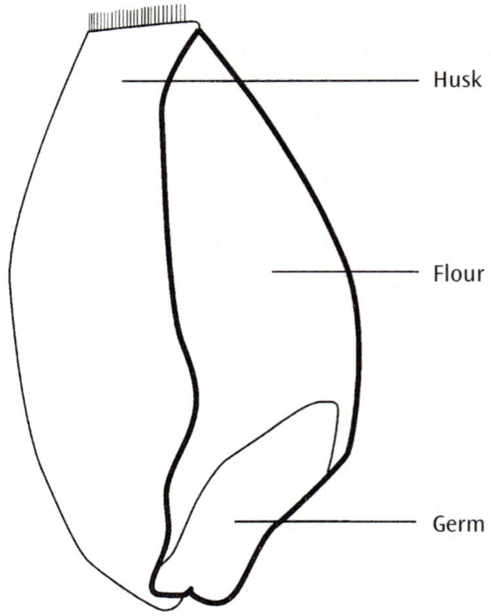

Figure 23.3 *The constituents of a wheat grain.*

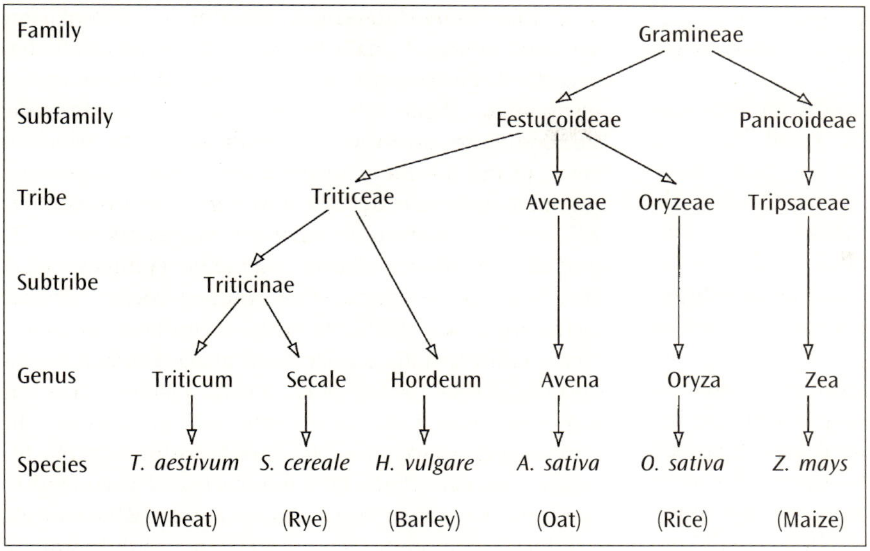

Figure 23.4 *Taxonomic relationships of major cereal grains.*

glutenins. Prolamins from the different cereals are termed gliadins from wheat, secalins from rye, hordeins from barley, avenins from oats, and zeins from coeliac non-toxic maize. The taxonomic relationship of the gramineae is shown in Fig. 23.4 and the classification of wheat proteins in Fig. 23.5. These are subdivided into classes according to their solubility characteristics: gliadins are soluble in 40–90 per cent ethanol, and glutenins are insoluble in neutral aqueous solution, saline and ethanol. The gliadins may be further subdivided either according to their relative electophoretic mobility into α, β, γ or ω, or in N-terminal amino-acid sequence α, γ and ω. Molecular masses rise from 32 to 58 kDa through α to ω gliadins (Autran *et al.*, 1979; Kasarda, 1981).

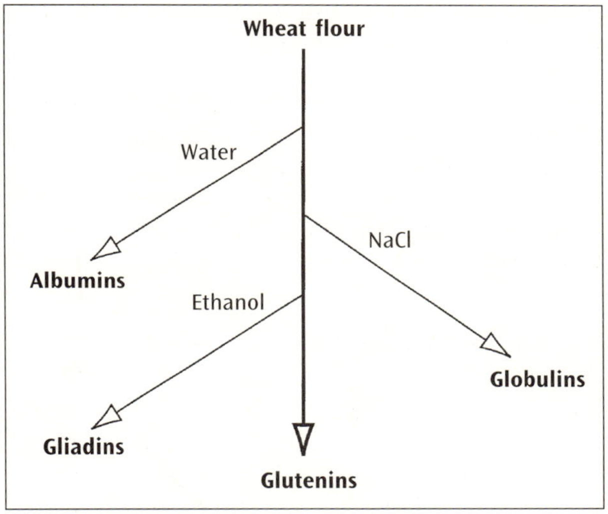

Figure 23.5 *The classification of wheat proteins.*

HYPOTHESIS FOR THE PATHOGENESIS OF COELIAC DISEASE

There are three main hypotheses for the pathogenesis of coeliac disease: (1) a small intestinal enzyme deficiency; (2) an enterocyte membrane defect, allowing lectin-like binding of gliadin to the small intestine enterocytes; and (3) a primary abnormal immune response to specific cereal peptides.

Enzyme deficiency hypothesis

It was postulated that an absence of a specific peptidase from the jejunal mucosa of coeliac patients results in an inability to digest gluten, which, in turn, damages the small intestinal mucosa. The finding of normal small intestinal brush-border enzymes in treated patients suggests this hypothesis is incorrect.

Lectin-binding hypothesis

It has been suggested that there is a defect in the cell surface of small intestinal enterocytes, which is either an abnormal glycoprotein or glycolipid structured element, or a reduced biosynthesis of one of these cell wall components (Rubin *et al.*, 1965; Weiser and Douglas, 1976). Lack of confirmation of the initial observations that gluten proteins bound selectively to coeliac small intestinal biopsy (Weiser and Douglas, 1976) suggests that this aetiology appears unlikely (Colyer *et al.*, 1986).

Primary immune hypothesis

It has been suggested that there may be an abnormal primary immune response of the small intestinal mucosa to gluten that results in allergic phenomena. There is considerable evidence to support this hypothesis. The rare occurrence of 'gluten shock', comprising vomiting, diarrhoea, tachycardia and cardiovascular collapse (von Krainick *et al.*, 1958) in a small number of treated patients after gluten challenge implies an immune aetiology.

It has been proposed that gliadin is initially presented by small intestinal dendritic cells in the lamina propria to the T-cell receptor of lamina propria helper cells (afferent limb), which generate immune products that damage the epithelial cells (efferent limb). The lymphocyte products also induce HLA-class II gene product expression on the small intestinal enterocytes that may then present further antigen to the sensitized lymphocytes. This is shown schematically in Fig. 23.6.

Tissue transglutaminase (tTG), a cytoplasmic enzyme for which gliadin is an excellent substrate, has recently been shown to be the antigen for endomysial antibodies (Dieterich *et al.*, 1997). Endomysial antibodies are unlikely to be essential for the development of the disorder, since patients with hypogammaglobulinaemia can develop the condition (Webster *et al.*, 1981). However, it has been suggested that tTG partially deamidates gliadin and the neoepitopes trigger the immune response that causes coeliac disease (Molberg *et al.*, 1998). Recently, it has been suggested that gliadin-specific T cells could provide help for tTG-specific B cells (Sollid *et al.*, 1997). I believe that the abnormal compartmentalization of gliadin in the enterocytes might be the predisposing factor for binding to tTG. Thus tTG might also be presented to the immune system in an abnormal way, which would produce antibodies against it. The withdrawal of gliadin from the diet would eliminate the abnormal presentation of tTG, by either of the above routes, to the immune system. This could explain the very high

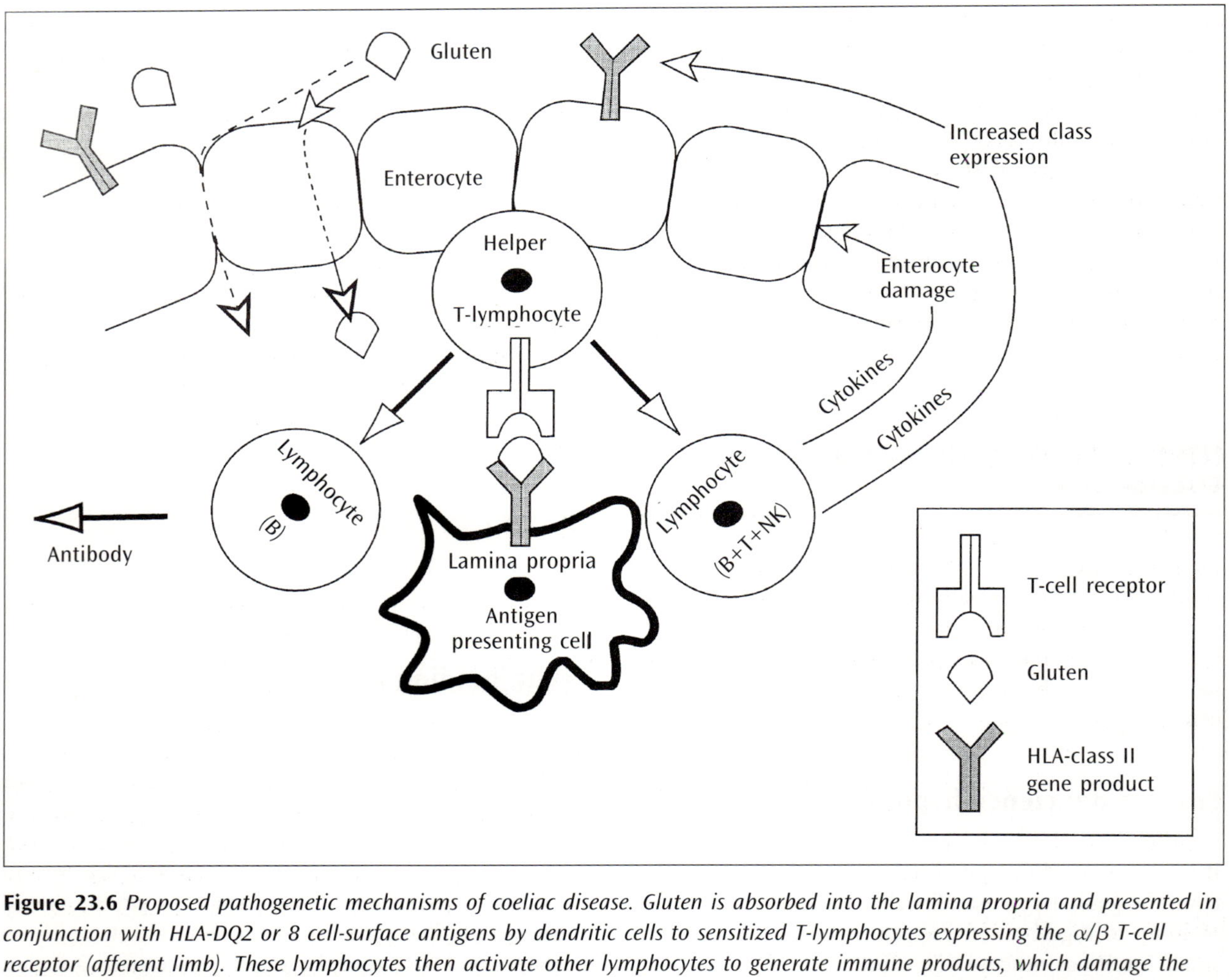

Figure 23.6 *Proposed pathogenetic mechanisms of coeliac disease. Gluten is absorbed into the lamina propria and presented in conjunction with HLA-DQ2 or 8 cell-surface antigens by dendritic cells to sensitized T-lymphocytes expressing the* α/β *T-cell receptor (afferent limb). These lymphocytes then activate other lymphocytes to generate immune products, which damage the enterocytes (efferent limb). Induction of aberrant HLA-class II cell-surface antigens on the enterocytes permits additional antigen presentation by these cells to the sensitized lymphocytes.*

sensitivity of endomysial antibodies for coeliac disease (Biagi *et al.*, 1999).

GENETICS OF COELIAC DISEASE

The precise inheritance of coeliac disease and dermatitis herpetiformis are unknown, although 10 per cent of first-degree relatives of coeliac patients are affected by the condition. Efforts to understand the mechanisms and genetics of polygenic human disease have focused on the identification of DNA and protein markers that segregate the diseases in populations and families. The most significant observation was the increased frequency of specific serologically defined lymphoid cell surface proteins, encoded in the HLA-D region of the major histocompatability complex and referred to as HLA-class II antigens. These comprise α- and β-chain transmembrane glycosylated heterodimers. The genes for these are organized into three subregions termed DR, DP and DQ (Trowsdale and Campbell, 1988).

The association of particular HLA-DR3 and DQ2 with coeliac disease and dermatitis herpetiformis has been well established (Tosi *et al.*, 1983; Hall *et al.*, 1990; Hall and Batt, 1991). Recently, a DQ-A gene (Bugawan *et al.*, 1989) and an HLA-DP locus association, although weaker, have also been demonstrated, although the strongest candidate for disease susceptibility to both coeliac disease and dermatitis herpetiformis is with DQ2. This suggested that the HLA molecule most likely to be involved in gluten-sensitive enteropathy is a specific DQα–DQβ heterodimer, encoded in a *cis* arrangement in DR3 haplotypes or *trans* in a DR5,7 haplotype.

CLINICAL FEATURES

The classical description by Gee (1888) described gross manifestations of the disorder. However, clinicians should not neglect the relatively mild symptomatology that represents the common presentation of the disorder as it is seen today. Patients may still have a severe illness, although it is now evident that many others have little or no symptoms. Diagnosis can be made by screening relatives of probands and placing a greater awareness of the disorder in the abnormalities encountered in haematological, biochemical and, more recently, HLA-class II profiles.

Infancy and childhood

The classical presentation of the condition in infancy occurs shortly after weaning and the introduction of dietary cereals. There is failure to thrive associated with apathy, pallor, anorexia, misery and muscle wasting. There is generalized hypotonia and abdominal distension with the child passing soft bulky, clay-coloured, offensive stools. Very young children may present with vomiting, which is often effortless, of large volume, and usually associated with abdominal distension and little or no diarrhoea. Abdominal pain may be so severe that the child undergoes laparotomy under the mistaken diagnosis of intestinal obstruction, which, in some cases, is precipitated by severe constipation. Multiple symptoms may see the patient presenting for advice and diagnosis, including rectal prolapse, which is much commoner in cystic fibrosis.

Older children tend to have more varied symptomatology, presenting with anaemia, rickets or failure to grow normally. Rickets is particularly common in Asian children. Unexplained short stature is an indication for jejunal biopsy, even when gastrointestinal symptoms are mild or absent. A study of 34 such patients revealed that eight had coeliac disease, of whom seven showed significant acceleration in height and weight gain when given a gluten-free diet (Groll *et al.*, 1980).

Gastrointestinal symptoms may date from birth in 25 per cent of children, while more than half become symptomatic in the first 6 months of life. The later presentation and diagnosis of coeliac disease in recent years can be ascribed to the current practice of introducing gluten in the form of cereals later, that is, after the age of 4 months. The exception is in Sweden, where infant-feeding practices have returned to the early introduction of gluten to infants within the first few weeks of life, which involves feeding flour mixed with milk. There has been an upsurge of cases presenting during infancy. It has been suggested that coeliac disease occurs predominantly in infants who had not been breast-fed; however, this has not been substantiated.

Adult life

Adults and adolescents with coeliac disease present with varied symptomatology to almost any hospital department. Diarrhoea is the usual presenting problem, while constitutional disturbances, such as lassitude, weight loss, glossitis and symptoms of anaemia form another group. A much smaller group present because of abnormal neurological or psychiatric symptoms, including schizophrenia. Patients may present with problems related to osteopenia, osteomalacia including spontaneous fractures and myopathy, skin complaints, bleeding diatheses or infertility (Cooke *et al.*, 1953; Comfort, 1958; Barry *et al.*, 1974).

Many patients have long-standing ill health for many years, never having had severe symptoms; they come to accept this as normal. Abdominal pain occurs in approximately 5 per cent of cases. Aphthous stomatitis may uncommonly be the sole presenting symptom and therefore coeliac disease should be excluded in cases of severe unexplained recurrent mouth ulceration. The stress of an operation or infection can occasionally induce severe diarrhoea. Pregnancy may precipitate macrocytic anaemia or the onset of unexplained diarrhoea. Following pregnancy, the symptoms may abate and the diagnosis be missed.

Presentation in patients with coeliac disease are non-specific and therefore a high diagnostic suspicion should be aroused with significant minor abnormalities on haematological or biochemical profiles. In a few patients investigated for an unrelated problem, the finding of a mild unexplained macrocytic anaemia with a persistent low serum or red-cell folate level will suggest further investigation and lead to a diagnosis of coeliac disease. A previous diagnosis in childhood can be overlooked with the patient re-presenting in later life. Clinicians should therefore explore childhood illnesses including short stature, anaemia or rickets.

There is a high prevalence of the condition amongst patients' relatives, with 10–15 per cent first-degree relatives of probands being similarly affected (Bolsover *et al.*, 1991).

Certain symptoms warrant particular mention, including lassitude, which may be attributed to mild psychiatric disturbances. Glossitis of varying severity may be found. Angular stomatitis may occur in a few patients and marked cheilosis may be present. Nausea and vomiting are common, particularly during episodes of diarrhoea and occur in 50 per cent of coeliac children. The appetite is usually lost, although it may be excessive in some patients. Failure to gain weight despite ingesting 6000–7000 calories a day has been reported (Green and Wallaeger, 1960).

Abdominal distension is common, often associated with flatulence and flatus. Symptoms of cramp and tetany may occur, usually associated with a low serum calcium level, although occasionally with hypomagnesaemia. Bowel disturbance is the most frequent problem, usually in the form of loose stools or diarrhoea. The motion may be paler than normal, sometimes offensive, occasionally frothy and sometimes difficult to flush away. The frequency of bowel action varies but is commonly 3–4 times a day, and rarely more than eight. However, pale stools can occur in other conditions. Normally formed and coloured stools do not preclude the diagnosis; indeed, some patients with steatorrhoea may have stools with a normal appearance. Physicians should not forget to enquire specifically about a subject's stools, since patients with long-standing bowel disturbances frequently have no complaints. It has been reported that 10 per cent of patients suffer incontinence, complicating nocturnal diarrhoea (Green and Wallaeger, 1960).

Many other factors can disturb bowel habit, including emotional problems. One study revealed that 10 per cent of patients attending a gastroenterology clinic and labelled as suffering from a functional non-organic bowel disorder were subsequently found to be suffering from coeliac disease. Constipation occurs in approximately 5–10 per cent of subjects with coeliac disease.

Abdominal pain is uncommon and may indicate the need for investigation to exclude intra-abdominal pathology complicating coeliac disease, such as volvulus, intussusception, mesenteric adenitis, cholelithiasis, peptic ulceration and pancreatitis.

Scurvy complicating coeliac disease has been reported. Bleeding into the skin and subcutaneous tissue, although uncommon, may reflect vitamin K deficiency. Prior to the discovery of the value of a gluten-free diet, purpura was reported to occur in l0 per cent of patients at some time and be the presenting feature in 2 per cent.

Osteopenia and osteomalacia, rickets or bone pains lead to the diagnosis of coeliac disease in an appreciable number of subjects, reflecting a failure of calcium and vitamin D absorption. Symptoms of rickets and osteomalacia tend to be insidious in onset and may become severe before being recognized. Negative calcium balances were shown to be associated with excessive endogenous faecal calcium and malabsorption of vitamin D; a gluten-free diet restores these abnormalities to normal.

Physical signs

PERSONALITY

Children with coeliac disease are usually irritable and miserable. Adults may suffer from depression, paranoia, Korsakov's syndrome and neurasthenia (Goldberg, 1970; Ross and Garabedian, 1970). The majority of patients do not appear abnormal when judged against their peers, although it is striking to note the significant change in outlook and mood experienced by most subjects when gluten is excluded from their diet.

HEIGHT

Coeliac patients frequently exhibit a short stature and occasionally dwarfism. Growth retardation in children is well documented and the return to normal growth rate is one of the criteria by which the effect of treatment can be judged. Coeliac patients are on average 8 cm shorter than their peers (Groll *et al.*, 1980). Tall patients do, however, exist and a height of over 1.8 m does not preclude the diagnosis.

WEIGHT

Loss of weight frequently affects both children and adults on initial presentation. Sixty per cent of newly diagnosed children with coeliac disease are below the third percentile for weight. The average weight loss in adults in one series was 12 kg; 90 per cent had lost more than 4.5 kg (Green and Wallaeger, 1960). An increase in weight of the order of 6 kg in adults is usually seen when a gluten-free diet is instituted. The occasional overweight patient can present with untreated coeliac disease.

TEETH

There may be a delay in the eruption of teeth in children and hypoplasia of dental enamel has been described.

FEVER

A low-grade fever associated with anaemia may be present in some individuals, but a recurrent marked pyrexia is frequently a manifestation of complications such as septicaemia or lymphoma.

FINGER CLUBBING AND KOILONYCHIA

Finger clubbing is reported in 10 per cent of cases of both children and adults. Koilonychia is usually associated with long-standing severe iron deficiency and anaemia, and responds to replacement therapy.

OEDEMA AND ASCITES

Oedema and ascites may be present in severe cases, reflecting hypoproteinaemia. Abdominal distension and general dilatation of the gastrointestinal tract are common in coeliac disease, making the abdomen feel like dough on physical examination and making the detection of ascites difficult.

SEXUAL CHARACTERISTICS

Menarche delay by 1 year has been reported in an untreated group of coeliac patients compared to controls (Sheldon, 1959). Amenorrhoea lasting more than 3 months, unrelated to pregnancy, occurs in a third of women of child-bearing age with coeliac disease, and menstrual loss is frequently shorter than normal, lasting 1–3 days. The average age of the menopause in untreated coeliac patients is 45 years compared to 53 in those on a gluten-free diet.

Many coeliac patients appear relatively infertile but usually conceive. The mean time for coeliac patients to conceive on a normal diet is 19 months, and is 12 months on a gluten-free diet. Infertile coeliac patients frequently become pregnant shortly after commencing a gluten-free diet. Spontaneous abortion is more common in untreated coeliac patients, occurring in 18–25 per cent of pregnancies, compared to coeliac patients on a gluten-free diet, where the frequency is reported to be 9 per cent. Recurrent abortions may be a presenting feature of the untreated condition.

There is sometimes a reduction in potency in men. Fertility and normal sperm counts are usually restored by a gluten-free diet after some years of oligospermia. Low levels of plasma testosterone, free testosterone and plasma 5-dihydrotestosterone have been reported; the plasma luteinizing hormone level is frequently raised (Farthing *et al.*, 1982). This may in part explain the frequently observed marked delay in puberty and late development of secondary sex characteristics in untreated male patients. These abnormalities usually revert to normal following prolonged treatment.

LYMPHADENOPATHY

This is unusual in coeliac disease and its presence should suggest the possibility of a complicating lymphoma. However, should lymphadenopathy occur, it may respond to a gluten-free diet.

METABOLIC ABNORMALITIES

Haematology

HAEMOGLOBIN

The characteristic blood picture in coeliac disease is that of a mild, hypochromic, macrocytic anaemia. Severe anaemia occurs uncommonly and should raise the suspicion of a superimposed complication, such as a malignancy. However, severe iron deficiency may be encountered during pregnancy.

The peripheral blood film may exhibit target cells, Howell–Jolly bodies, siderocytes, irregular and crenated red cells, Heinz bodies, microspherocytes, acanthocytes and occasional erythroblasts (Vaughan, 1936; Trowell, 1943; Fry *et al.*, 1967). An erythroblastic appearance with circulating nucleated red cells, pale ring cells and Howell–Jolly bodies suggests splenic atrophy, which invariably occurs in coeliac disease. Variation in the size and shape of the erythrocytes and the degree of haemoglobinization may give rise to the characteristic appearance of dimorphic anaemia, in which corpuscular volume varies, but is raised in a third of patients. In children, the predominant picture is that of hypochromic macrocytic anaemia which slowly responds to oral iron. The serum levels of iron and folic acid are normally low. A macrocytic megaloblastic anaemia may occasionally be seen in older children.

BONE MARROW

An examination in adult patients usually reveals megaloblastic erythropoiesis. Forty-five per cent have pure megaloblastic marrows, 55 per cent have megaloblastosis combined with lack of iron and a few have pure iron deficiency.

FOLIC ACID

A low serum folate level occurs in the majority of patients with untreated coeliac disease. However, red-cell folate is a better test for total body stores and a reduced level is present in 85 per cent of patients. The levels usually improve with a gluten-free diet, although it is often necessary to correct this therapeutically in the early stage of treatment.

VITAMIN B_{12}

Mean serum levels of vitamin B_{12} in patients with untreated coeliac disease are lower than in controls, although only 14 per cent have levels below normal values. Occasionally, patients may exhibit an anaemia due to a combined deficiency of vitamin B_{12} and folic acid, which requires combined therapeutic replacement. However, vitamin B_{12} levels usually rise to normal limits in most patients when treated with a gluten-free diet and folic acid.

IRON

Deficiency of iron is common in coeliac disease and may occur because of impaired absorption and increased loss into the intestinal tract, either as a result of rapid intraepithelial turnover or associated blood loss. Therapy with a gluten-free diet or corticosteroids increases the amount of iron absorbed, although initial iron replacement therapy may be required on commencing a gluten-free diet.

Biochemistry and immunology

GLIADIN ANTIBODIES

Patients with untreated coeliac disease have elevated antibody titres of immunoglobulin G (IgG), IgM and IgA circulating antibodies to wheat gliadin and other food proteins (Berger, 1958; Ciclitira *et al.*, 1983). Coeliac patients also have elevated circulating antibody titres to collagen, reticulin and endomysium, the significance of which is unclear. It has recently been shown that the antigen for antiendomysial antibodies is tissue transglutaminase (Dieterich *et al.*, 1997), the pathogenetic significance of which is not understood. Raised titres of endomysial reticulin or gliadin antibodies can be used to uncover intentional or inadvertent ingestion of gluten among coeliac patients who are ill. Raised antibody titres can also be used to screen for the condition, although raised titres alone should not be used to make a definitive diagnosis. This is because elevated antibody titres can occur in other disorders, including inflammatory bowel and liver disease, and patients with raised antibody titres to endomysium but without coeliac disease have been described.

CIRCULATING IMMUNE COMPLEXES

Elevated titres of circulating immune complex have been reported, but other groups have been unable to confirm this result and their diagnostic significance is unclear (Ciclitira *et al.*, 1979).

FAT MALABSORPTION

The majority of coeliac patients have steatorrhoea. To determine the amount of fat excreted over a fixed period, daily intake should be at least 50 g and preferably 100 g per day, the normal UK intake being 60–90 g. Patients with steatorrhoea and untreated coeliac disease frequently find that they can moderate their diarrhoea by reducing their fat intake; therefore, it is important to place subjects on a 100 g fat diet, which should commence 2 days prior to the study. Motions should be collected over a 3-day period, eliminating day to day variations. The generally accepted upper limit of fat excretion is 5 or 6 g per day (Stewart *et al.*, 1967). The estimation of faecal fat is relatively crude and is readily subject to errors of collection or measurement. Faecal fat determination was previously considered mandatory for the diagnosis; however, the introduction of jejunal biopsy has made quantification of faecal fats superfluous, particularly as 30 per cent of patients with untreated coeliac disease have a normal fat excretion.

BREATH TESTS

Hydrogen and ^{14}C bile acid breath tests may be mildly abnormal, reflecting a degree of bacterial overgrowth, which usually returns to normal when the condition is treated.

CARBOHYDRATE ABSORPTION TESTS

Untreated coeliac patients have characteristic flat glucose tolerance curves, although this is not of diagnostic value, since a significant proportion of the normal population exhibit this. The majority of untreated coeliac patients have a degree of lactose intolerance, which usually improves with treatment consisting of a gluten-free diet. A hypertonic lactulose sugar permeability test has been introduced as a method for assessing small intestinal permeability, which is invariably abnormal, with decreased absorption in the untreated condition.

PANCREATIC ENZYME

Pancreatic function tests may reveal low intraluminal trypsin and lipase concentrations. Intravenous stimulation by secretin and pancreozymin reveals that the pancreas is normally able to respond within normal limits in untreated coeliac disease.

GUT HORMONES

Cholecystokinin levels are reduced following a fatty meal in coeliac disease, which may explain the inertia of the gallbladder as well as the diminished pancreatic function responses to oral challenge that occur in this condition (Low-Bear *et al.*, 1971, 1975). A generalized reduction in many gut hormones is found in the condition, which tends to normalize following treatment with a gluten-free diet, except for a poor rise in plasma gastric inhibitory peptides following an oral stimulus. Grossly elevated levels of enteroglucogen and the abnormal responses to oral glucose are considered to be unique to this disorder (Besterman *et al.*, 1978; Bloom *et al.*, 1978).

SODIUM AND POTASSIUM

Individuals with persistent frequent loose stools may be at risk of developing sodium and potassium depletion, leading to loss of muscle power and fatigue. Should it become severe, signs suggestive of a peripheral neuropathy may appear. Potassium depletion may simulate a renal disorder with albuminuria, with oedema and tubular vacuolation, all of which can be reversed with potassium therapy.

CALCIUM AND MAGNESIUM

Untreated patients frequently have hypocalcaemia and hypomagnesaemia. Symptoms do not usually occur until the serum calcium level falls below 1.5 mEq/L (Bennett *et al.*, 1932). Clinical symptoms include personality changes, limb tremor, uncoordinated movements, convulsions, significant variation in reflexes, nausea, vomiting, abdominal pain and paralytic ileus. Vitamin D malabsorption may occur causing resistant osteomalacia and elevated serum parathormone levels; oral calcium and parenteral magnesium therapy may be required.

SERUM ALBUMIN

Untreated coeliac patients frequently exhibit hypoalbuminaemia, which occurs in a third of patients. It usually rectifies on introduction of a gluten-free diet. Persistent hypoalbuminaemia should suggest complications such as lymphoma of the gastrointestinal tract, possibly with jejunal ulceration.

ZINC AND COPPER

Zinc deficiency may occur in coeliac disease and zinc therapy has been reported to be complicated by the development of anaemia, apparently due to the induction of copper deficiency (Porter *et al.*, 1977).

INVESTIGATIONS

The diagnosis may be suspected on clinical grounds or as a result of screening tests. It is mandatory to proceed to a small intestinal biopsy.

Biopsy of the small intestine

A biopsy is indicated in any patient with a history suggestive of coeliac disease. This includes those with mild symptoms, particularly in relatives of probands; and all patients with dermatitis herpetiformis require biopsy. The commonest indications in childhood are diarrhoea, failure to thrive, anaemia and short stature.

Small intestinal biopsy is usually undertaken endoscopically or on rare occasions with a suction small intestinal biopsy capsule. It is preferable to estimate the haemoglobin concentration, platelet count and prothrombin time prior to biopsy because, in a significant number of patients, increased prothrombin time can be corrected with intravenous vitamin K. Anaemia should not be a contraindication to small intestinal biopsy unless it is very marked; the risk of haemorrhage with a normal prothrombin time is small.

Endoscopic biopsies should be obtained from the second part of the duodenum using a wide-bore channel endoscope with 'jumbo' forceps. It is advisable to take at least three biopsies to avoid difficulties in interpretation owing to the normal avillous mucosa overlying Brunner's glands in the duodenum. The macroscopic appearance of the duodenum at endoscopy should be noted, as duodenal ulcer or patchy duodenitis may produce a pattern of inflammation similar to that found in coeliac disease. Occasionally, the endoscopist may note a loss of the normal duodenal folds, which can be made more obvious by an injection of India ink via a fine-bore tube.

Ideally, a biopsy of the proximal jejunum should be obtained with some form of suction-guillotine biopsy capsule, commonly a Crosby–Krugler or Watson. An alternative capsule described by Bradburg *et al.* (1959) and termed a Quinton capsule, which is used to obtain multiple biopsies from the stomach, small intestine or colon, is considered to be for research purposes only.

Gastrointestinal permeability studies

Monosaccharide and disaccharide small intestinal permeability tests have been used to assess the absorptive capacity of the small intestine. The absorption of D-xylose, which is absorbed, then excreted in the urine within 5 hours, was for many years used as a diagnostic screening test. The 5 g oral loading test was found to be more discriminating than 25 g. A combination of measurements of the plasma level 1 hour after taking an oral load, considered in conjunction with the amount excreted in the urine within 5 hours, permits discrimination between coeliac disease and a normal small intestinal biopsy in 95 per cent of cases (Benson *et al.*, 1957). Many centres, however, only use the urinary value.

Screening can be undertaken by simultaneous measurement of the excretion of L-rhamnose and lactose after ingestion of a hypertonic solution containing both these sugars. One study revealed the lactulose per L-rhamnose urinary excretion ratio to be seven-fold higher in patients with untreated coeliac disease compared to controls; there was no overlap of values for patients and controls (Menzies *et al.*, 1979; Menzies, 1984). Tests can be useful for diagnostic management where peroral biopsy is contraindicated, for example, during pregnancy. They do not, however, replace the diagnostic value of peroral small intestinal biopsy, which remains the investigation of choice.

Radiology

Dilatation of the colon is an early radiological sign, although the commonest feature is dilatation of the small intestine. The upper limit for the diameter of the normal proximal small bowel on barium follow-through is 30 mm in adults, 24 mm in children aged 2 years and 14 mm up to the age of 6 months. The ileum does not exhibit much distension and measures up to 24 mm in the normal adult. In normal individuals, values of up to 50 mm for the diameter of the adult small intestine are found during enteroclysis or small bowel enema. Barium follow-through examination of the small intestine reveals a loss of the fine, feathery mucosal pattern with decreased mucosal folds in 85 per cent of subjects.

In small bowel enema or enteroclysis, there is usually a degree of straightening of the valvulae conniventes, thickening of the mucosal folds and an increase in their separation. Superimposed upon dilatation and thickening of the mucosal folds are varying degrees of flocculation, segmentation and clumping, which are more relevant when they occur early in the examination. These features are not specific to coeliac disease.

Whilst most patients with untreated coeliac disease have radiological findings suggesting the condition, others have findings resembling Crohn's disease or scleroderma, the latter of which should readily be differentiated on radiological screening because of decreased motility. Tropical sprue and, occasionally, chronic pancreatitis result in an abnormal appearance in a follow-through barium examination. A quarter of patients with untreated coeliac disease do not have any radiological abnormality. Radiological examination, however, remains important in the presence of abdominal pain to exclude complicating lesions, such as benign ulceration of the small intestine with strictures, lymphoma or carcinoma.

A dilated and often redundant colon is a feature that renders the untreated patient liable to develop volvulus with associated abdominal pain. Intussusception can complicate coeliac disease and may be diagnosed by its classical radiological appearance.

The recently introduced technique of computed tomography (CT) scanning and nuclear magnetic resonance imaging of the abdomen may also reveal the dilatation of the gastrointestinal tract, with splenic atrophy, which frequently occurs in this condition. Occasionally, mesenteric lymphadenopathy may be noted, possibly with cavitation of the nodes, which can be a prelude to the development of a gastrointestinal lymphoma.

DISEASE ASSOCIATIONS

Numerous diseases have been associated with coeliac disease as shown in Table 23.1 (Scott and Loskowsky, 1975). There is a high association with various autoimmune disorders, which have a high prevalence of the genes encoding HLA-DR3 and DQ2. The relationship with dermatitis herpetiformis has already been described above.

Diabetes mellitus

The coexistence of insulin-dependent diabetes and coeliac disease is well recognized in both children and adults. The prevalence has been reported to be between 6 and 8 per cent of diabetes in coeliac disease (Scott and Loskowsky, 1975). Diarrhoea is a symptom of both disorders.

Liver disease

A higher than expected incidence of chronic hepatitis, primary biliary cirrhosis and sclerosing cholangitis is found in coeliac disease (Logan *et al.*, 1978).

Table 23.1 *Factors and diseases associated with coeliac disease (reprinted from Scott and Losowsky, 1975)*

Disease	Approximate reported disease incidence (%)
First-degree relative of coeliac patients	10
Dermatitis herpetiformis	80
IgA deficiency	20
Hyposplenism	100
Aphthous ulceration	5
Cow's milk protein intolerance	10
Small intestinal T-cell lymphoma	6
Thyroid disease	U
Diabetes mellitus	U
Cutaneous vasculitis	U
Fibrosing alveolitis	U
Sjögren's syndrome	U
Polyarteritis	U
Addison's disease	U
Systemic lupus erythematosus	U
Ulcerative colitis	U
Rheumatoid arthritis	U
Idiopathic pulmonary haemosiderosis	U
Glomerulonephritis	U
Schizophrenia	U
Sarcoidosis	U
Histocompatibility antigens HLA-B8 and DR3	U

U, incidence unknown.

Pulmonary disorders

Chronic fibrosing alveolitis and other interstitial lung diseases, including idiopathic pulmonary haemosiderosis, have been reported in association with coeliac disease (Lancaster-Smith *et al.*, 1971).

Inflammatory bowel disease

There is a known association of coeliac disease with inflammatory bowel disease, particularly ulcerative proctocolitis (Kiln *et al.*, 1980). Patients with proctocolitis complicating coeliac disease invariably improve with a gluten-free diet and also therapy with oral salazoprine, mesalazine and corticosteroid enemas. The demonstration of an inflammatory infiltration of the rectal mucosa in response to local gluten challenge in coeliac disease suggests the aetiology of the proctocolitis is similar to that of the small intestinal enteropathy (Loft *et al.*, 1989, 1990). The relationship of these conditions to microscopic colitis, which may be associated with small bowel atrophy unresponsive to a gluten-free diet, remains obscure.

Jejunal ulceration and lymphoma

Ulcerative jejunitis is characterized by chronic, multiple, apparently benign ulcers, which are found most frequently in the jejunum, although occasionally the ileum may be affected (Bayless *et al.*, 1967). The condition affects those in the fifth and sixth decade of life and presents with fever, lassitude, anorexia, weight loss, abdominal pain and diarrhoea. Anaemia, both microcytic and macrocytic, are common, together with steatorrhea and a protein-losing enteropathy. The ulcers may be complicated by haemorrhage, perforation or stricture formation, frequently bringing the patient to laparotomy, which represents a common presentation of this complication. A flat jejunal mucosa is found on biopsy, similar to that found in coeliac disease. Patients may initially benefit from a gluten-free diet but the response is frequently lost. The nature of this entity is not entirely clear and is discussed later in this chapter.

The clinical features of both jejunal ulceration and lymphoma are similar, and both tend to occur in coeliac patients during mid-life. Some patients with ulceration proceed to develop malignancy. Isaacson and Wright have suggested that ulcerative jejunitis, intestinal pseudolymphoma and malignant lymphoma associated with villous atrophy of the adjacent small intestinal mucosa and malabsorption represent one condition, namely malignant lymphoma (Isaacson *et al.*, 1985).

Intestinal pseudo-obstruction

Intestinal pseudo-obstruction without any evidence of an organic lesion obstructing the lumen rarely occurs in coeliac disease and normally responds to a gluten-free diet (McClelland *et al.*, 1962).

Non-coeliac gluten intolerance

This disorder has been described in infants and young children, usually occurring in association with cow's milk intolerance. Ingestion of gluten-containing cereals is associated with diarrhoea, vomiting, and sometimes dermatitis, rhinitis and bronchitis occur. Investigations reveal a normal jejunal mucosa, and normal intraepithelial lymphocyte count and disaccharidase activity. This disorder may also affect adults with abdominal pain and diarrhoea, which can, on occasions, be incapacitating. Others suffer from headaches or recurrent apthous ulceration. All patients experience a dramatic relief with a gluten-free diet and relapse on challenge. Immunological disturbances, including immunoglobulin abnormalities, do not occur; gliadin, reticulin and endomysial antibody titres are all normal. The cause of intolerance is unknown. Sodium cromoglycate is unhelpful. Omitting cereals, particularly wheat bran, and replacing dietary fibre with regular ispaghula husks may prove useful.

TREATMENT

Coeliac disease should be treated with a gluten-free diet, avoiding products containing wheat, rye, barley and oats. There is disagreement concerning the toxicity of oats, resulting in some physicians permitting oats to be taken in the diet. However, in the UK the majority of commercial oat flours are contaminated with 10–15 per cent of wheat flour, as some mills are not cleaned after milling of the different cereals. Holmes *et al.* (1989) reported that a gluten-free diet decreases the incidence of small intestinal lymphoma in coeliac patients. For this reason and to protect against dietary deficiency, the author feels that even coeliac patients with relatively few symptoms should be advised to take a strict gluten-free diet.

Some patients improve well on a partially gluten-free diet; symptomatic sensitivity to gluten varies widely. It is not customary to discuss this with patients because it may provide a false impression of an easy way out of dealing with their condition. A small percentage of patients with untreated coeliac disease can become severely ill and require treatment with a short course of oral systemic steroids.

A gluten-free diet has a low roughage content and may lead to troublesome constipation. This usually responds to the addition of regular dietary rice bran and ispaghula husks, or ground psyllium seed husks, which should be taken twice daily. Patients may supplement their diet with commercial gluten-free products, which are available on prescription in many European countries. Any specific dietary deficiencies that occur should be corrected; these include iron, folic acid, calcium and, very rarely, vitamin B_{12} deficiency.

Following 4 months of treatment with a gluten-free diet, a repeat small intestinal biopsy should be undertaken to demonstrate improvement in the appearance of the small intestinal morphology. If this has not occurred, other possible causes of small intestinal villous atrophy, such as giardiasis or cow's milk allergy, should be considered and another small intestinal biopsy should then be performed after a further 6–9 months. Even if improvement in the small intestinal morphology is not observed, if symptomatic improvement has occurred, the diet should be continued and a further biopsy repeated after a year on a gluten-free diet.

Should an improvement in jejunal biopsy morphology have occurred, the author advocates further confirmation of the diagnosis by a deterioration of small intestinal morphology in a repeat biopsy after a gluten challenge. This is particularly important in children, where conditions such as infectious diarrhoea and cow's milk intolerance produce similar abnormalities in the small intestinal villous morphology. The most convenient way to give a gluten challenge is to ask the patient to ingest at least 10 g of gluten or four slices of normal bread a day for 4–6 weeks. In the case of adults, this may be reduced to a period of 1–2 weeks as many individuals become severely symptomatic. In this case arrangements to undertake a small intestinal biopsy should be brought forward.

The European Society of Paediatric Gastroenterology and Nutrition (ESPGAN) have recently suggested that it is not mandatory to proceed to a repeat jejunal biopsy following a gluten challenge, if a gluten-free diet has produced a good improvement in symptoms (with a fall in antibody titres for reticulin and endomysium) and morphology of the initial jejunal biopsy was characteristic. Many physicians do not practise gluten challenge.

The biopsy after the gluten challenge should exhibit relapse in small intestinal morphology, compared to the previous biopsy taken after at least 3 months of treatment with a gluten-free diet. Should the patient's symptoms persist or the jejunal biopsy morphology remain grossly abnormal while continuing a gluten-free diet, commercial gluten-free products based on wheat starch should be discontinued (this is termed a gluten-free wheat-free diet). The initial diagnosis should also be questioned. It should be stressed, however, that the commonest reason for a lack of response to a gluten-free diet is a lack of patient compliance with dietary therapy.

Failure to respond to a gluten-free diet

Patients who fail to adhere to a gluten-free diet frequently continue with ill-health and recurring symptoms, which can often be traced to dietary lapses that are either deliberate or accidental. The problem is frequently that food is not correctly labelled and contains gluten. Rarely, the development of a gastrointestinal lymphoma or jejunal ulceration may be the cause of persistent symptoms. Very rarely, a patient on treatment may deteriorate and die unaccountably.

Steroids

Coeliac disease can be controlled with systemic corticosteroids, with rapid improvement of diarrhoea, weight gain and improvement in faecal fat excretion, and deterioration within a few days of discontinuation of steroid treatment. Steroids are therefore indicated in the treatment of coeliac crisis with severe diarrhoea, dehydration, weight loss, acidosis, hypocalcaemia and hypoproteinaemia. They have also been used to treat gliadin shock, an anaphylactic reaction that rarely occurs in treated patients subject to gluten challenge (von Krainick *et al.*, 1958).

The necessity to use steroids in coeliac disease occurs rarely; they are given to complement a gluten-free diet when the serum albumin level is markedly depressed in an attempt to bring the associated protein-losing enteropathy under control. The use of azathiaprine as a steroid-sparing agent has been reported. There is a theoretical potential for the use of more specific immunotherapy in the form of cyclosporin A; however, in limited trials of this agent it has not been found to be useful.

The dose of steroids depends on each individual case. Should a patient require intravenous fluid, the normal dose is 100 mg hydrocortisone 6-hourly; with oral replacement, a dose of prednisolone 40 mg/day is usually adequate. This can gradually be reduced to a level of 5–7.5 mg a day. Failure to be able to discontinue systemic steroids implies either inadvertent gluten intake or a concomitant complication, such as malignancy.

Treatment of complications

The majority of patients with coeliac disease have lactose or sucrose intolerance at the time of diagnosis. A small percentage of patients continue to be troubled with persistent dissacharidase deficiency. Such patients develop diarrhoea and abdominal pain with lactose in the case of alactasia and with sucrose in the case of asucrasia. These conditions may be diagnosed either by enzyme assays of the mucosal part of the intestinal biopsy or by an appropriate sugar permeability study (Menzies, 1984). Should concomitant dissacharidase deficiency be diagnosed, the appropriate dissacharide should be excluded from the diet.

A small number of patients suffer from small intestinal bacterial overgrowth, diagnosable by an abnormal breath hydrogen or bile acid breath test, or an abnormal urinary indican excretion or an abnormally high small intestinal aspirate bacteriological count. Should bacterial overgrowth of the small intestine be a persistent problem, patients may be treated with antibiotics, such as oxytetracycline 250 mg four times a day, which may be rotated fortnightly with another agent, such as co-trimoxazole one tablet twice a day. A 10-day course of metronidazole, 200 mg three times a day, is frequently helpful if small bowel bacterial overgrowth is a problem, although this agent should not be used on a long-term basis because of neurological side-effects.

Neurological complications

Patients with coeliac disease may rarely exhibit severe neurological disease, including encephalopathy, cerebellar dysfunction, myelopathy, peripheral neuropathy or a combination of these, thought to be due to vitamin deficiency, the precise nature of which is unknown.

Malignant complications

Adult coeliac disease is associated with an increase in incidence of neoplasia, which includes lymphoma of the intestine, predominantly small intestinal, and carcinoma of the gastrointestinal tract, particularly small intestinal and oesophageal (Brzechwa-Ajdukiewicz *et al.*, 1966; Holmes *et al.*, 1989). This enhanced predisposition to malignancy extends to patients with dermatitis herpetiformis and associated enteropathy (Anderson *et al.*, 1971). In contrast, coeliac disease diagnosed and treated in childhood does not appear to be associated with a greater instance of neoplasia than the general population. The generally recorded incidences of malignancy in patients with coeliac disease is between 11 and 15 per cent. Adenocarcinoma of the small intestine has an incidence of 55 per 100 000 per year in adult coeliac patients, compared with less than 1 per 100 000 in the general population, and there is a relative risk of over 80. It has been suggested in earlier studies that there is a lifelong chance of a patient with adult coeliac disease developing lymphoma of the order of 1–7 per cent and a relative risk of 77 per cent.

CONCLUSION

Coeliac disease is thus a common genetic disorder that affects possibly 1:300 Europeans. The primary pathology is a loss of the normal small intestinal villous architecture, which leads to malabsorption. The condition rapidly responds to a gluten-free diet, involving avoidance of wheat, rye, barley and possibly oat-containing products.

GLUTEN-FREE DIET

Introduction

The treatment for people who have been diagnosed as having coeliac disease or dermatitis herpetiformis is a gluten-free diet. Gluten is a protein found in wheat, barley and rye, and a gluten-free diet is the avoidance of all these cereals, and foods containing them, e.g. cakes, bread and biscuits.

Oats

Oats are thought to be non-toxic to patients with coeliac disease, but are often contaminated with wheat flour in the milling process and should therefore be avoided unless they come from a dedicated miller.

Hidden gluten

Many tinned and packaged foods contain gluten. Possible gluten-containing ingredients on labels are: starch, modified starch, wheat starch, wheat germ, thickener, flour, cereal protein, rusk. In the UK, a booklet of manufactured products known to be gluten free is available from the UK Coeliac Society, which is updated every year. If unsure about a certain food, this is the best guide (see the end of this chapter for information on the UK Coeliac Society and how to obtain the booklet).

Gluten-free products

There are a variety of gluten-free products available, e.g. gluten-free flours, bread mixes, bread, rolls, biscuits and cakes. Many are available on prescription from general practitioners and can also be purchased over the counter, but are very expensive. Dietitians provide lists of gluten-free products that are obtainable on prescription. Non-prescribable gluten-free products can be purchased at health food stores and some chemists, or by mail order direct from the manufacturer.

For people who normally pay prescription charges, it may be easier and cheaper to obtain a season prepayment ticket, available from post offices, chemists or local social security offices on Form PP95.

Table 23.2 shows a variety of food categories and indicates which are gluten-free and which contain gluten.

Medicines

Some medicines and tablets, e.g. vitamin pills, contain gluten. Patients should check with their doctor or pharmacist before using any medicine.

Suggested meal plan

BREAKFAST

- Fruit or fruit juice
- Cereal, e.g. Cornflakes, Rice Krispies and milk
- Gluten-free bread (or toast)
- Butter/margarine and jam/marmalade and/or cooked breakfast
- Tea/coffee

MID-MORNING

- Tea/coffee/fruit juice/fresh fruit
- Gluten-free biscuit (if desired)

LUNCH OR SNACK MEAL

- Meat/fish/egg/cheese
- Salad or vegetables
- Potato, rice, gluten-free bread

MID-AFTERNOON

- Tea/coffee/fruit juice/fresh fruit
- Gluten-free biscuit (if desired)

EVENING OR MAIN MEAL

- Meat/fish/egg/cheese or vegetable dish
- Gluten-free gravy or sauce
- Vegetables or salad
- Potato, rice, gluten-free pasta
- Gluten-free pudding, e.g. homemade meringue and cream, yoghurt, fruit

BEDTIME

- Milk/tea/coffee
- Gluten-free bread/biscuit

General information

COOKING

It takes time to get used to baking with gluten-free flours. Don't worry if you start with a few failures. Keep experimenting and you will soon get it right. Cooking videos are available on loan from Scientific Hospital Supplies, Nutricia or from dietitians.

MEALS

Many family meals can be made gluten free by replacing wheat flour with cornflour. These are safe for the whole family to eat. For example, when thickening gravy or stews, or when making sauces.

CONSTIPATION

Constipation can be a problem on a gluten-free diet. Constipation can be avoided by eating high-fibre gluten-free products, brown rice, dried or fresh fruit, and vegetables and salads.

LACTOSE INTOLERANCE

Many people with coeliac disease initially experience an intolerance to milk, milk products and sugar. This usually resolves once a gluten-free diet is started.

EATING OUT

When eating out it is difficult to establish whether many items on the menu are gluten free. Therefore, choose foods that are known to be gluten free, e.g. Parma ham with melon, grilled steak, roast meats, fruit or fruit salad.

Table 23.2 *The gluten content of foods*

Food category	Gluten-free foods	Foods containing gluten
Flour and dried foods	Arrowroot, cornflour, potato flour, buckwheat flour, gluten-free flour, rice flour, soya flour, gram flour	Wheat flour, rye flour, barley flour
	Rice, millet, sago, tapioca, cornmeal, ground rice, rice pasta, rice noodles, gluten-free pasta, certain brands[a] of buckwheat pasta	Oats, barley, rye, semolina, bulgur wheat, couscous, wheat pasta, canned pasta, e.g. spaghetti, ravioli
Bread, biscuits and cakes	Gluten-free bread and crackers, gluten-free biscuits and cakes, rice cakes	Bread, biscuits, cakes made from wheat, barley, oats or rye, rye crispbreads, communion wafers
Breakfast cereals	Cornflakes, Crunchy Nut Cornflakes, Rice Krispies, Puffed Rice, Coco Pops, Frosties, rice bran, soya bran, beet bran	Cereals made from wheat, barley, oats or rye, e.g. muesli, Shredded Wheat, Sugar Puffs, All Bran, Weetabix, porridge, wheat bran, Bemax
Meat	All varieties prepared and cooked with suitable flour and breadcrumbs; certain brands of canned meats, continental sausage, sausages, burgers, meat pasties and pâtés	Savoury pies and puddings, and other pastry products, e.g. sausage rolls, spring rolls, samosas; sausages and burgers containing breadcrumbs or cereal protein
Fish	All varieties prepared and cooked with gluten-free flour and breadcrumbs; fish canned in oil or brine, e.g. tuna; certain brands of canned fish in sauce and certain brands of fish pastes	Fish in batter, breaded fish, fish fingers, fish cakes, frozen fish in sauce
Dairy products	All types of milk, e.g. fresh, canned, dried; soya milk, coffee creamers, most types of yoghurts, fresh cream, certain brands of artificial cream	Muesli yoghurts and yoghurts containing cereals
	All natural plain cheese, cream cheese, curd cheese; certain brands of cheese spreads	Roquefort cheese
Eggs	Boiled, poached, scrambled, fried, prepared and cooked with gluten-free flour and breadcrumbs	Scotch eggs
Fats and oils	All types of oils, butter, margarine, lard, dripping, low-fat spreads	Suet
Vegetables and pulses	All types of fresh, frozen and dried vegetables and pulses; vegetables and pulses canned in water or brine, mushy peas, marrowfat peas; certain brands of baked beans	Vegetable samosas, spring rolls; vegetables canned in sauce, e.g. potato salad, creamed mushroom
	Certain brands of vegetarian burgers and sausages	
	All plain chips, French fries, oven chips, microwave chips; certain brands of potato crisps	Potato croquettes and other potato products with breadcrumbs
Nuts	All plain and roasted nuts, peanut butter, certain brands of dry roasted nuts	
Fruit	All fresh, frozen, canned and dried fruit	Fruit pie fillings
Puddings and desserts	Sago, tapioca and rice pudding, certain brands of ice cream, certain brands of 'instant' desserts and custard, jelly, meringues (homemade), certain brands of shop-bought meringues	Semolina, ice cream cones and wafers, Arctic Roll, pies and crumbles using wheat flour
Sweets and chocolate	Certain brands of sweets and chocolates, plain ice lollies	Rock, liquorice, Smarties, Twix and other biscuit-containing chocolates; unwrapped boiled sweets
Drinks	Tea, coffee (fresh and instant), certain brands of herbal tea, fizzy drinks, fruit squashes, fruit juice, wines, spirits, Build Up, Complan, Nesquik, Crusha syrup	Barley-based coffee, e.g. Barley cup, orange and lemon barley drinks, barley water; beer, lager (see section on 'Alcohol'), malted milk drinks, e.g. Horlicks; hot drinks from vending machines, e.g. hot chocolate
Miscellaneous	Sugar, glucose, jam, marmalade, honey, treacle, syrup, certain brands of lemon curd and mincemeat; artificial sweeteners	
	Certain brands of tinned and packet soups	Soup containing wheat, barley, rye and pasta, e.g. chicken noodle, Scotch broth
	Salt, pure or fresh ground pepper, herbs; all types of vinegar, including malt vinegar; certain brands of herb mixes, spice mixes, curry powders and white pepper	
	Certain brands of stock cubes and powders; certain brands of gravy mixes, gravy salt, gravy browning; Bovril, Marmite	Bisto
	Tomato purée, garlic purée, certain brands of tomato ketchup, mayonnaise, salad cream and ready-mixed mustard	Mustard powder
	Fresh and dried yeast, bicarbonate of soda, cream of tartar, certain brands of baking powder	

Where 'certain brands' are indicated, check which brands are gluten-free using the Coeliac Society's list of gluten-free manufactured products.

ALCOHOL

Wines, spirits and ciders are all gluten free. Traditionally, beer, lagers and stouts were allowed on a gluten-free diet. However, modern analysis methods have shown that there is a small amount of barley protein in these drinks and they may need to be avoided.

The Coeliac Society (UK)

The Coeliac Society was formed in 1968 to promote the welfare of adults and children who have been medically diagnosed as having coeliac disease or dermatitis herpetiformis. There is no membership subscription at present. This may change. Those on the mailing list receive an introductory literature and copies of the Society's magazine *The Crossed Grain*, twice a year in April and October. In addition, a new list of gluten-free manufactured products (the food list) is sent to all on the mailing list, who are then asked to pay for it.

New members are advised to purchase from the Society:

- the coeliac handbook
- the list of gluten-free manufactured products.

There is also a telephone hotline dedicated to updating the food list, available 24 hours a day (recorded message). Tel: 01494 473510.

For further information contact:
The Coeliac Society
PO Box 220
High Wycombe
Bucks
HP11 2HY, UK

USEFUL ADDRESSES

Nutricia Dietary Products
Newmarket Avenue
White Horse Business Park
Trowbridge, Wiltshire
BA14 OQX
Tel: 01225 771801

Scientific Hospital Supplies
100 Wavertree Boulevard
Wavertree Technology Park
Liverpool
L7 9PQ
Tel: 0151 228 1992

Ultrapharm Ltd
PO Box 18
Henley on Thames
RG9 2AW
Tel: 01491 578016

Gluten Free Foods Ltd
PO Box 178
Stanmore,
Middlesex
HA7 4XN
Tel: 0181 954 7348

General Dietary Ltd
PO Box 38
Kingston upon Thames
Surrey
KT2 7YP
Tel: 0181 336 2323

Cantassium Co.
225–229 Putney Bridge Road
London
SW15 2PY
Tel: 0181 874 1130

Acknowledgement The author would like to acknowledge the contribution of the Department of Dietetics and Nutrition, Guy's and St Thomas' NHS Trust for the gluten-free diet.

REFERENCES

Anderson, H., Dotevall, G., Mobacken, H. 1971: Malignant mesenteric lymphoma in a patient with dermatitis herpetiformis. *Scandinavian Journal of Gastroenterology* 6, 397–400.

Autran, J.C., Ellen, J., Law, L. *et al.* 1979: N-terminal amino acid sequencing of prolamins of wheat and related species. *Nature* 282, 527–9.

Barry, R.E., Baker, P., Read, A.E. 1974: The clinical presentation. *Clinics in Gastroenterology* 3, 55–69.

Bayless, T.M., Kaplowitz, R.F., Shelley, W.M., *et al.* 1967: Intestinal ulceration, a complication of coeliac disease. *New England Journal of Medicine* 776, 996–1002.

Bennett, T.I., Hunter, D., Vaughan, J.M. 1932: Idiopathic steatorrhoea (Gee's disease): a nutritional disturbance associated with tetany osteomalacia and anaemia. *Quarterly Journal of Medicine* 1, 603–77.

Benson, J.A., Culver, P.J., Ragland, B. *et al.* 1957: The D-xylose absorption test in malabsorption syndromes. *New England Journal of Medicine* 256, 335–9.

Berger, E. 1958: Zur allerguchen pathogenese der coliakie; mit versuchenn aber die spaltung pathogenes antigene durch fermente. *Bibliotheca Paediatrica* 67, 1–55.

Besterman, H.S., Bloom, S.R., Sarson, D.L. *et al.* 1978: Gut-hormone profile in coeliac disease. *Lancet* 1, 785–8.

Biagi, F., Ellis, H.J., Parnell, N.D.J. *et al.* 1999: A non-toxic analogue of a coeliac activating gliadin peptide: a basis for immunomodulation. *Alimentary Pharmacology and Therapeutics* 13, 945–50.

Bloom, S.R, Polak, J.M., Besterman, H.S. 1978: Gut hormone profile in coeliac disease: a characteristic pattern of pathology. In McNicholl, B., Carthy, C.F., Fottrel, P.F. (eds) *Perspectives in coeliac disease*. Lancaster: MTP Press, 399–408.

Bolsover, W.J., Hall, M.A., Vaughan, R.W. *et al.* 1991: A family study confirms that the HLA-DP associations with coeliac disease are the result of an extended HLA-DR3 haplotype. *Human Immunology* 31, 100–8.

Booth, C.C. 1974: Definition of adult coeliac disease. In Hekkens, W.Th.J.M., Pena, A.S. (eds) *Coeliac disease*. Proceedings of the Second International Symposium. Leiden: Steinfoert Kroese, 17–22.

Bradburg, L.L., Rubin, C.E., Quinton, W.E. 1959: A multipurpose instrument for suction biopsy of the oesophagus, stomach, small bowel and colon. *Gastroenterology* 37, 1–16.

Brzechwa-Ajdukiewicz, A., McCarthy, C.F., Austad, W. *et al.* 1966: Carcinoma, villous atrophy and steatorrhoea. *Gut* 7, 572–7.

Bugawan, T.L., Angelini, G., Larrick, J. *et al.* 1989: A combination of a particular HLA-DPβ allele and an HLA-DQ heterodimer confers susceptibility to coeliac disease. *Nature* 339, 470–3.

Ciclitira, P.J., Harkiss, G.D., Hunter, J.O. 1979: The incidence of immune complexes by the Polyethylene Glycol Precipitation Complement Test (PEG-CC) in coeliac disease and inflammatory bowel disease. *Gut* 20, A909.

Ciclitira, P.J., Ellis, H.J., Evans, D.J. 1983: A solid phase radioimmunoassay for measurement of circulating antibody titres to wheat gliadin and its subfractions in patients with adult coeliac disease. *Journal of Immunological Methods* 62, 231–9.

Colyer, J., Farthing, M.J.G., Kumar, P.J. *et al.* 1986: Reappraisal of the lectin hypothesis in the aetiopathogenesis of coeliac disease. *Clinical Science* 71, 105–10.

Comfort, M.W. 1958: Non-tropical sprue: diagnosis and therapy. *Gastroenterology* 34, 476–83.

Cooke, W.T., Holmes, G.K.T. 1983: Coeliac disease definition and epidemiology. In Cooke, W.T., Holmes, G.K.T. (eds) *Coeliac disease*. London: Churchill Livingstone, 2–22.

Cooke, W.T., Holmes, G.K.T. 1984: Skin manifestation and dermatitis herpetiformis. In Cooke, W.T., Holmes, G.K.T. (eds) *Coeliac disease*. London: Churchill Livingstone, 204–24.

Cooke, W.T., Peeney, A.L.P., Hawkins, C.F. 1953: Symptoms, signs and diagnostic features of idiopathic steatorrhoea. *Quarterly Journal of Medicine* 22, 59–77.

Dicke, W.K., Weijers, N.A., Van Der Kamer, J.H. 1953: Coeliac disease. The presence in wheat of a factor having a deleterious effect in cases of coeliac disease. *Acta Paediatria* 42, 34–42.

Dieterich, W., Ehnis, T., Bauer, M. *et al.*, 1997: Identification of tissue transglutaminase as the autoantigen of celiac disease. *Nature Medicine* 3, 797–801.

Duhring, L.A. 1884: Dermatitis herpetiformis. *JAMA* 3, 225–9.

Farthing, M.J.G., Edwards, C.R.W., Rees, L.H. *et al.*, 1982: Male gonadal function in coeliac disease: I. Sexual dysfunction, infertility and semen quality. *Gut* 23, 608–14.

Freedman, A.R., Macartney, J.C., Nelufer, J.M. *et al.* 1987: Timing of infiltration of T-lymphocytes induced by gluten into the small intestine in coeliac disease. *Journal of Clinical Pathology* 40, 741–5.

Fry, L., Keir, P., McMinn, R.M.H. *et al.* 1967: Small intestinal structure and function and haemotological changes in dermatitis herpetiformis. *Lancet* 2, 729–34.

Gee, S. 1888: On the coeliac affection. *St Bartholomew's Hospital Report* 24, 17–20.

Goldberg, D. 1970: A psychiatric study of patients with disease of the small intestine. *Gut* 11, 459–65.

Green, P.A., Wallaeger, E.E. 1960: The clinical behaviour of sprue in The United States. *Gastroenterology* 38, 399–418.

Groll, A., Candy, B.C.A., Preece, M.A. *et al.* 1980: Short stature as the primary manifestation of coeliac disease. *Lancet* 2, 1097–9.

Hall, M.A., Batt, R.M. 1991: Abnormal permeability precedes the development of a gluten sensitive enteropathy in Irish setter dogs. *Gut* 32, 749–53.

Hall, M.A., Lanchbury, J.S.S., Bolsover, W.J. *et al.* 1990: Coeliac disease is associated with an extended HLA-DR3 haplotype which includes HLA-DPw1. *Human Immunology* 27, 220–8.

Holmes, G.K.T., Stokes, P.L., Sorahan, T.M. *et al.* 1976: Coeliac disease, gluten-free diet and malignancy. *Gut* 17, 612–19.

Holmes, G.K.T., Prior, P., Lane, M.R. *et al.* 1989: Malignancy in coeliac disease – effect of a gluten-free diet. *Gut* 30, 333–8.

Isaacson, P.G., O'Connor, N.T.J, Spencer, J.O. *et al.* 1985: Malignant histiocytosis of the intestine: a T-cell lymphoma. *Lancet* 2, 616–21.

Jenkins, D., Goodall, A., Scott, B.B. 1986: T-lymphocyte populations in normal and coeliac small intestinal mucosa defined by monoclonal antibodies. *Gut* 27, 1330–7.

Kasarda, D.D. 1981: Toxic proteins and peptides in coeliac disease; relations to cereal genetics in food nutrition and evolution. In Walcher, D., Kretchmer, H. (eds) *Food as an environmental factor in the genesis of human variability*. New York: Masson Publishing, 201–15.

Kiln, G., Holmes, G.K.T., Cooper, B.T. *et al.* 1980: Association of coeliac disease and inflammatory bowel disease. *Gut* 21, 636–41.

Lancaster-Smith, M.J., Benson, M.K., Strickland, I.D. 1971: Coeliac disease and diffuse intestinal lung disease. *Lancet* 1, 473–6.

Lancaster-Smith, M.J., Kumar, P., Marks, R. *et al.* 1974: Jejunal mucosa immunoglobulin containing cells and jejunal fluid immunoglobulins in adult coeliac disease and dermatitis herpetiformis. *Gut* 15, 371–6.

Loft, D.E., Marsh, M.N., Jandle, G.I. *et al.* 1989: Studies of intestinal lymhphoid tissue XII. Epithelial lymphocyte and mucosal responses to rectal gluten challenge in coeliac sprue. *Gastroenterology* 97, 29–37.

Loft, D.E., Marsh, M.N., Crowe, P.T. 1990: Rectal gluten challenge and diagnosis of coeliac disease. *Lancet* 335, 1293–5.

Logan, R.F.A., Ferguson, A., Finlayson, N.D.C. *et al.* 1978: Primary biliary cirrhosis and coeliac disease; an association? *Lancet* 1, 230–3.

Low-Bear, T.S., Heaton, K.W., Heaton, S.T. *et al.* 1971: Gall bladder inertia and sluggish enteropathic circulation of bile-salts in coeliac disease. *Lancet* 1, 991–4.

Low-Bear, T.S., Harvey, R.F., Davies, E.R. *et al.* 1975: Abnormalities of serum cholinystohime and gall bladder emptying in coeliac disease. *New England Journal of Medicine* 292, 961–3.

Marsh, M.N., Brown, A.C., Swift, J.A. 1970: The surface ultra-structure of the small intestinal mucosa of normal control human subjects and of patients with untreated and treated coeliac disease using the scanning electron microscope. In Booth, C.C. and Dowling, R.H. (eds) *Coeliac disease*. Edinburgh: Churchill Livingstone, 26–44.

McClelland, H.A., Lewis, M.J., Naish, J.M. 1962: Idiopathic steatorrhoea with intestinal pseudo-obstruction. *Gut* 3, 142–5.

Menzies, I.S. 1984: Transmucosal passage of inert molecules in health and disease. In Heintze, K., Sradhauge, E. (eds) *Intestinal absorption and secretion*. Lancaster: MTP Press.

Menzies, I.S., Laker, M., Pounder, R. *et al.* 1979: Abnormal intestinal permeability to sugar in villous atrophy. *Lancet* 2, 1107–9.

Molberg, Ø., McAdam, S.N., Körner, R. *et al.* 1998: Tissue transflutaminase selectively modifies gliadin peptides that are recognised by gut-derived T-cells in celiac disease. *Nature Medicine* 4, 713–17.

Mylotte, M., Egan-Mitchell, B., McCarthy, C.F. *et al.* 1973: Incidence of coeliac disease in Western Ireland. *British Medical Journal* 1, 703–5.

Porter, K.G., McMaster, D., Elmes, M.E. *et al.* 1977: Anaemia and low serum copper during zinc therapy. *Lancet* 2, 774.

Ross, J.R., Garabedian, M. 1970: Systemic manifestations of gluten enteropathies and gluten sensitivity in some other diseases. In Glass, G.B.J. (ed.) *Progress in gastroenterology* 2. New York: Grune and Stratton, 430–49.

Rubin, C.F., Brandborg, L.L., Flick, A.L. *et al.* 1962: Biopsy studies on the pathogenesis of coeliac sprue. In *Ciba Foundation study group,* Vol. 14. London: Ciba Foundation, 67–83.

Rubin, C.F., Cauci, A.S., Sleisenger, M.H. *et al.* 1965: Immunofluorescent studies in adult coeliac disease. *Journal of Clinical Investigation* 44, 475–85.

Scott, B.B., Losowsky, M.S. 1975: Coeliac disease: a cause of various associated diseases. *Lancet* 2, 956.

Scott, B.B., Losowsky, M.S. 1976: Patchiness and duodenal–jejunal variation of the mucosal abnormalities in coeliac disease and dermatitis herpetiformis. *Gut* 17, 984–92.

Sheldon, W. 1959: Coeliac disease. *Paediatrica* 23, 132–45.

Shiner, M., Doniach, I. 1960: Histopathological studies in steatorrhea. *Gastroenterology* 38, 419–40.

Sollid, L., Molberg, O., McAdam, S. *et al.* 1997: Autoantibodies in coeliac disease: tissue transglutaminase – guilt by association? *Gut* 41, 851–2.

Spencer, J., MacDonald, T.T., Diss, T.C. *et al.* 1989a: Changes in intra-epithelial lymphocyte subpopulations in coeliac disease and enteropathy associated T-cell lymphoma (malignant histocytosis of the intestine). *Gut* 30, 339–46.

Spencer, J., Isaacson, P.G., Diss, T.C. *et al.* 1989b: Expression of disulphide-linked and non-disulphide-linked forms of the T-cell receptor γ/δ heterodimer in human intra-epithelial lymphocytes. *European Journal of Immunology* 19, 1331–8.

Stewart, J.S., Pollock, D.J., Hoffbrand, A.V. *et al.* 1967: A study of proximal and distal intestinal structure and absorptive function in idiopathic steatorrhoea. *Quarterly Journal of Medicine* 36, 425–44.

Tosi, R., Vismara, D., Tanigaki, N. *et al.* 1983: Evidence that coeliac disease is intimately associated with a DC locus allelic specificity. *Clinical Immunology and Immunopathology* 28, 395–404.

Trowell, H.C. 1943: Dimorphic anaemia deficiency of iron associated with nutritional macrocytic anaemia. *Transactions of the Royal Society of Tropical Medicine and Hygiene* 37, 19–40.

Trowsdale, J., Campbell, R.D. 1988: Physical map of the human HLA region. *Immunology Today* 9, 2–34.

van de Kamer, J.H., Weijers, H.A., Dicke, W.K. 1953: Coeliac disease IV. An investigation into the injurious constituents of wheat in connection with their action on patients with coeliac disease. *Acta Paediatrica* 42, 223–31.

Vaughan, J.J. 1936: *The anaemias*, 2nd edn. London: Oxford University Press.

von Krainick, H.G., Debatin, F., Gautier, E. *et al.* 1958: Additional research on the injurious effect of wheat flour in coeliac disease I. Acute gliadin reactions (gliadin shock). *Helvetica Paediatrica Acta* 13, 432–54.

Webster, A.D.B., Slavil, G., Shiver, M. *et al.* 1981: Coeliac disease with severe hypogammaglobulinaemia. *Gut* 22, 153–7.

Weiser, M.M., Douglas, A.P. 1976: An alternative mechanism for gluten toxicity in coeliac disease. *Lancet* 1, 567–9.

24

Disaccharide intolerance

HEIKKI AROLA

INTRODUCTION

Hydrolysis of complex carbohydrates, such as glycogen, starch and its components, amylose and amylopectin, is initiated by the α-amylases (salivary and pancreatic), and results in maltose, maltotriose and α-limit dextrins (branched oligosaccharides). These glucose oligomers and sucrose are subsequently hydrolysed by the brush-border α-glucosidases, sucrase–isomaltase and glucoamylase (Heitlinger and Lebenthal, 1988). Lactose, a disaccharide unique to mammalian milks, is hydrolysed by lactase, a β-galactosidase, to glucose and galactose. Trehalose, mushroom sugar, is hydrolysed by trehalase to two molecules of glucose. The resulting glucose, galactose and fructose are then transported into the enterocyte by sodium-dependent active transport (glucose, galactose) and facilitated diffusion (fructose).

Disaccharides (lactose, maltose, sucrose and trehalose) are molecules composed of two monosaccharides, which need to be hydrolysed by specific enzymes, disaccharidases, in the small bowel mucosa before absorption (Table 24.1). Milk sugar, lactose, for example, is composed of one glucose and one galactose molecule, which both are readily absorbed after hydrolysis. If the activity of the disaccharidase is deficient, then malabsorption of the sugar in question will follow.

Disaccharide intolerances refer to abdominal symptoms that result from sugar malabsorption, such as flatulence, borborygmi, abdominal distension, pain and diarrhoea. The most common of these is lactose intolerance, creating abdominal symptoms after milk or milk product ingestion.

Table 24.1 *Disaccharidases of intestinal mucosa*

Enzyme	Substrates	Products
Lactase	Lactose	Glucose + galactose
Sucrase	Sucrose	Glucose + fructose
	Maltose	Glucose
Isomaltase	Isomaltose	Glucose
	α-Limit dextrins	Glucose oligomers
Glucoamylase	Glucose oligomers	Glucose
	Maltose	Glucose
Trehalase	Trehalose	Glucose

LACTOSE INTOLERANCE

Terminology

There have been many differences in the terminology used in this context. Sahi (1978) suggests the following terminology: primary, selective, adult-type *hypolactasia* means a low activity of lactase in the small bowel mucosa without any disturbance of the other disaccharides. *Lactose malabsorption* means that lactose is not absorbed. Flatz (1987) suggests the term *lactase restriction* (meaning low lactose digestion capacity) instead of hypolactasia and the term *lactase persistence* (meaning high lactose digestion capacity) to describe continuing lactase activity into adulthood. *Lactose intolerance* refers to the clinical symptoms caused by hypolactasia and is thus not synonymous with hypolactasia. This is because hypolactasia may occur without any symptoms, and lactose may not be tolerated, even though lactose is hydrolysed and absorbed. The term *milk intolerance* means that a person suffers from abdominal symptoms after milk ingestion, but this may be due to other ingredients of milk besides lactose.

Aetiology

It is generally accepted that the decline in the activity of intestinal lactase is determined by an autosomal recessive single gene (Sahi *et al.*, 1973; Flatz, 1987). The hypolactasia gene can be regarded as a normal developmental programme gene, which is ubiquitous in subhuman mammals and predominant in humans, resulting in the regular decline of lactase activity between the ages of 2 and 5 years (Simoons, 1980). Both transcriptional and post-transcriptional regulatory mechanisms are involved in the decline of lactase activity. The single overriding factor discriminating between subjects with high and low lactase activity is the increased rate of lactase biosynthesis in lactase persistence (Rossi *et al.*, 1997). It is not possible to induce lactase activity by drinking milk. With the generalized decline of lactase activity in essentially all mammals, lactase persistence, rather than lactase deficiency, should be considered abnormal.

Lactase deficiency can be either primary or secondary (Table 24.2). Secondary lactase deficiency occurs in any disease involving small bowel mucosal damage, such as coeliac disease and viral enteritis (Lebenthal, 1975).

Prevalence

The prevalence of adult-type hypolactasia varies considerably between different races and populations (Table 24.3). In White Europeans and their descendants (e.g. among the people in North America and Australia), the prevalence of hypolactasia is fairly low: typically less than 30 per cent. The lowest figures, 5 per cent or less, are reported for populations living in the north-western Europe (Sahi, 1994). The prevalences are much higher in southern Europe, Asia and in Africa. The highest prevalences have been reported from the countries of the Far East. In northern Thailand, a prevalence of 100 per cent has been found and, in central Thailand, 97 per cent (Flatz and Saengudom, 1969).

There are many theories explaining these wide differences in the prevalence rates in different countries. A cultural–historical hypothesis (Simoons, 1970) states that the longer the tradition of dairy farming among people under the conditions of nutritional stress, the lower the prevalence of lactase deficiency. This is based on the assumption that, compared to those with lactase deficiency, others in whom lactase activity persists

Table 24.2 *Classification of lactase deficiency*

Primary lactase deficiency
- Congenital
- Primary, adult-type lactase deficiency

Secondary lactase deficiency
- Small intestinal mucosal disease
  - Coeliac disease
  - Severe gastroenteritis
- Deficiency states
  - Prolonged starvation
  - Marasmus
  - Kwashiorkor
- Drugs
  - Neomycin
  - Kanamycin
  - Colchicine
- Anatomical
  - Short bowel syndrome
  - Postgastrectomy

Table 24.3 *Prevalence of lactase deficiency in different populations. (Adapted from Sahi, 1994)*

Country	Prevalence of lactase deficiency (%)
Europe	
Denmark	4
Great Britain	5
Sweden	5
Germany	15
Finland	17
Estonia	23–32
Poland	37
Hungary	37
Italy	40–70
Near East and Africa	
Turkey	71
Egypt	73
Most African countries	70–95
Nomadic Bedouins in Jordan	24
Asia, Oceania and Australia	
Thailand	97–100
China	86–92
Whites in Australia	6
Whites in New Zealand	9
Aborigines in Papua New Guinea	77–86
North and South America	
Whites in North America	6–19
Blacks in North America	80
Indians in North America	62–100
Eskimos	82
Mexico	66–74
Chile	70
Uruguay	65

throughout their lifetime can use all the nutrients of milk without suffering from diarrhoea, and are stronger and better equipped to survive. Thus the proportion of people with lactase persistence would increase in a population. In Northern Europe an additional theory (calcium absorption hypothesis) has been put forward (Flatz and Rotthauwe, 1973): pelvic deformity, rickets and osteomalacia were common in Northern Europe because of low solar irradiation, which caused a lack of cutaneous cholecalciferol production. Nutritional supply of vitamin D was also low. Lactose was found to be a stimulant of calcium absorption. Therefore, people with lactase persistence absorbed calcium better than people with hypolactasia; they also had less rickets and pelvic deformities and could bear more children. The result was a genetic selection in favour of the lactase persistence gene. These selective advantages have had enough time to explain the differences seen today (Cavalli-Sforza, 1973; Flatz, 1987).

Pathophysiology and the clinical picture

When lactose is ingested, it cannot be utilized as such, but must first be hydrolysed into its constituent sugars, glucose and galactose, by lactase. The highest lactase activity in the brush border of the enterocyte occurs in the jejunum, with lower levels of activity in the duodenum and ileum (Newcomer and McGill, 1966). After hydrolysis, galactose and glucose are readily absorbed by a common sodium-dependent carrier.

In hypolactasia, the activity of lactase diminishes to about 10 per cent of that of an infant (Dahlqvist and Semenza, 1985). Thus lactose remains unhydrolysed in the small intestine, where it causes an osmotic effect, retaining water in the intestinal lumen (Launiala, 1968). In the colon, lactose is metabolized by bacteria (a major part of the essential microflora is capable of fermenting lactose), leading to the formation of gases (hydrogen, carbon dioxide and methane), and various organic acids (mainly acetic, succinic, lactic and formic acids) (Arola and Tamm, 1994). This results in a second osmotic gradient between the plasma and the lumen with further movement of fluid into the lumen of the colon. These contribute to the symptoms caused by hypolactasia: diarrhoea (loose stools), flatulence (gas), borborygmi (rumbling) and abdominal distension. Pain is not a common symptom of lactose intolerance but may sometimes be present. The amount of lactose that provokes these symptoms varies considerably between different individuals (Cavalli-Sforza and Strata, 1986). Small amounts (< 7 g) do not usually cause symptoms (Vesa *et al.*, 1996a). This tolerance threshold does not seem to be correlated with the lactase activity left in the jejunum (Bedine and Bayless, 1973). The rate of gastric emptying (Vesa *et al.*, 1997a) and small intestinal passage as well as the ability of the colon to absorb gases and acids will modify the symptoms. Yoghurt is usually better tolerated than milk, which is partly due to bacterial lactase being activated at body temperature (Kolars *et al.*, 1984), and partly due to the slower gastric emptying of semi-solid milk products (Vesa *et al.*, 1996b). Neither the fat content (Vesa *et al.*, 1997b) nor viscosity (Vesa *et al.*, 1997a) of milk affect the symptoms of lactose intolerance. In general, the symptoms tend to be less severe when lactose is ingested with solid foods, presumably due to a slower rate of colonic fermentation (Solomons *et al.*, 1985), and when it is divided in several doses during the day.

Diagnosis and differential diagnosis

The diagnosis of hypolactasia is usually made based on a lactose tolerance test. It is possible to measure after an oral dose of lactose either the rise in blood glucose, blood or urinary galactose, or breath hydrogen. In hypolactasia, the rise in blood glucose is usually less than 1.1 mmol/L. This test is rather unreliable and many authors suggest using some other more reliable method when possible (Newcomer *et al.*, 1975).

A more reliable way is to measure blood galactose after an oral lactose load. Only one blood sample at 40 minutes is required (Isokoski *et al.*, 1972). In order to prevent the rapid metabolism of galactose to glucose in the liver, the test needs a small amount of ethanol (300 mg/kg), which can be regarded as a relative disadvantage, especially in children. In hypolactasia, blood galactose is less than 0.3 mmol/L at 40 minutes after lactose. A further simplification is obtained by determining urinary galactose concentration at 40 minutes, either quantitatively (Arola *et al.*, 1982) or qualitatively with a test strip (Arola *et al.*, 1987). Unfortunately, these strips are no longer available. In hypolactasia, urinary galactose is less than 2.0 mmol/L, and there is no colour change in the strip. The dose of ethanol needed can be diminished to 150 mg/kg. Ethanol can be omitted from the test by determining the urinary galactose/creatinine ratio or total galactose in pooled 3-hour urine samples after lactose (Grant *et al.*, 1989; Alvarez-Coca *et al.*, 1996). In hypolactasia, the urinary galactose/creatinine ratio is less than 0.125 and the total galactose excreted less than 19 mg. The sensitivity of total urinary galactose determination has been reported to be 94 per cent and specificity 100 per cent (Alvarez-Coca *et al.*, 1996). A simple visual screening method based on galactose dehydrogenase has recently been developed: in the presence of galactose in the urine, a darker red colour is observed in the test solution and colour is matched against the standard. The method is easy, convenient, inexpensive and ideally suited for field work (Buttery *et al.*, 1994).

Breath hydrogen tests are widely used today. Hydrogen production after lactose load takes place in the colon and 14–21 per cent of the hydrogen produced is exhaled through the lungs (Levitt, 1969). In hypolactasia, an increment in exhaled hydrogen of > 20 ppm is seen (Newcomer *et al.*, 1975). Suitable colonic flora capable of producing hydrogen are required (Levitt and Donaldson, 1970). A number of reports (Levitt and Donaldson, 1970; Newcomer *et al.*, 1975; Gilat *et al.*, 1978) have shown that 2–20 per cent of patients may be colonized with bacteria incapable of producing hydrogen. It has also been shown that, in some cases, colonic bacteria can consume hydrogen (Murphy and Calloway, 1972; Levitt *et al.*, 1974) to produce methane (Bjørneklett and Jenssen, 1982). That is why it is recommended that parallel measurement of breath hydrogen and methane is done (Bjørneklett and Jenssen, 1982). Sleeping, owing to a combination of hypoventilation and decreased colonic motility (Solomons and Viteri, 1976), and smoking, owing to gases in the tobacco smoke (Tadesse and Eastwood, 1977; Rosenthal and Solomons, 1983), will increase the rise in hydrogen not related to lactose. Thus the subjects in the test should not be allowed to sleep and should allow an interval of at least 15 minutes from the end of smoking to the collection of a breath sample. The prior use of antibiotics may increase (succinylsulphathiazole, neomycin, trimethoprim) or decrease (iodochlorohydroxyquin, neomycin) the rise in hydrogen, depending on the antibiotic used (Murphy and Calloway, 1972; Solomons *et al.*, 1978). The test is reliable when the abovementioned factors are taken into consideration (Newcomer *et al.*, 1975; Arola, 1994). A relative disadvantage is the need to take multiple samples for a long period of time.

While examining a patient with vague abdominal complaints, it is important to bear in mind that similar symptoms may be caused by many conditions other than hypolactasia. Hypolactasia is not a clinical entity but simply an enzyme deficiency that, even if present, may not be the cause behind the patient's symptoms. If the patient has lactose intolerance symptoms after lactose ingestion, these will disappear when lactose is removed or diminished from the diet for 2 weeks. If the symptoms disappear during the diet, lactose intolerance is probable and no further investigations are necessary. The diagnosis of hypolactasia may also be coincidential, which has nothing to do with the patient´s complaints. Patients with irritable bowel syndrome (IBS), especially females, seem to experience more symptoms after lactose than persons without this disease (Vesa *et al.*, 1998). In this Finnish study, among the subjects with IBS, the percentage of lactose maldigesters was the same as in the whole study group (24 per cent), but there were significantly more subjects who reported lactose intolerance (60 per cent versus 27 per cent). Whether these associations are of psychological or physiological origin remains to be determined. The possibility that lactose intolerance may also be associated with other illnesses that cause diarrhoea should be recognized and the dual aetiology of the diarrhoea borne in mind.

Recommended examinations include faecal examination for occult blood and bacteria, endoscopic examinations, possibly x-ray examinations, tests of liver and pancreatic functions, and ultrasonic scanning of the abdomen. The choice is determined by the patient's symptoms and the results of treatments, and examinations should be continued until the real cause behind the patient's symptoms is revealed.

Treatment and prognosis

Treatment is easy: elimination of milk and milk products from the diet to the level where they no longer cause symptoms. The lactose content of different milk products varies a lot (Table 24.4). Lactose tolerance is very variable and so the treatment is individual. Hard cheeses and butter can be used freely. Many patients tolerate fermented milk products much better than ordinary milk, which is partly due to bacterial lactase being activated at body temperature (Kolars *et al.*, 1984), and partly due to the slower gastric emptying of semi-solid milk products (Vesa *et al.*, 1996b). A large variety of lactose-hydrolysed milk products (milk, cream, yoghurt) is available nowadays, at least in Finland. In these products, the lactose content is

Table 24.4 *Lactose content in different milks and milk products. (Adapted from Tamm, 1994)*

Product	Lactose (g/100 g)
Milk	5
Low-fat milk	3.8–5.4
Skim milk	5.0–5.8
Buttermilk fluid	3.8–4.5
Chocolate milk	4.2–5.0
Sweetened condensed whole milk	11.4
Dried whole milk	37.5
Low-fat yoghurts	4.8–5.8
Acidophilus milk, skim	4.4
Kefir, part skim	4.0
Cheeses, various	0–5.7
Cottage cheese	2.4–2.9
Cottage cheese, low fat	3.0–3.5
Ripe cheeses	
Emmental	0
Edam	0–1.4
Camembert	0–1.8
Roquefort	2.0
Light cream	4
Whipping cream	2.8–3.0
Soured cream	3.4–4.3
Butter	1
Oleomargarine	0
Vanilla ice cream	7
French ice cream, soft	5.3

reduced to about 20 per cent of the usual milk product, and most lactose-intolerant subjects can use these products without symptoms. It is also possible to use exogenous lactase as tablets (Dairy Ease®), caplets (Lactaid®) or capsules (Lactrase®) before the meal to help to reduce the symptoms. However, these preparations differ in their ability to affect the symptoms after milk ingestion: Lactrase reduced pain, bloating and total symptomatic score; Dairy Ease reduced pain; while Lactaid did not reduce symptoms at all in one US study (Ramirez *et al.*, 1994).

The prognosis is excellent. If the need to reduce milk products from the diet is great, calcium intake should be ascertained.

CONGENITAL LACTASE DEFICIENCY

This form of lactase deficiency is very rare. It is most common in Finland, where two infants are born every year with this condition. It is also inherited in an autosomal recessive manner. Lactase was originally thought to be totally absent in this disease, but most probably lactase is present, albeit at trace levels much lower than in adult hypolactasia (Savilahti *et al.*, 1983).

A typical symptom is watery diarrhoea that the newborn child develops soon after ingesting breast milk or any other lactose-containing milk. At this stage, the newborn has a good appetite, and no vomiting occurs. The loss of nutrients due to diarrhoea is so considerable that the growth of the infant is retarded, and dehydration and acidosis will develop.

Diagnosis is ascertained by a lactose-free diet and later by jejunal biopsy, usually at the age of 6 months (Savilahti *et al.*, 1983). Lactase activity is very low.

Congenital lactase deficiency is not dangerous when the condition is diagnosed at an early stage. Infants must be fed with a lactose-free diet. Later in life, affected individuals may tolerate small amounts of lactose.

OTHER DISACCHARIDE INTOLERANCES

Sucrose–isomaltose intolerance

The prevalence of this disorder is also variable: it may occur in as many as 0.2 per cent of White North Americans (Welsh *et al.*, 1978), and in 10 per cent of Greenland Eskimos (Asp *et al.*, 1975). It produces osmotic diarrhoea after ingestion of sucrose and starch dextrins. A sucrose tolerance test will produce a flat glucose curve and the sucrose hydrogen breath test consistently demonstrates excessive H_2 excretion in the breath (Metz *et al.*, 1976). Treatment consists of the elimination of sucrose and starch from the diet in the first years of life. Restriction of starch intake is usually unnecessary after 2–3 years of age, although excessive amounts should be avoided.

Trehalose intolerance

Isolated trehalase deficiency was first described in a 71-year-old woman (Bergoz, 1971) and later in a family (Madzarovová-Nohejlová, 1973). The prevalence of trehalase deficiency has been reported to be 10–15 per cent in Greenland Eskimos (Asp *et al.*, 1975). The prevalence in most countries is unknown.

In practice, the only dietary source of trehalose is mushrooms. Trehalose intolerance is likely to go undetected, since ingestion of large quantities of food containing trehalose is uncommon. However, it is obvious that trehalose maldigestion can cause symptoms similar to those of lactose maldigestion and intolerance. Three factors control the genesis of symptoms: (1) the activity of small-bowel trehalase – if it is low, trehalose is maldigested and more trehalose is passed into the colon; (2) the maldigested trehalose, which causes osmotic water flow into the colon, resulting in loose stools and diarrhoea; and (3) most importantly, the microflora of the colon, from which symptoms will arise if there are bacteria capable of producing gases from maldigested trehalose. If colonic bacteria cannot produce gases, then distension of the abdomen and intestinal gas expulsion as eructations and flatus will not occur (Arola *et al.*, 1999).

Diagnosis is by trehalose tolerance test, resulting in increased hydrogen excretion after trehalose ingestion. Treatment is trehalose restriction to the level where they no longer cause symptoms.

SECONDARY DISACCHARIDE INTOLERANCES

Secondary disaccharidase deficiency can be caused by any condition or drug effect that damages the enterocytes of the small bowel mucosa. In acute bacterial or viral gastroenteritis, the microbe can damage the villous structure, especially in children. *Giardia lamblia* can also cause partial atrophy, particularly in chronic infection. In tropical sprue there may be severe villous damage and the activity of lactase can be near to nil (Sheehy and Anderson, 1965). Various drugs can cause damage to the mucosa causing secondary disaccharidase deficiency: neomysin, kanamycin (Dobbins, 1968), tetracycline (Mitchell *et al.*, 1982), colchicine (Longstreth and Newcomer, 1975) and many cytostatic drugs (Shaw *et al.*, 1979).

Coeliac disease in both children and adults is characterized by flat jejunal mucosa. The activities of all disaccharidases are decreased (Mercer *et al.*, 1990) and they return to normal when gluten is excluded from the diet.

GLUCOSE–GALACTOSE MALABSORPTION

Congenital glucose–galactose malabsorption is characterized by a selective defect in the intestinal transport of these two monosaccharides. It is rare – only little over 30 cases have been described. Infants suffer from profuse, chronic, watery diarrhoea that often leads to hypertonic dehydration. Successful treatment is possible with carbohydrate-free infant formula (Abad-Sinden *et al.*, 1997).

INTOLERANCE TO OTHER DIETARY CARBOHYDRATES

Fructose intolerance

Fructose is an important dietary carbohydrate found in its free form in fruit and as one of the component monosaccharides of sucrose. Figs contain 30 g, prunes 15 g, grapes 8 g and soft drinks 7 g of fructose per 100 g. In one study, fructose, 50 g as a 10 per cent solution, was incompletely absorbed by 37.5 per cent of healthy volunteers (Ravich *et al.*, 1983). In children under 6 years, all malabsorbed 2 g/kg fructose, with the highest peaks being observed between 1 and 3 years (Hoekstra *et al.*, 1993). There seems to be a correlation between fructose intolerance and the early signs of depression, especially in females (Ledochowski *et al.*, 1998). The background for this association is still unknown.

Apple juice contains fructose and sorbitol, substances that have been shown to be incompletely absorbed by most people. In young children (1–4 years of age) with chronic non-specific diarrhoea, the elimination of apple juice from the diet restored normal bowel function in a Dutch study. It was estimated that fructose accounted for 80 per cent and sorbitol for 20 per cent of the incomplete absorption (Kneepkens *et al.*, 1989). As little as 240 mL of apple juice caused significant carbohydrate malabsorption and diarrhoea in five children in an American study, and withdrawal of apple juice was curative in all cases (Hyams and Leichtner, 1985). This should be borne in mind, because an increase of fruit juice consumption by preschool children has been seen in recent years (Dennison, 1996). Honey contains fructose in excess of glucose and has also been shown to be able to cause fructose intolerance-related abdominal complaints (Ladas *et al.*, 1995).

Sorbitol intolerance

Sorbitol, a polyalcohol sugar, is the sweetener in most 'sugar-free' products and may produce an osmotic diarrhoea if ingested in moderate amounts. Ingestion of as little as 5 g of sorbitol was associated with a significant increase in breath hydrogen concentration. Most subjects experienced mild gastrointestinal distress (gas, bloating) after 10 g and severe symptoms (cramps, diarrhea) after 20 g in the study by Hyams (1983). In coeliac disease patients, 100 per cent malabsorbed as little as 5 g of sorbitol (Corazza *et al.*, 1988). Sorbitol is also a common natural constituent of fruit juices. Decreased carbohydrate absorption occurs more often after ingestion of juices that contain more sorbitol, a non-absorbable sugar, and higher concentrations of fructose over glucose than after ingestion of juices that lack sorbitol and contain equal amounts of fructose and glucose (Nobigrot *et al.*, 1997). It has been suggested that sorbitol might be the explanatory factor in the 'idiopathic' diarrhoea in diabetics (Badiga *et al.*, 1990). In one study (Jain *et al.*, 1985), clinical sorbitol intolerance was detected in 43 per cent of White and 55 per cent of non-White healthy volunteers after 10 g of sorbitol solution. Sorbitol absorption seems to be increased by the concomitant ingestion of glucose and lipids (Beaugerie *et al.*, 1995), probably by slowing the gastric emptying of sorbitol (Beaugerie *et al.*, 1996). Sorbitol can also cause the so-called chewing gum diarrhoea (Goldberg and Ditchek, 1978) and 'Halloween diarrhoea' caused by sorbitol-containing candies (Breitenbach, 1992). It seems that sorbitol and also fructose intolerance is common among patients with functional bowel disease (Rumessen and Gudmand-Høyer, 1988; Symons *et al.*, 1992), and recognition of these conditions might make it possible to separate and treat entities in this disease complex.

CONCLUDING REMARKS

Lactose intolerance is by far the most common disaccharide intolerance found in humans. It may be regarded as the normal condition for an adult human being. The diagnosis is often easy after suspicion has arised about sugar intolerance as the underlying cause. Final confirmation of the role of disaccharide intolerance in producing symptoms in an individual patient requires resolution of symptoms following elimination from the diet of the foods containing the offending disaccharide.

REFERENCES

Abad-Sinden, A., Borowitz, S., Meyers, R. *et al.* 1997: Nutrition management of congenital glucose–galactose malabsorption: a case study. *Journal of the American Dietetic Association* 97, 1417–21.

Alvarez-Coca, J., Pérez-Miranda, M., Iritia, M. *et al.* 1996: Usefulness of urinary galactose for the diagnosis of hypolactasia. *Journal of Clinical Gastroenterology* 23, 79–80.

Arola, H. 1994: Diagnosis of hypolactasia and lactose malabsorption. *Scandinavian Journal of Gastroenterology* 29(Suppl 202), 26–35.

Arola, H., Tamm, A. 1994: Metabolism of lactose in the human body. *Scandinavian Journal of Gastroenterology* 29(Suppl 202), 21–5.

Arola, H., Koivula, T., Jokela, H. *et al.* 1982: Simple urinary test for lactose malabsorption. *Lancet* 2, 524–5.

Arola, H., Koivula, T., Jokela, H. *et al.* 1987: Strip test is reliable in common prevalences of hypolactasia. *Scandinavian Journal of Gastroenterology* 22, 509–12.

Arola, H., Koivula, T., Karvonen, A.L. *et al.* 1999: Low trehalase activity is associated with abdominal symptoms caused by edible mushrooms. *Scandinavian Journal of Gastroenterology* 34, 898–903.

Asp, N.G., Berg, N.O., Dahlqvist, A. *et al.* 1975: Intestinal disaccharidases in Greenland Eskimos. *Scandinavian Journal of Gastroenterology*, 10, 513–19.

Badiga, M.S., Jain, N.K., Casanova, C., *et al.* 1990: Diarrhea in diabetics: the role of sorbitol. *Journal of the American College of Nutrition* 9, 578–82.

Beaugerie, L., Flourie, B., Lemann, M. *et al.* 1995: Sorbitol absorption in the healthy human small intestine is increased by the concomitant ingestion of glucose and lipids. *European Journal of Gastroenterology and Hepatology* 7, 125–8.

Beaugerie, L., Lemann, M., Jian, R. *et al.* 1996: Effect of glucose and lipids on intestinal absorption of sorbitol: role of gastric emptying. *Neurogastroenterology and Motility* 8, 235–9.

Bedine, M.S., Bayless, T.M. 1973: Intolerance of small amounts of lactose by individuals with low lactase levels. *Gastroenterology* 65, 735–43.

Bergoz, R. 1971: Trehalose malabsorption causing intolerance to mushrooms. Report of a probable case. *Gastroenterology* 60, 909–12.

Bjørneklett, A., Jenssen, E. 1982: Relationship between hydrogen and methane production in man. *Scandinavian Journal of Gastroenterology* 17, 985–92.

Breitenbach, R.A. 1992: 'Halloween diarrhea'. An unexpected trick of sorbitol-containing candy. *Postgraduate Medicine* 92, 63–6.

Buttery, J.E., Ratnaike, R.N., Chamberlain, B.R. 1994: A visual screening method for lactose maldigestion. *Annals of Clinical Biochemistry* 31, 566–7.

Cavalli-Sforza, L.T. 1973: Analytical review: some current problems of human population genetics. *American Journal of Human Genetics* 25, 82–104.

Cavalli-Sforza, L.T., Strata, A. 1986: Double-blind study on the tolerance of four types of milk in lactose malabsorbers and absorbers. *Human Nutrition, Clinical Nutrition* 40C, 19–30.

Corazza, G.R., Strocchi, A., Rossi, R., *et al.* 1988: Sorbitol malabsorption in normal volunteers and in patients with coeliac disease. *Gut* 29, 44–8.

Dahlqvist, A., Semenza, G. 1985: Disaccharidases of small intestinal mucosa. *Journal of Pediatric Gastroenterology and Nutrition* 4, 857–65.

Dennison, B.A. 1996: Fruit juice consumption by infants and children: a review. *Journal of the American College of Nutrition* 15(5 Suppl), 4–11S.

Dobbins, W.O. 1968: Drug-induced steatorrhea. *Gastroenterology* 54, 1193–5.

Flatz, G. 1987: Genetics of lactose digestion in humans. *Advances in Human Genetics* 16, 1–77.

Flatz, G., Rotthauwe, H.W. 1973: Lactose nutrition and natural selection. *Lancet* 2, 76–7.

Flatz, G., Saengudom, C. 1969: Lactose tolerance in Asians: a family study. *Nature* 224, 915–16.

Gilat, T., BenHur, H., Gelman-Malachi, E. *et al.* 1978: Alterations of the colonic flora and their effect on the hydrogen breath test. *Gut* 19, 602–5.

Goldberg, L.D., Ditchek, N.T. 1978: Chewing gum diarrhea. *American Journal of Digestive Diseases* 23, 568.

Grant, J.D., Bezerra, J.A., Thompson, J.H. *et al.* 1989: Assessment of lactose absorption by measurement of urinary galactose. *Gastroenterology* 97, 895–9.

Heitlinger, L.A., Lebenthal, E. 1988: Disorders of carbohydrate digestion and absorption. *Pediatric Clinics of North America* 35, 239–55.

Hoekstra, J.H., van Kempen A.A., Bijl, S.B. *et al.* 1993: Fructose breath hydrogen tests. *Archives of Diseases in Childhood* 68, 136–8.

Hyams, J.S. 1983: Sorbitol intolerance: an unappreciated cause of functional gastrointestinal complaints. *Gastroenterology* 84, 30–3.

Hyams, J.S., Leichtner, A.M. 1985: Apple juice. An unappreciated cause of chronic diarrhea. *American Journal of Diseases of Children* 139, 503–5.

Isokoski, M., Jussila, J., Sarna, S. 1972: A simple screening method for lactose malabsorption. *Gastroenterology* 62, 28–32.

Jain, N.K., Rosenberg, D.B., Ulahannan, M.J. *et al.* 1985: Sorbitol intolerance in adults. *American Journal of Gastroenterology* 80, 678–81.

Kneepkens, C.M., Jakobs, C., Douwes, A.C. 1989: Apple juice, fructose and nonspecific diarrhoea. *European Journal of Pediatrics* 148, 571–3.

Kolars, J.C., Levitt, M.D., Aouji, M. *et al.* 1984: Yoghurt – an autodigesting source of lactose. *New England Journal of Medicine* 310, 1–3.

Ladas, S.D., Haritos, D.N., Raptis, S.A. 1995: Honey may have a laxative effect on normal subjects because of incomplete fructose absorption. *American Journal of Clinical Nutrition* 62, 1212–15.

Launiala, K. 1968: The mechanism of diarrhoea in congenital disaccharide malabsorption. *Acta Paediatrica Scandinavica* 57, 425–32.

Lebenthal, E. 1975: Small intestinal disaccharidase deficiencies. *Pediatric Clinics of North America* 20, 757–66.

Ledochowski, M., Sperner-Unterweger, B., Widner, B. *et al.* 1998: Fructose malabsorption is associated with early signs of mental depression. *European Journal of Medical Research* 3, 295–8.

Levitt, M.D. 1969: Production and excretion of hydrogen gas in man. *New England Journal of Medicine*, 281, 122–7.

Levitt, M.D., Donaldson, R.M. 1970: Use of respiratory hydrogen (H_2) excretion to detect carbohydrate malabsorption. *Journal of Laboratory and Clinical Medicine* 75, 937–45.

Levitt, M.D., Berggren, T., Hastings, J. *et al.* 1974: Hydrogen (H_2) catabolism in the colon of the rat. *Journal of Laboratory and Clinical Medicine* 84, 163–7.

Longstreth, G.F., Newcomer, A.D. 1975: Drug-induced malabsorption. *Mayo Clinic Proceedings* 50, 284–93.

Madzarovová-Nohejlová, J. 1973: Trehalase deficiency in a family. *Gastroenterology* 65, 130–3.

Mercer, J., Eagles, M.E., Talbot, I.C. 1990: Brush border enzymes in coeliac disease: histochemical evaluation. *Journal of Clinical Pathology* 43, 307–12.

Metz, G., Jenkins, D.J.A., Newman, A. *et al.* 1976: Breath hydrogen in hyposucrasia. *Lancet* 1, 119.

Mitchell, T.H., Stamp, T.C.B., Jenkins, M.V. 1982: Steatorrhea after tetracycline. *British Medical Journal* 285, 780.

Murphy, E.L., Calloway, D.H. 1972: The effect of antibiotic drugs on the volume and composition of intestinal gas from beans. *American Journal of Digestive Diseases* 17, 639–42.

Newcomer, A.D., McGill, D.B. 1966: Lactose tolerance test in adults with normal lactase activity. *Gastroenterology* 50, 340–6.

Newcomer, A.D., McGill, D.B., Thomas, P.J. *et al.* 1975: Prospective comparison of indirect methods for detecting lactase deficiency. *New England Journal of Medicine* 293, 1232–5.

Nobigrot, T., Chasalow, F.I., Lifshitz, F. 1997: Carbohydrate absorption from one serving of fruit juice in young children: age and carbohydrate composition effects. *Journal of the American College of Nutrition* 16, 152–8.

Ramirez, F.C., Lee, K., Graham, D.Y. 1994: All lactase preparations are not the same: results of a prospective, randomized, placebo-controlled trial. *American Journal of Gastroenterology* 89, 566–70.

Ravich, W.J., Bayless, T.M., Thomas, M. 1983: Fructose: incomplete intestinal absorption in humans. *Gastroenterology* 84, 26–9.

Rosenthal, A., Solomons, N.W. 1983: Time-course of cigarette smoke contamination of clinical hydrogen breath-analysis tests. *Clinical Chemistry* 29, 1980–1.

Rossi, M., Maiuri, L., Fusco, M.I. *et al.* 1997: Lactase persistence versus decline in human adults: multifactorial events are involved in down-regulation after weaning. *Gastroenterology* 112, 1506–14.

Rumessen, J.J., Gudmand-Høyer, E. 1988: Functional bowel disease: malabsorption and abdominal distress after ingestion of fructose, sorbitol, and fructose-sorbitol mixtures. *Gastroenterology* 95, 694–700.

Sahi, T. 1978: Dietary lactose and the aetiology of human small-intestinal hypolactasia. *Gut* 19, 1074–86.

Sahi, T. 1994: Genetics and epidemiology of adult-type hypolactasia. *Scandinavian Journal of Gastroenterology* 29(Suppl 202), 7–20.

Sahi, T., Isokoski, M., Jussila, J. *et al.* 1973: Recessive inheritance of adult-type lactose malabsorption. *Lancet* 2, 823–6.

Savilahti, E., Launiala, K., Kuitunen, P. 1983: Congenital lactase deficiency. *Archives of Diseases in Childhood* 58, 246–52.

Shaw, M.T., Spector, M.H., Ladman, A.J. 1979: Effect of cancer radiotherapy and cytotoxic drugs on intestinal structure and function. *Cancer Treatment Reviews* 6, 141–51.

Sheehy, T.W., Anderson, P.R.A. 1965: Disaccharidase activity in normal and diseased small bowel. *Lancet* 2, 1–2.

Simoons, F.J. 1970: Primary adult lactose intolerance and the milking habit: a problem in biologic and cultural interrelations. II. A culture historical hypothesis. *American Journal of Digestive Diseases* 15, 695–710.

Simoons, F.J. 1980: Age of onset of lactose malabsorption. *Pediatrics* 66, 646–8.

Solomons, N.W., Viteri, F.E. 1976: Breath hydrogen during sleep. *Lancet* 2, 636.

Solomons, N.W., Viteri, F.E., Rosenberg, I.H. 1978: Development of an interval sampling hydrogen breath test for carbohydrate malabsorption in children: evidence for a circadian pattern of H_2 concentration. *Pediatric Research* 12, 816–23.

Solomons, N.W., Guerrero, A.-M., Torun, B. 1985: Dietary manipulation of postprandial colonic lactose fermentation. I. Effect of solid foods in a meal. *American Journal of Clinical Nutrition* 41, 199–208.

Symons, P., Jones, M.P., Kellow, J.E. 1992: Symptom provocation in irritable bowel syndrome. Effects of differing doses of fructose-sorbitol. *Scandinavian Journal of Gastroenterology* 27, 940–4.

Tadesse, K., Eastwood, M. 1977: Breath-hydrogen test and smoking. *Lancet* 2, 91.

Tamm, A. 1994: Management of lactose intolerance. *Scandinavian Journal of Gastroenterology* 29(Suppl 202), 55–63.

Welsh, J.D., Poley, J.R., Bhatia, M. *et al.* 1978: Intestinal disaccharidase activities in relation to age, race, and mucosal damage. *Gastroenterology* 75, 847–55.

Vesa, T.H., Korpela, R.A., Sahi, T. 1996a: Tolerance to small amounts of lactose. *American Journal of Clinical Nutrition* 64, 197–201.

Vesa, T.H., Marteau, P., Zidi, S. *et al.* 1996b: Digestion and tolerance of lactose from yoghurt and different semi-solid fermented dairy products containing *Lactobacillus acidophilus* and bifidobacteria in lactose maldigesters – Is bacterial lactase important? *European Journal of Clinical Nutrition* 50, 730–3.

Vesa, T.H., Marteau, P.R., Briet, F.B. *et al.* 1997a: Effects of milk viscosity on gastric emptying and lactose tolerance in lactose maldigesters. *American Journal of Clinical Nutrition* 66, 123–6.

Vesa, T.H., Lember, M., Korpela, R. 1997b: Milk fat does not affect the symptoms of lactose intolerance. *European Journal of Clinical Nutrition* 51, 1–4.

Vesa, T.H., Seppo, L.M., Marteau, P.R. *et al.* 1998: Role of irritable bowel syndrome in subjective lactose intolerance. *American Journal of Clinical Nutrition* 67, 710–15.

25

Crohn's disease of the small bowel

IAN C ROBERTS-THOMSON, GITANJALI PAWAR

INTRODUCTION

Crohn's disease takes the name of Dr Burrill B. Crohn, a physician from the Mount Sinai Hospital, New York. In 1932, Crohn, Ginzburg and Oppenheimer described 14 patients, mostly young adults, with ileal inflammation associated with strictures and fistulae, which they called 'regional ileitis'. Although previous descriptions had appeared in the medical literature, notably by Dalzeil (1913), the description by Crohn *et al.* (1932) captured the attention of the medical establishment. The next step was the recognition that Crohn's disease could also involve the colon and that Crohn's colitis could be distinguished from ulcerative colitis. This process was largely completed by Lockhart-Mummery and Morson (1960) in a classical paper that described pathological differences between the two forms of colonic inflammation.

As the cause of Crohn's disease is unknown, current definitions focus on pathological changes, which often involve the small bowel but may affect any part of the gastrointestinal tract. The histological finding is that of chronic inflammation, often granulomatous in nature, which extends through all layers of the bowel wall and typically includes diseased segments separated by apparently healthy segments. At a clinical level, the disease is characterized by an indolent course, often with exacerbations and remissions, and with a variety of gastrointestinal symptoms as well as extraintestinal manifestations.

The past two decades have witnessed an exponential increase in the number of medical reports on various aspects of Crohn's disease. Most reports, however, have considered Crohn's disease as a single entity without consideration of the possibility of heterogeneity, based on the site of the disease or other clinical or pathological variables. This contribution will focus on Crohn's disease of the small bowel, and will attempt to highlight differences between involvement of the small bowel and other areas of the gastrointestinal tract.

EPIDEMIOLOGY

Demographics

Estimates of the annual incidence of Crohn's disease rely on satisfactory methods for case identification. For example, hospital admission and mortality rates may not be reliable markers of incidence, while outpatient statistics and results of investigations are notoriously difficult to collect. Nevertheless, persuasive evidence exists for a substantial increase in the incidence of Crohn's disease in many countries in the period 1935–1985. This incidence may have peaked at about 6–7 per 100 000 population per year in the USA, UK and Scandinavia (Logan, 1998). In contrast, the mean annual incidence was estimated at 1.9 per 100 000 in Olmsted County, Minnesota, during the period

1935–1954 (Sedlack *et al.*, 1980), and 0.2 per 100 000 in Cardiff, Wales, during the period 1935–1945 (Rose *et al.*, 1988).

Other countries with a relatively high incidence of Crohn's disease include Australia and several countries in Western Europe. Incidence rates for Crohn's disease in many developing countries in Asia, Africa and South America remain unclear, but appear to be extremely low. There is little information on the incidence of Crohn's disease in migrant populations, although the disease appears to be less common in the Jewish population in Israel than in Jewish populations in the USA and Northern Europe. In high-incidence countries, some ethnic minorities appear to have lower incidence rates including African Americans, Hispanics and Asians in the USA, and Maoris in New Zealand. Furthermore, lower incidence rates have been reported in Blacks than in Whites in South Africa. Variation between racial groups seems more likely to reflect true differences in incidence than artefactual differences related to access to quality health-care facilities (Ekbom and Adami, 1992).

A consistent observation in several studies is a higher incidence of Crohn's disease in urban than in rural communities. Again, this does not appear to be explained by better access to health care. In high-risk countries, socioeconomic variables do not appear to have a significant influence on incidence, although there has been a trend towards a higher incidence in individuals of higher educational attainment. Jewish ethnicity has also been associated with higher risk for Crohn's disease, particularly in those individuals born in North America and Western Europe.

Few studies have been large enough to examine changes in the site of Crohn's disease over time, but a study from Stockholm, which covered the period 1955–1989, showed similar proportions of patients with ileal disease, an increase in the proportion with colitis (from 15 to 32 per cent) and a decrease in the proportion with ileo-caecal disease (from 58 to 41 per cent) (Lapidus *et al.*, 1997).

Gender and age

Most studies have shown a higher incidence rate for Crohn's disease in women than in men with a female:male ratio of approximately 1.3:1. In high-risk populations, incidence rates peak between the ages of 20 and 40 years, whereas there is no such peak in low-risk populations. Some studies have shown a second, smaller incidence peak between the ages of 60 and 70 years, perhaps because of a higher proportion of elderly patients with Crohn's colitis. In the Stockholm study (Lapidus *et al.*, 1997), the mean age for diagnosis of Crohn's disease increased from 25 years in 1960–1964 to 32 years in 1985–1989. In children, however, increases in the incidence of Crohn's disease have paralleled that in adults with a threefold increase between the 1960s and 1980s (Logan, 1998).

There is little information on changes over time in the age- and gender-specific incidence rates in Crohn's disease at specific sites, apart from the likelihood of an increase in the incidence of colitis in older women.

Infection

The role of infections as precipitating factors for the onset of disease or the occurrence of relapse remains unclear. There have been no consistent findings for seasonality for onset of disease, clustering of cases among neighbours and friends, or a higher than expected frequency of disease in spouses of affected patients.

However, the existence of birth cohorts with a higher cumulative incidence of Crohn's disease has raised the possibility of the importance of factors operating early in childhood. Such factors are difficult to study but Crohn's disease has been associated with a higher than expected frequency of gastroenteritis during the first 6 months of life and with a higher than expected frequency of various infections early in life (Ekbom *et al.*, 1990). One infection of interest is that of measles and the possibility that Crohn's disease is associated with a persistent measles virus infection in the intestinal microvascular endothelium. However, a recent study showed similar antibody titres to measles virus in peripheral blood in patients with Crohn's disease to those in control subjects (Fisher *et al.*, 1997).

Smoking

One of the most intriguing observations in the epidemiology of inflammatory bowel disease is the association of smoking with Crohn's disease and non-smoking with ulcerative colitis. Risks for Crohn's disease increase twofold in individuals who smoke, with similar risks in heavy and light smokers and an intermediate risk in ex-smokers. This association may be more prominent for ileal and ileo-caecal disease than for colonic disease. Furthermore, smoking appears to have an adverse effect on outcome with more aggressive disease, more frequent relapses and a higher frequency of surgical resection (Timmer *et al.*, 1998).

One possibility is that smoking influences the expression of inflammatory bowel disease (either Crohn's disease or ulcerative colitis) in individuals who are susceptible to the disorder because of genetic or other environmental factors. Whether the effect of smoking is mediated by changes in intestinal permeability, immune function or intestinal blood flow remains unclear.

Drugs

A weak association between oral contraceptive use and Crohn's disease has been found in several studies. In one study, however, the higher risk was confined to patients with Crohn's colitis (Rhodes *et al.*, 1984). In another study, patients taking oral contraceptives were at higher risk for relapse of Crohn's disease and this risk increased in smokers (Timmer *et al.*, 1998).

The possibility that non-steroidal anti-inflammatory drugs increase the risk of Crohn's disease, particularly in the ileum, has not been clarified. One of the difficulties is differentiation of ileal ulceration with haemorrhage (and sometimes perforation) due to non-steroidal anti-inflammatory drugs alone from that due to Crohn's disease.

Diet

Although variation in diet is an attractive explanation for Crohn's disease, few positive associations have been described. A higher than expected intake of refined sugar has been reported in some studies, but this could be secondary to the development of Crohn's disease and has been associated with smoking. The consumption of margarine, fast foods, alcohol and coffee does not appear to influence risk for Crohn's disease (Ekbom and Adami, 1992; Reif *et al.*, 1997). Despite the above, there is some evidence that elemental and exclusion diets are of benefit in Crohn's disease, perhaps because of their effects on intestinal permeability.

Associations with other diseases

Associations between inflammatory bowel disease and autoimmune disorders are stronger for ulcerative colitis than for Crohn's disease. Indeed, a large study by Snook *et al.* (1989) showed a similar frequency of autoimmune disorders in Crohn's disease (1.9 per cent) to that in control subjects (2.0 per cent). Other reports have linked Crohn's disease with Turner syndrome, Hermansky–Pudlak syndrome, multiple sclerosis and pachydermoperiostosis (a rare, hereditary form of hypertrophic osteoarthropathy). In contrast to ulcerative colitis, appendectomy has not been associated with a decreased risk for Crohn's disease (Russel *et al.*, 1997; Sandler, 1998).

GENETIC STUDIES

There is now persuasive data to support the importance of genetic factors in the pathogenesis of Crohn's disease (Satsangi *et al.*, 1997; Cho and Brant, 1998). The first clues came from family studies. Up to 20 per cent of patients with Crohn's disease have an affected family member, often a first-degree relative. For siblings, this increase in risk has been estimated at 30-fold in relation to the general community. A more accurate reflection of risk can be made by adjusting for age. In high-risk communities, such as Ashkenazi Jews in the USA, age-adjusted risks for siblings, parents and offspring were 8.8 per cent, 3.5 per cent and 8.9 per cent, respectively (Roth *et al.*, 1989).

Another useful genetic index is concordance of inflammatory bowel disease in monozygotic and dizygotic twins, particularly when twins have lived apart for many years before the onset of symptoms. Such studies have shown higher concordance rates (i.e. both twins affected) for Crohn's disease than ulcerative colitis, and higher concordance rates for monozygotic twins than dizygotic twins. In Sweden, for example, concordance for Crohn's disease was found in 8 of 18 monozygotic twins but in only 1 of 26 dizygotic twins (Tysk *et al.*, 1988). There is also consistency in the nature of inflammatory bowel disease in monozygotic twins; no pair has been described where one has Crohn's disease and the other ulcerative colitis.

Another issue is concordance in site and type (inflammatory, stricturing or fistulizing) of Crohn's disease in affected family members. Studies in this area have shown concordance rates of about 80 per cent for site, type of disease and extraintestinal manifestations. Such studies, however, do not necessarily support genetic factors, since there may be sharing of environmental factors including concordance for smoking.

The first genes to be examined in inflammatory bowel disease were the HLA genes. Despite several studies in this area, no consistent patterns have been observed, although a recent study showed a strong association between HLA-DRB3*0301 and Crohn's disease (Forcione *et al.*, 1996). In sib-pair studies, there has been no consistent evidence of linkage of inheritance of the disease to HLA-A or HLA-B loci.

Other studies have examined the possibility of associations between Crohn's disease and inherited variation (polymorphism) in genes which might influence other immunological or metabolic characteristics. Again, no consistent associations have been observed, although polymorphisms affecting cytokine genes and their receptors remain of interest (Viney, 1998). Another approach uses DNA from affected and non-affected family members to identify linkages between genetic regions and inflammatory bowel disease. Such studies appear to confirm a link between a genomic region (IBD1) on chromosome 16 and Crohn's disease, and have raised the possibility of linkages with regions on chromosomes 3, 7 and 12 (Cho and Brant, 1998).

The above observations are consistent with the hypothesis that several genes are associated with inflammatory bowel disease; some are common to both

Crohn's disease and ulcerative colitis, while others may be exclusively associated with Crohn's disease. Whether these genes affect various pathways involved in mucosal immunity or aspects of intestinal physiology, such as permeability, have not been clarified.

PATHOGENESIS

Despite a substantial research effort, the pathogenesis of Crohn's disease is still poorly understood. The most persuasive hypothesis is that the disease is due to changes in mucosal immunity with loss of tolerance to components of the faecal stream, perhaps enteric bacteria. This hypothesis is supported by human studies showing induction of inflammation by luminal contents in postoperative patients with segments of excluded ileum (D'Haens *et al.*, 1998). If bacteria are involved, however, responses to antibiotics with effects on anaerobic and other bacteria have been disappointing. An alternative explanation is that the faecal stream effect is related to dietary components including various food additives.

The nature of the abnormal immune response has been difficult to determine by studies on mucosal lymphocytes *in vitro*. More recently, there has been considerable interest in transgenic or 'knockout' rodents, which develop bowel inflammation after suppression or deletion of a gene for cytokines or other immunoregulatory molecules. In many of these models, however, bowel inflammation has resembled ulcerative colitis rather than Crohn's disease. Nevertheless, the models have emphasized the importance of immune regulation in bowel inflammation, and may help to clarify the relative importance of a number of pro-inflammatory and anti-inflammatory cytokines (Fiocchi, 1998). In Crohn's disease, a central role has been proposed for Th1 (helper) lymphocytes and their pro-inflammatory cytokines, interleukin-2 and interferon-γ. One possibility is that Th1 lymphocytes are stimulated to produce cytokines by interleukin-12, a cytokine which is produced by macrophages and is present at higher concentrations in Crohn's tissue than in mucosa from normal subjects or patients with ulcerative colitis (Pallone and Monteleone, 1998).

Another immunological aspect of inflammatory bowel disease is the potential role of autoantibodies in the pathogenesis of bowel inflammation (Shanahan, 1997; Rutgeerts and Vermeire, 1998). Although a variety of autoantibodies have been described, some, such as anticolon antibodies and perinuclear antineutrophil cytoplasmic antibody (pANCA), are more common in ulcerative colitis than in Crohn's disease. In contrast, anti-*Saccharomyces cerevisiae* antibody (ASCA) and antierythrocyte antibody appear to have some specificity for Crohn's disease. However, such autoantibodies seem unlikely to be involved in bowel inflammation, although ASCA may reflect abnormal intestinal permeability, particularly as the autoantibody can be detected in about 20 per cent of healthy relatives of patients with Crohn's disease.

Other cells relevant to inflammatory bowel disease may include non-immune cells, such as epithelial cells, mesenchymal cells, nerve cells and endothelial cells, and their interactions with more typical local immune cells, such as lymphocytes and macrophages. Much of this work has involved epithelial cells and enhanced expression of class II antigens and cytokine receptors in the presence of inflammatory bowel disease. Furthermore, there is some evidence that epithelial cells in patients with inflammatory bowel disease preferentially activate CD4+ helper T cells rather than CD8+ suppressor T cells (MacDermott, 1998).

The potential role of growth factors, eicosanoids, and reactive oxygen and nitrogen metabolites in the pathogenesis of inflammatory bowel disease is still being clarified (Dotan and Rachmilewitz, 1998). Thus far, there is no clear evidence that Crohn's disease is related to a deficiency of protective growth factors, such as transforming growth factor-β or trefoil peptide. Faecal concentrations of eicosanoids appear to be higher in ulcerative colitis than in Crohn's disease but suppression of eicosanoids associated with inflammation (COX-2) does not appear to result in improvement in symptoms. Mucosal concentrations of oxygen and nitrogen metabolites are increased in both Crohn's disease and ulcerative colitis, and are associated with an increase in nitric oxide synthetase activity. However, since nitric oxide can have both protective and toxic effects, the contribution of reactive metabolites to epithelial cell damage remains unclear. On the other hand, several of the drugs that are helpful in inflammatory bowel disease have antiradical activity.

The above observations have led to various hypotheses for the pathogenesis of Crohn's disease. One hypothesis proposes that patients with Crohn's disease have an inherited or acquired defect in the intestinal mucosal barrier, perhaps involving specialized epithelial cells (M cells), which overlie Peyer's patches. This defect in permeability may be aggravated by other factors, such as infections, toxins and the use of non-steroidal anti-inflammatory drugs. In this setting, there is increased access of luminal antigens into the lamina propria, including food antigens and bacterial antigens, such as *n*-formyl-methionyl-leucyl-phenylalanine, peptidoglycan-polysaccharide polymers and lipopolysaccharide. These antigens invoke an inflammatory response, which may be down-regulated and result in resolution of inflammation, or up-regulated with persistent chronic inflammation and scarring. In this model, genetic factors could operate at a number of stages, including immune responses to

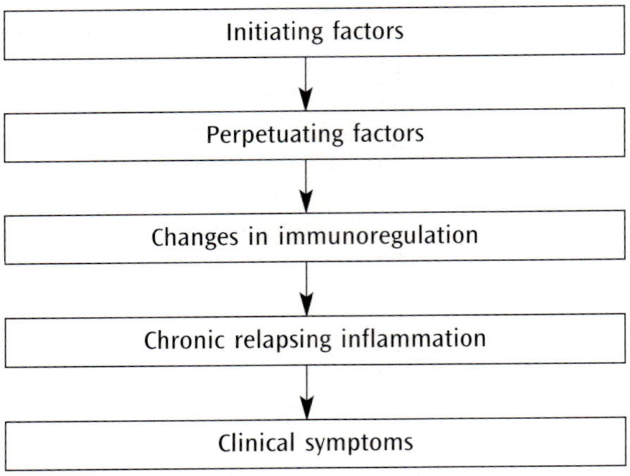

Figure 25.1 *Proposed pathogenesis of Crohn's disease.*

luminal antigens, and, in particular, in the area of suppression or amplification of the inflammatory reaction (Fig. 25.1).

Another hypothesis for the pathogenesis of Crohn's disease is that of a persistent infection of the bowel due to *Mycobacterium* species, viruses, mycoplasma or cell-wall defective bacteria. Indeed, similarities between Crohn's disease and Johne's disease (a mycobacterial infection initially described in cattle) were noted early this century by Dalziel (1913). Despite several positive reports, however, chronic enteritis due to a persistent infection of some type remains unproven. For many organisms, including *Mycobacterium paratuberculosis*, this includes the use of the polymerase chain reaction (PCR) to detect microbial DNA in Crohn's disease tissue (Riggio *et al.*, 1997).

CLINICAL FEATURES

The clinical features of small intestinal Crohn's disease are largely determined by the site, type and severity of bowel inflammation. Most patients (95 per cent) have macroscopic involvement of the distal ileum and, of these, approximately 50 per cent have extension of inflammation into the right colon. Approximately 5 per cent of patients have atypical disease with diffuse jejuno-ileitis or focal lesions in the jejunum, duodenum, stomach or oesophagus.

The major symptoms of Crohn's disease of the small bowel are abdominal pain, diarrhoea, fever and weight loss. Typically, abdominal pain is located in the right iliac fossa or lower abdomen, fluctuates in severity and may be more prominent 1–2 hours after meals. Diarrhoea varies in severity depending on the extent and severity of bowel inflammation, but may not be prominent when inflammation is restricted to short segments of terminal ileum. The identification of blood in stools is uncommon in ileal disease, although many patients have mild iron-deficiency anaemia at presentation. A low-grade fever up to 38.5°C is also a common feature of active disease but higher spiking fevers should raise the possibility of an associated abscess. Weight loss is usually of the order of 10–20 per cent of body weight and is partly dependent on the duration of symptoms. For example, there was a mean interval of 2.3 years between the onset of symptoms and the diagnosis of small bowel Crohn's disease in a large series from the UK (Andrews and Allan, 1990).

Additional clinical features are determined by the nature of the inflammatory process, the development of various local complications and the presence of extraintestinal manifestations. For example, some patients appear to have a form of Crohn's disease that largely involves mucosal inflammation (inflammatory form), while others have inflammation that often results in strictures (fibrostenotic form) or fistula formation (fistulous form). However, these forms are not mutually exclusive, since manifestations may change over time, at least in some patients. In the inflammatory form, the major symptom is that of diarrhoea, often associated with abdominal cramps. Diarrhoea is usually due to bowel inflammation, but may be aggravated by drug therapy, previous bowel resections (short bowel syndrome), enteric fistulas or malabsorption of bile acids or lactose. Small bowel strictures may result in symptoms of a partial or complete small bowel obstruction, and can be caused by localized acute inflammation or a healed lesion with a focal fibrous stricture. In contrast, extension of inflammation through the bowel wall may result in a localized abscess or in a fistula involving adjacent loops of ileum (enteroenteric fistula), ascending colon (enterocolic fistula) or other adjacent structures, such as the bladder (enterovesical fistula). Abscesses and fistulas have been estimated to complicate the course of small bowel Crohn's disease in about 20 per cent and 40 per cent of patients, respectively.

Physical findings vary with the site and severity of disease, and may include local complications and extraintestinal manifestations. Abdominal tenderness, usually in the right lower quadrant, is common in Crohn's ileitis and may be accompanied by fullness in the region or a definite mass. The latter is usually due to adherent loops of small bowel but can also reflect a coexisting abscess. Anal examination may reveal features of perianal disease, including skin tags, fissures and fistulas.

The extraintestinal manifestations of Crohn's disease are listed in Table 25.1. These appear to be more frequent when Crohn's disease involves the large bowel than when Crohn's disease is restricted to the small bowel (O'Brien, 1992). Some manifestations, such as those involving the skin, eyes, joints and mouth, are

Table 25.1 *Extraintestinal manifestations of Crohn's disease*

Joints	Monoarthritis, oligoarthritis, ankylosing spondylitis
Skin	Erythema nodosum, pyoderma gangrenosum
Mouth	Aphthous ulcers, stomatitis
Eyes	Uveitis, episcleritis
Renal tract	Oxalate stones, hydronephrosis
Liver–bile duct	Sclerosing cholangitis, pericholangitis, steatosis, gallstones
Miscellaneous	Amyloidosis, venous thrombosis

associated with active bowel inflammation and respond to medical or surgical management directed at the underlying bowel disease. Other manifestations, such as sclerosing cholangitis, ankylosing spondylitis and uveitis, are associated with Crohn's disease but pursue a course that is unrelated to the severity of bowel inflammation. A third group of extraintestinal manifestations is secondary to small bowel disease with malabsorption, and includes renal stones, metabolic bone disease and gallstones.

Although the frequency of extraintestinal manifestations in Crohn's disease has been debated, common manifestations include peripheral arthritis (10 per cent), erythema nodosum (10 per cent), aphthous ulcers (10 per cent), renal stones (5 per cent), ureteric obstruction with hydronephrosis (5 per cent) and episcleritis (4 per cent). Erythema nodosum is more frequent in children than in adults and appears to be more common in females than in males. Axial arthropathies including sacro-ileitis and ankylosing spondylitis can be detected by plain x-ray in up to 20 per cent of patients with Crohn's disease, but only about one-third have clinical symptoms, such as backache or morning stiffness.

The pathogenesis of many extraintestinal manifestations remains unclear. Those manifestations associated with active bowel inflammation are thought to be due to the presence of immune complexes in serum with specificity for extraintestinal tissues. Renal stones in patients with Crohn's disease of the small bowel are largely composed of calcium oxalate. This reflects binding of calcium to fatty acids rather than oxalate in the lumen of the small bowel, which then permits the absorption of free oxalate in the colon. Other factors may also be relevant, including dehydration, bed rest and steroid administration. Ureteric obstruction is usually due to involvement of the ureter in an inflammatory mass in the retroperitoneal space, while gallstones may form because of a relative deficiency of bile acids, sometimes aggravated by the effects of parenteral nutrition. Thromboembolic events may be secondary to bed rest or to effects on various coagulation factors, including fibrinogen, factor V, factor VIII, antithrombin III and platelets.

INVESTIGATIONS

The diagnosis of Crohn's disease of the small bowel can be supported by a variety of investigations, including blood tests, small bowel radiology, small bowel endoscopy and histopathology. Supplementary investigations can also include computed tomography (CT) and labelled leucocyte scans.

Blood tests

Results from various blood tests are helpful markers of small bowel inflammation. For example, ileitis is often associated with mild anaemia due to chronic disease or blood loss, and is occasionally associated with deficiencies of folic acid or vitamin B_{12}. A modest leucocytosis may be due to active disease or steroid therapy, but a marked leucocytosis should raise the possibility of a coexisting abscess. Other non-specific markers of active inflammation include an elevated erythrocyte sedimentation rate (ESR) and C-reactive protein, an elevated platelet count and a low plasma albumin. Abnormal liver enzymes can be due to a fatty liver (steatosis), pericholangitis or sclerosing cholangitis. Anti-*Saccharomyces cerevisiae* antibody tests are not readily available at present, but appear to have reasonable sensitivity and specificity for Crohn's disease, particularly in children. In adults, about 60–70 per cent of patients with Crohn's disease have positive tests compared to 10–15 per cent of patients with ulcerative colitis and 0–5 per cent of control subjects (Rutgeerts and Vermeire, 1998).

Small bowel imaging

Barium studies of the small bowel are the most common method for diagnosing small bowel involvement by Crohn's disease. This can be achieved by small bowel follow-through, small bowel enteroclysis or barium enema with reflux into the terminal ileum. Although small bowel enteroclysis has been promoted as being superior to follow-through, a comparative study showed that follow-through was preferred by patients, and gave similar or superior results to enteroclysis (Bernstein *et al.*, 1997).

A variety of radiological abnormalities have been described, which reflect oedema, ulceration, fistulas, strictures and pseudopolyps. Signs of oedema include changes in valvulae conniventes with straightening, blunting, distortion and nodule formation. Oedema of the deep layers of the bowel wall can lead to wall thickening and to separation of barium-filled bowel loops. Superficial (aphthoid) ulcers appear as a speck of barium surrounded by mucosal oedema, while deep penetrating ulcers often have a spike or 'rosethorn' appearance,

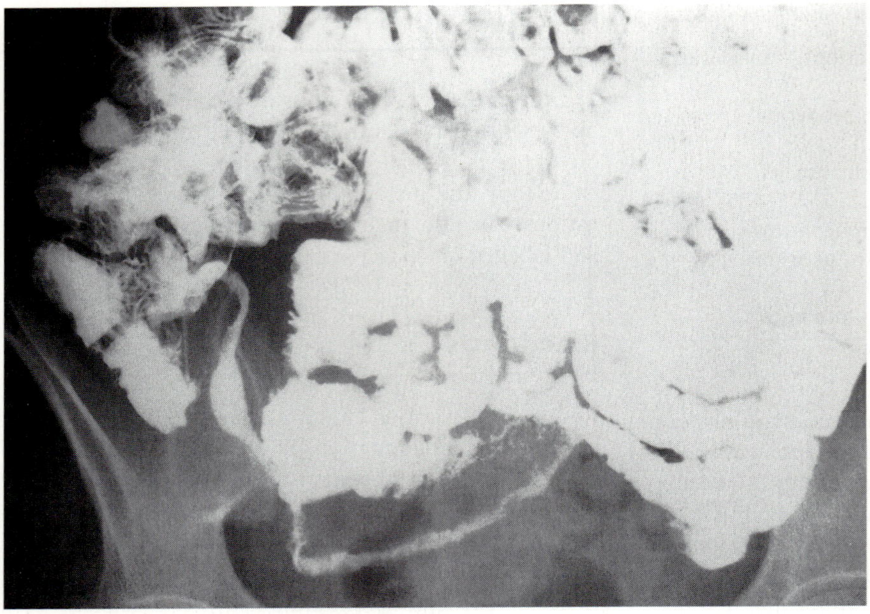

Figure 25.2 *A barium follow-through x-ray of Crohn's ileitis showing a long segment of terminal ileum, which is narrow, irregular and separated from other ileal loops.*

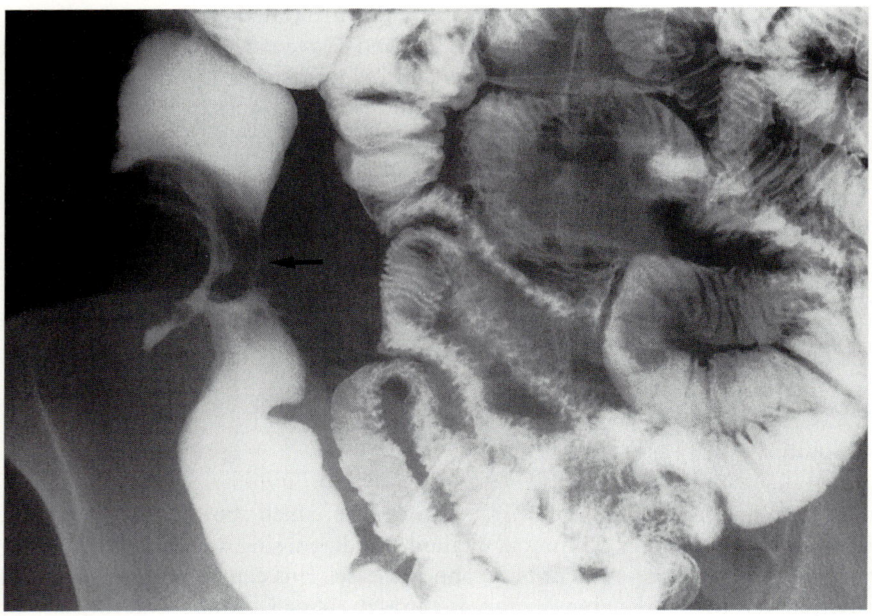

Figure 25.3 *A barium follow-through x-ray of Crohn's ileitis showing a deep ulcer in the terminal ileum, a fistula between the terminal ileum and caecum (arrow), and mild dilatation of the ileum proximal to the diseased segment.*

sometimes associated with 'collar stud' lesions due to undermining of the mucosa. Other appearances include large deep ulcers and extensive denuded areas, often both linear and transverse, leading to a cobblestone appearance. Narrow regions can reflect oedema, fibrosis or spasm (Fig. 25.2). The presence of spasm can sometimes be inferred by a reduction in narrowing after use of smooth muscle relaxants, such as glucagon. As fibrosis is often asymmetrical and predominantly involves the mesenteric border, a degree of shortening of the bowel may occur, sometimes with pseudosacculation. Most fistulas arise from the terminal ileum, and involve adjacent loops of small bowel or the ascending colon (Fig. 25.3). Large fistulas can usually be demonstrated by a barium study but this may not apply to small fistulas, such as enterovesical fistulas.

Computed tomography has a particular role in the demonstration of abdominal and psoas abscesses, which may complicate the course of Crohn's disease (Fig. 25.4). The investigation may also reveal thickening of the bowel wall, adherent loops of small bowel and helpful information on complications such as fistulas. Leucocyte scans can be used to detect ileitis, particularly in the setting of known Crohn's disease, where persisting symptoms might be due to active inflammation or to a coexisting irritable bowel syndrome. Such scans, however, appear to be more sensitive and specific for colitis than for small bowel disease.

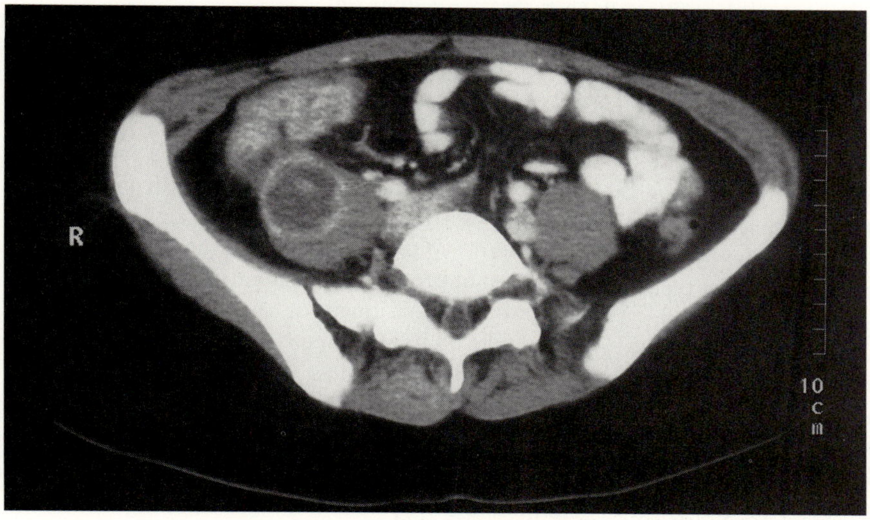

Figure 25.4 *Computed tomography scan of the lower abdomen showing an abnormality in the right psoas muscle due to an abscess associated with Crohn's ileitis.*

Small bowel endoscopy

Experienced endoscopists can visualize the terminal ileum in the majority of patients, while, in unusual settings, helpful information may be obtained by upper gastrointestinal endoscopy or enteroscopy. The endoscopic features of small bowel Crohn's disease have been described previously (Chapter 13.1), but include patchy inflammation, aphthous ulcers, longitudinal ulcers, a cobblestone appearance and small bowel strictures. An advantage of endoscopy is the ability to take mucosal biopsies for histological evaluation.

Histopathology

Specimens for histological evaluation can be obtained by small bowel endoscopy or by operative resection. The macroscopic appearance of a typical operative specimen resembles a 'garden hose' with thickening and oedema of the bowel wall, often associated with mucosal ulceration and a variable degree of stenosis (Plate 25.1). The mesentery is often thick, fatty and oedematous while adjacent lymph nodes are enlarged and firm, and may form an irregular mass. Additional features may include fistulas and abscesses.

Microscopic findings are influenced, in part, by the nature of the tissue specimen (endoscopic or operative) but always include a chronic inflammatory infiltrate. This is often associated with ulceration, oedema, lymphoid hyperplasia, microabscesses and crypt abscesses. In addition, operative specimens may reveal sinuses, fistulas and hyperplasia of the muscularis mucosa. Granulomas can be identified in about 60 per cent of operative specimens but in only about 10 per cent of endoscopic specimens. The presence of granulomas is helpful for the diagnosis of Crohn's disease but is not specific for Crohn's disease, since similar lesions may occur in tuberculosis, yersiniosis and fungal infections. Histological features of arteritis can also be found in about 10 per cent of operative specimens (Thompson, 1990).

Activity indices

The severity of disease is assessed intuitively by most physicians on the basis of symptoms, signs and results from laboratory tests. However, a quantitative scale is sometimes helpful, particularly in the setting of a controlled trial of a therapeutic intervention. One such scale is the Crohn's Disease Activity Index (Best *et al.*, 1976), a relatively complex scale which assesses a variety of features for up to 1 week. Simpler scales more suited to clinical practice have been proposed by Van Hees *et al.* (1980), Harvey and Bradshaw (1980) and the 'Oxford Index' outlined by Myren *et al.* (1984). These simpler indices correlate fairly well with the Crohn's Disease Activity Index apart from that proposed by Van Hees *et al.* (1980).

Differential diagnosis

In many patients, Crohn's disease of the small bowel is one of a number of possible diagnoses. When the duration of symptoms is relatively short, diagnoses which may need to be considered include acute appendicitis, acute diverticulitis, infection with *Yersinia enterocolitica* and various gynaecological disorders, including pelvic inflammatory disease, ectopic pregnancy and complications of ovarian cysts. When symptoms are of longer duration, the differential diagnosis may include coeliac disease, ileo-caecal tuberculosis, eosinophilic gastroenteritis, radiation enteritis and various tumours including caecal cancer, carcinoid tumours and ileo-caecal lymphoma.

MANAGEMENT

Therapy for Crohn's disease is directed at reducing bowel inflammation and providing symptomatic relief. Approaches in individual patients will be determined by the site, severity and duration of the disease process, as well as the presence of various gastrointestinal complications and extraintestinal manifestations. There may also be variations in approach in response to the type of disease, with corticosteroids and 5–aminosalicylic acid (5-ASA) preparations for the inflammatory type, immunomodulating drugs for the fistulous type and earlier surgery for the fibrostenotic type. Another consideration is the mode of action of individual drugs. For example, sulphasalazine is unlikely to be helpful for Crohn's disease of the small bowel as the active component, 5-ASA, is largely released in the colon owing to the action of bacterial azoreductases. In contrast, drugs such as budesonide, which are released in the distal small bowel, may be more effective in ileitis than in colitis.

5-ASA products

There is only a limited role for 5-ASA preparations in the treatment of acute Crohn's disease of the small bowel. Sulphasalazine seems unlikely to be helpful on theoretical grounds and was ineffective in the National Cooperative Crohn's Disease Study (Summers *et al.*, 1979). This led to the development of a variety of different 5-ASA formulations designed to increase drug concentrations in the terminal ileum by the use of capsules that disintegrate slowly or in response to changes in luminal pH. Thus far, however, the role of these drugs in the treatment of active small bowel inflammation remains unclear. In one study, which compared mesalazine (mesalamine) and budesonide in active Crohn's disease involving the ileum or ascending colon, mesalazine at a dose of 4 g/day was less effective than budesonide, 9 mg/day, at inducing remission (Thomsen *et al.*, 1998).

For maintenance of remission, mesalazine has been superior to placebo in some but not all studies. One relatively large study from Canada (Sutherland *et al.*, 1997) showed a trend in favour of treatment with mesalazine (3 g/day) rather than placebo, but differences reached statistical significance only in ileo-caecal disease and in women. However, a meta-analysis of 15 controlled trials showed a reduction in the probability of relapse with mesalazine, particularly in patients with ileal disease, recent bowel surgery and disease of prolonged duration (Camma *et al.*, 1997). Despite these studies, the use of delayed-release preparations of 5-ASA for maintenance of remission does not appear to have been widely adopted.

Corticosteroids

Corticosteroids used orally or intravenously are of established benefit for the treatment of acute inflammation, particularly if it is judged to be moderate or severe. A typical regimen will begin with moderate to high doses (e.g. prednisolone or prednisone, 40–60 mg/day), followed by tapering of the dose as symptoms improve. In most patients, corticosteroids will need to be continued for several weeks. Remissions can be induced in 80–90 per cent of patients, but some patients relapse as the dose is tapered or after the drug has been ceased. Avoidance of long-term therapy with corticosteroids is desirable but a minority of patients appear to be steroid-dependent and are at higher risk for a variety of adverse events, particularly adrenal suppression and osteoporosis.

These adverse events have led to the development of new products, which deliver corticosteroids to the inflamed bowel but minimize systemic concentrations of active drugs. One such product is budesonide. It is formulated to be released into the terminal ileum and, after absorption, is largely (90 per cent) converted by the liver into metabolites with low corticosteroid activity. In Crohn's disease of mild to moderate activity, budesonide at a dose of 9 mg/day was as effective as prednisolone, 40 mg/day (Campieri *et al.*, 1997), or prednisone at a tapering dose (Bar-Meir *et al.*, 1998). The efficacy of budesonide for maintenance of remission has not been clarified, although results in one study were disappointing (Gross *et al.*, 1998).

Immunomodulating drugs

Immunomodulating drugs are widely used in the management of patients with difficult Crohn's disease. This includes patients who respond poorly to 5-ASA compounds or corticosteroids, patients with steroid-dependent or relapsing disease, and patients with fistulas. The most commonly used drugs are azathioprine and its active metabolite, 6-mercaptopurine (Pearson *et al.*, 1995). These drugs are of limited benefit for active disease since improvement in symptoms may only occur after 3–6 months of continuous therapy. However, a number of longer term studies support their use for chronic active disease and maintenance of remission. One of these studies specifically addressed ileal recurrence after previous surgery (D'Haens *et al.*, 1997). Azathioprine is usually given at a dose of 2 mg/kg per day while 6-mercaptopurine is given at a dose of 1–2 mg/kg per day. Side-effects are uncommon, but include leucopaenia, pancreatitis, hepatitis and rashes. There is no evidence that use of these drugs during pregnancy increases the rate of birth defects.

Other immunomodulating drugs include cyclosporin A and methotrexate. Cyclosporin A given intravenously may be helpful for acute inflammation associated with fistulas but longer term therapy with oral medication has been ineffective (Feagan *et al.*, 1994). Methotrexate can be given as a weekly dose either orally or intramuscularly. Intramuscular methotrexate (25 mg) has been associated with improvement in symptoms and steroid-sparing effects but withdrawal of the drug is often associated with relapse. The longer term use of oral medication appears to be less effective for active disease and is of doubtful benefit for maintenance of remission. Furthermore, a variety of adverse events have been described, including leucopaenia, nausea, vomiting, hepatotoxicity and pneumonitis (Feagan *et al.*, 1995).

Newer therapeutic developments have targeted a number of pro-inflammatory cytokines that are thought to be involved in the pathogenesis of Crohn's disease. One promising form of therapy is a monoclonal antibody to the pro-inflammatory cytokine, tumour necrosis factor-α (TNF-α). Single intravenous injections of monoclonal antibody have been associated with improvement in symptoms, an effect which often lasts for 3–6 months (Targan *et al.*, 1997). Furthermore, monoclonal antibody to TNF-α may have a particular role in the management of fistulas, one of the most difficult complications of the disease. Other therapeutic strategies are also being examined, which could impair the effects of pro-inflammatory cytokines or promote the effects of anti-inflammatory cytokines. Monoclonal antibodies have also been developed against cell adhesion molecules, such as intercellular adhesion molecule 1 (ICAM-1), which has enhanced expression in inflammatory processes (Yacyshyn *et al.*, 1998).

Antibiotics

The possibility that Crohn's disease is due to loss of tolerance to luminal bacteria has led to renewed interest in the longer term use of antibiotics (Peppercorn, 1993). Metronidazole is helpful for anorectal sepsis and is of similar efficacy to sulphasalazine for colitis, but appears to be ineffective for treating active inflammation in the small bowel. There is no data on the role of metronidazole for maintenance of remission in ileal disease. Metronidazole is usually given at a dose of 10–20 mg/kg per day, a dose which has a number of adverse events including nausea, a metallic taste and peripheral neuropathy. The role of other antibiotics, such as ciprofloxacin, also remains unclear, particularly in small bowel disease. Furthermore, trials of antituberculous drugs have failed to support the proposed link between Crohn's disease and *Mycobacterium* species (Thomas *et al.*, 1998).

Nutritional therapy

The concept that Crohn's disease was due to an exaggerated immune response to dietary antigens led to a variety of trials of parental and enteral nutrition. These studies showed that parental nutrition and bowel rest did not provide a therapeutic advantage over the administration of nutritional support by an enteral route (Greenberg *et al.*, 1988). However, parental nutrition may be indicated in particular circumstances, such as bowel obstruction and various postoperative problems.

Enteral nutrition can involve various formula diets (amino-acid based, peptide based or polymer based), which may be used for total dietary intake or as a supplement to the diet. Although the place of nutritional supplements in the treatment of active disease is debated, one study showed that aggressive enteral nutrition was of similar efficacy to oral corticosteroids (O'Morain *et al.*, 1984). The role of nutritional supplements in the maintenance of remission remains unclear but various preparations have been helpful when Crohn's disease in children is complicated by growth retardation. These supplements are sometimes given overnight through nasogastric feeding tubes.

Nutritional problems in Crohn's disease are common and include weight loss, growth retardation and a low plasma albumin, as well as various micronutrient deficiencies involving iron, folate, magnesium, zinc and various other vitamins. These can be corrected, at least in part, by enteral supplements with some improvement in disease activity (Harries *et al.*, 1983). Dietary modification may also be appropriate in some patients, including diets low in fat, fibre, lactose and oxalate.

NATURAL HISTORY

Most patients with Crohn's disease of the small bowel have episodes of ileal inflammation, often associated with complications, such as obstruction, fistula or abscess formation. Indeed, one study showed that 80 per cent of patients required surgical treatment at some stage during the course of their disease after a mean follow-up period of 18.8 years (Andrews and Allan, 1990). Recurrence rates after surgery increase in a linear fashion over time, with rates of 50–80 per cent after 15 years. Patients who have a short interval between the onset of symptoms and first resection are more likely to have an early recurrence and further surgery, presumably because they have more aggressive disease. Recurrence rates do not appear to be influenced by age of onset of disease. The site of recurrent disease after surgery is usually in the region of the anastomosis or just proximal to the anastomosis (Higgens and Allan, 1980).

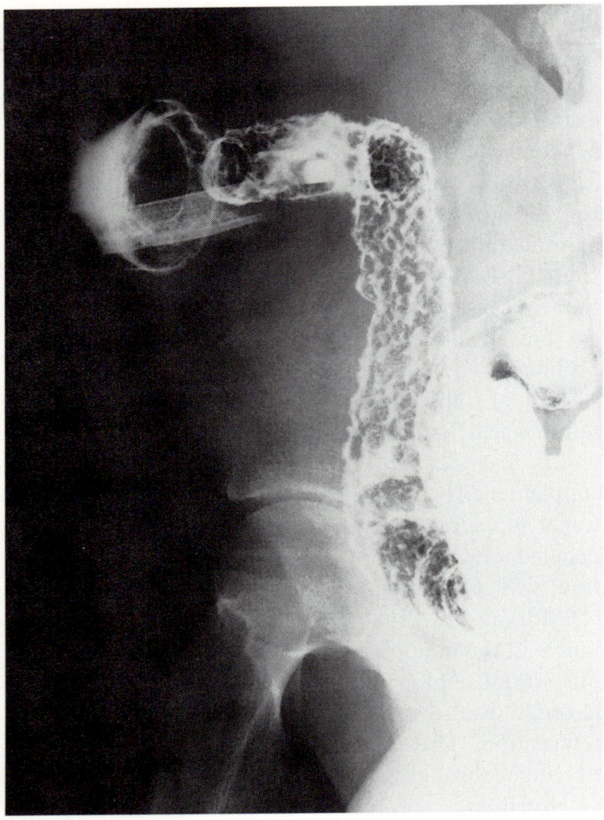

Figure 25.5 *A barium follow-through x-ray showing a previous iliostomy and recurrent ileitis with 'rosethorn' ulcers and linear and transverse ulcers creating a 'cobblestone' appearance.*

Recurrent disease in the small bowel is readily identified in most patients on the basis of recurrent symptoms and the development of new radiological and/or endoscopic abnormalities (Fig. 25.5). In a minority of patients, however, recurrent symptoms can be due to a coexisting irritable bowel syndrome or to variable symptoms largely due to previous surgery including a short bowel syndrome. The latter is associated with important nutritional and metabolic issues but occurs in only about 10 per cent of patients followed for more than 20 years (Cooke *et al.*, 1980).

The natural history described above largely reflects the role of surgery for management of complications. The influence of medical therapy on recurrence rates and surgical rates in the longer term still remains unclear, although 5-ASA preparations and some immunomodulating drugs appear to be helpful over 1–2 years.

MANAGEMENT OF COMPLICATIONS

The management of small bowel obstruction, fistula formation and abscess formation will be discussed briefly as these complications are common in small bowel disease. Other complications, which largely apply to colonic disease, include toxic dilatation, perforation and massive haemorrhage. Anorectal manifestations, such as fissures and fistulas, may coexist with small bowel disease but their management is outside of the scope of this report.

Small bowel obstruction

Small bowel obstruction may be due to acute inflammation associated with relapse or to established fibrosis. The former may respond to intravenous fluids, nasogastric suction and medical treatment, but the latter will require treatment by surgery. At laparotomy, the obstruction can be relieved by resection of a diseased segment or by a strictureplasty, where the stricture is divided longitudinally and then sutured transversely. The latter minimizes the loss of small bowel and does not appear to be associated with a higher incidence of recurrent obstruction. Procedures designed to bypass loops of small bowel are largely avoided as ongoing inflammation may result in fistulas and abscesses. There is also little support for major small bowel resections where frozen sections are used in an endeavour to clear all small bowel tissue that is histologically abnormal.

Fistulas

Barium studies may show fistulas between loops of small bowel, or between the small bowel and the right colon. Some of these fistulas are asymptomatic and, in this setting, specific treatment is often unnecessary. However, treatment will be required for symptomatic enteroenteric fistulas or fistulas that are enterovesical, enterovaginal or enterocutaneous. Some symptomatic fistulas can be managed medically, usually with a combination of antibiotics, immunomodulating drugs and drugs that reduce the volume of intestinal secretions, such as the somatostatin analogue, octreotide. This can be effective in up to 50 per cent of patients. Others require a surgical resection, particularly if the fistula is associated with a stricture or abscess. Enterovesical fistulas are normally treated by surgery because of the risk of recurrent urinary tract infections. After surgery, total parental nutrition with bowel rest may promote healing and may decrease the risk of fistula recurrence and postoperative complications.

Abscesses

The presence of an abscess is usually an indication for drainage, either percutaneously or operatively. Percutaneous drainage may be appropriate in patients who are seriously ill but the majority of patients eventually require a small bowel resection. In addition, some abscesses are multiloculated and are difficult to drain by percutaneous methods.

RISK OF CANCER

Patients with Crohn's disease have been reported to be at higher risk for a variety of cancers localized to the gastrointestinal tract (small intestine, colorectal and pancreas) as well as extraintestinal cancers, such as skin cancers and lymphomas. In a cohort study from Sweden, however, the overall risk of cancer in Crohn's disease was only marginally higher than that observed in the general population. This was largely due to an increased incidence of cancer of the small bowel and bladder (Persson *et al.*, 1994). In another large study of Crohn's disease of the small bowel from the UK, however, there were no cases of ileal cancer, perhaps because of an aggressive surgical policy as well as avoidance of small bowel bypass (Andrews and Allan, 1990).

PROGNOSIS

For many patients, Crohn's disease requires long-term drug therapy and ongoing medical supervision. Although this is sometimes associated with impaired quality of life, death from Crohn's disease is uncommon. Overall mortality increases about twofold in relation to the general population. For example, in longer term follow-up studies by Farmer *et al.* (1985) and Andrews and Allan (1990), death was directly attributed to Crohn's disease in 6 per cent and 7 per cent of patients, respectively. In another study, mortality rates were high in the first 3 years after diagnosis but were subsequently similar to those observed in the general population (Mayberry *et al.*, 1980). The most common causes of death were sepsis, malnutrition, amyloidosis and hypertension induced by corticosteroids.

In relation to quality of life, some patients with Crohn's disease have longer term symptoms with effects on employment, lifestyle and family dynamics. Furthermore, there is a financial burden for medical and surgical care, which impacts both on the family and the health-care system. These annual costs were estimated at $1.0–1.2 billion in the USA in 1990 with an annual cost per patient of $6600 (Hay and Hay, 1992). Whether these costs can be reduced by basic or applied research remains unclear. The hope is for an innovative solution similar to *Helicobacter pylori* and peptic ulceration, but a more likely outcome is a gradual improvement in medical therapy resulting from new products and well-designed clinical trials.

REFERENCES

Andrews, H.A., Allan, R.N. 1990: Crohn's disease of the small intestine. In Allan R.N., Keighley M.R.B., Alexander-Williams J., Hawkins C. (eds) *Inflammatory bowel diseases*, 2nd edn. Edinburgh: Churchill Livingstone, 329–38.

Bar-Meir, S., Chowers, Y., Lavy, A. *et al.* and the Israeli Budesonide Study Group 1998: Budesonide versus prednisone in the treatment of active Crohn's disease. *Gastroenterology* 115, 835–40.

Bernstein, C.N., Boult, I.F., Greenberg, H.M., Van Der Putten, W., Duffy, G., Grahame, G.R. 1997: A prospective randomized comparision between small bowel enteroclysis and small bowel follow-through in Crohn's disease. *Gastroenterology* 113, 390–8.

Best, W.R., Becktel, J.M., Singleton, J.W., Kern, F. 1976: Development of a Crohn's disease activity index. *Gastroenterology* 70, 439–44.

Camma, C., Giunta, M., Rosselli, M., Cottone, M. 1997: Mesalamine in the maintenance treatment of Crohn's disease: a meta-analysis adjusted for confounding variables. *Gastroenterology* 113, 1465–73.

Campieri, M., Ferguson, A., Doe, W., Persson, T., Nilsson, L.-G. and the Global Budesonide Study Group 1997: Oral budesonide is as effective as oral prednisolone in active Crohn's disease. *Gut* 41, 209–14.

Cho, J.H., Brant, S.R. 1998: Genetics and genetic markers in inflammatory bowel disease. *Current Opinion in Gastroenterology* 14, 283–8.

Cooke, W.T., Mallas, E., Prior, R., Allan, R.N. 1980: Crohn's disease; course, treatment, and long-term prognosis. *Quarterly Journal of Medicine* 49, 363–84.

Crohn, B.B., Ginzburg, L., Oppenheimer, G.D. 1932: Regional ileitis: a pathologic and clinical entity. *JAMA* 99, 1323–9.

Dalziel, T.K. 1913: Chronic interstitial enteritis. *British Medical Journal* 2, 1068–70.

D'Haens, G., Geboes, K., Ponette, E., Penninckx, F., Rutgeerts, P. 1997: Healing of severe recurrent ileitis with azathioprine therapy in patients with Crohn's disease. *Gastroenterology* 112, 1475–81.

D'Haens, G.R., Geboes, K., Peeters, M., Baert, F., Penninckx, F., Rutgeerts, P. 1998: Early lesions of recurrent Crohn's disease caused by infusion of intestinal contents in excluded ileum. *Gastroenterology* 114, 262–7.

Dotan, I., Rachmilewitz, D. 1998: Inflammatory mediators in inflammatory bowel disease. *Current Opinion in Gastroenterology* 14, 295–9.

Ekbom, A., Adami, H.-O. 1992: The epidemiology of inflammatory bowel disease. In MacDermott, R.P., Stenson, W.F. (eds) *Inflammatory bowel disease*. New York: Elsevier, 1–15.

Ekbom, A., Adami, H.O., Helmick, C.G., Jonzon, A., Zack, M.M. 1990: Perinatal risk factors for inflammatory bowel disease: a case-control study. *American Journal of Epidemiology* 132, 1111–19.

Farmer, R.G., Whelan, G., Fazio, V.W., 1985: Long-term follow-up of patients with Crohn's disease. Relationship of the clinical pattern and diagnosis. *Gastroenterology* 88, 1818–25.

Feagan, B.G., McDonald, J.W.D., Rochon, J. *et al.* for the Canadian Crohn's Relapse Prevention Trial Investigators 1994: Low-dose cyclosporine for the treatment of Crohn's disease. *New England Journal of Medicine* 330, 1846–51.

Feagan, B.G., Rochon, J., Fedorak, R.N. *et al.* for the North American Crohn's Study Group Investigators 1995: Methotrexate for the treatment of Crohn's disease. *New England Journal of Medicine* 332, 292–7.

Fiocchi, C. 1998: Inflammatory bowel disease: etiology and pathogenesis. *Gastroenterology*, 115, 182–205.

Fisher, N.C., Yee, L., Nightingale, P., McEwan, R., Gibson, J.A. 1997: Measles virus serology in Crohn's disease. *Gut* 41, 66–9.

Forcione, D.G., Sands, B., Isselbacher, K.J., Rustgi, A., Podolsky, D.K., Pillai, S. 1996: An increased risk of Crohn's disease in individuals who inherit the HLA class 11 DRB3*0301 allele. *Proceedings of the National Academy of Sciences USA* 93, 5094–8.

Greenberg, G.R., Fleming, C.R., Jeejeebhoy, K.N., Rosenberg, I.H., Sales, D., Tremaine, W.J. 1988: Controlled trial of bowel rest and nutritional support in the management of Crohn's disease. *Gut* 29, 1309–15.

Gross, V., Andus, T., Ecker, K.W. *et al.* and the Budesonide Study Group 1998: Low dose oral pH modified release budesonide for maintenance of steroid induced remission in Crohn's disease. *Gut* 42, 493–6.

Harries, A.D., Jones, L.A., Danis, V., Fifield, R., Heatley, R.V., Newcombe, R.G., Rhodes, J. 1983: Controlled trial of supplemented oral nutrition in Crohn's disease. *Lancet* 1, 887–90.

Harvey, R.F., Bradshaw, J.M. 1980. A simple index of Crohn's disease activity. *Lancet* 1, 514–15.

Hay, A.R., Hay, J.W. 1992: Inflammatory bowel disease: medical cost algorithms. *Journal of Clinical Gastroenterology* 14, 318–27.

Higgens, C.S., Allan, R.N. 1980: Crohn's disease of the distal ileum. *Gut* 21, 933–40.

Lapidus, A., Bernell, O., Hellers, G., Persson, P.-G., Löfberg, R. 1997: Incidence of Crohn's disease in Stockholm county 1955–1989. *Gut* 41, 480–6.

Lockhart-Mummery, H.E., Morson, B.C. 1960: Crohn's disease (regional enteritis) of the large intestine and its distinction from ulcerative colitis. *Gut* 1, 87–105.

Logan, R.F.A 1998: Inflammatory bowel disease incidence: up, down, or unchanged? *Gut* 42, 309–11.

MacDermott, R.P., 1998: Immunology of inflammatory bowel disease. *Current Opinion in Gastroenterology* 14, 289–94.

Mayberry, J.F., Newcombe, R.G., Rhodes, J. 1980: Mortality in Crohn's disease. *Quarterly Journal of Medicine* 49, 63–8.

Myren, J., Bouchier, I.A.D., Watkinson, G., Softley, A., Clamp, S.E., de Dombal, F.T. 1984. The OMGE Multinational Inflammatory Bowel Disease Survey 1976–1982. A further report on 2657 cases. *Scandanavian Journal of Gastroenterology* 19(Suppl 95), 1–27.

O'Brien, J. 1992: Extraintestinal manifestations of inflammatory bowel disease. In MacDermott R.P., Stenson W.F. (eds) *Inflammatory bowel disease*. New York: Elsevier, 387–403.

O'Morain, C., Segal, A.W., Levi, A.J. 1984: Elemental diet as primary treatment of acute Crohn's disease: a controlled trial. *British Medical Journal* 288, 1859–62.

Pallone, F., Monteleone, G. 1998: Interleukin 12 and Th1 responses in inflammatory bowel disease. *Gut* 43, 735–6.

Pearson, D.C., May, G.R., Fick, G.H., Sutherland, L.R. 1995: Azathioprine and 6-mercaptopurine in Crohn's disease: a meta-analysis. *Annals of Internal Medicine* 123, 132–42.

Peppercorn, M.A. 1993: Is there a role for antibiotics as primary therapy in Crohn's ileitis? *Journal of Clinical Gastroenterology* 17, 235–7.

Persson, P.G., Karlen, P., Bernell, O., Leijonmarck, C.E., Brostrom, O., Ahlbom, A., Hellers, G. 1994: Crohn's disease and cancer: a population-based cohort study. *Gastroenterology* 107, 1675–9.

Reif, S., Klein, I., Lubin, F., Farbstein, M., Hallak, A., Gilat, T. 1997: Pre-illness dietary factors in inflammatory bowel disease. *Gut* 40, 754–60.

Rhodes, J.M., Cockel, R., Allan, R.N., Hawker, P.C., Dawson, J., Elias, E. 1984: Colonic Crohn's disease and use of oral contraception. *British Medical Journal* 288, 595–6.

Riggio, M.P., Gibson, J., Lennon, A., Wray, D., MacDonald, D.G. 1997: Search for *Mycobacterium paratuberculosis* DNA in orofacial granulomatosis and oral Crohn's disease tissue by polymerase chain reaction. *Gut* 41, 646–50.

Rose, J.D.R., Roberts, G.M., Williams, G., Mayberry, J.F., Rhodes, J. 1988: Cardiff Crohn's disease jubilee: the incidence over 50 years. *Gut* 29, 346–51.

Roth, M.-P., Peterson, G.M., McElree, C., Vadheim, C.M., Panish, J.F., Rotter, J.I. 1989: Familial empiric risk estimates of inflammatory bowel disease in Ashkenasi Jews. *Gastroenterology* 96, 1016–20.

Russel, M.G., Dorant, E., Brummer, R.-J.M. *et al.* and the South Limburg Inflammatory Bowel Disease Study Group 1997: Appendectomy and the risk of developing ulcerative colitis or Crohn's disease: results of a large case-control study. *Gastroenterology* 113, 377–82.

Rutgeerts, P., Vermeire, S. 1998: Clinical value of the detection of antibodies in the serum for diagnosis and treatment of inflammatory bowel disease. *Gastroenterology* 115, 1006–22.

Sandler, R.S. 1998: Appendicectomy and ulcerative colitis. *Lancet* 352, 1797–8.

Satsangi, J., Jewell, D.P., Bell, J.I. 1997: The genetics of inflammatory bowel disease. *Gut* 40, 572–4.

Sedlack, R.E., Whisnant, J., Elveback, L.R., Kurland, L.T. 1980: Incidence of Crohn's disease in Olmsted county, Minnesota, 1935–1975. *American Journal of Epidemiology* 112, 759–63.

Shanahan, F. 1997: Antibody 'markers' in Crohn's disease: opportunity or overstatement? *Gut* 40, 557–8.

Snook, J.A., De Silva, H.J., Jewell, D.P. 1989: The association of autoimmune disorders with inflammatory bowel disease. *Quarterly Journal of Medicine* 72, 835–40.

Summers, R.W., Switz, D.M., Sessions, J.T., Jr, Becktel, J.M., Best, W.R., Kern, F., Jr, Singleton, J.W. 1979: National Cooperative Crohn's Disease Study: results of drug treatment. *Gastroenterology* 77, 847–69.

Sutherland, L.R., Martin, F., Bailey, R.J. *et al.* and The Canadian Mesalamine for Remission of Crohn's Disease Study Group 1997: A randomized, placebo-controlled, double-blind trial of mesalamine in the maintenance of remission of Crohn's disease. *Gastroenterology* 112, 1069–77.

Targan, S.R., Hanauer, S.B., van Deventer, S.J.H. *et al.* 1997: A short-term study of chimeric monoclonal antibody cA2 to tumour necrosis factor α for Crohn's disease. *New England Journal of Medicine* 337, 1029–35.

Thomas, G.A.O., Swift, G.L., Green, J.T. *et al.* 1998: Controlled trial of antituberculous chemotherapy in Crohn's disease: a five year follow up study. *Gut* 42, 497–500.

Thompson, H. 1990: Histopathology of Crohn's disease. In Allan R.N., Keighley, M.R.B., Alexander-Williams, J., Hawkins, C. (eds) *Inflammatory bowel diseases*, 2nd edn. Edinburgh: Churchill Livingstone, 263–85.

Thomsen, O.O., Cortot, A., Jewell, D. *et al.* for the International Budesonide-Mesalamine Study Group 1998: A comparison of budesonide and mesalamine for active Crohn's disease. *New England Journal of Medicine* 339, 370–4.

Timmer, A., Sutherland, L.R., Martin, F. and The Canadian Mesalamine for Remission of Crohn's Disease Study Group 1998: Oral contraceptive use and smoking are risk factors for relapse in Crohn's disease. *Gastroenterology* 114, 1143–50.

Tysk, C., Lindberg, E., Jarnerot, G., Floderus-Myrhed, B. 1988. Ulcerative colitis and Crohn's disease in an unselected population of monozygotic and dizygotic twins. A study of heritability and the influence of smoking. *Gut* 29, 990–6.

Van Hees, P.A., Van Elteren, P.H., Van Lier, H.J.J., Van Tongeren, J.H.M. 1980: An index of inflammatory activity in patients with Crohn's disease. *Gut* 21, 279–86.

Viney, J.L. 1998: Altering cytokine soups: a recipe for inflammatory bowel disease? *Gut* 42, 607–8.

Yacyshyn, B.R., Bowen-Yacyshyn, M.B., Jewell, L., Tami, J.A., Bennett, C.F., Kisner, D.L., Shanahan, W.R., Jr 1998: A placebo-controlled trial of ICAM-1 antisense oligonucleotide in the treatment of Crohn's disease. *Gastroenterology* 114, 1133–42.

26

Pathology of small bowel tumours

SVEN WIDGREN, IPATIA DOUSSIS-ANAGNOSTOPOULOU

INTRODUCTION

The small bowel has a length of 300–900 cm, depending on whether it is measured at operation or during necropsy. The duodenum is 20–25 cm long, has a retroperitoneal course until the angle of Treitz, and is followed by the jejunum and the ileum, which are attached to the mesentery. The mucosa has large circumferential folds, which are shorter in the jejunum and nearly non-apparent in the ileum. The macroscopical surface accounts for 90 per cent of the whole gastrointestinal tract.

Small bowel tumours (SBT) are rare, representing about 1.5 per cent of all the tumours of the gastrointestinal tract. The true incidence of both benign and malignant tumours is difficult to establish for several reasons (Fenoglio-Preiser *et al.*, 1990): the ampulla of Vater was not always considered a site of intestinal tumours; in older series, there was often no clear definition of 'polyps' (see below); non-neoplastic conditions were included; there was uncertainty whether multiple tumours occurring in one single patient should be registered as single or separate lesions; neuroendocrine tumours (carcinoids) were variously classified as benign or malignant; some series were made up of autopsy material, others of surgical specimens, and still others of both; and, in some cases, it was difficult to state whether a tumour was originating in the small bowel or was due to an infiltration from a neighbouring organ.

Many tumours, benign or malignant, present as polyps. A polyp is defined as a structure protruding into the lumen of a hollow space (cavity or tube). This eponym does not signify anything about its structure (inflammatory, neoplastic, etc.) or behaviour (benign or malignant). The term 'pseudo-polyp' is inadequate and must be avoided.

The *frequency of benign tumours* is very difficult to assess for the reasons enumerated above; moreover, they are not included in the data collected by tumour registries. They are truly rare. In a review of the literature, about 1000 cases were recorded, gastrointestinal stromal tumours (GIST) being excluded (Widgren, 1995).

Malignant tumours are rare. Their age-standardized incidence rate according to the Geneva Registry of Tumours is 0.6 per 100 000 for males and 0.4 for females, while in the USA it is 1.2 for White males, 2.1 for Black males and 2.3 in Hawaiian males (IARC, 1997). Adenocarcinomas are the most frequent tumours (25–50 per cent), followed by carcinoids, malignant lymphomas and sarcomas in decreasing order. The following protective mechanisms have been suggested as an explanation for the rarity of small bowel malignant tumours: the fluid content of the small bowel tends to reduce the intensity of exposure of the mucosa to oral carcinogens; the rapid small bowel transit reduces the contact time with ingested carcinogens; the small bowel content is relatively sterile; the high levels of immunoglobulins, especially IgA, have a protective effect; and ingested carcinogens are detoxified by enzymatic activity, e.g. benzopyrene-hydrolase (Lowenfels, 1973).

The *aetiology* of malignant small bowel tumours remains obscure, but the protective factors enumerated may play a role. The fact that about 50 per cent of carcinomas are located in the duodenum (ampulla of Vater and periampullary region) suggests that bile is involved in the pathogenesis of carcinomas of this region (Lowenfels, 1978).

Clinically, most benign small bowel tumours are discovered at necropsy or incidentally during a laparotomy performed for another cause. If large, benign tumours may produce symptoms and signs similar to those of malignant tumours: abdominal discomfort; pain; cramps, often related to obstruction or intussusception; jaundice and bleeding; and diarrhoea or perforation. Neuroendocrine tumours may be recognized by a specific syndrome, e.g. the carcinoid syndrome, or the Zollinger–Ellison syndrome. The clinical diagnosis is thus difficult to establish because of the non-specific symptoms and signs. Various techniques are helpful.

Endoscopy of the duodenum to the angle of Treitz is easy to perform and biopsies may be taken; the same is possible for the distal ileum, which can be reached through colonoscopy. Enteroscopy is used for the jejunum and the ileum, a diagnosis being made in 50 per cent of patients (Lewis *et al.*, 1991). However, the procedure does not permit biopsies to be taken. Biopsies are sometimes difficult to evaluate because the tissue has been teased, crushed or fragmented. Radiological techniques have been considerably improved. Double-contrast enema and enteroclysis allow better imaging than plain barium studies. A computed tomography (CT) scan is useful for detecting transmural extension and metastases, thus being helpful for staging of the tumour. Ultrasound and magnetic resonance imaging are of limited value according to some authors. Angiography may identify the source of massive bleeding. These methods are useful in the diagnosis of small bowel tumours, but only in a fraction of patients, e.g. in 31 per cent in a series of 35 jejuno-ileal cases (Desa *et al.*, 1991).

The staging of tumours has been defined by the International Union Against Cancer (UICC, 1997) (Table 26.1). For malignant tumours the prognosis varies with the histological type. Neuroendocrine tumours (carcinoids), even with metastases, may have a long survival. Carcinomas, malignant stromal tumours and lymphomas have a worse prognosis. DiSario *et al.* (1994) gave a 5-year survival of 54 per cent, compared with the 20 per cent in the literature they cited.

HANDLING OF BIOPSIES AND OPERATION SPECIMENS

Importance of good clinical information

At the first meeting of the European Gastrointestinal Pathology Group in Brussels in March 1996, a symposium was dedicated to quality reporting in gastrointestinal pathology. The *pathologist is a member of the team* responsible for the diagnosis, treatment and well-being of the patient. Therefore, all clinical information is mandatory for the pathologist to interpret biopsies or surgical specimens. Without the necessary information, the pathologist is exposed to diagnostic misinterpretation with subsequent serious harm to the patient (Morson and Dawson, 1990a). The *pathologist's report* should be the basis of the patient's treatment, hence good clinical information is indispensable on the request form. In the case of biopsies, the endoscopist should give a clinical summary and findings on endoscopy, the site of biopsies and appearance. *Printed sheets*, derived from those recommended in the guidelines for inflammatory bowel disease by the British Society of Gastroenterology (Jenkins *et al.*, 1997) are strongly recommended. The surgeon should state the reasons for the operation, the principal operative findings, the identification and orientation of the specimens, as well as identification marks (threads), e.g. the proximal vascular ligature or places that are of special interest or are a problem.

The *pathology report* must fulfil several aims: firstly, diagnosis and prognosis, as well as providing pre- and postgraduate teaching, and providing information for epidemiology and research, a medical audit, for quality control and evaluation of cost effectiveness. A weekly *clinicopathological meeting* is also very useful to clinicians, surgeons and pathologists to discuss problems or to organize further treatment strategies, especially for oncological cases. *Check-lists* are helpful for a valuable pathology report for clinicians, surgeons and oncologists (Kempson, 1992). The 'Joint National Guidelines Minimum Data Set Colorectal Cancer Histopathology Report' recommended by Shepherd and Quirke (1997) represents the best available pro forma and will

Table 26.1 *TNM staging of small intestinal tumours according to UICC (1997)*

pT0	No evidence of primary
pTis	Carcinoma *in situ*
pT1	Tumour invades lamina propria or submucosa
pT2	Invades muscularis propria
pT3	Extends < 2 cm into subserosa or into non-peritonealized perimuscular tissue (mesentery of jejunum or ileum) or retroperitoneum (duodenum)
pT4	Perforates visceral peritoneum, or directly invades adjacent structures > 2 cm
pNX	Regional lymph nodes (LN) not assessed
pN0	No regional LN metastasis
pN1	Regional LN metastasis
pMX	Presence of distant metastasis not assessed
pM0	No distant metastasis
pM1	Distant metastasis

p, pathologic stage; T, tumour extension; N, involvement of lymphatic nodes; M, presence of distant metastases.

probably be adopted by the European Gastrointestinal Pathology Group (Shepherd, 1997). Presently no check-lists are available for the duodenum and small bowel, apart from the one proposed by Rosai (1993) for Whipple resection specimens; those for the colorectum might be used by analogy. The report should also include prognostic indications. This is best established by using the TNM classification of malignant tumours under the auspices of the UICC (Table 26.1). Finally, one has to give results of newer prognostic factors (proliferation markers, ploidy results and molecular biology data), which should be interpreted presently with caution, although they may be of help in the near future.

Handling of biopsies

Until recently, the small bowel was a kind of white zone on geographic maps of the nineteenth century. The Crosby capsule, conducted under fluoroscopic control, is now obsolete. Enteroscopy, developed during the last decade (Lewis *et al.*, 1991), permits the inspection of the bowel beyond the angle of Treitz but no biopsies. All other endoscopic methods allow the harvest of biopsies of 2–3 mm in size. Textbooks on biopsy pathology of the digestive tract (Whitehead, 1985; Talbot and Price, 1987; Day and Dixon, 1995) all give similar indications on how to handle this material. They are also the subject of Chapter 13.2.

We must, however, emphasize two points of utmost importance.

1. Inadequate handling of specimens and delay in fixation should be avoided.
2. Adequate fixation is of major importance; in our experience, mercury-formalin (Zenker's fluid) permits good routine stains and also the majority of immunohistochemistry.

When there is doubt on the handling of biopsies for peculiar techniques, a discussion with the pathologist is mandatory before the endoscopy is undertaken.

Handling of polyps

Polyps may present as small knobs on the surface of the mucosa, and may be excised *in toto* and handled like a mucosal biopsy. If larger, polyps with a stalk should be resected at the base with a snare or a cautery (hot biopsy). A long stalk will permit the pathologist to take adequate sections in the correct plane to establish the relationship between the lesion and the head, the stalk and the resection site (Fenoglio-Preiser and Noffsinger, 1995). More often, the stalk is rather short and retracts into the head, so that it becomes quite imperceptible, and inserting a needle into that site may allow the pathologist to locate it. Placing polyps as soon as possible into the container with adequate fixative will allow optimal preservation. Larger polyps are best put into buffered formaldehyde; other fixatives (Bouin's and Zenker's solutions) should be avoided because of their slow penetration of tissues.

Handling of operation specimens

Textbooks and various articles (Morson and Dawson, 1990a; Sheffield and Talbot, 1992; Widgren, 1996) give indications on the handling of colorectal specimens. These recommendations can be used, by extension, for duodenal (Whipple's operation) or small intestinal surgical specimens. Good histological results depend on *rapid fixation* of specimens. Optimally, they should be brought immediately, fresh and untouched, to the pathology laboratory. This allows the pathologist to open them *lege artis*, take photographs, and, if necessary, take unfixed tissues for special requirements. Specimens should not be separated in several pieces and sent to various pathologists with the idea of assuring the diagnosis; the interesting lesion may not be present in these various parts and this procedure is contrary to medical ethics. If the surgeon is especially interested in a lesion, the specimen should be opened on its anti-mesenteric side and markers placed on it or a diagram made. If immediate transportation is not possible, the specimen can be placed into a plastic bag and kept in a refrigerator (but not in a deep freeze) and sent on the next morning to the laboratory. If such a procedure is not possible, one may consider immediate fixation in a sufficient quantity of formaldehyde, after having properly opened the specimen. Orientation of specimens by marker threads is important. It is preferable not to open specimens when strictures are present. They should be gently rinsed with water, tied up at each end and inflated with formalin, then floated in a container with a sufficient quantity of formalin. This procedure will allow the pathologist to take adequate sections of the lesion of interest and to collect appropriate material for a thorough histological study.

EPITHELIAL TUMOURS

Benign epithelial tumours

ADENOMAS

Adenomas are benign epithelial tumours arising from the epithelium of glands or villi. The classification used in this chapter is that adopted by the WHO (Jass and Sobin, 1989): *tubular adenomas*, composed of glands or tube-like structures resembling normal Lieberkühn's

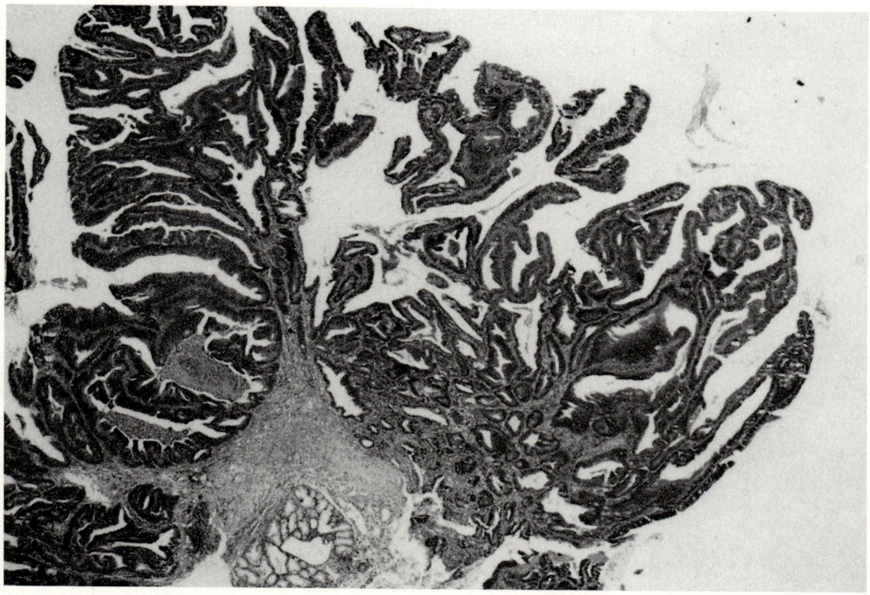

Figure 26.1 *Villous adenoma of the duodenum; low-power histology (haematoxylin and eosin; H&E).*

glands; *villous* (*papillary*), made up of villous structures resembling normal small intestinal villi; and *tubulovillous*, made up of a mixture of tubular and villous structures.

Adenomas of the small intestine are rare. Few series have documented more than 50 cases (Perzin and Bridge, 1981; Seifert *et al.*, 1992). Macroscopically (and endoscopically), duodenal adenomas are usually sessile and have a villous appearance. Those situated in other parts of the small bowel are mainly polypoid (Plate 26.1). Histologically, small intestinal adenomas are similar to those seen in the colon. Duodenal tumours are predominantly villous (papillary) (Fig. 26.1). Like those of the colon, adenomas may follow the dysplasia–carcinoma sequence, which will be discussed below. So-called Brunner's glands adenomas (hyperplasia) will be dealt with in the section entitled 'Other polypoid lesions.'

The treatment of duodenal adenomas may be either endoscopic resection or total resection through duodenotomy. Those of the jejunum and the ileum can be resected by enterotomy.

FAMILIAL ADENOMATOUS POLYPOSIS (FAP)

Multiple adenomas associated with familial adenomatous polyposis (FAP) of the colon may also be found in various parts of the small intestine, especially in the duodenum, the most frequent extra-colonic localization of FAP. According to Franzin *et al.* (1995) this site is found in 50 per cent of cases in Western publications and up to 100 per cent in Japanese ones. This may be due to a racial incidence, possibly modulated by the kind of surveillance of asymptomatic postcolectomized patients (Lynch, 1995). These adenomas are similar to the colonic ones, i.e. they are essentially tubular. Adenomas after colectomy may be found in ileo-anal continent pouches or in continent ileostomy reservoirs (Shepherd and Bussey, 1990). It is generally agreed that a rigorous postcolectomy surveillance is necessary, since adenomas of the small intestine may undergo the same adenoma–dysplasia–carcinoma sequence as colonic adenomas.

DYSPLASIA IN ADENOMAS

Since small bowel tumours are rare, biopsies can seldom be performed in search of a dysplasia and systematic studies on the dysplasia–carcinoma sequence, to the best of our knowledge, have not been performed in this location. However, this is highly probable for the duodenum, since remnants of adenomas within adenocarcinomas have been described by several authors (Perzin and Bridge, 1981; Sellner, 1990; Seifert *et al.*, 1992).

Epithelial dysplasia replaces the term 'atypia' found in the older literature, which basically applies only to modifications of the nucleus. According to Konishi and Morson (1982), the word dysplasia is used in the description of histopathological precursor lesions for cancer in various epithelial surfaces, both within and outside the gastrointestinal tract. The St Mark's group has established three grades of dysplasia for the colorectum, according to the severity of nuclear, cellular and architectural changes: *mild, moderate* (Fig. 26.2) and *severe dysplasia.* The latter is also referred to as *in situ carcinoma* but should be avoided because of its misleading significance. Unfortunately, this term is used in the World Health Organisation (WHO) classification of intestinal tumours (Jass and Sobin, 1989). Another classification of dysplasia has been established by the Inflammatory Bowel Disease–Dysplasia Morphology Study Group (Riddell *et al.*, 1983). It has been extended to the adenoma–carcinoma sequence of

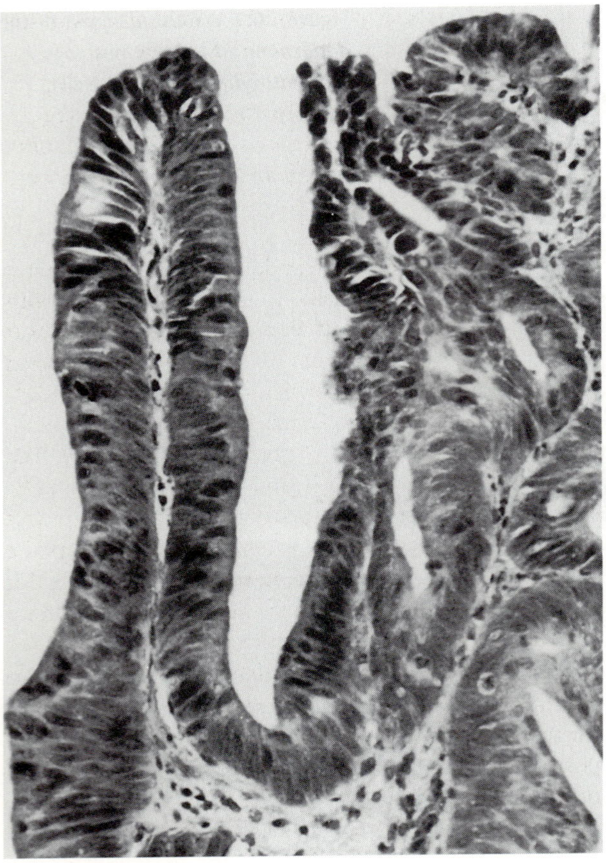

Figure 26.2 *Detail of Fig. 26.1 showing moderate dysplasia: distorted crypts with pleomorphic, pseudostratified nuclei (H&E).*

the colorectum, as well as to Barrett's oesophagus and the stomach, and has gained extending recognition in the literature. However, it is not easy to grasp for pathologists unfamiliar with the problems of digestive pathology. Histological modifications are described as *negative, indefinite,* or *positive for dysplasia,* which is divided into *low* and *high grade.* Low-grade dysplasia corresponds to low and moderate dysplasia of the St Mark's grading, which requires repeat biopsies. High-grade dysplasia is a condition in which colectomy should be considered, according to this Working Group.

Malignant epithelial tumours

ADENOCARCINOMAS

As already mentioned in the 'Introduction', malignant tumours of the small intestine are rare and less than 1 per cent of gastrointestinal carcinomas are located in the small intestine (Morson and Dawson, 1990b). Series on carcinomas of the small bowel rarely exceed 50 cases (Bridge and Perzin, 1975; Perzin and Bridge, 1981). Clinically, the symptoms and signs are those described in the introduction of this chapter.

Macroscopically, adenocarcinomas of the small intestine have the same appearance as those of the colon: polypoid, annular or ulcerating (Fig. 26.3). Invasion of neighbouring organs or tissues may be found in advanced stages. *Histologically,* the tumours are also similar to adenocarcinomas of the colon, either well or moderately differentiated (Plate 26.2). Often, remnants of adenomas may be seen at the proximity of, or within, the carcinoma (Lioe and Biggart, 1990) indicating that the (adenoma)–dysplasia–carcinoma sequence is also valid in this location.

The prognosis depends on the depth of invasion and the presence of lymph node metastases. The overall 5-year survival is between 20 and 30 per cent (Ouriel and Adams, 1984; Morson and Dawson, 1990b; Gore, 1997).

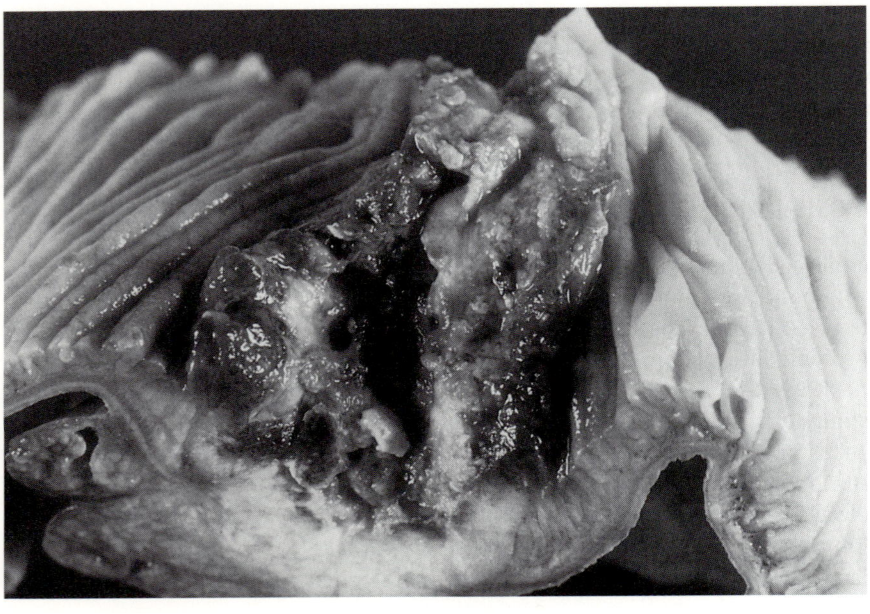

Figure 26.3 *Adenocarcinoma of the jejunum; circumferential ulcerated tumour.*

OTHER HISTOLOGICAL TYPES OF CARCINOMA

Anaplastic, adenosquamous and small cell carcinomas have been reported as single case reports or very small series, and are quoted in textbooks (Rosai, 1995; Whitehead, 1995).

ADENOCARCINOMA ARISING IN PECULIAR CONDITIONS

Familial adenomatous polyposis

It is well known that, if untreated, FAP patients will die of colonic carcinoma during the fifth decade of their life. There are numerous reports of duodenal carcinomas, predominantly periampullary, occurring in FAP (Jagelman *et al.*, 1988; Shepherd and Bussey, 1990). Most of the tumours had remnants of adenomas or were associated with one or more adenomas. In a prospective study performed on 1391 subjects of 157 families, Offerhaus *et al.* (1992) found upper gastrointestinal tract carcinoma in 14 cases, showing that cancers in this location are not uncommon in FAP, and that these patients should undergo close follow-up, before as well as after colectomy.

Hereditary non-polyposis colorectal cancer

Hereditary non-polyposis colorectal cancer (HNPCC, Lynch syndrome) is characterized by the early appearance of colorectal cancer associated or not with carcinomas of various other organs: endometrium, urinary tract, small bowel, etc. (McMunnick and Nelson, 1998). These cases represent between 1–3 per cent (Burt, 1991) and 5–10 per cent (Vasen *et al.*, 1991), respectively, of all Western colorectal cancers. The disease is familial autosomal dominant and is characterized by one or more adenocarcinomas, mostly mucinous, appearing between 40 and 45 years of age in the proximal colon, synchronous or metachronous (Marra and Boland, 1995). They are associated with the mutation of four genes with defects in the DNA mismatch repair (Burt, 1991; Marra and Boland, 1995). Small intestinal carcinomas may occur in this condition (Watson and Lynch, 1993). The possibility of the existence of HNPCC should be kept in mind when small intestinal carcinoma is diagnosed. The patients with this syndrome and their families should also be, like those of FAP, submitted to screening and genetic counselling. This syndrome has been recently remarkably well updated by Lynch *et al.* (1997).

Peutz–Jeghers syndrome

Peutz–Jeghers syndrome is a rare condition discussed under 'Other polypoid lesions' later in this chapter. Small intestinal carcinomas are found in 3–6 per cent of these patients (Ryan, 1996), most before the age of 40 years. There is controversy about the pathogenesis of these carcinomas. Cochet *et al.* (1979) found dysplastic foci, without associated adenomas, within polyps of the small and large intestine. However, Franzin *et al.* (1995) are of the opinion that these carcinomas develop in adenomas found in hamartomatous polyps and suggest that this condition occurs in zones of cellular replication, which may become dysplastic and then carcinomatous.

Coeliac disease

After isolated cases of carcinomas and malignant lymphomas of the small intestine associated with coeliac disease were recorded, a collaborative study was set up in the UK (Swinson *et al.*, 1983), which reported 235 patients with lymphomas and carcinomas, including 19 carcinomas of the small intestine. Marsch *et al.* (1990) recently collected 39 cases in the literature. The adenocarcinomas are moderately to poorly differentiated. In some cases the diagnosis of coeliac disease was only established on the mucosa surrounding the tumour on the resected specimen (Gander *et al.*, 1993; MacGowan *et al.*, 1996). Carcinomas may develop in up to 15 per cent of patients with undiagnosed, untreated or refractory coeliac disease (Halsted, 1996). The association is now well known and should be searched for when a patient with coeliac disease on a gluten-free diet shows worsening of their symptoms. Conversely, coeliac disease should be suspected in the case of adenocarcinoma of the small bowel.

Crohn's disease

Adenocarcinoma of the small intestine associated with Crohn's disease is very rare, supervening in an equally rare disease. The first case of carcinoma in the small intestine was reported in 1956 by Ginzburg (Gilmour, 1995). Since then, publications in the 1960s and 1970s confirmed this relationship, the relative risk for the small intestine being between 6 and 20 times that of the colon, according to Morson and Dawson (1990b), and up to 6–320 according to Ribeiro *et al.* (1991). Carcinomas in Crohn's disease occur at a median age of 46 years, compared to 64.6 years for sporadic intestinal cancer (Lashner, 1992). The *risk factors* for small bowel carcinoma occurring in Crohn's disease are long-standing disease with an early-onset and bypassed section of small bowel. The symptoms are non-specific, obstruction being the most frequent presentation. The diagnosis of the carcinoma is often made only by the examining pathologist. It occurs frequently in strictured segments, so that its macroscopical recognition during laparotomy or at the pathology laboratory may be difficult. The location of carcinoma of the small bowel is the inverse of that of *de novo* carcinoma, the most frequent being the ileum. Histologically, most tumours are poorly differentiated adenocarcinomas. Dysplasia may be found in the surrounding mucosa, either intact or diseased. The prognosis is poor, corresponding to a survival of 25 per cent at 36 months (Ribeiro *et al.*, 1991). Because of the rarity of the condition, there is no consensus about follow-up of long-standing Crohn's disease patients, as the small bowel lesions are most often beyond the reach of endoscopy, or hidden in stenotic or excluded parts of the intestine.

ADENOCARCINOMAS ARISING IN UNCOMMON SITES

Isolated case reports of adenomas and carcinomas have been documented in patients with ileo-anal continent pouches after coloproctectomy for FAP. Low-grade or moderate dysplasia in pouches of ulcerative colitis patients have also been documented (Widgren and Cox, 1997).

Adenocarcinomas may develop in ileostomies. Gilson and Sollenberger (1992) have collected 18 cases, including their own: 14 after ulcerative colitis and 3 after FAP. The exact location of the tumours (at the margin of the stomy or within the efferent ileal loop) was not indicated. Thus the pathogenesis is difficult to establish and has been attributed to local recurrence of FAP, to dysplasia in 'colonized' small bowel mucosa, or to an atypical response to chronic irritation by the faeces. The mean duration between the establishment of the ileostomy and the occurrence of the carcinoma is approximately 25 years, so that surveillance of the stomata is suggested by the above-mentioned authors from the 20th year onwards.

Ileal conduits performed after cystectomies may be the site, at long term, of an adenocarcinoma. The condition is, however, very rare, since patients die mostly after a few years from urinary complications or recurrence of the bladder tumour (Sakano *et al.*, 1995).

There have been reports of adenocarcinomas developing in Meckel's diverticulum (Kusumoto *et al.*, 1992). They are surrounded by gastric heterotopic mucosa, but the relationship between the latter and a tumour is difficult to understand, since the usual intestinal metaplasia–dysplasia–carcinoma sequence is not mentioned, nor has intestinal metaplasia been described by the authors cited above.

NEUROENDOCRINE TUMOURS (CARCINOIDS)

In 1907 Oberndorfer gave the name 'carcinoid' to a peculiar type of ileal tumour, which resembled a carcinoma. Later the term was applied to tumours occurring with a typical clinical syndrome, the carcinoid syndrome, or to tumours that had certain staining features with silver salts (argentafin and argyrophilic). The term APUD tumours (amine production, uptake and decarboxylation) has now been abandoned, as well as the terms foregut, midgut and hindgut tumours (for a short historical review, *see* Capella *et al.*, 1995). The eponym carcinoid, used in the WHO classification (Williams *et al.*, 1980), is inappropriate because of the uncertainty about prognosis and the restricted meaning of the term. A group of European pathologists proposed a *new classification* considering the morphological, functional and biological features for each localization with the global heading of neuroendocrine tumours (Capella *et al.*, 1994, 1995; Klöppel, 1997). They are grouped in three categories: well-differentiated neoplasms (benign), or with uncertain behaviour, presenting with or without functional signs; well-differentiated carcinomas; and poorly differentiated endocrine carcinomas. The tumours are classified according to their morphology, biology and prognosis, taking into account the criteria of the site, histological differentiation, size, vascular invasion, and proliferative and functional activity (Klöppel, 1997).

The term *neuroendocrine tumours* (NETs) is now used, with indications of the type of peptide or hormone they produce. Functioning tumours may have the same histological and immunohistochemical patterns as non-functioning ones, so that they cannot be differentiated by their morphological features. The haematoxylin and eosin histological features suggest the diagnosis of a NET, which is then confirmed by immunohistochemical features and subsequent clinical investigations. For scanning, neurone-specific enolase (NSE), chromogranins and synaptophysin are commonly used, followed by the specific identification of the peptide(s) or hormone(s) contained in the tumour cells. Solcia *et al.* (1995) have emphasized that the use of functional labellings like 'gastrinoma' should be restricted to tumours with a clinical syndrome; those which have no clinical functional signs should be labelled according to the predominance of the peptide(s) or hormone(s) found on immunohistochemical evidence, e.g. 'gastrin-producing NET'. Some tumours may contain more than one secretory product, either in various parts of the tumour, or sometimes in the same cells. The reasons why some tumours produce a clinical syndrome and others remain silent have been attributed to various factors (Dayal, 1991), such as the small amount of secretion, the intermittent release into the circulation, the rapid degradation of the product or molecular heterogeneity.

NETs are rare (Vinik *et al.*, 1989); they account for 13–34 per cent of all malignant tumours of the small intestine in the USA and 41 per cent in Geneva (Registre Genevois des Tumeurs, personal communication). The incidence has risen since the 1980s because of the increased accuracy of the diagnostic methods, especially those using immunohistochemistry. *Macroscopically*, they are most often found in the submucosa where they produce isolated or multiple nodules or plaques, which may bulge into the mucosa and the lumen (Plate 26.3) and extend towards the serosa. In the majority the colour is beige–yellow, which is more apparent after formalin fixation. They are often accompanied by marked fibrosis and muscular hyperplasia of

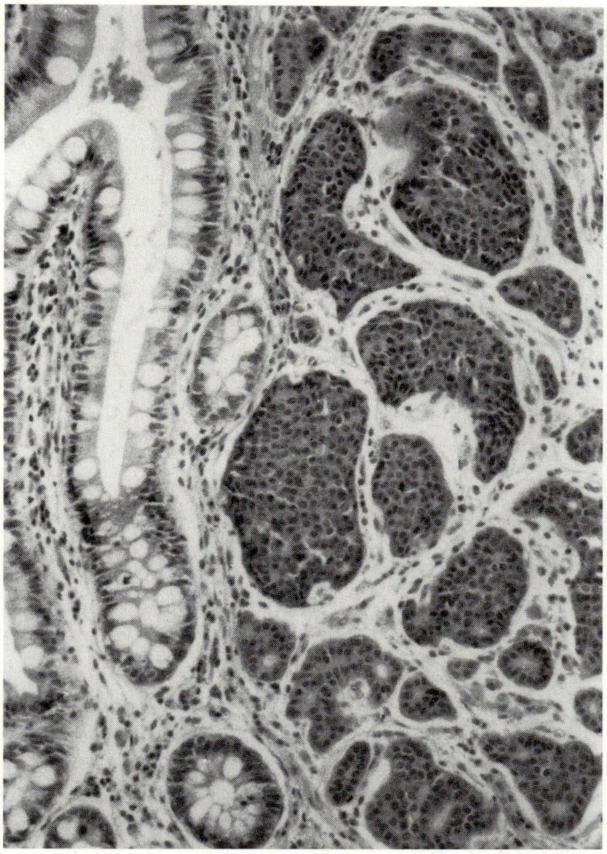

Figure 26.4 *Neuroendocrine tumour; histology showing solid and gland-like structures (H&E.)*

the bowel wall (Plate 26.4), which may be responsible for obstruction, intussusception, or compression of blood vessels with ischaemic complications.

From a purely histological point of view, NETs were subdivided into five groups by Soga and Tazawa (1971) according to their architectural pattern: insular, trabecular, glandular, mixed and undifferentiated (Fig. 26.4 and Plate 26.5). Most NETs are located in the appendix. In the material by Fenoglio-Preiser *et al.* (1990), which included extradigestive sites, this location accounts for 92 per cent of all NETs, followed by the ileum (23 per cent), the jejunum (4 per cent) and the duodenum (5 per cent). They will be described in the following section dealing with the various segments of the small intestine according to the most recent classification (Capella *et al.*, 1995; Klöppel, 1997).

Tumours of the duodenum

There are five groups of NETs that occur in the duodenum. These are listed below.

1 *Gastrin-producing tumours* present as solitary or multiple nodules, the latter being associated in about a third of cases with the clinical gastrinoma syndrome characteristic of the Zollinger–Ellison syndrome (refractory peptic ulcer disease, gastric hypersecretion, large gastric mucosal folds, hypergastrinaemia), which may be part of the MEN-1 syndrome. As these tumours are often small, they may be overlooked during laparotomy, and may necessitate transillumination or duodenotomy (Pipeleers-Marichal *et al.*, 1993), or will only manifest through lymph node metastases.
2 *Somatostatin-producing tumours* occur almost exclusively in the ampulla of Vater, where they are usually malignant with bile duct obstruction. A true somatostatinoma syndrome is not described.
3 *Serotonin-producing tumours* are rare and usually do not produce a carcinoid syndrome in this location.
4 *Gangliocytic paragangliomas* are included in this group by Pipeleers-Marichal *et al.* (1993). They are usually polypoid and benign. They have characteristic appearances forming cell nests (Zellballen) intermingled with spindle cells and ganglion cells.
5 *Poorly differentiated neuroendocrine carcinomas* are exceptional and composed of small undifferentiated cells, the endocrine nature of which is established by immunohistochemistry.

Tumours of the jejunum and ileum

These tumours may be multiple and identical to those found in the duodenum. The classically described carcinoid tumours occur in the ileum and secrete serotonin, substance P and various other amines, and metastases to the liver produce the carcinoid syndrome in approximately 20 per cent of malignant tumours. This syndrome consists of diarrhoea, facial flushing and right-sided valvular heart disease. Locally, the tumour (situated in the submucosa) is nodular, sometimes multifocal, tan-yellow and may bulge into the lumen causing obstruction or intussusception. Long survival may be observed even when the tumour is metastatic.

NON-EPITHELIAL TUMOURS

Benign non-epithelial tumours

Non-epithelial tumours of the small intestine are rare. The incidence varies between 0.04 per cent and 6.5 per cent of all gastrointestinal tract tumours (Widgren, 1995). There is a slight male predominance. Epidemiological conditions are not known. The majority of these tumours are ileal lesions (43.1 per cent in our review), the remnant being evenly distributed between the

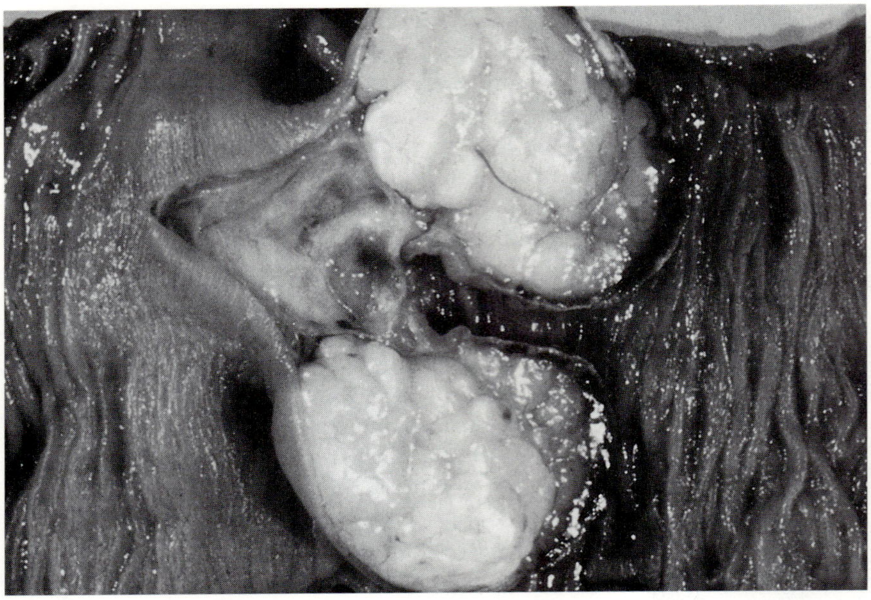

Figure 26.5 *Submucosal pedunculated lipoma; the section shows lobulated adipose tissue.*

duodenum and the jejunum. About half of them were lipomas; haemangiomas and neurogenic tumours made up approximately the other half.

Clinically, there is no major difference between the various histological types, as already mentioned. Macroscopically, the tumours may be intraluminal (Plate 26.6), intraparietal or subserosal. They may appear flat, sessile or polypoid, and spherical or ovoid. The colour is related to the histological type: lipomas are pale yellow (Fig. 26.5); angiomas, cherry red or violet; and lymphangiomas, whitish and translucent. Microscopically, *lipomas* are made up of a mass of well-encapsulated mature adipocytes, which may be mixed with a variable quantity of collagen (fibrolipomas) or blood vessels (angiolipomas). *Haemangiomas* are capillary or cavernous, according to the calibre of their constituent vessels, which are lined by flat endothelial cells. They must be distinguished from angiodysplasia, which is rarely found in the small intestine, being characteristically located in the ascending colon. *Lymphangiomas* are predominantly cystic, the spaces lined by an inconspicuous endothelium. They are distinguished from dilated lymphatics filled with lipid-laden macrophages, the chylangiomas, appearing on the mucosa as small isolated or grouped yellow spots. They are classically associated with obstruction of larger lymphatics of the mesentery by tumours (primary or metastatic to lymph nodes).

Gastrointestinal stromal tumours

Non-epithelial mesenchymal tumours other than lipomas or vascular tumours have been considered for years as smooth muscle tumours (leiomyomas and leiomyosarcomas) or of the neural type (schwannomas and neurofibromas). However, it became evident that the majority of these tumours could not be identified as 'smooth muscle' or 'neural' in origin, from either an immunohistochemical or ultrastructural point of view, so it was suggested that they be classified as gastrointestinal tract stromal tumours (GIST) (for a review, *see* Basson *et al.*, 1992).

GISTs constitute 1 per cent of all gastrointestinal tract tumours, the stomach being the most frequent site, followed by the jejunum and ileum, the rectum and the duodenum (Fenoglio-Preiser *et al.*, 1990). There is a slight male predominance without any ethnic incidence, with a peak between the 5th and the 7th decade; there are no recognized aetiological factors.

Macroscopically, the size varies from a few millimetres up to 30 cm in diameter. The smaller tumours are located in the muscularis mucosae, the submucosa or muscularis propria. If larger, they may bulge under the mucosa, which may become ulcerated, or under the serosa (Fig. 26.6). Most often they are single, rounded, occasionally dumb-bell shaped, and may be easily enucleated. On the cut surface they appear white or yellowish, with a rubbery consistency, malignant tumours being more often pink–tan and fleshy. Larger tumours may show central necrosis, followed by cavitation due to ulceration of the surface.

Histologically, they are made up of spindle cells arranged in interlacing or whorled bundles, or intermingled with collagen tracts, occasionally with palisading of the nuclei, which are elongated, blunt or pointed (Fig. 26.7). GISTs lack a true capsule and may be slightly interdigitated with the adjacent tissues. According to Kempson and Hendrickson (1995), 80–90 per cent of these tumours show affinities with muscle actin, smooth muscle actin and desmin, and are therefore considered as differentiated towards smooth muscle cells. Other tumours show differ-

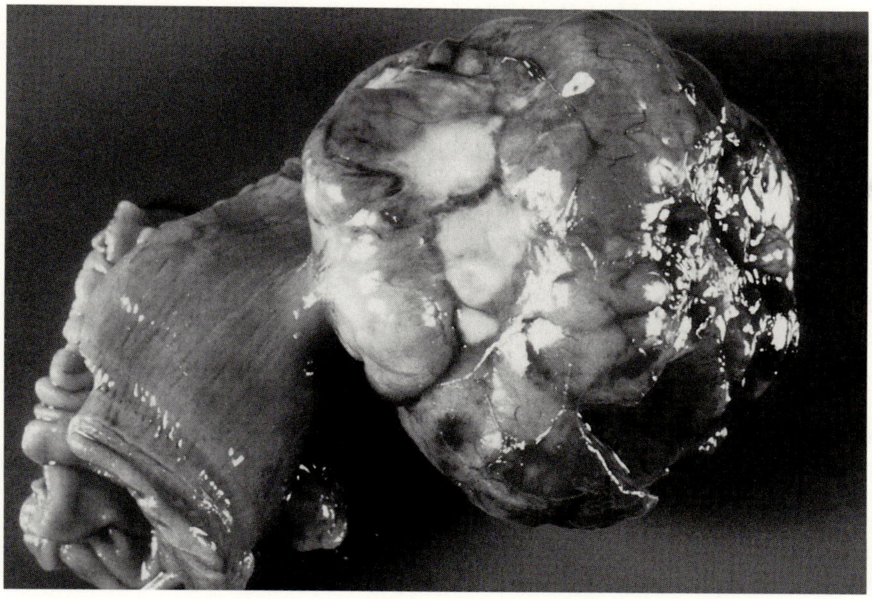

Figure 26.6 *Subserosal pedunculated stromal tumour.*

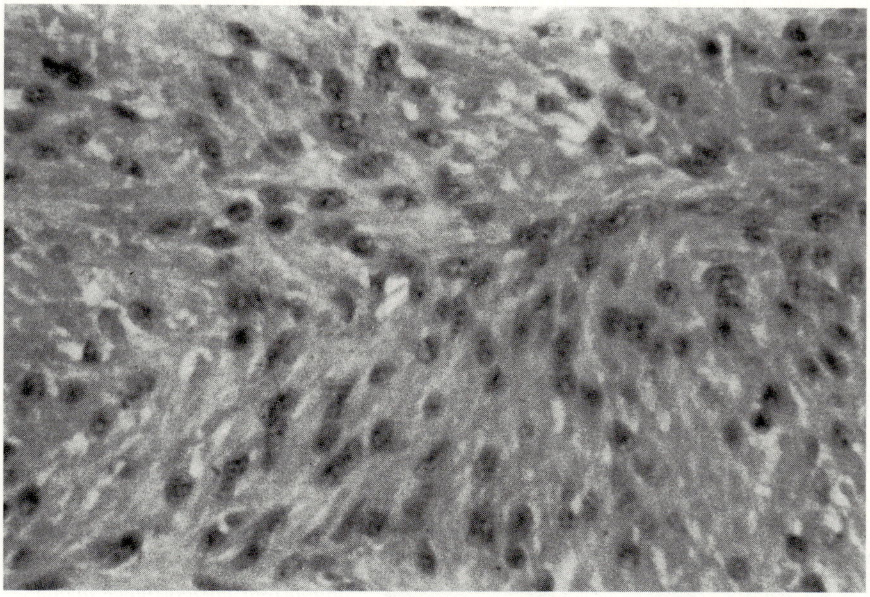

Figure 26.7 *Stromal tumour; histological appearance showing spindled interlacing cells with regular nuclei (H&E).*

entiation towards neural elements, their cells being positive with neurone-specific enolase and S-100 protein, and may be designated as gastrointestinal tract autonomic nerve tumours (GANT). Still others show lack of any of the immunohistochemical features described, with the exception of CD34, an antibody originally described in leukaemias and vascular tumours, which may be present in most of the GISTs (Plate 26.7) and are considered as 'uncommitted' (Rosai, 1995).

Electron microscopy is of value in differentiating the two major types of cells involved in GISTs, but is not suitable for routine diagnosis. Skeinoid fibres, which are peculiar deposits of collagen with a characteristic ultrastructural appearance, are distinguished in some neural-type tumours.

The benign and the malignant variants of these tumours were (and still are) difficult to separate, especially from the point of view of their prognosis and the survival of affected patients. It is a truism to state that invasion of neighbouring structures and metastases are the essential features of malignancy. Size, necrosis, cellular density, nuclear pleomorphism and anaplasia are features found more often in malignant than in benign tumours.

According to Kempson and Hendrickson (1995), intestinal stromal tumours more than 4 cm in diameter are diagnosed as sarcomas and designated as low grade when they present less than 10 mitotic figures (MF)/10 high-power fields (HPF), or high grade when there are more than 10 MF/10 HPF. Tumours from 1 to 4 cm are diagnosed as of 'uncertain malignant potential' if they are bland hypocellular and mitotically inactive (less that 10 MF/50 HPF); otherwise they are regarded as sarcomas. The use of immunohistochemical proliferation markers, such as MiB1 (Ki-67 antigen) (Ma *et al.*, 1997), will probably be helpful in the future, but has to be tested on further series of cases.

Small intestinal stromal tumours, although morphologically similar to those of the stomach, are more aggressive. Metastases of malignant stromal tumours are mainly haematogenous (liver and lungs) but rarely spread to regional lymph nodes.

SMOOTH MUSCLE TUMOURS IN HIV-POSITIVE CHILDREN

Leiomyomas and leiomyosarcomas have been described in human immunodeficiency virus (HIV)-positive children with visceral involvement (Chadwick *et al.*, 1990), which either remained asymptomatic and were found at necropsy, or were responsible for severe disease (pulmonary or intestinal involvement). *In situ* hybridization showed positivity for the Epstein–Barr virus (EBV) in tumour cells (Prévot *et al.*, 1994; McClain *et al.*, 1995), suggesting that EBV may contribute to the pathogenesis of these tumours.

Gastrointestinal autonomic nerve tumours

Shanks *et al.* (1996) added nine of their own to 42 cases described in the literature of a type of tumour that has also been termed plexosarcoma. They often present like other stromal tumours of the gastrointestinal tract, both macroscopically and histologically, but have peculiar ultrastructural features: cellular processes and dense-core granules; skeinoid fibres were also found in some of these tumours. Immunohistochemically, they are distinguished by their positive staining with NSE, PGP 9.5 (a marker of neuroendocrine/neuronal cells) and vimentin, and less frequently with smooth muscle actin (alpha-SMA), vaso-active intestinal peptide (VIP) and CD34.

Kaposi's sarcoma

Kaposi's sarcoma (KS) is a multicentric neoplastic disease due to the proliferation of spindle cells of mesenchymal origin (Wang *et al.*, 1995), which has recently been attributed to a virus named Kaposi's sarcoma herpes virus (KSVH) or human herpes virus 8 (HHV-8) (Knowles and Cesarman, 1997). Since the acquired immunodeficiency syndrome (AIDS) was first reported in 1981, the frequency of KS has become more prevalent and is a major complication of the syndrome.

Involvement of the gastrointestinal tract is found in more than 50 per cent of HIV-positive patients (Clayton and Clayton, 1997). Patients may have bleeding, diarrhoea, abdominal pain or protein-losing enteropathy owing to extensive intestinal involvement (Wang *et al.*, 1995). KS may remain asymptomatic and be an incidental necropsy finding (Meyer and Schneider, 1991; Ioachim *et al.*, 1995; Widgren, 1995). Endoscopically and macroscopically, the lesions have a characteristic appearance of submucosal, reddish-violaceous, mulberry-like nodules about 1 cm in diameter, which occasionally may be ulcerated (Fig. 26.8).

The tumour is made up of spindle cells and vascular structures. The spindle cells are arranged in loose or dense bundles ('stromal' pattern), with varying pleomorphic or atypical nuclei and mitoses. The

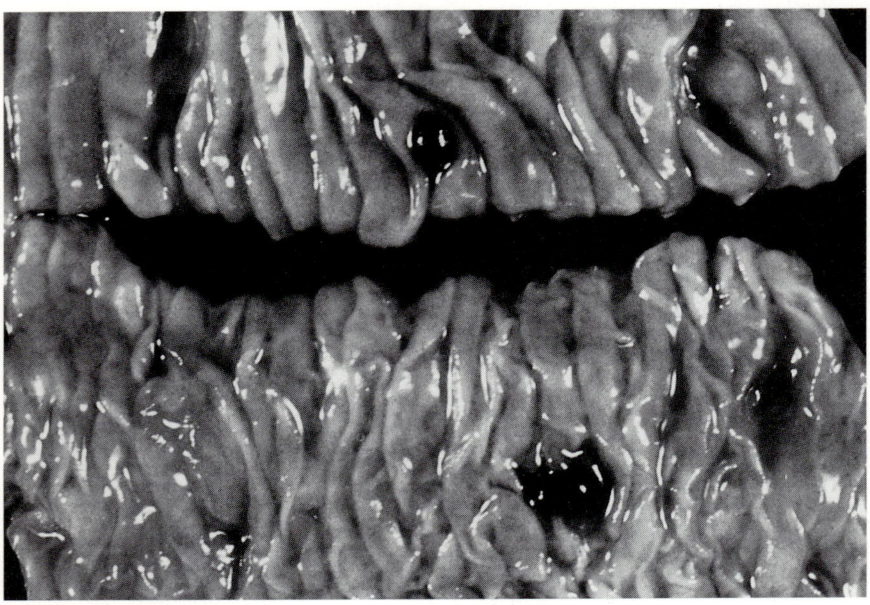

Figure 26.8 *Kaposi's sarcoma; submucosal haemorrhagic nodules. (Reprinted with permission of Professor Richard Whitehead and Harcourt Brace & Co., Australia from* Rare and secondary tumours, *1995, R. Whitehead (ed.), Ch. 40, Part II, Churchill Livingstone.)*

vascular spaces may range from capillary and slit patterns to ectatic vessels, lined by endothelium that may be stratified and atypical, and contain blood cells. In biopsy samples, KS is diagnosed in only 30 per cent of cases. In the early stages, the accompanying inflammatory cells may falsely lead to interpreting the lesion as granulation tissue (Fenoglio-Preiser *et al.*, 1990). Immunohistochemically, the endothelial cells are positive with factor VIII and *Ulex europaeus*, while spindle cells are variably identified with smooth muscle markers.

The prognosis depends on the extension and speed of progression of KS, and is also determined by other AIDS-related manifestations: the presence of systemic symptoms, the severity of immunosuppression and opportunistic infections (Levine, 1993).

MALIGNANT LYMPHOMAS AND RELATED DISORDERS

Normal structure of the small intestine and the concept of mucosa-associated lymphoid tissue

The small bowel is one of the organs that contain, in the normal state, organized lymphoid tissue, called mucosa-associated lymphoid tissue (MALT). This consists of B- and T-cell lymphocytes, natural killer (NK) cells and macrophages. In the intestinal mucosa MALT is mainly organized in Peyer's patches and mesenteric lymph nodes. Immunocompetent cells can also be found isolated, either in the surface epithelium or within the lamina propria.

Peyer's patches are lymphoid aggregates that extend through the mucosa and submucosa of the small intestine and are formed by four different zones. The *follicle-associated epithelium* contains specialized epithelial cells, the membranous or M cells, which absorb and transport intraluminal antigens, allowing access to immunocompetent cells. The *dome*, situated beneath the surface epithelium, is populated mainly by B lymphocytes (the centrocyte-like cells) and is equivalent to the marginal zone of the spleen and lymph nodes. The *lymphoid follicle* is the area where the B lymphocytes proliferate and the *interfollicular zone* corresponds to the thymo-dependent zone of the T-lymphocyte proliferation. The cells that are present in the Peyer's patches circulate in the blood stream, mature and then return to the digestive mucosa, probably due to 'homing' properties.

The lamina propria contains both plasma cells, which secrete mainly IgA, and T-cell lymphocytes, which are CD4+. Intraepithelial lymphocytes are mainly CD8+ T cells, expressing the monoclonal antibody HML-1 (CD103) (Cerf-Bensussan *et al.*, 1987), specific for lymphocytes associated with epithelia. A population of natural killer cells is also present.

Malignant lymphomas

Gastrointestinal lymphomas are the most common type of primary extranodal lymphomas. Primary small bowel lymphomas account for approximately 5–7 per cent of all lymphomas, and represent the third most common malignancy after adenocarcinomas and NETs (Freeman *et al.*, 1972; O'Riordan *et al.*, 1996). In Western populations, only 20–30 per cent of the primary gastrointestinal tract lymphomas arise in the small bowel (Dragosics *et al.*, 1985; Herrmann *et al.*, 1980; Weingrad *et al.*, 1982), gastric lymphomas being the most frequent, while in the Middle East more than half of gastrointestinal tract lymphomas are localized in the small bowel (Al-Bahrani *et al.*, 1983; Al-Mondhiry, 1986). The possibility of a lymphoma of a systemic nature should always be excluded, as 10 per cent of patients with non-Hodgkin's lymphoma (NHL) present with gastrointestinal tract involvement at the time of the initial evaluation (Lewin *et al.*, 1978).

The most common presenting symptoms are abdominal pain, weight loss and bowel obstruction, followed by the presence of an abdominal mass, diarrhoea, nausea and vomiting (Domizio *et al.*, 1993).

In order to classify primary malignant gastrointestinal tract lymphomas, criteria to take into consideration are the B- or T-cell lineage, the presence of a predisposing condition, and the histological and phenotypic similarities with the normal MALT. Based on these elements, Isaacson *et al.* (1988) proposed a classification of primary gastrointestinal tract lymphomas that we find the most appropriate to follow: this is shown in Table 26.2.

Table 26.2 *Classification of primary gastrointestinal lymphomas. Reprinted with permission from Isaacson, P.G., Spenser, J., Wright, D.H. 1988: Classifying primary gut lymphomas.* Lancet *2, 1148–9. © by The Lancet Ltd.*

B-cell lymphoma
Low-grade B-cell lymphoma of MALT
High-grade B-cell lymphoma of MALT, with or without a low-grade component
IPSID (Mediterranean lymphoma, α-chain disease)
Mantle cell lymphoma (lymphomatoid polyposis)
Burkitt's lymphoma and Burkitt-like
Other types of low- or high-grade lymphoma (corresponding to peripheral lymph node equivalents)
T-cell lymphoma
Enteropathy-associated T-cell lymphoma (EATCL)[a]
Other types, unassociated with enteropathy[a]

[a]With or without eosinophilia.
MALT, mucosa-associated lymphoid tissue; IPSID, immunoproliferative small intestinal disease.

B-CELL NON-HODGKIN'S LYMPHOMAS

The majority of gastrointestinal tract lymphomas are of B-cell origin and arise from the MALT. This concept, first proposed by Isaacson and Wright (1983), has now won world-wide acceptance and has been incorporated in the Revised European–American classification of Lymphoid neoplasms (REAL) under the designation 'extranodal marginal zone B-cell lymphoma' (Harris *et al.*, 1994).

B-cell lymphomas are exophytic, polypoid, annular, diffusely infiltrating or bulky ulcerated, usually single tumour masses, 25 per cent being multifocal (Fig. 26.9) (Domizio *et al.*, 1993). The ileum is more commonly affected, followed by the jejunum and duodenum.

Low-grade B-cell lymphoma of MALT type

The low-grade B-cell lymphoma of MALT type is less frequent in the small bowel than in the stomach. The diagnosis is based on the presence of a diffuse infiltrate of small lymphocytes with indented or cleaved nuclei and abundant clear cytoplasm, the *centrocyte-like* cells, which selectively invade epithelial structures forming *lymphoepithelial lesions*, and the presence of reactive lymphoid follicles. A monocytoid population and a lymphoplasmacytic infiltrate can be associated. A high-grade component may be present.

The monoclonal character of the lesion can be demonstrated by the immunohistochemical expression of B-cell markers by the lymphoid cells. No rearrangement of the *bcl*-2 gene could be demonstrated in a series of gastrointestinal tract lymphomas, arguing against a centrofollicular origin (Pan *et al.*, 1989).

Low-grade lymphomas of MALT type often remain confined to the initial localization and, when they progress, they tend to invade other MALT localizations, probably due to their particular 'homing' capacities.

High-grade B-cell lymphoma

High-grade B-cell lymphomas are the most frequent lymphomas of the small intestine, representing 62 per cent (Domizio *et al.*, 1993). They are diffuse, high-grade, centroblastic, immunoblastic or large-cell anaplastic, with or without a low-grade component of MALT type. The diffuse lymphoid infiltrate is composed of large cells with a basophilic cytoplasm and round non-cleaved nuclei, of either centroblastic or immunoblastic type (Plate 26.8). A plasmacytoid differentiation may sometimes be present. The B-cell nature of the tumour is demonstrated immunohistochemically by the positivity of the tumour cells for the leucocyte common antigen (LCA), and the B-cell markers CD20 and CD79a (Plate 26.9).

Immunoproliferative small intestinal disease

Immunoproliferative small intestinal disease (IPSID) is a spectrum of disorders that affects young adults, who suffer from diarrhoea, malabsorption, weight loss and abdominal pain (WHO, 1976). There is an association with lower socioeconomic status, where the frequency of intestinal infections is particularly high.

This disease is known as Mediterranean or Middle Eastern lymphoma (Khojasteh *et al.*, 1983), or α-heavy chain disease, since in the early stages the cells of the lymphoplasmacytic infiltrate contain a monoclonal α-heavy chain in their cytoplasm, without a light chain. This infiltrate is originally reactive, the response of some cases to tetracycline treatment supporting a probable infectious origin (Asselah *et al.*, 1983). The disease may evolve into an overt B-cell lymphoma (Galian *et al.*, 1977) of low or high grade, and often the two components may coexist. The same immunohistochemical staining pattern for α chain has been demonstrated on the small lymphoplasmacytic cells and the

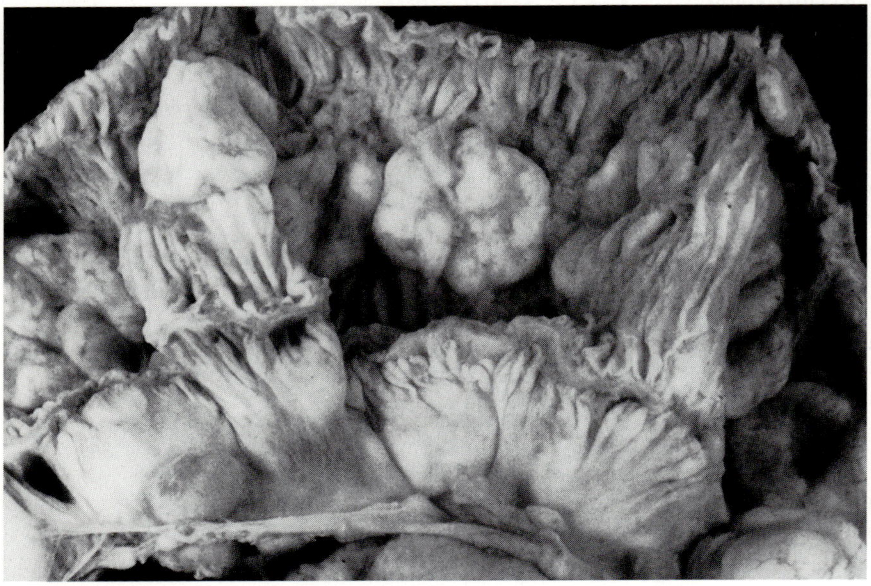

Figure 26.9 *Malignant lymphoma; multiple tumours, polypoid and sessile.*

large blastic cells, suggesting a common origin (Pangalis and Rappaport, 1977). A minority of cases express monotypic light chain.

IPSID presents with a diffuse uninterrupted thickening of a long segment of the proximal part of the small intestine (Nassar *et al.*, 1978). Three stages of the disease have been described: in stage A, the lesion is confined to the mucosa, and consists of mature plasma cells and centrocyte-like lymphocytes; in stage C, it corresponds to a high-grade immunoblastic lymphoma, with frequent plasmacytic differentiation and involvement of mesenteric lymph nodes; and stage B is between the two.

The clinical course is typically prolonged and fatal, the lymphoma remaining confined to the abdomen for many years. Death occurs as a complication of malabsorption, cachexia or of the tumour.

Follicular lymphoma

Follicular lymphoma is rare in the gastrointestinal tract, with a predilection for the terminal ileum, where it presents as multiple mucosal polyps. Expression of the bcl-2 protein can be useful in the differential diagnosis with prominent lymphoid hyperplasia (LeBrun *et al.*, 1992).

Mantle cell lymphoma

Mantle cell lymphoma is formed by a monotonous population of medium-sized lymphoid cells that can involve any part of the gastrointestinal tract, but is usually located in the ileo-caecal region. The most common presentation is that of small polypoid masses throughout the bowel, known as lymphomatoid polyposis (O'Briain *et al.*, 1989), a term first used by Cornes (1960) to describe a polypoid mucosal involvement of long segments of the gastrointestinal tract by lymphoma. Various types of lymphomas can produce this clinical presentation, with mantle cell and follicular lymphomas being the most frequent (Moynihan *et al.*, 1996), and it is more appropriate to classify each case according to the standard lymphoma classification (Chan, 1996).

Burkitt's lymphoma

The non-endemic form of Burkitt's lymphoma is a rare disease, more frequently encountered in Africa and the Middle East than in Western countries (Anaissie *et al.*, 1985). Children are usually affected, and the disease is often located in the small bowel with a predilection for the ileum and the ileo-caecal valve (van Krieken *et al.*, 1992). The morphology of the tumour is characteristic, with a monotonous population of medium-sized tumour cells, a high mitotic rate and a prominent 'starry-sky' pattern owing to the presence of benign macrophages. The clinical course is aggressive and chemotherapy is the treatment of choice.

T-CELL NON-HODGKIN'S LYMPHOMAS

T-cell malignant lymphomas are less frequent in the gastrointestinal tract than their B-cell counterparts. They represent 34 per cent of small intestinal lymphomas and 83 per cent are high-grade tumours (Domizio *et al.*, 1993).

In the small intestine, T-cell lymphomas are usually associated with malabsorption and are referred to as *enteropathy-associated T-cell lymphomas* (EATCL) (O'Farrelly *et al.*, 1986). However, cases without enteropathy have also been reported (Chott *et al.*, 1992; Domizio *et al.*, 1993), so in the REAL classification the term *intestinal T-cell lymphoma with or without enteropathy* was proposed rather than EATCL (Harris *et al.*, 1994). They may present as jejunal ulcers, which may perforate, or as a tumour mass. Histologically, a variable admixture of small, medium and large or anaplastic tumour cells may be present, associated with a high content of intraepithelial T cells in the adjacent mucosa. Villous atrophy may also be present and the development of the lymphoma as a complication of coeliac disease is now generally accepted (for a review, *see* Isaacson, 1995). Considered for a long time as malignant histiocytosis, the neoplastic cells have a characteristic T-cell phenotype (CD3+, CD8+/–, CD103+), favouring an intraepithelial T-cell origin of these tumours (Spenser *et al.*, 1988; Chott *et al.*, 1992). A spectrum of cytological atypia and degree of infiltration exist, ranging from intramucosal spread of small tumour cells to neoplastic tumours composed of CD30+ pleomorphic cells (Schmitt-Gräff *et al.*, 1996). The clinical course is aggressive and death usually occurs from multifocal intestinal perforation caused by refractory malignant ulcers.

T-cell lymphoma associated with eosinophilia is a rare, distinctive type of small intestinal lymphoma of middle-aged and elderly patients (Shepherd *et al.*, 1987). The jejunal lesions predominate, may be multiple, and present either as ulcerated tumour-like masses or as diffuse areas of mucosal 'cobblestoning', ulceration and serosal fibrosis, reminiscent of Crohn's disease. Tumour cells are large and pleomorphic, and may be rare. Eosinophils predominate in the inflammatory infiltrate and their presence has been considered secondary to the secretion of a chemotactic agent by the tumour cells. Complete local surgical excision is the treatment of choice.

HODGKIN'S DISEASE

Primary gastrointestinal tract Hodgkin's disease is a rarity, and a localization in the small bowel is exceptional, with very few cases reported in the literature (Lewin *et al.*, 1978; Manning, 1987). Most of the cases reported in the past were examples of B- or T-cell lymphomas, as proven later by immunohistochemistry.

A diagnosis of gastrointestinal tract Hodgkin's disease should always be supported by both classical histopathologic features and a typical immunohistochemical profile (Devaney and Jaffe, 1991).

Post-transplant lymphoproliferative disorders

The post-transplant lymphoproliferative disorders (PTLDs) represent a spectrum of lymphoid proliferations occurring in a setting of exogenous immunosuppression following solid organ or bone marrow transplantation. They range from early lesions, corresponding to polymorphic, polyclonal lesions resembling a viral infection, to monomorphic monoclonal proliferations consistent with non-Hodgkin's lymphomas, usually of B-cell origin and EBV associated (for reviews, *see* Swerdlow, 1992; Harris *et al.*, 1997). Gastrointestinal involvement was of the order of 12–21 per cent in various reported series, with a predominance of multiple lesions of the distal part of the small bowel (Nalesnic, 1990). Primary treatment includes surgical resection of the lesion and reduction of the immunosuppression.

True histiocytic tumours

Most of the tumours designated in the past as 'histiocytic' are now classified as B- or T-cell lymphomas as demonstrated by immunohistochemistry. Malignancies of true histiocytic origin, while very rare, do exist in the small bowel (Milchgrub *et al.*, 1992; Kamel *et al.*, 1995). They occur in middle-aged patients, causing intestinal obstruction. The neoplastic cells demonstrate histological evidence of histiocytic lineage, and an immunohistochemical profile of histiocytes or of interdigitating reticulum cells (Miettinen *et al.*, 1993).

Follicular dendritic cell tumours

These are extremely rare tumours and can present as a small bowel mass (Hollowood *et al.*, 1995). They display a biphasic pattern, composed of large cells with indistinct cytoplasmic borders, admixed with spindle cells presenting a storiform or fascicular pattern, and associated with numerous small T lymphocytes. The characteristic immunohistochemical profile, positive for CD21 and CD35 and negative for cytokeratin, permits the formal identification of the tumour that has a significant recurrence and metastatic potential (Chan *et al.*, 1997).

Granulocytic sarcoma

Granulocytic sarcoma may present as a small bowel mass, preceding the development of acute granulocytic leukaemia (Brugo *et al.*, 1975). A bacterial infection may also mimic this condition (Kraemer *et al.*, 1981) and should be ruled out by special stains. A cytogenetic–clinicopathologic association of a small bowel presentation of granulocytic sarcoma, with acute myelomonocytic leukaemia with abnormal eosinophils and inversion of chromosome 16, has been established (Russell *et al.*, 1988; Hamilton *et al.*, 1992).

Lymphoid hyperplasia

This condition is characterized by large reactive germinal centres and a diffuse infiltrate of lymphoid cells and eosinophils, which can extend through the muscularis propria. It has been a cause of confusion, mainly in the past when the term 'pseudolymphoma' was used (Jacobs, 1963). The ileo-caecal region is the most common location, with abdominal pain or a palpable mass as presenting symptoms. The bowel wall is usually thickened and may be accompanied by mesenteric lymphadenopathy. There may be close morphological resemblance to a low-grade lymphoma of the MALT type. Immunohistochemistry can demonstrate polyclonality for light chains, proving the reactive nature of the process (Rubin and Isaacson, 1990). Focal lymphoid hyperplasia is more common in children, and it can lead to intussusception (Montgomery and Popek, 1994).

SECONDARY TUMOURS

Secondary tumours of the small intestine may be the consequence of either direct extension of tumours of neighbouring organs, or of metastases of organs or tissues located at a distance from the gut. Clinically, in both conditions, obstructive signs are the most frequent, followed by anaemia, pain or abdominal discomfort; ascites may be frequent.

Direct extension

The duodenum is frequently involved by carcinoma of the pancreas, stomach and biliary tract. The jejunum and the ileum may be implicated by tumours of the colon, bladder and female genital organs.

Metastases

Although it is classically assumed that small intestinal metastases are rare, it appears from our data and the comparison with those of the literature that they are not uncommon (Widgren, 1995).

Table 26.3 *The frequency of small intestinal metastases from various organs.*[a] *A comparison with data in the literature*

Organ/tissue of origin	Total primaries	Number with metastases	Data in the literature (%)
Lung/bronchi	1217	39 (3.2 per cent)	2–11
Melanomas	72	23 (32 per cent)	58
Lymphomas	230	19 (8.2 per cent)	—
Colon and rectum	742	19 (2.6 per cent)	0.75
Ovaries	170	12 (7 per cent)	70–89
Stomach	370	11 (2.9 per cent)	12.8–37.9
Leukaemias	340	10 (2.9 per cent)	14.8–25
Pancreas	333	9 (2.7 per cent)	3.8–9.3
Breast	489	8 (1.6 per cent)	1–18
Gallbladder and bile duct	138	6 (4.3 per cent)	4–32.8

[a]Material from the University Department of Pathology, Geneva: 16 814 necropsies performed between July 1971 and December 1989. (Reprinted with permission of Professor Richard Whitehead and Harcourt Brace & Co., Australia from *Rare and secondary tumours*, 1995, R. Whitehead (ed.), Ch. 40, Part II, Churchill Livingstone.)

When intramural, submucosal or mucosal, metastases form nodules or masses, which are sessile or pedunculated. Sometimes necrosis, fistulae or perforations with peritonitis may occur. Adenocarcinomas may be mucoid, grey and translucent. The origins of the metastatic disease are shown in Table 26.3. It appears that proportionally malignant melanoma is the most frequent cause of intestinal metastases (Fig. 26.10), followed by tumours of the lungs, ovaries, stomach and colorectum, pancreas and breast. Immunohistochemistry may be helpful in distinguishing the origin of the tumour. Histologically, the diagnosis is not a major problem, especially if the site of the primary tumour of the patient is known. However, an ulcerated mucosal metastasis may mimic a primary tumour.

OTHER POLYPOID LESIONS

Inflammatory fibroid polyp

Inflammatory fibroid polyp (IFP) is an infrequent tumour-like condition, formerly known as eosinophilic granuloma, which may be found in various parts of the digestive tract (Kolodziejczyk *et al.*, 1993; Widgren and Cox, 1997), including the small intestine. Among odd locations, two cases situated in continent ileal pouches have been described (Tysk *et al.*, 1994; Widgren and Cox, 1997). It may appear as a polyp or as an intraparietal mass of a size between 1 and 12 cm. On microscopy, it is made up of a fibroblast-like cellular

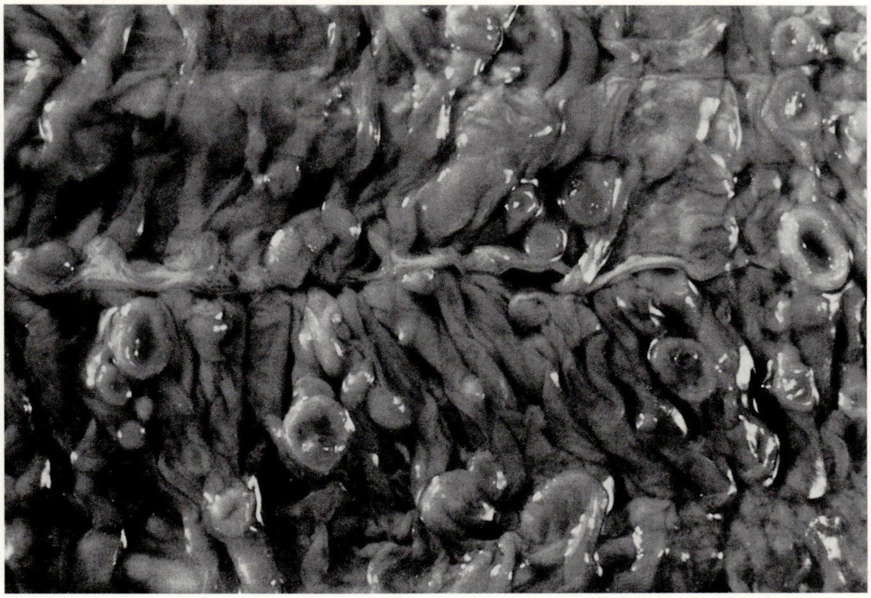

Figure 26.10 *Multiple metastases of malignant melanoma with polypoid and buttercup appearance. (Reprinted with permission of Professor Richard Whitehead and Harcourt Brace & Co., Australia from* Rare and secondary tumours, *1995, R. Whitehead (ed.), Ch. 40, Part II, Churchill Livingstone.)*

population, with scattered lymphocytes, plasma cells, and often numerous eosinophils, in a myxoid or collagenized stroma with a prominent vascular component. Myofibroblasts are also present (Widgren and Pizzolato, 1987; Kolodziejczyk *et al.*, 1993). IFP is considered as a peculiar type of granulation tissue and is an entirely benign condition. The treatment is merely surgical by single resection of the mass.

Brunner's glands hyperplasia

Brunner's glands hyperplasia (BGH) is a rare condition found mostly in the first part of the duodenum. It is considered by various authors to be either a hamartoma or an adenoma; it may cause haemorrhages. Endoscopically and microscopically, BGH appears with two patterns, either as single or multiple sessile polyps, or as diffuse small mucosal elevations. BGH is composed of lobules of glands that appear normal, separated by smooth muscle bands. In rare cases of larger polyps, the diagnosis between hyperplasia and adenoma may be difficult to establish. The aetiology is not known, but BGH is found in association with high gastric acid secretion in renal failure, duodenitis or hypergastrinaemia (Järvinen, 1991).

Heterotopic tissues in the small bowel

Heterotopia is the presence of a particular tissue where it is normally not found. It has to be distinguished from metaplasia, which is a change of one type of tissue into another, usually as the result of tissue injury (inflammation or erosion). Gastric and pancreatic heterotopias are the most common ones, and are found mainly in the duodenum and in Meckel's diverticulum.

GASTRIC HETEROTOPIA

Gastric heterotopia (GH) is typically found in the first part of the duodenum in 1–3 per cent of endoscopies, where it appears as few or multiple nodules, pink to red, less than 1 cm in diameter. They may be found incidentally in biopsies or in the duodenal cuff of gastric resection specimens. When small, they are clinically silent; larger nodules may produce symptoms, such as bleeding and, less often, obstruction. Histologically, they are composed of clusters of normal-appearing fundic mucosa with parietal and chief cells. GH is considered as a developmental abnormality. It should be distinguished from gastric metaplasia of the duodenum characterized by the presence of gastric-type goblet cells covering a part or the whole surface of duodenal villi, which is now recognized as one of the histological features of the duodenitis often associated with duodenal ulcer. Dysplasia or malignant change in GH are not known. Thus there is no treatment, apart from resection of the larger nodules.

PANCREATIC HETEROTOPIA

Pancreatic heterotopia (PH) is not uncommon. It may be found in 0.6–14 per cent of autopsies, depending on the pathologist's diligence. It is a remnant of the pancreas after rotation of the foregut during the embryologic development. Radiologically, endoscopically and macroscopically, PH presents as a single hemispherical sessile nodule in the wall of the duodenum, often with a superficial dimple (umbilication), of yellowish to tan colour, which may be mistaken for a stromal or neuroendocrine tumour. The size may attain 3–4 cm, but it is mostly an incidental histological finding. Microscopically, it is composed of regular pancreatic lobules, canaliculi (sometimes cystically dilated), which may lead to the lumen of the duodenum at the level of the umbilication. Islets of Langerhans may be present. No documented case of carcinoma arising in ectopic pancreatic tissue has been reported in the literature (Fenoglio-Preiser *et al.*, 1990). Endoscopic or surgical resection is the treatment of choice.

Juvenile polyposis syndrome

Juvenile polyposis syndrome (JPS) is a very rare, ill-defined condition (Jass *et al.*, 1988; Shepherd and Bussey, 1990). Multiple juvenile polyps appear during the first and second decade of life with a predilection for the colon and rectum, although sometimes the whole gastrointestinal tract is affected, including the small bowel. Their true nature is controversial, considered either as hamartomatous or inflammatory. The familial JPS is an autosomal dominant condition. There is an association with increased incidence of colorectal cancer, but no case of small intestinal carcinoma has been reported (Jass *et al.*, 1988).

Peutz–Jeghers syndrome

Peutz–Jeghers syndrome (PJS) is a rare condition with a familial autosomal dominance and variable penetrance, presenting at an early age and characterized by mucocutaneous pigmentation associated with gastrointestinal tract hamartomatous polyps. The polyps are located throughout the gastrointestinal tract, with a predominance in the jejunum and ileum, producing abdominal pain, mostly due to intussusception or obstruction, warranting repeated resections throughout the patient's lifetime. These operations may in turn be responsible for adhesions with obstructive episodes (Franzin *et al.*, 1995). Macroscopically, there are numerous polyps (from a few up to about

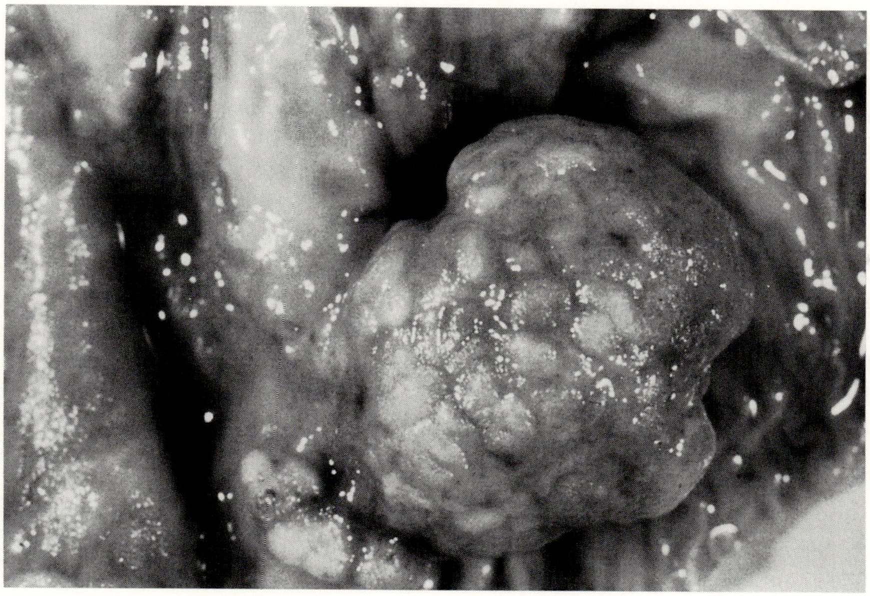

Figure 26.11 *Peutz–Jeghers polyp; macroscopical appearance. (Courtesy of Professor F. Gloor, St Gallen, Switzerland.)*

100), showing a coarse lobulation (Fig. 26.11). Microscopically, the most characteristic feature is the branching of smooth muscle bundles in a tree-like fashion, extending from the muscularis mucosae into the branches of the polyp. These villus-like structures are covered with a normal-appearing mucosa, and glands sometimes situated between muscle fibres (misplaced epithelium) may closely mimic invasive malignancy (Shepherd and Bussey, 1990) (Plate 26.10). This pattern must be distinguished from true adenocarcinoma developing in PJS (*see* earlier text in section entitled 'Epithelial tumours').

Other rare polyposis syndromes

COWDEN'S DISEASE

Cowden's disease, also known as multiple hamartoma syndrome, is a rare autosomal dominant inherited disorder and about 130 cases have been described (Haibach *et al.*, 1992). It is characterized by numerous cutaneous lesions (trichilemmomas, papules, molluscum pendulum) associated with oral modifications (pebble tongue, papillomas, fibromas). About 35 per cent of patients have polyps of the digestive tract, mostly hamartomatous, similar to those of PJS (Marra *et al.*, 1994). Adenomas are usually not found. In eight members of two Geneva families, hamartomatous polyps in the stomach and colon, juvenile polyps in the duodenum and colon, fundic gastric heterotopia in the duodenum and a lipomatous polyp in the colon were observed (Laugier *et al.*, 1979; Hauser *et al.*, 1980). Until recently, molecular genetic analyses have not shown DNA amplification or rearrangement (Williard *et al.*, 1992). It is important to recognize this syndrome, as breast tumours, both benign and malignant, and thyroid lesions may be found in 30–50 per cent and 67 per cent, respectively, of affected patients (Williard *et al.*, 1992; Schrager *et al.*, 1998).

CRONKHITE–CANADA SYNDROME

Cronkhite–Canada syndrome is a rare, sporadic, non-familial, non-neoplastic polyposis located in the stomach, the small intestine and the colon, associated with protein loss, diarrhoea, alopecia, nail dystrophy and skin pigmentation, occurring at the seventh decade of life. The gastrointestinal tract polyps are often indistinguishable from those in juvenile polyposis. The association with dysplasia and colorectal cancer is controversial. The morbidity and mortality are severe, mainly due to nutritional deficiency.

Acknowledgements The authors would like to thank: Dr Rudolf Peter Baumann, Director of the Institut Neuchâtelois d'Anatomie Pathologique, for logistical support; Dr Jeremiah N. Cox, FRCPath., for reviewing the manuscript and for friendly criticism; Professor Jacques Diebold for reviewing the section on lymphomas; Dr Reymond de Peyer for providing the endoscopical pictures; our colleagues at the Registre Genevois des Tumeurs, Dr Christine Bouchardy (Director), Dr Myriana Obradovic and Mr Gerald Fioretta, for providing epidemiological data; Mrs Isabelle Gerardi, Mrs Elisabeth Colin and Mrs Alberte Politchouk for secretarial work; Mrs Barbara Borer for help with the literature search; and Mr Jean-Claude Rumbeli and Mr Etienne Denkinger for the photographs.

REFERENCES

Al-Bahrani, Z.R., Al-Mondhiry, H., Bakir, F., Al-Saleem, T. 1983: Clinical and pathological subtypes of primary intestinal lymphoma. Experience with 132 patients over a 14-year period. *Cancer* 52, 1666–72.

Al-Mondhiry, H. 1986: Primary lymphomas of the small intestine: East–West contrast. *American Journal of Hematology* 22, 89–105.

Anaissie, E., Geha, S., Allam, C., Jabbour, J., Khalyl, M., Salem, P. 1985: Burkitt's lymphoma in the Middle East. A study of 34 cases. *Cancer* 56, 2539–43.

Asselah, F., Slavin, G., Sowter, G., Asselah, H. 1983: Immunoproliferative small intestinal disease in Algerians. I. Light microscopic and immunohistochemical studies. *Cancer* 52, 227–37.

Basson, M.C., Modlin, I.M., Flynn, S.D. 1992: Current clinical and pathologic perspectives on gastric stromal tumors. *Surgery, Gynecology and Obstetrics* 175, 477–89.

Bridge, M.F., Perzin K.H. 1975: Primary adenocarcinoma of the jejunum and ileum. *Cancer* 36, 1876–87.

Brugo, E.A., Larkin, E., Molina-Escobar, J., Costanzi, J. 1975: Primary granulocytic sarcoma of the small bowel. *Cancer* 35, 1333–40.

Burt, R.W. 1991: Familial risk and colorectal cancer. *Gastroenterology Clinics of North America* 25, 793–805.

Capella, C., Heitz, P.U., Höfler, H. *et al.* 1994: Revised classification of neuroendocrine tumours of the lung, pancreas and gut. *Digestion* 55(Suppl. 3), 11–23.

Capella, C., Heitz, P.U., Höfler, H. *et al.* 1995: Revised classification of neuroendocrine tumours of the lung, pancreas and gut. *Virchows Archiv* 425, 547–60.

Cerf-Bensussan, N., Jarry, A., Brousse, N. *et al.* 1987: A monoclonal antibody (HML-1) defining a novel membrane molecule present on human intestinal lymphocytes. *European Journal of Immunology* 17, 1279–85.

Chadwick, E.G., Connor, E.J., Guerra Handon, C. *et al.* 1990: Tumors of smooth-muscle origin in HIV-infected children. *JAMA* 263, 3182–4.

Chan, J.K.C. 1996: Gastrointestinal lymphomas: an overview with emphasis on new findings and diagnostic problems. *Seminars in Diagnostic Pathology* 13, 260–96.

Chan, J.K., Fletcher, C.D., Nayler, S.J., Cooper, K. 1997: Follicular dendritic cell sarcoma. Clinicopathologic analysis of 17 cases suggesting a malignant potential higher than currently recognized. *Cancer* 79, 294–313.

Chott, A., Dragosics, B., Radaszkiewicz, T. 1992: Peripheral T-cell lymphomas of the intestine. *American Journal of Pathology* 141, 1361–71.

Clayton, F., Clayton, C.H. 1997: Gastrointestinal pathology in HIV-infected patients. *Gastroenterology Clinics of North America* 26, 191–240.

Cochet, B., Carrel, J., Desbaillets, L., Widgren, S. 1979: Peutz–Jeghers syndrome associated with gastrointestinal carcinoma. Report of two cases in a family. *Gut* 20, 169–75.

Cornes, J.S. 1960: Multiple lymphomatous polyposis of the gastrointestinal tract. *Cancer* 14, 249–57.

Day, D.W., Dixon, M.F. 1995: *Biopsy pathology of the oesophagus, stomach and duodenum*, 2nd edn. London: Chapman and Hall Medical.

Dayal, Y. 1991: Neuroendocrine cells and their proliferative lesions. In Norris, T.H. (ed.), *Pathology of the colon, small intestine and anus*, 2nd edn. Contemporary Issues in Surgical Pathology, Vol. 17. New York: Churchill Livingstone, 305–65.

Desa, L.A.J., Bridger, J., Grace, P.A. *et al.* 1991: Primary jejunoileal tumors: a review of 45 cases. *World Journal of Surgery* 15, 81–7.

Devaney, K., Jaffe E.S. 1991: The surgical pathology of gastrointestinal Hodgkin's disease. *American Journal of Clinical Pathology* 95, 794–801.

DiSario, J.A., Burt, R.W., Vargas, H., McWhorter, W.P. 1994: Small bowel cancer: epidemiological and clinical characteristics from a population-based registry. *American Journal of Gastroenterology* 89, 699–701.

Domizio, P., Owen, R.A., Shepherd, N.A., Talbot, I.C., Norton, A.J. 1993: Primary lymphoma of the small intestine. A clinicopathological study of 119 cases. *American Journal of Surgical Pathology* 17, 429–42.

Dragosics, B., Bauer, P., Radaszkiewicz, T. 1985: Primary gastrointestinal non-Hodgkin's lymphomas. A retrospective clinicopathologic study of 150 cases. *Cancer* 55, 1060–73.

Fenoglio-Preiser, C.M., Noffsinger, A.E. 1995: Epithelial tumours and tumour-like conditions. In Whitehead R. (ed.), *Gastrointestinal and oesophageal pathology*, 2nd edn. Edinburgh: Churchill Livingstone, Ch. 41, Part I, 863–92.

Fenoglio-Preiser, C.M., Pascal, R.R., Perzin, K.H. 1990: Tumors of the intestine. In *Atlas of tumor pathology*, 2nd series, fascicle 27. Washington, D.C.: Armed Forces Institute of Pathology.

Franzin, G., Zamboni, G., Scarpa, A. 1995: Polyposis syndromes. In Whitehead R. (ed.), *Gastrointestinal and oesophageal pathology*, 2nd edn. Edinburgh: Churchill Livingstone, Ch. 41, Part II, 892–909.

Freeman, C., Berg, J.W., Cutler, S.J. 1972: Occurrence and prognosis of extranodal lymphomas. *Cancer* 29, 252–60.

Galian, A., Lecestre, M.J., Scotto, J. *et al.* 1977: Pathological study of alpha-chain disease with special emphasis on evolution. *Cancer* 39, 2081–101.

Gander, M., Leyvraz, S., Widgren, S. 1993: Adenocarcinoma of the small bowel associated with coeliac disease. *Bulletin Suisse du Cancer* 13, 141–3.

Gilmour, H.M. 1995: The large intestine: Crohn's disease. In Whitehead R. (ed.), *Gastrointestinal and oesophageal pathology*, 2nd edn. Edinburgh: Churchill Livingstone, Ch. 27, Part II, 604–13.

Gilson, T.P., Sollenberger, L.L. 1992: Adenocarcinoma of an ileostomy in a patient with familial adenomatous polyposis, report of a case. *Diseases of Colon and Rectum* 35, 261–5.

Gore, R.M. 1997: Small bowel cancer, clinical and pathologic features. *Radiologic Clinics of North America* 35, 351–60.

Haibach, H., Burns, T.W., Carlson, H.E. *et al.* 1992: Multiple hamartoma syndrome (Cowden's disease) associated with renal cell carcinoma and primary neuroendocrine carcinoma of the skin (Merkel cell carcinoma). *American Journal of Clinical Pathology* 97, 705–12.

Halsted, C.H. 1996: The many faces of celiac disease. *New England Journal of Medicine* 334, 1190–1.

Hamilton, M.S., Sheperd, P., Porter, J., Richards, J.D. 1992: Granulocytic sarcoma of small intestine and brain are associated with acute myelomonocytic leukaemia with abnormal eosinophils and inversion of chromosome 16. *Leukemia Lymphoma* 8, 409–13.

Harris, N.L., Ferry, J.A., Swerdlow, S.H. 1997: Posttransplant lymphoproliferative disorders: summary of Society for Hematopathology Workshop. *Seminars in Diagnostic Pathology* 14, 8–14.

Harris, N.L., Jaffe E.S., Stein, H. *et al.* 1994: A revised European–American classification of lymphoid neoplasms: a proposal from the International Lymphoma Study Group. *Blood* 84, 1361–92.

Hauser, H., Ody, B., Plojoux, O., Wettstein, P. 1980: Radiological findings in multiple hamartoma syndrome (Cowden disease), a report of three cases. *Radiology* 137, 317–23.

Herrmann, R., Panahon, A.M., Barcos, M.P., Walsh, D., Stutzman, L. 1980: Gastrointestinal involvement in non-Hodgkin's lymphoma. *Cancer* 46, 215–22.

Hollowood, K., Stamp, G., Zouvani, I., Fletcher, C.D. 1995: Extranodal follicular dendritic cell sarcoma of the gastrointestinal tract. Morphologic, immunohistochemical and ultrastructural analysis of two cases. *American Journal of Clinical Pathology* 103, 90–7.

IARC 1997: *Cancer incidence in five continents,* Vol. VII. Lyon: IARC.

Ioachim, H.L., Adsay, V., Giancotti, F.R. *et al.* 1995: Kaposi's sarcoma of internal organs. A multiparameter study of 86 cases. *Cancer* 75, 1376–85.

Isaacson, P.G. 1995: Intestinal lymphoma and enteropathy. *Journal of Pathology* 177, 111–13.

Isaacson, P.G., Wright, D.H. 1983: Malignant lymphoma of mucosa-associated lymphoid tissue. A distinctive type of B-cell lymphoma. *Cancer* 52, 1410–16.

Isaacson, P.G., Spenser, J., Wright, D.H. 1988: Classifying primary gut lymphomas. *Lancet* 2, 1148–9.

Jacobs, D.S. 1963: Primary gastric malignant lymphoma and pseudolymphoma. *American Journal of Clinical Pathology* 40, 379–94.

Jagelman, D.G., DeCosse, J.J., Bussey, H.J.R. 1988: Upper gastrointestinal cancer in familial adenomatous polyposis. *Lancet* 1, 1149–51.

Järvinen, H.J. 1991: Other gastrointestinal polyps. *World Journal of Surgery* 15, 50–6.

Jass, J.R., Sobin, L.H. 1989: *Histological typing of intestinal tumours*, 2nd edn. Berlin: Springer-Verlag.

Jass, J.R., Williams, C.B., Bussey, H.J.R., Morson, B.C. 1988: Juvenile polyposis – a precancerous condition. *Histopathology* 13, 619–30.

Jenkins, D., Balsitis, M., Gallivan, S. *et al.* 1997: Guidelines for the initial biopsy diagnosis of suspected chronic idiopathic inflammatory bowel disease. The British Society of Gastroenterology Initiative. *Journal of Clinical Pathology* 50, 93–105.

Kamel, O.W., Gocke, C.D., Kell, D.L., Cleary, M.L., Warnke, R.A. 1995: True histiocytic lymphoma: a study of 12 cases based on current definition. *Leukemia Lymphoma* 18, 81–6.

Kempson, R.L. 1992: The time is now. Checklists for surgical pathology reports. Editorial. *Archives of Pathology and Laboratory Medicine* 116, 1107–8.

Kempson, R.L., Hendrickson, M.R. 1995: Gastrointestinal stromal (smooth muscle) tumours. In Whitehead R. (ed.), *Gastrointestinal and oesophageal pathology*, 2nd edn. Edinburgh: Churchill Livingstone, Ch. 35, 727–39.

Khojasteh, A., Haghshenass, M., Haghighi, P. 1983: Immunoproliferative small intestinal disease. A 'Third-World lesion'. *New England Journal of Medicine* 308, 1401–5.

Klöppel, G. 1997: Classification of neuroendocrine tumors. *Verhandlungen der Deutschen Gesellschaft für Pathologie* 81, 111–17.

Knowles, D.M., Cesarman, E. 1997: The Kaposi's sarcoma-associated herpesvirus (human herpesvirus-8) in Kaposi's sarcoma, malignant lymphoma, and other diseases. *Annals of Oncology* 8(Suppl 2), S123–9.

Kolodziejczyk P., Yao, T., Tsuneyoshi M. 1993: Inflammatory fibroid polyp of the stomach. A special reference to an immunohistochemical profile of 42 cases. *American Journal of Surgical Pathology* 17, 1159–68.

Konishi, F., Morson, B.C. 1982: Pathology of colorectal adenomas: a colonoscopic survey. *Journal of Clinical Pathology* 35, 830–41.

Kraemer, B.B., Foucar, K., Osborn, B., Butler, J.J. 1981: Bacterial infection simulating granulocytic sarcoma of the small bowel. *American Journal of Clinical Pathology* 76, 227–31.

Kusumoto, H., Yoshitake, H., Mochida, K. *et al.* 1992: Adenocarcinoma in Meckel's diverticulum: report of a case and review of 30 cases in the English and Japanese literature. *American Journal of Gastroenterology* 87, 910–13.

Lashner, B.A. 1992: Risk factors for small bowel cancer in Crohn's disease. *Digestive Diseases and Sciences* 37, 1179–84.

Laugier, P., Kuffer, R., Olmos, L. *et al.* 1979: Maladie de Cowden: à propos de 8 cas familiaux. *Annales de Dermatologie et Vénéréologie (Paris)* 106, 453–63.

LeBrun, D.P., Kamel, O.W., Cleary, M.L., Dorfman, R.F., Warnke, R.A. 1992: Follicular lymphoma of the gastrointestinal tract. Pathologic features in 31 cases and bcl-2 oncogenic protein expression. *American Journal of Pathology* 140, 1327–35.

Levine, A.M. 1993: AIDS-related malignancies: the emerging epidemic. Review. *Journal of the National Cancer Institute* 85, 1382–97.

Lewin, K.J., Ranchod, M., Dorfman, R.F. 1978: Lymphomas of the gastrointestinal tract: a study of 117 cases presenting with gastrointestinal disease. *Cancer* 42, 693–707.

Lewis, B.S, Kornbluth, A., Waye, J.D. 1991: Small bowel tumours: yield of enteroscopy. *Gut* 32, 763–5.

Lioe, T.F., Biggart, J.D. 1990: Primary adenocarcinoma of the jejunum and ileum: clinicopathological review of 25 cases. *Journal of Clinical Pathology* 43, 533–6.

Lowenfels, A.B. 1973: Why are small-bowel tumours so rare? Hypothesis. *Lancet* 1, 24–6.

Lowenfels, A.B. 1978: Does bile promote extra-colonic cancer? Hypothesis. *Lancet* 2, 239–41.

Lynch, H.T., Smyrk, T., Lynch J. 1997: An update of HNPCC (Lynch syndrome). *Cancer Genetics and Cytogenetics* 93, 84–99.

Lynch, P.M. 1995: Polyposis syndromes. In Haubrich, W.S., Schaffner, F. (eds), *Bockus: Gastroenterology*, Vol. 2, 5th edn. Philadelphia: W.B. Saunders Co, 1731–43.

Ma, C.K., De Peralta, M.N., Amin, M.B. *et al.* 1997: Small intestinal stromal tumors: a clinicopathologic study of 20 cases with immunohistochemical assessment of cell differentiation and the prognostic role of proliferation antigens. *American Journal of Clinical Pathology* 108, 641–51.

MacGowan, D.J.L., Hourihane, D.O'B., Tanner, W.A., O'Morain, C. 1996: Duodeno-jejunal adenocarcinoma as a first presentation of coeliac disease. *Journal of Clinical Pathology* 49, 602–4.

Manning, R.J. 1987: Hodgkin's disease presenting as diffuse nonspecific inflammation of small bowel. *Journal of Clinical Gastroenterology* 9, 701–4.

Marra, G., Armelao, F., Vecchio, F.M. *et al.* 1994: Cowden's disease with extensive gastrointestinal polyposis. *Journal of Clinical Gastroenterology* 18, 42–7.

Marra, G., Boland, C.R. 1995: Hereditary nonpolyposis colorectal cancer: the syndrome, the genes, and historical perspectives. *Review Journal of the National Cancer Institute* 87, 1114–25.

Marsch, S.C.U., Heer, M., Sulser, H., Hany A. 1990: Das Adenokarzinom des Dünndarms bei Zöliakie. Kasuistik und Literaturübersicht. *Schweizerische medizinische Wochenschrift* 120, 135–41.

McClain, K.L., Leach, C.T., Jenson, H.B. *et al.* 1995: Association of Epstein–Barr virus with leiomyosarcomas in young people with AIDS. *New England Journal of Medicine* 332, 12–18.

McMunnick, P.J., Nelson, H. 1998: Managing the patient with hereditary nonpolyposis colon cancer. *Current Opinion in Gastroenterology* 14, 21–6.

Meyer, M., Schneider J. 1991: Pathologie des Verdauungstraktes bei HIV-Patienten. *Schweizerische medizinische Wochenschrift* 121, 1308.

Miettinen, M., Fletcher, C.D., Lasota, J. 1993: True histiocytic lymphoma of the small intestine. Analysis of two S-100 protein-positive cases with features of interdigitating reticulum cell sarcoma. *American Journal of Clinical Pathology* 100, 285–92.

Milchgrub, S., Kamel, O.W., Wiley, E., Vuitch, F., Cleary, M.L., Warnke, R.A. 1992: Malignant histiocytic neoplasms of the small intestine. *American Journal of Surgical Pathology* 16, 11–20.

Montgomery, E.A., Popek, E.J. 1994: Intussusception, adenovirus, and children: a brief reaffirmation. *Human Pathology* 25, 169–74.

Morson, B.C., Dawson, I.M.P. 1990a: Reception and examination of biopsy and surgical specimens. In Morson, B.C., Dawson, I.M.P. (eds), *Morson and Dawson's gastrointestinal pathology*, 3rd edn. Oxford: Blackwell Scientific Publications, 3–7.

Morson, B.C., Dawson, I.M.P. 1990b: Malignant epithelial tumours. In *Morson and Dawson's gastrointestinal pathology*, 3rd edn. Oxford: Blackwell Scientific Publications, Ch. 26, 360–71.

Moynihan, M.J., Bast, M.A., Chan, W.C. *et al.* 1996: Lymphomatous polyposis. A neoplasm of either follicular mantle or germinal center cell origin. *American Journal of Surgical Pathology* 20, 442–52.

Nalesnic, M.A. 1990: Involvement of the gastrointestinal tract by Epstein–Barr virus-associated posttransplant lymphoproliferative disorders. *American Journal of Surgical Pathology* 14(Suppl 1), 92–100.

Nassar, V.H., Salem, P.A., Shahid, M.J. *et al.* 1978: 'Mediterranean abdominal lymphoma' or immunoproliferative small intestinal disease. Part II: Pathological aspects. *Cancer* 41, 1340–54.

O'Briain, D.S., Kennedy, M.J., Daly, P.A. *et al.* 1989: Multiple lymphomatous polyposis of the gastrointestinal tract. A clinicopathologically distinctive form of non-Hodgkin's lymphoma of B-cell centrocytic type. *American Journal of Surgical Pathology* 13, 691–9.

O'Farrelly, C., Feighery, C., O'Briain, D.S. *et al.* 1986: Humoral response to wheat protein in patients with coeliac disease and enteropathy associated T cell lymphoma. *British Medical Journal* 293, 908–10.

O'Riordan, B.G., Vilor, M., Herrera, L. 1996: Small bowel tumors: an overview. *Digestive Diseases* 14, 245–57.

Offerhaus, J.G.A., Giardiello, F.M., Krush, A.J. *et al.* 1992: The risk of upper gastrointestinal cancer in familial adenomatous polyposis. *Gastroenterology* 102, 1980–2.

Ouriel, K., Adams, J.T. 1984: Adenocarcinoma of the small intestine. *American Journal of Surgery* 147, 66–71.

Pan, L., Diss, T.C., Cunningham, D., Isaacson, P.G. 1989: The bcl-2 gene in primary B-cell lymphoma of mucosa-associated lymphoid tissue (MALT). *American Journal of Pathology* 135, 7–11.

Pangalis, G.A., Rappaport, H. 1977: Common clonal origin of lymphoplasmacytic proliferation and immunoblastic lymphoma in intestinal α-chain disease. *Lancet* 2, 880.

Perzin, K.H., Bridge, M.F. 1981: Adenomas of the small intestine: a clinicopathologic review of 51 cases and a study of their relationship to carcinoma. *Cancer* 48, 799–819.

Pipeleers-Marichal, M., Donow, C., Heitz, P.U., Klöppel G. 1993: Pathologic aspects of gastrinomas in patients with Zollinger–Ellison syndrome with and without multiple endocrine neoplasia type 1. *World Journal of Surgery* 17, 481–8.

Prévot, S., Néris. J., de Saint Maur, P.O. 1994: Detection of Epstein Barr virus in an hepatic leiomyomatous neoplasm in an adult human immunodeficiency virus 1-infected patient. *Virchows Archiv* 425, 321–5.

Ribeiro, M.B., Greenstein, A.J., Heimann, T.M. *et al.* 1991: Adenocarcinoma of the small intestine in Crohn's disease. *Surgery, Gynecology and Obstetrics* 173, 343–9.

Riddell, R.H., Goldmann, H., Ransohoff, D.F. *et al.* 1983: Dysplasia in inflammatory bowel disease: standardized classification with provisional clinical applications. *Human Pathology* 14, 931–68.

Rosai, J. 1993: Standardized reporting of surgical pathology diagnoses for the major tumour types. *American Journal of Clinical Pathology* 100, 240–55.

Rosai, J. 1995: *Ackerman's surgical pathology*, 8th edn. St Louis: Mosby.

Rubin, A., Isaacson, P.G. 1990: Florid reactive lymphoid hyperplasia of the terminal ileum in adults: a condition bearing a close resemblance to low-grade malignant lymphoma. *Histopathology* 17, 19–26.

Russell, S.J., Giles, F.J., Thompson, D.S., Scanlon, D.J., Walker, H., Richards, J.D. 1988: Granulocytic sarcoma of the small intestine preceding acute myelomonocytic leukemia with abnormal eosinophils and inv (16). *Cancer Genetics and Cytogenetics* 35, 231–5.

Ryan, J.C. 1996: Premalignant conditions of the small intestine. *Seminars in Gastrointestinal Diseases* 7, 88–93.

Sakano, S., Yoshihiro, S., Joko, K. *et al.* 1995: Adenocarcinoma developing in an ileal conduit. *Journal of Urology* 153, 146–8.

Schmitt-Gräff, A., Hummel, M., Zemlin, M. *et al.* 1996: Intestinal T-cell lymphoma: a reassessment of cyto-morphological and phenotypic features in relation to patterns of small bowel remodelling. *Virchows Archiv* 429, 27–36.

Schrager, C.A., Schneider, D., Gruener, A.C. *et al.* 1998: Clinical and pathological features of breast disease in Cowden's syndrome: an underrecognized syndrome with an increased risk of breast cancer. *Human Pathology* 29, 47–53.

Seifert, E., Schulte F., Stolte, M. 1992: Adenoma and carcinoma of the duodenum and papilla of Vater: a clinicopathologic study. *American Journal of Gastroenterology* 87, 37–42.

Sellner, F. 1990: Investigations on the significance of the adenoma–carcinoma sequence in the small bowel. *Cancer* 66, 702–15.

Shanks, J.H., Harris, M., Banerjee, S.S., Eyden, B.P. 1996: Gastrointestinal autonomic nerve tumours: a report of nine cases. *Histopathology* 29, 111–21.

Sheffield, J.P., Talbot, I.C. 1992: Gross examination of the large intestine. ACP Broadsheet 132. *Journal of Clinical Pathology* 45, 751–5.

Shepherd, N.A. 1997: *Pathology section report for members.* London: British Society of Gastroenterology.

Shepherd, N.A., Blackshaw, A.J., Hall, P.A. *et al.* 1987: Malignant lymphoma with eosinophilia of the gastrointestinal tract. *Histopathology* 11, 115–30.

Shepherd, N.A., Bussey, J.H.R. 1990: Polyposis syndromes: an update. In Berry, C.L., Grundmann, E. (eds), *Current topics in pathology*, Vol. 81. Berlin: Springer Verlag, 323–51.

Shepherd, N.A., Quirke P. 1997: Correspondence. *Journal of Clinical Pathology* 50, 881–2.

Soga, J., Tazawa, K. 1971: Pathologic analysis of carcinoids. Histologic re-evaluation of 62 cases. *Cancer* 28, 990–8.

Solcia, E., Fiocca, R., Rindi, G. *et al.* 1995: Endocrine tumors of the small and large intestine. *Pathology Research and Practice* 191, 366–72.

Spenser, J., Cerf-Bensussan, N., Jarry, A. *et al.* 1988: Enteropathy-associated T cell lymphoma (malignant histiocytosis of the intestine) is recognized by a monoclonal antibody (HML-1) that defines a membrane molecule on human mucosal lymphocytes. *American Journal of Pathology* 132, 1–5.

Swerdlow, S.H. 1992: Post-transplant lymphoproliferative disorders: a morphologic, phenotypic and genotypic spectrum of disease. *Histopathology* 20, 373–85.

Swinson, C.M., Slavin, G., Coles, E.C., Booth C.C. 1983: Coeliac disease and malignancy. *Lancet* 1, 111–15.

Talbot, I.C., Price, A.B. 1987: *Biopsy pathology in colorectal disease.* London: Chapman and Hall.

Tysk, C., Schnürer, L.-B., Wickbom, G., 1994: Obstructing inflammatory fibroid polyp in pelvic ileal reservoir after restorative proctocolectomy in ulcerative colitis, report of a case. *Diseases of Colon and Rectum* 37, 1034–7.

UICC 1997: *TNM Classification of malignant tumours*, 5th edn. Sobin, L.H., Wittekind, Ch. (eds) New York: Wiley-Liss.

van Krieken, J.H.J.M., Medeiros, J., Pals, S.T., Raffeld, M., Kluin, P.M. 1992: Diffuse aggressive B-cell lymphomas of the gastrointestinal tract. An immunophenotypic and gene rearrangement analysis of 22 cases. *American Journal of Clinical Pathology* 97, 170–8.

Vasen, H.F.A., Mecklin, J.-P., Meera Khan, P., Lynch, H.T. 1991: The International Collaborative Group on Hereditary Non-Polyposis Colorectal Cancer (ICG-HNPCC). *Diseases of Colon and Rectum* 34, 424–5.

Vinik, A.I., McLeod, M.K., Fig, L.M. *et al.* 1989: Clinical features, diagnosis, and localization of carcinoid tumors and their management. *Gastroenterology Clinics of North America* 18, 865–96.

Wang, C.-Y.E., Schroeter, A.L., Su, W.P.D. 1995: Acquired immunodeficiency syndrome-related Kaposi's sarcoma. *Mayo Clinic Proceedings* 70, 869–79.

Watson, P., Lynch, H.T. 1993: Extracolonic cancer in hereditary nonpolyposis colorectal cancer *Cancer* 71, 677–85.

Weingrad, D.N., Decosse, J.J., Sherlock, P., Straus, D.,

Lieberman, P.H., Filippa, D.A. 1982: Primary gastrointestinal lymphoma: a 30-year review. *Cancer* 49, 1258–65.

Whitehead, R. 1985: *Mucosal biopsy of the gastrointestinal tract*. In Bennington, J.L. (ed.), *Major problems in pathology*, Vol. 3, 3rd edn. Philadelphia: W.B. Saunders Co., xi–xiii.

Whitehead, R. 1995: Other tumours of the small intestine: epithelial tumours. In Whitehead R. (ed.), *Gastrointestinal and oesophageal pathology*, 2nd edn. Edinburgh: Churchill Livingstone, Ch. 40, Part I, 847–9.

WHO 1976: Alpha-chain disease and related lymphoma. *Bulletin WHO* 54, 615–24.

Widgren, S. 1995: Rare and secondary (metastatic) tumours. In Whitehead, R. (ed.), *Gastrointestinal and oesophageal pathology*, 2nd edn. Edinburgh: Churchill Livingstone, Ch. 40, Part II, 849–61.

Widgren, S. 1996: Reporting small intestinal and colonic surgical specimens. Some guidelines for a high quality pathology report. *Acta Endoscopica* 26, 107–18.

Widgren, S., Cox, J.N. 1997: Inflammatory fibroid polyp in a continent ileo-anal pouch after colectomy for ulcerative colitis – case report. *Pathology Research and Practice* 193, 643–7.

Widgren, S., Pizzolato, G.P. 1987: Inflammatory fibroid polyp of the gastrointestinal tract: possible origin in myofibroblasts? A study of twelve cases. *Annales de Pathologie (Paris)* 7, 184–92.

Williams, E.D., Siebenmann, R.E., Sobin, L.H. 1980: *Histological typing of endocrine tumours*. International Histological Classification of Tumours, no. 23. Geneva: WHO.

Williard, W., Borgen, P., Bol, R. *et al*. 1992: Cowden's disease. A case report with analyses at the molecular level. *Cancer* 69, 2969–74.

27

Miscellaneous conditions and small intestinal manifestations of systemic disease

NAJIB Y HABOUBI, NADIM Y HABOUBI, PAUL HOADLEY

RADIATION ENTEROPATHY

Radiation therapy is an important treatment for many solid tumours. When radiation is directed towards the abdomen or pelvis, the malignancy may be controlled or eliminated. However, an accompanying injury to the surrounding intestine may result in a serious short- or long-term morbidity, or mortality. The intestinal complication was first documented only 2 years after Roentgen rays were first used (Walsh, 1897). We can only estimate the magnitude of radiation injury if we realize that approximately 50 per cent of all patients with malignancy will at some time undergo radiation therapy as part of their treatment (Bloomer and Hellman, 1975), irrespective of whether it is curative or palliative.

Radiation-induced intestinal injury occurs clinically in three stages. The first stage is during or immediately after treatment, and is manifested clinically as abdominal pain, diarrhoea or tenesmus. These symptoms usually resolve in 2–6 months. Histologically, they are characterized by the presence of transient epithelial injury, which characteristically shows meganucleosis and eosinophilic abscess, which is followed within weeks by the vascular-type injury that is characterized by destructive vasculopathy, with or without inflammation, and usually with thrombosis of the arteries, arterioles and venules.

The second stage is the chronic stage, which manifests itself after a delayed period of 6–24 months after completion of radiotherapy and has been estimated to occur in approximately 2–5 per cent of patients receiving radiation therapy to their pelvic organs (Russell and Welch, 1979). This is probably on the increase (Allen-Mersh *et al.*, 1986; Galland and Spencer, 1987). It is not known, however, why only a minority of patients progress to the late disease. This phase is characterized by abdominal pain, bleeding, diarrhoea, malabsorption, vomiting and abdominal distension. The diagnosis should be suspected whenever the patient has gastrointestinal symptoms and has a previous history of radiation to the pelvis or abdomen. Absorptive studies such as ^{14}C-labelled bile-acid breath tests and the Schilling test can be useful. Plain x-ray of the abdomen may show dilated intestinal loops with fluid levels. Barium studies show various fissures, such as fistulae, nodular filling defects and fissuring. The most interesting finding is the very low perfusion pattern seen in the affected segment when infused by radio-opaque material (Carr *et al.*, 1984) (Fig. 27.1). Pathologically, there could be ulcerations, stricture formations and sometimes perforations. Histologically, there is significant fibrosis with vascular telangiectasia of the postpapillary venules and significant narrowing of the arterioles, arteries, and medium- and large-sized vessels. Sometimes appearances of bizarre multinucleated giant cells, probably of fibroblastic origin, can occur.

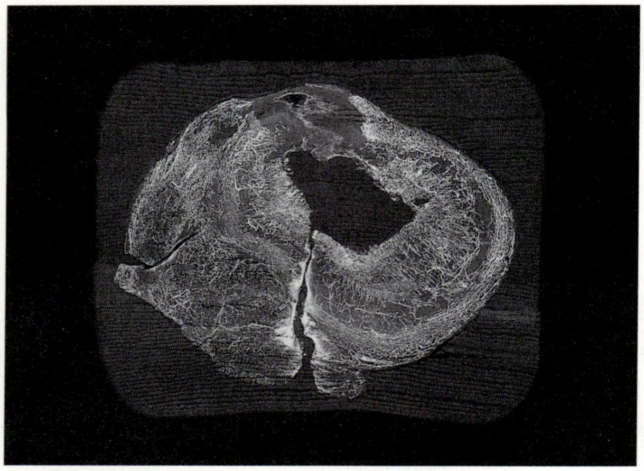

Figure 27.1 *Perfusion study in radiation. This is the small intestine from a case of late-phase radiation disease. There is a segmental loss of perfusion due to occlusive vascular lesions, which are characteristic of the disease. (Courtesy of Professor P.F. Schofield.)*

The third stage is latent injury, which appears after years or decades. This is due to subtle abnormality of the DNA, which may lead, in the future, to a mutation, carcinogenesis and teratogenesis (Pearson *et al.*, 1992).

The predisposing factors for radiation-induced injury include hypertension, atherosclerosis, arterial disease, diabetes, coincident chemotherapy and prior surgery (Schofield, 1989). Surgery is a predisposing factor for radiation-induced disease because adhesions may lead to entrapment of the terminal ileum in the pelvic organs and therefore exposure to a higher dosage of radiation than necessary.

Usually early changes are short and self-limiting. However, supportive measures are desirable and, in children who have had total abdominal radiotherapy for lymphoma or other malignancies, a low-residue, low-fat, no milk and a gluten-free diet regime has been said to improve symptoms (Donaldson *et al.*, 1975).

Medical treatment of small intestinal disease is principally directed towards the correction of any abnormalities that involve the gut, e.g. giving a low-fat diet or cholestyramine or loperamide if diarrhoea develops. Vitamin B_{12} injections should be given periodically if the terminal ileum is involved. Medium-chain triglyceride supplements, and a low-residue, high-calorie liquid diet are other measures that may be of benefit. Surgical treatment is only indicated in cases of fistula formation, perforation, severe hemorrhage or intestinal obstruction.

As far as the treatment for late disease is concerned, there appear to be no successful medical measures that materially affect the progression of late radiation bowel disease. Sulphasalazine, steroids, antifibrinolytic drugs and dietary manipulations both of high- and low-residue diets are still used in the medical management, but there is no objective evidence to support their use (Schofield, 1989). Medical management, therefore, should be largely symptomatic and supportive.

On rare occasions, surgery is necessary for acute enteritis with perforation. Such patients with a free perforation should not have a primary anastomosis because the extent of the disease is difficult to define. A resection with exteriorization of the segment is the safest procedure, leaving reconstruction to be carried out when the acute resection and illness are overcome. In late ileal disease, Carr *et al.* (1984) advocated wide excision of the involved small bowel because of the diffuse nature of the radiation damage. They found it appropriate to resect 50–60 cm of small bowel so that the anastomosis will be well above the dead area and well into the vascularized small bowel. If an adequate resection is carried out, there seems to be no greater risk of leakage than from other small bowel anastomoses with a varied degree of leakage: 0–6 per cent in more recent series (Schofield *et al.*, 1986). The terminal ileum may be involved alone but in a significant minority of cases there is also injury to the sigmoid colon and rectum. It is therefore important in these circumstances to correct the recto-sigmoid lesions at the same time as the ileal lesions are resected because this obstruction would be a factor in increasing the chance of an anastomotic leak. The indications for bypass are rare. Although mobilization of the involved ileum is frequently difficult due to adhesions, it is usually possible with experience and patience.

DRUG-INDUCED DISORDERS

The effect of various medications on the small intestine has received wide publicity in the last two decades. It is not uncommon for symptoms, especially nausea, vomiting, diarrhoea and constipation, to be encountered with various medications.

Non-steroidal anti-inflammatory drugs

Several non-steroidal anti-inflammatory drugs (NSAIDs) can produce characteristic small bowel lesions in animals. In rats, indomethacin leads to multiple small bowel ulcers, mostly seen at the ileum (Kent *et al.*, 1969; Fang *et al.*, 1977). The pathogenesis of these lesions is not very clear. They can, however, be prevented by treatment with prostaglandins and antibiotics. It was suggested that reduction in the mucosal synthesis of prostaglandins induced by NSAIDs disrupts mucosal integrity with a subsequent ulceration and bacterial invasion (Robert and Ansano, 1977; Whittle, 1981; Satoh *et al.*, 1983). This damage is likely to affect the intercellular junction between enterocytes. Long-term treatment with NSAIDs in patients with rheumatoid arthritis and osteoarthritis is associated with inflammation of the small intestine (Bjarnason *et al.*, 1984, 1986). It has been shown by epidemiological and experimental data that NSAIDs are associated with clinically significant gastrointestinal blood and protein loss (Bjarnason *et al.*, 1987).

Pathologically, the changes are inflammation, ulceration, perforation and strictures (Day, 1983; Neoptolemos and Lock, 1983; Saverymuttu *et al.*, 1986).

A 'diaphragm disease' was first described in 1988, affecting the small intestine (Lang *et al.*, 1988). These diaphragms are in fact made up of exaggerated mucosal folds, composed of thin folds of muscularis mucosa and submucosa, which show extensive fibrosis. The muscularis propria is not affected. These diaphragms can occlude the lumen, although this is infrequent. There is no good explanation for the appearances of these lesions but the suggestion by Lang's group is that it is possibly multifactorial. There was a strong correlation between these features and the long history of NSAID prescription. The intestinal diaphragms are difficult to identify at the time of surgery because the serosal surface of the bowel appears normal. On transillumination, however, the diaphragm-like structures may be seen. It is important that the clinician and the pathologist are aware of the possible diagnosis and that the bowel is fixed by formalin insufflation. These changes will appear much more readily when there is proper fixation. These diaphragms can have superficial ulcerations, chronic inflammation, vascular prominence and characteristic submucosal vertical fibrosis. On occasions it could be misdiagnosed as Crohn's disease but the absence of transmural inflammation in diaphragm disease can differentiate between the two conditions.

Drug-induced malabsorption

NEOMYCIN

This drug is poorly absorbed (3–6 per cent) from the gastrointestinal tract, which makes it well suited for its principal use – suppression of bacterial growth in the gut lumen, particularly in patients with hepatic encephalopathy. Early reports (Faloon *et al.*, 1958; Jacobson *et al.*, 1960a, 1962; Hayman *et al.*, 1964) documented reversible malabsorptive defects associated with the oral administration of neomycin. These included depressed absorption of fat, nitrogen, carotene, iron, vitamin B_{12}, xylose and glucose, as well as hypocholesterolaemia. Parenterally administered neomycin in doses of 200 mg daily does not cause malabsorption (Leveille *et al.*, 1963). Hvidt and Kjeldsen (1963) reported that mild steatorrhoea (maximum 20 g fat/day) developed in six out of ten normal men who were taking small doses of neomycin (3 g daily) for 10 days; the stool fat excretion reverted to normal within 1 week afterwards. There is limited evidence to suggest that malabsorption of fat is related to the dose (Rogers *et al.*, 1966) but that malabsorption of xylose is not (Hvidt and Kjeldsen, 1963).

In addition, neomycin causes histological changes in the small bowel mucosa, such as clubbing of intestinal villi, increased lymphocytes and plasma cells in the lamina propria, ballooning of microvilli, and fragmentation of the brush border (Jacobson *et al.*, 1960b; Cain *et al.*, 1968). The pigment seen in the macrophages of the lamina propria is thought to represent cell breakdown products caused by neomycin toxicity (Dobbins *et al.*, 1968). The toxic effect of neomycin is rapid: within 6 hours, a small dose (2 g) can cause histological evidence of damage to intestinal epithelial cells as well as diminished absorption of xylose and sucrose (Keusch *et al.*, 1970). A gluten-free diet or treatment with corticosteroids has no ameliorative effect on the degree of steatorrhoea (Jacobson *et al.*, 1962).

COLCHICINE

The use of colchicine, whether orally or intravenously, as treatment for an attack of acute gouty arthritis is frequently associated with diarrhoea. Ordinarily, this is of little significance because high-dose therapy is maintained for only a few hours and the diarrhoea soon ceases. Gastrointestinal symptoms are much less common with the lower doses of colchicine used on a daily basis to prevent flares. Although the usual prophylactic dosage of colchicine (0.5–1.0 mg/day) does not cause steatorrhoea or megaloblastic anaemia secondary to vitamin B_{12} malabsorption, a reversible malabsorption syndrome does develop in patients who take 1.9–3.9 mg/day (Race *et al.*, 1970). Steatorrhoea occurs and is proportional to the amount of drug used. In addition, abnormal absorption of xylose and carotene and hypocholesterolaemia may occur. Malabsorption of vitamin B_{12} appears to be secondary to mucosal damage in the ileum and not from any of the following mechanisms: depressed intrinsic factor, abnormal binding of intrinsic factor to vitamin B_{12} and defective attachment of the intrinsic factor vitamin B_{12} complex to ileal mucosa (Webb *et al.*, 1968). Faloon and Chodos (1969) showed that the effect on vitamin B_{12} absorption occurs with intravenous as well as oral administration of colchicine and also that neomycin accentuates the effect of oral colchicine on vitamin B_{12} absorption. The hypocholesterolaemic effect is not correlated with the degree of steatorrhoea (Faloon *et al.*, 1967). Colchicine can depress activities of the brush-border enzymes such as alkaline phosphatase (Herbst *et al.*, 1970) and the disaccharidases (Levin 1966; Faloon *et al.*, 1967; Herbst *et al.*, 1970).

CHOLESTYRAMINE

Cholestyramine is an anion exchange resin that binds bile acids and causes increased faecal excretion of these acids. This ability to interrupt the enterohepatic circulation of bile salts and to deplete the body bile salt pool has led to its use in the treatment of pruritus caused by liver disease (Van Itallie *et al.*, 1961). In addition, the drug is used in treatment of hypercholesterolaemia (Levy *et al.*, 1973) and cholerrhoeic diarrhoea resulting from disease or resection of the ileum (Hofmann and Poley, 1969).

Normal persons taking cholestyramine have constipation and a slight increase in faecal fat (Hofmann and Kern, 1971). When the drug is given to patients with limited ileal resection and mild steatorrhoea, faecal fat excretion doubles (Hofmann and Poley, 1969). Malabsorption of fat-soluble vitamins may occur, and hypoprothrombinaemia resulting from vitamin K deficiency may be severe enough to cause bleeding complications (Gross and Brotman, 1970). Osteomalacia occurred in a patient during the second year of cholestyramine therapy for postiliectomy diarrhoea, and she responded to therapy with vitamin D (Heaton *et al.*, 1972). Fat-soluble vitamins, and possibly calcium, should be provided to patients taking cholestyramine.

BIGUANIDES

The biguanide group (metformin, phenformin, buformin) of oral hypoglycaemic agents has been shown to cause malabsorption of glucose, xylose, vitamin B_{12}, amino acids and probably fat. The postulated mechanisms by which the biguanides decrease blood glucose levels included enhanced insulin action on tissues (Butterfield *et al.*, 1961) and an interference with mitochondrial oxidative phosphorylation (Falcone *et al.*, 1962). In addition, evidence is accumulating that intestinal malabsorption of glucose may be a major mechanism of action (Czyzyk *et al.*, 1968; Arvanitakis *et al.*, 1973). Weight loss commonly occurs when patients take biguanides and, although drug-induced anorexia plays a part, Stowers and Bewsher (1969) found glucose malabsorption to be the primary mechanism in causing negative caloric balance. Xylose absorption was also impaired in these studies.

In addition to this effect on glucose absorption, both phenformin and metformin can cause reversible malabsorption of vitamin B_{12} (Willms and Creutzfeldt, 1970; Berchtold *et al.*, 1971; Tomkin *et al.*, 1971; Herbert, 1972). Abnormal Schilling tests occur within 7–14 days of the start of therapy (Herbert, 1972).

ANTACIDS

Antacids can inhibit the absorption of dietary phosphate, which has led to the use of aluminium hydroxide in hyperphosphataemia and metabolic bone disease owing to renal failure. A rare syndrome of phosphorus depletion can occur in patients taking long-term antacid therapy (Bloom and Flinchum, 1960; Lotz *et al.*, 1968; Ansari, 1970; Dent and Winter, 1974). The metabolic features of the syndrome include hypophosphataemia, hypophosphaturia, increased gastrointestinal absorption of calcium and hypercalciuria leading to negative calcium balance. These abnormalities eventually lead to osteomalacia. Severe debility, weakness and anorexia occur, and may be related to lack of the phosphorus necessary for intermediary metabolism. Patients described as having this syndrome had been taking 240–360 mL of antacid preparation per day (aluminium hydroxide) for periods ranging from 1 month to 5 years.

Antacids may affect absorption of orally administered drugs by changing their physicochemical states or by affecting the physiological function of the gastrointestinal tract (Hurwitz, 1971). The depressed absorption of tetracycline that has been noted when the drug is taken with antacids has been attributed to several factors. Tetracycline forms poorly absorbed chelates with polyvalent cations, such as calcium, magnesium and aluminium contained in antacids (Bessman and Doorenbos, 1957). In addition, Barr *et al.* (1971) showed that sodium bicarbonate can greatly decrease tetracycline absorption even though chelation does not occur. They postulated that increasing the gastric pH decreases the rate of dissolution of the drug. The absorption of two related antibiotics, chlortetracycline (Waisbren and Hueckel, 1950) and demethylchlortetracycline (Scheiner and Altemeier, 1962), and vitamin A (Hoffman and Dyniewicz, 1945) is also inhibited by aluminium antacids. Iron absorption is depressed by magnesium trisilicate, perhaps secondary to the formation of insoluble compounds (Hall and Davis, 1969). Other drugs whose absorption in man may be inhibited by antacids include chlorpromazine (Forrest *et al.*, 1970; Fann *et al.*, 1973) and enteric-coated salicylate (Feldman and Carlstedt, 1974).

ORAL CONTRACEPTIVES

Shojania *et al.* (1971) found decreased folate levels in serum and erythrocytes in women taking oral contraceptive agents. However, other authors (Spray, 1968; McLean *et al.*, 1969; Stephens *et al.*, 1972) have failed to confirm this. Shojania *et al.* reported that the serum folate concentration was low in 9 per cent of women who were on the regimen less than 1 year and in 40 per cent of those on the regimen more than 4 years. Megaloblastic anaemia secondary to folate deficiency in women taking oral contraceptive has been reported but it is rare (Holmes, 1970; Necheles and Snyder, 1970; Streiff, 1970; Ryser *et al.*, 1971; Salter, 1972), perhaps because in well-developed countries the diet usually contains considerably more folate than the minimum requirement.

PARA-AMINOSALICYLIC ACID

Gastrointestinal side-effects commonly occur with the use of para-aminosalicylic acid. The standard therapeutic dose of sodium para-aminosalicylic acid generally does not cause steatorrhoea but this complication has been reported in six patients (Akhtar *et al.*, 1968; Coltart, 1969; Halsted and McIntyre, 1972; Longstreth *et al.*, 1972). Various combinations of malabsorption of vitamin B_{12}, folate, xylose and iron also occurred, and disappeared when the drug regimen was stopped.

LAXATIVES

The widespread belief that a daily bowel movement is necessary for good health frequently leads to laxative abuse. Laxative dependence is a common result but, occasionally, more serious consequences occur. Mild steatorrhoea (9–15 g/day) has occasionally been reported as a complication of chronic laxative abuse (Rawson, 1966; Heizer *et al.*, 1968; Cummings *et al.*, 1974). Other abnormalities include protein-losing gastroenteropathy (Heizer *et al.*, 1968), osteomalacia (Meulengracht, 1939; Frame *et al.*, 1971), diminished xylose (Meulengracht, 1939; Heizer *et al.*, 1968; Frame *et al.*, 1971; Cummings *et al.*, 1974) and glucose absorption (Hart and McColl, 1968), and a syndrome of weakness, hypokalaemia, alkalosis, azotaemia, and hypocalcaemia (Staffurth and Allott, 1962; Rawson, 1966; Cummings *et al.*, 1974). Only laxatives from the irritant group (for example, phenolphthalein, bisacodyl, cascara and oxyphenisatin) have been associated with these problems.

MEFENAMIC ACID

Steatorrhoea as a complication of mefenamic acid treatment should be considered in all cases presenting with diarrhoea, which is a common and well-recognized adverse reaction.

Heavy metals

GOLD-INDUCED ENTERITIS

A small number of patients receiving gold therapy, usually for rheumatoid arthritis, may develop enterocolitis, usually within 3 months of the start of the treatment. The usual presenting features of the disease begin with diarrhoea, pain, fever and sometimes eosinophilia. Both the small and large intestine may be involved showing haemorrhage, oedema and thickening on endoscopy. The biopsies show features of ulceration and diffuse inflammatory changes, which, on occasions, may show features similar to Crohn's disease (Jackson *et al.*, 1986).

Chemotherapy

Studies on patients receiving cyclophosphamide, methotrexate and 5-fluorouracil for breast cancer show normal small intestinal mucosa on light microscopy. However, on an electron microscopical level, there is stunted growth of the enterocytes and the crypt cells show focal vacuolation, which may correspond to secondary lysosomes ingesting fragments of damaged crypts (Cunningham *et al.*, 1985).

Ethanol

Disturbances in digestive physiology are common in alcoholics (Small *et al.*, 1959). Multiple defects in absorption have been observed and are secondary to a number of factors, including deficiency of folate and other dietary nutrients, abnormalities in small bowl function, liver disease, pancreatic insufficiency and neomycin treatment (Marin *et al.*, 1969; Roggin *et al.*, 1969).

The folate deficiency commonly seen in alcoholics results from multiple factors, including poor dietary intake of the vitamin, diminished absorption of folate, and the effects of alcohol on the liver (Cherrick *et al.*, 1965) and bone marrow (Sullivan *et al.*, 1964). In addition, malabsorption of xylose, glucose and fat occurs in alcoholics. Interpretation of the causes of small bowel malabsorption is complicated by the interaction of the toxic effect of alcohol and the deficiency of folate as well as of other dietary nutrients.

Morphological changes in the small bowel have been observed secondary to either alcohol intake or folate deficiency. For example, alcohol alone, in the absence of nutritional deficiencies, can cause striking electron microscopic changes in the small intestine of man, such as abnormalities of the mitochondria, endoplasmic reticulum and Golgi apparatus, as well as focal cytoplasmic degradation. The tissue is generally normal under light microscopy (Rubin *et al.*, 1972). Studies in ethanol-fed rats, however, revealed haemorrhagic erosions of small bowel mucosa, villous changes by light microscopy, and decreased jejunal oxygen consumption and enzyme activities (Baraona *et al.*, 1974).

Folate deficiency with or without alcohol can cause the following changes in the small intestine: decreased mitotic figures in crypts; shortened crypts and villi; and enlarged epithelial cells and nuclei (Hermos *et al.*, 1972). Halsted *et al.* (1971) demonstrated that the absorption of folic acid is decreased in malnourished, actively drinking alcoholics. Their data suggested that the functional defect is caused by poor nutrition rather than by a toxic effect of alcohol on the jejunum. In a later study (Halsted *et al.*, 1973), the same authors, on the basis of preliminary data, concluded that the malabsorption of folic acid, xylose and glucose in alcoholics required a combination of both folate deficiency and prolonged ethanol administration. Ethanol or folate deficiency alone caused only mild net secretion of water and sodium in the small intestine. Ethanol directly inhibits absorption of amino acids and glucose in rats (Chang *et al.*, 1967; Israel *et al.*, 1968), perhaps because it decreases ATP content in the small intestine (Carter and Isselbacher, 1973).

Lindenbaum and Lieber (1969) reported that vitamin B_{12} absorption is inhibited by ethanol in humans on a nutritious diet. In alcohol-fed well-nourished rats, several defects in vitamin B_{12} absorption have been demonstrated, including deficiency of intrinsic factor and depressed uptake of intrinsic factor-vitamin B_{12} complex by the small intestine (Lindenbaum *et al.*, 1973).

It has been suggested that changes in intestinal permeability may be important in the pathophysiology of various gastrointestinal diseases and that increased permeability to antigens may account for some of the extraintestinal manifestations seen in these disorders. Gastrointestinal function is disturbed in chronic alcoholic patients by several interacting and interrelated factors, including poor dietary intake, maldigestion and malabsorption, which may all contribute to the malnutrition so common in these patients. Ethanol ingestion may also be associated with increased permeation of macromolecules, at least in animals.

Potassium-related enteropathy

The pathological lesions in this condition are mostly ulcerations and strictures. They have been recognized for some time (Davies and Brightmore, 1970; Leyonmarck and Ralf, 1985; Thomas and Williamson, 1985). These ulcers occur mostly in the ileum and affect both sexes at any age. The usual presenting features are haemorrhage or obstruction, which could be due to stricture or perforation. The ulcers are usually circumferential, short and have a punched-out appearance resembling simple peptic ulceration. Most often they are single but can be found in small groups. Sometimes they can produce an hour-glass deformity. Histologically, the features are non-specific. There is a mucosal necrosis with flattening of the adjacent villi and mild inflammatory changes in the lamina propria. The muscularis mucosa is often hypertrophied. The submucosa shows fibrosis and a variable degree of mixed inflammatory cell infiltrate. The causes of these changes are uncertain; however, ischaemia must play an important part. Potassium tablets probably adhere locally to the bowel and liberate a high concentration of potassium chloride, which may exert direct constrictive effect on local vessels leading to an acute ischaemic ulcer. These features have been seen experimentally in dogs (Boley *et al.*, 1965). Slow-release potassium chloride has reduced the incidence of this complication.

PNEUMATOSIS INTESTINALIS

These are gas-filled cysts in the wall of the small bowel. They are basically of two types: the infantile type and the adult type.

Infants who have developed necrotizing enterocolitis are sometimes found to have gas-filled cysts in the submucosa at autopsy. They mostly occur in the ileum and the serosa is rarely affected. Histologically, the cysts are not lined by epithelium and later become surrounded by a brisk inflammatory cell infiltrate. The aetiology is unknown but gas-forming organisms are implicated.

The adult type is more common and is more often seen in men than women. This condition is mostly associated with chronic obstructive airway disease and, in the past, with pyloric stenosis (Koss, 1952), although the latter is much less frequent as an aetiological factor. More recently, reports have appeared in association with coeliac disease (Sackier *et al.*, 1988), after bone marrow transplantation (Bates *et al.*, 1989), after jejuno-ileal bypass and after kidney transplantation (Van der Jaget *et al.*, 1987).

The clinical presentation varies according to the underlying pathology. Frequently, they are discovered incidentally after radiological examination or at laparotomy. Sometimes the presentation is with diarrhoea or rectal bleeding. Pathologically, the gas cysts appear in the small and large intestine in the submucosa, serosa or both. They can give a spongy feel to the bowel, and can be single or multiple, sessile or pedunculated polypoidal structures that may involve one or more regions of the bowel. Microscopically, the mucosa is essentially normal, but, in one study, the submucosa and cysts or spaces were lined by endothelial cells. Haboubi *et al.* (1984) suggested that these cysts are mainly made up of lymphatic channels that became dilated. The inflammatory infiltrate is due to leakage of lymphatic contents into the surrounding tissue to initiate a brisk chronic inflammatory cell infiltrate.

The treatment in the uncomplicated case is conservative with intermittent high-flow oxygen therapy. This therapeutic modality is effective but relapses are common. The principal complications are spontaneous ruptures of the serosal cysts and also the development of intestinal obstruction. Surgical resection is reserved for the complicated cases.

VASCULAR DISORDERS

Apart from the first part of the duodenum, the rest of the small intestine receives a blood supply from the superior mesenteric artery. Under normal circumstances, the artery runs a curved course through the mesentery and gives branches to form intestinal arteries, which arise from the convex aspect of the curve. They unite with each other to form arcades and from these arcades short straight branches, which usually do not anastomose significantly, supply the jejunum and most of the duodenum. Each branch ramifies in the serosa and passes through the muscle coat to the submucosa. Arterioles arise from the small branches inside the muscle coat to supply the villi. The venous drainage is through the portal system via the superior mesenteric vein.

As elsewhere in the body, the essential factors in ischaemia apply: the affected segment receives less blood than it requires to maintain its proper structure and function. The difference, however, is twofold. When ischaemia occurs, a rapid chain of events starts with a breach of the surface epithelium and direct exposure of the subepithelial tissue to the small intestine flora. This may lead to rapid dissemination of infection.

Ischaemia

Ischaemia can be divided broadly into two main categories: occlusive, and non-occlusive or slow flow.

OCCLUSIVE ISCHAEMIA

Arterial occlusion

It has been estimated that approximately 50 per cent of cases of intestinal ischaemia have an associated vascular block mostly due to atheroma (Kairaluoma *et al.*, 1977). This vascular block is due to atheroma but may be complicated by thrombus or embolus. Occasionally, vasculitis could be the cause (Kumar and Dawson, 1972). In a carefully conducted autopsy study, atheromatous change appeared to be more common and severe in the proximal 2.0 cm of the superior and inferior mesenteric arteries, leaving the most distal vessels relatively uninvolved (Croft *et al.*, 1981). It has been suggested that, for ischaemia to ensue, the lumen of the proximal 1.0 cm of the mesenteric artery should be narrowed by at least two thirds. What is more important is a balance between the blood pressure and the patency of the vessel as both affect the state of perfusion. Thrombosis on its own has been shown to account for approximately one-quarter of cases of acute ischaemia (Wilson *et al.*, 1987). Occasionally, ischaemia of the small bowel can occur after an aortic graft operation.

Venous occlusion

Small bowel ischaemia secondary to venous occlusion accounts for approximately 5–10 per cent of cases (Hilderband and Zieler, 1980). Causes include: extramural pressure, for example, incarcerated hernia or large abdominal mass; intravascular thrombosis, mostly due to internal sepsis (a rarity these days owing to the efficacy of antibiotics); oral contraceptives (Civetta and Kolodny, 1970; Cotton and Thomas, 1971); cirrhosis and hepatic tumour, which initiate portal vein thrombosis that propagates back to the mesenteric vein (Marston, 1962). There is some evidence that haemoconcentration and polycythaemia may predispose to ischaemic lesions, presumably by increasing blood viscosity (Schwartz *et al.*, 1961). Ischaemia can also be a manifestation of disseminated intravascular coagulation (Whitehead, 1971).

NON-OCCLUSIVE ISCHAEMIA

This, by and large, is due to a drop in arterial blood pressure, which is seen in left ventricular failure, aortic insufficiency and cases of shock. To understand this phenomenon it is important to realize that the arterial pressure, at the origin of the superior mesenteric artery, is approximately the same as in the aorta. The portal venous pressure, however, is about 10 per cent of that. There is considerable peripheral resistance in the splanchnic bed. The vessels of this bed are sensitive to pressor amines. In any situation, therefore, which causes hypotension or low flow states, the splanchnic vessels are likely to constrict in an attempt to maintain normal blood pressure. Therefore, both the initial hypotension and the subsequent vascular constriction reduce, markedly, the effective flow to the bowel. It has been shown that, in a quarter to half of all patients with clinical and pathological evidence of bowel ischaemia, no significant organic vascular block is demonstrable, and the cause is attributed to hypotension. The majority of patients in whom shock is associated with bowel infarction are elderly people, who are more likely to have an accompanying mesenteric vessel atheroma. Therefore, any major hypotensive episode is more likely to precipitate the mucosal damage and allows invasion by intestinal bacterial flora and particularly the *Clostridium* species.

PATHOLOGY OF INTESTINAL ISCHAEMIA

Initially the bowel becomes oedematous and plum coloured. The mucosa is necrotic and congested, and has a nodular surface appearance due to extensive submucosal haemorrhage and oedema. The deep muscular layers may initially escape injury in the acute phase. However, this may proceed to tissue necrosis and perforation. When the entire bowel is infarcted, the serosa becomes deeply congested and dull, and sometimes full-blown gangrene may occur. At any stage, perforation may result. In some cases, however, only the mucosa is affected, with good preservation of the deeper layers of the wall. This is characteristic of the low-flow non-occlusive cases. In these cases, the bowel may be of normal colour externally, and only on opening the bowel does severe congestion and necrosis of the mucosa become apparent. Sometimes pseudomembranous enteritis can be seen.

HISTOLOGICAL APPEARANCES

The early mucosal lesions are usually patchy. Almost normal mucosa surrounds the diseased area, in which the villi appear normal. The affected segments appear initially congested with separation of the surface epithelium from the subjacent tissue, followed by a mummification of the surface epithelium with formation of haemorrhagic necrosis (Plate 27.1). Once this phase appears, the subsequent phases of necrosis and perforation will ensue, with no characteristic histological appearances.

If the patient survives the initial episode, and the damage is confined to the mucosa, then complete recovery is expected. Indeed, the entire episode may pass unnoticed. In the event of repeated insults or if the damage has extended beyond the mucosa, then a more chronic fibrotic state will appear, which is characterized by a fibrotic stricture, affecting mostly the submucosa, but which may involve the muscularis propria, depending on the degree and depth of the initial damage. Ulceration may complicate chronic ischaemia.

Vasculitis

The small intestine is frequently involved in systemic vasculitis and also involvement has been reported in polyarteritis nodosa, Wegener's granulomatosis, collagenous disorders and other syndromes.

Abdominal pain, often of the anginal type, together with bloody diarrhoea is a common symptom of polyarteritis nodosa. The intraoperative or necropsy findings will show nodules along the course of the mesenteric vessels together with localized ulcers, usually along the antimesenteric borders, which can penetrate deeply and may perforate to produce haemorrhagic infarctions. Histologically, the typical appearance of polyarteritis nodosa consists of severe intimal and subintimal proliferation of endothelial and subendothelial cells, producing narrowing of the lumen, sometimes occlusion, with or without thrombus formation. The rest of the vessel wall shows active inflammation with or without giant cell formation. The inflammation sometimes extends into the perivascular tissue. In Churg–Strauss syndrome, there is granulomatous reaction in the vessel wall, which has a similar clinical picture to polyarteritis nodosa, but which is associated with asthma and eosinophilia (Chumbley *et al.*, 1977).

Minor causes of angiitis are seen in progressive systemic sclerosis, systemic lupus, thromboangiitis obliterans, Kohlmier–Degos syndrome (progressive arterio-occlusive disease) and rheumatoid arthritis (Morson and Dawson, 1991). In rheumatoid arthritis, approximately 1 per cent of the patients show vasculitis and a fifth of these will demonstrate gastrointestinal involvement, which usually involves the colon (Burt *et al.*, 1983).

Behçet's syndrome

This syndrome, which is characterized by buccal and genital mucosal ulcerations, may affect the gastrointestinal tract (Kasahara *et al.*, 1981). Other organs that may be involved are the skin, nervous system, joints and classically the eyes. It has been reported that approximately 22 per cent of patients with Behçet's syndrome will have appendicitis-like symptoms indicative of the involvement of the terminal ileum and the right colon (Kodama, 1977). The involvement of the small intestine is seen more in Japan than in Western countries, where there is more involvement of the colon. Pathologically, there is intestinal mucosal ulceration, which can be solitary but more commonly multiple. It could be localized to one segment, or occur throughout the small and large intestine. The ulcerations, when present, are often punched out, sometimes fissural, sometimes superficial and aphthoid, and on occasions linear ulcers up to 5.0 cm in length occur. The intervening mucosa, however, appears normal. Histologically, there is nonspecific ulceration with inflammation of the small veins and venules with lymphocytic infiltrates and occasional granulomata (Baba *et al.*, 1976).

Aorto-enteric fistula

This is a condition described in patients with an infected aortic prosthesis. They usually present either with severe and recurrent upper gastrointestinal tract bleeding, or sometimes with septicaemia, anaemia and leucocytosis with a high erythrocyte sedimentation rate. The diagnosis is made at upper gastrointestinal tract endoscopy, or by a barium meal and follow-through. Treatment is usually surgical by replacing the aortic prosthesis under antibiotic cover.

AMYLOIDOSIS

Amyloid is a pathological proteinaceous substance deposited between cells of various organs of the body in a wide variety of clinical settings. It has special biochemical and chromatic characteristics (Robins *et al.*, 1989). Macroscopically, painting the cut surface of the affected organs with iodine solution imparts a yellow–red discoloration. This changes to violet or blue after treatment with diluted sulphuric acid. Microscopically, it represents areas of amorphous pink extracellu-

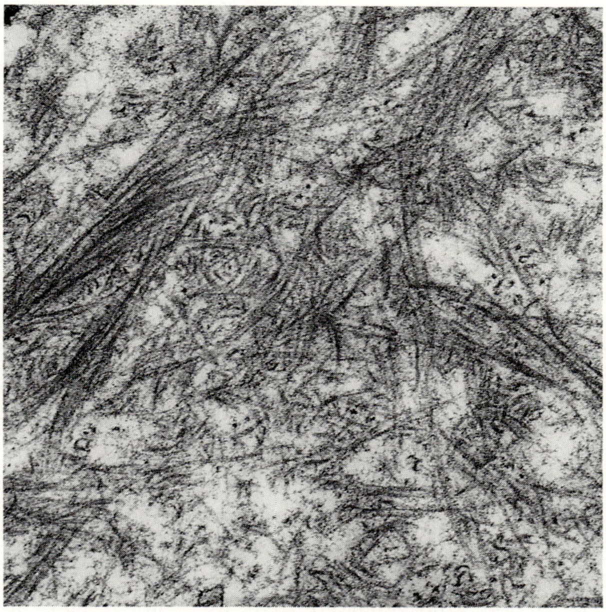

Figure 27.2 *The typical ultrastructural appearance of amyloidosis in which the fibrils are deposited in an irregular pattern.*

lar deposits. This material can be differentiated from other amorphous materials by a variety of stains, the most widely used being Congo red, which gives the affected tissue red discoloration, and on polarization will transform into a characteristic apple-green pattern. Ultrastructurally, however, it appears as aggregates of non-branching fibrils of approximately 7.5–10 nm (Fig. 27.2). Biochemically, it has been shown that approximately 90 per cent of the material consists of fibril protein and the other 10 per cent is a glycoprotein called P component (Glenner, 1980).

There are two chemically distinct major classes of amyloid fibril protein, AL (amyloid light chain), which is an immunoglobulin produced by the plasma cells, and AA (amyloid associated), which is a non-immunoglobulin and is produced by the liver.

Clinically, there are four main types of amyloidosis, often with overlapping patterns, which are listed below.

1 Primary amyloidosis occurs without recognizable predisposing factors.
2 Secondary amyloidosis is a form of systemic amyloidosis, which is associated with recognized predisposing conditions such as chronic inflammation or neoplasia.
3 Heredofamilial forms, which include amyloidosis seen in familial Mediterranean fever.
4 Single-organ amyloidosis.

The gastrointestinal tract is commonly involved in patterns 1, 2 and 3. The small bowel will gradually thicken and become waxy in appearance, and converts into a rigid tube with walls up to 1.0 cm thick. Microscopically, there is a pericollagenous distribution predominantly in the walls of the blood vessels. Amyloid can also be found between the muscle fibres. Local symptoms can occur, particularly perforation and haemorrhage.

ULCERATIVE NON-GRANULOMATOUS CHRONIC JEJUNO-ILEITIS

This is a controversial entity, which is characterized by widespread non-specific ulceration of the small bowel in association with malabsorption. Mills *et al.* (1980) showed that this interesting condition of unknown aetiology presents like coeliac disease and most patients have subtotal villous atrophy but without any response to the gluten-free diet (Mills *et al.*, 1980). These patients have chronic small intestinal non-specific ulcerations. The diagnosis can only be firmly established by laparotomy and histological examination following resection. Melaena, intestinal obstruction and perforation often complicate this condition. The latter complication resulted in death in three out of the five patients reported by Mills *et al.* (1980). The management of these patients is extremely difficult and the long-term outcome is poor. It seems that surgical resection of the worst affected segment is the most effective course of action. One series suggested that there is an association between this condition and intestinal lymphoma (Isaacson and Wright, 1978). This view, however, is not uniformly supported.

PRIMARY CHRONIC INTESTINAL PSEUDO-OBSTRUCTION SYNDROME (CIPS)

Intestinal pseudo-obstruction is defined as a syndrome characterized by symptoms and signs of intestinal obstruction in the absence of mechanical blockage (Faulk and Anuras, 1978; Schuffler, 1981). This syndrome can be purely functional with no recognizable morphological abnormalities. Alternatively, light or electron microscopical changes are sometimes seen.

In its acute form, it is mostly self-limiting and is associated with a variety of conditions. This is usually known as paralytic ileus, ileus or spastic ileus. The pathogenesis is not known. The chronic form may, in addition to the signs and symptoms of intestinal obstruction, have features of malabsorption. The aetiology is a primary disorder of the smooth muscle or the myenteric plexus. The classification in Table 27.1 is based partly on the clinical presentation and partly on the distinct morphological features.

The familial visceral myopathies are rare genetic diseases characterized by degeneration and fibrous replacement of the smooth muscle of the gastrointestinal

Table 27.1 *Classification of chronic intestinal pseudo-obstruction*

I. Primary chronic intestinal pseudo-obstruction
A. Familial type
  1. Familial visceral myopathies
  2. Familial visceral neuropathies
B. Non-familial (or sporadic) type
  1. Visceral myopathies
  2. Visceral neuropathies
  3. Normal histology

II. Secondary chronic intestinal pseudo-obstruction
A. Disease involving the intestinal smooth muscle
  1. Collagen diseases: scleroderma, dermatomyositis, and systemic lupus erythematosus
  2. Muscular dystrophies: myotonic dystrophy, Duchenne's muscular dystrophy
  3. Amyloidosis
B. Neurological diseases
  1. Chagas' disease
  2. Ganglioneuromatosis of the intestine
  3. Visceral neuropathy in carcinomatosis
C. Endocrine disorders
  1. Myxoedema
  2. Hypoparathyroidism
D. Pharmacologic agents
  1. Phenothiazines
  2. Tricyclic antidepressants
  3. Anti-Parkinsonian medications
  4. Ganglionic blockers
  5. *Amanita* (mushroom) poisoning
  6. Narcotics (morphine and meperidine)
E. Miscellaneous
  1. Non-tropical sprue
  2. Jejuno-ileal bypass
  3. Small intestinal diverticulosis
  4. Porphyria
  5. Eosinophilic gastroenteritis
  6. Radiation enteritis
  7. Sclerosing mesenteritis
  8. Diffuse lymphoid infiltration of the small intestine

tract and, in some families, the urinary tract. Several families with visceral neuropathies (FVN) have been reported (Kern and Harris, 1973; Royer *et al.*, 1974; Tanner *et al.*, 1976; Schuffler *et al.*, 1978; Roy *et al.*, 1980; Mayer *et al.*, 1986).

Three categories are identified:

1 CIPS with myenteric plexus abnormalities (Dyer *et al.*, 1969; Cocker *et al.*, 1973; Schuffler *et al.*, 1978; Schuffler and Jonak, 1982).
2 CIPS with smooth muscle fibre abnormalities (Schuffler *et al.*, 1977; Faulk *et al.*, 1978; Jacobs *et al.*, 1979; Fitzgibbons and Chandrasome, 1987).
3 CIPS, apparently idiopathic, without any detectable morphological changes.

With respect to the second category, Shuffler *et al.* (1977) reported the first cases of intestinal myopathy under the name of hollow visceral myopathy (HVM) (Schuffler *et al.*, 1977; Faulk *et al.*, 1978; Jacobs *et al.*, 1979; Fitzgibbons and Chandrasome, 1987). One year later, a similar condition, called familial visceral myopathy (FVM), was reported by Faulk *et al.* (1978). Subsequent studies underlined the frequent association of urological abnormalities and the various clinical aspects of this condition (Faulk *et al.*, 1978; Schuffler *et al.*, 1988). Its occurrence in infancy and childhood has only recently been recognized (Kaschula *et al.*, 1987; Vargas *et al.*, 1988).

The clinical manifestations of primary intestinal myopathy include repeated obstructive episodes, permanent or intermittent constipation alternating with periods of diarrhoea, dysphagia, nausea, vomiting and painful abdominal distension. In most reported cases, the first symptoms usually appear in adolescence or early adulthood. Because the condition is now more readily recognized, early forms, beginning in the neonatal period and characterized by some delay in meconium passage, are now clearly identified (Schuffler *et al.*, 1988; Vargas *et al.*, 1988).

In many cases, the smooth muscle abnormalities are not restricted to the gastrointestinal tract but may also involve the urinary tract with repeated urinary infections, uretero-hydronephrosis and abnormalities on cystometrogram (Schuffler *et al.*, 1977; Faulk *et al.*, 1978). The combination of cystogram and cystomanometry has been of value in determining the presence of urological involvement. Other non-gastrointestinal manifestations, in particular ophthalmoplegia (Anuras *et al.*, 1983), mental retardation (Fitzgibbons and Chrandrasome, 1987) and cardiac involvement responsible for sudden death during parenteral nutrition have been reported (Anuras *et al.*, 1982).

Among the additional investigations, only abdominal x-ray and manometric studies seem to be of value (Arhan *et al.*, 1979).

Medical treatment is usually ineffective. Acute obstructive episodes often lead to exploratory laparotomy and ileostomy or colostomy that may be effective in decreasing intraluminal pressure. However, most surgical procedures appear to be of limited value or even useless. At least in children, parenteral nutrition appears to offer more comfort as well as those nutrients essential for growth. Cisapride improves measurements of intestinal transit but has little effect on patients' symptomatology. Steatorrhoea may improve with long-term treatment with antibiotics. Surgery should be carried out on a few selected cases, such as gastrojejunostomy for patients with severe duodenal obstruction, caecostomy or ileostomy for severe colonic dilatation, and subtotal enterectomy when the small intestine is involved extensively.

The differential diagnosis of intestinal myopathy includes all the usual causes of CIPS. Because the changes are restricted to the muscular layers and spare the myenteric plexus, it is easy to eliminate the usual cause of CIPS, namely abnormalities of intrinsic innervation, such as aganglionosis, hypoganglionosis, hypertrophy and hyperplasia of the myenteric plexus, deficiency of argyrophilic neurons (Tanner *et al.*, 1976) and Chagas' disease. However, endocrine disorders (hypothyroidism), neurological disorders (Schuffler and Jonak, 1982), intestinal myositis (Nezelof *et al.*, 1985), short bowel syndrome associated with pyloric stenosis and various malformations (Royer *et al.*, 1974; Nezelof *et al.*, 1976), and megacystis-microcolon intestinal hypoperistalsis syndrome (Puri *et al.*, 1983) deserve mention. Drug- or diet-induced constipation should also be considered. Kaschula *et al.* (1987) reported 25 cases of degenerative leiomyopathy with marked chronic abdominal distension in indigenous Africans. This condition, which is in some ways similar to intestinal myopathy, is sporadic and linked to a particular diet and repeated ritual rectal enemas.

PHLEGMONOUS JEJUNITIS

This is a rare entity of unknown aetiology, which can affect the duodenum, stomach and the intestine in middle-aged and elderly people. The stomach is most often involved. It occurs more frequently in patients with alcoholic liver disease and cirrhosis (Rosen and On, 1978). It is usually an autopsy diagnosis with a mortality rate of 60–70 per cent (Kneafsy *et al.*, 1987). The presenting symptoms are similar to intestinal obstruction with nausea and vomiting followed by absolute constipation. Commonly there is fever, tachycardia and hypotension. The bacterial culture from the blood and, less commonly, from the peritoneal fluid usually grows *Streptococcus pneumoniae* or group A haemolytic streptococci. To the naked eye the inflamed loop of bowel is sharply demarcated, oedematous, inflamed and distended (Plate 27.3). Histologically, it is characterized by diffuse acute inflammation of the submucosa leaving the surface epithelium intact (Plate 27.4). In addition, there is widespread lymphangitis and regional lymphadenitis. It is postulated that the organisms, which invade the submucosa and blood, are normal inhabitants of the small intestine. Under certain circumstances these organisms breach the mucosal lining in a small area to invade the submucosa and spread haematogenously from this point.

BROWN BOWEL SYNDROME

This is a rare condition characterized by the deposition of lipofuscin pigments in the smooth muscles of the gastrointestinal tract. The number of reported cases is small but the majority are associated with malabsorption. Foster (1979) suggested that the condition represents a smooth muscle mitochondrial myopathy. The brown pigment lipofuscin is deposited in the mitochondria of the intestinal smooth muscle and therefore interferes with the cellular energy system. The association of brown pigments with malabsorption and vitamin E deficiency was recognized by Pappenheimer and Victor (1946). Vitamin E exerts a high degree of protection to the membrane lipids from the free radicals. When vitamin E deficiency occurs, as in malabsorption, there is peroxidation of unsaturated membrane lipids with accumulation of lipofuscin. The loss of energy supply within the muscle and the deposition of the brown pigment lipofuscin result in the dilated atonic brown bowel seen in this condition.

SMALL BOWEL MANIFESTATIONS OF SYSTEMIC DISEASE

Chronic renal failure

Uraemia affects the gastrointestinal tract, and the level of uraemia correlates with gastrointestinal disease. Symptoms include anorexia, hiccups, nausea and vomiting. Patients with chronic renal failure receiving haemodialysis exhibit fewer upper gastrointestinal pathologies (Chachati and Godon, 1987). In well-managed patients with chronic renal failure, the absorptive capacity of the small bowel is essentially normal (el-Lakany *et al.*, 1990).

In chronic renal failure, upper gastrointestinal bleeding is a significant problem, and the commonest causes are peptic ulcer disease (Zuckerman *et al.*, 1985) and angiodysplasia (Zuckerman *et al.*, 1985; Marcuard and Weinstock, 1988; Richardson and Lordon, 1993). Vascular ectasia (Chalasani *et al.*, 1996) also contributes.

Endocrine disease

ADRENAL INSUFFICIENCY

Addison's disease commonly involves gastrointestinal symptoms, including anorexia, nausea and vomiting in almost all advanced cases, as well as abdominal pain and diarrhoea (Tobin *et al.*, 1989).

PHAEOCHROMOCYTOMA

Phaechromocytoma can present with nausea and vomiting, and, less frequently, watery diarrhoea and steatorrhoea. Gastrointestinal pseudo-obstruction (Turner, 1983) and gastrointestinal bleeding (Vazquez-Quintana *et al.*, 1995) have also been reported. The aetiology of these clinical findings is not known.

HYPOPARATHYROIDISM

Hypoparathyroidism is associated with mild to moderate steatorrhoea (Heubi *et al.*, 1983), diarrhoea (Peracchi *et al.*, 1998), and recurrent or chronic intestinal pseudo-obstruction (Anuras and Christensen, 1981). Correction of hypocalcaemia is the treatment for these symptoms.

HYPERPARATHYROIDISM

Gastrointestinal symptoms in primary hyperparathyroidism are common, and include nausea, vomiting, abdominal pain and constipation (Gardner and Hersh, 1981). Hypercalcaemia has been implicated in increased gastric acid secretion, and may account for exacerbation of peptic ulcer disease and associated pain. The explanation for the other symptoms is not clear.

Fabry's disease

Fabry's disease is an X-linked recessive disorder of glycosphingolipid metabolism due to a deficiency or absence of alpha-galactosidase A. The pathological lesion is sphingolipid deposition in all tissues. Gastrointestinal symptoms are common in patients with Fabry's disease (Sheth *et al.*, 1981), and include impaired motility and complaints of crampy abdominal pain and frequent liquid stools. Ischaemic bowel can result from thrombotic lesions in small bowel vessels due to glycolipid deposition.

Haemophilia and iatrogenic bleeding diatheses

The gastrointestinal tract is a common site for haemorrhage in haemophilia, with peptic ulcer being the primary cause (Mittal *et al.*, 1985). In patients overanticoagulated with heparin or warfarin (Griffin *et al.*, 1986), or with vitamin K deficiency, intramural haemorrhage may present clinically as an acute abdomen, but surgical intervention is not necessary (Griffin *et al.*, 1986). Radiological features of an intramural bleed in the small intestine include thickened mucosal folds, rigidity and luminal narrowing. Treatment is conservative and aimed at replacement of clotting factors (Griffin *et al.*, 1986).

Neoplastic disease

LEUKAEMIA

A small proportion of patients with leukaemia suffer from gastrointestinal symptoms, either as a direct consequence of the disease (consequences of direct invasion of the bowel), immunodeficiency and coagulation defects, or associated with chemotherapy.

During some chemotherapeutic regimes, gastrointestinal infection rates, particularly fungal infections, can be as high as 28 per cent (Micozzi *et al.*, 1996). Various agents, for example, cytosine-arabinoside, can cause paralytic ileus, pneumatosis intestinalis, thickened loops of small bowel, bowel wall erosions, necrosis and transmural or submucosal haemorrhage (Tjon *et al.*, 1990).

Intestinal perforation occurs in the small intestine only marginally less frequently than in the large intestine in patients receiving chemotherapy alone or in combination with corticosteroids for treatment of various tumours including leukaemias (Torosian and Turnbull, 1988).

Small bowel function has been shown to be impaired in children receiving treatment for acute lymphoblastic leukaemia, leading to various malabsorption syndromes (Pearson *et al.*, 1984).

BONE MARROW TRANSPLANTATION

The process of bone marrow transplantation (BMT) can affect the small bowel due to chemotherapy and chemoradiotherapy, which cause damage to the small bowel mucosa. The subsequent increase in mucosal permeability may persist for up to 4 weeks (Fegan *et al.*, 1990). Other problems that involve the small bowel are acute graft-versus-host disease (GVHD), which develops in about 30–50 per cent of allogeneic BMT recipients, and 10–20 per cent of these patients present with either haemorrhage or perforation (Chirletti *et al.*, 1998). Diarrhoea is common, and severe protein-losing enteropathy suggests the presence of GVHD (Papadopoulou *et al.*, 1996). Overt gastrointestinal haemorrhage is uncommon (Kaur *et al.*, 1996). Opportunistic infections due to immunosuppression are widely prevalent (McDonald, 1984).

MULTIPLE MYELOMA

Multiple myeloma can involve the gastrointestinal tract due to amyloidosis or plasmacytomas. Myelomatous involvement of the gut may histologically mimic malignant lymphoma (Griffiths *et al.*, 1997), and plasmacytomas can cause small intestinal obstruction (Benson *et al.*, 1983) and are a rare cause of massive gastrointestinal haemorrhage (Pimentel and van Stolk, 1993).

WALDENSTROM'S MACROGLOBULINAEMIA

Involvement of the gastrointestinal tract in macroglobulinaemia is rare (Veloso *et al.*, 1988), but can include cellular and immunoglobulin infiltration of the lamina propria and mesenteric nodes. Symptoms include diarrhoea, steatorrhoea, intestinal pseudo-obstruction, and dilatation of the small bowel (Heenan *et al.*, 1976; Brandt *et al.*, 1981; Veloso *et al.*, 1988).

Sarcoidosis

Although gastrointestinal involvement in sarcoidosis is uncommon, symptoms result from infiltration or indirectly via lymph node involvement. Sarcoidosis has been reported to cause protein-losing enteropathy (Godeau *et al.*, 1992), duodenal obstruction (Stampfl *et al.*, 1990), granulomatous enterocolitis resembling Crohn's disease (Bulger *et al.*, 1988), fatal gastrointestinal haemorrhage (Briley *et al.*, 1980; Munker and Sharma, 1987), and can present as malabsorption (Sprague *et al.*, 1984).

REFERENCES

Akhtar, A.J., Crompton, G.K., Schonell, M.E. 1968: Para-aminosalicylic acid as a cause of intestinal malabsorption. *Tubercle* 49, 328–31.

Allen-Mersh, T.G., Wilson, E.J., Hope-Stone, F.H., Mann, C.V. 1986: Has the incidence of radiation-induced bowel damage following treatment of uterine carcinoma changed in the last 20 years? *Journal of the Royal Society of Medicine* 79, 387–90.

Ansari, A. 1970: Antacid-induced phosphorus depletion and repletion. *Minnesota Medicine* 53, 837–8.

Anuras, S., Christensen, J. 1981: Recurrent or chronic intestinal pseudo-obstruction. *Clinics in Gastroenterology* 10, 177–89.

Anuras, S., Mitros, F.A., Shirazi, S.S., Soper, R.T., Younoszai, K., Green, J.B. 1982: Cardiac arrest in two children with non-familial chronic intestinal pseudo-obstruction on total parenteral nutrition. *Journal of Pediatric Gastroenterology and Nutrition* 1, 137–44.

Anuras, S., Mitros, F.A., Nowak, T.W. *et al.* 1983: A familial visceral myopathy with external ophthalmoplegia and autosomal recessive transmission. *Gastroenterology* 84, 346–53.

Arhan, P., Devroede, G., Pellerin, D. 1979: Physiology of motility in the terminal intestine. *Gastroenterologie Clinique et Biologique* 3, 911–18.

Arvanitakis, C., Lorenzsonn, V., Olsen, W.A. 1973: Phenformin-induced alterations of small intestinal function and mitochondrial structure in man. *Journal of Laboratory Clinical Medicine* 92, 195–200.

Baba, S., Maruta, M., Ando, K., Teramoto, T., Endo, I. 1976: Intestinal Behcet's disease, a report of five cases. *Diseases of the Colon and Rectum* 9, 428–40.

Baraona, E., Pirola, R.C., Lieber, C.S. 1974: Small intestinal damage and changes in cell population produced by ethanol ingestion in the rat. *Gastroenterology* 66, 226–34.

Barr, W.H., Adir, J., Garrettson, L. 1971: Decrease of tetracycline absorption in man by sodium bicarbonate. *Clinical Pharmacology and Therapeutics* 12, 779–84.

Bates, F.T., Gurney, J.W., Goodman, L.R., Santamaria, J.J., Hansen, R.M., Ash, R.C. 1989: Pneumatosis intestinalis after bone marrow transplants. *American Journal of Gastroenterology* 152, 991–4.

Benson, W.J., Scarffe, J.H., Houwen, B., Crowther, D. 1983: Gastrointestinal involvement with myeloma. *Medical and Pediatric Oncology* 11, 256–62.

Berchtold, P., Dahlqvist, A., Gustafson, A. *et al.* 1971: Effects of a biguanide (metformin) on Vitamin B12 and folic acid absorption and intestinal enzyme activities. *Scandinavian Journal of Gastroenterology* 6, 751–4.

Bessman, S.P., Doorenbos, N.J. 1957: Chelation (editorial). *Annals of Internal Medicine* 47, 1036–41.

Bjarnason, I., Williams, P., So, A. *et al.* 1984: Intestinal permeability and inflammation in rheumatoid arthritis; effect of non-steroidal anti-inflammatory drugs. *Lancet* ii, 1171–4.

Bjarnason, I., Williams, P., Smethurst, P., Peters, T.J., Levy, A.J. 1986: The effect of non-steroidal anti-inflammatory drugs and prostaglandins in the permeability of the human small intestine. *Gut* 27, 1292–7.

Bjarnason, I., Zeanelli, G., Prouse, P. *et al.* 1987: Blood and protein loss via small intestinal inflammation induced by NSAID. *Lancet* ii, 711–14.

Bloom, W.L., Flinchum, D. 1960: Osteomalacia with pseudofractures caused by the ingestion of aluminium hydroxide. *JAMA* 174, 1327–30.

Bloomer, W.D., Hellman, S. 1975: Normal tissue responses to radiation therapy. *New England Journal of Medicine* 293, 80–3.

Boley, S.J., Schultz, L., Krieger, H., Schwartz, S., Elguezabala, S., Allen, A.C. 1965: Experimental evaluation of thiazides and potassium as a cause of small bowel ulcer. *JAMA* 192, 763–5.

Brandt, L.J., Davidoff, A., Bernstein, L.H., Biempica, L., Rindfleisch, B., Goldstein, M.L. 1981: Small-intestine involvement in Waldenstrom's macroglobulinemia. Case report and review of the literature. *Digestive Diseases and Sciences* 26, 174–80.

Briley, C.A., Jr, Jackson, D.C., Johnsrude, I.S., Mills, S.R. 1980: Acute gastrointestinal hemorrhage of small-bowel origin. *Radiology* 136, 317–19.

Bulger, K., O'Riordan, M., Purdy, S., O'Brien, M., Lennon, J. 1988: Gastrointestinal sarcoidosis resembling Crohn's disease. *American Journal of Gastroenterology* 83, 1415–17.

Burt, R.W., Berenson, M.M., Samuelson, C.O., Cathy, W.J. 1983: Rheumatoid vasculitis of the colon presenting as acute pan colitis. *Digestive Diseases and Sciences* 28, 183–8.

Butterfield, W.J.H., Fry, I.K., Whichelow, M.J. 1961: The hypoglycaemic action of Phenformin: studies in diabetics after short-term therapy. *Lancet* 2, 563–7.

Cain, G.D., Reiner, E.B., Patterson, M. 1968: Effects of neomycin on disaccharidase activity of the small bowel. *Archives of Internal Medicine* 122, 311–14.

Carr, N.D., Pullen, B.R., Haselton, P.S., Schofield, P.F. 1984: Microvascular studies in human radiation bowel disease. *Gut* 25, 448–54.

Carter, E.A., Isselbacher, K.H. 1973: Effect of ethanol on intestinal adenosine triphosphate (ATP) content. *Proceedings of the Society of Experimental Biology and Medicine* 142, 1171–3.

Chachati, A., Godon, J. 1987: Effect of haemodialysis on upper gastrointestinal tract pathology in patients with chronic renal failure. *Nephrology Dialysis Transplantation* 1, 233–7.

Chalasani, N., Cotsonis, G., Wilcox, C.M. 1996: Upper gastrointestinal bleeding in patients with chronic renal failure: role of vascular ectasia. *American Journal of Gastroenterology* 91, 2329–32.

Chang, T., Lewis, J., Glazko, A.J. 1967: Effect of ethanol and other alcohols on the transport of amino acids and glucose by everted sacs of rat small intestine. *Biochemica et Biophysica Acta* 135, 1000–7.

Cherrick, G.R., Baker, H., Frank, O. *et al.* 1965: Observations on hepatic avidity for folate in Laennec's cirrhosis. *Journal of Laboratory Clinical Medicine* 66, 446–51.

Chirletti, P., Caronna, R., Arcese, W., Iori, A.P., Calcaterra, D., Cartoni, C., Sammartino, P., Stipa, V. 1998: Gastrointestinal emergencies in patients with acute intestinal graft-versus-host disease. *Leukemia and Lymphoma* 29, 129–37.

Chumbley, L.C., Harrison, E.G., de Rernee, R.A. 1977: Allergic granulomatosis angitis (Church–Strauss syndrome). Report and analysis of thirty cases. *Mayo Clinic Proceedings* 52, 477–84.

Civetta, J.M., Kolodny, M. 1970: Mesenteric venous thrombosis association with oral contraceptives. *Gastroenterology* 58, 713–16.

Coltart, D.J. 1969: Malabsorption induced by para-aminosalicylate. *British Medical Journal* 1, 825–6.

Cotton, P.B., Thomas, M.L. 1971: Ischaemic colitis and contraceptive pills. *British Medical Journal* 3, 27–8.

Croft, R.J., Menon, G.P., Marston, A. 1981: Does intestinal angina exist? A critical study of obstructed visceral arteries. *British Journal of Surgery* 68, 316–18.

Cummings, J.H., Sladen, G.E., James, O.F.W. *et al.* 1974: Laxative-induced diarrhoea: a continuing problem. *British Medical Journal* 1, 537–41.

Cunningham, D., Morgan, R.J., Mills, P.R. *et al.* 1985: Functional and structural changes in the human proximal small intestine after cytotoxic therapy. *Journal of Clinical Pathology* 38, 265–70.

Czyzyk, A., Tawecki, J., Sadowshi, J. *et al.* 1968: Effect of biguanides on intestinal absorption of glucose. *Diabetes* 17, 492–8.

Davies, D.R., Brightmore, T. 1970: Idiopathic and drug induced ulceration of the small intestine. *British Journal of Surgery* 57, 134–9.

Day, P.K. 1983: Intestinal perforation associated with osmotic low release indomethacin capsules. *British Medical Journal* 287, 167–72.

Dent, C.E., Winter, C.S. 1974: Osteomalacia due to phosphate depletion from excessive aluminium hydroxide ingestion. *British Medical Journal* 1, 551–2.

Dobbins, W.O., III, Herrero, B.A., Mansback, C.M. 1968: Morphologic alterations associated with neomycin induced malabsorption. *American Journal of Medical Science* 255, 63–77.

Donaldson, S.S., Jundt, S., Ricour, C. *et al.* 1975: Radiation enteritis in children: a retrospective review. Clinico-pathological correlation and dietary management. *Cancer* 35, 1167–78.

Dyer, N.H., Dawson, A.M., Smith, B., Todd, I.P. 1969: Obstruction of bowel due to lesion in the myenteric plexus. *British Medical Journal* 1, 686–9.

el-Lakany, S., Eagon, P.K., Gavaler, J.S., Schade, R.R., Whiteside, T., Van Thiel, D.H. 1990: Gastrointestinal function, morphology, and immune status in uremia. *Nutrition* 6, 461–8.

Falcone, A.B., Mao, R.L., Shrago, E. 1962: A study of the action of hypoglycemia-producing biguanide and sulfonylurea compounds on oxidative phosphorylation. *Journal of Biological Chemistry* 237, 904–9.

Faloon, W.W., Chodos, R.B. 1969: Vitamin B12 absorption studies using colchicine, neomycin and continuous 57Co B12 administration (abstract). *Gastroenterology* 56, 1251.

Faloon, W.W., Fisher, C.J., Duggan, K.C. 1958: Occurrence of a sprue-like syndrome during neomycin therapy (abstract). *Journal of Clinical Investigation* 37, 893.

Faloon, W.W., Webb, D.I., Race, T.F. 1967: Cholesterol lowering effect of colchicine (abstract). *Annals of Internal Medicine* 66, 1058.

Fang, W.-F., Broughton, A., Jacobson, E.D. 1977: Indomethacin-induced intestinal inflammation. *American Journal of Digestive Disease* 22, 49–60.

Fann, W.E., Davis, J.M., Janowski, D.S. *et al.* 1973: The effects of antacids on the blood levels of chlorpromazine (abstract). *Clinical Pharmacology and Therapeutics* 14, 135.

Faulk, D.L., Anuras, C.J. 1978: Chronic intestinal pseudo-obstruction. *Gastroenterology* 74, 922–31.

Faulk, D.L., Anuras, S., Gardner, G.D., Mitros, F.A., Summers, R.W., Christensen, J. 1978: A familial visceral myopathy. *Annals of Internal Medicine* 89, 600–6.

Fegan, C., Poynton, C.H., Whittaker, J.A. 1990: The gut mucosal barrier in bone marrow transplantation. *Bone Marrow Transplantation* 5, 373–7.

Feldman, S., Carlstedt, B.C. 1974: Effect of antacid on absorption of enteric-coated aspirin (letter to the editor). *JAMA* 227, 660–1.

Fitzgibbons, P.L., Chandrasome, P.T. 1987: Familial visceral myopathy. Evidence of diffuse involvement of intestinal smooth muscle. *American Journal of Surgical Pathology* 11, 846–54.

Forrest, F.M., Forrest, I.S., Serra, M.T. 1970: Modification of chlorpromazine metabolism by some other drugs frequently administered to psychiatric patients. *Biological Psychiatry* 2, 53–8.

Foster, C.S. 1979: The brown bowel syndrome: a possible smooth muscle mitochondrial myopathy. *Histopathology* 3, 1–17.

Frame, B., Guiang, H.L., Frost, H.M. *et al.* 1971: Osteomalacia induced by laxative (phenolphthalein) ingestion. *Archives of Internal Medicine* 128, 794–6.

Galland, R.B., Spencer, J. 1987: Natural history and surgical management of radiation enteritis. *British Journal of Surgery* 74, 742.

Gardner, E.C., Jr, Hersh, T. 1981: Primary hyperparathyroidism and the gastrointestinal tract. *Southern Medical Journal* 74, 197–9.

Glenner, G.G. 1980: Amyloid deposits and amyloidosis. The B-fibriloses. *New England Journal of Medicine* 302, 1333–43.

Godeau, B., Farcet, J.P., Delchier, J.C., Xuan, D.H., Chaumette, M.T., Gaulard, P. 1992: Protein-losing enteropathy in gastrointestinal sarcoidosis associated with malignant lymphoma. *Journal of Clinical Gastroenterology* 14, 78–80.

Griffin, P.H., Schnure, F.W., Chopra, S., Brooks, D.C., Gilliam, J.I. 1986: Intramural gastrointestinal hemorrhage. *Journal of Clinical Gastroenterology* 8, 389–94.

Griffiths, A.P., Shepherd, N.A., Beddall, A., Williams, J.G. 1997: Gastrointestinal tumour masses due to multiple myeloma: a pathological mimic of malignant lymphoma. *Histopathology* 31, 318–23.

Gross, L., Brotman, M. 1970: Hypoprothrombinemia and haemorrhage associated with cholestyramine therapy. *Annals of Internal Medicine* 72, 95–6.

Haboubi, N.Y., Honan, R.P., Hasleton, P.S. *et al.* 1984: *Pneumotosis coli.* A case report with ultra-structural study. *Histopathology* 8, 145–55.

Hall, G.J.L., Davis, A.E. 1969: Inhibition of iron absorption by magnesium trisilate. *Medical Journal of Australia* 2, 95–6.

Halsted, C.H., McIntyre, P.A. 1972: Intestinal malabsorption caused by aminosalicylate acid therapy. *Archives of Internal Medicine* 130, 935–9.

Halsted, C.H., Robles, E.S., Mezey, E. 1971: Decreased jejunal uptake of labeled folic acid (^{3}H-PGA) in alcoholic patients: roles of alcohol and nutrition. *New England Journal of Medicine* 285, 701–6.

Halstead, C.H., Robles, E.S., Mezey, E. 1973: Intestinal malabsorption in folate-deficient alcoholics. *Gastroenterology* 64, 526–32.

Hart, S.L., McColl, I. 1968: The effect of the laxative oxyphenisatin on the intestinal absorption of glucose in rat and man. *British Journal of Pharmacology* 32, 683–6.

Hayman, H., Fisher, C.J., Duggan, K.C. *et al.* 1964: Effect of fat-poor diet upon neomycin induced malabsorption. *Gastroenterology* 47, 161–5.

Heaton, K.W., Lever, J.V., Barnard, D. 1972: Osteomalacia associated with cholestyramine therapy for post-ilectomy diarrhoea. *Gastroenterology* 62, 642–6.

Heenan, P.J., Mason, D.Y., Skinner, J.M., Taylor, C.R. 1976: Waldenstrom's disease of the jejunum. *Beitrage zur Pathologie* 157, 76–83.

Heizer, W.D., Warshaw, A.L., Waldmann, T.A. *et al.* 1968: Protein-losing gastroenteropathy and malabsorption associated with factitious diarrhoea. *Annals of Internal Medicine* 68, 839–52.

Herbert, V. 1972: Metformin and B12 malabsorption (editorial). *Annals of Internal Medicine* 76, 140–1.

Herbst, J.J., Hurwitz, R., Sunshine, P. *et al.* 1970: Effect of colchicine on intestinal disaccharidases: correlation with biochemical aspects of cellular renewal. *Journal of Clinical Investigation* 49, 530–6.

Hermos, J.A., Adams, W.H., Liu, Y.K. *et al.* 1972: Mucosa of small intestine in folate-deficient alcoholics. *Annals of Internal Medicine* 76, 957–65.

Heubi, J.E., Partin, J.C., Schubert, W.K. 1983: Hypocalcemia and steatorrhea – clues to etiology. *Digestive Diseases and Sciences* 28, 124–8.

Hilderband, H.D., Zierler, R.E. 1980: Mesenteric vascular disease. *American Journal of Surgery* 139, 188–92.

Hoffman, W.S., Dyniewicz, H.A. 1945: The effect of alumina gel upon the absorption of Vitamin A from the intestinal tract. *Gastroenterology* 5, 512–22.

Hofmann, A.F., Kern, F., Jr 1971: The significance of bile acids in gastrointestinal and hepatic disease. *DM* 1–38.

Hofmann, A.F., Poley, J.R. 1969: Cholestyramine treatment of diarrhoea associated with ileal resection. *New England Journal of Medicine* 281, 397–402.

Holmes, R.P. 1970: Megaloblastic anemia precipitated by the use of oral contraceptives: a case report. *North Carolina Medical Journal* 31, 17–18.

Hurwitz, A. 1971: The effects of antacids on gastrointestinal drug absorption. Effect on sulfadiazine and quinine. *Journal of Pharmacology and Experimental Therapeutics* 179, 485–9.

Hvidt, S., Kjeldsen, K. 1963: Malabsorption induced by small doses of neomycin sulphate. *Acta Medica Scandinavica* 173, 699–705.

Isaacson, P., Wright, D. 1978: Malignant histocytosis of the intestine: its relationship to malabsorption and ulcerative jejunitis. *Human Pathology* 9, 661–77.

Israel, Y., Salazar, I., Rosenmann, E. 1968: Inhibitory effects of alcohol on intestinal amino acid transport in vivo and in vitro. *Journal of Nutrition* 96, 499–504.

Jackson, C.W., Haboubi, N.Y., Whorewell, P.J., Schofield, P.F. 1986: Gold-induced enterocolitis. *Gut* 27, 452.

Jacobs, E., Ardichvili, D., Perissino, A., Gottignies, P., Nanssens, J.F. 1979: A case of familial visceral myopathy with atrophy and fibrosis of the longitudinal muscle layer of the entire small bowel. *Gastroenterology* 77, 745–50.

Jacobson, E.D., Chodos, R.B., Falcon, W.W. 1960a: An experimental malabsorption syndrome induced by neomycin. *American Journal of Medicine* 28, 524–33.

Jacobson, E.D., Prior, J.T., Faloon, W.W. 1960b: Malabsorption syndrome induced by neomycin: morphologic alterations in the jejunal mucosa. *Journal of Laboratory Clinical Medicine* 56, 245–50.

Jacobson, E.D., Hibbs, S., Faloon, W.W. 1962: Effect of adrenal steroids and of gluten upon malabsorption induced by neomycin. *American Journal of Clinical Nutrition* 10, 325–31.

Kairaluoma, M.I., Karkola, P., Heikkinen, E., Huttunen, R., Mokka, R.E.M., Larmi, T.K.I. 1977: Mesenteric infarction. *American Journal of Surgery* 133, 188–93.

Kasahara, Y., Tanaka, S., Nishino, M., Umemura, H., Shiraha, S., Kuyama, T. 1981: Intestinal involvement in Behcet's disease. A review of 136 surgical cases in the Japanese literature. *Diseases of the Colon and Rectum* 24, 103–6.

Kaschula, R.O., Cywes, S., Katz, A., Louw, J.H. 1987: Degenerative leiomyopathy with massive megacolon. Myopathic form of chronic intestinal pseudo-obstruction occurring in indigenous Africans. *Perspectives in Paediatric Pathology* 11, 193–213.

Kaur, S., Cooper, G., Fakult, S., Lazarus, H.M. 1996: Incidence and outcome of overt gastrointestinal bleeding in patients undergoing bone marrow transplantation. *Digestive Diseases and Sciences* 41, 598–603.

Kent, T.H., Cardelli, R.M., Stammler, F.W. 1969: Small intestinal ulcers and intestinal flora in rats given indomethacin. *American Journal of Pathology* 54, 237–45.

Kern, I.B., Harris, M.J. 1973: Congenital short bowel. *Australian and New Zealand Journal of Surgery* 42, 283–5.

Keusch, G.T., Troncale, F.J., Plaut, A.G. 1970: Neomycin-induced malabsorption in a tropical population. *Gastroenterology* 58, 197–202.

Kneafsy, P.D., Kelly, J.K., Church, D.L., Rapp, E.F., Lafreniere, R. 1987: Phlegmonous duodenitis complicating multiple myeloma: a successful treated case. *American Journal of Gastroenterology* 82, 1322–5.

Kodama, H. 1977: Intestinal Behcet's disease (in Japanese). *Surgery and Therapy* 37, 51–18.

Koss, L.G. 1952: Abdominal gas cysts, pneumatosis intestinalis hominis: an analysis with a report of a case and a critical review of the literature. *Archives of Pathology* 53, 523–49.

Kumar, P.J., Dawson, A.M. 1972: Vasculitis of the alimentary tract. *Clinical Gastroenterology* 1, 719–22.

Lang, J., Price, A.B., Levi, A.J., Burke, M., Gumpel, J.M., Bjarnason, I. 1988: Diaphragm disease: pathology of disease of the small intestine induced by non-steroidal anti-inflammatory drugs. *Journal of Clinical Pathology* 41, 516–26.

Leveille, G.A., Powell, R.C., Sauberlich, H.E. *et al.* 1963: Effect of orally and parenterally administered neomycin on plasma lipids of human subjects. *American Journal of Clinical Nutrition* 12, 421–6.

Levin, R.J. 1966: Effect of colchicine on intestinal function in the rat. *Gut* 7, 250–7.

Levy, R.I., Frederickson, D.S., Stone, N.J. *et al.* 1973: Cholestyramine in Type II hyperlipoproteinemia: a double-blind trial. *Annals of Internal Medicine* 79, 51–8.

Leyonmarck, C.E., Ralf, L. 1985: Ulceration of the small intestine due to slow-release potassium chloride tablets. *Acta Chirurgica Scandinavica* 151, 273–6.

Lindenbaum, J., Lieber, C.S. 1969: Alcohol-induced malabsorption of Vitamin B12 in man (letter to the editor). *Nature* 224, 806.

Lindenbaum, J., Saha, J.R., Shea, N. *et al.* 1973: Mechanism of alcohol-induced malabsorption of Vitamin B12 (abstract). *Gastroenterology* 64, 762.

Longstreth, G.F., Newcomer, A.D., Westbrook, P.R. 1972: Para-aminosalicylate acid-induced malabsorption. *American Journal of Digestive Diseases* 17, 731–4.

Lotz, M., Zisman, E., Bartter, F.C. 1968: Evidence for a phosphorus-depletion syndrome in man. *New England Journal of Medicine* 278, 409–15.

Marcuard, S.P., Weinstock, J.V. 1988: Gastrointestinal angiodysplasia in renal failure. *Journal of Clinical Gastroenterology* 10, 482–4.

Marin, G.A., Clark, M.L., Senior, J.R. 1969: Studies on malabsorption occurring in patients with Laennec's cirrhosis. *Gastroenterology* 56, 727–36.

Marston, A. 1962: The bowel in shock. *Lancet* ii, 365–9.

Mayer, E.A., Schuffler, M.D., Rotter, J.I., Hanna, P., Mogard, M. 1986: Familial visceral neuropathy with autosomal dominant transmission. *Gastroenterology* 91, 1528–35.

McDonald, G.B. 1984: Gastrointestinal problems in bone-marrow transplant patients. In Bayless, T.M. (ed.) *Current therapy in gastroenterology and liver disease.* New York: B.C. Decker, 188–94.

McLean, F.W., Heine, M.W., Held, B. *et al.* 1969: Relationship between the oral contraceptive and folic acid metabolism: serum folate concentrations. *American Journal of Obstetrics and Gynecology* 104, 745–7.

Meulengracht, E. 1939: Osteomalacia of the spinal column from deficient diet or from disease of the digestive tract. III. Osteomalacia abuse laxantium. *Acta Medica Scandinavica* 101, 187–210.

Micozzi, A., Cartoni, C., Monaco, M., Martino, P., Zittoun, R., Mandelli, F. 1996: High incidence of infectious gastrointestinal complications observed in patients with acute myeloid leukemia receiving intensive chemotherapy for first induction of remission. *Support Care Cancer* 4, 294–7.

Mills, P.R., Brown, I.L., Watkinson, G. 1980: Idiopathic chronic ulcerative enteritis. *Quarterly Journal of Medicine* 194, 133–49.

Mittal, R., Spero, J.A., Lewis, J.H., Taylor, F., Ragni, M.V., Bontempo, F.A., Van Thiel, D.H. 1985: Patterns of gastrointestinal hemorrhage in hemophilia. *Gastroenterology* 88, 515–22.

Morson, B.C., Dawson, I.P. 1991: Vascular disorders. In Morson, B.C., Dawson, I.P., Day, D.W., Jas, J.R., Price,

A.B., Williams, G.T. (eds), *Gastrointestinal pathology*, 3rd edn., Oxford: Blackwell Scientific Publications, 344–7.

Munker, M., Sharma, O.P. 1987: Fatal gastrointestinal haemorrhage in sarcoidosis: a previously unreported occurrence. *Sarcoidosis* 4, 55–7.

Necheles, T.F., Snyder, L.M. 1970: Malabsorption of folate polyglutamates associated with oral contraceptive therapy. *New England Journal of Medicine* 282, 858–9.

Neoptolemos, J.P., Locke, T.J. 1983: Recurrent small bowel obstruction associated with phenylbutazone. *British Journal of Surgery* 70, 244–5.

Nezelof, C., Jaubert, F., Lyon, G. 1976: Familial syndrome combining short small intestine, intestinal malrotation, pyloric hypertrophy and brain malformation. Three anatomoclinical case reports. *Annual of Anatomic Pathology* 21, 401–12.

Nezelof, C., Vivien, E., Bigel, P. *et al.* 1985: Idiopathic myositis of the small intestine. An unusual cause of chronic intestinal pseudo-obstruction in children. *Archives of French Paediatrics* 42, 823–8.

Papadopoulou, A., Lloyd, D.R., Williams, M.D., Darbyshire, P.J., Booth, I.W. 1996: Gastrointestinal and nutritional sequelae of bone marrow transplantation. *Archives of Disease in Childhood* 75, 208–13.

Pappenheimer, A.M., Victor, A. 1946: Ceroid pigment in human tissue. *American Journal of Pathology* 22, 395–412.

Pearson, A.D., Craft, A.W., Pledger, J.V., Eastham, E.J., Laker, M.F., Pearson, G.L. 1984: Small bowel function in acute lymphoblastic leukaemia. *Archives of Disease in Childhood* 59, 460–5.

Pearson, J.M., Kumar, S., Butterworth, D.M., Schofield, P.F., Haboubi, N.Y. 1992: Flow cytometric DNA characteristic of radiation colitis. A preliminary study. *Anti-cancer Research* 12, 1647–9.

Peracchi, M., Bardella, M.T., Conte, D. 1998: Late-onset idiopathic hypoparathyroidism as a cause of diarrhoea. *European Journal of Gastroenterology and Hepatology* 10, 163–5.

Pimentel, R.R., van Stolk, R. 1993: Gastric plasmacytoma: a rare cause of massive gastrointestinal bleeding. *American Journal of Gastroenterology* 88, 1963–4.

Puri, P., Lake, B.D., Gorman, F., O'Donnell, B., Nixon, H.H. 1983: Megacystis-microcolon-intestinal hypoperistalsis syndrome: a visceral myopathy. *Journal of Paediatric Surgery* 18, 64–9.

Race, T.F., Paes, I.C., Faloon, W.W. 1970: Intestinal malabsorption induced by oral colchicine: comparison with neomycin and cathartic agents. *American Journal of Medical Science* 259, 32–41.

Rawson, M.D. 1966: Cathartic colon. *Lancet* 1, 1121–4.

Richardson, J.D., Lordon, R.E. 1993: Gastrointestinal bleeding caused by angiodysplasia: a difficult problem in patients with chronic renal failure receiving hemodialysis therapy. *American Surgeon* 59, 636–8.

Robert, A., Ansano, T. 1977: Resistance of germ free rats to indomethacin induced intestinal lesions. *Prostaglandins* 14, 331–41.

Robins, S.L., Cotran, Kumar (eds) 1989: *Robins pathologic basis of disease*, 4th edn. Philadelphia: W.B. Saunders, 212–16.

Rogers, A.I., Vloedman, D.A., Bloom, E.C. *et al.* 1966: Neomycin-induced steatorrhoea: a preliminary report on the in vivo hydrolysis of a long-chain unsaturated fat. *JAMA* 197, 185–90.

Roggin, G.M., Iber, F.L., Kater, R.M.H. *et al.* 1969: Malabsorption in the chronic alcoholic. *Johns Hopkins Medical Journal* 125, 321–30.

Rosen, Y., On, W. 1978: Phlemonous enterocolitis. *Digestive Diseases and Sciences* 23, 248–56.

Roy, A.D., Bharucha, H., Nevin, N.C., Odling-Smec, G.W. 1980: Idiopathic intestinal pseudo-obstruction: a familial visceral neuropathy. *Clinical Genetics* 18, 291–7.

Royer, P., Ricour, C., Nihou-Fekete, C., Pellerin, D. 1974: Le syndrome familial de grele court avec malrotation intestinale et stonose hypertrophique du pylore chez le nourrisson. *Archive Francais de Pediatries* 31, 223–39.

Rubin, E., Ryback, B.J., Lindenbaum, J. *et al.* 1972: Ultrastructural changes in the small intestine induced by ethanol. *Gastroenterology* 63, 801–14.

Russell, J.C., Welch, J.P. 1979: Operative management of radiation injuries of the intestinal tract. *American Journal of Surgery* 137, 433–42.

Ryser, J.E., Farquet, J.J., Petite, J. 1971: Megaloblastic anemia due to folic acid deficiency in a young woman on oral contraceptives. *Acta Haematologica (Basel)* 45, 319–24.

Sackier, J.M., Smith, E.J., Wood, C.B. 1988: Cystic pneumatosis in coeliac disease. *Gut* 29, 852–5.

Salter, W.M. 1972: Megaloblastic anemia and oral contraceptives. *Minnesota Medicine* 55, 554–5.

Satoh, H., Guth, P.H., Grossman, M.I. 1983: Role of bacteria in gastric ulceration produced by indomethacin in rats, cytoprotective action of antibodies. *Gastroenterology* 84, 483–9.

Saverymuttu, S.H., Thomas. A., Grundy, A., Maxwell, J.D. 1986: Ileal stricturing after long-term indomethacin treatment. *Postgraduate Medical Journal* 62, 967–8.

Scheiner, J., Altemeier, W.A. 1962: Experimental study of factors inhibiting absorption and effective therapeutic levels of Declyomycin. *Surgery, Gynecology and Obstetrics* 114, 9–14.

Schofield, P.F. 1989: Treatment of radiation bowel disease. In *The causation and clinical management of pelvic radiation disease.* Berlin: Springer-Verlag, 95–103.

Schofield, P.F., Carr, N.D., Holden, D. 1986: The pathogenesis and treatment of radiation bowel disease. *Journal of the Royal Society of Medicine* 79, 30–2.

Schuffler, M.D. 1981: Chronic intestinal pseudo-obstruction syndromes. *Medical Clinics of North America* 65, 173–96.

Schuffler, M.D., Jonak, Z. 1982: Chronic idiopathic intestinal pseudo-obstruction caused by a degenerative disorder of the myenteric pelxus: the use of Smith's method to define the neuropathology. *Gastroenterology* 82, 475–86.

Schuffler, M.D., Lowe, M.C., Bill, A.H. 1977: Studies of idiopathic intestinal pseudo-obstruction. I. Hereditary hollow visceral myopathy: clincial and pathological studies. *Gastroenterology* 73, 327–38.

Schuffler, M.D., Bird, T.D., Sumi, M., Cook A. 1978: A familial neuronal disease presenting as intestinal pseudo-obstruction. *Gastroenterology* 75, 889–98.

Schuffler, M.D., Pagon, R.A., Schwartz, R., Bill, A.H. 1988: Visceral myopathy of the gastrointestinal and genito-urinary tracts in infants. *Gastroenterology* 94, 892–8.

Schwartz, C.J., Acheson, E.D., Webster, C.V. 1961: Chronic mid-gut ischaemia with steatorrhoea in polycythaemia rubra vera. *American Journal of Medicine* 32, 950–5.

Sheth, K.J., Werlin, S.L., Freeman, M.E., Hodach, A.E. 1981: Gastrointestinal structure and function in Fabry's disease. *American Journal of Gastroenterology* 76, 246–51.

Shojania, A.M., Hornady, G.J., Barnes, P.H. 1971: The effect of oral contraceptives on folate metabolism. *American Journal of Obstetrics and Gynecology* 111, 782–91.

Small, M., Longarini, A., Zamcheck, N. 1959: Disturbances of digestive physiology following acute drinking episodes in 'skid row' alcoholics. *American Journal of Medicine* 27, 575–85.

Sprague, R., Harper, P., McClain, S., Trainer, T., Beeken, W. 1984: Disseminated gastrointestinal sarcoidosis. Case report and review of the literature. *Gastroenterology* 87, 421–5.

Spray, G.H. 1968: Oral contraceptives and serum-folate levels (letter to the editor). *Lancet* ii, 110–11.

Staffurth, J.S., Allott, E.N. 1962: Paralysis and tetany due to simultaneous hypokalemia and hypocalcemia, with other metabolic changes. *American Journal of Medicine* 33, 800–6.

Stampfl, D.A., Grimm, I.S., Barbot, D.J., Rosato, F.E., Gordon, S.J. 1990: Sarcoidosis causing duodenal obstruction. Case report and review of gastrointestinal manifestations. *Digestive Diseases and Sciences* 35, 526–32.

Stephens, M.E.M., Craft, I., Peters, T.J. *et al.* 1972: Oral contraceptives and folate metabolism. *Clinical Science* 42, 405–14.

Stowers, J.M., Bewsher, P.D. 1969: Studies on the mechanism of weight reduction by Phenformin. *Postgraduate Medical Journal* 45(Suppl), 13–16.

Streiff, R.R. 1970: Folate deficiency and oral contraceptives. *JAMA* 214, 105–8.

Sullivan, L.W., Herbert, V. 1964: Supervision of hematopoiesis by ethanol. *Journal of Clinical Investigations* 43, 2048–62.

Tanner, M.S., Smith, B., Lloyd, J.K. 1976: Functional intestinal obstruction due to deficiency of argyrophil neurones in the myenteric plexus. Familial syndrome presenting with short small bowel, malrotation, and pyloric stenosis. *Archives of Diseases in Children* 51, 837–41.

Thomas, W.E.G., Williamson, R.C.N. 1985: Non-specific small bowel ulceration. *Postgraduate Medical Journal* 61, 587–91.

Tjon, A., Tham, R.T., Vlasveld, L.T., Willemze, R. 1990: Gastrointestinal complications of cytosine-arabinoside chemotherapy: findings on plain abdominal radiographs. *American Journal of Roentgenology* 154, 95–8.

Tobin, M.V., Aldridge, S.A., Morris, A.I., Belchetz, P.E., Gilmore, I.T. 1989: Gastrointestinal manifestations of Addison's disease. *American Journal of Gastroenterology* 84, 1302–5.

Tomkin, G.H., Hadden, D.R., Weaver, J.A. *et al.* 1971: Vitamin B12 status of patients on long-term metformin therapy. *British Medical Journal* 2, 685–7.

Torosian, M.H., Turnbull, A.D. 1988: Emergency laparotomy for spontaneous intestinal and colonic perforations in cancer patients receiving corticosteroids and chemotherapy. *Journal of Clinical Oncology* 6, 291–6.

Turner, C.E. 1983: Gastrointestinal pseudo-obstruction due to pheochromocytoma. *American Journal of Gastroenterology* 78, 214–17.

Van der Jaget, E.J., Van Son, W.J., Van der Woude, F.J., Meijet, S., Sloof, M.J., Tegzess, A.M. 1987: Pneumatosis intestinalis related to cytomegalovirus infection. A new aetiology. *European Journal of Radiology* 7, 28–9.

Van Itallie, T.B., Hashim, S.A., Crampton, R.S. *et al.* 1961: The treatment of pruritus and hypercholesteremia of primary biliary cirrhosis with cholestyramine. *New England Journal of Medicine* 265, 469–74.

Vargas, J.H., Sachs, P., Ament, M.E. 1988: Chronic intestinal pseudo-obstruction syndrome in paediatrics. Results of a national survey by members of the North American Society of Paediatric Gastroenterology and Nutrition. *Journal of Paediatric Gastroenterology and Nutrition* 7, 323–32.

Vazquez-Quintana, E., Vargas, R., Perez, M., Porro, R., Gomez Duarte, C., Tellado, M., Marcial, M. 1995: Pheocromocytoma and gastrointestinal bleeding. *American Surgeon* 61, 937–9.

Veloso, F.T., Fraga, J., Saleiro, J.V. 1988: Macroglobulinemia and small intestinal disease. A case report with review of the literature. *Journal of Clinical Gastroenterology* 10, 546–50.

Waisbren, B.A., Hueckel, J.S. 1950: Reduced absorption of aureomycin caused by aluminium hydroxide gel (Amphojel). *Proceedings of the Society of Experimental Biology and Medicine* 73, 73–4.

Walsh, D. 1897: Deep tissue traumatism from Roentgen ray exposure. *British Medical Journal* 2, 272–3.

Webb, D.I., Chodos, R.B., Mahar, C.Q. *et al.* 1968: Mechanism of vitamin B12 malabsorption in patients receiving colchicine. *New England Journal of Medicine* 279, 845–50.

Whitehead, R. 1971: Ischaemic entrocolitis, an expression of intra-vascular coagulation syndrome. *Gut* 12, 912–17.

Whittle, B.J.R. 1981: Temporal relation between cyclooxygenase inhibition as measured by prostacyclin biosynthesis and the gastrointestinal damage induced by indomethacin in rats. *Gastroenterology* 80, 94–8.

Willms, B., Creutzfeldt, W. 1970: Contribution to the intestinal resorption of Vitamin B12 (Schilling Test) and of d-xylose in biguanide treatment (abstract). *Diabetologia* 6, 652.

Wilson, C., Gupta, R., Gilmour, D.G., Imrie, C.W. 1987: Acute superior mesenteric ischaemia. *British Journal of Surgery* 74, 279–81.

Zuckerman, G.R., Cornette, G.L., Clouse, R.E., Harter, H.R. 1985: Upper gastrointestinal bleeding in patients with chronic renal failure. *Annals of Internal Medicine* 102, 588–92.

28

Surgical conditions of the small intestine

BOOSHANAM V MOSES

INTESTINAL OBSTRUCTION

Intestinal obstruction is defined as obstruction to the forward movement of the intestinal contents. It can be classified based on the presence or absence of peristalsis (dynamic obstruction, and adynamic obstruction or paralytic ileus), according to the site of obstruction (high and low), and according to the type of clinical presentation (acute, chronic and acute on chronic).

Dynamic obstruction (synonym: mechanical obstruction)

In this case, intestinal peristalsis is present and tries to overcome the obstruction.

AETIOLOGY

Obstruction in the lumen:

- meconium (inspissated)
- bolus, which may be trichobezoars or phytobezoars, or partially digested food particles
- gallstones
- worms
- enterolith.

Lesions of the bowel wall:

- congenital – atresia and stenosis, megacolon (Hirschsprung's disease), Meckel's diverticulum, imperforate anus
- traumatic (intramural haematoma following blunt trauma)
- inflammatory – tuberculosis, Crohn's disease, diverticulitis
- neoplastic
- miscellaneous, e.g. radiation fibrosis.

Outside the wall:

- adhesions
- volvulus
- hernia
- intussusception.

Table 28.1 lists the common causes of dynamic obstruction according to age at presentation.

TYPES OF DYNAMIC OBSTRUCTION

Dynamic obstruction can be further classified as follows.

1. Simple mechanical obstruction, in which there is obstruction to the passage of intestinal contents but the blood supply to the intestine remains intact.
2. Strangulated obstruction. In addition to intestinal obstruction, the blood supply to the intestine is compromised. This leads to gangrene, perforation and peritonitis.
3. Closed-loop obstruction (Fig. 28.1) occurs when both the proximal and distal loops of bowel are obstructed, for example, a mechanical obstruction by a constricting growth in the recto-sigmoid, with

a proximal physiological obstruction due to the competent ileo-caecal valve. The pressure within the transverse and ascending colon increases progressively to result in caecal blow-out or stercoral ulcer perforation of the colon proximal to the recto-sigmoid.

Table 28.1 *Common causes of dynamic obstruction according to age at presentation*

Neonate	Congenital atresia Volvulus neonatorum Meconium ileus Hirschsprung's disease[a] Imperforate anus[a]
Infants	Strangulated inguinal hernia Intussusception Complications of a Meckel's diverticulum Hirschsprung's disease[a]
Young adult	Adhesions and bands Strangulated inguinal hernia
Middle age	Adhesions and bands Strangulated inguinal hernia Strangulated femoral hernia Carcinoma of the colon[a]
Elderly	Adhesions and bands Strangulated inguinal hernia Strangulated femoral hernia Carcinoma of the large bowel[a] Diverticulitis Impacted faeces[a]

[a]Included for the sake of completion, as these occur in the large intestine.

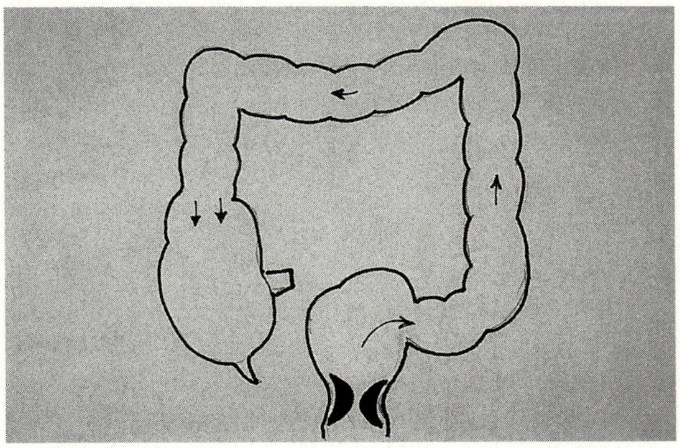

Figure 28.1 *Closed-loop obstruction.*

Table 28.2 *Gastrointestinal secretions and their contents*

Secretion	Volume (mL)	Contents
Saliva	1500	Predominantly [HCO_3^-], [Na^+], [Cl^-] ions
Gastric juice	2500	Predominantly [Na^+] and [Cl^-] ions
Bile and pancreatic juice	1000	Predominantly [HCO_3^-] ions
Succus entericus	3000	Predominantly [Na^+], [K^+], [HCO_3^-] ions

PATHOPHYSIOLOGY (Fig. 28.2)

There is progressive distension of the intestine proximal to the level of obstruction caused by both gas and fluids. Sources of gas are swallowed atmospheric air (68 per cent), diffusion from blood into the bowel lumen (22 per cent), and the products of digestion and bacterial activity (10 per cent). Of these gases, oxygen and carbon dioxide are absorbed into the blood stream, and the residual mixture in the intestine will contain hydrogen sulphide and nitrogen (Mann *et al.*, 1995). Fluid proximal to the obstruction consists of secretions into the gastrointestinal tract (Table 28.2).

Hence, both the level and the duration of obstruction will determine the extent and severity of electrolyte abnormalities. In strangulated obstruction, there is in addition a loss of blood volume, which is directly related to the length of the bowel involved. Unlike simple obstruction, the obstructed segment of the bowel alone distends. When distension occurs, there is translocation of bacteria through the devitalized bowel and peritonitis ensues.

CLINICAL FEATURES

The cardinal symptoms and signs of acute intestinal obstruction are abdominal pain, vomiting, distension, and failure to pass faeces or gas.

Abdominal pain

This is the first symptom. It is often colicky in nature and is usually experienced near the centre of the abdomen. The spasmodic cramp-like pain is due to the vigorous peristalsis of the small intestine trying to overcome the obstruction. In between the attacks of pain, the patient lies down quietly. If the obstruction is not relieved, a steady generalized abdominal pain replaces the colicky pain.

Vomiting

In high obstruction, vomiting is early and occurs with each bout of colic. In low ileal obstruction, vomiting does not follow each attack of pain but, as time goes on, the frequency of vomiting increases and vomitus changes from bilious to faeculent. This is because of bacterial proliferation and its action on the static contents of the obstructed segment.

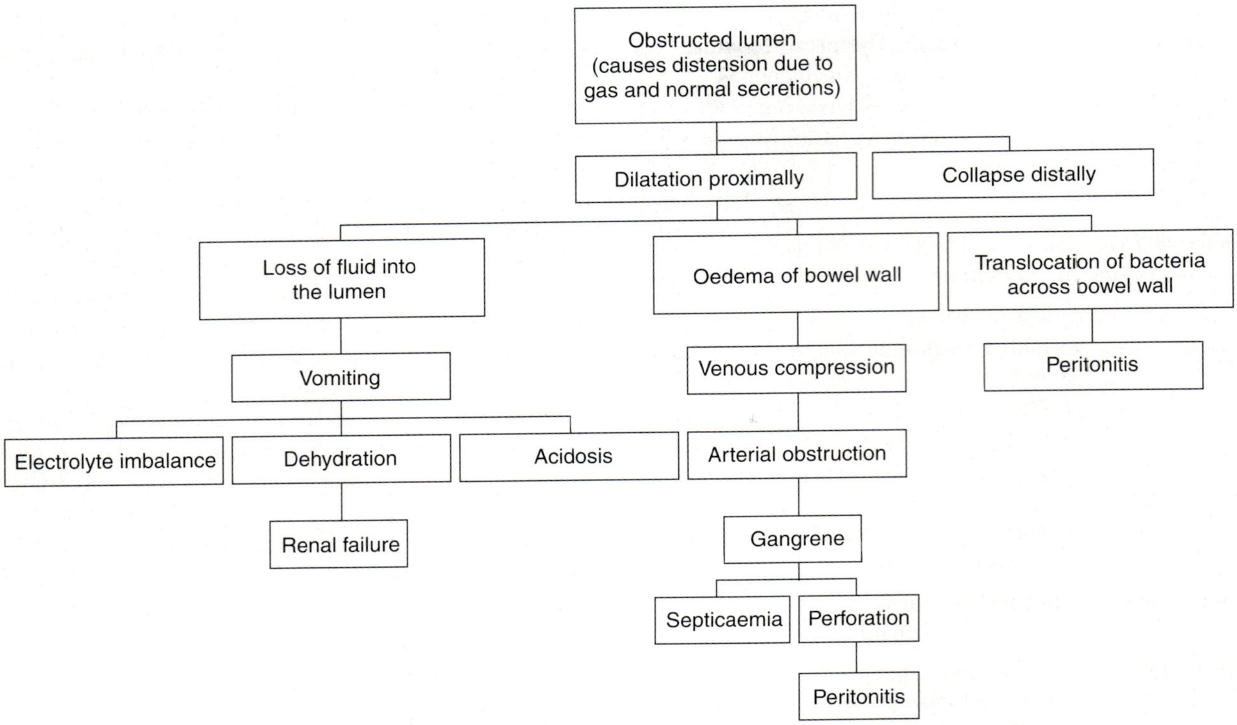

Figure 28.2 *Pathophysiology of dynamic intestinal obstruction.*

Distension

This gradually increases and is centrally located.

Constipation

At the onset of intestinal obstruction, the bowel distal to the site of obstruction, being normal, will empty its contents. However, once it is empty, there is no passage of faeces or gas per rectum.

DIFFERENTIATION BETWEEN STRANGULATED AND NON-STRANGULATED OBSTRUCTION

Even experienced clinicians can find it difficult to make a preoperative diagnosis of non-viable bowel or strangulation confidently. However, fever, tachycardia, tenderness and rebound tenderness, leucocytosis and unexplained acidosis (especially when a combination of these are present) can be considered as indicative of strangulation. Experimental studies in animal models have shown decreased absorption of intraperitoneally instilled xenon-133 in the presence of strangulation (Bulkley *et al.*, 1981). This may be of value in confirming the existence of gangrene preoperatively.

INVESTIGATIONS

Plain x-rays of the abdomen, erect and supine views, are taken. The erect view demonstrates air–fluid levels and the supine view shows the character of the distended bowel.

Jejunal shadows are characterized by valvulae conniventes producing a concertina effect (Figs 28.3 and 28.4). Ileal shadows are plain and characterless. The large bowel has prominent haustral folds that are incomplete circumferentially and are not opposite to each other. Typically, small bowel shadows occupy the centre of the film while colonic shadows will be in the periphery. It must be remembered that the dilated loop is proximal to the obstruction. Air–fluid levels are seen in the advanced stage of obstruction when air and fluid separate in the dilated loops of bowel. In high obstruction, few or no air–fluid levels are seen. Double bubble appearance is diagnostic of duodenal obstruction. In low ileal obstruction, there will be multiple air–fluid levels (Fig. 28.5). In strangulated obstruction, only one loop may be seen.

Use of barium studies for diagnosis of intestinal obstruction has been reported and may be of particular value when plain films are not diagnostic (Fig. 28.6). Barium can be used either as a small bowel series or enteroclysis (Dunn *et al.*, 1984). In mechanical obstruction, barium studies will demonstrate dilated proximal intestine and progression of barium to the level of obstruction in 1 hour or less. The danger of a barium leak through a perforation into the peritoneal cavity will have to be weighed against the benefit obtained. In obstruction distal to the ileo-caecal valve, a barium enema may be of use.

Haematocrit, blood sugar, electrolyte studies, serum creatinine, etc., need to be performed for the correction

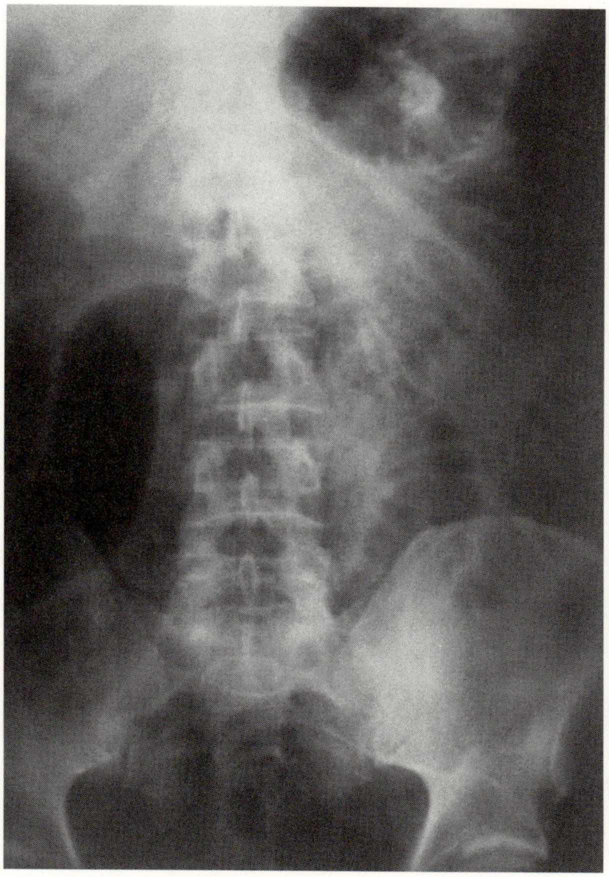

Figure 28.3 *Plain x-ray of the abdomen showing jejunal and ileal shadows.*

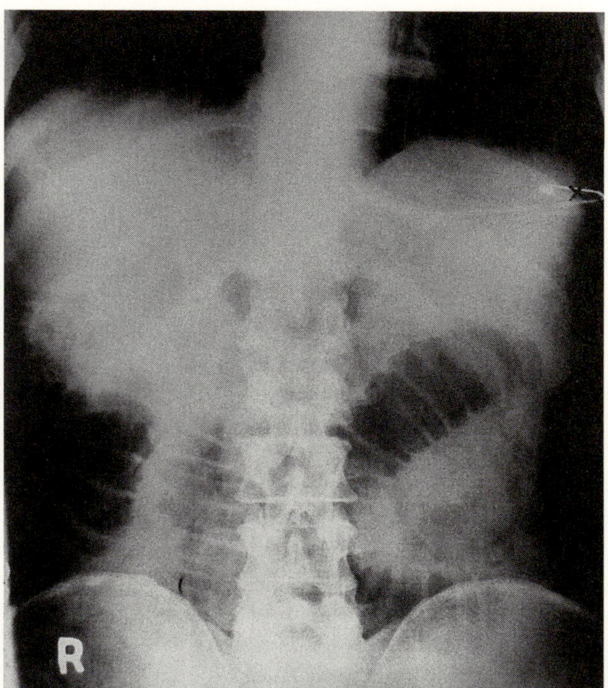

Figure 28.4 *Plain x-ray of the abdomen showing valvulae conniventes.*

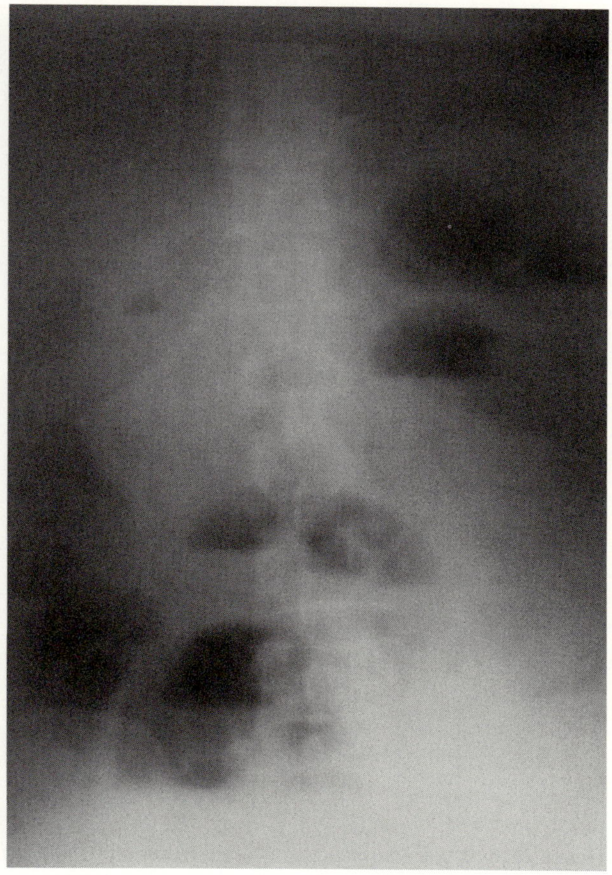

Figure 28.5 *Plain x-ray of the abdomen showing multiple air–fluid levels.*

of related abnormalities and in the preparation for surgery.

MANAGEMENT

The principles of management are: (1) fluid and electrolyte administration; (2) nasogastric suction – decompression; (3) administration of antibiotics to combat possible translocation of bacteria; and (4) relief of the obstruction.

Fluid and electrolyte therapy

A large central venous catheter is inserted for rapid administration of fluid and measurement of central venous pressure, and an indwelling urinary catheter is inserted for accurate measurement of urine output. Patients with bowel obstruction are likely to be depleted of water, sodium, chloride and potassium, and hence intravenous therapy with isotonic sodium chloride should be started. Large quantities of fluid may have to be infused to maintain a central venous pressure of 7–10 cm of saline. Monitoring of central venous pressure and urine output are the best controls for the rate of administration of fluids. Potassium

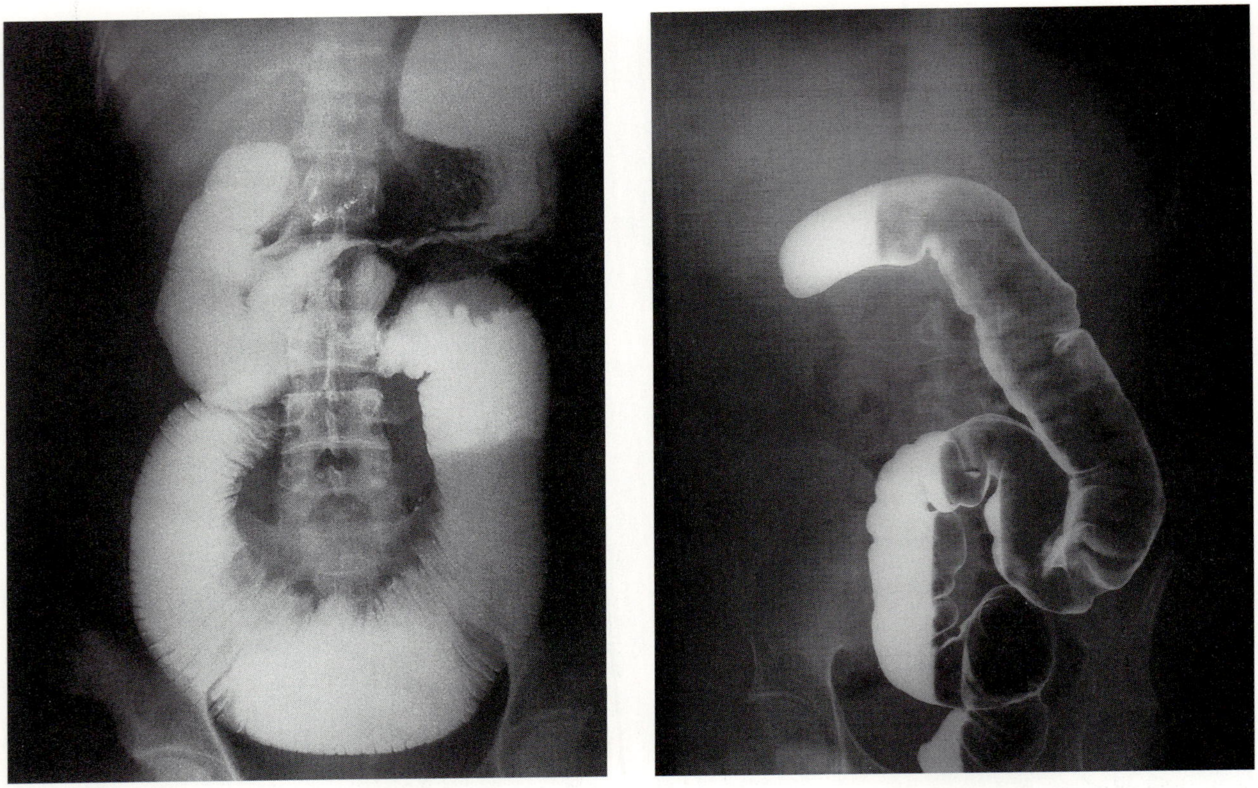

(a) (b)

Figure 28.6 *(a) Barium meal showing obstruction of the proximal jejunum due to a band. (b) Barium enema showing obstruction of the transverse colon due to stricture at the site of closure colostomy.*

chloride can be added only after ensuring adequate urinary output

Decompression of the Bowel

Nasogastric decompression using a Levine tube is the most commonly employed technique even though complete decompression is not possible as only gas and fluid from the upper intestine may regurgitate into the stomach for aspiration. Nevertheless, it is quite efficient in reducing the hazard of pulmonary aspiration as well as in minimizing further intestinal distension from swallowed air. Although long intestinal tubes, such as the Miller–Abbott tube, are available, their use is not popular owing to the difficulty in placing them accurately.

Operative treatment for intestinal obstruction

Indications for operation are:

- suspicion of strangulation
- closed-loop obstruction
- worsening of patient's condition on conservative management
- no improvement on conservative management for 48 hours.

Operation for intestinal obstruction should be performed under general anaesthesia administered through an endotracheal tube. In the absence of external hernia, abdominal exploration is performed through a midline vertical incision. On opening the peritoneum, the presence of free fluid is noted. Clear straw-coloured fluid is found in simple obstruction, while blood-stained fluid denotes strangulation. The point of obstruction is best found by looking at the caecum. If the caecum is distended, the obstruction is in the colon. If the caecum is collapsed, the intestine is followed back to the point of obstruction. Once the affected segment is identified, the viability of that segment is decided by its colour, peristalsis and arterial pulsation. Administration of 100 per cent oxygen to the patient and local application of warm sponges will help in deciding about the viability when the colour is dusky. In simple mechanical obstruction, division of a peritoneal band, or reduction of an internal hernia or untwisting of incomplete volvulus may be all that is necessary. However, when bowel is not viable, the options available are primary resection and anastomosis, or resection and exteriorization of the ends of the two loops as ostomies. In all cases, decompression of proximal dilated bowel is necessary and could be done through the bowel that is to be resected. Another satisfactory method of decompression, without spilling toxic intestinal contents into the peritoneal cavity, is to milk the intestinal contents into the stomach from where it can be aspirated with a nasogastric tube. When the diseased segment cannot be removed, as in neoplastic infiltration of adjacent structures, or in obstructive ileocaecal tuberculosis with very poor general condition of the patient, a short-circuiting procedure to bypass the obstruction can be performed.

Adynamic obstruction (synonyms: paralytic ileus, neurogenic ileus)

In this condition there is loss of normal propulsive activity in all or part of the alimentary canal.

The local causes of adynamic obstruction are:

- postoperative state
- peritonitis
- spinal injuries
- retroperitoneal haemorrhage.

The systemic causes of adynamic obstruction are:

- electrolyte imbalance, e.g. hypokalaemia
- metabolic disturbances, e.g. uraemia, myxoedema, diabetic coma
- septicaemia.

PATHOPHYSIOLOGY

Once there is bowel distension, the same mechanisms that appear in the later stages of dynamic obstruction operate in this case also. The mechanism of injury in paralytic ileus is summarized in Fig. 28.7.

CLINICAL FEATURES

The typical features are painless abdominal distension, effortless vomiting or copious nasogastric aspirate and absolute constipation. On auscultation, bowel sounds may be absent, or occasional high-pitched tinkling sounds due to shifting of fluid from one distended loop to another may be present. Succussion splash may be heard. Repeated clinical examination will be of great value in making the diagnosis.

INVESTIGATIONS

Plain x-rays will show multiple air–fluid levels, distended small bowel and air in a non-distended colon. Other investigations are carried out to confirm or rule out the conditions mentioned earlier.

TREATMENT

Supportive measures, such as nasogastric aspiration, antibiotics as and when required, intravenous fluids with electrolytes, and correction of predisposing causes, may be all that is required to treat this condition.

POSTOPERATIVE ILEUS

Postoperative ileus is believed to be related to neurotransmitters. After uncomplicated laparotomy, stomach function returns within 24–48 hours postoperatively. Small intestinal functions return within 16–24 hours and colonic functions within 48–72 hours. It is prudent to

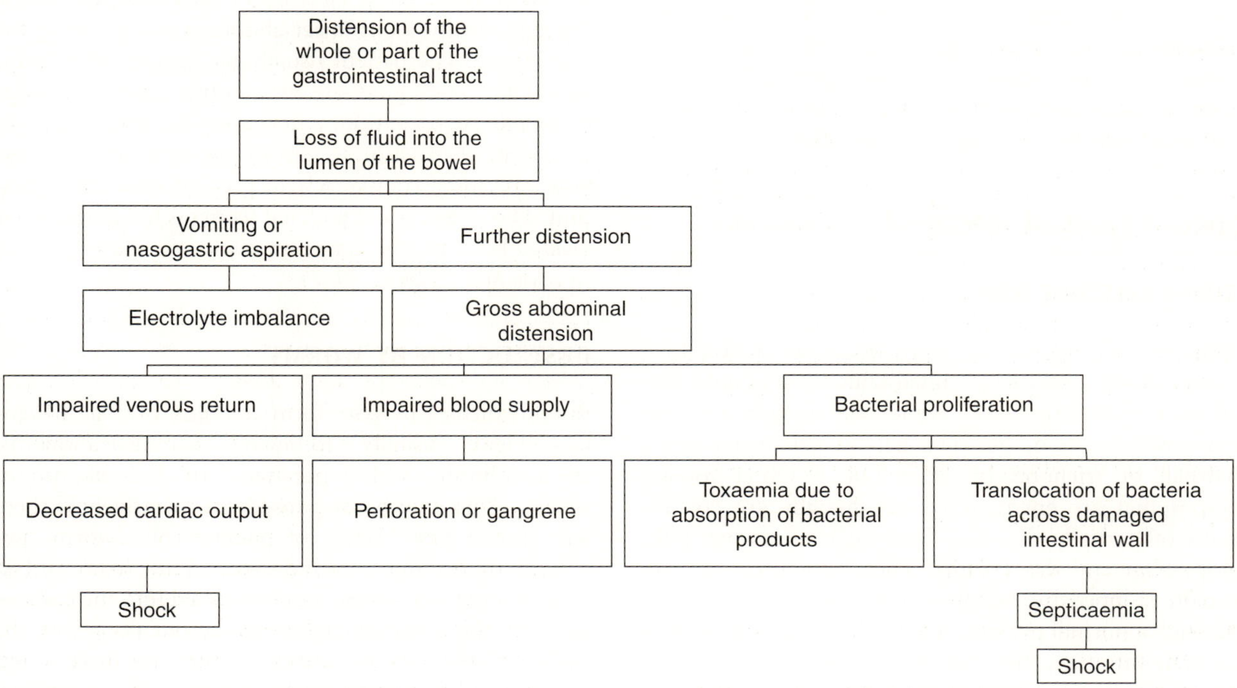

Figure 28.7 *Pathophysiology of paralytic ileus.*

Table 28.3 *Features of high and low intestinal obstruction*

Feature	High obstruction	Low obstruction
Vomiting	Severe, incessant	Present but late onset
Dehydration	Early	Late
Distension	Very little	Marked in the centre of the abdomen
Visible peristalsis	Left to right	Stepladder pattern
Plain x-ray	Few or no air–fluid levels	Many air–fluid levels

wait for 24–48 hours postoperatively before starting the patient on enteral feeds, as patients with upper gastrointestinal ileus may be at an increased risk of aspiration. Minimal and gentle handling of the intestine during laparotomy helps to prevent or minimize postoperative paralytic ileus. Postoperative ileus lasting more than 4 days will warrant further evaluation and a possibility of mechanical obstruction should be suspected.

High versus low obstruction

Intestinal obstruction can also be classified further into high or low small bowel obstruction. The main features of each are shown in Table 28.3.

Clinical types

Intestinal obstruction can be acute, chronic or acute on chronic. Acute obstruction usually involves the small bowel, and the onset and progression are rapid. Colicky abdominal pain, vomiting, distension and constipation are the sequence of events. Chronic obstruction usually involves the large bowel. Constipation, abdominal distension, pain and vomiting are the sequence of events. Acute on chronic obstruction primarily starts as large intestinal obstruction and progresses to involve the small intestine, e.g. sigmoid volvulus.

Special types of intestinal obstruction

BOLUS OBSTRUCTION

Intraluminal obstruction may occur as a result of foreign body ingestion by small children and individuals with psychiatric illness. A mentally disturbed person may swallow his or her own hair, which turns into a hairball or trichobezoar (Plate 28.1). Other foreign bodies that are encountered occasionally are concretions of partially digested food, such as orange pith, grape skin and dried fruits. These 'phytobezoars' are usually stopped by the pylorus but at times may pass through a normal pylorus. If the bezoars manage to pass into the intestine, they may be arrested in the narrowest part of ileum, which is 60 cm proximal to the ileocaecal junction. If conservative management does not relieve the intestinal obstruction, enterotomy and removal of the bezoars with stricturoplasty will have to be performed (Ward-McQuaid, 1950; Billings and Farrington, 1987).

ENTEROLITH

These are usually formed inside a diverticulum or proximal to a small bowel stricture. The nidus is usually an undigested seed, e.g. seeds of pomegranate, custard apple, etc. (Plate 28.2). Obstruction by enterolith is similar to obstruction by foreign bodies. This is managed by enterotomy or resection of the segment of bowel along with the stricture and enteroliths (Phillips, 1953; Ottinger and Edwin, 1975).

GALLSTONE OBSTRUCTION

For a gallstone to obstruct the small intestine, it has to be more than 2.5 cm in diameter. The only way such a large stone could enter the small intestine is through a cholecysto-duodenal fistula. These patients are usually elderly women who are known to have had gallstones for many years. Plain x-ray of the abdomen may reveal the stone in the right lower abdomen and/or air in the biliary tree. The patient usually has recurrent abdominal colic and gradually the obstruction becomes complete. At operation, enterotomy is performed over the site of obstruction to remove the stone and then the bowel is closed transversely to prevent stricture formation. The cholecysto-duodenal fistula is left alone, to be tackled later, if it becomes symptomatic (Turner, 1932; Brockis and Gilberg, 1957).

OBSTRUCTION BY WORMS

Roundworms can also form a bolus or ball by entanglement, usually following administration of antihelminthic, which paralyses the musculature of worms. This may be diagnosed preoperatively if there has been a past history of passing roundworms per rectum or finding a roundworm in the vomitus. At laparotomy these worms can be pushed into the caecum and then the worms would be passed out along with the faeces. If the ball of worms cannot be broken up, enterotomy is performed to remove them (Gupta, 1996).

OBSTRUCTION BY ADHESIONS

Peritoneal irritation, irrespective of the cause, results in exudation of fibrin locally and leads to adhesion formation between the apposed surfaces (Ellis, 1962). These adhesions may disappear by themselves or may become vascularized and later replaced by fibrous tissue. Various factors that seem to produce adhesions are infection, foreign material introduced into the peritoneal cavity, such as talcum powder used in gloves, suture material, drain tubes, and contrast material, such as barium.

Types of adhesions (Mann *et al.*, 1995)

Fibrinous adhesions, called bread and butter adhesions, are a reaction to handling of the intestine at surgery. They resolve completely without treatment and can be separated easily at operation.

Fibrous adhesions usually occur at sites of vascular compromise. Whenever there is deficient blood supply to an organ, it tends to become attached to the omentum, parietal peritoneum or an adjacent structure to obtain an additional blood supply. This attachment develops into strong fibrous adhesions that can be lysed only by sharp dissection.

Inflammatory adhesions occur when omentum and loops of bowel become adherent to an inflamed organ, such as the appendix, or a tubo-ovarian mass.

Treatment of obstruction due to adhesions

Most of the adhesive obstructions may resolve with conservative measures. If obstruction is not relieved by these measures, or if there is suspicion of strangulation, laparotomy should be performed. At laparotomy, even though many adhesions may be found, usually only one of them will be responsible for obstruction. This should be released. Recurrent adhesive intestinal obstruction may be treated by Noble's plication or Child–Phillip's transmesenteric plication (Noble, 1937; Child and Phillips, 1960). Baker tube intubation also might help in reducing the chances of recurrent adhesive obstructions.

BANDS AND INTERNAL HERNIA

Bands

Bands may be congenital, e.g. persistent vitello-intestinal duct or transduodenal band of Ladd, or acquired (occurring after peritonitis). These bands cause obstruction by direct compression of the bowel. The obstruction thus produced may be partial or complete. Strangulation of bowel can also occur. If conservative measures fail, laparotomy should be performed and the offending band/omentum should be divided.

Obstruction due to internal hernia

A loop of small bowel enters a pre-existing opening or the peritoneal fossa and may become obstructed. Examples are congenital diaphragmatic hernia, defects in the mesentery, and peritoneal fossae near the duodenum, caecum and sigmoid colon. This condition is often diagnosed only at operation. As some of these fossae have important vessels in their boundaries, extreme care should be taken while releasing the intestines from these fossae.

CROHN'S DISEASE

Crohn's disease, a chronic non-specific inflammatory disease, may present with either perforation or intestinal obstruction. It produces transmural inflammation of the bowel, which results in stricture formation. Treatment is conservative resection of the involved area.

TUBERCULOSIS OF SMALL INTESTINE

Tuberculosis may produce obstruction due to transmural involvement and stricture or through adhesions (Plate 28.3). Pulmonary tuberculosis may coexist in some of these patients. Barium examination will show dysmotility, barium retention, or irregularity and strictures. Treatment will be resection of the stricture followed by antituberculous therapy. Ileo-caecal tuberculosis may require only a limited resection. A right hemicolectomy may be required in rare instances when the ascending colon is also involved or when an ileo-transverse colon bypass operation had been done earlier (Prakash, 1978; Addison, 1983).

INTESTINAL OBSTRUCTION IN THE PREGNANT PATIENT

Intestinal obstruction can occur in pregnancy and is associated with 5 per cent maternal and 20–25 per cent foetal mortality. Presenting symptoms are the same as seen in non-pregnant patients. However, as vomiting and constipation are common complaints during pregnancy, these symptoms are likely to be ignored. Abdominal distension may be difficult to assess in the presence of an enlarged uterus. Early surgery will improve the chances of survival of the mother and foetus.

INTESTINAL OBSTRUCTION IN AIDS PATIENTS

Apart from the general causes of intestinal obstruction, these patients may present with obstruction secondary to unusual conditions, such as *Mycobacterium avium* complex, non-Hodgkin's lymphoma, histoplasmosis and Kaposi's sarcoma (La Raja *et al.*, 1989; Wilson *et al.*, 1989).

CANCER AND SMALL BOWEL OBSTRUCTION

Surgeons are generally reluctant to operate on patients after any previous surgery for abdominal malignancies because they attribute the obstruction to recurrence or spread of cancer. However, many now feel that resection or bypass of the obstructing lesions, if feasible, improves the quality of life and increases survival.

ACUTE INTESTINAL OBSTRUCTION IN THE NEWBORN

Congenital atresia and stenosis are common causes of obstruction in the newborn. The other causes include volvulus neonatorum, meconium ileus, anorectal malformations, intussusception and Hirschsprung's disease.

Congenital atresia and stenosis

The common sites in the descending order of frequency of occurrence are duodenum, ileum, jejunum and ascending colon. Atresia may also occur at multiple sites. Congenital atresia can be classified as in Fig. 28.8.

Duodenal atresia

Duodenal atresia presents with persistent vomiting and upper abdominal distension. The presence or absence of bile in vomitus depends on whether the obstruction is proximal or distal to the ampulla of Vater, and whether the obstruction is complete or incomplete. Visible gastric peristalsis may be seen. Plain x-rays reveal double bubble gas shadows. Gastrografin studies will demonstrate obstruction. Duodenal atresia can be differentiated from oesophageal atresia by the absence of constant dribbling of saliva and from congenital pyloric stenosis by the absence of a lump. Duodeno-duodenostomy is the recommended operation. If this is not possible, duodeno-jejunostomy should be performed.

Jejuno-ileal atresia (Plate 28.4)

The prominent features are central abdominal distension, jaundice, bilious vomiting and failure to pass meconium in the first 24 hours of life. Polyhydramnios may be noted in a quarter of the cases. Vomitus usually contains bile. The diagnosis is based mainly on the presence of a distended abdomen and multiple air–fluid levels shown on plain x-ray of the abdomen.

Treatment

Treatment depends on the type of obstruction, its level and the extent of dilatation of the proximal intestine. Parenteral vitamin K, intravenous antibiotics and intravenous fluids may be started in preparation for surgery. Possible procedures include excision of the obstructing diaphragm, and resection of the atretic segment and

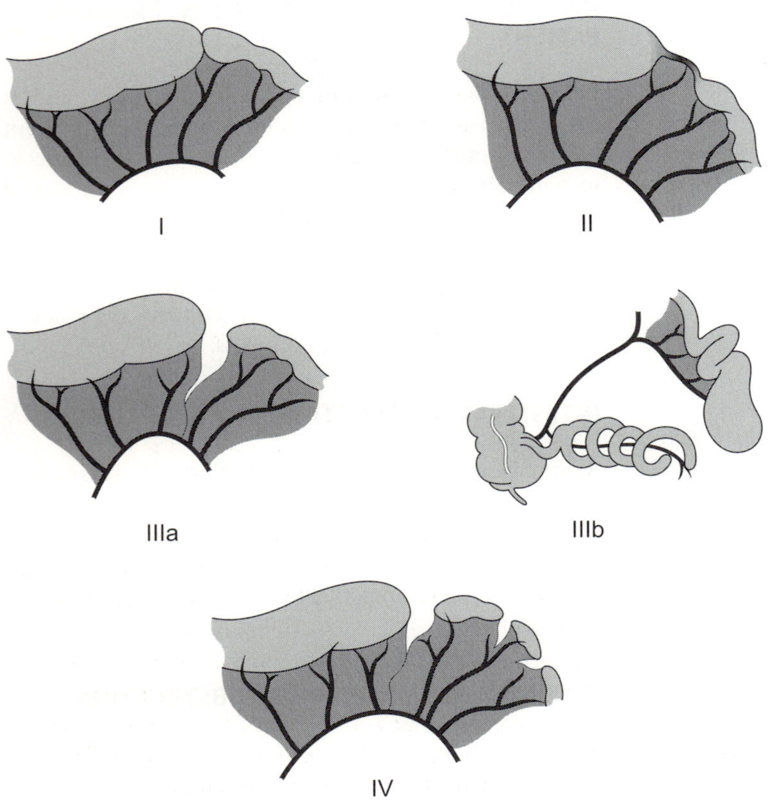

Figure 28.8 *Classification of intestinal atresia; Type I – membraneous atresia with intact bowel and mesentery; Type II – blind ends are separated by a fibrous cord; Type IIIa – blind ends are separated by a V-shaped mesenteric defect; Type IIIb – apple peel atresia; Type IV – multiple atresia. (Reprinted with permission from Grosfield, J.L., Ballantine, T.V.N., Shoemakier, R. 1979: Operative management of intestinal atresia and stenosis based on pathologic findings.* Journal of Pediatric Surgery *14, 368.)*

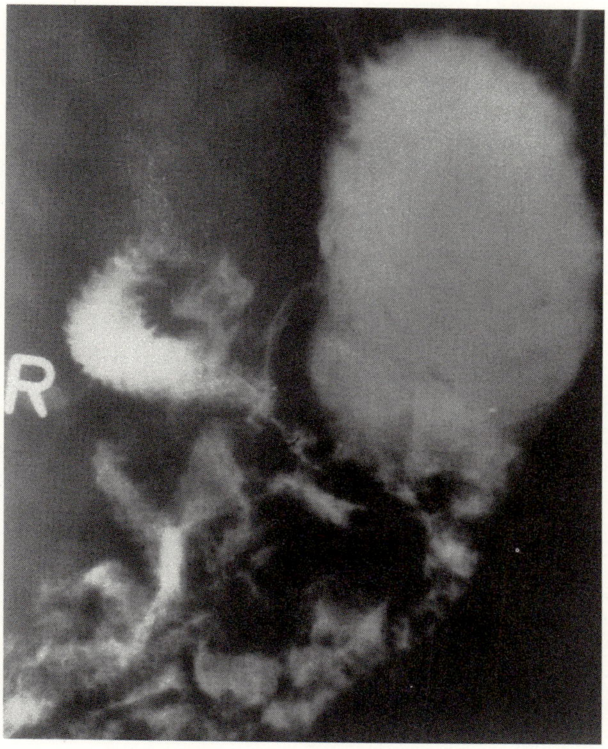

Figure 28.9 *Contrast study showing arrested rotation. Note the absence of the C loop of duodenum and presence of most of the small intestine on the right side of the abdomen.*

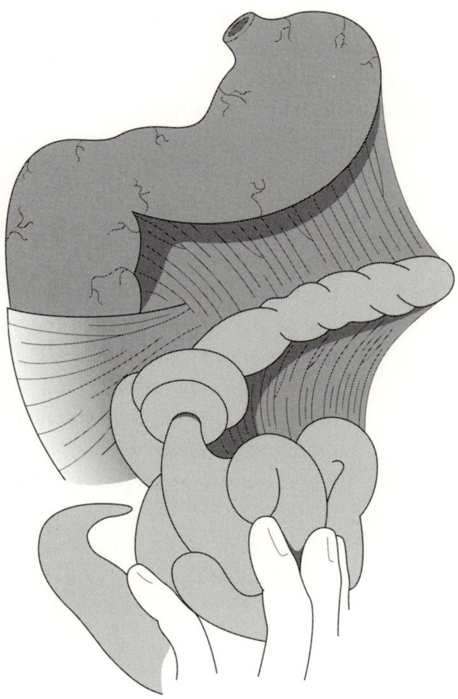

Figure 28.10 *Arrested rotation of the intestine. The entire intestinal mass is drawn out of the abdomen showing a narrow mesentery. (Reprinted with permission from Ladd, W.E., Gross, R.E. 1941:* Abdominal surgery of infancy and childhood. *Philadelphia: W.B. Saunders.)*

anastomosis. In ileal atresia with volvulus, when vascular integrity is in question, it would be better to resect and bring out both the ends, proximal as an ileostomy and distal as a mucous fistula. In jejunal atresia, resection and end-to-end anastomosis is the treatment of choice, as infants do not tolerate loss of fluid and electrolytes of even a temporary fistula.

Arrested rotation (Figs 28.9 and 28.10)

The transduodenal band of Ladd, a peritoneal band running from the undescended caecum in the central abdomen across the duodenum, causes duodenal obstruction and the clinical features are identical to that of duodenal stenosis. The transduodenal band and the often-present second peritoneal band over the proximal jejunum are divided. The caecum and colon are mobilized to lie on the left side of abdomen while keeping the small bowel to the right. This procedure is combined with appendicectomy and is known as Ladd's procedure (Fig. 28.11).

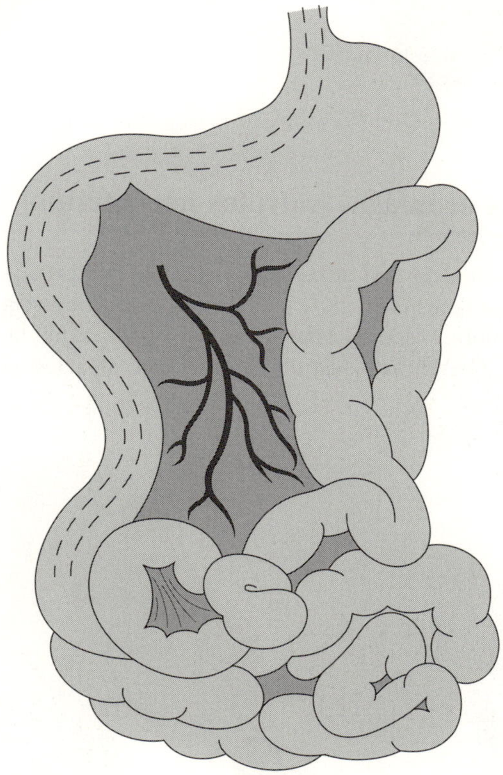

Figure 28.11 *Ladd's procedure completed. The duodenum descends along the right gutter. The small intestine lies on the right side of the abdomen, and the caecum and ascending colon are on the left side or on the midline. The superior mesenteric artery and its branches are left exposed as shown. A nasogastric tube has been passed into the jejunum to rule out intrinsic obstruction. (Reprinted with permission from Ladd, W.E., Gross, R.E. 1941:* Abdominal surgery of infancy and childhood. *Philadelphia: W.B. Saunders.)*

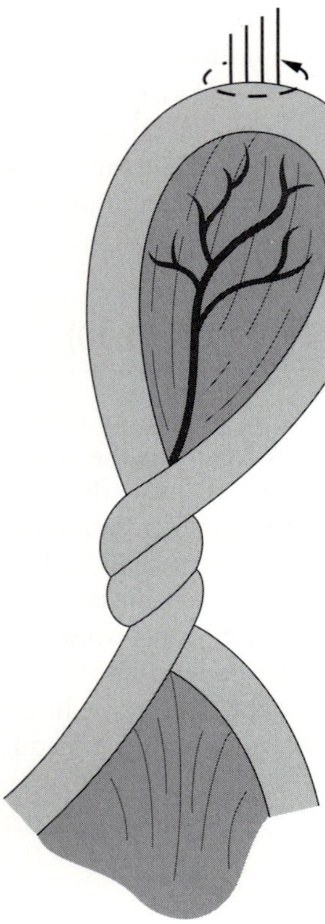

Figure 28.12 *Volvulus due to arrested rotation of the midgut. (Redrawn with permission from Mann, C.Y., Russel, R.C.G., Williams, N.S. (eds) 1995:* Bailey and Love's short practice of surgery. *London: Chapman and Hall.)*

Volvulus of midgut (volvulus neonatorum)

Arrested rotation and adhesion to the parietes predisposes to volvulus (Fig. 28.12). The small intestine along with the mobile caecum rotates clockwise producing the volvulus. The clinical features are as that of arrested rotation, but the onset is acute and the condition of the infant worsens rapidly. Laparotomy should be performed early, and the volvulus derotated anticlockwise, along with division of the transduodenal band and Ladd's procedure.

Meconium ileus (Plate 28.5)

Mucoviscidosis (fibrocystic disease) presents as meconium ileus in the neonatal period. In this condition the terminal ileum becomes filled with viscid mucus. Later this mucus becomes hard (Fig. 28.13) and intestinal obstruction can occur even at birth. A plain x-ray shows a distended, mottled, small intestine and a typical soap-bubble or ground-glass appearance in the right iliac fossa. Failure to digest a sensitized coat of an x-ray plate by the vomitus of an infant is diagnostic of mucoviscidosis, as there is a deficiency of trypsin. If the diagnosis is not clear, Gastrografin enema is diagnostic and may be therapeutic (Fig. 28.14). Since Gastrografin (diatrizoate meglumine) is hyperosmolar, fluid is drawn into the lumen of the intestine. This fluid dislodges the hard meconium, relieving the obstruction (Noblett, 1969). Failed Gastrografin enema treatment and complicated meconium ileus will need operation. At laparotomy, resection and anastomosis of bowel (end-to-side) with exteriorization of either the proximal (Santulli) or distal (Bishop–Koop) ileum as a mucous fistula is performed (Figs 28.15 and 28.16). The distal ileum is utilized to eliminate the meconium. The mucous fistula needs to be closed at a later date. Infants with this condition may develop pulmonary complications and require treatment with antibiotics, mucolytics and oxygen.

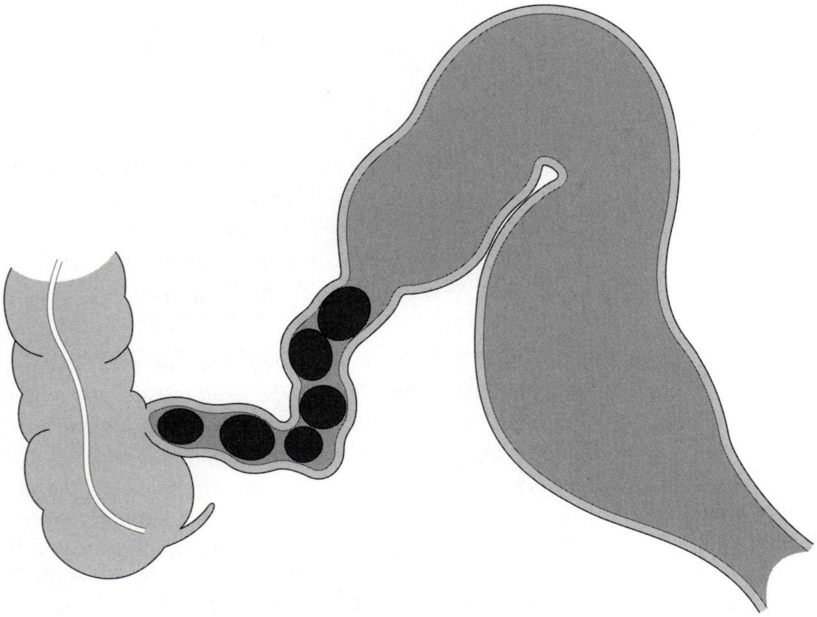

Figure 28.13 *Uncomplicated meconium ileus with obstruction due to inspissated pellets in the terminal ileum. (Reprinted with permission from Rescorla, F.J., Grosfeld, J.L. 1993: Contemporary management of meconium ileus.* World Journal of Surgery *17, 318.)*

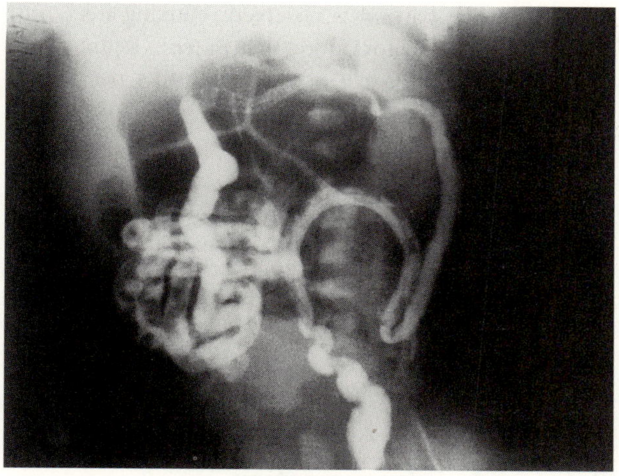

Figure 28.14 *Gastrografin enema showing pellets of meconium, in meconium ileus.*

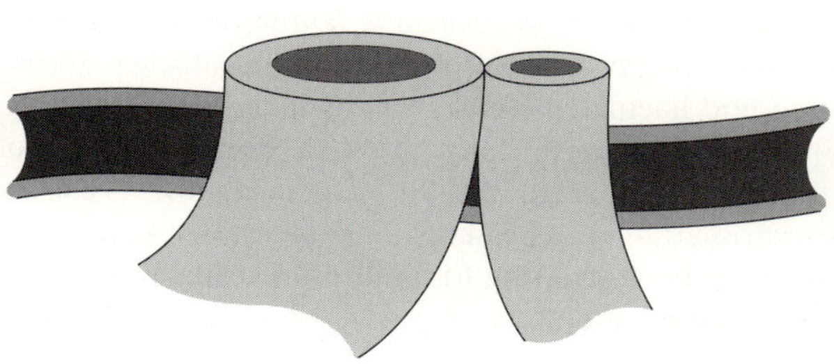

Figure 28.15 *The double-barrel side by side (modified Mikulicz) enterostomy.*

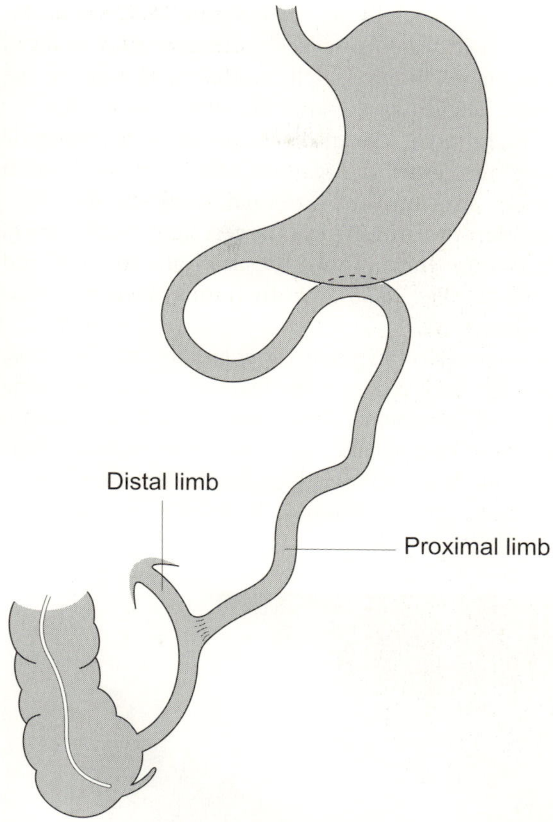

Figure 28.16 *Bishop–Koop operation.*

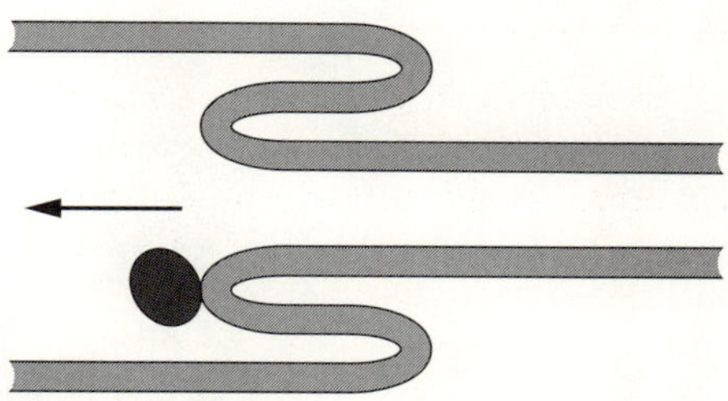

Figure 28.17 *Intussusception showing a lead point.*

INTUSSUSCEPTION

Intussusception is invagination of one loop of bowel into the adjacent loop. It is usually anterograde but can be retrograde also. The entering and middle tube are together called the intussusceptum and the outer tube is called the intussuscipiens. The neck is the junction of the entering tube with the bowel mass of intussusception. There may be a polyp or lipoma at the apex or leading point of the intussusception. External constriction of the mesentery at the neck by the outer layer is likely to compromise the blood supply of the inner layer and gangrene will supervene. The various types of intussusception are ileo-ileal, ileo-colic, ileo-ileo-colic, colocolic and multiple intussusceptions.

Aetiology

This may be idiopathic or secondary. Polyps, submucous lipoma and papilliferous carcinoma, which protrude intraluminally, start off an intussusception in the secondary type. In the idiopathic variety, no such lesions are found. There are various theories about the cause of primary or idiopathic intussusception. Changes in intestinal flora, consequent to weaning or adenovirus/rotavirus upper respiratory tract infection, may cause a hypertrophy of the lymphatic follicles in the intestinal wall (Ross *et al.*, 1962). These submucosal bulges in turn form the lead point or apex of the intussusception (Fig. 28.17).

Clinical features

Usually a male child of 4–12 months of age is brought with a history of sudden paroxysms of abdominal pain and vomiting. The attacks of colic occur at 15-minute intervals and the child may be quiet in between attacks. Redcurrant-jelly stools replace normal stools. Usually, a sausage-shaped lump is felt in the right side of the abdomen lateral to the umbilicus or just under the costal margin. In rare instances, it can even protrude through the anus. Unrelieved, the condition soon progresses to complete intestinal obstruction. Ultrasound often reveals a typical 'target' sign (Daniel *et al.*, 1977). Barium enema shows the classical 'claw' sign and is diagnostic (Fig. 28.18). Treatment may be non-operative or operative.

Non-operative treatment for colo-colic and ileo-colic intussusception is reduction by hydrostatic pressure using saline or barium enema. For barium reduction, a column of barium should be held 30 cm above the buttocks of the patient. For hydrostatic reduction, the pressure should not exceed 120 cm of water. Reduction is considered complete when barium is observed refluxing freely into the small intestine for more than 5 cm. Reduction is followed by free passage of gas and faeces per rectum (Ravitch and Robert, 1948).

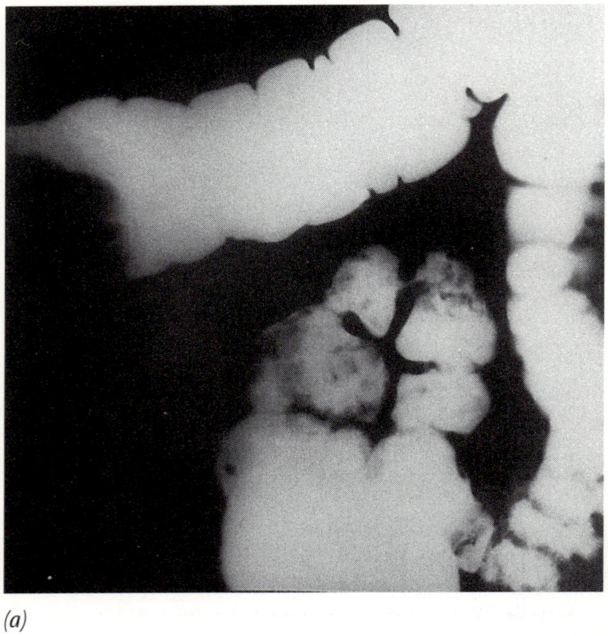

(a)

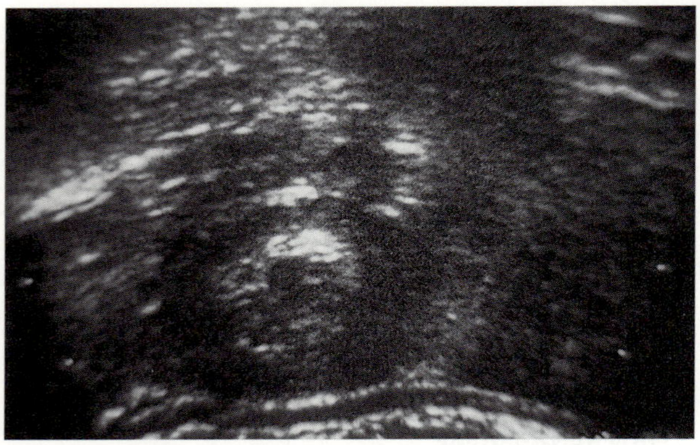

(b)

Figure 28.18 *(a) Barium enema in intussusception showing claw sign. (b) Ultrasound showing typical target sign in intussusception.*

Operative reduction

After laparotomy through a right paramedian incision, the apex of the intussusception should be pushed. The entering tube should never be pulled. Identification of a specific lead point lesion or non-viable bowel will need resection and anastomosis (Zachary, 1955).

Retrograde intussusception

This is rare but may occur in any part of the intestine. A special form of this occurs after Polya or Billroth type II gastrectomy or gastrojejunostomy. The efferent or afferent loop projects into the stomach causing obstruction and haematemesis.

A barium meal x-ray shows a doughnut type of filling defect (Fig. 28.19). The diagnosis can be confirmed by gastroscopy. A permanent cure is achieved by converting to a Billroth I using an interposition jejunal loop.

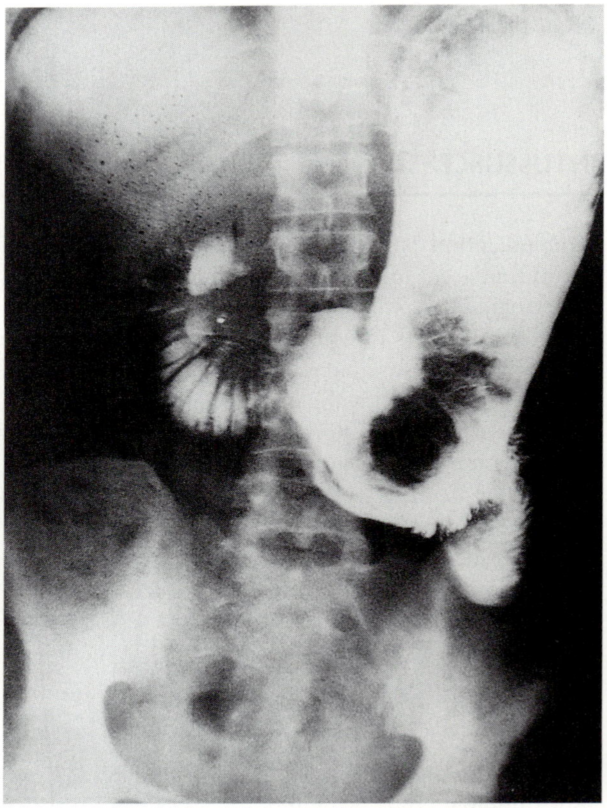

Figure 28.19 *Barium meal x-ray showing retrograde jejuno-gastric intussusception.*

DIVERTICULA OF THE SMALL INTESTINE

These may be congenital or acquired. The congenital type has all the coats of bowel in the wall of the diverticulum, e.g. Meckel's diverticulum (Plate 28.6). The acquired diverticulum lacks the muscular coat. Most alimentary tract diverticula are thought to be acquired. It is presumed that small intestinal diverticula are due to herniation of mucosa at the point of entry of the blood vessels (the weakest part of the bowel wall). Chronic intestinal motility disorders with increased intraluminal pressures predispose to these diverticula (pulsion diverticula) (Shoba *et al.*, 1983).

Diverticula can be single or multiple, and they occur in the mesenteric border, mostly in the jejunum and to a lesser extent in the ileum. Jejunal diverticula are often associated with colonic and other gastrointestinal diverticula. They vary greatly in size. The symptoms of small bowel diverticula are vague epigastric or paraumbilical discomfort, abdominal pain, early satiety, flatulence and borborygmi. Most often, the onset of complications reveals their presence. Diverticulosis may also be discovered while investigating a case of malabsorption syndrome. Barium meal studies, particularly late films, often reveal small bowel diverticula.

Complications

DIVERTICULITIS

Diverticulitis presents with pain, vomiting and signs of intra-abdominal sepsis owing to perforation producing either localized or generalized peritonitis. Preoperative diagnosis is rarely possible (Donald, 1979).

OBSTRUCTION

Mechanical obstruction usually occurs from adhesions that follow diverticulitis. Enteroliths arising from diverticula may also cause obstruction. Adhesions between the bowel and the parietes may predispose to volvulus (Ottinger and Edwin, 1975; Billings and Farrington, 1987).

HAEMORRHAGE

Diverticular disease often produces recurrent bouts of massive lower gastrointestinal bleeding. Angiography and a red-cell tagged scan is useful in the diagnosis and localization of lesions. Laparotomy is sometimes required and the segment involved is resected (Shackelford and Marcus, 1960; Hugo and John, 1978).

MALABSORPTION

Small bowel diverticulosis is one of the common causes of malabsorption or stagnant bowel syndrome. Stasis induces bacterial overgrowth. This leads to lysis of vitamin B_{12}, producing megaloblastic anaemia. Bacterial hydrolysis of the conjugated bilirubin leads to diarrhoea. Weight loss, hypoproteinaemia and neuropathy are associated problems. Colonic bacteria in the duodenal aspirate, along with malabsorption and the presence of diverticula on the barium x-rays, clinch the diagnosis. Parenteral vitamin B_{12} and oral broad-spectrum antibiotics cure most of the cases. Resection of the affected segment of bowel is necessary if medical therapy fails (Brian and Stair, 1985).

BILIARY PANCREATIC COMPLICATIONS

Periampullary diverticula have been implicated in the pathogenesis of calculus formation and obstructive biliary tract disease, and can be considered as a differential diagnosis for postcholecystectomy symptoms (Donald, 1979). This may also be a rarer cause for acute pancreatitis.

Management

Diverticula are primarily managed by non-surgical methods with a trial of antacids, antispasmodics, low-fat diets and small meals. Periampullary diverticula causing biliary obstruction may be managed with endoscopic papillotomy. Surgery is reserved for patients with complications and for those who do not improve with an adequate period of conservative treatment. Resection offers the best treatment, especially in localized disease. Other operative modalities include local excision and inversion.

NEONATAL ENTEROCOLITIS (NECROTIZING ENTEROCOLITIS) (Plate 28.7)

Premature infants with perinatal hypoxia are usually affected. It is more likely to occur when such infants are fed formula (high osmotic) feeds. It is suggested that blood is diverted to vital organs during a hypoxic episode, thus causing ischaemia of the bowel mucosa, which is then invaded by bacteria from within the bowel lumen. The terminal ileum and caecum are commonly involved with gross mucosal hemorrhage, ulceration and necrosis. Microscopically, there is a marked vascular congestion and oedema with mucosal necrosis. A pseudomembrane of necrotic mucosa is frequently present. Clinical presentation includes abdominal distension, high nasogastric aspirate, vomiting, diarrhoea, haematochaezia and, occasionally, pallor or skin mottling. Gas bubbles in the submucosa (pneumatosis intestinalis) seen on x-ray aids in the diagnosis. Portal vein air, if seen, is a bad prognostic sign. Indications for surgery are the presence of pneumo-peritoneum, worsening of the general condition of the infant while on conservative treatment, erythema of abdominal wall, an abdominal mass, a fixed dilated loop of intestine, portal vein air and a positive paracentesis. Operative treatment may be exteriorization and creation of mucous fistula, or resection and primary anastomosis (if the disease is well demarcated with good general condition of the patient) (Kosloske, 1994).

VASCULAR LESIONS OF THE SMALL INTESTINE

Vascular lesions of the small intestine can be classified as congenital or acquired, and consist mainly of haemangiomas/arteriovenous malformations, and angiodysplasias.

Haemangiomas represent sequestration of mesoangial tissue and are present from birth. They are subdivided into capillary, cavernous and mixed types.

Capillary haemangiomas involve only the capillaries. They have a well-differentiated endothelium and appear as non-ectatic mucosal lesions.

Cavernous haemangiomas consist of vascular spaces lined by many layers of endothelial cells. These lesions are usually large and often project into the bowel lumen as polypoidal masses visualized by conventional barium x-rays or endoscopy. Angiography may also be helpful (Plate 28.8). At laparotomy, serosal involvement may be visible, but enteroscopy is essential for the definitive diagnosis and treatment. Resection of the affected segment is curative.

Angiodysplasia or vascular ectasia

These acquired vascular lesions of the small intestine are one of the frequent causes of gastrointestinal bleeding in people over 60 years of age. These are too small to be seen and require a special technique using latex rubber perfusion/angiogram of the resected bowel segment (Fig. 28.20) to demonstrate their presence. The angiodysplasias are not new growths but distortion of existing vessels by the ageing process. It is postulated that there could be partial obstruction of submucosal veins leading to dilatation of the capillaries (Boley *et al.*, 1977). Such dilated capillaries make the precapillary sphincters incompetent, producing arteriovenous communication, and they are responsible for early filling of veins in the angiograms.

The lesions are made up of dilated tortuous submucosal veins and, on histology, appear as dilated, distorted, thin-walled vessels lined by endothelium only, with very little muscular coat (Eastman *et al.*, 1994). These lesions are only a few millimetres thick and appear as reddish raised areas endoscopically.

Angiodysplasias of the small intestine are seen usually after 60 years of age but may be found in a younger age group in developing countries (Jesudason *et al.*, 1985). Angiodysplasia also occurs in the colon either as single or multiple lesions, or as pan-gastrointestinal lesions in elderly patients with heart disease. Angiodysplasia of the small intestine are not associated with skin lesions. These may present as acute gastrointestinal bleeding or chronic occult blood loss. The diagnosis is mainly by endoscopy, angiography and intraoperative enteroscopy. Diagnostic features on angiography are the presence of vascular tufts and early venous filling (Figs 28.21 and 28.22). However, in small bowel angiodysplasia, angiographic demonstration may be difficult because of the length of the bowel, the large number of the branches of the superior mesenteric artery and the small size of the lesions (Duray *et al.*, 1984). Radioactive technetium (^{99m}Tc) scanning may reveal the source of haemorrhage, but most cases require intraoperative enteroscopy for diagnosis (Lau *et al.*, 1989). Angiodysplasia in a well-defined segment is suitable for resection. Recurrence may be as high as 20 per cent when multiple lesions are present. The lesions accessible by endoscope can be coagulated. Pan-intestinal lesions can be treated effectively in older patients by oral administration of the oestrogen–progesterone combination (the 'pill') (Richardson, 1991).

Vasculitis

Vasculitis is a multisystem disorder that involves mainly the gastrointestinal, musculoskeletal and renal systems. In the gastrointestinal system it may present as mesenteric or visceral vasculitis.

Mesenteric vasculitis affects the splanchnic blood vessels of all sizes, including arteries, veins, the vasa-recta, arterioles and venules. Symptoms are largely due to bowel ischaemia. Abdominal pain, fever, bleeding, diarrhoea and intestinal obstruction are the common symptoms. Occasionally perforation and stricture are also seen.

Deposition of immune complexes leads to activation of the inflammatory response leading to injury of the vessels. Most of these are part of systemic diseases like polyarteritis nodosa, rheumatoid arthritis, Henoch–Schonlein purpura, Churg–Strauss syndrome, systemic lupus erythematosis, Degos and other collagen vascular disease.

Once confirmed by cutaneous biopsy, a search for the aetiology and associated disease is carried out. Patients with gastrointestinal involvement may benefit from corticosteroids (Callen, 1994). Surgery is indicated only when complications arise.

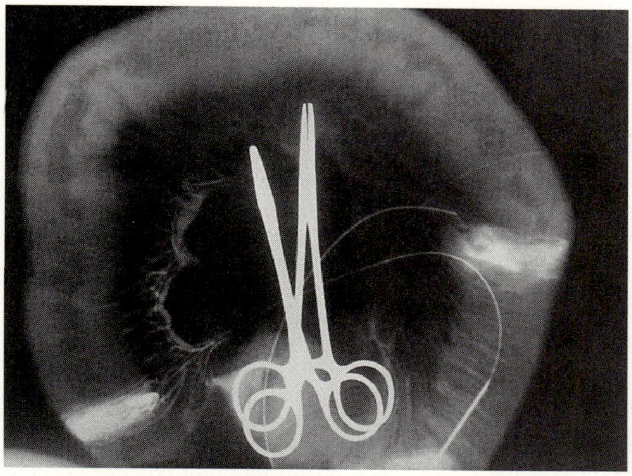

Figure 28.20 *Specimen angiogram of the resected segment of jejunum showing two localized patches of pooling of contrast material.*

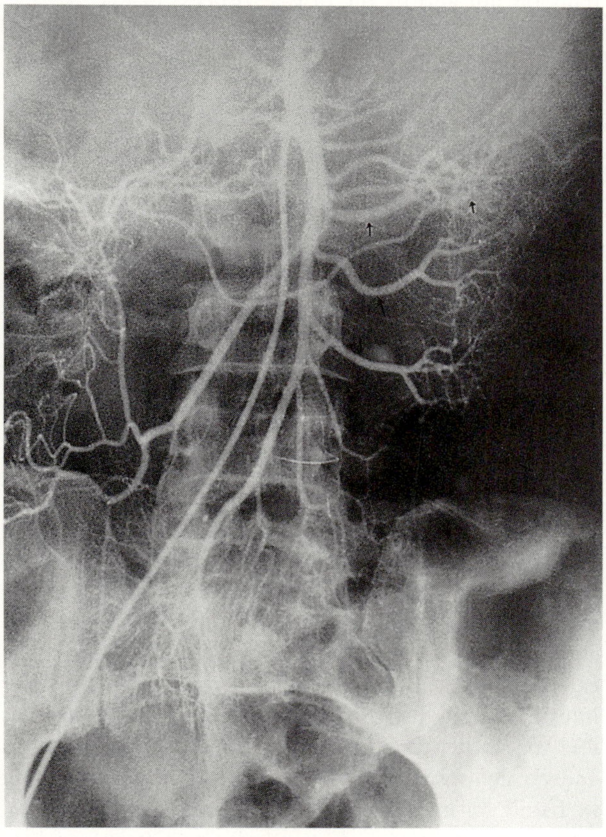

Figure 28.21 *Hypertrophied upper jejunal arteries and accumulation of contrast material in vascular tufts in the region of the distribution (arrows).*

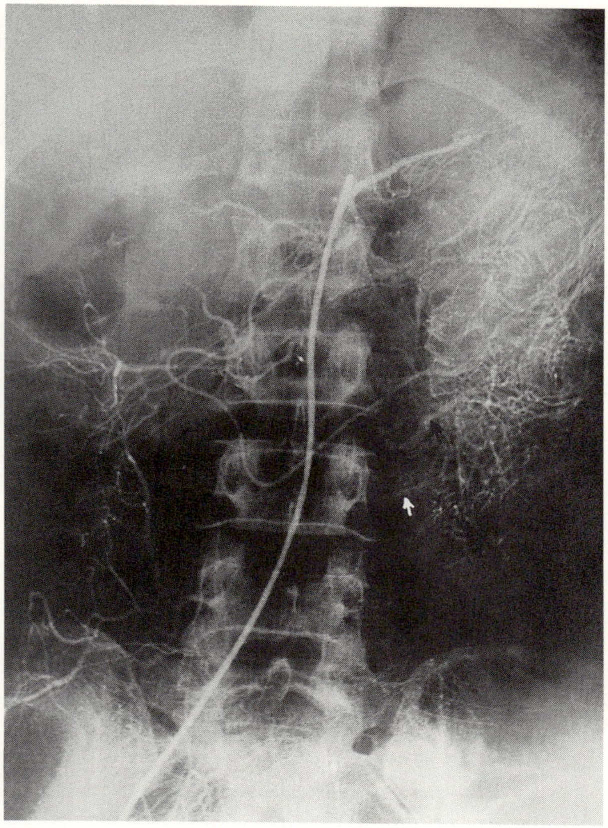

Figure 28.22 *Early filling of drainage veins in the capillary phase (arrows).*

SMALL INTESTINAL TRAUMA

Injury to the small bowel can be due to penetrating or blunt injury. Penetrating injuries are usually due to bullets, knives or sharp objects piercing the abdomen. These are easily diagnosed by their typical history, signs of peritoneal irritation and the presence of gas under the diaphragm on plain x-rays. These are managed by suturing the perforation (after trimming the edges) or resection of the bowel if it has multiple holes in it. In blunt injury to the abdomen, the three most common mechanisms are: (1) a crush injury between the vertebrae and anterior abdominal wall; (2) a sudden increase in the intraluminal pressure of the bowel; and (3) tangential tears at relatively fixed points, such as the duodeno-jejunal flexure, the ileo-caecal junction, etc., as described by Vance (1928) (Fig. 28.23). Here again the diagnosis is based on the history, signs of peritoneal irritation, gas under the diaphragm on x-rays, a positive ultrasound examination for fluid and a peritoneal aspiration containing bile and intestinal contents. Treatment is by resection and anastomosis.

Foreign bodies

The types of foreign body in the intestine are varied, and can be exogenous (swallowed) or endogenous, such as enteroliths or gallstones. The exogenous foreign bodies are ingested intentionally or accidentally.

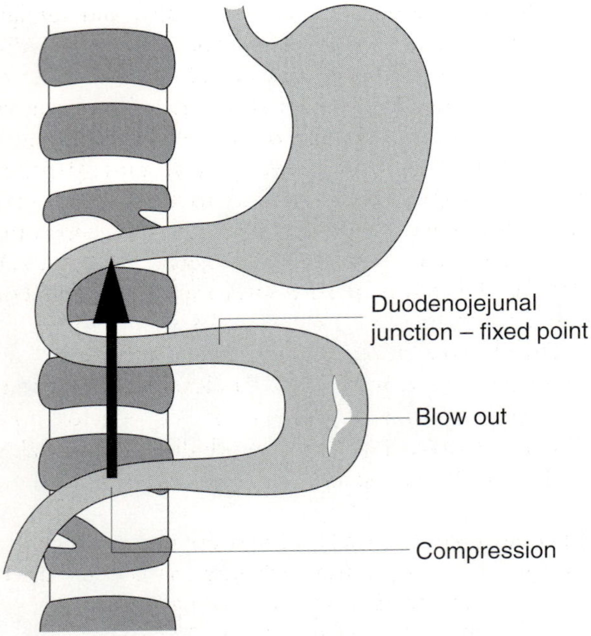

Figure 28.23 *Mechanism of injury to the small intestine in blunt trauma.*

Examples of intentional ingestion are:

- Ingestion of gold biscuits and narcotics in condoms by professional smugglers (Caruna *et al.*, 1984)
- Ingestion of razor blades, pins, nuts and bolts by psychiatric patients (Carp, 1950)
- Ingestion of toys, pencils and button batteries by children.

Examples of accidental ingestion are:

- Dentures, toothpicks, coins, sewing needles
- Seeds of fruits, e.g. mango
- Glass pieces, e.g. glass tumbler breaking while drinking.

Once they pass the pylorus, most foreign bodies transit the gastrointestinal tract safely by the so-called mural withdrawal reflex (Carp, 1927). Sometimes obstruction occurs if the object is large. Sharp objects, such as needles and open safety pins, may cause perforation of the small bowel. Chemicals from alkaline batteries and narcotics from condoms may cause local or systemic effects by virtue of their chemically active substances, which require appropriate treatment. Most foreign bodies, including glass pieces, which contain lead as impurity, are seen on plain x-rays. Treatment is usually expectant but operation is necessary when complications occur.

SMALL INTESTINAL FISTULAS

These are abnormal communications between the lumen of the bowel to another hollow organ or to the skin. These fistulas are classified according to the aetiology, site of origin and termination of the fistula, by the daily output and by the disease process (Table 28.4).

Table 28.4 *Classification of fistulas*

According to aetiology
1 Congenital, e.g. patent vitellointestinal duct
2 Acquired
   (a) Primary (spontaneous), e.g. Crohn's disease, diverticulitis and neoplasms
   (b) Secondary, e.g. postoperative, postirradiation

According to site of termination of discharge
1 External, e.g. entero-cutaneous
2 Internal, e.g. cholecysto-enteric, aorto-enteric

According to volume of output
1 Low – less than 200 mL/day
2 Medium – 200–500 mL/day
3 High – more than 500 mL/day

Aetiology

Small intestinal fistulas arise owing to a variety factors. The most common cause is operative damage to the integrity of the intestinal wall. Another important cause is a leaking bowel anastomosis. Pathological changes in the bowel, such as neoplasm, radiation enteritis or inflammatory bowel disease, may cause spontaneous gastrointestinal fistulas (Galland and Spencer, 1980; Berry and Fischer, 1996).

Natural history

When the anastomotic site is the cause, the leak leads to the formation of an abscess, which will result in a fistula if the abscess is drained or if it leaks to the exterior. Spontaneous fistulas also present initially as abdominal abscesses, which finally break out to the external surface, initially discharging pus and later intestinal contents. In contrast, gastrointestinal fistulas due to synthetic material begin as perigraft infections and collections, which erode into the bowel, resulting in fistula formation, e.g. prolene mesh of abdominal wall hernia repairs and prosthetic aortic grafts. Most fistulas close spontaneously if factors at the intestinal end of the tract are favourable. The unfavourable factors that keep the fistula persistent are a large adjacent abscess, intestinal discontinuity, lateral duodenal fistula, ileal fistula, diseased bowel, fistulous tract of < 2 cm and distal obstruction (Berry and Fischer, 1996).

Management of a fistula is directed at inducing a spontaneous closure. If conservative steps fail, surgery is needed. Most fistulas close by 4–6 weeks if conditions are favourable.

Principles of management

STABILIZATION

Stabilization is achieved in the following ways.

1. Correction of electrolytes and fluid imbalance and blood volume replacement.
2. Control of sepsis, instituting adequate drainage and appropriate antibiotics (Soeters *et al.*, 1979).
3. Nutritional support. Total parenteral nutrition (TPN) is started immediately and is continued as long as the situation demands and may spontaneously heal the fistula (Agirre *et al.*, 1974). If the fistula is distal and adequate small bowel (jejunum) of at least 90 cm is present, enteral feeding could start with a low-residue diet after 2–3 weeks of TPN.
4. Protection of the skin and containment of cutaneous discharge.

EVALUATION OF THE FISTULA

This would include a detailed study of the probable aetiology and condition of the patient. Common bedside investigations are checking the pH of the discharge and looking for bluish staining of a gauze piece kept at the fistulous opening after oral administration of methylene blue. Contrast computed tomography (CT) and ultrasound scans of the abdomen will help to localize the abscess and to drain it. (Lambiase *et al.*, 1992). A sinusogram is the most important investigation for accurate delineation of the fistulous tract and, in addition, diagnoses the nature of the bowel, its continuity, the presence of distal obstruction and the length of the tract (Tassiopoulos *et al.*, 1996). Barium meal may be useful in selected cases.

TREATMENT

Treatment is essentially conservative, which would include nasogastric suction, adequate drainage of the abscess, sump suction drain close to the intestinal end of the tract and administration of drugs, such as H-2 inhibitors and octreotide. Surgical treatment would include laparotomy, drainage of any residual abscess and resection of the bowel with the fistulous tract (Coutsoftides and Fazio, 1979).

Aorto-enteric fistula

Aorto-enteric fistula (AEF) is another form of small bowel fistula that may be further classified as primary or secondary. The primary AEFs are more often due to an atheromatous aneurysmal dilatation of the aorta eroding commonly into adjacent third and fourth parts of the duodenum (Reckless *et al.*, 1972) and occasionally due to infections, radiation therapy, and foreign body or gallstone erosion into the aorta. Secondary AEF occurs when a proximal suture line of the aorto-femoral bypass or a pseudoaneurysm at the site of anastomosis erodes into the duodenum, or, less often, the jejunum or ileum (Peck and Larry, 1992). The diagnosis depends primarily on the degree of clinical suspicion, which may be further aided by oesophago-gastro-duodenoscopy, angiography and contrast CT (Higgins *et al.*, 1991). Other useful studies include isotope scans and magnetic resonance imaging.

Once confirmed, emergency laparotomy is performed with closure of the duodenal rent and extra-anatomic bypass after removal of the infected graft (Kleinman *et al.*, 1979). The morbidity and mortality are high with this fistula.

Acknowledgements I hereby acknowledge the help of my colleagues in the Department of Surgery Unit III at the Christian Medical College Hospital, Vellore: Dr David Sadhu, Dr Sunil Agarwal, Dr Philip Joseph, Dr Sabu Thomas and Dr Sajjan Mathew in the preparation of this article, and Mrs Vasanthi Shanmugham for secretarial assistance. Dr S.R.B Jesudason of Surgery Unit II, Dr Sudipta Sen of the Department of Paediatric Surgery and the Department of Pathology, all at Christian Medical College, Vellore, and Dr A. Pavai and Dr K.E. Mammen, Department of Paediatric Surgery, Coimbatore Medical College, Coimbatore, provided some pictures from their collections. The medical illustration department of this hospital helped with the preparation of illustrations.

REFERENCES

Addison, N.V. 1983: Abdominal tuberculosis, a disease revived. *Annals of the Royal College of Surgeons of England* 65, 105–11.

Agirre, A., Fischer, J.E., Welch, C.E. 1974: The role of surgery and hyperalimentation in therapy of gastrointestinal cutaneous fistulae. *Annals of Surgery* 180, 393–401.

Berry, S.M., Fischer, J.E. 1996: Classification and pathophysiology of enterocutaneous fistulas. *Surgical Clinics of North America* 76, 1009–18.

Billings, P.J., Farrington, G.H. 1987: Small bowel obstruction caused by bezoars from intestinal diverticuli. *British Journal of Surgery* 74, 1186.

Boley, S.J., Sammartano, R., Adams, A. *et al.* 1977: On the nature and etiology of vascular ectasia of the colon. *Gastroenterology* 72: 650–60.

Brian, J.E., Stair, J.M. 1985: Non colonic diverticular disease. *Surgery, Gynecology and Obstetrics* 161, 189–95.

Brockis, J.G., Gilberg, M.C. 1957: Intestinal obstruction by gall stones – a review of 179 cases. *British Journal of Surgery* 44, 461–6.

Bulkley, G.B., Gharagozloo, F., Alderson, P.D. *et al.* 1981: Use of intraperitoneal xenon 133 for imaging of intestinal strangulation in small bowel obstruction. *American Journal of Surgery* 141, 128–35.

Callen, J.P. 1994: Skin manifestations of digestive disease. In Hanbrick, W.S., Schaffner, F., Berk, J.E. (eds) *Gastroenterology*. Philadelphia: W.B. Saunders.

Carp, L. 1927: Foreign bodies in the intestine. *Annals of Surgery* 85, 575–91.

Carp, L. 1950: Foreign bodies in the gastrointestinal tracts of psychiatric patients. *Archives of Surgery* 60, 1055–75.

Caruna, B.D.S., Weinback, B., Georg, D. *et al.* 1984: Cocaine-packet ingestion. *Annals of Internal Medicine* 100, 73.

Child, W.A., Phillips, R.B. 1960: Experience with intestinal plication and a proposed modification. *Annals of Surgery* 152, 258–65.

Coutsoftides, T., Fazio, V.W. 1979: Small intestinal cutaneous fistulas. *Surgery, Gynecology and Obstetrics* 149, 333–6.

Daniel, L.W., Williams, S., George, R.L. 1977: Ultrasonographic appearance of adult intussusception. *Radiology* 124, 791–2.

Donald, J.W. 1979: Major complications of small bowel diverticula. *Annals of Surgery* 190, 183–8.

Dunn, J.T., Halls, J.M., Berne, T.V. 1984: Roentgenographic contrast studies in acute small bowel obstruction. *Archives of Surgery* 119, 1305–8.

Duray, P.H., Marcal, J.M., Jr, Livolsi, U.A., Fisher, R. *et al.* 1984: Small intestinal angiodysplasia in the elderly. *Journal of Clinical Gastroenterology* 6, 311–19.

Eastman, J., Nazek, M., Mangels, D. 1994: Localized arterio-venous malformation of the jejunum. *Archives of Pathology and Laboratory Medicine* 118, 181–3.

Ellis, H. 1962: The aetiology of post-operative abdominal adhesions – an experimental study. *British Journal of Surgery* 50, 10–16.

Galland, R.B., Spencer, J. 1980: Radiation-induced gastrointestinal fistulae. *Annals of the Royal College of Surgeons of England* 68, 5–7.

Grosfield, J.L., Ballantyne, T.V.N., Schoemakier, R. 1979: Operative management of intestinal atresia and stenosis based on pathological findings. *Journal of Paediatric Surgery* 14, 368–75.

Gupta, R.L. 1996: *Textbook of surgery*. New Delhi: Jaypee Publications of India.

Higgins, R.S.D., Steed, D.L., Zajko, A.B. *et al.* 1991: Computed tomographic scan confirmation of paraprosthetic enteric fistula. *American Journal of Surgery* 162, 36–8.

Hugo, L.M., John, O.V. 1978: Jejunal diverticulosis with massive hemorrhage. *American Journal of Gastroenterology* 70, 657–9.

Jesudason, S.R.B., Devasia, A., Mathan, V.I., Bhaktaviziam, A. 1985: The pattern of angiodysplasia of the gastrointestinal tract in a tropical country. *Surgery, Gynecology and Obstetrics* 161, 525–31.

Kleinman, L.H., Towne, J.B., Bernard, V.M. 1979: A diagnostic and therapeutic approach to aortoenteric fistulas. Clinical experience with twenty patients. *Surgery* 86, 868–80.

Kosloske, A.M. 1994: Indications for operation in necrotizing enterocolitis revisited. *Journal of Pediatric Surgery* 29, 663–6.

La Raja, R.D., Rothenberg, R.E., Odom, J.E. *et al.* 1989: The incidence of intra-abdominal surgery in acquired immune deficiency syndrome: a statistical review of 904 patients. *Surgery* 105, 175–9.

Ladd, W.E., Gross, R.E. 1941: *Abdominal surgery of infancy and childhood.* Philadelphia: W.B. Saunders.

Lambiase, R.E., Deyoe, L., Cronan, J.J. *et al.* 1992: Percutaneous drainage of 335 consecutive abscesses; results of primary drainage with 1 year follow-up. *Radiology* 184, 167–79.

Lau, W.Y., Wong, S.Y., Yuen, W.K., Weng, K.K. 1989: Intraoperative enteroscopy for bleeding angiodysplasias of small intestine. *Surgery, Gynecology and Obstetrics* 168, 341–4.

Mann, C.V., Russel, R.C.G., Williams, N.S. (eds) 1995: *Bailey and Love's short practice of surgery*. London: Chapman and Hall.

Noble, T.B. 1937: Plication of small intestine as prophylaxis against adhesions. *American Journal of Surgery* 35, 41–4.

Noblett, H.R. 1969: Treatment of uncomplicated meconium ileus by Gastrografin enema: a preliminary report. *Journal of Paediatric Surgery* 4, 190–7.

Ottinger, L.N., Edwin, L.C. 1975: Obturation of the ileum by a jejunal diverticular enterolith. *Gastroenterology* 68, 1596–7.

Peck, J.J., Larry, R.E. 1992: Aortoenteric fistula. *Archives of Surgery* 127, 1191–4.

Phillips, J.H.C. 1953: Jejunal diverticulosis – some clinical aspects. *British Journal of Surgery* 40, 350–4.

Prakash, A. 1978: Ulceroconstrictive tuberculosis of bowel. *Indian Journal of Surgery* 63, 23–9.

Ravitch, M.M., Robert, M.M. 1948: Reduction of intussusception by barium enema. *Annals of Surgery* 128, 904–17.

Reckless, J.P.D., McColl, I., Taylor, G.W. 1972: Aortoenteric fistulae: an uncommon complication of abdominal aortic aneurysm. *British Journal of Surgery* 59: 458–62.

Rescorla, F.J., Grosfield, J.L. 1993: Contemporary management of meconium ileus. *World Journal of Surgery* 17, 318.

Richardson, J.D. 1991: Vascular lesions of the intestines. *American Journal of Surgery* 161, 284–92.

Ross, J.G., Potter, C.W., Zachary, R.B. 1962: Adenovirus infection in association with intussusception in infancy. *Lancet* 2, 221–3.

Shackelford, R.T., Marcus, W.Y. 1960: Jejunal diverticulum. A cause of gastrointestinal hemorrhage. *Annals of Surgery* 151, 930–8.

Shoba, K., Mary, M.K., Charles, A.R., Michael, D.S. 1983: Jejunal diverticulosis: a heterogenous disorder caused by a variety of abnormalities of smooth muscle or myenteric plexus. *Gastroenterology* 85, 538–47.

Soeters, P.B., Ebeid, A.M., Fischer, J.E. 1979: Review of 404 patients with gastrointestinal fistulas. *Annals of Surgery* 190, 189–202.

Tassiopoulos, A.K., Baum, G., Halverson, J.D. 1996: Small bowel fistulas. *Surgical Clinics of North America* 76, 1175–81.

Turner, G. 1932: A giant gall stone impacted in the colon and causing acute obstruction. *British Journal of Surgery* 20, 26–33.

Vance, B.M. 1928: Subcutaneous injuries of the abdominal viscera. *Archives of Surgery* 16, 631–9.

Ward-McQuaid, N. 1950: Intestinal obstruction due to food. *British Medical Journal* 1, 1106–9.

Wilson, S.E., Robinson, G., Williams, R.A. *et al.* 1989: Acquired immune deficiency syndrome (AIDS): indications for abdominal surgery, pathology and outcome. *Annals of Surgery* 210, 428–34.

Zachary, R.B. 1955: Acute intussusception in childhood. *Archives of Diseases of Childhood* 30, 32–6.

29

Short bowel syndrome

ANDREAS FRENZER

DEFINITION AND INTRODUCTION

Short bowel syndrome (SBS) is defined as malabsorption following massive resection of a significant portion of the small intestine (Vanderhoof, 1996). This definition implies that significant malabsorption has to be present and that mechanisms of the small intestine are not able to compensate for the loss of length.

The incidence of SBS is difficult to estimate owing to a lack of epidemiological prospective studies. In the UK, Lennard-Jones (1990) estimated the incidence of severe SBS requiring long-term parenteral nutrition to be two per million inhabitants per year. The prevalence is certainly increasing owing to advances in surgical techniques, postoperative care and nutritional support. There are also an increasing number of children surviving extensive small bowel resection, who enter adulthood. With the improvement of anaesthetic, surgical, postoperative and nutritional support techniques, an increasing number of patients survive extensive intestinal resection, and currently several thousands of such patients survive in the USA (Howard *et al.*, 1986).

In adults, resection of 40–50 per cent of the small intestine is usually well tolerated. However, the percentage of resected bowel is difficult to estimate because the total length of small bowel may vary from person to person from 300 cm to 850 cm (Backman and Hallberg, 1974; Cook and Carruthers, 1974). In practice, a small bowel length of 200 cm is approximately the length of small intestine that is necessary to maintain adequate nutrition without supplementation (Lennard-Jones, 1994). However, malabsorption is highly variable from patient to patient, and depends on the extent, the site of resection and whether the colon is still present or not.

AETIOLOGY

Crohn's disease accounts for about two-thirds of SBS and intestinal resections after ischaemic insults of the mesenteric vascular system are the other major cause in adults (Hylander *et al.*, 1981; Nightingale *et al.*, 1992) (Table 29.1). After jejuno-ileal bypass surgery for morbid obesity, patients can present with all the symptoms and signs of SBS. However, owing to malabsorption and diarrhoea, this operation is now largely abandoned.

In the paediatric population, neonates are most commonly affected by SBS. The indications for surgery in this age group in about two-thirds of cases are congenital malformations, such as intestinal atresia, abdominal wall defects or agangliosis. Necrotizing enterocolitis accounts for about one-third of the cases

Table 29.1 *Causes of short bowel syndrome in adults*

Vascular insults	Miscellaneous
Thrombosis or embolus of the superior mesenteric vein or artery, including the coagulopathies: deficiency of antithrombin III, protein C and S, mutation of factor V (Leiden)	Crohn's disease
Volvulus of the small intestine	Radiation enteritis
Strangulated hernia	Resection after abdominal trauma
	Jejuno-ileal bypass for morbid obesity

(Grosfeld *et al.*, 1986). Rarer causes that affect older children are Hirschsprung's disease involving the small bowel, mesenteric vascular embolism, thrombosis due to hypercoagulable state, mesenteric vascular embolism due to cardiac vegetations, abdominal trauma, radiation enteritis or Crohn's disease.

Volvulus, resulting in vascular compromise and massive bowel resection, can affect all age groups (Table 29.2).

Table 29.2 *Causes of short bowel syndrome in children*

Prenatal	Postnatal
Vascular accidents	Necrotizing enterocolitis
Intestinal atresia	Volvulus
Abdominal wall defects	Crohn's disease
Midgut or segmental volvulus (associated with malrotation, intra-abdominal bands)	Hirschsprung's disease
	Radiation enteritis
	Venous thrombosis
	Arterial thrombosis or embolism
	Abdominal trauma

INFLUENCING FACTORS

Extent and site of resected bowel

About half the small intestine can be resected to sustain normal nutritional requirements (Weser, 1976). This redundancy of intestine may be explained in an evolutionary sense as a protective mechanism against the formerly common occurrence of infectious diarrhoea.

On average, 2000 mL of fluid is ingested and about 7000 mL of fluid is secreted by the liver, pancreas and the gastrointestinal mucosa. Only about 100–150 mL of this fluid is excreted (5 per cent) and the rest is reabsorbed in the intestine: about 5500 mL in the jejunum, 2000 mL in the ileum and the rest in the colon (Ganong, 1983).

Two groups of patients with SBS have to be distinguished: (1) patients with only small intestine and no colon in continuity and (2) patients with small intestine and some colon in continuity (Tables 29.3 and 29.4). The latter group can be divided into a group of patients with the ileo-caecal valve present and a group of patients without the ileo-caecal valve. It was thought that to survive without parenteral nutrition, at least 120 cm of small bowel without colon or at least 70 cm of small bowel with a portion of colon in continuity have to be present at the time of resection (Gouttebel *et al.*, 1986; Wilmore *et al.*, 1971). However, later Wilmore *et al.* (1997) were able to wean permanently 40 per cent of patients with less than 50 cm of small bowel in continuity with the colon. Patients with a structural bowel disorder, such as Crohn's disease or radiation enteritis, tolerate less extensive resection owing to diminished function of the remaining intestine (Table 29.5).

The duodenum is fixed in the retroperitoneum and is only rarely resected in patients with SBS. The intraperitoneal jejunum–ileum is most vulnerable to injury and disease. The relative length of the jejunum is approximately two-fifths and that of the ileum about three-fifths. The function and morphology of the small intestine changes from proximal to distal. The jejunum has a larger diameter and thicker circular folds (i.e. valvulae conniventes) than the ileum. The villi are taller and the crypts are deeper in the proximal than in the distal small intestine.

Table 29.3 *Clinical differences for the two main types of short bowel syndrome*

	Jejunostomy	Jejunal–colonic anastomosis
Water and sodium loss, magnesia deficiency	Common	Uncommon
Nutrient malabsorption	Common	Common[a]
Renal stones (%)	0	25
Gallstones (%)	45	45
D-Lactic acidosis	0	Rare, but possible

[a]In patients with the colon *in situ*, carbohydrates can be utilized in the colon by transformation to short-chain fatty acids.

Table 29.4 *Site-specific long-term consequences in patients with short bowel syndrome*

Resection	Effects
Ileum	
Resection > 60 cm	Malabsorption of bile acids and vitamin B_{12}
Resection > 100 cm	Steatorrhoea
Ileo-caecal valve	Decreased transit time Bacterial overgrowth
Colon	Loss of electrolytes and water Decreased transit time

Table 29.5 *Prognostic factors after massive bowel resection that help to predict a poor outcome*

Older age
Short length of residual bowel
Distal versus proximal resection
Absence of ileo-caecal valve and colon
Disease of the residual intestine
Lack of small bowel adaptation

Absorption of nutrients is many times greater in the jejunum than in the ileum. Therefore, resection of jejunum results initially in more severe malabsorption than resection of ileum. However, the jejunum, unlike the ileum, shows little capacity for structural and functional changes following resection of the ileum

(Porus, 1965; O'Keefe *et al.*, 1992). In the ileum, enhanced absorption occurs after an adaptation period (Dowling and Booth, 1966; Gouttebel *et al.*, 1989; O'Keefe *et al.*, 1992).

The ileum slows intestinal transit markedly. This phenomenon is called the 'ileal break'. Indeed, jejunal motility is inhibited by perfusing the ileum with fat (Spiller *et al.*, 1984).

The presence of the ileo-caecal valve is a favourable factor, especially in children. Patients after resection of this valve have decreased intestinal transit time, which leads to increased diarrhoea. Since the function of this valve is to separate the colonic from the ileal contents, its removal results in bacterial overgrowth of the small bowel. This can worsen absorption of several nutrients, especially vitamin B_{12} and fat. The bacteria deconjugate the bile salt–fat complexes, which reduces absorption of fat and fat-soluble vitamins. In addition, bacterial overgrowth by itself can cause diarrhoea by several mechanisms.

In contrast to the jejunum, the ileum and the colon are able to absorb sodium against a steep concentration gradient. Thus, the distal small bowel and colon conserve both salt and water. As a result, in patients with jejunal resection only, water and sodium absorption is less compromised than in patients with ileal resection. If the volume is in excess in relation to the absorptive capacity, diarrhoea with loss of electrolytes and nutrients will result. In mesenteric infarction, a major portion of the mid-small bowel is resected and the proximal jejunum is anastomosed to the terminal ileum. The outcome is generally favourable for the reasons mentioned above. If the entire ileum is removed, usually with the ileo-caecal valve, patients are more likely to suffer from diarrhoea and malabsorption.

Vitamin B_{12} and the bile acids are only absorbed in the ileum. All the other nutrients, such as carbohydrates, fats, proteins, vitamins and minerals are mainly absorbed in the proximal small bowel, duodenum and jejunum (*see* Chapters 9 and 10). However, these nutrients can also be absorbed by the distal small intestine in case of resection of the proximal small intestine. After ileal resection, the jejunum can compensate bile acid loss only partially by increased diffusion across its mucosa (Weser, 1976).

In the case of ileal resection, it is important to distinguish clinically between cholerrhoeic and steatorrhoeic diarrhoea. As a rule of thumb, 100 cm of resected ileum is the cut-off line; if less than 100 cm are resected, the faecal bile acid loss is compensated by an increase of hepatic synthesis and there is no steatorrhoea. However, an increased amount of bile acids enter the colon and this leads to a secretory diarrhoea. If more than 100 cm of ileum is resected, the faecal bile acid loss cannot be compensated and steatorrhoea results. Therefore, the former can be treated with cholestyramine and patients with ileal resections of more than 100 cm have to be treated with a low-fat diet. If patients with steatorrhoea are treated with cholestyramine, their faecal fat excretion and diarrhoea may increase.

Resection of less than 60 cm of ileum does not result in a vitamin B_{12} malabsorption (Dowling, 1988). If more than 60 cm are resected, megaloblastic anaemia, peripheral neuropathy and ultimately degeneration of the spinal cord will result unless parenteral substitution of vitamin B_{12} occurs.

The colon is very important in patients with SBS. It can digest carbohydrates and therefore salvage calories. Malabsorbed carbohydrates are fermented by colonic bacteria to short-chain fatty acids (e.g. acetate, propionate and butyrate), which are absorbed to provide 5–10 per cent additional calories (Nordgaard *et al.*, 1994). In addition, the colon can increase its absorptive capacities for water up to 5 L per day, and, finally, patients with SBS and the colon *in situ* have a slower intestinal transit time (Nightingale *et al.*, 1993).

Intestinal adaptation

Intestinal adaptation encompasses structural and functional changes of the intestine. In 1912, Flint performed intestinal resections of varying lengths in dogs. He demonstrated that absorption improved with time after resection and that this correlated with hypertrophy of the intestinal mucosa. He concluded that up to 80 per cent of the small intestine could be resected without increased mortality.

The adaptive process begins within 12–24 hours after resection and continues for 1–2 years (Wilmore *et al.*, 1997). This process is characterized by elongation and dilatation of the remnant bowel, and an increase in villus height, crypt depth (Fig. 29.1), cell proliferation and increased brush-border enzyme activity (McCarthy and Kim, 1973). Remington *et al.* (1983) showed changes in the gut migrating motor complexes (MMC) in patients with SBS, leading to a slowing of gastrointestinal transit. In addition, massive intestinal resection results in delayed gastroduodenal emptying, which is a major factor in adaptive increased intestinal transit time (Johnson *et al.*, 1996). Finally, patients with SBS and a

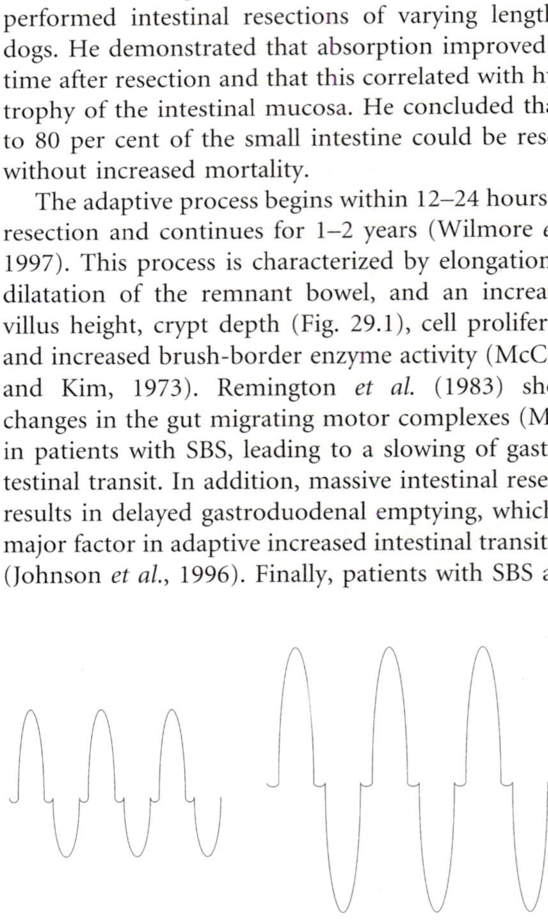

Figure 29.1 *Adaptive changes after massive resection of bowel: elongation of the crypts and the villi.*

colon in continuity have qualitative and quantitative changes in colonic flora that result in an increased capacity to metabolize carbohydrate (Briet *et al.*, 1995).

The mechanisms of these adaptive changes are poorly understood. However, three different factors are thought to influence this process: (1) luminal factors in the diet; (2) factors that are triggered by the provision of enteral feeding; and (3) growth factors that are extrinsic to the bowel.

Standard total parenteral nutrition without oral nutrition after extensive bowel resection results in mucosal hypoplasia (Hughes and Dowling, 1980). Bowel compensation only occurs after enteral feeding is introduced (Feldman *et al.*, 1976); therefore, an intestinal stimulus is necessary for this process. Indeed, Levy *et al.* (1988) have shown that aggressive luminal feeding with a polymeric formula during the postoperative phase increases the probability of enteral autonomy in patients with relatively short segments of small bowel.

MANAGEMENT

Introduction

The treatment of SBS can be divided into three phases: (1) the initial postoperative period, (2) the adaptation period, and (3) the maintenance period.

In the immediate postoperative phase, no oral nutrition is tolerated by the patient. In the adaptive phase, diarrhoea starts to stabilize and the patient can increase fluid and electrolyte balance with oral intake. Malabsorption and malnutrition are the major clinical problems in this phase. Gradually, the phase of full intestinal adaptation is achieved. Many patients absorb about two-thirds of their energy intake. Therefore, they increase their calorie intake usually about by half to maintain a nutritional balance. This is often done by eating larger meals or by having snacks.

Initial postoperative period

In this phase, life-saving measures such as substitution of fluids and electrolytes, as well as antibiotic therapy, are of paramount importance. Water and electrolyte losses have to be carefully assessed and parenterally replaced. This phase may last up to 10 days and premature attempts at oral feeding result in increased diarrhoea. During the early adaptive phase, since eating often results in increased diarrhoea, cramping and bloating, many patients will avoid oral nutrient intake. However, after about the fourth or fifth postoperative day, as the patients recover from the operation, controlled oral intake should be started. Only small volumes of isotonic fluids (salt and glucose-containing solutions, such as Gatorade® or Pedialyte®) should be administered in small frequent portions along with small meals or snacks of complex carbohydrates and proteins (600–1000 kcal/day). Care should be taken to give the patient initially only a minimal oral input to keep the diarrhoea and abdominal pain as little as possible. In patients with a high jejunostomy, sodium concentration should be at least 90 mmol/L or more.

Balance studies in patients have shown that drinking isotonic glucose–sodium solutions leads to sodium and water loss if the sodium concentration is 60 mmol/L, but absorption occurs when the concentration is 90 mmol/L or more (Rodrigues *et al.*, 1988). A mixture of 120 mmol sodium chloride and 50 mmol glucose is recommended to take advantage of the coupled transport of sodium with glucose in the small bowel. This type of solution has a poor palatability. An alternative, sodium chloride capsules, can be given with the meals. Foods such as oatmeal, rice, baked potatoes and pasta should form the basis of the patient's diet. Since glutamine is the main nutrient for the enterocytes, small amounts of this amino acid (5–10 g) dissolved in water can be started at this time and administered 2–3 times a day (Wilmore *et al.*, 1997). Even when patients are able to tolerate a greater intake, this should be initially discouraged, because in this phase higher intake results in more severe diarrhoea and possibly abdominal pain. Total parenteral nutrition alone results in hypoplasia of the intestinal mucosa (Hughes and Dowling, 1980). However, if parenteral and enteral nutrition are combined, intestinal adaptation occurs faster than on enteral nutrition alone (Wilmore *et al.*, 1997).

Adaptive and maintenance period

Average daily electrolyte and trace element losses in patients with high jejunostomies are very important. These losses have to be replaced intravenously in patients on parenteral nutrition and in the other patients orally in dosages that take account of the malabsorption. The most dangerous situation in SBS patients with a high jejunostomy is sodium depletion with corresponding fluid losses. A life-threatening situation with hypotension and prerenal uraemia may develop within a few days, unless adequate intravenous supplementation occurs. Chronic sodium depletion is more difficult to recognize. Typically, these patients have a low serum value, minimal urinary sodium excretion and increased plasma aldosterone (Ladefoged and Olgaard, 1985). In contrast, the colon absorbs sodium effectively and patients with the colon in continuity rarely suffer from sodium depletion.

A fat-reduced diet with 20–40 g/day has been reported to decrease the number of stools, stool weight and steatorrhoea while increasing body cell mass (Anderson *et al.*, 1974). However, the composition of the nutrient solution in jejunostomy patients on oral intake can be liberal, because the amount of absorbed energy does not depend on the relative amount of fat and carbohydrates (Woolf *et al.*, 1983, 1987; McIntyre *et al.*, 1986); therefore, the fat content of the diet in patients with a jejunostomy does not have to be reduced. One small study of five jejunostomy patients documented that net calcium, magnesium, zinc and copper losses on a high-fat diet were reversed to net absorption on a low-fat diet (Ovesen *et al.*, 1983). Patients with the colon in continuity can benefit from a low fat (30 per cent of calories) and high carbohydrate diet (50–60 per cent of calories), owing to stimulation of colonic water and electrolyte excretion by fatty acids (Nordgaard *et al.*, 1994). In addition, the colonocytes can metabolize carbohydrates to short-chain fatty acids. Owing to a poor palatability, patients do not like this diet on a long-term basis.

Medium-chain (C8–C10) triglycerides (MCT) do not require the presence of bile acids for digestion and are rapidly absorbed in the small intestine. MCT can also be absorbed by the colon (Jeppesen and Mortensen, 1997). Despite these theoretical advantages, MCT have been shown to increase faecal volume without a beneficial effect on absorption of magnesium and calcium in patients with SBS (Hadersley *et al.*, 1998). In addition, MCT have an unpleasant taste, which reduces their acceptability.

Lactose has only to be restricted in patients with a lactase deficiency (*see* Chapter 10). In most patients with SBS, lactose is well tolerated (Arrigoni *et al.*, 1994).

When parenteral nutrition is discontinued, because of uncertain absorption, nutrient deficiency states are actually more likely to develop. Severe calcium deficiency seems to be associated with the very short bowel syndrome (Colette *et al.*, 1986). Hypocalcaemia will be aggravated by steatorrhoea, magnesium and vitamin D deficiency. These deficiencies can lead to severe osteopenia, which can result in debilitating fractures (Hylander *et al.*, 1981). A generous calcium intake of about 1000–1500 mg/day with vitamin D seems to be indicated, despite the lack of clinical studies. Since 1,25-dihydroxy vitamin D has a substantial toxicity, serum levels of 25-hydroxy vitamin D, as well as serum and urinary calcium concentrations, should be monitored. In postmenopausal women with SBS, oestrogen replacement therapy should be prescribed generously. Biphosphonates are promising agents in preventing and treating osteopenia in patients with SBS, and clinical studies will probably follow.

Hypomagnesaemia is often present in patients with SBS, which can lead to muscle cramps, tetany, cardiac rhythm disturbance and other symptoms. A number of these patients have depletion of magnesium on the cellular level assessed by measuring magnesium in muscle biopsies (Hessov *et al.*, 1983). This can lead to muscle weakness, fatigue, renal stones and depression. Decreased urinary magnesium excretion is more sensitive for magnesium depletion than the serum magnesium (Fleming *et al.*, 1996). Owing to the cathartic effect of oral magnesium, parenteral supplementation is often necessary, for example, as frequent administration of 2 mL of 50 per cent $MgSO_4$ in each buttock or a larger amount directly intravenously. In case of a severe magnesium deficiency, hypocalcaemia cannot be treated, unless magnesium is administered first.

Iron deficiency has been noted in 25–50 per cent of patients with SBS, and is particularly prevalent in those with Crohn's disease (Compston and Creamer, 1977). If oral iron supplementation is not tolerated, intravenous replacement is required.

Clinically evident zinc deficiency (*see* Chapter 9) with acral skin lesions is rare in patients with SBS (McClain *et al.*, 1980). However, many patients have a marginal zinc status and are in a negative zinc balance (Sturniolo *et al.*, 1980). Since zinc losses parallel the faecal volume, zinc deficiency should especially be considered in patients with severe diarrhoea (Wolman *et al.*, 1979). Assessment of zinc status is difficult, because serum levels are affected by factors such as serum albumin and inflammatory mediators (Ainley *et al.*, 1988). Newer methods, such as white blood cell zinc and measurement of zinc-dependent enzymes, seem to be promising methods (Jones *et al.*, 1981).

Deficiencies of other traces elements, such as copper, molybdenum, selenium and chromium have been reported in patients with SBS (Table 29.6).

Therapy with a combined multivitamin and mineral preparations is usually adequate to prevent trace element and water-soluble vitamin deficiency. However, in patients with severe diarrhoea or losses via a fistula, zinc losses can be enormous and parenteral substitution is required. The fat-soluble vitamins A, E and K might require additional oral replacement by commercial liquid preparations.

Patients who fail to tolerate or meet their nutritional requirements with an oral diet should be on a constant infusion of an enteral formula. To improve the quality of life of the patients, additional feeding through a nasogastric tube or a percutaneous endoscopic gastrostomy (PEG) can often be limited to night-time application only.

Glutamine and growth factors

Glutamine is the major nutrient for the small bowel. Parenteral feedings that contain this amino acid support mucosal growth under a variety of conditions (O'Dwyer *et al.*, 1989), including mucosal hypertrophy that occurred after extensive small bowel resection (Tamada *et al.*, 1993).

Both animal and human studies have demonstrated that growth hormone stimulates intestinal growth

Table 29.6 *Nutrient deficiencies of vitamins and trace elements of patients on home parenteral nutrition*

Nutrient	Clinical effects	Reference
Chromium	Glucose intolerance, peripheral neuropathy	Brown *et al.* (1986) Verhage *et al.* (1996)
Selenium	Muscle weakness, liver dysfunction, haematology abnormalities	Fleming *et al.* (1984)
Copper	Anaemia, neutropenia	Dunlap *et al.* (1974)
Molybdenum	Encephalopathy, hypouricaemia, tachycardia, tachypnoea	Abumrad *et al.* (1981)
Zinc	Acral skin lesions	Okada *et al.* (1976)
Biotin	Alopecia, skin rash, lethargy, organic aciduria	Khalidi *et al.* (1984)
Vitamin D	Metabolic bone disease	Klein *et al.* (1980)
Vitamin E	Neurological deficits, muscle weakness	Howard *et al.* (1982)
Thiamine	Wernicke's encephalopathy, cardiac failure, refractory lactic acidosis	Kishi *et al.* (1979)
Vitamin B_{12}	Weakness, diarrhoea, anaemia, combined degeneration of the posterolateral columns	Hoffbrand (1967)
Essential fatty acids	Eczemoid dermatitis	Abushufa *et al.* (1995)

(Shulman *et al.*, 1992) and enhances transport of nutrients across the small bowel (Inoue *et al.*, 1994). Byrne *et al.* (1995) examined the influence of L-glutamine and recombinant growth hormone in association with a diet high in carbohydrate and low in fat on patients with SBS who have been on long-term parenteral nutrition. L-Glutamine was supplemented in doses of 0.6 g/kg per day enterally and/or parenterally, and recombinant growth hormone in doses of 0.11 mg/kg per day subcutaneously for 3 weeks.

Intensive nutritional counselling and surveillance of the patients was also a part of the study protocol. Forty-seven patients with severe SBS were examined: 40 per cent of the patients could be weaned completely from parenteral nutrition and, in 40 per cent, the need for parenteral nutrition during a mean follow-up of 1 year was reduced. In a preliminary part of the study, it was shown that neither the diet, nor the glutamine nor the growth hormone, when administered alone, improved intestinal absorption. However, when all were combined, the requirements for total parenteral nutrition diminished dramatically in most patients.

In a similar study, however, only the body weight, the absorption of sodium and potassium, and the gastric emptying time improved after a 3-week course of growth hormone, glutamine and a high-carbohydrate and low-fat diet. In this study, no improvement in small bowel morphology, stool losses or macronutrient absorption were noted (Scolapio *et al.*, 1997). In rats, no structural adaptation of the small intestine occurred when glutamine and growth hormone were applied concomitantly (Vanderhoof, 1996). Hence, administration of growth hormone and glutamine is controversial, and should only be applied in the setting of clinical studies.

Epidermal growth factor (Chaet *et al.*, 1994) and insulin-like growth factor 1 (Zhang *et al.*, 1994) improve epidermal function and structure in the rat. Therefore, these substances might prove beneficial in the future for clinical use in patients with SBS. Other substances, such as glucagon-like peptide 2, hepatocyte growth factor, keratinocyte growth factor, prostaglandin E_2, insulin, testosterone and neurotensin have also been shown to stimulate small bowel adaptation on an experimental basis.

Home parenteral nutrition

If daily energy or sodium intake are insufficient, or jejunostomy output is so large that it results in social disability, parenteral supplementation is indicated. If patients absorb only about one-third of their oral energy intake, adequate nutrition is not possible and parenteral nutrition is required (Rodrigues *et al.*, 1989). Gouttebel *et al.* (1986) reported that patients with 60 cm of small bowel and no colon in continuity, and patients with as little as 30–50 cm of healthy small bowel and with most or their colon in continuity, can be successfully weaned off parenteral nutrition. Others have reviewed this issue in depth (Fleming *et al.*, 1980; Stokes *et al.*, 1988; Howard and Hassan, 1998) and only the most important points are considered here.

Home parenteral nutrition (HPN) is usually administered through a Silastic central venous catheter, which has been tunnelled subcutaneously to reduce the risk of catheter infection. As an alternative, arteriovenous fistulas similar to those used for haemodialysis have been used. Most patients infuse their nutrient solution overnight, and assume an active normal life during the day.

Adequate training of patients in aseptic techniques and active help by a nutritional support team are crucial. Patients must also be instructed how to manage accidents, such as catheter rupture, to prevent possibly fatal air embolism. Patients should be able to control urinary sugar and ketones. By paying attention to these measures, adequate nutrition and hydration is possible. For example, Lin *et al.* (1987) has described children with normal growth and development on parenteral nutrition.

However, HPN is associated with many complications. The most common and most severe are related to catheter use. Organisms that typically reside on the skin, especially *Staphylococcus* species, and fungi are usually involved in catheter infection (Steiger and Srp, 1983). The skin and the environment of patients with ostomies are colonized with Gram-negative bacteria. Therefore, these bacteria infect the catheter most commonly in this patient group. Infection occurs by non-adequate catheter manipulation and migration of the organism along the catheter tract. With good aseptic techniques, infection rates of as few as one episode per 3 years have been described (Fuchs *et al.*, 1984). Bacterial catheter-related infections can often be treated with antibiotics without removal of the catheter; however, fungal infections usually require catheter removal (Schuman *et al.*, 1985).

Thrombosis of the catheter is another severe complication, which often requires catheter removal. However, thrombolytic therapy with urokinase can successfully restore catheter patency (Smith *et al.*, 1985).

Patients with SBS have an increased risk of gallbladder disease and parenteral nutrition itself increases this risk considerably. Indeed, patients on total parenteral nutrition after ileal resection for Crohn's disease have a higher prevalence of gallstones than patients who receive oral nutrition (Roslyn *et al.*, 1983). After 4–6 weeks of parenteral nutrition, most patients have gallbladder sludge when examined by ultrasound (Messing *et al.*, 1983). Roslyn *et al.* (1983) reported a prevalence of mostly symptomatic gallstone in 35 per cent of patients on home parenteral nutrition and described cases of acalculous cholecystitis. Three factors are implicated as causes for biliary disease secondary to parenteral nutrition: (1) gallbladder stasis; (2) use of medication that diminishes gallbladder contraction, such as narcotics, anticholinergics and octreotide (Roslyn *et al.*, 1983); and (3) effects of total parenteral nutrition on bile composition affecting lithogenicity (Gimmon *et al.*, 1982).

Cholestasis that evolved into biliary cirrhosis has been described in children on parenteral nutrition (Whitington, 1985), whereas adults are at greater risk for non-alcoholic steatohepatitis, which can also progress to hepatic cirrhosis (Bowyer *et al.*, 1985).

Severe metabolic bone disease is a well-known complication in patients on HPN. Osteopenia and osteomalacia have been noted in these patients. Osteopenia is often already present in patients with Crohn's disease on prolonged treatment with corticosteroids. Osteoporosis in patients on HPN has been associated with a low bone turnover rate (De Vernejoul *et al.*, 1985; Shike *et al.*, 1986). Others described a negative calcium balance with hypercalciuria, which might be influenced by the amino acid, phosphate or acetate content of the nutritional solution (Bengoa *et al.*, 1983; Berkelhammer *et al.*, 1988). Osteomalacia with severe bone pain, which was apparently caused by aluminium contamination of the protein hydrolysate, has been observed (Klein *et al.*, 1980). Newer nutritional solutions do not contain aluminium. However, certain additives (i.e. calcium gluconate) may contain aluminium. Toxicity of the intravenously administered vitamin D has been suggested as a causative factor for osteomalacia by others (Shike *et al.*, 1986).

Several deficiencies of vitamins and trace elements are described in patients on long-term parenteral nutrition (Table 29.6). Essential fatty-acid deficiency is another common problem, which can be prevented by giving 500 mL Intralipid® once a week (Jeppesen *et al.*, 1998).

HPN is extremely expensive and costs have been estimated to be around US$100 000 per year not including hospitalizations, nursing and laboratory costs (Howard and Hassan, 1998).

Long-term prognosis on HPN is best predicted by the primary disease. The respective 5-year survival rates in a recent study were: inflammatory bowel disease 90 per cent; ischaemic bowel 64 per cent; radiation enteritis 48 per cent; and cancer 30 per cent (Scolapio *et al.*, 1997).

Once HPN is started, this certainly does not mean lifelong dependency on intravenous nutrition. Despite the limited adaptive capacity, especially of the jejunum, about 50 per cent of patients on HPN are able to switch completely to oral intake after 1–2 years (Lennard-Jones, 1990).

Medical management

The primary goal of medical treatment of the patient with SBS is the control of diarrhoea. It is important to reduce faecal losses of nutrients and fluids by increasing the contact time of the nutrients and the bowel mucosa. It is equally important to increase the patient's quality of life.

Codeine and loperamide are the most effective drugs to reduce intestinal transit time, and have been shown to diminish ileostomy output effectively (Sandhu *et al.*, 1981; Schiller *et al.*, 1982). It is advisable to start treatment with loperamide, which does not have an addiction potential. If this medication fails, codeine or tincture of opium should be used. Liquid forms of medication are preferred, because transit time might be so short that solid forms might not dissolve.

In severe cases, parenteral narcotics can be effective (Weser, 1976). In patients with mild diarrhoea, kaolin–pectin mixtures or psyllium fibre preparations may be used alone or in conjunction with the above drugs. Cholestyramine can be effective to reduce diarrhoea in patients after ileal resection and the colon in continuity. However, it might increase steatorrhoea. Owing to further depletion of the bile acid pool, this substance will increase the already high risk of cholelithiasis (Sherlock and Dooley, 1997).

Octreotide, a synthetic, long-acting analogue of somatostatin, has been used effectively in patients with SBS to treat diarrhoea. Doses of 50–100 μg twice a day significantly reduced diarrhoea and electrolyte losses (Cooper *et al.*, 1986; Ladefoged *et al.*, 1989; Rosen, 1992); greater doses were not effective. However, octreotide has important side-effects. Pain at the injection site and even intestinal obstruction have been reported (Rosen, 1992). In addition, octreotide increases further the risk of cholelithiasis in patients with SBS and it decreases the availability of amino acids for splanchnic protein synthesis (O'Keefe *et al.*, 1994). In rabbits, octreotide diminished luminal nutrient transport activity after massive small bowel resection, although this negative effect could be inhibited by administering epidermal growth factor (Seydel *et al.*, 1996). The mechanisms of octreotide are complex, as it decreases intestinal motility, reduces fluid secretion and alters mucosal electrolyte transport (Shulkes, 1994).

To reduce gastric secretion and to diminish the risk of stress ulcerations, usually H-2 blockers or omeprazole are given intravenously postoperatively. However, these drugs may also reduce diarrhoea in the stable ambulatory patient (Aly *et al.*, 1980; Jacobsen *et al.*, 1986). Even in patients without gastric hypersecretion, these drugs can reduce faecal or ostomy fluid and electrolyte losses (Williams *et al.*, 1985; Dowling, 1988).

A few patients with severe SBS may have functional pancreatic insufficiency owing to a blunted release of secretin and cholecystokinin. These patients will benefit from pancreatic enzyme replacement therapy (Table 29.7).

Surgical treatment

INTRODUCTION

The main goal of the initial operation must be preservation of maximal intestinal length to prevent SBS. After SBS has been established, at least 1 year should be allowed for the bowel to adapt before surgery is considered (Thompson *et al.*, 1995). Surgical procedures to increase absorption in patients with SBS can be divided into procedures that optimize intestinal function and those that prolong intestinal transit time (Table 29.8).

Several surgical techniques allow avoidance of intestinal resection. For example, tapering a dilated segment of small bowel to improve its function, stricturoplasty for benign strictures, and serosal patches for perforation or for certain strictures are other established techniques (Thompson, 1994). Depending on previous operations, patients have occasionally segments that can

Table 29.7 *Drug treatment for short bowel syndrome*

Drug function	Drug	Recommended daily dose
Inhibition of gastrointestinal motility	Loperamide[a]	4–16 mg orally
	Codeine phosphate[a]	30–40 mg
	Octreotide	50–(100) μg subcutaneously, twice daily
Decrease of gastric secretion	Ranitidine	300–600 mg orally
	Famotidine	40–80 mg orally
	Omeprazole	20–40 mg orally
	Lansoprazole	30–60 mg orally
	Pantoprazole	40–80 mg orally
Binding of bile acids	Cholestyramine	4–12 g orally
Antibiotics	Metronidazole	800–1500 mg orally
	Amoxicillin	375–650 mg three times daily

[a]Loperamide and codeine phosphate are ideally given 1 hour before meals and at bedtime. Dosages may be increased if required due to malabsorption.

Table 29.8 *Surgical procedures for improvement of malabsorption in patients with short bowel syndrome*

Optimizing intestinal function	Prolonging intestinal transit
Prevention of SBS	Interposition of reversed intestinal segments
Tapering of dilated segments	Colonic interposition
Stricturoplasty for strictures	Artificial valves and sphincters
Serosal patches for strictures and perforations	Recirculating loops
Established SBS	
Tapering and lengthening of dilated intestine	

be recruited into continuity at the time of reoperation (Kaveggia *et al.*, 1991).

OPTIMIZING INTESTINAL FUNCTION IN PATIENTS WITH SBS

Dilated intestine secondary to chronic obstruction or the adaptive process often develops in patients with SBS. This may lead to stasis and bacterial overgrowth, which further increase malabsorption. Chronic obstruction should always be excluded in these patients. This is often due to a stenosed anastomosis, adhesions or strictures due to the underlying disease.

Tapering of dilated segments by simple imbrication improves motility by permitting closure of the lumen during contraction of the wall (Weber *et al.*, 1982). Numerous anecdotal reports have described improvement of intestinal function in infants (Weber *et al.*, 1982; Borgstein *et al.*, 1991). Bianchi (1997) described a surgical procedure that tapers and duplicates dilated intestinal segments simultaneously to increase intestinal length. Intestinal lengthening of segments as long as 35 cm has been reported in more than 20 children. Postoperatively, the children suffered from prolonged ileus but significant improvement of malabsorption occurred in most cases. However, patients must be very carefully selected, because potential complications, such as segmental necrosis or anastomotic leaks can have disastrous consequences. The intestinal diameter should be at least 4 cm to provide an adequate lumen size after tapering. The procedure is most likely to be successful if bacterial overgrowth or other signs of malabsorption that appear to be related to the dilated segment are identified.

PROCEDURES TO PROLONG INTESTINAL TRANSIT TIME

Three surgical procedures have been described to prolong intestinal transit time: (1) reversed intestinal segments, (2) colon interposition, and (3) artificial sphincters.

Reversed intestinal segments of generally 10–15 cm have been used for many years for a variety of motility problems, including the dumping syndrome (Fink and Olson, 1967; Pertsemlidis and Kark, 1974; Williams and King, 1985; Pigot *et al.*, 1990). This reversed segment causes peristalsis into the opposite direction. Panis *et al.* (1997) reported successful segmental reversal of the small bowel in eight patients with SBS. However, if the segment is too long, it will cause pseudo-obstruction, and some manometric and radiological studies questioned long-term efficacy. The reversed segment may not function properly and an actual increase of malabsorption might ensue.

Since colonic transit is slower than small intestinal transit, colon interposition has been attempted in both an isoperistaltic and an antiperistaltic fashion (Carner and Raju, 1981; Glick *et al.*, 1984; Brolin, 1986). Only a few have been reported in the literature and the overall success seems to be about 50 per cent (Thompson, 1994).

Several types of artificial valves and sphincters have been reported on an experimental basis in a few case reports but are not of proven benefit (Ricotta *et al.*, 1983). Also on an experimental basis, a variety of recirculating loops and pouches has been constructed in an attempt to promote repeated contact of the luminal contents with the bowel surface. However, owing to a high morbidity and mortality in animals, these procedures have not been evaluated in humans.

In summary, all the surgical procedures mentioned have only been applied in a few patients and need further study. The only curative surgical procedure is small bowel transplantation (*see* Chapter 30).

COMPLICATIONS AND THEIR MANAGEMENT

Gastric hypersecretion

Gastric hypersecretion occurs in as many as one-third of patients after massive bowel resection (Weser, 1976; Cortot *et al.*, 1979). This leads to increased faecal fluid and electrolyte loss, and can cause severe peptic ulcer disease. In addition, the increased acidity inhibits the function of the pancreatic digestive enzymes, damages the remaining bowel mucosa and impairs micelle formation, all factors which increase malabsorption (Weser, 1976). In patients with leaks of the surgical anastomosis, gastric hypersecretion is a common phenomenon (Weser, 1976). Gastric hypersecretion occurs within 24 hours after resection and almost always gradually decreases with time; hence, long-term medical treatment is usually not necessary (Williams and King, 1985; Dowling, 1988). Gastric hypersecretion can be effectively treated conservatively by either H-2 blockers or proton pump inhibitors. Gastric operations should be avoided.

It seems that gastric hypersecretion is proportional to the length of bowel resected. The exact mechanisms involved in this phenomenon are unknown and some patients even manifest hypochlorhydria after massive bowel resection (Dowling, 1988). Elevated levels of serum gastrin have been reported in humans and dogs (Buxton, 1974). It is not clear whether the increased gastrin concentrations are due to increased synthesis or decreased catabolism of this hormone. In some patients with gastric hypersecretion, normal serum gastrin values have been observed (Murphy *et al.*, 1979), which makes the involvement of hormones other than gastrin likely.

Gallstones

The incidence of gallstones both among patients with a jejunostomy and those with a short gut in continuity with the colon is increased by about 2–3-fold (Hill *et al.*, 1975; Nightingale *et al.*, 1992). Both pigment and cholesterol stones occur more commonly and the pathophysiological mechanisms have not been elucidated as yet. It has been suggested that interruption of the enterohepatic cycle results in increased hepatic cholesterol synthesis, thereby producing supersaturation of bile with cholesterol (Dowling, 1988). However, 40 per cent of patients with ileostomy have radio-opaque calcium-containing gallstones rather than radiolucent (cholesterol-rich) stones (Heaton and Read, 1975). Others have suggested that the bile actually becomes hyposaturated with cholesterol, with increasing loss of bile acids in the faeces (Farkkila, 1988).

Ileal resection seems to predispose to formation of pigment stones (Farkkila, 1988; Bickerstaff and Moossa, 1983; Pitt *et al.*, 1984). Thompson (1996) defined the following risk factors in 50 adults with SBS for developing gallstones over a follow-up period of 15 years: intestinal remnant of less than 120 cm (incidence of 47 per cent versus 13 per cent), an absent ileo-caecal junction (41 per cent versus 0 per cent), long-term total parenteral nutrition (45 per cent versus 13 per cent), and Crohn's disease (67 per cent versus 24 per cent). He concluded that prophylactic cholecystectomy is indicated in patients with benign conditions and anticipated long-term survival.

In summary, patients with SBS have a clearly increased incidence of gallstones; however, the mechanisms involved in this phenomenon require further elucidation.

Oxalate kidney stones

Long-chain fatty acids in the colon inhibit water reabsorption and decrease transit time (Spiller *et al.*, 1986). Steatorrhoea also leads to increased absorption of oxalate and hyperoxaluria (Dobbins and Binder, 1977). Long-chain fatty acids combine with the divalent cations magnesium and calcium, contributing to the deficiency of both ions (Booth *et al.*, 1964). Under normal circumstances, calcium and oxalate form calcium oxalate, which cannot be absorbed. Owing to the relative deficiency of calcium in patients with steatorrhoea, an increased amount of free oxalate is present, which can easily be absorbed. In addition, bile salts are thought to increase the colonic permeability, which further increases absorption of oxalate (Lennard-Jones, 1994). It is important to note that hyperoxaluria only occurs in patients with a colon in continuity. In one study, a quarter of patients with less than 200 cm of jejunum anastomosed to the colon developed symptomatic renal stones, whereas a comparable group of patients with a jejunostomy did not experience this problem (Nightingale *et al.*, 1992).

In patients at risk for kidney stones, urinary oxalate excretion should be monitored. Oxalate kidney stones can be prevented by sufficient hydration and by reducing oxalate content in the diet of the patients with a jejunum anastomosed to the colon. Foods rich in oxalate are spinach, parsley, rhubarb, beetroot, cocoa, celery, carrots, chocolate and tea (Nelson *et al.*, 1994). Tea is the most important source of oxalate in the average person (Zarembski and Hogkinson, 1962). An oxalate-reduced diet effectively reduces the rate of stone formation; however, many patients find long-term adherence to this diet difficult (Hodgkinson, 1981). Calcium restriction is contraindicated as this increases oxalate absorption. Also, since oxalate is the end product of ascorbic acid metabolism, not more than 1 g of vitamin C should be given in the diet (Nelson *et al.*, 1994). Calcium supplements in the form of citrate are recommended (Pak, 1998).

D-Lactic acidosis

D-Lactic acidosis is a rare complication that only occurs in patients with a colon *in situ*. D-Lactate is the right-turning isomer of the normally occurring L-lactate. Malabsorbed carbohydrate is metabolized by colonic bacteria to short-chain fatty acids and lactate; the latter lowers the colonic pH. The acid pH in the colon promotes the growth of acid-resistant Gram-positive anaerobes such as *Lactobacillus* and *Eubacterium*, which have the ability to produce D-lactate. D-Lactate is absorbed from the gut but, owing to a lack of D-lactate dehydrogenase, humans have only a limited capacity to metabolize this substance. Provocation of attacks with an oral carbohydrate load (Hudson *et al.*, 1990) and the beneficial effect of antibiotics support the above-mentioned theory. In some patients with SBS, the consumption of live lactobacilli or the use of broad-spectrum antibiotics have been followed by D-lactic acidosis with encephalopathy (Oh *et al.*, 1979; Perlmutter *et al.*, 1983; Forsyth *et al.*, 1991), which also speaks for this hypothesis. D-lactic acidosis has been described in relation to bacterial overgrowth of the small intestine (Scully *et al.*, 1989). One case of D-lactic acidosis associated with the use of medium-chain triglycerides has been published (Jover *et al.*, 1995).

Infusion of D-lactate in healthy subjects does not trigger neurological symptoms (Oh *et al.*, 1985; Forsyth *et al.*, 1991). In patients with D-lactic acidosis, normalization of the acidosis with bicarbonate does not improve the symptomatology (Oh *et al.*, 1985). Therefore, D-lactic acid might only be a marker of another unidentified toxic substance. Abnormal phenylalanine or tyrosine absorption has been suggested (Schoorel *et al.*, 1980). In another case, thiamine deficiency has been demonstrated by elevated red cell transketolase levels and a thiamine supplement prevented recurrence (Hudson *et al.*, 1990). This is of considerable interest, because the symptomatology of D-lactic acidosis resembles Wernicke's encephalopathy.

Patients develop neurological symptoms including headache, drowsiness, stupor, confusion, behavioural disturbance, ataxia, blurred vision, ophthalmoplegia, or nystagmus. Associated ileus has been described (Hudson *et al.*, 1990; Forsyth *et al.*, 1991). However, this is probably a consequence of the metabolic disturbance rather than its cause. If neurological symptoms occur, D-lactic acidosis should be suspected. Laboratory findings show a metabolic acidosis with an increased anion gap. It is important to note that standard lactate determinations do not detect D-lactic acid. Testing for D-lactate requires the use of the enzyme D-lactate dehydrogenase.

No proven treatment of D-lactic acidosis exists. Some patients have improved when carbohydrate, particularly excessive sugar or glucose, were restricted (Perlmutter *et al.*, 1983; Scully *et al.*, 1989; Hudson *et al.*, 1990), but others have not (Forsyth *et al.*, 1991). One patient was helped by the substitution of starch by monosaccharides or oligosaccarides in the diet. This patient's bacteria were only able to metabolize oligosaccarides up to a chain length of five but not starch (Mayne *et al.*, 1990). Cultures of stools tend to yield mainly lactobacilli or other Gram-positive anaerobes (Coronado *et al.*, 1995; Caldarini *et al.*, 1996).

In several cases, clinical improvement has been noted after one or more treatment courses of neomycin (Perlmutter *et al.*, 1983; Scully *et al.*, 1989; Hudson *et al.*, 1990; Forsyth *et al.*, 1991) or vancomycin (Stohlberg *et al.*, 1982). However, response to antibiotics is unpredictable (Bongaerts *et al.*, 1997) as they can even induce D-lactic acidosis (Coronado *et al.*, 1995). One child was successfully treated by recolonization of the gut with a modified faecal flora given orally over a period of 5 days (Schoorel *et al.*, 1980) and three other children were effectively treated by a probiotic therapy with live *Lactobacillus plantarum* 299V (Young and Vandenhoof, 1997).

Bacterial overgrowth

Bacterial overgrowth (*see* Chapter 12) is a common complication of SBS and it occurs in most patients. Bacterial counts normally reach from 10^3 organisms/mL in the proximal intestine to higher levels in the distal intestine. The cause for bacterial overgrowth is probably multifactorial. The loss of the ileo-caecal valve has been suggested as a possible explanation (Weser, 1976); however, this valve is certainly not bacteriologically competent. Dowling (1988) suggested the motility disturbances in relation to SBS are responsible for bacterial overgrowth.

Bacterial overgrowth results in exacerbation of malabsorption by several mechanisms (Gracey, 1979). Inflammation of the small intestine damages the absorptive surface and limits nutrient transport. In case of severe inflammation, gastrointestinal blood loss may even occur (Drenick *et al.*, 1977; Taylor, 1991). In addition, bacteria deconjugate bile salts, resulting in bile salt loss and decreased fat absorption. Bacteria also compete with the host for vitamin B_{12} and maybe other nutrients (Vanderhoof *et al.*, 1992). Symptoms encompass bloating, abdominal cramps and diarrhoea. Rarely, bacterial overgrowth may result in colitis or ileitis with ulcerations resembling Crohn's disease (Taylor *et al.*, 1991). Kaufman *et al.* (1997) have recently shown that bacterial overgrowth prolongs the time of administration of parenteral nutrition in children with SBS.

Diagnosis of bacterial overgrowth may be confirmed by aspiration and culture of the small intestinal fluid in an anaerobic culture medium. As a screening test, breath hydrogen measurement after oral ingestion of glucose is useful (*see* Chapter 13.3). However, owing to the decreased intestinal transit time in patients with SBS, the breath test is often difficult to interpret.

Antibiotic therapy is usually effective. Intermittent treatment courses for 7–14 days with either metronidazole, trimethoprim–sulphamethoxazole, tetracycline or amoxicillin are recommended. Combinations can be administered as well. Antibiotics should be rotated to avoid development of resistant strains. After antibiotic treatment, recolonization of the colon with acidophilus or other non-pathogenic organisms may be helpful (Wilmore *et al.*, 1997).

REFERENCES

Abumrad, N.N., Schneider, A.J., Steel, D. *et al.* 1981: Amino acid intolerance during prolonged total parenteral nutrition reversed by molybdate therapy. *American Journal of Clinical Nutrition* 34, 2551–9.

Abushufa, R., Reed, P., Weinkove, C. *et al.* 1995: Essential fatty acid status in patients on long-term home parenteral nutrition *JPEN: Journal of Parenteral and Enteral Nutrition* 19, 286–90.

Ainley, C.C., Cason, J., Carlsson, L.K. *et al.* 1988: Zinc status in inflammatory bowel disease. *Clinical Science* 75, 277–83.

Aly, A., Barany, F., Kollberg, B. *et al.* 1980: Effect of an H2-receptor blocking agent on diarrhoeas after extensive small bowel resection in Crohn's disease. *Acta Medica Scandinavica* 207, 119–22.

Anderson, H., Isaksson, B., Sjogren, B. 1974: Fat reduced diet in the symptomatic treatment of small bowel disease. *Gut* 15, 351–9.

Arrigoni, E., Marteau, P., Briet, F. *et al.* 1994: Tolerance and absorption of lactose from milk and yogurt during short-bowel syndrome in humans. *American Journal of Clinical Nutrition* 60, 926–9.

Backman, L., Hallberg, D., 1974: Small-intestinal length: an intraoperative study in obesity. *Acta Chirurgica Scandinavica* 140, 57–63.

Bengoa, J.M., Sitrin, M.D., Wood, R.J. *et al.* 1983: Amino acid induced hypercalciuria in patients on total parenteral nutrition. *American Journal of Clinical Nutrition* 38, 264–9.

Berkelhammer, C.H., Wood, R.J., Sitrin, M.D. *et al.* 1988: Acetate and hypercalciuria during total parenteral nutrition. *American Journal of Clinical Nutrition* 48, 1482–9.

Bianchi A, 1997: Longitudinal intestinal lengthening and tailoring: results in 20 children. *Journal of the Royal Society of Medicine* 90, 429–32.

Bickerstaff, K., Moossa, A.R. 1983: Effects of resection or by-pass of the distal ileum on the lithogenicity of bile. *American Journal of Surgery* 145, 34–40.

Bongaerts, G.P.A., Tolboom, J.J.M., Naber, A.H.J. *et al.* 1997: Role of bacteria in the pathogensis of short bowel syndrome-associated D-lactic acidemia. *Microbial Pathogenesis* 22, 285–93.

Booth, C.C., MacIntyre, I., Mollin, D.L. 1964: Nutritional problems associated with extensive lesions of the distal small intestine in man. *Quarterly Journal of Medicine* 33, 401–20.

Borgstein, E.S., Munro, A., Youngston, G.G. 1991: Intestinal plication: an alternative to tapered jejunostomy in functional small bowel obstruction. *British Journal of Surgery* 78, 1075–6.

Bowyer, B.A., Fleming, C.R., Ludwig, J. *et al.* 1985: Does long-term home parenteral nutrition in adult patients cause chronic liver disease? *JPEN: Journal of Parenteral and Enteral Nutrition* 9, 11–17.

Briet, F., Lourie, B., Achour, L. *et al.* 1995: Bacterial adaptation in patients with short bowel and colon in continuity. *Gastroenterology* 109, 1446–53.

Brolin, R.E. 1986: Colon interposition for extreme short bowel syndrome: a case report. *Surgery* 100, 576–80.

Brown, R.O., Forloines-Lynn, S., Cross, R.E. *et al.* 1986: Chromium deficiency after long-term total parenteral nutrition. *Digestive Diseases and Sciences* 31, 661–4.

Buxton, B. 1974: Small bowel resection and gastric acid hypersecretion. *Gut* 15, 229–38.

Byrne, T.A., Persinger, R.L., Young, L.S. *et al.* 1995: A new treatment for patients with short-bowel syndrome: growth hormone, glutamine, and a modified diet. *Annals of Surgery* 222, 243–55.

Caldarini, M.I., Pons, S., D'Agostino, D. *et al.* 1996: Abnormal fecal flora in a patient with short bowel syndrome. An in vitro study on effect of pH on D-lactic acid production. *Digestive Diseases and Sciences* 41, 1649–52.

Carner, D.V., Raju, S. 1981: Failure of antiperistaltic colon interpositions to ameliorate short bowel syndrome. *American Surgeon* 47, 538–40.

Chaet, M.S., Arya, G., Ziegler, M.M., Warner, B.W., Sith, S. 1994: Epidermal growth factor enhances intestinal adaptation after massive small bowel resection. *Journal of Pediatric Surgery* 29, 1035–9.

Colette, C., Gouttebel, M.C., Monnier, L.H. *et al.* 1986: Calcium absorption following small bowel resection in man: evidence for an adaptive response. *European Journal of Clinical Investigation* 16, 271–6.

Compston, J.E., Creamer, B. 1977: The consequences of small intestinal resection. *Quarterly Journal of Medicine* 46, 485–97.

Cook, G.C., Carruthers, R.H. 1974: Reaction of human small intestine to an intraluminal tube and its importance in jejunal perfusion studies. *Gut* 15, 545–8.

Cooper, J.C., Williams, N.S., King, R.F.G.J. *et al.* 1986: Effects of a long-acting somatostatin analogue in patients with severe ileostomy diarrhoea. *British Journal of Surgery* 73, 128–31.

Coronado, B.E., Opal, S.M., Yoburn, D.C. 1995: Antibiotic-induced D-lactic acidosis. *Annals of Internal Medicine* 122, 839–42.

Cortot, A., Fleming, R., Malagelada, J.R. 1979: Improved nutrient absorption after cimetidine in short bowel syndrome with gastric hypersecretion. *New England Journal of Medicine* 300, 79–80.

De Vernejoul, M.C., Messing, B., Modrowski, K. *et al.* 1985: Multifactorial low remodeling bone disease during cyclic total parenteral nutrition. *Journal of Clinical Endocrinology and Metabolism* 60, 109–13.

Dobbins, J.W., Binder, H.J. 1977: Importance of the colon in enteric hyperoxaluria. *New England Journal of Medicine* 296, 298–301.

Dowling, R.H. 1988: The short bowel syndrome. *Endoscopy Review* 1, 47–54.

Dowling, R.H., Booth, C.C. 1966: Functional compensation after small bowel resection in man. *Lancet* 2, 146–7.

Drenick, E.J., Ament, M.E., Finegold, S.M. *et al.* 1977: Bypass enteropathy: an inflammatory process in the excluded segment with systemic complications. *American Journal of Clinical Nutrition* 30, 76–89.

Dunlap, W.M., James, J.C., Hume, D.M. 1974: Anemia and neutropenia caused by copper deficiency. *Annals of Internal Medicine* 80, 470–6.

Farkkila, M.A. 1988: Biliary cholesterol and lithogeneity of bile in patients after ileal resection. *Surgery* 104, 18–25.

Feldman, E.J., Dowling, R.H., McNaughton, J., Peters, T.J. 1976: Effects of oral versus intravenous nutrition on intestinal adaptation after small bowel resection in the dog. *Gastroenterology* 70: 712–19.

Fink, W.J., Olson, J.D. 1967: The massive bowel resection syndrome: treatment with reversed intestinal segments. *Archives of Surgery* 94, 700–6.

Fleming, C.R., Beart, R.W., Berkner, S. *et al.* 1980: Home parenteral nutrition for management of the severely malnourished adult patients. *Gastroenterology* 79, 11–18.

Fleming, C.R., McCall, J.T., O'Brien, J.F. *et al.* 1984: Selenium status in patients receiving home parenteral nutrition. *JPEN: Journal of Parenteral and Enteral Nutrition* 8, 258–62.

Fleming, C.R., George, L., Stoner, G.L. *et al.* 1996: The importance of urinary magnesium values in patients with gut failure. *Mayo Clinic Proceedings* 71, 21–4.

Flint, J.M. 1912: The effect of extensive resection of the small intestine. *Bulletin of the Johns Hopkins Hospital* 23, 127–44.

Forsyth, R.J., Moulden, A., Hull, D. 1991: D-Lactate associated encephalopathy in short bowel syndrome: management with long-term non-absorbable oral antimicrobials. *Clinical Nutrition* 10, 352–5.

Fuchs, P.C., Gustafson, M.E., King, J.T. *et al.* 1984: Assessment of catheter associated infection risk with the Hickman right atrial catheter. *Infection Control* 5, 226–30.

Ganong, W.F. 1983: Gastrointestinal secretions and motility. In *Review of Medical Physiology*, 11th edn. Los Altos: Lange Medical Publications, 387–413.

Gimmon, Z., Kelley, R.E., Simko, V. *et al.* 1982: Total parenteral nutrition solution increases bile lithogenicity in rats. *Journal Surgical Research* 32, 256–63.

Glick, P.L., de Lorimier, A.A., Adzick, N.S. *et al.* 1984: Colon interposition: an adjuvant operation for short gut syndrome. *Journal of Pediatric Surgery* 19, 719–25.

Gouttebel, M.S., Saint-Aubert Astre, C. *et al.* 1986: Total parenteral nutrition needs in different types of short bowel syndrome. *Digestive Diseases and Sciences* 31, 718–23.

Gouttebel, M.C., Aubert, B.S., Colette, S. *et al.* 1989: Intestinal adaptation in patients with short bowel syndrome. *Digestive Diseases and Sciences* 34, 709–15.

Gracey, M. 1979: The contaminated small bowel syndrome: pathogenesis, diagnosis and treatment. *American Journal of Clinical Nutrition* 32, 234–43.

Grosfeld, J.L., Rescorla, F.J., West, K.W. 1986: Short bowel syndrome in infancy and childhood. *American Journal of Surgery* 151, 41–6.

Hadersley, K., Mortensen, P.B., Jorgensen, J. *et al.* 1998: Absorption of sodium, potassium, calcium and magnesium in short bowel patients treated with medium-chain fatty acids (abstract). *Gastroenterology* 114, G1535.

Heaton, K.W., Read, A.E. 1975: Gallstones in patients with disorders of the terminal ileum and disturbed bile salt metabolism. *British Medical Journal* 3, 494–6.

Hessov, I., Hasselblad, C., Fasth, S. *et al.* 1983: Magnesium deficiency after ileal resection for Crohn's disease. *Scandinavian Journal of Gastroenterology* 18, 643–9.

Hill, G.L., Mair, W.S.H., Goligher, J.C. 1975: Gallstones after ileostomy and ileal resection. *Gut* 16, 932–6.

Hodgkinson, A. 1981: Comment: Is there a place for a low-oxalate diet? *Journal of Human Nutrition* 35, 136–8.

Hoffbrand, A.V. 1967: Vitamin B_{12} and folic acid. In Krinkler, D.M. (ed.) *Postgastrectomy nutrition*. London: Lloyd-Luke, 1–15.

Howard, L., Hassan, N. 1998: Home parenteral nutrition – 25 years later. *Gastroenterology Clinics of North America* 27, 481–512.

Howard, L., Ovesen, L., Satya-Murti, S. *et al.* 1982: Reversible neurological symptoms caused by vitamin E deficiency in a patient with short bowel syndrome. *American Journal of Clinical Nutrition* 36, 1243–9.

Howard, L., Heaphey, L.L., Timchalk, M. 1986: A review of the current national status of home parenteral and enteral nutrition from the provider and consumer perspective. *JPEN: Journal of Parenteral and Enteral Nutrition* 10, 416–24.

Hudson, M., Pocknee, R., Mowat, N.A.G. 1990: D-Lactic acidosis in short bowel syndrome: an examination of possible mechanisms. *Quarterly Journal of Medicine* 74, 157–63.

Hughes, C.A., Dowling, R.H. 1980: Speed of onset of adaptive mucosal hypoplasia and hypofunction in the intestine of parenterally fed rats. *Clinical Science* 59, 317–27.

Hylander, E., Ladefoged, K., Madsen, S. 1981: Calcium balance and bone mineral content following small-intestinal resection. *Scandinavian Journal of Gastroenterology* 16, 167–76.

Inoue, Y., Copeland, E.M., Souba, W.W. 1994: Growth hormone enhances amino acid uptake by the human small intestine. *Annals of Surgery* 219, 715–24.

Jacobsen, O., Ladefoged, K., Stage, J.G. *et al.* 1986: Effects of cimetidine on jejunostomy effluents in patients with severe short-bowel syndrome. *Scandinavian Journal of Gastroenterology* 21, 824–8.

Jeppesen, P.B., Mortensen, P.B. 1997: Colonic digestion of medium-chain fat in patients with short bowel (abstract). *Gastroenterology* 112, 882.

Jeppesen, P.B., Hoy, C.E., Mortensen, P.B. 1998: Essential fatty acid deficiency in patients receiving home parenteral nutrition (abstract). *Gastroenterology* 114, G2629.

Johnson, C.P., Sarna, S.K., Zhu, Y.R. *et al.* 1996: Delayed gastroduodenal emptying is an important mechanism for control of intestinal transit in short gut syndrome. *American Journal of Surgery* 171, 90–5.

Jones, R.B., Keeling, P.W.N., Hilton, P.J. *et al.* 1981: The relationship between leucocyte and muscle zinc in health and disease. *Clinical Science* 60, 237–9.

Jover, R., Leon, J., Palazon, J.M., Dominguez, J.R. 1995: D-Lactic acidosis with use of medium-chain triglycerides (letter). *Lancet* 346, 314.

Kaufman, S.S., Loseke, C.A., Lupo, J.V. *et al.*. 1997: Influence of bacterial overgrowth and intestinal inflammation on duration of parenteral nutrition in children with short bowel syndrome. *Journal of Pediatrics* 131, 356–61.

Kaveggia, F.F., Thompson, J.S., Taylor, R.J. 1991: Placement of an ileal loop urinary diversion back into continuity with the intestinal tract. *Surgery* 110, 557–60.

Khalidi, N., Wesley, J.R., Thoene, J.G. *et al.* 1984: Biotin deficiency in a patient with short bowel syndrome during home parenteral nutrition. *JPEN: Journal of Parenteral and Enteral Nutrition* 8, 311–14.

Kishi, H., Nishii, S., Ono, T. *et al.* 1979: Thiamin and pyridoxine requirements during intravenous hyperalimentation. *American Journal of Clinical Nutrition* 32, 332–8.

Klein, G.L., Ament, M.E., Bluestone, R. *et al.* 1980: Bone disease associated with total parenteral nutrition. *Lancet* 2, 1041–4.

Ladefoged, K., Olgaard, K. 1985: Sodium homeostasis after small-bowel resection in man. *Scandinavian Journal of Gastroenterology* 20, 361–9.

Ladefoged, K., Christensen, K.C., Hegnhoj, J. *et al.* 1989: Effect of a long acting somatostatin analogue SMS 201–995 on jejunostomy effluents in patients with severe short bowel syndrome. *Gut* 30, 943–9.

Lennard-Jones, J.E. 1990: Indications and need for long-term parenteral nutrition: implications for intestinal transplantation. *Transplant Proceedings* 22, 2427–9.

Lennard-Jones, J.E. 1994: Review article: Practical management of the short bowel. *Alimentation, Pharmacology and Therapy* 8, 563–77.

Levy, E., Frileux, P., Sandrucci, S. *et al.* 1988: Continuous enteral nutrition during the early adaptive stages of the short bowel syndrome. *British Journal of Surgery* 75, 549–53.

Lin, C.H., Rossi, T.M., Heitling, L.A. *et al.* 1987: Nutritional assessment of children with short-bowel syndrome receiving home parenteral nutrition. *American Journal of Diseases of Childhood* 141, 1093–8.

Mayne, A.J., Handy, D.J., Preece, M.A. *et al.* 1990: Dietary management of D-lactic acidosis in short bowel syndrome. *Archives of Diseases of Childhood* 65, 229–31.

McCarthy, D., Kim, Y.S. 1973: Changes in sucrase, enterokinase, and peptide hydrolase after intestinal resection. The association of cellular hyperplasia and adaptation. *Journal of Clinical Investigations* 52, 942–51.

McClain, C., Soutor, C., Zieve, L. 1980: Zinc-deficiency: a complication of Crohn's disease. *Gastroenterology* 78, 272–9.

McIntyre, P.B., Fitchew, M., Lennard-Jones, J.E. 1986: Patients with a high jejunostomy do not need a special diet. *Gastroenterology* 91, 25–33.

Messing, B., Bories, C., Kunstlinger, F. *et al.* 1983: Does total parenteral nutrition induce gallbladder sludge formation and lithiasis? *Gastroenterology* 84, 1012–19.

Murphy, J.P., King, D.R., Dubois, A. 1979: Treatment of gastric hypersecretion with cimetidine in the short bowel syndrome. *New England Journal of Medicine* 300, 80–1.

Nelson, K.J., Moxness, K.E., Jensen, M.D., Gastineau, C.F. 1994: Renal diseases and disorders. In Laura De Young ed. *Mayo Clinic diet manual*, 7th edn. St Louis: Mosby, 315–64.

Nightingale, J.M.D., Lennard-Jones, J.E., Gertner, D.F. *et al.* 1992: Colonic preservation reduces need for parenteral therapy, increases incidence of renal stones, but does not change high prevalence of gall stones in patients with a short bowel. *Gut* 33, 1493–7.

Nightingale, J.M.D., Kamm, M.A., van der Sijp, J.R.M. *et al.* 1993: Disturbed gastric emptying in the short bowel syndrome. Evidence for a "colonic brake". *Gut* 34, 1171–6.

Nordgaard, I., Hansen, B.S., Mortensen, P.B. 1994: The colon as a digestive organ in patients with short bowel. *Lancet* 343, 373–6.

O'Dwyer, S.O., Smith, R.J., Hwang, T.L., Wilmore, D.W. 1989: Maintenance of small bowel mucosa with glutamine-enriched parenteral nutrition. *JPEN: Journal of Parenteral and Enteral Nutrition* 13, 579–85.

O'Keefe, S.J.D., Shroter, R.G., Bennet, W.M., Haymond, M.W. 1992: Villous hyperplasia is uncommon in patients with massive intestinal resection (abstract). *Gastroenterology* 102, A231.

O'Keefe, S.J.D., Haymond, M.W., Bennet, W.M. *et al.* 1994: Long-acting somatostatin analogue therapy and protein metabolism in patients with jejunostomies. *Gastroenterology* 107, 379–88.

Oh, M.S., Phelps, K.R., Traube, M. *et al.* 1979: D-Lactic acidosis in a man with the short-bowel syndrome. *New England Journal of Medicine* 301, 249–52.

Oh, M.S., Uribarri, J., Alveranga, D.L. *et al.* 1985: Metabolic utilization and renal handling of D-lactate in men. *Metabolism: Clinical & Experimental* 34, 621–5.

Okada, A., Takagi, Y., Itakura, T. *et al.* 1976: Skin lesions during intravenous hyperalimentation: zinc deficiency. *Surgery* 80, 629–35.

Ovesen, L., Chu, R., Howard, L. 1983: The influence of dietary fat on jejunostomy output in patients with severe short bowel syndrome. *American Journal of Clinical Nutrition* 38, 270–7.

Pak, C.Y.C. 1998: Kidney stones. *Lancet* 351, 1797–801.

Panis, Y., Messing, B., Rivet, P. *et al.* 1997: Segmental reversal of the small bowel as an alternative to intestinal transplantation in patients with short bowel syndrome. *Annals of Surgery* 225, 401–7.

Perlmutter, D.H., Boyle, J.T., Campos, J.M. *et al.* 1983: D-Lactic acidosis in children: an unusual metabolic complication of small bowel resection. *Journal of Pediatrics* 102, 234–8.

Pertsemlidis, D., Kark, A. 1974: Antiperistaltic segments for the treatment of short bowel syndrome. *American Journal of Gastroenterology* 62, 526–30.

Pigot, F., Messing, B., Chaussade, S. *et al.* 1990: Severe short bowel syndrome with a surgically reversed small bowel segment. *Digestive Diseases and Sciences* 35, 137–44.

Pitt, H.A., Lewinski, M.A., Muller, E.L. *et al.* 1984: Ileal resection-induced gallstones: altered bilirubin or cholesterol metabolism? *Surgery* 96, 154–62.

Porus, R.L. 1965: Epithelial hyperplasia following massive small bowel resection in man. *Gastroenterology* 48, 753–7.

Remington, M., Malagelada, J.R., Zinsmeister, A., Fleming, C.R. 1983: Abnormalities in gastrointestinal motor activity in patients with short bowels: effect of a synthetic opiate. *Gastroenterology* 85, 629–36.

Ricotta, J., Zuidema, F.D., Gadacz, T.R. *et al.* 1983: Construction of an ileocecal valve and its role in massive resection of the small intestine. *Surgical Gynecology and Obstetrics* 152, 310–14.

Rodrigues, C.A., Lennard-Jones, J.E., Thompson, D.G., Farthing, M.J.G. 1988: What is the ideal sodium concentration of oral rehydration solutions for short bowel patients? *Clinical Science* 74(Suppl. 18), 69P.

Rodrigues, C.A., Lennard-Jones, J.E., Thompson, D.G., Farthing, M.J.F. 1989: Energy absorption as a measure of intestinal failure in the short bowel syndrome. *Gut* 30, 176–83.

Rosen, G. 1992: Somatostatin and its analogs in the short bowel syndrome. *Nutrition in Clinical Practice* 7, 81–5.

Roslyn, J.J., Pitt, H.A., Mann, L.L. *et al.* 1983: Gallbladder disease in patients on long-term parenteral nutrition. *Gastroenterology* 84, 148–54.

Sandhu, B.K., Tripp, J.H., Candy, C.A. *et al.* 1981: Loperamide: studies on its mechanism of action. *Gut* 22, 658–62.

Schiller, L.R., Davis, G.R., Santa Ana, C.A. *et al.* 1982: Studies of the mechanism of the antidiarrheal effect of codeine. *Journal of Clinical Investigation* 70, 999–1008.

Schoorel, E.P., Giesberts, M.A.H., Blom, W., Van Gelderen, H.H. 1980: D-Lactic acidosis in a boy with short bowel syndrome. *Archives of Diseases of Childhood* 55, 810–12.

Schuman, E.S., Winters, V.N., Gross, G.F. *et al.* 1985: Management of Hickman catheter sepsis. *American Journal of Surgery* 149, 627–8.

Scolapio, J., Camilleri, M., Fleming, C.R. *et al.* 1997: Effect of growth hormone, glutamine and diet on adaptation in short-bowel syndrome: a randomized controlled study. *Gastroenterology* 113, 1074–81.

Scully, T.B., Kraft, S.C., Carr, W.C., Harig, H.M. 1989: D-Lactate associated encephalopathy after massive small-bowel resection. *Journal of Clinical Gastroenterology* 11, 448–51.

Seydel, A.S., Miller, J.H., Sarac, T.P. *et al.* 1996: Octreotide diminishes luminal nutrient transport activity, which is reversed by epidermal growth factor. *American Journal of Surgery* 172, 267–71.

Sherlock, S., Dooley, J. 1997: *Diseases of the liver and biliary tract.* London: Blackwell Science, 594–603.

Shike, M., Shils, M.E., Heller, A. *et al.* 1986: Bone disease in prolonged parenteral nutrition: osteopenia without mineralization defect. *American Journal of Clinical Nutrition* 44, 89–98.

Shulkes, A. 1994: Somatostatin: physiology and clinical application. *Bailliere's Clinical Endocrinology and Metabolism* 8, 215–36.

Shulman, D.I., Hu, C.S., Duckett, G., Lavallee-Grey, M. 1992: Effects of short-term growth hormone therapy in rats undergoing 75 per cent small intestinal resection. *Journal of Pediatric Gastroenterology and Nutrition* 14, 3–11.

Smith, N.L., Ravo, B., Soroff, H.S. *et al.* 1985: Successful fibrinolytic therapy for superior vena cava thrombosis secondary to long-term total parenteral nutrition. *JPEN: Journal of Parenteral and Enteral Nutrition* 9, 55–7.

Spiller, R.C., Trotman, I.F., Higgins, B.E. *et al.* 1984: The ileal brake – inhibition of jejunal motility after ileal fat perfusion in man. *Gut* 25, 365–74.

Spiller, R.C., Brown, M.L., Philips, S.F. 1986: Decreased fluid tolerance, accelerated transit, and abnormal motility of the human colon induced by oleic acid. *Gastroenterology* 91, 100–7.

Steiger, E., Srp, F. 1983: Morbidity and mortality related to home parenteral nutrition in patients with gut failure. *American Journal of Surgery* 145, 102–5.

Stohlberg, L., Rolfe, R., Gitlin, N. *et al.* 1982: D-Lactic acidosis due to abnormal gut flora. *New England Journal of Medicine* 306, 1344–8.

Stokes, M.A., Almond, D.J., Pettil, S.H. *et al.* 1988: Home parenteral nutrition: a review of 100 patient years of treatment in 76 consecutive cases. *British Journal of Surgery* 75, 481–3.

Sturniolo, G., Molukhia, M.M., Shields, R. *et al.* 1980: Zinc absorption in Crohn's disease. *Gut* 21, 387–91.

Tamada, H., Nezu, R., Matsuo, Y. *et al.* 1993: Alanyl glutamine-enriched total parenteral nutrition restores intestinal adaptation after either proximal or distal massive resection in rats. *JPEN: Journal of Parenteral and Enteral Nutrition* 17, 236–42.

Taylor, S.F., Sondheimer, J.M., Sokol, R.J. *et al.* 1991: Noninfectious colitis associated with short gut syndrome in infants. *Journal of Pediatrics* 119, 24–8.

Thompson, J.S. 1994: Management of the short bowel syndrome. *Gastroenterology Clinics of North America* 23, 403–20.

Thompson, J.S. 1996: The role of prophylactic cholecystectomy in the short-bowel syndrome. *Archives of Surgery* 131, 556–9.

Thompson, J.S., Langnas, A.N., Lewis, W. *et al.* 1995: Surgical approach to short-bowel syndrome, experience in a population of 160 patients. *Annals of Surgery* 222, 605–7.

Vanderhoof, J.A. 1996: Short bowel syndrome in children and small intestinal transplantation. *Pediatric Clinics of North America* 43, 533–50.

Vanderhoof, J.A., Langnas, A.N., Pench, L.W. *et al.* 1992: Invited review: Short bowel syndrome. *Journal of Pediatric Gastroenterology* 14, 359–70.

Verhage, A.H., Cheong, W.K., Jeejeebhoy, K.N. 1996: Neurologic symptoms due to possible chromium deficiency in long-term parenteral nutrition that closely mimic metronidazole-induced syndromes. *JPEN: Journal of Parenteral and Enteral Nutrition* 20, 123–7.

Weber, T.R., Vane, D.W., Grosfield, J.L. 1982: Tapering enteroplasty in infants with bowel atresia and short gut. *Archives of Surgery* 117, 684–8.

Weser, E. 1976: The management of patients after small bowel resection. *Gastroenterology* 71, 146–50.

Whitington, P.F. 1985: Cholestasis associated with total parenteral nutrition in infants. *Hepatology* 5, 693–6.

Williams, N.S., King, R.F.G. 1985: The effect of a reversed ileal segment and artificial valve on intestinal transit and absorption following colectomy and low ileorectal anastomosis in the dog. *British Journal of Surgery* 72, 169–74.

Williams, N.S., Evans, P., King, R.J.F.J. 1985: Gastric acid secretion and gastrin production in the short bowel syndrome. *Gut* 26, 914–19.

Wilmore, D.W., Dudrick, S.J., Daly, J.M., Vars, H.M. 1971: The role of nutrition in the adaptation of the small intestine after massive resection. *Surgery, Gynecology and Obstetrics* 134, 673–80.

Wilmore, D.W., Byrne, T.A., Pesringer, R.L. 1997: Short bowel syndrome: new therapeutic approaches. *Current Problems in Surgery* 34, 391–44.

Wolman, S.L., Anderson, G.H., Marliss, E.B. *et al.* 1979: Zinc in total parenteral nutrition: requirements and metabolic effects. *Gastroenterology* 76, 458–67.

Woolf, G.M., Miller, C., Kurian, R., Jeejeebhoy, K.N. 1983: Diet for patients with a short bowel: high fat or high carbohydrate?. *Gastroenterology* 84, 823–8.

Woolf, G.M., Miller, C., Kurian, R. *et al.* 1987: Nutritional absorption in short bowel syndrome. *Digestive Diseases and Sciences* 32, 8–15.

Young, R.J., Vandenhoof, J.A. 1997: Probiotic therapy in children with short bowel syndrome and bacterial overgrowth (abstract). *Gastroenterology* 112, A916.

Zarembski, P.M., Hodgkinson, A. 1962: The oxalic acid content of English diets. *British Journal of Nutrition* 16, 627–34.

Zhang, W., Fraukel, W.L., Roth, J. *et al.* 1994: Insulin-like growth factor I improves mucosal structure and function in small bowel transplantation in the rat. *Transplant Proceedings* 26, 1458–9.

30

Small bowel transplantation

DAVE L BIGAM, DAVID R GRANT

INTRODUCTION

Patients with intestinal failure are unable to maintain their nutrition and/or fluid and electrolyte balance on an enteral diet. They experience dehydration, weight loss and malnutrition. The short bowel syndrome, which follows extensive bowel resection, is the most common cause of intestinal failure. In children, gastroschisis, intestinal atresia, midgut volvulus and necrotizing enterocolitis are the common causes of short bowel syndrome. In adults, mesenteric infarction, Crohn's disease and locally invasive tumors involving the superior mesenteric artery are the common causes of the short bowel syndrome (Table 30.1). Intestinal failure may also be due to functional disorders, such as radiation enteritis, microvillous inclusion disease and pseudo-obstruction (Kocoshis, 1994; Kocoshis *et al.*, 1997).

Table 30.1 *Etiology of intestinal failure*

Mechanical (short bowel)	Functional
Children	
Gastroschisis	Idiopathic pseudo-obstruction
Intestinal atresia	Microvillous inclusion disease
Malrotation/midgut volvulus	Intestinal aganglionosis
Necrotizing enterocolitis	Visceral myopathy
	Autoimmune enteritis
Adults	
Mesenteric ischemia	Crohn's disease
Volvulus	Radiation enteritis
Trauma	Idiopathic pseudo-obstruction
Desmoid tumor	
Gardner's disease/familial polyposis	

Treatment for intestinal failure is aimed at maintaining hydration and nutrition until the patient can be sustained on an enteral diet. Oral nutrition is provided to promote mucosal adaptation and to maintain gut barrier function. Iso-osmolar tube feeds that contain glutamine, an essential gut nutrient, are administered. Medications, such as narcotics, cholestyramine, histamine antagonists and somatostatin analogs, are used to slow intestinal transit and to decrease luminal fluid losses. Surgical procedures that increase the absorptive capacity of the remaining bowel may be attempted in some patients (Thompson *et al.*, 1995).

Many patients require total parenteral nutrition for prolonged periods of time. Adults with more than 60 cm of small bowel, or 30 cm of small bowel plus an intact ileo-cecal valve, can usually be weaned off parenteral nutrition once the remaining small bowel has adapted. Accurately predicting the requirement for lifelong parenteral nutrition is difficult, as some children have been weaned off parenteral nutrition with as little as 10 cm of small bowel (Kurkubasche *et al.*, 1993).

Long-term home parenteral nutrition is effective in most cases, but this therapy is expensive and it interferes with normal daily activities (Howard *et al.*, 1995). Many patients lose their venous access sites because of recurrent line infections and thrombosis. In addition, some patients develop severe cholestatic liver disease.

Successful small bowel transplantation allows patients with intestinal failure to resume a normal lifestyle.

Success in small bowel transplantation has been more difficult to achieve than with other organs due in large part to three unique and inter-related problems: (1) the large amount of immunocompetent donor lymphocytes transplanted with the graft; (2) microbial colonization of the graft; and (3) the lack of a reliable, non-invasive method to diagnose rejection. Expression of MHC class II antigens on the intestinal epithelium and lymphocytes within the graft provides a strong stimulus for rejection (Bland, 1988). Intense immune suppression is required to prevent rejection, which in turn leads to a higher risk of infectious complications. If gut barrier function is compromised by preservation injury or graft rejection, bacterial translocation occurs, completing the vicious circle of events that have contributed to the high morbidity and mortality rates associated with intestinal transplantation.

HISTORY OF SMALL BOWEL TRANSPLANTATION

In 1902, Dr Alexis Carrel successfully transplanted segments of canine small bowel to the great vessels of the neck (Carrel, 1902). Lillehei later demonstrated that canine small bowel allografts could provide normal nutrition, despite disruption of the normal lymphatic and neural connections of the bowel (Lillehei *et al.*, 1959, 1967). In the 1960s, the success of renal transplantation stimulated attempts at bowel transplantation in humans, but these procedures were unsuccessful owing to rejection, sepsis and graft failure. Interest in the procedure waned in the early 1970s, when total parenteral nutrition became available as a treatment for patients with intestinal failure. It was revived in the late 1980s following reports of successful isolated clinical small bowel transplantation, and combined liver and small bowel transplantation, using cyclosporine immunosuppression (Goulet *et al.*, 1990; Grant *et al.*, 1990).

These cases were followed by successful isolated intestinal grafting using tacrolimus (Prograf®) (Todo *et al.*, 1995). Currently, there are more than 30 programs worldwide performing up to 100 intestinal transplants per year.

INDICATIONS AND RECIPIENT SELECTION

At present, intestinal transplantation is reserved for patients who have failed conventional therapy of intestinal failure. Patients who cannot be weaned off long-term parenteral nutrition and have lost venous access due to repeated catheter infections or thrombosis are candidates for isolated intestinal grafting. A combined liver and small bowel transplant is reserved for patients who develop complications of cholestatic liver disease secondary to parenteral nutrition. Occasionally, a combined liver and small bowel transplant is offered when a new liver can correct the underlying etiology of the intestinal failure. For example, mesenteric venous thrombosis and subsequent massive small bowel resection associated with protein C deficiency would be best dealt with by a combined transplant. As the results of isolated small bowel transplantation have improved, there has been a move towards earlier transplantation in an effort to avoid parenteral nutrition-induced liver disease and the increased morbidity of a combined transplant. Motility disorders and locally invasive tumors are potential indications for multivisceral grafting that may include the liver, small bowel, duodenum, pancreas, stomach, colon and kidneys (Alessiani *et al.*, 1995).

The initial step in recipient selection is to confirm that conventional treatments for intestinal failure, including aggressive attempts at enteral feedings, have truly failed. A barium swallow with small bowel follow-through is performed to visualize the extent of remaining bowel. Doppler studies are performed to assess the abdominal vasculature. Motility studies are ordered for patients with pseudo-obstruction to confirm that there will be adequate intestinal motility into and out of the bowel graft. The complete work-up includes cardiopulmonary and renal assessments as well as a psychosocial evaluation.

It can be difficult to predict if a patient on long-term parenteral nutrition with elevated liver function tests is best treated with a combined liver and small bowel transplant or an isolated small bowel transplant. The cholestasis associated with parenteral nutrition will usually resolve with a successful small bowel transplant (Grant *et al.*, 1989). Moreover, a failed isolated intestinal graft can be removed and the patient can survive on parenteral nutrition, whereas a failed combined transplant will result in patient death if retransplantation is not an option. Thus, patients with cholestasis or mild fibrosis but no portal hypertension are offered isolated intestinal grafting, which usually normalizes liver function.

Incurable malignancy, significant co-morbid conditions, such as cardiopulmonary disease or advanced age, and systemic infection are contraindications to intestinal transplantation.

DONOR SELECTION

Although the small bowel could be retrieved from most multiorgan cadaveric donors, most centers currently only use 'ideal' donors in an effort to maximize favorable patient outcomes. Previous bowel resections leave many recipients with smaller than expected abdominal cavities (loss of domain). Therefore, a donor who weighs 20–30 per cent less than the recipient is used whenever possible. Preoperatively, donors are given oral non-absorbable and intravenous antibiotics to decontaminate the bowel lumen. We no longer use mechanical bowel preparation since it produces a fluid-filled graft that can be difficult to manipulate.

Identical blood group (ABO) match is preferred because of the risk of hemolysis due to antibodies produced by B cells within the graft (Cohen *et al.*, 1986). HLA typing is performed for future reference but does not change the clinical decision making. The benefit of administering antilymphocyte products to the donor to deplete immune cells from the graft in an attempt to decrease graft versus host disease is unproven. Living-related small bowel transplants have been performed and, as outcomes improve, the indications for living-related transplantation may expand as they have for kidney transplantation (Pollard *et al.*, 1996).

PROCUREMENT PROCEDURE

Isolated small bowel donor procurement is usually performed as part of a multiorgan retrieval. The procurement procedure begins by examining the bowel to ensure suitability for transplant. The bowel should be free from trauma with no evidence of intrinsic pathology. The superior mesenteric vein and portal vein are separated from the pancreas, which is divided at its neck. The proximal jejunum and distal ileum are stapled. Clips are placed along the cut edge of the small bowel mesentery to prevent chylous ascites in the recipient. A cannula is inserted above the aortic bifurcation. The graft is perfused with University of Wisconsin solution and cooled topically. The origin of the superior mesenteric artery, with a Carrel patch of aorta, is taken to complete the retrieval. When the liver is also being retrieved, the liver and small bowel are removed *en bloc* with careful division of the vasculature on the back table. Aberrant right hepatic arteries, originating from the superior mesenteric artery, are retained with the liver. An iliac artery interposition graft can then be used to lengthen the foreshortened superior mesenteric artery supplying the bowel. We try to keep the cold ischemic time less than 6–10 hours.

The techniques for combined liver and small bowel retrieval continue to evolve. Previously, the jejunum and ileum were removed *en bloc* with the liver, connected by the portal vein/superior mesenteric vein and an aortic conduit, with the celiac and superior mesenteric artery as well as a length of thoracic aorta. The University of Nebraska has recently recommended including the donor duodenum and head of the pancreas as part of this graft to obviate the need for biliary reconstruction and facilitate orientation of the transplanted bowel.

In the donor procurement procedure for a multivisceral transplant, the abdominal organs anterior to the kidneys (if they are not being retrieved as well) are eviscerated along with generous lengths of vena cava and the thoracic aorta. A donor splenectomy is performed, taking care to avoid injury to the tail of the pancreas, to minimize the risk of graft versus host disease in the recipient.

RECIPIENT SURGERY

Isolated intestinal transplantation (Fig. 30.1)

The donor superior mesenteric artery is anastomosed to the recipient's infrarenal or supraceliac aorta, or to the superior mesenteric artery. This anastomosis can be technically difficult owing to the short length of the donor artery, the depth of the wound and suboptimal exposure with the donor bowel obscuring the field. Exposure can be improved by first anastomosing an iliac artery graft to the aorta and then anastomosing the donor superior mesenteric artery to the iliac interposition graft (Alan Langnas, University of Nebraska, personal communication). The donor superior mesenteric vein can be anastomosed to the recipient's superior mesenteric vein, portal vein or inferior vena cava. Theoretical advantages of portal venous drainage over systemic venous drainage include the delivery of hepatotrophic substances from the bowel directly to the liver, the filtering of organisms and toxins from the graft by the native liver, and immune protection from rejection (Grant *et al.*, 1990).

After completion of the vascular anastomoses, the proximal end of the graft is anastomosed to the native bowel. A segment of the donor colon may be retained in continuity with the small bowel to increase the absorptive capacity of the graft and to potentially decrease ileostomy output, but some centers believe including the colon may be associated with increased graft loss (Black *et al.*, 1994; Reyes *et al.*, 1998). The distal end of the intestinal graft can be anastomosed to the native bowel, with the creation of a diverting loop ileostomy, or exteriorized as a stoma. The ileostomy is closed once the patient has stabilized with no evidence of rejection or infection, usually 3–6 months after the transplant.

Small bowel and liver transplantation (Fig. 30.2)

The recipient operation for combined liver and small bowel transplant begins with the standard suprahepatic

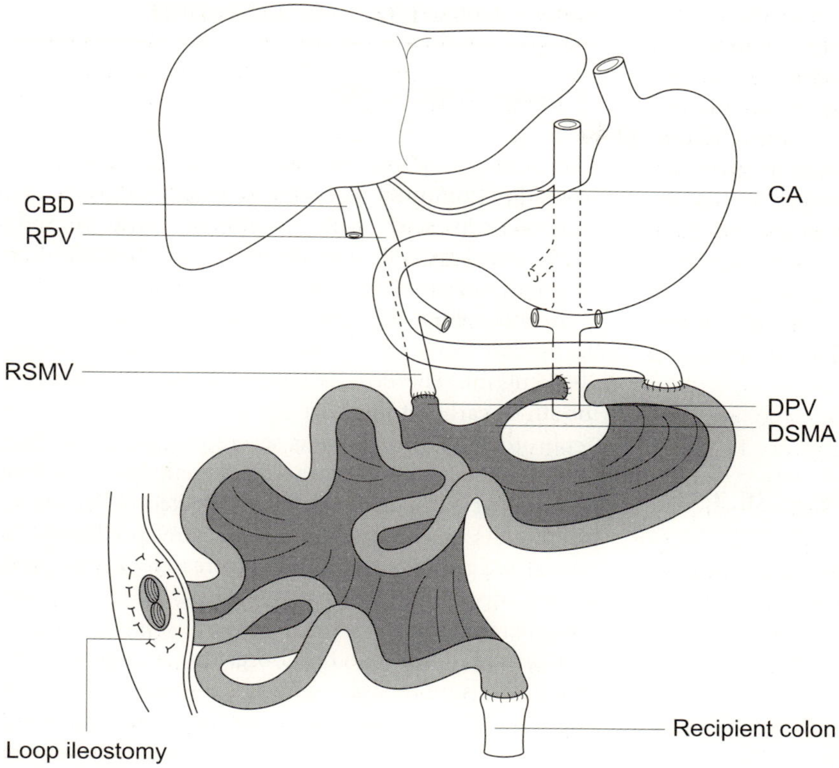

Figure 30.1 *Isolated small bowel recipient operation. The donor superior mesenteric artery is anastomosed to the infrarenal aorta while the donor portal vein is anastomosed to the recipient superior mesenteric vein. The proximal and distal ends of the bowel are anastomosed to the native bowel with a diverting loop ileostomy. CA, celiac artery; CBD, common bile duct; DPV, donor portal vein; DSMA, donor superior mesenteric artery; RPV, recipient portal vein; RSMV, recipient superior mesenteric vein.*

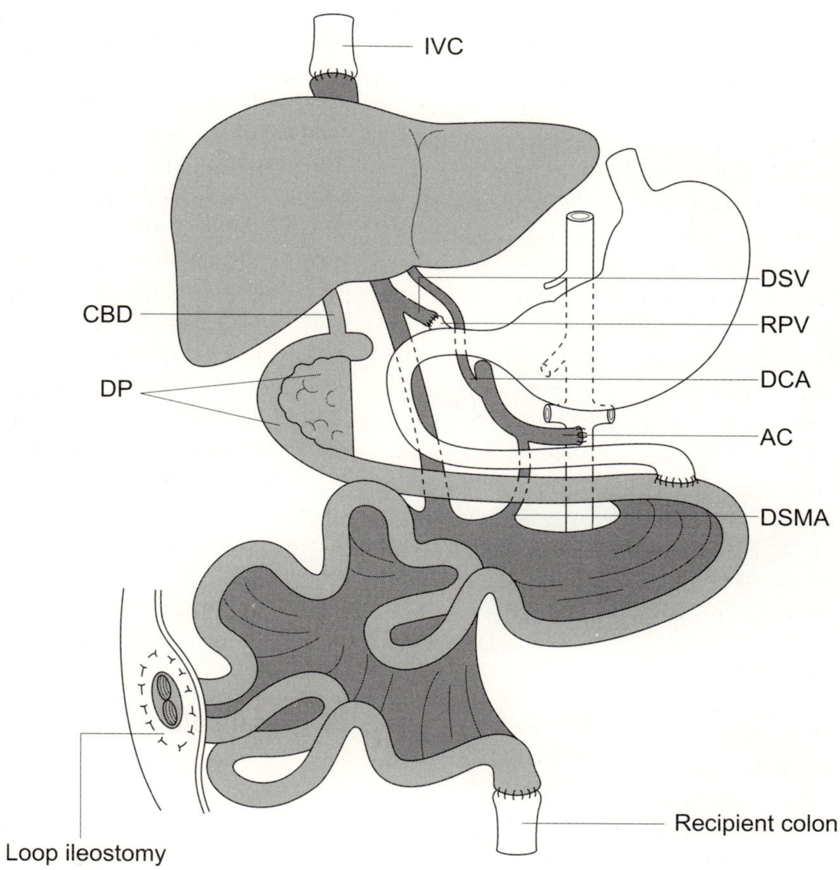

Figure 30.2 *Combined small bowel/liver recipient operation. The suprahepatic and infrahepatic caval anastomoses are performed as in isolated liver transplantation. The aortic conduit is anastomosed to the infrarenal aorta. The recipient portal vein is anastomosed to the donor splenic vein. Biliary reconstruction is not required because the duodenum and head of the pancreas are included with the graft. AC, aortic conduit; CBD common bile duct; DCA, donor celiac artery; DP, duodenum and head of pancreas; DPV, donor portal vein; DSMA, donor superior mesenteric artery; DSV, donor splenic vein; IVC, inferior vena cava; RPV, recipient portal vein.*

and infrahepatic caval anastomoses, as in isolated liver transplantation. The native portal vein, draining the stomach, duodenum, pancreas and spleen, is anastomosed end-to-side to the donor portal vein or end-to-end to the donor splenic vein. The donor aortic conduit is anastomosed to the infrarenal or suprarenal aorta. When the common bile duct is divided during the retrieval, biliary continuity is restored via a Roux-en-Y hepaticojejunostomy with the donor bowel. No biliary reconstruction is required if the duodenum and head of the pancreas are preserved with the graft. The bowel anastomoses are performed as in isolated intestinal transplantation.

Multivisceral transplantation (Fig. 30.3)

The recipient operation begins with an evisceration of the abdominal organs. The graft can include the liver, small bowel, pancreas, duodenum, stomach, colon and kidneys. The caval anastomoses proceed as for liver transplantation. The end of the donor aortic conduit is anastomosed to the side of the recipient's infrarenal or suprarenal aorta. A portal venous anastomosis is not required. Intestinal continuity is restored as in isolated intestinal transplantation.

POST-TRANSPLANT MANAGEMENT

Immune suppression

The immunosuppressive regimen for intestinal transplantation continues to evolve. Currently, most recipients are induced with tacrolimus and steroids. Mycophenolate mofetil (CellCept®) and prostaglandins are often added to this regimen.

At our center, we start oral tacrolimus at a dose of 0.3 mg/kg per day, aiming for serum levels of 20–25 ng/ml. The dose is tapered down after the first month or earlier if there are signs of cardiac-, neuro- or nephrotoxicity, or if there is severe glucose intolerance (Atkinson *et al.*, 1995). Intravenous methylprednisolone is started at 1 mg/kg per day, and tapered to 0.3 mg/kg per day. As bowel function returns, oral prednisone is started and the dose is gradually decreased over the next several months. Muromonab-CD3 (OKT®3) is given intraoperatively and for the first two postoperative days. One unit of donor blood is also given for its potentially immune suppressive effect. Prostaglandin E1 (0.6–0.8 μg/kg per day) is given intravenously for 2 weeks for its immune suppressive, renal protective and vasodilatory effects. Thereafter, patients receive oral misoprostol (200 μg three times daily).

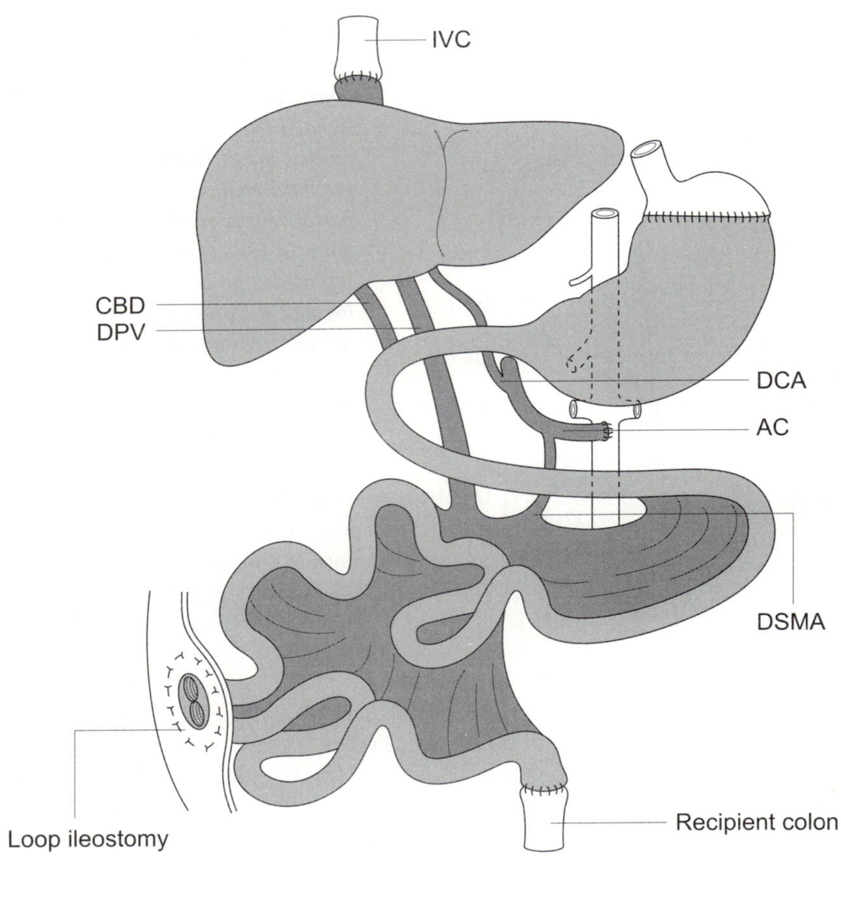

Figure 30.3 *Multivisceral recipient operation. The suprahepatic, infrahepatic and aortic conduit anastomoses are performed as in combined small bowel/liver transplantation. Neither portal venous nor biliary reconstruction is required. The pancreas is not shown but is included in the graft. AC, aortic conduit; CBD, common bile duct; DCA, donor celiac artery; DPV, donor portal vein, DSMA, donor superior mesenteric artery; IVC, inferior vena cava.*

Rejection

Acute rejection can be difficult to diagnose. Patients may be asymptomatic or have symptoms ranging from mild fever and non-specific abdominal pain to vomiting, ileus, increased stomal output, acidosis, bacteremia and septic shock. There are currently no sensitive, specific, non-invasive tests for intestinal rejection. Increased intestinal permeability is an early, non-specific sign of graft rejection and can be screened for by performing chromium-labeled EDTA (ethylenediaminetetraacetic acid) intestinal permeability studies (Lillehei *et al.*, 1967).

The diagnosis of rejection requires histological confirmation. Endoscopic mucosal biopsies are performed via the ileostomy twice weekly for 1 month or longer to screen for rejection. The endoscopic appearance of mild to moderate rejection reveals dusky mucosa with edema, hyperemia and decreased peristalsis. Severe rejection presents endoscopically with ulceration, mucosal sloughing, friability, bleeding and loss of peristalsis. Microscopically, early acute rejection reveals cryptitis and blunting of the villi, which may progress to vasculitis with a mononuclear cell infiltrate. Microscopic evidence of severe rejection includes mucosal sloughing, inflammation and graft necrosis (Lee *et al.*, 1996). The bowel graft may undergo active rejection without any evidence of hepatic rejection. Sampling error is always a potential problem as the endoscopic biopsies may be normal at one site with severe rejection occurring at another area in the graft.

Refractory diarrhea and weight loss are signs of chronic rejection. Endoscopy may reveal loss of mucosal folds, pseudomembrane formation and decreased peristalsis. Microscopic findings include villous atrophy, subintimal vascular thickening and fibrosis. A full-thickness biopsy may be required to confirm chronic rejection.

Initial treatment of rejection consists of increasing the dose of tacrolimus and giving short-term high-dose steroids. Treatment with OKT®3 (5 mg/day for 7–10 days) or antithymocyte gammaglobulin (Atgam®, beginning at 500 mg/day with the dose titrated to a CD2 count of 100 cells/mm^3 for 7–10 days) is used for severe rejection. Mycophenolate mofetil may be added to reduce the risk of subsequent rejection episodes. The graft may need to be removed if rejection remains refractory to treatment.

Results from the Intestinal Transplant Registry suggest that a combined transplant is associated with less rejection than an isolated small bowel transplant (Grant, 1999). It should be noted, however, that these results are not yet definitive and there is an increased mortality with combined transplants.

Graft versus host disease

Graft versus host disease was expected to be a major problem in clinical intestinal transplantation because of the large amount of immunocompetent cells transplanted with the bowel. Fortunately, it has not been a common complication after clinical small bowel transplantation despite being well documented in experimental intestinal transplantation (Grant *et al.*, 1989; Langnas *et al.*, 1996). Graft versus host disease presents with dermatologic, hepatic or pulmonary changes. Dermatologic involvement ranges from a maculopapular rash to exfoliative dermatitis. If the liver is affected, jaundice develops and biopsies show cholestasis, ductopenia, fibrosis and a portal mononuclear cellular infiltration. Interstitial pneumonitis is the characteristic finding if there is pulmonary involvement. Diagnosis is confirmed with a tissue biopsy. Short-term, high-dose steroids are used to treat graft versus host disease.

Infection

Most small bowel transplant recipients have one or more bacterial, viral or fungal infections during the first 3 months after transplant. To reduce the risk of sepsis, recipients are given prophylactic perioperative antibiotics, antivirals and antifungals. We avoid excessive immune suppression by insisting on biopsy confirmation of graft rejection prior to antirejection treatment.

The increased intestinal permeability associated with graft rejection results in bacterial translocation and systemic sepsis. Therefore, the most important step in preventing bacterial sepsis is close observation for rejection and prompt treatment if diagnosed. Other measures to reduce the risk of bacterial infection include: (1) bowel decontamination with oral and intravenous antibiotics; and (2) early enteral feeds to stimulate mucosal growth and to preserve gut barrier function.

Bacterial infections of central venous lines can be difficult to treat. Patients requiring intestinal transplantation have limited venous access due to long-term parenteral therapy and it may be difficult to remove an infected line for lack of another venous access site. Fortunately, systemic antibiotic therapy is usually successful in treating these infections.

The combination of small bowel transplantation and multiorgan failure places patients at an increased risk for fungal sepsis. Perioperative antifungal prophylaxis is provided with agents such as fluconazole. Treatment of established fungal infection requires prolonged courses of antifungal therapy and supportive care.

Cytomegalovirus (CMV) and Epstein–Barr virus (EBV) are the most common causes of viral illness complicating intestinal transplantation. The requirement for increased immune suppression to treat acute rejection and donor–recipient mismatches (CMV-seropositive donor into CMV-seronegative recipient) are risk factors for CMV disease. Prophylactic ganciclovir and gammaglobulin are given for the first post-transplant month to most patients. Grafts from CMV-serologically negative donors are implanted into serologically negative recipients whenever possible. In addition, only CMV-seronegative blood products are used, if available.

CMV infection may present with fever, leukopenia, gastrointestinal complications, hepatitis or interstitial pneumonia. If active disease is diagnosed, treatment includes reducing immune suppression and administering intravenous ganciclovir. It can be difficult, and sometimes impossible, to eradicate established CMV infection from intestinal grafts. This is likely to be because the bowel acts as a massive reservoir for the virus.

There are various presentations of EBV infection ranging from a non-specific fever or mononucleosis-like syndrome to generalized lymphadenopathy, atypical lymphocytosis, or hepatitis. After EBV infection, the virus is maintained within B lymphocytes in a latent state. EBV-stimulated B-cell proliferation results in polyclonal reactive lymphoid hyperplasia that can eventually progress to a monoclonal large-cell lymphoma (Nalesnik, 1996).

The risk of developing post-transplant lymphoproliferative disorders appears to be greater following intestinal transplantation than after other organ transplants, possibly because of the increased amount of immune suppression required for these patients. Rates as high as 29 per cent in children or infants with small bowel grafts have been reported by the Pittsburgh program (Reyes *et al.*, 1998). Primary EBV infection carries a higher risk of developing a post-transplant lymphoproliferative disorder compared to EBV reactivation or reinfection and this may explain the high rates in children. Methods to decrease the risk of post-transplant lymphoproliferative disorders include minimizing immune suppression whenever possible, giving prophylactic treatment with gammaglobulin containing high titers of anti-EBV antibodies, and using pre-emptive ganciclovir when polymerase chain reaction testing reveals high titers of EBV genome in the peripheral blood lymphocytes. The diagnosis of post-transplant lymphoproliferative disorders can be difficult and a high index of suspicion must be maintained. A careful review of the microscopic features of tissue biopsies is essential as early changes of post-transplant lymphoproliferative disorder may resemble rejection and lead to inappropriate therapy. The initial treatment for post-transplant lymphoproliferative disorder is to reduce immune suppression and administer intravenous acyclovir or ganciclovir. Systemic chemotherapy is reserved for patients who do not respond to these initial therapeutic maneuvers.

Nutrition

Enteral feedings are begun after transplantation via a nasoduodenal feeding tube placed at the time of surgery. Patients are initially started on an elemental formula tube feed with added glutamine. Once the patient tolerates this regimen, it is changed to a non-elemental formula. The early enteral feedings provide luminal nutrients that prevent the villous atrophy and increased intestinal permeability that occur with prolonged parenteral nutrition. Oral intake is encouraged and, once the daily caloric oral intake is satisfactory, tube feeding is discontinued. Some young children have difficulty learning, or relearning, to take oral nutrition. Parenteral nutrition is gradually weaned off and the majority of patients are able to resume full enteral nutrition within 4–6 weeks post-transplant.

Complications

Rejection, infection and post-transplant lymphoproliferative disorders are the major complications after intestinal transplantation. Other potentially significant complications involve the vascular, gastrointestinal, renal and pulmonary systems.

Arterial and venous thrombosis, the two most significant vascular complications, can lead to loss of graft and patient death. Potential risk factors for arterial and venous thrombosis include increased postoperative abdominal pressure, pre-existing hypercoagulable states, the use of interposition aortic or iliac artery conduits and the small size of the arteries, particularly in the pediatric recipients. Increased postoperative abdominal pressure may develop when there is a size mismatch between the donor organ and the recipient's abdominal cavity, leading to the abdominal compartment syndrome. The risk of this complication can be reduced by selecting donors that weigh 20–30 per cent less than the recipient and using synthetic mesh to close the abdomen when the donor organs are larger than anticipated, so that the abdomen is never closed under tension. The use of magnifying loupes or an operating microscope may improve vascular anastomotic patency rates. A pre-existing hypercoagulable state may be corrected by a combined liver and small bowel transplant. If recipients are still deemed to be at high risk for a thrombotic event post-transplant, they receive low-molecular-weight heparin, coumadin or enteric coated aspirin.

Risk factors for impaired healing at the gastrointestinal anastomotic sites include graft preservation damage, exogenous steroid administration and malnutrition. Strategies to limit these risks include minimizing graft ischemic time, avoiding excessive steroid administration, and optimizing nutritional status before and after transplant. Endoscopic biopsies are performed under direct vision with minimal insufflation of air in an attempt to avoid iatrogenic bowel perforation. Spontaneous perforation of the graft has been seen with transmural rejection. Anastomotic leaks or bowel perforations can usually be managed by primary repair with or without fecal diversion. Enteral feeding is resumed as soon as possible.

Fluid and electrolyte imbalances are common in the postoperative period. Rejection, infection and medication toxicity can lead to diarrhea, and subsequent dehydration and metabolic acidosis. Treatment includes parenteral fluids, bicarbonate and medications, such as codeine, ranitidine and somatostatin, to slow intestinal transit and to decrease fluid losses. Renal insufficiency is a risk post-transplant, particularly with the high doses of tacrolimus used for intestinal transplantation. Impaired renal function places the patient at risk for fluid overload and pulmonary edema. This combination may lead to a requirement for prolonged ventilation. Patient management in this setting is often complicated by inadequate venous access, which can make ultrafiltration or hemodialysis technically impossible.

GRAFT FUNCTION

A marked improvement in quality of life follows successful small bowel transplantation with freedom from the 8–12 hours required each day for parenteral nutrition (Asfar *et al.*, 1996; Langnas *et al.*, 1996; Reyes *et al.*, 1998). Adults regain the ability to enjoy meals and young children may begin to eat normally for the first time in their lives. Intestinal graft function is demonstrable in the early postoperative period. Tacrolimus is given orally immediately post-transplant and adequate serum levels are attained quickly. Enteral intake is gradually increased until patients are able to maintain their hydration and nutrition without parenteral support. Most patients are converted to purely enteral feedings, with 95 (77 per cent) of the 126 patients surviving intestinal transplant followed in the Intestinal Transplant Registry having been successfully weaned off parenteral nutrition (Grant, 1999).

Preservation damage, neural and lymphatic disruption, rejection, infection, medication toxicity, and recurrent disease are all potential risk factors for poor graft function. Preservation injury to the graft appears to lead to temporary mucosal dysfunction with resolution expected within the first few days after transplant. Neural disruption in rats results in significant changes in the transport characteristics of the bowel, but these changes have little impact on the well-being of the animal (Sigalet *et al.*, 1992). In humans, bowel motility is altered on manometry testing, but these changes do not appear to be clinically significant as peristalsis is maintained and intestinal motility has not been a problem in the postoperative period (Pernthaler *et al.*, 1996). The lymphatic drainage of the bowel is disrupted when the mesentery is divided. Immediately post-transplant, the lymph drains into the peritoneal cavity where it is absorbed. In animal models, lymphatic regeneration into the retroperitoneum and subsequently to the cysterna chyli appears to be complete by 2–4 weeks post-transplant (Lillehei *et al.*, 1967). Although a potential risk, chylous ascites has not been a significant clinical problem. If chylous ascites develops, patients are started on a low-fat enteral intake or total parenteral nutrition and a somatostatin analog.

Graft function may rarely become compromised by recurrent disease. There has been one report of recurrent Crohn's disease involving an intestinal graft, which ultimately contributed to graft failure (Sustento-Reodica *et al.*, 1997).

PATIENT AND GRAFT SURVIVAL

An international Intestinal Transplant Registry has been developed to track the outcomes of clinical bowel transplantation (Grant, 1996). To the end of February 1997, 273 transplants had been performed on 260 patients in 33 programs (Grant, 1999). Approximately two-thirds of the recipients were children or teenagers. The types of transplants included isolated small bowel with or without the colon (41 per cent), combined liver and small bowel (48 per cent), and multivisceral grafts (11 per cent). Tacrolimus-based immune suppression was used for the majority of the grafts (212; 78 per cent), while cyclosporine was used for 51 grafts (19 per cent). Several of these patients also received mycophenolate mofetil.

A total of 131 of the 260 intestinal transplant recipients have died. The majority (73 per cent) of recipient mortality was accounted for by sepsis and multisystem organ failure. Other common causes of mortality were vascular complications (10 per cent) and post-transplant lymphomas (10 per cent). The registry results reveal a steady improvement in outcome as experience is gained. Transplants performed after 1991 and at centers that had performed at least 10 transplants had significantly higher graft survival rates. The 1-year graft survival for all types of intestinal transplants performed between February 1995 and February 1997 was approximately 60 per cent.

The first report from the Intestinal Transplant Registry analysed graft and patient survival of 180 transplants in 170 patients (Grant, 1996). For isolated small bowel transplantation, 3-year graft survival under cyclosporine immune suppression was only 11 per cent (Table 30.2), while tacrolimus-based immune suppression gave a 29 per cent survival (Table 30.3). The majority of the early intestinal transplants were performed under cyclosporine immune suppression and this may bias the results to a degree as there does appear to be a learning curve in intestinal transplantation. Neverthe-

Table 30.2 *Three-year graft and patient survival rates using cyclosporine-based immune suppression*

	Graft survival (%)	Patient survival (%)
Isolated small bowel	11	50
Combined liver/small bowel	28	28
Multivisceral	41	41

Table 30.3 *Three-year graft and patient survival rates using tacrolimus-based immune suppression*

	Graft survival (%)	Patient survival (%)
Isolated small bowel	29	47
Combined liver/small bowel	38	40
Multivisceral	37	43

less, these improved results have led the majority of programs to use tacrolimus-based immune suppression. The 3-year patient survival for isolated intestinal transplantation was similar in the two groups, approximately 50 per cent, reflecting the fact that patients with failed isolated small bowel transplants can survive graft removal and possibly undergo a second attempt at transplantation. It should be noted that the survival in this group is higher than in the combined liver and small bowel transplant group.

There was an improved graft survival in combined transplants over isolated transplants. This may be due to a protective effect of the liver against rejection. In 1969, Calne reported that liver transplantation induces donor-specific tolerance in pigs (Calne *et al.*, 1969). More recently, it has been reported that simultaneous liver and renal transplantation in humans can prevent kidney graft damage by cytotoxic antibodies and that the combined transplant may protect both organs from rejection (Gonwa *et al.*, 1988). Although the immunologic mechanism remains unclear, the protective effect of a combined transplant is further evidenced in the upcoming report from the intestinal Transplant Registry (Grant, 1999). This report shows that acute graft rejection for isolated small bowel, combined liver and small bowel, and multivisceral transplants was 79 per cent, 71 per cent and 56 per cent, respectively. Chronic rejection for isolated small bowel, and combined liver and small bowel was 13 per cent and 3 per cent, respectively, with no chronic rejection in the multivisceral transplant group.

Tables 30.2 and 30.3 show that patient survival is basically equivalent to graft survival in combined transplants as a failed graft in this setting is very difficult to manage. This factor, combined with the improved results of isolated intestinal grafting, has led to a trend toward earlier isolated small bowel transplant prior to the onset of parenteral nutrition-induced liver disease.

CONCLUSIONS AND FUTURE PROSPECTS

While patients can be palliated for a time with parenteral nutrition, intestinal transplantation is the only method available that will cure intestinal failure. Currently, intestinal transplantation is recommended only for patients who have failed conventional therapy but, as results improve, it will become the treatment of choice for intestinal failure, as renal transplantation has for the treatment of chronic renal failure. Long-term results for patient and graft survival are currently lacking, but will be available over the next few years as patients are followed in the transplant registry. The intestinal transplant registry allows for close follow-up of all transplant recipients and will hopefully continue to show improved survival rates over time.

The challenge now is to reduce the morbidity and mortality of the procedure. There is ongoing laboratory and clinical research in several areas. Immunomodulation of the donor bowel using radiation or antilymphocyte products is being investigated. The role of HLA matching will be determined as these data are collected in a prospective manner. New immunosuppressive regimens are being evaluated, including infusion of donor bone marrow and different medications, such as cyclophosphamide. The search for a sensitive, specific and non-invasive test to diagnose rejection continues. Long-term graft function, including nutrient absorption and motility, is being evaluated. The debate over whether or not to include the colon in intestinal transplants should be answered as the numbers of recipients increases. Finally, research into tolerance induction of the intestinal graft may lead to the most significant improvement in patient outcomes.

Acknowledgements The authors thank Ms Cate Abbott for editorial assistance and Mr George Moogk for preparing the figures.

REFERENCES

Alessiani, M., Tzakis, A., Todo, S., Demetris, A.J., Fung, J.J., Starzl, T.E. 1995: Assessment of five-year experience with abdominal organ cluster transplantation. *Journal of the American College of Surgeons* 180, 1–9.

Asfar, S., Atkison, P., Ghent, C. *et al.* 1996: Small bowel transplantation. A life-saving option for selected patients with intestinal failure. *Digestive Diseases and Sciences* 41, 875–83.

Atkinson, P., Joubert, G., Barron, A. *et al.* 1995: Hypertrophic cardiomyopathy associated with tacrolimus in paediatric transplant patients. *Lancet* 345(8945), 894–6.

Black, R.T., Hashimoto, T., Zhong, R.Z. *et al.* 1994:

Transplantation of segmental rat intestinal grafts including the ileocecal valve and the ascending colon. *Transplantation* 57, 997–1002.

Bland, P. 1988: MHC class II expression by the gut epithelium. *Immunology Today* 9, 174–8.

Calne, R.Y., Sells, R.A., Pena, J.R. *et al.* 1969: Induction of immunological tolerance by porcine liver allografts. *Nature* 223, 472–6.

Carrel, A. 1902: La technique operatoire des anastomoses vasculaire et la transplantation des visceres. *Lyon Med* 98, 859.

Cohen, Z., Silverman, R.E., Wassef, R. *et al.* 1986: Small intestinal transplantation using cyclosporine. Report of a case. *Transplantation* 42, 613–21.

Gonwa, T.A., Nery, J.R., Husberg, B.S., Klintmalm, G.B. 1988: Simultaneous liver and renal transplantation in man. *Transplantation* 46, 690–3.

Goulet, O., Revillon, Y., Jan, D. *et al.* 1990: Small-bowel transplantation in children. *Transplantation Proceedings* 22, 2499–500.

Grant, D. 1996: Current results of intestinal transplantation. *Lancet* 347(9018), 1801–3.

Grant, D. 1999: Intestinal transplantation: 1997 Report of the international registry. Intestinal Transplant Registry. *Transplantation* 67, 1061–4..

Grant, D., Sommerauer, J., Mimeault, R. *et al.* 1989a: Treatment with continuous high-dose intravenous cyclosporine following intestinal transplantation. *Transplantation* 48, 151–2.

Grant, D., Zhong, R., Gunn, H. *et al.* 1989b: Graft-versus-host disease associated with intestinal transplantation in the rat. Host immune function and general histology. *Transplantation* 48, 545–9.

Grant, D., Wall, W., Mimeault, R. *et al.* 1990: Successful small-bowel/liver transplantation. *Lancet* 335(8683), 181–4.

Howard, L., Ament, M., Fleming, C.R., Shike, M., Steiger, E. 1995: Current use and clinical outcome of home parenteral and enteral nutrition therapies in the United States. *Gastroenterology* 109, 355–65.

Kocoshis, S.A. 1994: Small bowel transplantation in infants and children. *Gastroenterology Clinics of North America* 23, 727–42.

Kocoshis, S.A., Reyes, J., Todo, S., Starzl, T.E. 1997: Small intestinal transplantation for irreversible intestinal failure in children. *Digestive Diseases and Sciences* 42, 1997–2008.

Kurkubasche, A.G., Row, M.I., Smith, S.D. 1993: Adaptation in short bowel syndrome: reassessing old limits. *Journal of Pediatric Surgery* 28, 1069–71.

Langnas, A.N., Shaw, B.W., Jr, Antonson, D.L. *et al.* 1996: Preliminary experience with intestinal transplantation in infants and children. *Pediatrics* 97, 443–8.

Lee, R.G., Nakamura, K., Tsamandas, A.C. *et al.* 1996: Pathology of human intestinal transplantation. *Gastroenterology* 110, 1820–34.

Lillehei, R.C., Goott, B., Miller, F.A. 1959: Homografts of the small bowel. *Surgical Forum* 10, 197–201.

Lillehei, R.C., Idezuki, Y., Feemster, J.A. *et al.* 1967: Transplantation of stomach, intestine, and pancreas: experimental and clinical observations. *Surgery* 62, 721–41.

Nalesnik, M.A. 1996: Posttransplantation lymphoproliferative disorders (PTLD): current perspectives. *Seminars in Thoracic and Cardiovascular Surgery* 8, 139–48.

Pernthaler, H., Nehoda, H., Riedmann, B., Aichberger, C., Margreiter, R. 1996: Altered but preserved motility of a human small bowel allograft. *Transplantation Proceedings* 28, 2794.

Pollard, S.G., Lodge, P., Selvakumar, S., Heatley, R.V., Wyatt, J., Wood, R. 1996: Living related small bowel transplantation: the first United Kingdom case. *Transplantation Proceedings* 28, 2731–2.

Reyes, J., Bueno, J., Kocoshis, S. *et al.* 1998: Current status of intestinal transplantation in children. *Journal of Pediatric Surgery* 33, 243–54.

Sigalet, D.L., Kneteman, N.M., Fedorak, R.N., Kizilisik, A.T., Thomson, A.B.R. 1992: Intestinal function following allogeneic small intestinal transplantation in the rat. *Transplantation* 53, 264–71.

Sustento-Reodica, N., Ruiz, P., Rogers, A., Viciana, A.L., Conn, H.O., Tzakis, A.G. 1997: Recurrent Crohn's disease in transplanted bowel. *Lancet* 349(9053), 688–91.

Thompson, J.S., Langnas, A.N., Pinch, L.W., Kaufman, S., Quigley, E.M.M., Vanderhoof, J.A. 1995: Surgical approach to short-bowel syndrome. *Annals of Surgery* 222, 600–7.

Todo, S., Reyes, J., Furukawa, H. *et al.* 1995: Outcome analysis of 71 clinical intestinal transplantations. *Annals of Surgery* 222, 270–82.

Index

NOTE: All entries relate to the small intestine unless otherwise stated. Entries have been kept to a minimum under 'small intestine' and readers are advised to seek more specific entries. This index is in letter-by-letter order whereby the hyphens and spaces in main entries are ignored in the alphabetization. *vs* denotes differential diagnosis or comparisons